FOOD AND NUTRITION BOARD, INSTITUTE OF MEDICINE—NATIONAL ACADEMY

DIETARY REFERENCE INTAKES: RECOMMENDED LEVELS FOR INDIVIDUAL INTAKE

Life-Stage Group	Calcium (mg/d)	Phosphorus (mg/d)	Magnesium (mg/d)	D (μg/d)†,‡	Fluoride (mg/d)	Thiamin (mg/d)	Riboflavin (mg/d)	Niacin (mg/d)§	B_6 (mg/d)	Folate (μg/d)‖	B_{12} (μg/d)	Pantothenic Acid (mg/d)	Biotin (μg/d)	Choline# (mg/d)
Infants														
0–5 mo	210*	100*	30*	5*	0.01*	0.2*	0.3*	2*	0.1*	65*	0.4*	1.7*	5*	125*
6–11 mo	270*	275*	75*	5*	0.5*	0.3*	0.4*	4*	0.3*	80*	0.5*	1.8*	6*	150*
Children														
1–3 yr	500*	460	80	5*	0.7*	0.5	0.5	6	0.5	150	0.9	2*	8*	200*
4–8 yr	800*	500	130	5*	1*	0.6	0.6	8	0.6	200	1.2	3*	12*	250*
Males														
9–13 yr	1300*	1250	240	5*	2*	0.9	0.9	12	1.0	300	1.8	4*	20*	375*
14–18 yr	1300*	1250	410	5*	3*	1.2	1.3	16	1.3	400	2.4	5*	25*	500*
19–30 yr	1000*	700	400	5*	4*	1.2	1.3	16	1.3	400	2.4	5*	30*	550*
31–50 yr	1000*	700	420	5*	4*	1.2	1.3	16	1.3	400	2.4	5*	30*	550*
51–70 yr	1200*	700	420	10*	4*	1.2	1.3	16	1.7	400	2.4**	5*	30*	550*
> 70 yr	1200*	700	420	15*	4*	1.2	1.3	16	1.7	400	2.4**	5*	30*	550*
Females														
9–13 yr	1300*	1250	240	5*	2*	0.9	0.9	12	1.0	300	1.8	4*	20*	375*
14–18 yr	1300*	1250	360	5*	3*	1.0	1.0	14	1.2	400††	2.4	5*	25*	400*
19–30 yr	1000*	700	310	5*	3*	1.1	1.1	14	1.3	400††	2.4	5*	30*	425*
31–50 yr	1000*	700	320	5*	3*	1.1	1.1	14	1.3	400††	2.4	5*	30*	425*
51–70 yr	1200*	700	320	10*	3*	1.1	1.1	14	1.5	400††	2.4**	5*	30*	425*
> 70 yr	1200*	700	320	15*	3*	1.1	1.1	14	1.5	400	2.4**	5*	30*	425*
Pregnancy														
≤ 18 yr	1,300*	1250	400	5*	3*	1.4	1.4	18	1.9	600‡‡	2.6	6*	30*	450*
19–30 yr	1,000*	700	350	5*	3*	1.4	1.4	18	1.9	600‡‡	2.6	6*	30*	450*
31–50 yr	1,000*	700	360	5*	3*	1.4	1.4	18	1.9	600‡‡	2.6	6*	30*	450*
Lactation														
≤ 18 yr	1,300*	1250	360	5*	3*	1.5	1.6	17	2.0	500	2.8	7*	35*	550*
19–30 yr	1,000*	700	310	5*	3*	1.5	1.6	17	2.0	500	2.8	7*	35*	550*
31–50 yr	1,000*	700	320	5*	3*	1.5	1.6	17	2.0	500	2.8	7*	35*	550*

μg = microgram; mg = milligram

NOTE: This table presents Recommended Dietary Allowances (RDAs) and Adequate Intakes (AIs) followed by an asterisk (*). RDAs and AIs may both be used as goals for individual intake. RDAs are set to meet the needs of almost all (97% to 98%) individuals in a group. For healthy breastfed infants, the AI is the mean intake. The AI for other life stage groups is believed to cover their needs, but lack of data or uncertainty in the data prevent clear specification of this coverage.

† As cholecalciferol. 1 μg cholecalciferol = 40 IU vitamin D.

‡ In the absence of adequate exposure to sunlight.

§ As niacin equivalents. 1 mg of niacin = 60 mg of tryptophan; 0–5 months = preformed niacin (not mg NE).

‖ As dietary folate equivalents (DFE). 1 DFE = 1 μg food folate = 0.6 μg of folic acid (from fortified food or supplement) consumed with food = 0.5 μg of synthetic (supplemental) folic acid taken on an empty stomach.

Although AIs have been set for choline, there are few data to assess whether a dietary supply of choline is needed at all stages of the life cycle, and it may be that the choline requirement can be met by endogenous synthesis at some of these stages.

** Since 10% to 30% of older people may malabsorb food-bound B_{12}, it is advisable for those older than 50 years to meet their RDA mainly by consuming foods fortified with B_{12} or a B_{12}-containing supplement.

†† In view of evidence linking folate intake with neural tube defects in the fetus, it is recommended that all women capable of becoming pregnant consume 400 μg of synthetic folic acid from fortified foods and/or supplements in addition to intake of food folate from a varied diet.

‡‡ It is assumed that women will continue taking 400 μg of folic acid until their pregnancy is confirmed and they enter prenatal care, which ordinarily occurs after the end of the periconceptional period—the critical time for formation of the neural tube.

Fourth Edition

CONTEMPORARY NUTRITION

ISSUES AND INSIGHTS

Gordon M. Wardlaw, Ph.D., R.D., L.D., C.N.S.D.
Division of Medical Dietetics
School of Allied Medical Professions
The Ohio State University

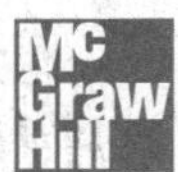

Boston Burr Ridge, IL Dubuque, IA Madison, WI New York San Francisco St. Louis
Bangkok Bogotá Caracas Lisbon London Madrid
Mexico City Milan New Delhi Seoul Singapore Sydney Taipei Toronto

McGraw-Hill Higher Education

A Division of The ***McGraw-Hill*** *Companies*

Contemporary Nutrition: Issues and Insights, Fourth Edition

 This book is printed on recycled, acid-free paper containing 10% postconsumer waste.

1 2 3 4 5 6 7 8 9 0 QPD/QPD 0 9 8 7 6 5 4 3 2 1 0

ISBN 0-07-109368-0

Vice president and editorial director: *Kevin T. Kane*
Publisher: *Colin H. Wheatley*
Senior developmental editor: *Lynne M. Meyers*
Senior marketing manager: *Pamela S. Cooper*
Senior project manager: *Marilyn Rothenberger*
Senior production supervisor: *Sandra Hahn*
Coordinator of freelance design: *Michelle D. Whitaker*
Photo research coordinator: *John C. Leland*
Supplement coordinator: *David A. Welsh*
Compositor: *GAC—Indianapolis*
Typeface: *10/12 Giovanni Book*
Printer: *Quebecor Printing Book Group/Dubuque, IA*

Freelance cover/interior design: *Kristyn A. Kalnes*
Cover image: *© Zane B. Williams*
Cover photograph: *Photo taken in mid-August; Dane County Farmer's Marker, on the square; Cart owned/operated by Kingsfield Gardens in Blue Mounds, WI*

The credits section for this book begins on page c-1 and is considered an extension of the copyright page.

Library of Congress Cataloging-in-Publication Data

Wardlaw, Gordon M.
Contemporary nutrition : issues and insights / Gordon M. Wardlaw.
—4th ed.
p. cm.
Includes bibliographical references and index.
ISBN 0-07-109368-0
1. Nutrition. I. Title.
QP141.W378 2000 99-18616
613.2—dc21 CIP

www. mhhe.com

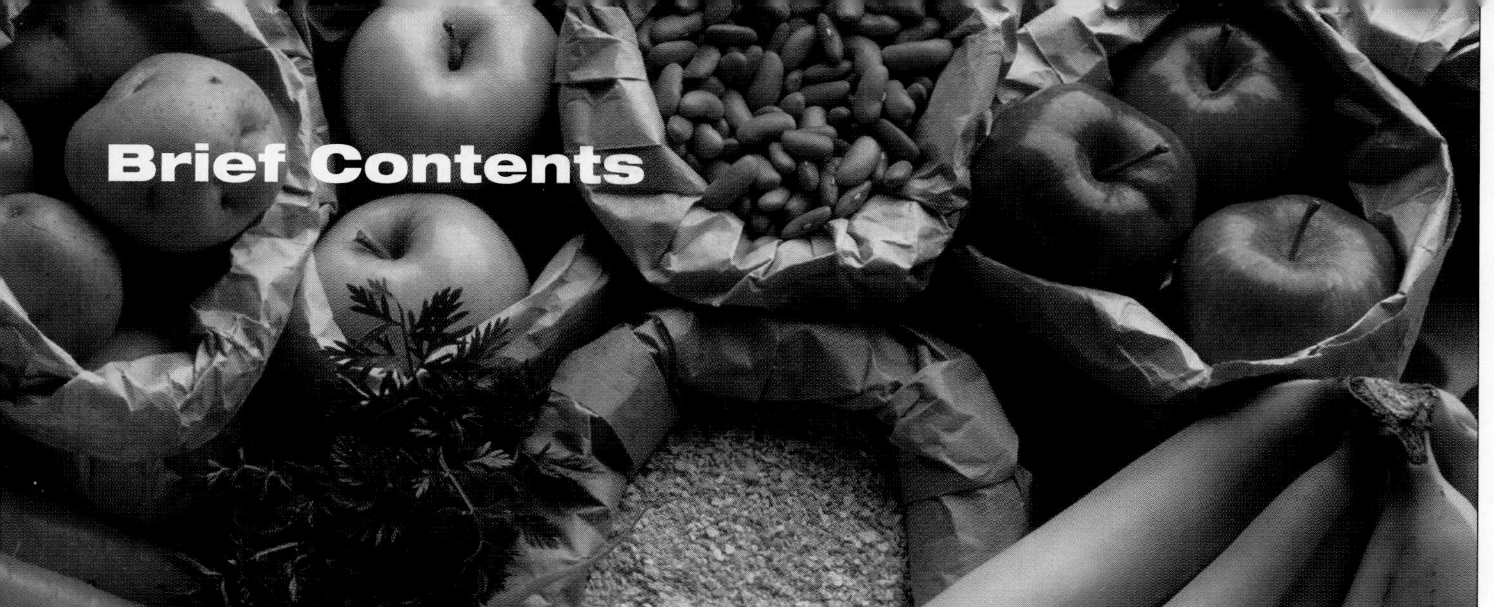

Brief Contents

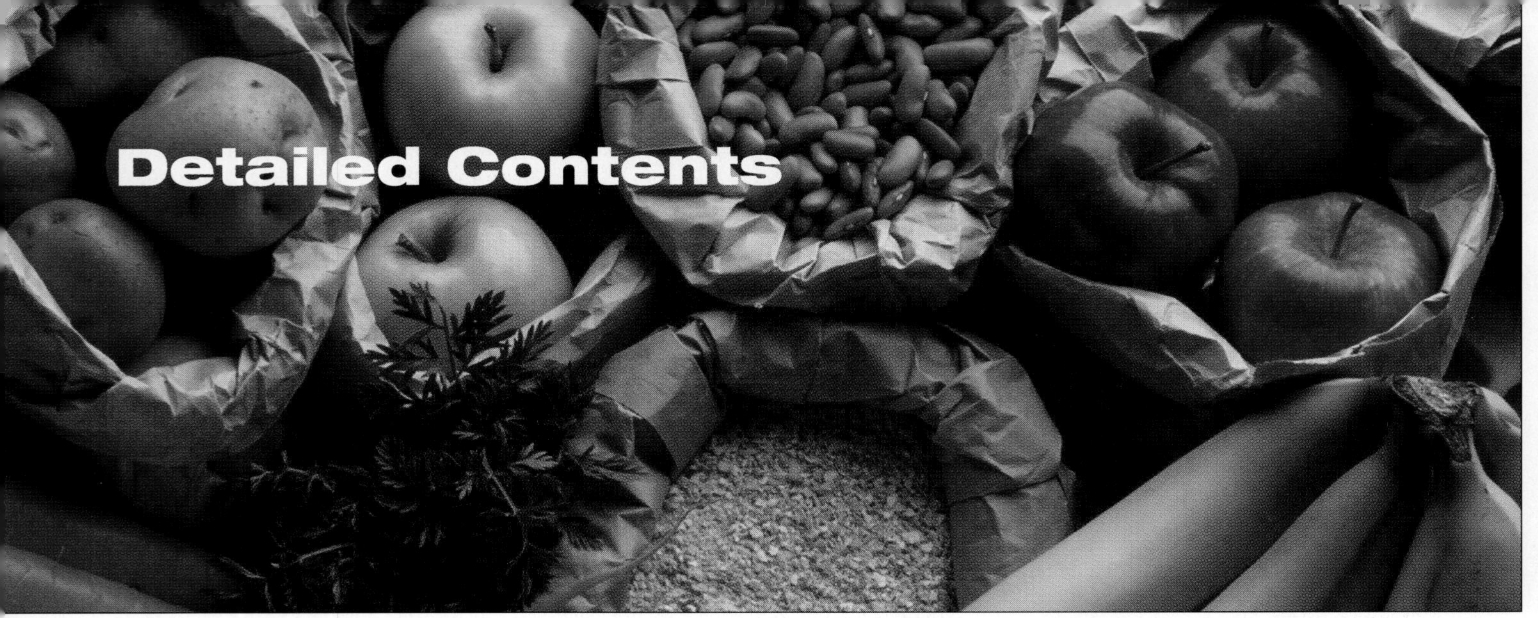

Detailed Contents

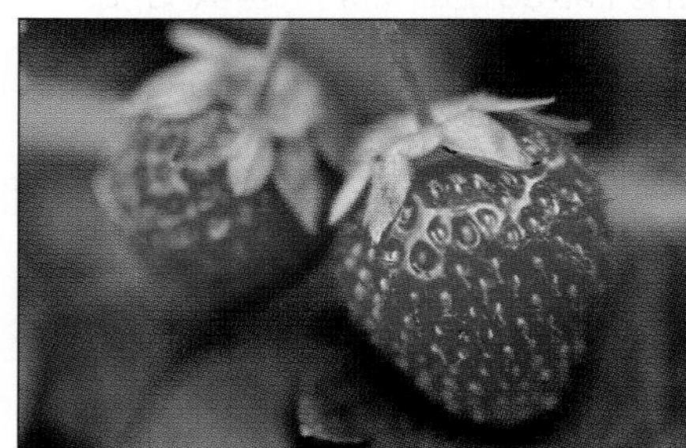

PART 2
NUTRIENTS
The Heart of Nutrition

4 Carbohydrates, 102

5 Lipids, 134

6 Proteins, 174

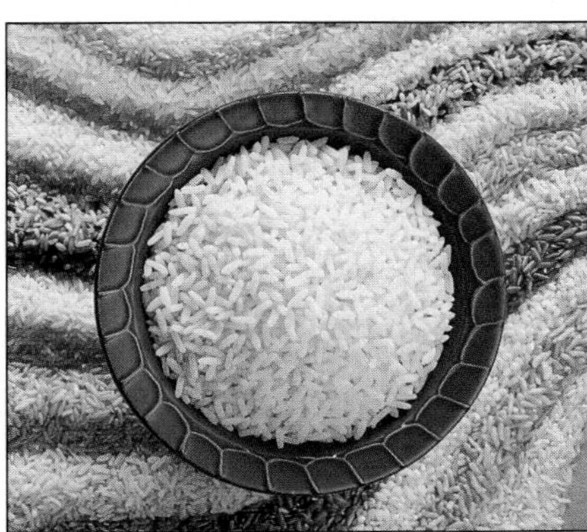

7 Vitamins, 206

8 Water and Minerals, 256

PART 3

ENERGY BALANCE AND IMBALANCE

9 Weight Control, 308

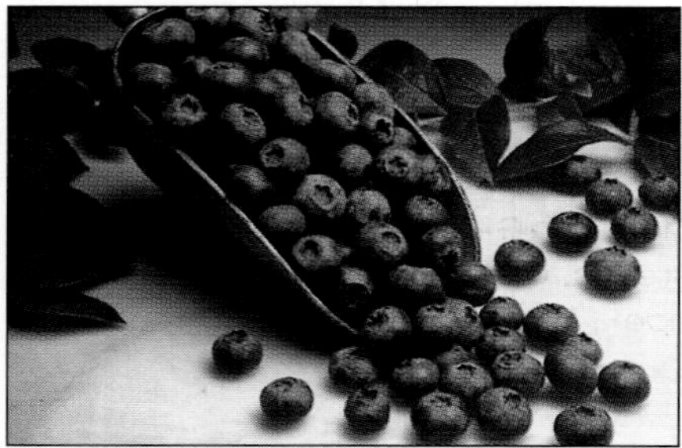

10 Nutrition: Fitness and Sports, 356

11 Eating Disorders: Anorexia Nervosa and Bulimia Nervosa, 384

PART 4

NUTRITION
A Focus on Life Stages

12 Pregnancy and Breastfeeding, 412

13 Nutrition from Infancy Through Adolescence, 444

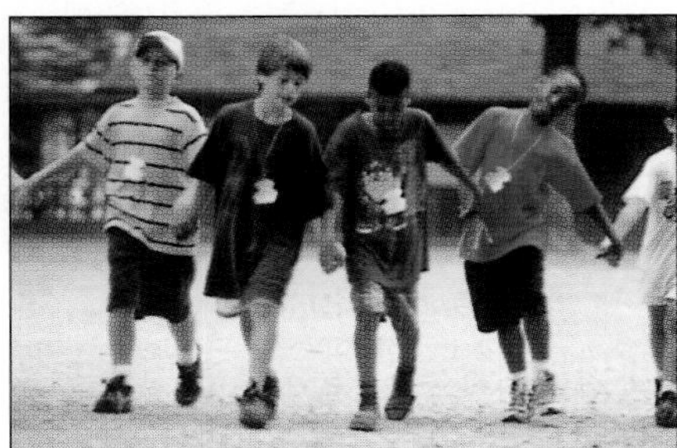

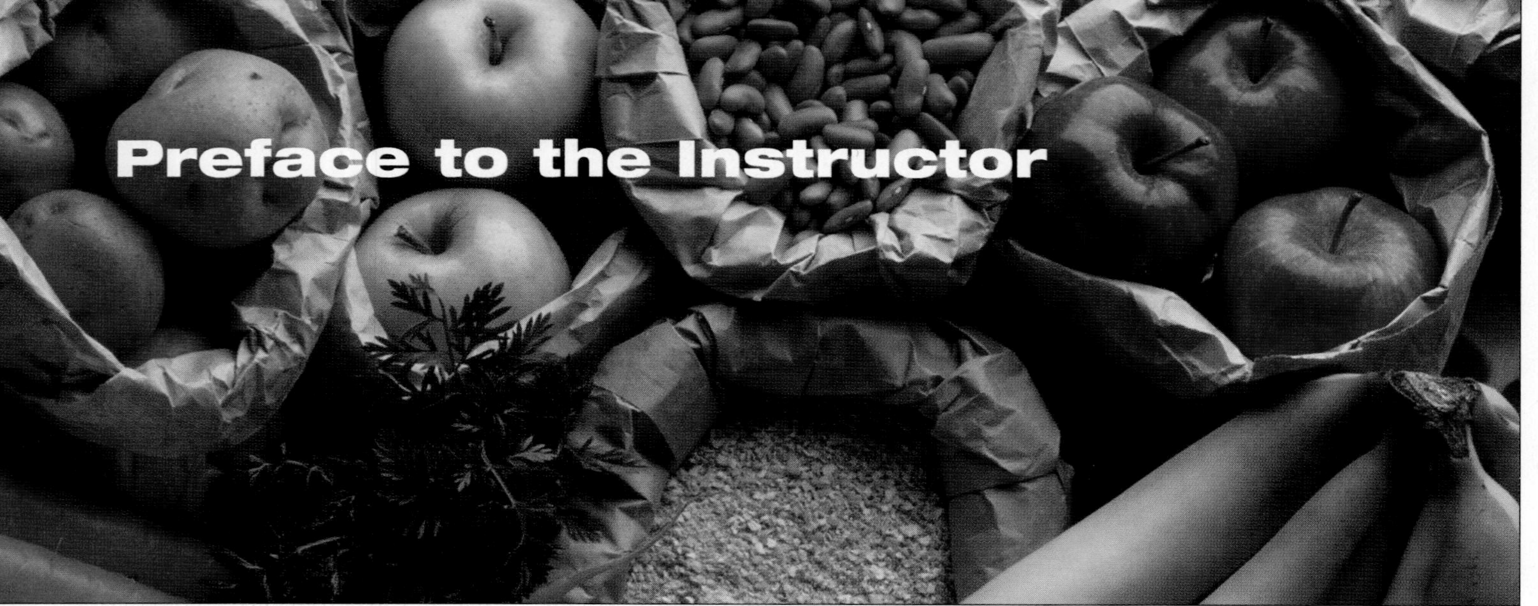

Preface to the Instructor

If you teach nutrition, you undoubtedly already find it a fascinating topic. However, nutrition can also be quite frustrating to teach. Claims and counterclaims abound regarding the need for certain constituents in our diets. Sodium is a good example. One group of researchers promotes a low-sodium diet for the general population as an effective preventive measure for high blood pressure. Other groups state that this is much less of a concern compared to other habits; such as inactivity and adult weight gain.

As an author, I too am aware of conflicting opinions in our field and thus draw on as many sources as possible in the continual updating of this textbook, now in its fourth edition. I have incorporated much new material, especially from recently published articles in major nutrition and medical journals; supplements to the *American Journal of Clinical Nutrition;* the 9th edition of *Modern Nutrition in Health and Disease,* edited by Shils, Olson, Shike; and *Present Knowledge in Nutrition,* edited by Ziegler and Filer. In addition, available information on the latest Dietary Reference Intake revisions to the 1989 RDA are incorporated where appropriate.

In all, the book strives to present many perspectives in current nutrition research so that you and your students can better understand and participate in debates about current nutrition issues.

Personalizing Nutrition

One prominent theme in nutrition research today is *individuality.* Not all of us, for example, find that saturated fat in our diets raises our blood cholesterol values above recommended standards. Each person responds individually, often idiosyncratically, to nutrients, and that is something I continually point out in this textbook.

Moreover, even at this basic level the book discussions do not assume that all nutrition students are alike. Chapter content repeatedly asks students to learn more about themselves and their health status and to use this new knowledge to improve their health. After reading this textbook, students will understand much more clearly how the nutrition information given on the evening news, on cereal box labels, in popular magazines, and by government agencies applies to them. They will become sophisticated consumers of both nutrients and nutrition information. They will understand that their knowledge of nutrition allows them to personalize information, rather than follow every guideline issued for an entire population. After all, a population by definition consists of individuals with varying genetic and cultural backgrounds, and these individuals have varying responses to diet.

In addition, the book covers important questions that students often raise concerning ethnic diets, eating disorders, nutrient supplements, phytochemicals, vegetarianism, diets for athletes, food safety, and fad diets, with an overall emphasis on the importance of understanding one's food choices and changing one's diet as needed.

Audience

This book has been designed for a nonmajors audience. The chemistry has been kept to a minimum, and more so than in previous editions. Health majors, home economics majors, nursing students, physical education students, and students in other health-related areas will also find this text appropriate. Because of the flexible chapter organization and content, this book can be adopted for students of diverse educational backgrounds. Although it is not absolutely necessary, most students will find that having an understanding of basic biological concepts provides a helpful background when using this book.

Organization

The book is most suitable for a semester-length course; it can also be used in a quarter-length course by omitting chapters or by skipping various sections. A useful feature of this text is that it is presented in five segments:

PART 1 NUTRITION: A Key to Health
PART 2 NUTRIENTS: The Heart of Nutrition
PART 3 ENERGY: Balance and Imbalance
PART 4 NUTRITION: A Focus on Life Stages
PART 5 NUTRITION: Beyond the Nutrients

This organization makes it easy to tailor the text to specific course needs.

New to This Edition

The changes I've made to the fourth edition of *Contemporary Nutrition: Issues and Insights* are designed to enhance student learning and understanding; many of them are a direct result of the feedback I received from instructors who team the introductory nutrition course.

Updated Content

To give students an accurate picture of nutrition today, it's important to provide the most up-to-date information available. So I've gone carefully through recent research and updated the text throughout.

Updated *Readings for Further Study*

Of course, as the content throughout the text has been updated, so too has the list of readings at the end of each chapter. Current texts and journal articles are contained in a list of relevant citations at the end of each chapter, as well as discussions from leading nutrition newsletters. Should you or your students want additional information about a particular topic, these lists will point you in the right direction. I decided not to directly cite references in the body of the text because of the basic level of content. Much of the discussions are very introductory in nature. If you would like a specific literature citation to support text material, please contact me and I will provide the reference.

Fewer Chapters

Now with 16 chapters instead of 18, I consider this to be a more streamlined edition. Many instructors told me that while Chapter 2 and 12 from the third edition contained useful information, it was not necessary to devote entire chapters to them. As a result these chapters have been deleted, and most of the information from them has been shifted to other chapters.

Nutrition Web

Key chapter concepts at the beginning of each chapter are now in a web format. Unlike the list of key concepts in the previous edition, this new format allows students to see how one concept is related to another, and because it is more visually interesting, it is more likely to pique students' interest.

Expanded Rate Your Plate Activities

Each Rate Your Plate activity at the end of each chapter is now in a two-part format. This provides the student with more opportunities to put their acquisition of nutrition knowledge into practice.

Addresses for Nutrition-Related Web Sites

Because of the abundance of information contained on the World Wide Web today, addresses (URLs) for a variety of credible nutrition-related web sites are now included in each chapter. These URLs will also be included as hot links from the text's web site. I've also included toll-free telephone numbers and other resources whenever available.

Richest Source of Each Nutrient in the Margins

To make this information more easily accessible, the richest sources of each nutrient discussed in Chapters 7 and 8 are now listed in numerical format in the margins.

Updated Illustration Program

New photos and illustrations help to better convey important concepts, and also help to keep the text current and fresh.

Pedagogy

The following pedagogical features continually reinforce the learning process—enhancing students' learning and understanding.

Nutrition Web

This new format for illustrating key chapter concepts allows students to see how one concept is related to another, and because it is more visually interesting, it is more likely to pique students' interest.

Margin Notes

Margin notes throughout the book clarify concepts and provide further details about them; they also provide interesting examples and references to other chapters.

Margin Definitions

Important terms are set in boldface type at first mention and, when possible, they are defined in the text's margins (all are defined in the glossary at the end of the book).

Concept Check Boxes

These boxes provide a summary of chapter content every few pages, which reinforces students' understanding of the material.

Nutrition Insight Boxes

Short essays, often on controversial topics in nutrition, are located in each chapter.

Summary

At the end of each chapter is an overall summary of the chapter's main points.

Study Questions

Approximately 10 questions at the end of each chapter encourages students to probe deeper into the chapter content.

Further Readings

Each chapter contains an up-to-date list of readings that will direct you and your students to resources for further information about a particular topic.

Critical Thinking Questions

Within each chapter are two questions found in the margins of the text, which allow students to apply information to practical situations.

Rate Your Plate

Similar to the Critical Thinking Questions, these activities at the end of each chapter allow students to put theory into practice. The suggested assignments are usually proactive, and sometimes ask students to carefully analyze part of their current diet or lifestyle.

Nutrition Issue Boxes

These essays at the end of each chapter take a more detailed look at a specific topic relevant to the chapter.

Glossary

Located at the end of the text, this comprehensive glossary of key terms is included for students' reference, and includes pronunciation keys for unfamiliar words.

Supplementary Materials

Numerous supplementary materials are available to you and your students, which will expand on the concepts presented in this text, and increase the overall value of this text.

Instructor's Manual and Test Bank

This comprehensive teaching aid is available to adopters of the book. It includes chapter summaries with suggestions for teaching difficult material: activities; suggested readings; activities to use with *NutriQuest*™ 2.0, and a "survival" section that discusses class organization, scheduling, and problem areas such as cheating. The test bank features multiple-choice, short-answer, and matching test questions.

Microtest III Computerized Test Bank

Instructors who adopt this text can receive the computerized test bank for Windows or Macintosh. This software allows the instructor to select, edit, delete, or add questions, and print tests and answer keys.

Transparency Acetates

Text adopters may receive a package of 185 full-color transparency acetates featuring key illustrations from this text, and others.

Visual Resource Library (VRL)

This CD-ROM for Windows and Macintosh contains a PowerPoint presentation based on *Contemporary Nutrition*, fourth edition, as well as a separate section of key illustrations, photographs, and animations. The PowerPoint presentation can be used as is, or portions can be imported into instructor's own PowerPoint presentation. Illustrations can also be imported into another program.

Student Study Guide

This student aid is prepared by Gordon Wardlaw, and was developed in consultation with a learning theory expert. This comprehensive guide reinforces concepts presented in the text and integrates them with study activities to emphasize key concepts. It features vocabulary review and sample examinations structured to reflect the actual examinations students will face in the classroom.

NutriQuest™ 2.0—Dietary Analysis Software

Students will learn more about their own personal health habits with this upgraded dietary analysis software program that allows users to track energy intake and expenditure, set weight goals, and more. Improvements to this version includes more foods (approximately 4000), better printing options for reports, and the ability to save data to another disk. The software is available on CD-ROM for Macintosh and Windows, disks for Windows, or you can purchase a site license so you can place it on your school's network. NutriQuest 2.0 also has its own web site for related on-line information—http://www.mhhe.com/hper/nutrition/nutriquest/.

INNOVATIONS Newsletter

This newsletter, produced in partnership with Novartis Pharmaceuticals, offers students an in-depth look at important issues in nutritional science..

NutriNews

Upon request, adopters are given the password to this electronic newsletter made up of nutrition-related articles. You'll find the newsletter, as well as several other features, on WCB/McGraw-Hill's nutrition web site at http://www.mhhe.com/hper/nutrition/.

Annual Editions: Nutrition

Supplement any of your nutrition texts with this annually updated compilation of carefully selected nutrition-related articles from magazines, newspapers, and journals.

Diet and Fitness Log

This convenient paper-and-pencil system allows students to keep a handwritten record of their diet and exercise program so they can assess their eating and physical activity habits.

Nutrition Videos

Two 10- to 12-minute videotapes are available to qualified adopters: *Issues in Nutrition: Eating Disorders* and *Issues in Nutrition: Obesity and Weight Control.* Both videos incorporate interviews with professionals in their respective fields.

Web Resources

This text is supported by a variety of on-line resources, such as the McGraw-Hill Nutrition web site (http://www.mhhe.com/hper/nutrition) and a web site designed specifically for CONTEMPORARY NUTRITION (http://www.mhhe.com/hper/nutrition/wardlaw). See p. xix–xx for more information on the on-line resources available from McGraw-Hill.

Text Web Site and Online Learning Center

This textbook is supported by a specially developed web site, designed to help students get the most out of their first nutrition course. One component of the web site, the Online Learning Center, contains a variety of chapter-correlated resources from web links to on-line quizzes and flash cards. http://www.mhhe.com/hper/nutrition/wardlawcon/

Questions About These Supplements?

If you have questions about these supplements, please contact your McGraw-Hill sales representative, or call Customer Service at (800) 338-3987.

Special Acknowledgments

I would like to personally thank those individuals who contributed their expertise to the project. Janet Haworth, R.D., and Sally Smith, R.D., participated in key phases of the revision, as well as Regina Stachowiak, who helped with proofreading and preparing the final manuscript. My editors, Kassi Radomski and Lynne Meyers, supported and assisted me through the revision, and facilitated the difficult decisions that frequently arose. Beatrice Sussman and Marilyn Rothenberger did excellent copyediting and production work.

Reviewers

As with earlier editions, my goal is to provide the most accurate, up-to-date, and useful introductory nutrition text available. I, along with my editors, would like to recognize and thank those people whose direction and insight guided this fourth edition:

Wendy Hunt
American River College

Kaye Stanek
University of Nebraska, Omaha

Robert D. Reynolds
University of Illinois, Chicago

Joelle E. Romanchik
Georgia Southern University

Marlene McCall
Community College of Allegheny County

Rao V. Ivaturi
Indiana State University

Cherie Moore
Cuesta College

Prisca Nemapare
Ohio University

Bahram Faraji
University of Texas, Pan American

Sofi Boutros
Western Illinois University

Richard P. Dowdy
University of Missouri, Columbia

John S. Avens
Colorado State University

Marjorie T. Hagerman
Ohio University

LuAnn Soliah
Baylor University

Amelia Finan
Anne Arundel Community College

Laura Nihan
Eastern Kentucky University

Richard D. Mattes
Purdue University

William Helfrich
University of Illinois, Urbana-Campaign

Millicent Owens
College of the Sequoias

David Gee
Central Washington University

Marcia C. Miller
Queens College, CUNY

C. Alan Titchenal
University of Hawaii

Beverly A. Benes
University of Nebraska, Lincoln

Michael Olpin
Concord College

Pat Brown
Cuesta College

Cindy Beck
The Evergreen State College

Ethan A. Bergman
Central Washington University

Cynthia Gossage
Prince George's Community College

Nancy Harris
East Carolina University

Carmen L. Nochera
Grand Valley State University

Janet Colson
Middle Tennessee State University

Marie A. Caudill
California State Polytechnic University

Marilyn Mook
Michigan State University

Carol A. Higginbotham
Barat College

Richard A. Ahrens
University of Maryland

Janice K. Goodwin
University of North Dakota

Marsha H. Read
University of Nevada, Reno

Sharlene Holladay
George Mason University

Liz Applegate
University of California, Davis

Judith D. Fraser Arsenault
Mount Saint Vincent University, Halifax

Carolyn Lara-Braud
University of Iowa

Thaddeus Osmolski
University of Massachusetts, Lowell

The dietary analysis software, NutriQuest 2.0, is a valuable extension to this text. We would also like to thank those individuals whose feedback and suggestions have made NutriQuest 2.0 an even more effective and reliable nutrition assessment tool:

Sara Long Anderson
Southern Illinois University

Rosalie Barretta
Charles County Community College

Beverley Benes
University of Nebraska—Lincoln

Louise Berner
California Polytechnic and State University

Blakley Brown
University of Minnesota

Pat Brown
Cuesta College

Dorothy Cope
Phoenix College

Denise Eagan
Marshall University

Jill Golden
Orange Coast College

Michael Hamrick
University of Memphis

Annamarie Herndon
Purdue University

Patti Marincic
College of St. Benedict/
St. John's University

Judy Paisley
Ryerson Polytechnic University

Stephanie Raach
Rock Valley College

Barbara Reynolds
College of the Sequoias

Thaxton Springfield
St. Petersburg Junior College

Kathryn Timmons
Murray State University

Elaine Turner
University of Florida

Jane Vincent
Indiana University

Dana Wassmer
California State University, Sacramento

This book began with a dream. Each new edition is fostered by the excitement that improvements bring, and ends with the revision of an innovative textbook that continues to set a standard for introductory nutrition textbooks.

Gordon M. Wardlaw

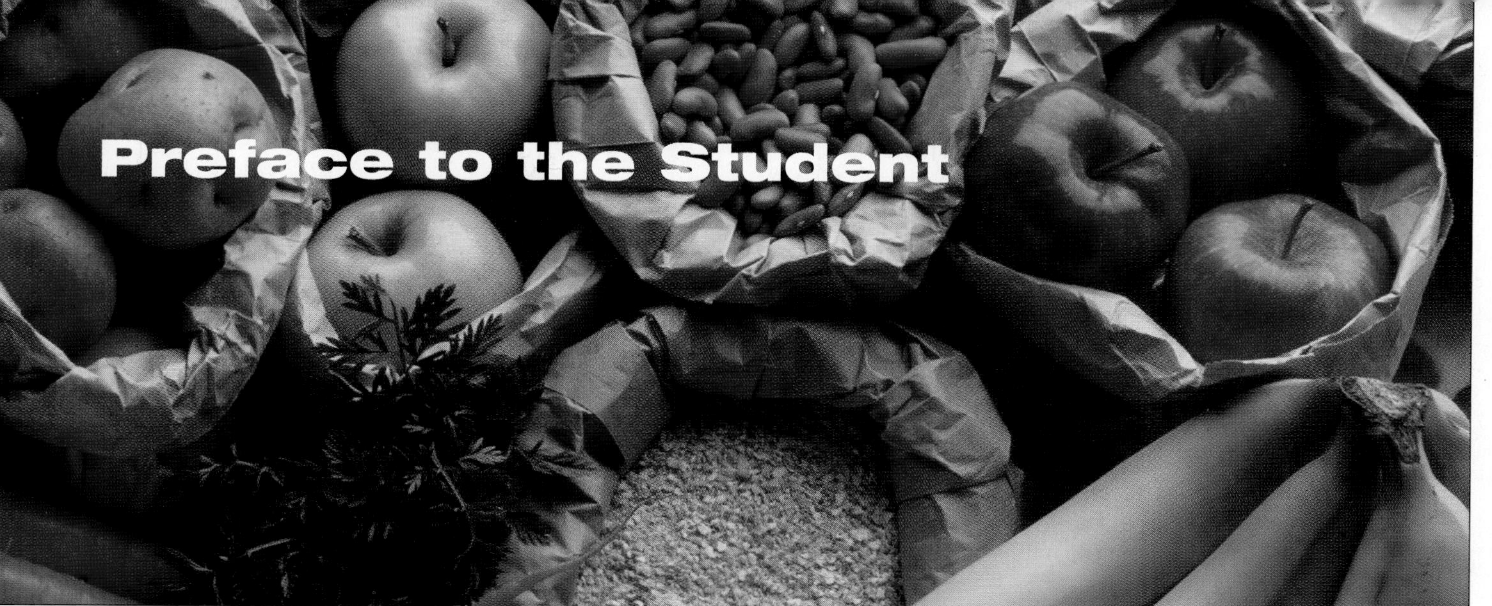

Preface to the Student

Cholesterol, sports drinks, food labeling, bulimia nervosa, alternative sweeteners, vegetarianism, and *Salmonella* foodborne illness—I suspect you have heard about these topics. Which of them are important enough to be a consideration in your life or in the life of someone you know?

Americans pride themselves on their individuality. Nutritional advice should be given accordingly. For example, not all of us have high blood cholesterol and other significant risk factors for premature development of heart disease. The need to tailor dietary advice to each person's individual nature is the basic approach of this book. First you are given a brief introduction to the study of nutrition; then, how to be a knowledgeable consumer is discussed. With so much information floating around—both accurate and inaccurate—you should know how to make informed decisions about your nutritional well-being. Then you are encouraged to learn the basic principles of nutrition and to discover how to apply the concepts in this book that pertain specifically to you.

The text discusses some of the most interesting and important elements of nutrition and food consumption to help you understand both how your body works and how your food choices affect your health.

Features

Planning a New Way of Eating

Early in the text, many of the basic guidelines for planning a healthy diet are presented, including a description of the USDA Food Guide Pyramid, in Chapter 2. Later in Chapter 9, the steps involved in setting nutritional goals and designing a diet plan to attain those goals are reviewed.

Understanding the World Around Us

In a college environment, it is often difficult to envision how real the problem of world hunger is. Chapter 16 examines the problem of undernutrition and the conditions that created it. The chapter allows you to explore possible solutions that offer hope for the future of our world.

Pedagogy

The fourth edition of *Contemporary Nutrition: Issues and Insights* incorporates some important tools (called pedagogy) to help you learn the nutrition concepts in this text. Following is a guide to those tools:

1. Each chapter begins with a Nutrition Web. This will help you focus your attention on key ideas in the chapter.
2. Throughout each chapter are **boldfaced key terms,** many of which are defined in the margin. All boldfaced terms appear with their definitions and pronunciations in the glossary at the end of the text.
3. Also throughout each chapter are **margin notes,** which further explain ideas, provide references to other chapters, and provide the URLs to nutrition-related web sites.
4. The numerous **tables** throughout the text summarize major points.
5. The **Concept Checks** that follow the major sections within each chapter summarize key points. If you don't understand the material in the Concept Check, you should reread the preceding section.
6. Each chapter ends with a **summary,** which conveys the main ideas in the chapter, and **study questions**—both provide excellent review for examinations.

7. **Further Readings** are provided to support material presented in the chapter. Much of this has been published since the last edition of the text. If you are preparing a research paper for your class, or would just like more information on specific topics, consult these sources.
8. Also at the end of each chapter is a **Rate Your Plate box** that makes major concepts presented in the chapter relevant to your own life. For example, you may be asked to look more carefully at your own diet, examine your family history, or apply information you've learned to friends or family.
9. **Nutrition Insight boxes** allow you to explore current topics that your instructor may not have time to cover but that may be of interst to you.
10. **Critical Thinking questions** ask you to apply information as you learn it. This fosters understanding of the material.
11. **Nutrition Issue essays** at the end of each chapter develop current topics in nutrition, often covered earlier in the chapter, in greater detail.
12. A variety of supplements to this text, including **Student Study Guide,** and ***NutriQuest™ 2.0,*** dietary analysis software, are available to you. These instructional aids are designed to help you learn the major concepts developed in the text and prepare for class examinations.

Student Study Guide

The valuable Student Study Guide, written by your textbook author, reinforces concepts presented in the text and integrates them with activities to facilitate learning. Sample examinations reflect the actual tests you will face in the classroom. Vocabulary reviews increase your knowledge of the terminology. Activities include fill-in tables, labeling, and matching terms. These activities follow the text discussion and are anchored with quotations and page citations from the text.

NutriQuest™ 2.0—Dietary Analysis Software

This user-friendly dietary analysis program provides a variety of useful features, which allow you to track daily food intake, energy expenditure, and establish weight or body mass index (BMI) goals. Several different reports and pie charts allow users to see how calories from a specific food, meal, day, or daily average break out. For example, you can click on the USDA Pyramid to determine how many servings from the fruit or grain group you have consumed on a given day; or on the fat pie chart to see what percentage of calories from saturated, monounsaturated, or polyunsaturated fat were in this morning's breakfast.

Features

- *NutriQuest's* 2.0 database of nearly 4000 foods allows you to accurately record their intake, and analyze a specific food, meal, day or average.
- *NutriQuest* 2.0 calculates recommended daily calories and body mass index (BMI) based on height, weight, and other information entered in the Personal Profile.
- You can track your daily activities—from sleeping to jogging—and *NutriQuest* 2.0 will calculate daily energy expenditure.
- You can view a "personalized" food label in standard food label format for a given food.
- This colorful program is intuitively designed, making it easy to maneuver from one screen to another.
- Additional features include: an easily accessible "Help" function; and an Explore Center with recipes, how to read standard food labels, answers to common dietary myths, a link to the *NutriQuest* 2.0 web site, and so on.

A Request to Professors and Students Who Use This Book

As you might imagine, it is difficult to range across the vast areas of nutrition science, following all of the various controversies and new developments. I try my best but realize that sometimes I miss a side of an argument that deserves attention. If as you read this book you find content that you question or believe warrants a more detailed or broader look, fee free to contact me.

Dr. Gordon M. Wardlaw
The Ohio State University
516H School of Allied Medical Professions
1583 Perry Street
Columbus, OH 43210
Phone: (614) 292-8142
Fax: (614) 292-0210
E-mail: wardlaw.1@osu.edu

Ghadeer -

Thanks so much for letting me borrow your nutrition book. It helped out a lot. Good luck on finals

-Lisa

ristmas Dinner to be served on Wednesday, hed flyer provides all the details.

the holiday spirit with your Mercy family.

Chapter 2 Tools for Diet Design 41

generally reliable. However, an in-depth examination of nutritional health is impossible without the rather expensive process of biochemical assessment. This involves the measurement of specific blood enzyme activities and of the concentrations of nutrients and nutrient by-products in the blood.

A clinical examination would follow, during which a health professional would search for any physical evidence of diet-related diseases. Last, a diet history, documenting at least the previous few days' intake, is an invaluable took for insight into possible problem areas. Together these activities form the **ABCDs** of nutritional assessment: **a**nthropometric measurements, **b**iochemical assessment, **c**linical examination, and **d**iet history.

Recognizing the Limitations of Nutritional Assessment

As mentioned, a long time may elapse between the initial development of poor nutritional health and the first clinical evidence of a problem. Recall that a diet high in saturated (typically solid) fat often increases blood **cholesterol** concentration, but without producing any clinical evidence for years. However, when the blood vessels become sufficiently blocked by cholesterol and other materials, chest pain during physical activity or a **heart attack** may occur. Much current nutrition research aims to develop better methods for early detection of nutrition-related problems such as this.

Another example in the delay of evidence that serious consequences are occurring is with a calcium deficiency, a particularly relevant issue for adolescent females. Many young women consume well below the needed amount of calcium but often suffer no ill effects in their younger years. However, women whose bone structures do not reach full potential during the years of growth are likely to face an increased risk for osteoporosis later in life.

Furthermore, clinical evidence of nutritional deficiencies is often not very specific, such as diarrhea, an irregular walk, and facial sores. These may have different causes. Long lag times and vague evidence often make it difficult to establish a link between an individual's current diet and nutritional state.

Table 1–4 in Chapter 1 showed the close relationship of nutrition and health. The rest of this current chapter helps you plan a diet to maximize your health and minimize the development of nutrition-related diseases.

Cholesterol
A waxy lipid found in all body cells. It has a structure containing multiple chemical rings that is found only in foods that contain animal products (see Chapter 5).

Heart attack
Rapid fall in heart function caused by reduced blood flow through the heart's blood vessels. Often part of the heart dies in the process (see Chapter 5). Technically called a myocardial infarction.

ConceptCheck

Variety, balance, and moderation are the foundations of a healthy diet. A desirable nutritional state results when the body has enough nutrients to function fully and contains stores to use in times of increased needs. When nutrient intake fails to meet body needs, undernutrition develops. Symptoms of such an inadequate nutrient intake can take months or years to develop. Overloading the body with nutrients, leading to overnutrition, is another potential problem to avoid. Nutritional state can be assessed by using anthropometric measurements, biochemical evidence, clinical evaluation, and diet history.

Critical Thinking

Tom loves to eat hamburgers, fries, and lots of pizza with doul amounts of cheese. He rare eats any vegetables and fru but instead snacks on cook and ice cream. He insists that he has no problems w his health, is rarely ill, and doesn't see how his diet co cause him any health risks. How would you explain to Tom that despite his curren good health, his diet could predispose him to future health problems?

The Food Guide Pyramid— A Menu-Planning Tool

Since the early twentieth century, researchers have worked on various food plans to simplify nutrition science into practical terms so that people with no special training could estimate whether their nutritional needs were being met. In recent years

Throughout each chapter are **boldfaced key terms.** These are terms you will need to be familiar with throughout your study. The more difficult terms include a **definition in the text's margins.** All boldfaced terms appear with their definitions and pronunciations in the **glossary** at the end of the text.

Nutrition Webs help you visualize a mental map of the relationship between key nutrition concepts.

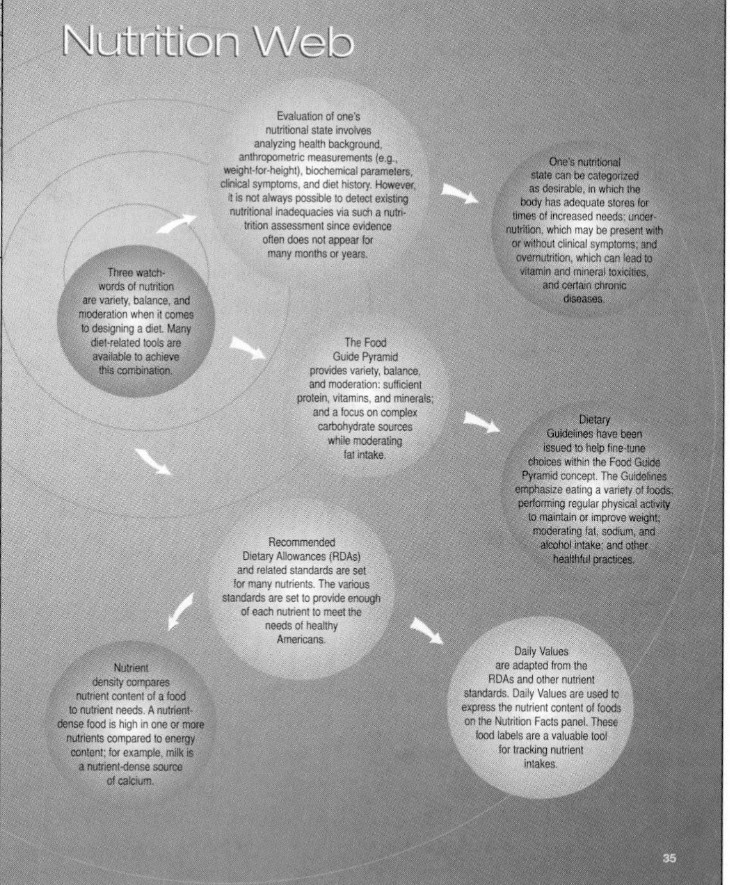

You'll find that the numerous full-color, 3-dimensional illustrations almost jump off the page and will help nutrition "come alive" for you.

360 Part 3 Energy Balance and Imbalance

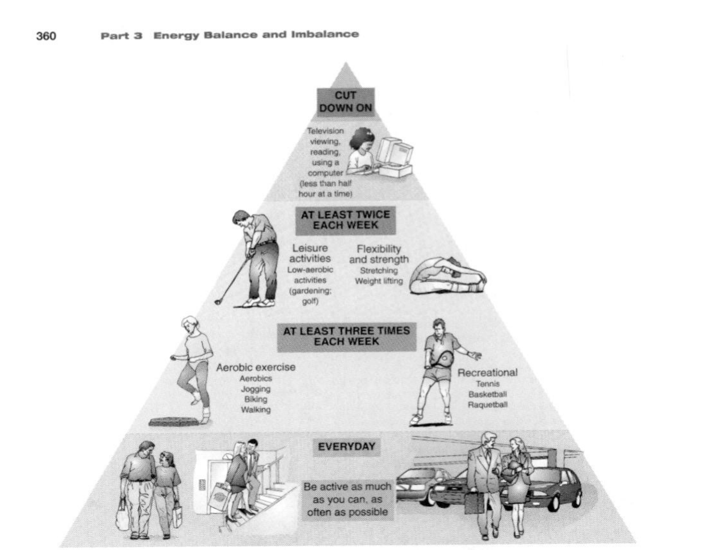

Figure 10-2 *Using the concept of the Food Guide Pyramid, health educators at Park Nicollet Medical Foundation in Minneapolis have created an easy reference—the Physical Activity Pyramid. The recommendations in the pyramid are based on American College of Sports Medicine guidelines.*

into each day's tasks. If there is not much time for activity, one can go for more intensity in the activities that can fit in to get the same benefits (Figure 10–2). Note that only about 1 in 10 adults practices vigorous activities daily, and about half of all adults quit their exercise plan within 3 months of the onset.

The easiest way to increase physical activity is to make it part of a daily routine, similar to other regular activities, such as eating. One does not need to join a gym or attend aerobic classes. Daily activities can meet the Phase 1 goal. Many people find that the best time to exercise is when they need an energy pick-me-up or a break from work. Rather than abandon an exercise program entirely when obstacles impede, one can strive to use any small periods of available time. Once reaping the benefits of exercise, a person will tend to spend more time at it.

Clearly, many of the activities recommended for Phase 1 are not very vigorous. By recommending Phase 1 for those starting an exercise program, fitness experts have not given up on the value of more vigorous physical activity. They're just making concessions to human nature.

Chapter 8 Water and Minerals 269

TABLE 8-2

Questionnaire for Evaluating Your Sodium Habits with Respect to Typically Rich Sources

HOW OFTEN DO YOU:	Rarely	Occasionally	Often	Regularly (daily)
1. Eat cured or processed meats, such as ham, bacon, sausage, frankfurters, and other luncheon meats?	☐	☐	☐	☐
2. Choose canned or frozen vegetables with sauce?	☐	☐	☐	☐
3. Use commercially prepared meals, main dishes, or canned or dehydrated soups?	☐	☐	☐	☐
4. Eat cheese, especially processed cheese?	☐	☐	☐	☐
5. Eat salted nuts, popcorn, pretzels, corn chips, or potato chips?	☐	☐	☐	☐
6. Add salt to cooking water for vegetables, rice, or pasta?	☐	☐	☐	☐
7. Add salt, seasoning mixes, salad dressings, or condiments—such as soy sauce, steak sauce, catsup, and mustard—to foods during preparation or at the table?	☐	☐	☐	☐
8. Salt your food before tasting it?	☐	☐	☐	☐
9. Ignore labels for sodium content when buying foods?	☐	☐	☐	☐
10. When dining out, choose foods at restaurants with sauces, or foods that are obviously salty?	☐	☐	☐	☐

The more checks you have in the last two columns, the higher your dietary sodium intake.

Adapted from USDA *Home and Garden Bulletin* No. 232-6, April 1986.

The numerous tables throughout the text provide convenient capsules of information for your reference.

Concept Check

Sodium is the major positive ion of extracellular fluid. It is important for maintaining fluid balance and conducting nerve impulses. Sodium depletion is unlikely, since the typical American's diet has abundant sources of sodium and most of it gets absorbed. The more foods we prepare at home, the more control we have over our sodium intake. The minimum sodium requirement for adults is 500 milligrams per day. The average adult consumes 3000 to 6000 milligrams or more daily. About 10% to 15% of the population is sensitive to sodium. In these people, high blood pressure can develop as a result of high-sodium diets, but many other lifestyle habits are more important. Many scientific groups suggest that for all adults sodium intake should be limited to about 3 grams (3000 milligrams). Sodium in the American diet is provided predominantly through processed foods and salt added in cooking and at the table.

Potassium (K)

Potassium performs many of the same functions as sodium, such as fluid balance and nerve impulse transmission. However, it operates inside, rather than outside, cells. Intracellular fluids—those inside cells—contain 95% of the potassium in the body. Also, unlike sodium, potassium is associated with lower rather than higher blood pressure values. We absorb about 90% of the potassium we eat.

The CONCEPT CHECKS appear every few pages and summarize content. If you don't understand what the Concept Check says, you should reread the preceding section in the textbook.

Vitamin A in Foods and Needs

Preformed vitamin A is found in liver, fish oils, vitamin A–fortified milk and breakfast cereals, and eggs. Butter and margarine are also sources because they are fortified with vitamin A. Provitamin A is found mainly in dark green and orange vegetables and some fruits. Carrots, spinach, winter squash, broccoli, papayas, and apricots are examples of sources. Consuming a varied diet rich in green vegetables and carrots ensures sufficient sources for meeting vitamin A needs (Figure 7–2). About half of the vitamin A in the American diet comes from animal sources, the other half from plants.

Recently, derivatives of vitamin A have been put into creams (Renova) that reduce some effects of aging on the skin. Note that if the skin is already deeply wrinkled, these creams are ineffective.

ANOTHER Bite *Most nutrient amounts in foods, including vitamin A, were formerly expressed in less precise* ***international units (IU)****. Some supplement labels still show the older IU values for vitamin A. For vitamin A the current unit of measurement is the retinol equivalent (RE). In this system, all potential forms of vitamin A are scaled based on their activity. Based on a mixture of preformed and provitamin A, 1 RE of vitamin A is equivalent to 5 IU of vitamin A.*

International unit (IU) *A crude measure of vitamin activity, often based on the growth rate of animals. Today these units have largely been replaced by more precise milligram and microgram measures.*

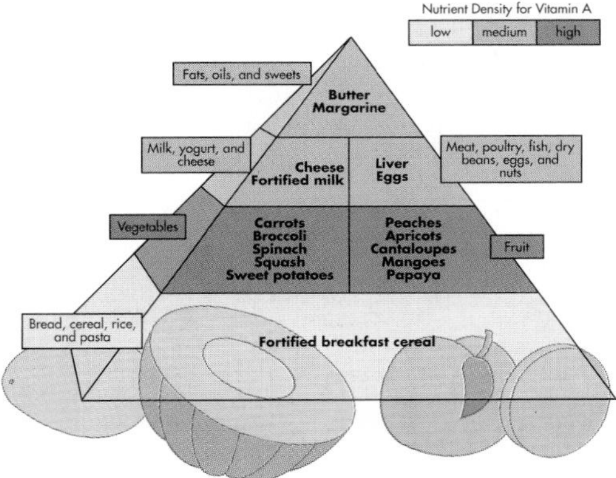

Figure 7–2 *Food sources of vitamin A from the Food Guide Pyramid. The fruit and vegetable groups supply abundant carotenoids if they have an intense yellow-orange or green color. Some of these carotenoids yield vitamin A. Liver is the richest source of preformed vitamin A, because that is the major site of vitamin A storage in animals. Milk is often fortified with vitamin A. The background color of each food group indicates the average nutrient density (RE per kcal) for vitamin A in that group.*

Leading food sources for major nutrients are identified in 20 colorful variations of the USDA Food Guide Pyramid. These illustrations will enable you to gain a further understanding of the distribution of nutrients among food groups.

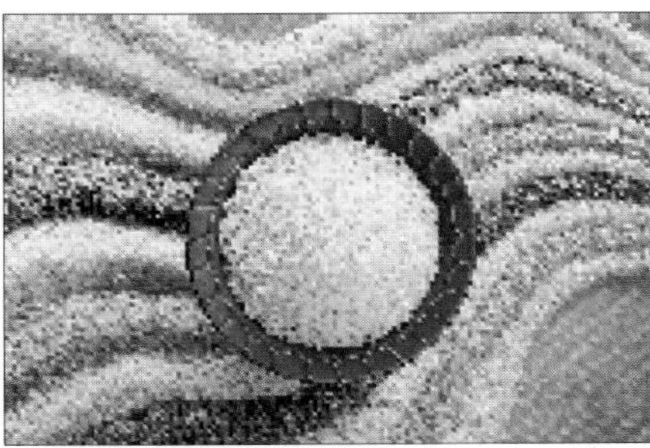

Rice is a rich source of carbohydrates.

Pyramid—fat intake should automatically decrease, as long as added fat is kept to a minimum and foods are prepared and served without additional fat.

Only in cases where a person's blood triglycerides are high is a carbohydrate-rich diet not recommended. (This will be covered further in Chapter 5.) Actually the chief culprits in this case are excessively large meals full of foods both rich in simple sugars and low in dietary fiber, and these aren't practices that should form the basis of a diet. But unfortunately, they often do.

Keep in mind, however, that any nutrient can lead to health problems when consumed in excess, including complex carbohydrate and dietary fiber. The contribution of high-carbohydrate foods to total energy intake still needs to be watched. Generally speaking, though, Americans are becoming fatter not because they are eating too much bread and pasta but because they are physically inactive and their diets are high in fat and simple sugars. In fact, added sugars, such as those in soft drinks, comprise about 16% of energy intake of adults. That corresponds to about 20 teaspoons (85 grams) per day. Recall from Chapter 2 that the Food Guide Pyramid suggests considerably lower intakes for many of us: 1600 kcal, 8 teaspoons; 2200 kcal, 12 teaspoons; 2800 kcal, 18 teaspoons. These allotments work out to 10% or less of total calories, a typical recommendation made by many health authorities. Overall, most adults are not active enough to warrant current use of added sugars (Figure 4–9).

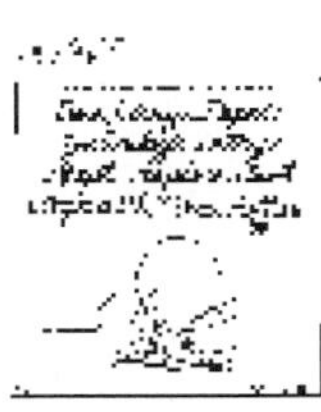

Figure 4–9
Ziggy.

ANOTHER Bite *During food processing, the sugar content is often increased. Usually, the more processed the food, the higher the sugar content. An apple has 0 grams of added sugar, canned apples in heavy syrup have 10 to 15 grams, and one sixth of a 9-inch apple pie has 30 grams of added sugar. For comparison purposes, 1 teaspoon of sugar is 4 grams.*

ANOTHER BITE boxes are short paragraphs within the text designed to provide you with a different perspective on chapter material or more detail. You'll discover new and different ways to apply information.

To briefly clarify and expand concepts presented, **margin notes** are provided for you. These help reinforce concepts you'll learn in every chapter. **Critical Thinking** questions also appear in the margins to give you the opportunity to apply chapter content to real-life situations. Answers are in the back of the book.

Chapter 3 The Human Body 89

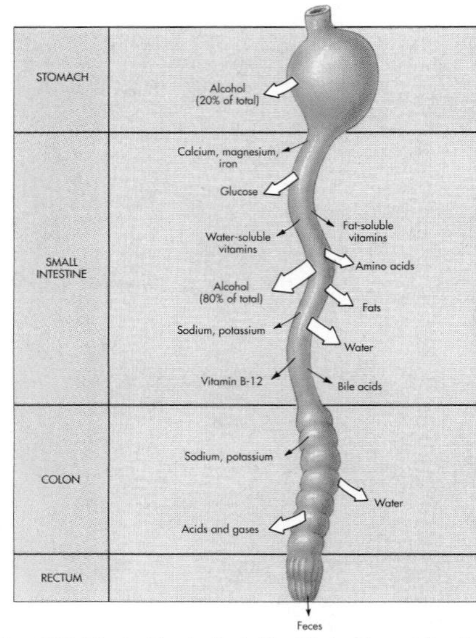

Figure 3-10 *Major sites of absorption along the GI tract. The size of the arrow indicates the relative amount of absorption at that site.*

Critical Thinking

The medical history of a young girl who is greatly underweight shows that she had three quarters of her small intestine removed after she was injured in a car accident. Explain how this accounts for her underweight condition, even though her medical chart shows that she eats well.

The Large Intestine Completes Absorption

When the intestinal contents enter the large intestine, little of the original foodstuff eaten still remains. Only a minor amount (5%) of carbohydrate, protein, and fat has escaped absorption (Figure 3-10). Some water is still present because the small intestine absorbs only 85% to 90% of the fluid it receives, which includes large amounts of GI-tract secretions produced during digestion. The remnants of the meal also include some minerals and what we call dietary fiber.

In the upper half of the large intestine, much of the remaining water and the minerals—mostly sodium and potassium—are absorbed. The unabsorbed water

Nutrient intake also directly influences nutrient absorption. For example, vitamin C in a meal modestly increases iron absorption in the same meal because it changes iron into a more absorbable state.

NUTRITION INSIGHTS are boxes within the text that allow you to learn more about timely topics that should be of interest to you.

376

Nutrition Insight

Sports Drinks: Most Helpful for Endurance Athletes

A question that often arises is whether to drink water or a sports-type drink, such as All Sport, Exceed Energy Drink, Gatorade, PowerAde, and Amino Force, during competition. For sports that require less than 30 minutes of exertion or when total weight loss is less than 5 to 6 pounds, the primary concern is replacing the water lost in sweat, because losses of body carbohydrate stores and electrolytes (sodium, chloride, potassium, and other minerals) are not usually too great. Although electrolytes are lost in sweat, the quantities lost in exercise of brief to moderate duration can easily be replaced later by consuming normal foods, such as orange juice, potatoes, and tomato juice. Keep in mind that sweat is about 99% water and only 1% electrolytes and other substances.

The use of sports drinks is most critical for athletes engaged in sports events lasting longer than 60 to 90 minutes. Prolonged exercise results in large sweat losses and some of the fluid for sweating comes from the bloodstream. If plain water is used to replace the fluid lost from the blood, the concentration of essential electrolytes in the bloodstream may become too diluted. Thus when sports drinks are used to help maintain blood volume, they must contain small amounts of sodium and potassium to avoid electrolyte imbalance. Generally speaking, beverages for the endurance athlete must provide water for hydration, electrolytes to both enhance water and glucose absorption from the intestine and help maintain blood volume, and carbohydrate to provide energy. Beyond 2 to 4 hours of exertion, electrolyte and carbohydrate replacement become increasingly important, especially in hot weather. In fact, sports drinks that contain carbohydrate have been found to delay fatigue during endurance sports with exercise intensities of a 3-hour marathon pace.

The following is but one possible protocol for using sports drinks as part of fluid replacement:

- About 2 hours before endurance exercise, consume 2 cups of water
- Once exercise begins, consume ½ to ¾ cup of a 6% to 8% carbohydrate solution (14 to 19 grams per cup of fluid) about every 15 minutes. The fluid should be cool to enhance palatability. The carbohydrate concentration of many common sports drinks is 6% to 8%, but check the label to be sure (Figure 10-5). If the exercise session is to last more than one hour, the goal for fluid replacement is to yield between 2½ to 5 cups (1600 to 1200 milliliters) of this fluid per hour.

Comparisons of drinks containing **glucose polymers** (glucoses linked together, more properly known as *maltodextrins*), glucose, and sucrose show that all of these carbohydrates have similar positive effects on exercise performance and physiologial function as long as the carbohydrate concentration is in the 6% to 8% range. Drinks in which fructose is the only carbohydrate source are the only exception to this rule. Fructose is absorbed from the intestine more slowly than glucose and often causes bloating and diarrhea.

For the most part, then, the decision to use a sports drink depends primarily on the duration of the activity. As the duration of continuous activity approaches 60 minutes or longer, the advantages from use of a sports drink over plain water begin to emerge.

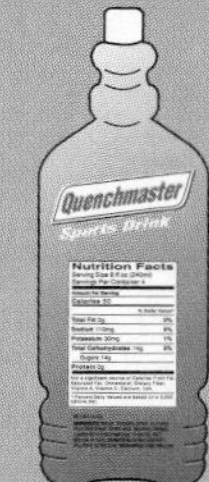

Figure 10-5 *Sports drinks for fluid and electrolyte replacement typically contain a form of simple carbohydrate plus sodium and potassium. The various sugars in this product total 14 grams per 1 cup (240 ml) serving. In percentage terms based on weight, the sugar content is about 6% ([14 grams sugar per serving ÷ 240 grams per serving] × 100 = 5.8%). Sports drinks typically contain about 6% to 8% sugar. This provides ample glucose and other monosaccharides to aid in fueling working muscles, and it is well tolerated. Drinks with a higher sugar content may cause stomach distress.*

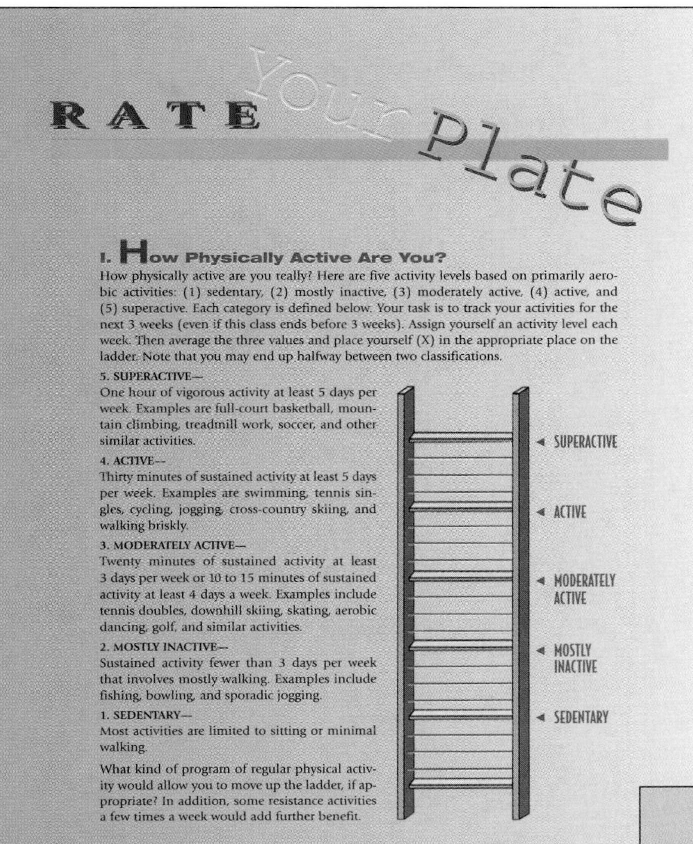

RATE Your Plate

I. How Physically Active Are You?

How physically active are you really? Here are five activity levels based on primarily aerobic activities: (1) sedentary, (2) mostly inactive, (3) moderately active, (4) active, and (5) superactive. Each category is defined below. Your task is to track your activities for the next 3 weeks (even if this class ends before 3 weeks). Assign yourself an activity level each week. Then average the three values and place yourself (X) in the appropriate place on the ladder. Note that you may end up halfway between two classifications.

5. SUPERACTIVE—
One hour of vigorous activity at least 5 days per week. Examples are full-court basketball, mountain climbing, treadmill work, soccer, and other similar activities.

4. ACTIVE—
Thirty minutes of sustained activity at least 5 days per week. Examples are swimming, tennis singles, cycling, jogging, cross-country skiing, and walking briskly.

3. MODERATELY ACTIVE—
Twenty minutes of sustained activity at least 3 days per week or 10 to 15 minutes of sustained activity at least 4 days a week. Examples include tennis doubles, downhill skiing, skating, aerobic dancing, golf, and similar activities.

2. MOSTLY INACTIVE—
Sustained activity fewer than 3 days per week that involves mostly walking. Examples include fishing, bowling, and sporadic jogging.

1. SEDENTARY—
Most activities are limited to sitting or minimal walking.

What kind of program of regular physical activity would allow you to move up the ladder, if appropriate? In addition, some resistance activities a few times a week would add further benefit.

At the end of each chapter is a **RATE YOUR PLATE** section that will help you apply a major concept in each chapter to your own life. The activity encourages you to look more carefully at your diet, examine your family history, or apply information to help other people you know.

NUTRITION ISSUES are boxes at the end of chapters that develop current topics in nutrition in greater detail than can be done in the chapter. Topics include nutrition and alcohol, heart disease, cancer, fad diets, and food labeling.

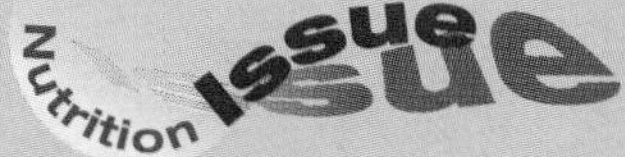

381

Evaluating Ergogenic Aids to Enhance Athletic Performance

Diet manipulation to improve athletic performance is not a recent innovation. As long as 30 years ago, American football players were encouraged on hot practice days to "toughen up" for competition by liberally consuming salt tablets before and during practice and by not drinking water. Now it is widely recognized that this practice can be fatal. Today's athletes are as likely as their predecessors to experiment; artichoke hearts, bee pollen, dried adrenal glands from cattle, seaweed, freeze-dried liver flakes, gelatin, and ginseng are just some of the ineffective substances now used by athletes in hopes of gaining an **ergogenic** (work-producing) edge.

Still, today's athletes can benefit from recent scientific evidence documenting the ergogenic properties of a few dietary substances. These ergogenic aids include sufficient water, lots of carbohydrates, and a balanced and varied diet consistent with the Food Guide Pyramid. Protein and amino acid supplements are not among those aids, because athletes can easily meet protein needs from foods, as Table 10-4 demonstrated. Clearly, changing average athletes into champions is not possible simply by altering their diets. The use of nutrient supplements should be designed to meet a specific dietary weakness, such as an inadequate iron intake. These and other aids, which often have dubious benefits and may pose health risks, must be given close scrutiny before use. The risk-benefit ratio of these ergogenic aids especially needs to be examined.

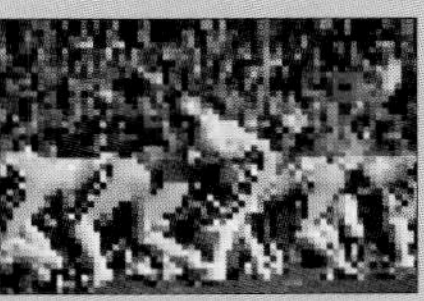

Attention to carbohydrate and fluid needs—along with meeting overall nutrient needs—is the most important ergogenic aid.

As summarized in Table 10-6, no scientific evidence supports the effectiveness of many substances touted as performance-enhancing aids. Many are useless; some are dangerous. Athletes should be skeptical of any substance until it's ergogenic effect is scientifically verified. FDA has a limited ability to regulate these dietary supplements (see the Nutrition Issue in Chapter 1). Even substances whose ergogenic effects have been supported by systematic scientific studies should be used with caution, as the testing conditions may not match those of the intended use. Finally, rather than waiting for a magic bullet to enhance performance, athletes are advised to concentrate their efforts on improving their training routines and sport technique and consuming well-balanced diets as described in this chapter. Adequate fluid and carbohydrate are the primary diet-related ergogenic aids.

Sodium bicarbonate
An alkaline substance basically made of sodium and carbon dioxide ($NaHCO_3$).

Anabolic steroids
A general term for hormones that stimulate development in male sex organs and such male characteristics as facial hair (for example, testosterone).

Growth hormone
A pituitary hormone that produces body growth and release of fat from storage, among other effects.

Carnitine
A compound used to shuttle fatty acids into the cell mitochondria. This allows for the fatty acids to be burned for energy.

Summary

- Regular physical activity is a vital part of a healthy lifestyle, ideally constituting a total of at least 30 minutes per day, including some aerobic and resistance activities. People over 35 years should first discuss plans with a physician. Physically active people show lower risks of heart disease, diabetes, obesity, and other common chronic diseases.
- Adenosine triphosphate (ATP) is the major form of energy used by cells. Human metabolic pathways are able to extract that energy from foodstuffs and store it as ATP energy. Phosphocreatine (PCr) can also provide the energy needed to form ATP in a human cell.
- In carbohydrate fuel use, glucose is broken down into three-carbon compounds, yielding some ATP. The three-carbon compounds can then proceed to an aerobic pathway to form carbon dioxide (CO_2) and water (H_2O) or to an anaerobic pathway to form lactic acid.
- At low workloads, muscle cells use mainly fat for fuel, forming CO_2 and H_2O. For high-output exercise of short duration, muscles use PCr and glucose for energy.
- For endurance exercise, fat and carbohydrate are used as fuels; carbohydrate is used increasingly as activity intensifies. Little protein is used to fuel muscles.
- Anyone who exercises regularly needs to consume a diet that is moderate to high in carbohydrates and consistent with the Food Guide Pyramid. Vitamin and mineral supplements are indicated primarily if a low energy intake makes it difficult to meet nutrient needs or a nutrient deficiency exists.
- Carbohydrate loading can increase usual stores of muscle glycogen. Participants in endurance events that last more than 2 hours benefit most from carbohydrate loading, which basically involves eating a diet very high in carbohydrate for about 3 days before the event.
- Athletes should consume enough fluid both to minimize loss of body weight from fluid loss during exercise and to ultimately restore preexercise weight. A sports-type drink can be helpful for endurance athletes participating in activities lasting more than 60 minutes.

Study Questions

1. How does greater physical fitness contribute to greater overall health? Explain the process.
2. The store of ATP in muscle is rapidly depleted once contraction begins. For physical activity to continue, ATP must be resupplied immediately. Describe how this occurs after initiation of exercise and at various times thereafter.
3. What is the difference between anaerobic and aerobic exercise? Explain why aerobic metabolism is increased by a regular exercise routine.
4. What is glycogen? How does the body obtain it? How is it used during exercise?
5. Are fat stores used as an energy source during exercise? If so, when?
6. What are some typical measures used to assess whether an athlete's energy intake is adequate.
7. List five specific nutrients that athletes need and appropriate food sources from which these nutrients can be obtained.
8. If an athlete wanted to help meet these needs with supplements, what guidelines could you provide to promote safe use.
9. What advice would you give your neighbor, who is planning to run a 50-kilometer (km) race, concerning fluid intake before and during the event?
10. One of your friends, a competitive athlete, asks your opinion about a nutritional supplement sold in a local sporting-goods store. She has read that such supplements, which contain amino acids, can help improve athletic performance. What would you tell her about the general effectiveness of such products?

Each chapter ends with a **SUMMARY.** These summary points convey the major ideas of each chapter.

There are approximately ten **STUDY QUESTIONS** per chapter. These provide an excellent review for studying for examinations.

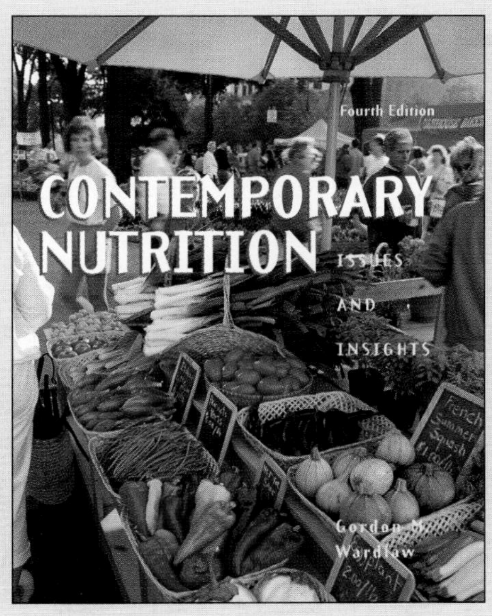

MCGRAW-HILL IS PROUD TO OFFER AN EXCITING NEW SUITE OF MULTIMEDIA PRODUCTS AND SERVICES CALLED COURSE SOLUTIONS.

Designed specifically to help you with your individual course needs, **Course Solutions** will assist you in integrating your syllabus with our premier titles and state-of-the-art new media tools that support them.

AT THE HEART OF COURSE SOLUTIONS YOU'LL FIND:

- Fully integrated multimedia
- A full-scale Online Learning Center
- A Course Integration Guide

AS WELL AS THESE UNPARALLELED SERVICES:

- McGraw-Hill Learning Architecture
- McGraw-Hill Course Consultant Service
- Visual Resource Library (VRL) Image Licensing
- McGraw-Hill Student Tutorial Service
- McGraw-Hill Instructor Syllabus Service
- PageOut Lite
- PageOut: The Course Web Site Development Center
- Other Delivery Options

COURSE SOLUTIONS truly has the solutions to your every teaching need. Read on to learn how we can specifically help you with your classroom challenges.

SPECIAL ATTENTION *to your specific needs.*

These "perks" are all part of the extra service delivered through McGraw-Hill's **Course Solutions**:

McGRAW-HILL LEARNING ARCHITECTURE

Each McGraw-Hill *Online Learning Center* is ready to be ported into our *McGraw-Hill Learning Architecture*—a full course management software system for Local Area Networks and Distance Learning Classes. Developed in conjunction with Top Class software, *McGraw-Hill Learning Architecture* is a powerful course management system available upon special request.

McGRAW-HILL COURSE CONSULTANT SERVICE

In addition to the *Course Integration Guide*, instructors using **Course Solutions** textbooks can access a special curriculum-based *Course Consultant Service* via a web-based threaded discussion list within each *Online Learning Center.* A **McGraw-Hill Course Solutions Consultant** will personally help you—as a text adopter—integrate this text and media into your course to fit your specific needs. This content-based service is offered in addition to our usual software support services.

VISUAL RESOURCE LIBRARY (VRL) IMAGE LICENSING

Most of our **Course Solutions** titles are accompanied by a *Visual Resource Library (VRL) CD-ROM,* which features text figures in electronic format. Previously, use of these images was restricted to in-class presentation only. Now, McGraw-Hill will license adopters the right to use appropriate VRL image files—**FREE OF CHARGE**—for placement on their local Web site! Some restrictions apply. Consult your McGraw-Hill sales representative for more details.

McGRAW-HILL INSTRUCTOR SYLLABUS SERVICE

For *new* adopters of **Course Solutions** textbooks, McGraw-Hill will help correlate all text, supplement, and appropriate materials and services to your course syllabus. Simply call your McGraw-Hill sales representative for assistance.

PAGEOUT LITE

Free to **Course Solutions** textbook adopters, *PageOut Lite* is perfect for instructors who want to create their own Web site. In just a few minutes, even novices can turn their syllabus into a Web site using *PageOut Lite*.

PAGEOUT: THE COURSE WEB SITE DEVELOPMENT CENTER

For those that want the benefits of *PageOut Lite's* no-hassle approach to site development, but with even more features, we offer *PageOut: The Course Web Site Development Center.*

PageOut shares many of *PageOut Lite's* features, but also enables you to create links that will take your students to your original material, other Web site addresses, and to *McGraw-Hill Online Learning Center* content. This means you can assign *Online Learning Center* content within your syllabus-based Web site. *PageOut's* gradebook function will tell you when each student has taken a quiz or worked through an exercise, automatically recording their scores for you. *PageOut* also features a discussion board list where you and your students can exchange questions and post announcements, as well as an area for students to build personal Web pages.

OTHER DELIVERY OPTIONS

Online Learning Centers are also compatible with a number of full-service online course delivery systems or outside educational service providers. For a current list of compatible delivery systems, contact your McGraw-Hill sales representative.

And for your students . . .

McGRAW-HILL STUDENT TUTORIAL SERVICE

Within each *Online Learning Center* resides a **FREE** *Student Tutorial Service*. This web-based "homework hotline"—available via a threaded discussion list—features guaranteed, 24-hour response time on weekdays.

www.mhhe.com/hper/nutrition/wardlaw

Nutrition: A Key to Health

part 1

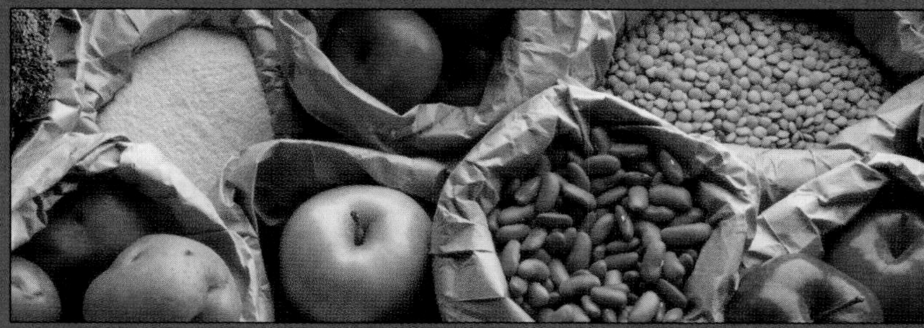

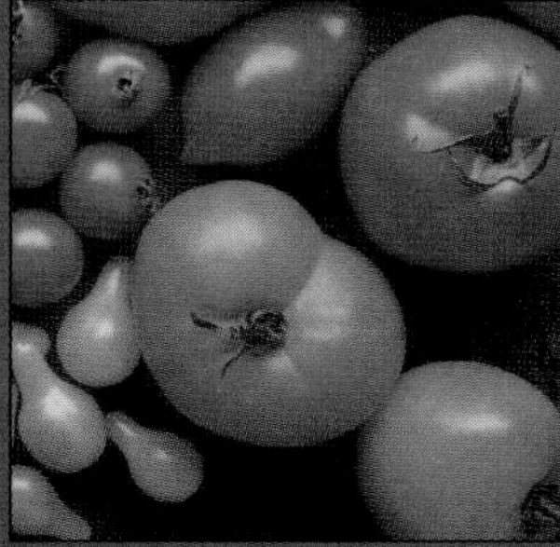

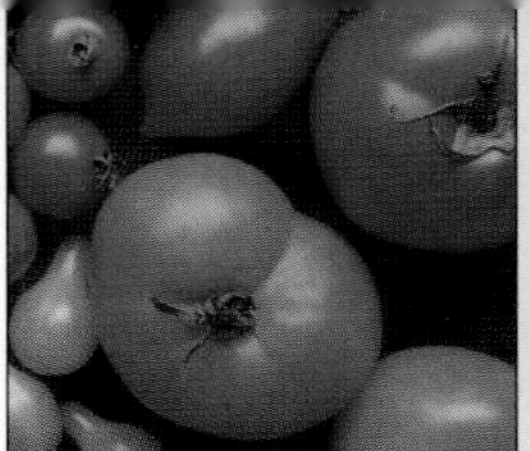

chapter 1

Nutrition: A Key to Health
What You Eat and Why

Do you need vitamin and mineral supplements? Are you eating too much fat and cholesterol? Is much of what you eat unsafe? Are some foods actually *junk foods?* Should you become a vegetarian? If you're confused about what you should eat, welcome to what is probably the fastest-growing club in the country. This chapter will help you begin to sort out some of these issues as you are introduced to the science of nutrition.

And as you begin this study of nutrition, keep in mind what nutrition expert Dr. Irwin Rosenberg recently provided as his "bottom line" for a healthy lifestyle: "Research has shown no better way to slow or even reverse the progress of aging itself and of all the age-related degenerative conditions than through the combination of aerobic and strength building exercise and a balanced, nutritious diet." Overall, it is clear that the nutritional lifestyles of some Americans are out of balance with their physiology. And since we live longer than our ancestors, preventing the nutrition-related diseases that develop later in life is more important than in the past.

By changing our "problem" food and related lifestyle habits, we can strive to bring the goal of a healthy life within our reach. This is a primary theme not just in this chapter but throughout this entire book.

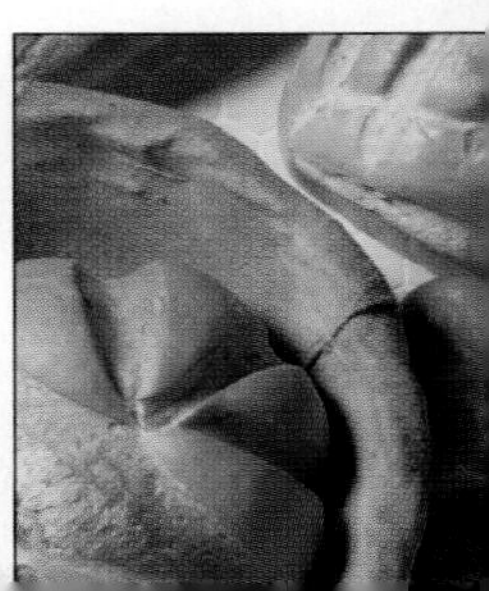

Nutrition Web

Nutrition is the study of food and nutrients and their influence on the health of the body.

To some degree, we can influence our long-term health by eating a varied diet, performing regular physical activity, not smoking, getting adequate fluid and sleep, and limiting alcohol intake and stress.

Results from large nutrition surveys suggest that some Americans do not consume enough vitamin A, certain B vitamins, vitamin C, calcium, iron, zinc, and dietary fiber. Thus for many of us our diets need improvements.

The six classes of nutrients include carbohydrates, proteins, lipids, water, vitamins, and minerals.

On average, fat provides 9 kcal per gram, while carbohydrates and protein provide 4 kcal per gram.

The hypothalamus, along with other brain regions, affect hunger. In addition, hormones and hormone-like compounds trigger hunger and eventually satiety.

The body transforms the energy trapped in carbohydrate, protein, and fat into other forms of energy to allow the body to function.

A variety of external (appetite-related) forces affect satiety. Hunger cues combine with appetite cues to promote feeding.

Water, vitamins and minerals are essential for proper body functioning, though they do not supply any energy to the body.

Our daily food choices are mainly controlled by flavor and texture. In addition, personal preferences and lifestyle, past experiences, cultural factors, economics, and health influence food choices.

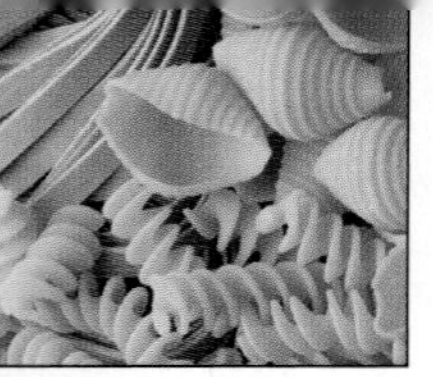

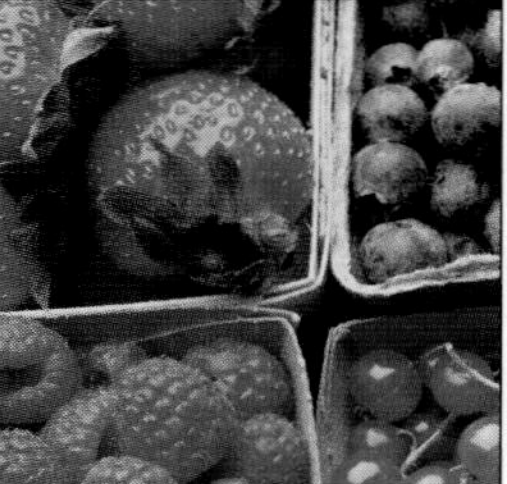

Nutrition and Your Health

Although the science of nutrition is relatively young, we already know much about what nutrients are needed for an adequate diet and what foods provide them. You are likely already familiar with some of this nutrition knowledge. Reading food labels and watching one's weight are two common adult pursuits. Still, you will benefit by learning even more about nutrition, especially its role in contributing to overall health.

In this opening chapter you will take a close look at your eating habits and discover the underlying reasons for them. This is an important first step. Ironically, people often have good intentions about healthy food choices but fail to act on them. However, if you make even small changes in your behavior toward food (and physical activity), you can increase your chances for enjoying a long and vigorous life.

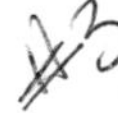

Recent evidence points to poor diet as a **risk factor** for **chronic** diseases that are the leading causes of adult deaths: **heart disease, stroke, high blood pressure, diabetes,** and some forms of **cancer** (Table 1–1). Together, these disorders account for two-thirds of all deaths in the United States (Table 1–2). Not consuming enough **nutrients** also makes us more likely to suffer consequences of poor nutrition habits

TABLE 1-1

Glossary Terms to Aid Your Introduction to Nutrition*

cancer A condition characterized by uncontrolled growth of abnormal cells.

chronic Long-standing, developing over time; slow to develop or resolve. When referring to disease, this term indicates that the disease process, once developed, is slow and tends to remain; a good example is heart disease.

cirrhosis of the liver Anything that is toxic to liver cells can lead to cirrhosis. The most common cause is a chronic, excessive alcohol intake.

diabetes A disease characterized by high blood glucose resulting from either insufficient insulin release by the pancreas or general inability of insulin to act on certain body cells, such as muscle cells.

heart disease A disease characterized by the deposition of fatty material and related hardening in the blood vessels that serve the heart. These deposits restrict blood flow through the heart, which in turn can lead to heart damage and death. Also termed *coronary heart disease* (CHD), as the vessels of the heart are the primary site of disease.

high blood pressure A condition in which blood pressure remains persistently elevated, especially when the heart is between beats.

nutrients Chemical substances in food that are essential parts of a diet. Nutrients nourish us by providing energy, materials for building body parts, and factors to regulate necessary chemical processes in the body. The body either can't make these nutrients or can't make them fast enough for its needs.

osteoporosis Decreased bone mass and bone mineral density where no outward causes can be found. Related to effects of aging, poor diet, and hormonal effects of postmenopausal status in women.

risk factor A term used frequently when discussing diseases and factors contributing to their development. A risk factor is an aspect of our lives—such as heredity, lifestyle choices (i.e., smoking), or nutritional habits—that may make us more likely to develop a disease.

stroke The loss of body function that results from a blood clot or other change in the brain that affects blood flow. This in turn causes the death of brain tissue. Also called a *cerebrovascular accident.*

*All bold terms in the book are defined in a glossary that follows Chapter 16. Many of these key terms are also defined in the chapter margin.

in later years, such as bone fractures from the disease **osteoporosis.** At the same time, taking too much of a nutrient supplement—such as vitamin A, vitamin D, vitamin B-6, calcium, or copper—can be harmful. Another dietary problem, drinking too much alcohol, is associated with **cirrhosis of the liver,** some forms of cancer, accidents, and suicides. All of these consequences of modern living are partly an "affliction of affluence."

The great tragedy is that these diseases are often preventable. Government scientists have calculated that a poor diet combined with a lack of sufficient physical activity account for 300,000 fatal cases of heart disease, cancer, and diabetes each year. Smoking makes matters even worse. (But quitting smoking quickly begins to reduce health risks.)

As you gain understanding about your nutritional habits and increase your knowledge about nutrition, you have the opportunity to dramatically cut your risk for many of these problems. To help, the federal government provides a web site that can link you to many sites providing health information (http://www.healthfinder.gov).

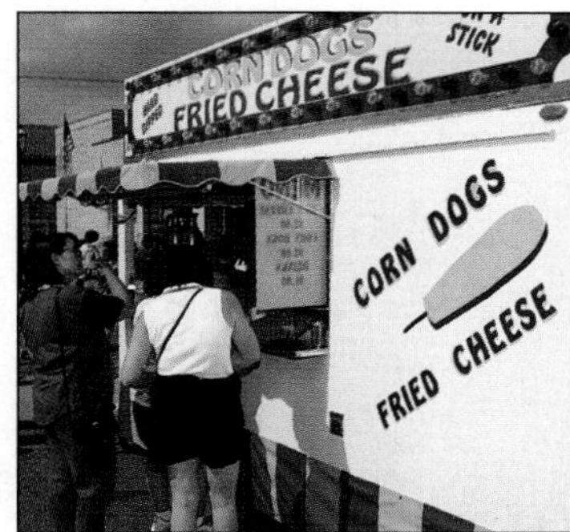

Many major health problems in the United States are largely caused by a poor diet, excessive calorie intake, and lack of physical activity.

What Is Nutrition?

The Council on Food and Nutrition of the American Medical Association defines ***nutrition*** as "The science of food, the nutrients and the substances therein, their action, interaction, and balance in relation to health and disease, and the process by which the organism ingests, digests, absorbs, transports, utilizes, and excretes food substances."

Some nutrients that perform life-sustaining functions can be produced by the body if they are missing from the diet. The essential nature of such nutrients sometimes is not clear-cut. For example, the body requires a regular source of vitamin D, but the skin is capable of synthesizing its own vitamin D upon receiving sunlight. This reduces the need from dietary sources.

Nutrients Come from Food

What is the difference between food, nutrients, and nutrition? Food provides both the energy and the materials needed to build and maintain all body cells. Nutrients

TABLE 1-2

Ten Leading Causes of Death in the United States

Rank	Cause of death	Percent of total deaths
	All causes	100.0
1	Heart disease (primarily **heart attacks**)*	31
2	Cancer*	23
3	Cerebrovascular diseases (stroke)*	7
4	Chronic obstructive pulmonary diseases and allied conditions (lung diseases)	5
5	Accidents and adverse effects†	
	Motor vehicle accidents	2
	All other accidents and adverse effects	2
6	Pneumonia and influenza	4
7	Diabetes*	3
8	Suicide†	1
9	Kidney disease*	1
10	Liver disease†	1

From Centers for Disease Control and Prevention, *National Vital Statistics Report,* October 7, 1998.
*Causes of death in which diet plays a part.
†Causes of death in which excessive alcohol consumption plays a part.

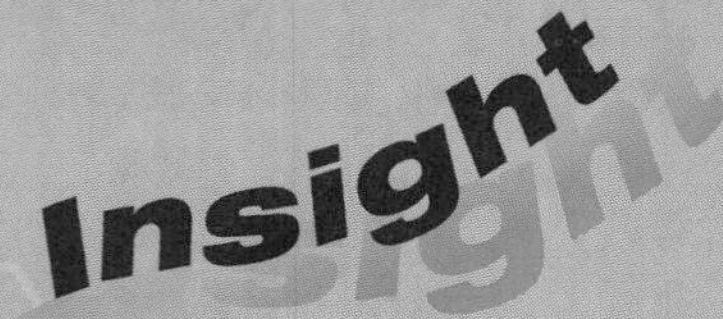

Math Tools for Nutrition

You will use a few mathematical concepts in studying nutrition. Besides performing addition, subtraction, multiplication, and division, you need to know how to calculate percentages and convert English units of measurement to metric units.

Percentages

The term *percent* (%) refers to a part of the total when the total represents 100 parts. For example, if you earn 80% on your first nutrition examination, you will have answered the equivalent of 80 out of 100 questions correctly. This equivalent could be 8 correct answers out of 10; 80% also describes 16 of 20 (16/20 = 0.80 or 80%). The best way to master this concept is to calculate some percentages. Some examples are given below:

Question	Answer
What is 6% of 45?	$0.06 \times 45 = 2.7$
What is 32% of 8?	$0.32 \times 8 = 2.6$
What percent of 16 is 6?	$\frac{6}{16} = 0.375$ or 37.5%
What percent of 99 is 3?	$\frac{3}{99} = 0.03$ or 3%

Joe ate 15% of the adult Recommended Dietary Allowance (RDA) for vitamin C at lunch. How many milligrams did he eat? (RDA = 60 milligrams)

0.15 × 60 milligrams = 9 milligrams

It is difficult to succeed in a nutrition course unless you know what a percentage means and how to calculate one. Percentages are used frequently when referring to menus and nutrient composition.

The Metric System

The basic units of the metric system are the meter, which indicates length; the gram, which indicates weight; and the liter, which indicates volume. The inside cover of this textbook lists conversions from the metric system to the English system (pounds, feet, cups) and vice versa. Here is a brief summary:

One meter is 39.4 inches long, or about 3 inches longer than 1 yard (3 feet).
A meter can be divided into 100 units of centimeters, or into 1000 units of millimeters.
A millimeter is about the thickness of a dime.
There are 2.54 centimeters in 1 inch and about 30 centimeters in 1 foot.
A person 6 feet tall is equivalent to 183 centimeters tall.
A gram is about 1/30 of an ounce (28 grams to the ounce).
Five grams of sugar or salt is about 1 teaspoon.
  A pound weighs 454 grams.
A kilogram is 1000 grams, equivalent to 2.2 pounds.
  To convert your weight to kilograms, divide it by 2.2.
  A 154-pound man weighs 70 kilograms (154/2.2 = 70).
  A gram can be divided into 1000 milligrams or 1,000,000 micrograms.
  15 milligrams of zinc (approximately the adult RDA) would be a few grains of zinc oxide.
Liters are divided into 1000 units called milliliters.
  One teaspoon equals about 5 milliliters, 1 cup is about 240 milliliters, and 1 quart (4 cups) equals almost 1 liter (0.946 liter to be exact).

If you plan to work in any scientific field, you will need to learn the metric system. **For now, remember that a kilogram equals 2.2 pounds, an ounce weighs 28 grams, 2.54 centimeters equals 1 inch, and a liter is almost the same as a quart.** In addition, know what the prefixes micro (1/1,000,000), milli (1/1000), centi (1/100), and kilo (1000) represent.

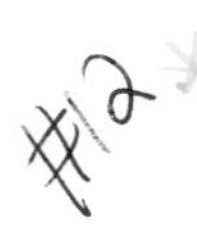

are the nourishing substances we must obtain from food. These essential substances are vital for growth and maintenance from infancy to adulthood. For a nutrient to be considered essential, two characteristics are needed. First, its omission from the diet must lead to a decline in certain aspects of human health, such as function of the nervous system. Second, if the omitted nutrient is restored to the diet before permanent damage occurs, those aspects of human health hampered by its absence should regain normal function.

TABLE 1-3

Essential Nutrients in the Human Diet and Their Classes*

ENERGY-YIELDING NUTRIENTS

Carbohydrate	Fat (lipids)†	Protein (amino acids)	Water
Glucose‡ (or a carbohydrate that yields glucose)	Linoleic acid (omega-6)	Histidine	Water
	α-Linolenic acid (omega-3)	Isoleucine	
		Leucine	
		Lysine	
		Methionine	
		Phenylalanine	
		Threonine	
		Tryptophan	
		Valine	

VITAMINS		MINERALS		
Water-soluble	**Fat-soluble**	**Major**	**Trace**	**Questionable**
Thiamin	A	Calcium	Chromium	Arsenic
Riboflavin	D§	Chloride	Copper	Boron
Niacin	E	Magnesium	Fluoride ‖	Cobalt
Pantothenic acid	K	Phosphorus	Iodide	Lithium
Biotin		Potassium	Iron	Nickel
B-6		Sodium	Manganese	Silicon
B-12		Sulfur	Molybdenum	Tin
Folate			Selenium	
C			Zinc	

*This table includes nutrients that the 1989 RDA publication lists for humans. Some disagreement exists over the questionable and other minerals not listed. Dietary fiber could be added to the list of essential substances, but it is not a nutrient (see Chapter 4). Alcohol is a source of calories, but is not a nutrient per se.
†The lipids listed are needed only in slight amounts, about 2% of total energy needs (see Chapter 5).
‡To prevent ketosis and thus the muscle loss that would occur if protein was used to synthesize carbohydrate (see Chapter 4).
§Sunshine on the skin also allows the body to make vitamin D for itself (see Chapter 7).
‖Primarily for dental health (see Chapter 8).

The vitamin-like compound choline plays essential roles in the body but is not listed under the vitamin category at this time. Rough estimates of human needs for this water-soluble compound recently have been set (see the inside cover of the text). Note, however, that body synthesis suffices during most states of life (see Chapter 7 for details).

Classes and Sources of Nutrients

You have probably heard the terms **carbohydrates, proteins, lipids** (fats and oils), **vitamins** and **minerals** (Figure 1–1). These, plus **water,** make up the six classes of nutrients found in food (Table 1–3). Today we know that the minimum diet for human growth, development, and maintenance must contain about 45 essential nutrients.

Nutrients can be further sorted into three groups: (1) those that primarily provide us with energy, (2) those that are important for growth, development, and maintenance, and (3) those that act to keep body functions running smoothly. Some overlap exists between these groupings. The energy-yielding nutrients make up a major portion of most foods.

Provide energy	Promote growth and development	Regulate body processes
carbohydrates	proteins	proteins
proteins	lipids	lipids
lipids (fats and oils)	vitamins	vitamins
	minerals	minerals
	water	water

Carbohydrate
A compound containing carbon, hydrogen, and oxygen; most are known as sugars, starches, *and* dietary fibers. *Yield on average 4 kcal per gram.*

Protein
Food components made of amino acids; amino acids contain carbon, hydrogen, oxygen, nitrogen, and sometimes other chemical elements, in a specific configuration. Proteins contain the form of nitrogen most easily used by the human body. Yield on average 4 kcal per gram.

Carbohydrate

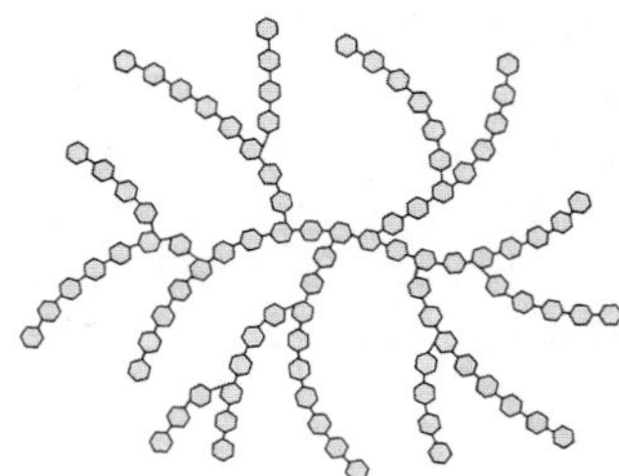

Each yellow circle represents one glucose molecule.

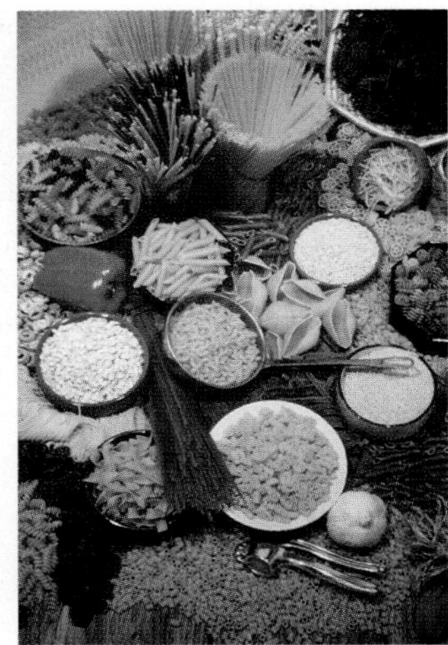

Lipid

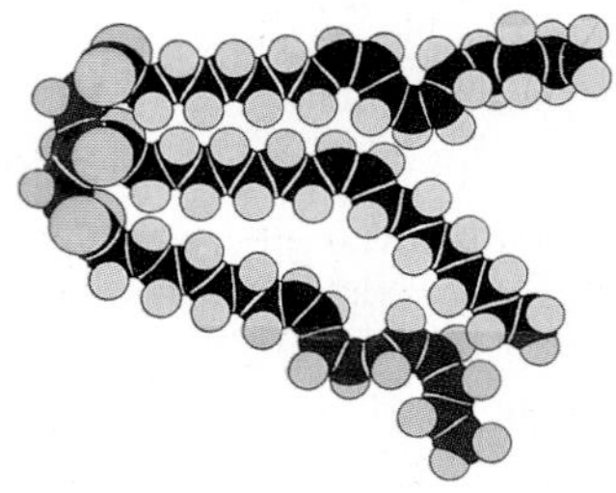

The black, blue, and yellow circles represent carbon, hydrogen, and oxygen, respectively, in the triglyceride structure.

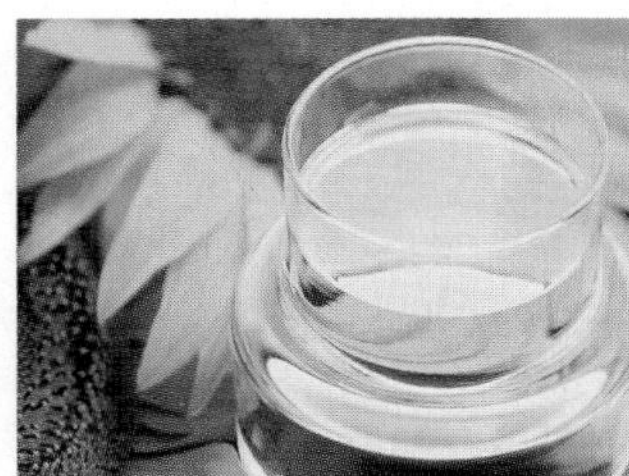

Protein

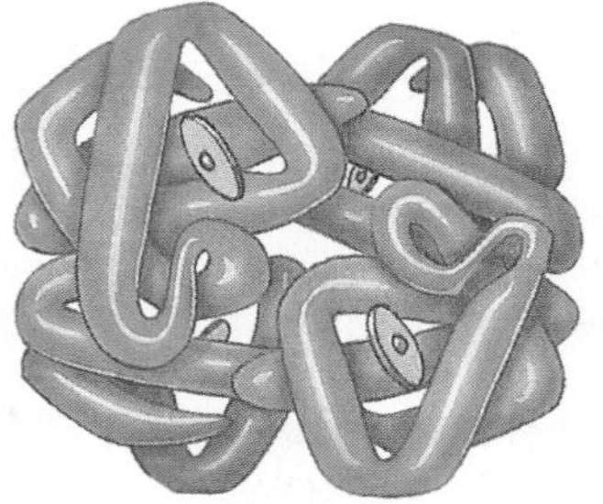

This protein found in a red blood cell is a structure formed primarily of linked amino acids.

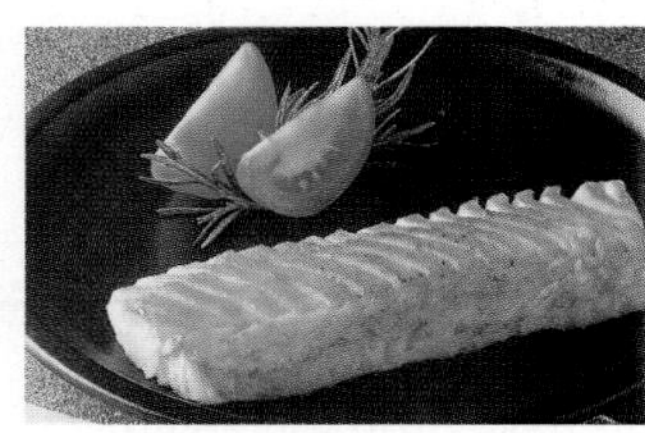

Figure 1–1 *Two views of carbohydrates, lipids, and proteins—chemical and dietary perspectives.* Illustrations by William Ober.

Lipid
A compound containing much carbon and hydrogen, little oxygen, and sometimes other chemical elements. Lipids dissolve in ether or benzene and include fats, oils, and cholesterol. Yield on average 9 kcal per gram.

Vitamins
Compounds needed in very small amounts in the diet to help regulate and support chemical reactions in the body.

Minerals
Chemical elements used in the body to promote chemical reactions and to form body structures.

Kilocalorie (kcal)
The heat needed to raise the temperature of 1000 grams (1 liter) of water 1°C. This is the same as raising the temperature of about 4 cups of water by 2°F.

Glucose
A six-carbon carbohydrate found in blood and in table sugar bound to fructose; also known as dextrose, *it is one of the simple sugars.*

Carbohydrates

Carbohydrates are composed mainly of carbon, hydrogen, and oxygen. Carbohydrates provide a major source of fuel for the body, on average 4 **kilocalories** (kcal) per gram. Small carbohydrate structures are called sugars or simple sugars. Table sugar (sucrose) is an example. Some simple sugars such as **glucose**, can link chemically to form large storage carbohydrates, called polysaccharides or complex carbohydrates (see Figure 1–1). An example is the **starch** in potatoes.

Aside from enjoying their taste, we need sugars and other carbohydrates in our diets primarily to satisfy the energy needs of body cells. Glucose, which the body can produce from most carbohydrates, is the primary source of energy for many cells. When not enough carbohydrate is eaten to supply sufficient glucose, the body is forced to make glucose from proteins. However, a typical diet contains more than enough carbohydrate to prevent this from happening.

The links between the sugar molecules in certain complex carbohydrates cannot be broken down by human digestive processes. These carbohydrates are part of what is called **dietary fiber.** Such dietary fiber passes through the small intestine undigested and provides bulk for the stool (feces), which is formed in the large intestine (colon). Chapter 4 focuses on carbohydrates, including the health benefits of dietary fiber.

Dietary fiber
Substances in food (essentially from plants) that are not digested by the processes that take place in the stomach or small intestine. These add bulk to feces.

Triglyceride
The major form of lipid in the body and in food. It is composed of three fatty acids linked to glycerol, an alcohol.

Fatty acid
Major part of most lipids; composed of a chain of carbons flanked by hydrogen with an acid group

$$\begin{array}{c} O \\ \| \\ (-C-OH) \end{array}$$

at one end and a methyl group ($-CH_3$) at the other (see Chapter 5).

Lipids

Lipids (mostly fats and oils) contain carbon and hydrogen; they contain less oxygen than carbohydrates. Because of this difference in composition, lipids yield more energy per gram than carbohydrates, on average 9 kcal per gram.

One form of lipids, **triglycerides,** are a key energy source for the body, the major form of fat in foods, and the major form for energy storage in the body.

In this book the more familiar terms fats and oils will generally be used rather than lipids or triglycerides. Roughly speaking, fats are lipids that are solid at room temperature, and oils are lipids that are liquid at room temperature.

Fats are separated into two basic types—saturated and unsaturated—based on the chemical structure of their dominant **fatty acids.** This property determines whether a fat is solid or liquid at room temperature. Plant oils tend to contain many unsaturated fatty acids, which makes them liquid. Animal fats are often rich in saturated fatty acids, which makes them solid. Many foods contain both saturated and unsaturated fats.

Certain unsaturated fatty acids are essential nutrients. These key fatty acids that the body can't produce, called essential fatty acids, perform several important functions in the body: they help regulate blood pressure and play a role in the synthesis and repair of vital cell parts. Thus, some fat is needed in the diet. However, we need only about 1 tablespoon of a common vegetable oil (such as corn oil found in supermarkets) each day to supply the essential fatty acids. The average American diet supplies about three times the amount of essential fatty acids needed daily.

Much attention has been given to saturated fat in the past few years. This is because saturated fat bears a great deal of the responsibility for raising blood cholesterol. High blood cholesterol leads to clogged arteries, and so can eventually lead to heart disease. For this reason, it is recommended that adults generally limit the amount of saturated fat in their diets.

Adding fish in a diet about twice a week adds to this benefit derived from some inclusion of vegetable oil. The fatty acids in fish complement the healthy aspects of vegetable oil. This will be developed in greater detail in Chapter 5, which focuses on lipids.

Proteins

Like carbohydrates and fats, proteins are composed of carbon, oxygen, and hydrogen; in contrast to the other energy-yielding nutrients, all proteins also contain nitrogen. Proteins are the main structural building blocks of the body (see Figure 1-1). For example, proteins constitute a major part of bone and muscle; they are also important components in blood, cell membranes, **enzymes,** and immune factors. Furthermore, proteins can also provide energy for the body, on average 4 kcal per gram. Typically, little protein is used for that purpose in terms of daily energy use. Proteins are formed by the linking of **amino acids.** Twenty common amino acids are found in food; nine of these are essential nutrients for adults.

Enzyme
A compound that speeds the rate of a chemical process but is not altered by the process. Almost all enzymes are proteins (see Chapter 3 for details).

Most of us eat about one and a half to two times more protein than the body needs to maintain health. In a healthy person this amount of extra protein in the diet is generally not harmful—it simply reflects the standard of living and the dietary habits that most Americans enjoy. The excess is mostly used for fuel; some may be made into fat or carbohydrate. Chapter 6 focuses on proteins.

Amino acid
The building block for proteins containing a central carbon with a nitrogen and other chemical elements attached.

Three other classes of nutrients are vitamins, minerals, and water. Although vitamins and minerals are vital to good health, they are needed only in small amounts in the diet and provide no direct source of energy for the body.

Vitamins

Vitamins exhibit a wide variety of chemical structures and can contain carbon, hydrogen, nitrogen, oxygen, phosphorus, sulfur and other chemical elements. The main function of vitamins is to enable many chemical processes in the body to occur. Some of these processes help release the energy trapped in carbohydrates, lipids, and proteins. Keep in mind, however, that vitamins themselves provide no usable energy for the body.

The 13 vitamins are divided into two groups: four that are fat soluble (vitamins A, D, E, and K) and nine that are water soluble (vitamin C and the B vitamins). The two groups of vitamins often act quite differently. For example, cooking destroys water-soluble vitamins much more readily than it does fat-soluble vitamins. Water-soluble vitamins are also excreted from the body much more readily than are fat-soluble vitamins. Thus the fat-soluble vitamins, especially vitamins A and D, are much more likely to build up in excessive amounts in the body, which then can cause toxicity. The vitamins are the focus of Chapter 7.

Minerals

Minerals typically function as such in the body (Na^+, K^+), or as parts of simple mineral combinations, such as in bone mineral [Ca_{10} $(PO_4)_6$ OH_2]. Because of their simple structure, minerals are not destroyed during cooking, but they can still be lost if they leak into the water used for cooking and then are discarded if that water is not consumed. Although minerals themselves yield no energy as such for the body, they are critical players in nervous system functioning, other cellular processes, water balance, and structural (e.g., skeletal) systems.

The amounts of the 16 or more essential minerals that are required in the diet for good health vary enormously. Thus they are divided into two groups: major minerals and trace minerals. The actual dietary requirement for some trace minerals has yet to be determined. Minerals are the focus of Chapter 8.

Water
The solvent of life; chemically H_2O. The body is composed of about 60% water. Water (fluid) needs are about 6–8 cups per day.

Water

Water is the sixth and last class of nutrients. Although sometimes overlooked as a nutrient, water (chemically, H_2O) has numerous vital functions in the body. It acts as a **solvent** and lubricant, as a medium for transporting nutrients and waste, and as a medium for temperature regulation and chemical processes. For these reasons, and because the human body is approximately 60% water, we require about 2 liters (L)—equivalent to 2000 grams. That is why we often hear the recommendation to consume 6 to 8 cups of fluid every day. Water is examined in detail in Chapter 8.

Nutrient Composition of Diets and the Human Body Differ

The quantities of the various nutrients that people consume vary widely, and the nutrient amounts present in different foods also vary a great deal. The total daily intake of protein, fat, and carbohydrate amounts to about 500 grams (slightly more than 1 pound). In contrast, the typical daily mineral intake totals about 20 grams, and the daily vitamin intake totals less than 300 milligrams. Although each day we require nearly a gram of some minerals, such as calcium and phosphorus, we need

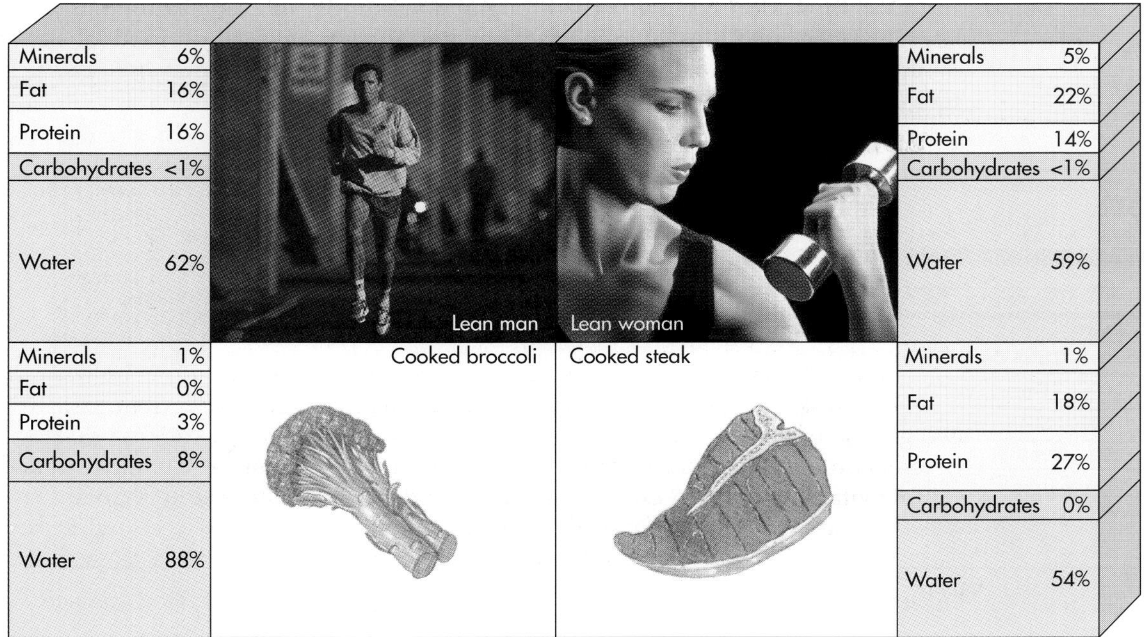

Figure 1–2 *You aren't what you eat! The proportions of nutrients in the human body do not match those found in typical foods—animal or vegetable.*

only a few milligrams or less of other minerals. For example, we need about 15 milligrams of zinc per day, which is just a few specks of the mineral.

The nutrient composition of the body differs from the nutritional profiles of the foods we eat (Figure 1–2). This is because growth, development, and later maintenance of the human body are directed by the genetic material (**genes**) inside body **cells.** This genetic blueprint determines how each cell uses the nutrients to perform body functions. These nutrients can come from a variety of sources. Cells are not concerned whether the amino acids available come from animal or plant sources. The carbohydrate glucose can come from sugars or starches. Thus, you aren't what you eat. Instead, what you eat provides cells with the ability to function as directed by the genetic material housed in the cell.

Gene
The genetic material on chromosomes that makes up DNA. Genes provide the blueprint for the production of cell proteins.

Alcohol
Refers to ethyl alcohol or ethanol, CH_3CH_2OH; yield about 7 kcal per gram.

Energy Sources and Uses

We get the energy to perform body functions and do work from carbohydrates, fats, and proteins. Foods generally provide more than one energy source. Vegetable oils and shortenings are two of a few exceptions; these are 100% fat.

Alcohol is also an energy source for some of us, supplying 7 kcal per gram. It is not considered a nutrient, however, because it has no required function. Still, alcoholic beverages—generally also rich in carbohydrate—are a leading contributor of energy to the American diet.

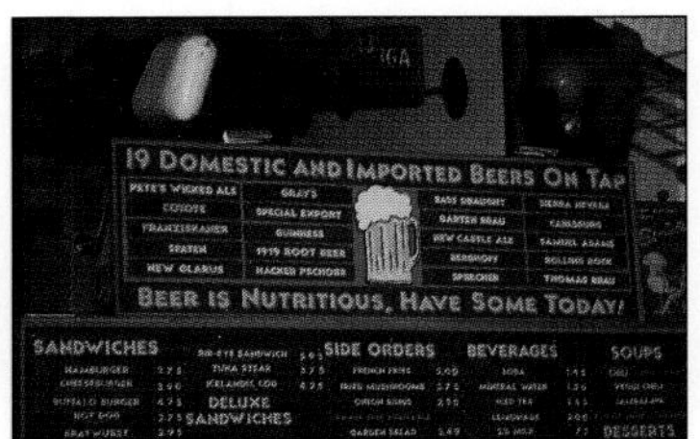

Alcoholic beverages are calorie-rich, but alcohol is not a nutrient per se.

The body transforms the energy trapped in carbohydrate, protein, fat, and alcohol into other forms of energy to allow the body to function. Chapter 10 describes how that energy is released from these sources and then used by body cells.

As noted earlier, the energy in food is often measured in terms of kilocalories, or calories. Technically, a calorie is the amount of heat it takes to raise the temperature of 1 gram of water by 1 degree Celsius (1°C, centigrade scale). Because a calorie is such a tiny measure of heat, food energy is more often expressed in terms of the kilocalorie, or kcal, which equals 1000 calories. A kcal is the amount of heat it takes to raise the temperature of 1000 grams (1 liter) of water by 1°C. The term *kilocalorie* and its abbreviation *kcal* are used throughout this book. In everyday life the word *calorie* is often used loosely to mean *kilocalorie.* The values given on food labels in calories are actually in kilocalories (Figure 1–3). A suggested intake of 2000 calories on a food label is really 2000 kcal.

Nutrition Facts

Serving Size 1 slice (36g) Servings Per Container 19

Amount Per Serving

Calories 80 Calories from Fat 10

	% Daily Value*		% Daily Value*
Total Fat 1g	**2%**	**Total Carbohydrate** 15g	**5%**
Saturated Fat 0g	**0%**	Dietary Fiber 2g	**8%**
Cholesterol 0mg	**0%**	Sugars less than 1g	
Sodium 200mg	**8%**	**Protein** 3g	

Vitamin A 0% Vitamin C 0% Calcium 0% Iron 4%

*Percent Daily Values (DV) are based on a 2,000 calorie diet. Your daily values may be higher or lower depending on your calorie needs:

	Calories:	2,000	2,500
Total Fat	Less than	65g	80g
Sat Fat	Less than	20g	25g
Cholesterol	Less than	300mg	300mg
Sodium	Less than	2,400mg	2,400mg
Total Carbohydrate		300g	375g
Dietary Fiber		25g	30g

INGREDIENTS: WHOLE WHEAT, WATER, ENRICHED WHEAT FLOUR [FLOUR, MALTED BARLEY, NIACIN, REDUCED IRON, THIAMINE MONONITRATE (VITAMIN B1) AND RIBOFLAVIN (VITAMIN B2)], CORN SYRUP, PARTIALLY HYDROGENATED COTTONSEED, OIL, SALT, YEAST.

HONEY WHEAT BREAD

Figure 1–3 *Food labels use the term calories, but these are actually kilocalorie (kcal) amounts.*

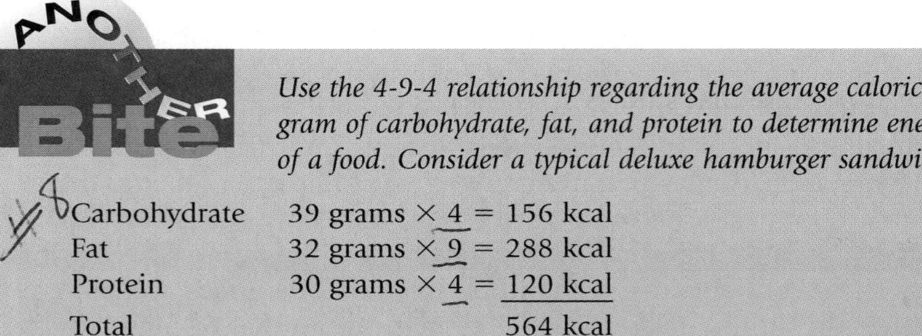

Use the 4-9-4 relationship regarding the average caloric yield per gram of carbohydrate, fat, and protein to determine energy content of a food. Consider a typical deluxe hamburger sandwich:

Carbohydrate	39 grams × 4 =	156 kcal
Fat	32 grams × 9 =	288 kcal
Protein	30 grams × 4 =	120 kcal
Total		564 kcal

You can also use the 4-9-4 relationship to determine what portion of total energy intake is contributed by the various energy-yielding nutrients. Assume that one day you consume 290 grams of carbohydrates, 60 grams of fat, and 70 grams of protein. This consumption yields a total of 1980 kcal ([290 × 4] + [60 × 9] + [70 × 4] = 1980). The percentage of your total energy intake derived from each nutrient can then be determined:

% of kcal as carbohydrate = (290 × 4) ÷ 1980 = 0.586 or 59%
% of kcal as fat = (60 × 9) ÷ 1980 = 0.273 or 27%
% of kcal as protein = (70 × 4) ÷ 1980 = 0.141 or 14%

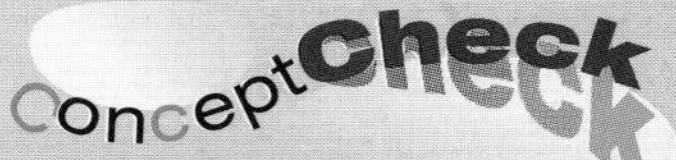

Nutrition is the study of food and nutrients, their digestion, absorption and metabolism, and their effect on health and disease. The six classes of nutrients include carbohydrates, lipids, proteins, water, vitamins, and minerals. On average, carbohydrates and protein provide 4 kcal per gram of energy to the body, while lipids provide 9 kcal per gram. The other classes of nutrients do not supply energy but are essential for proper body functioning.

The American Diet

For most of us living in America, our main dietary sources of energy are carbohydrates, fats, and proteins. If we ignore alcohol, adults consume about 16% of their kcal as proteins, 50% as carbohydrates, and 33% as fats. These percentages are estimates and vary slightly from year to year and from person to person. As a rough estimate, changing to a 15%, 55% to 60%, and 25% to 30% distribution for protein, carbohydrate, and fat is widely advocated. Note that recommendations for different distributions of calories between proteins, carbohydrates, and fats come and go in the popular press. The pros and cons of these patterns will be reviewed in future chapters.

Animal sources supply about two-thirds of protein intake for most Americans; plant sources supply only about one-third. In many other parts of the world, it is just the opposite: plant proteins—from rice, beans, and corn, and other vegetables—dominate protein intake. About half the carbohydrate in American diets comes from simple sugars; the other half comes from starches (such as in pastas, breads, and potatoes). About 60% of our dietary fat comes from animal sources, and 40% from vegetable sources.

Profiling the American Diet

To find out what and when people eat, information about American food habits is gathered in large surveys, such as the Continuing Survey of Food Intakes of Individuals by the United States Department of Agriculture (USDA). Results from these surveys and other studies show that we eat a wide variety of foods. Some people are meeting their nutrient needs; others are not. Chapter 2 will look at this situation in more detail. For now, note that studies show that some of us should choose more foods that are rich in iron, calcium, vitamin A, various B vitamins, vitamin C, zinc, and dietary fiber.

Many experts also recommend that we pay more attention to matching energy intake with energy output. Eating somewhat less fat and increasing physical activity would help with this. In addition African-Americans may need to pay special attention to the amount of sodium (**salt** is a mixture of sodium and chloride) and alcohol in their diets because they have a greater chance of developing high blood pressure than other ethnic groups in America, and these substances are linked to that health problem. Actually, a careful look at sodium and alcohol intake—along with saturated and total fat intake—is a useful task for all adults.

Salt
Generally refers to a compound of sodium and chloride in a 40:60 ratio.

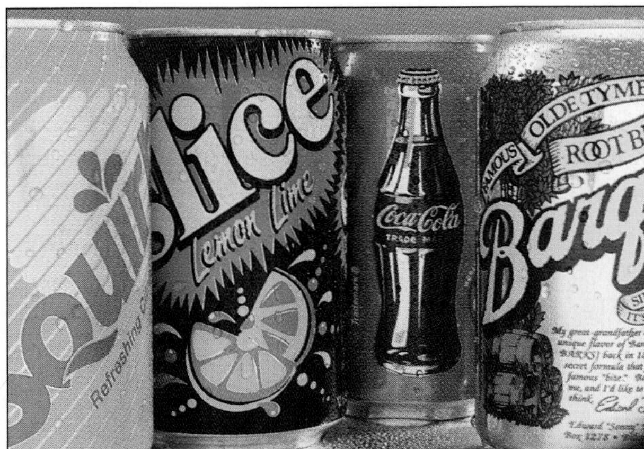

Today, soft drinks are more popular than milk, although not as beneficial to the diet. These products account for 10% of the energy intake of teenagers, and in turn contribute to generally poor calcium intakes seen in this age group.

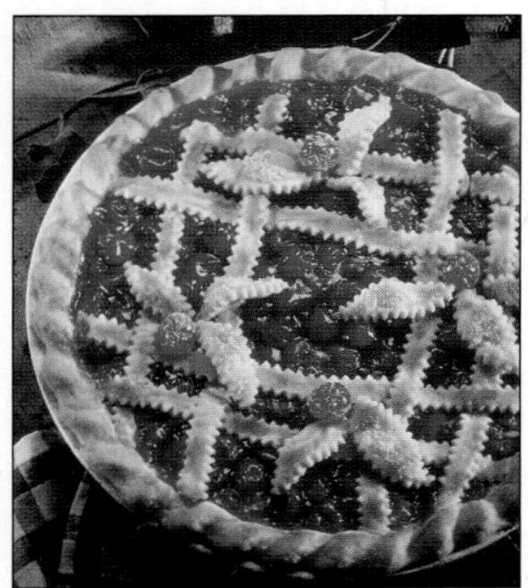

All foods can fit into a healthy diet—cherry pie included. Frequency and amount are the most important considerations.

How Aware Are We of Our Nutritional Health?

Judging from the responses in the Food Marketing Institute's 1997 Trend Report, more than 9 out of 10 shoppers say they are very or somewhat concerned about the nutritional content of what they eat. Many Americans have a general awareness of possible health hazards from overeating, especially the problems of too much fat, sodium, and energy in a diet. However, although they may be concerned, they often don't make changes to significantly improve their diets.

Our overall population is getting fatter, probably due to an increasingly sedentary lifestyle with no decrease in total energy intake. Most Americans would benefit from a closer examination of a healthful balance of foods in their diet—greater moderation in the intake of some foods is needed, while increasing variety in other foods, such as fruits and vegetables, needs attention. Few adults meet the minimum daily servings for these food groups—2 fruit and 3 vegetable servings—even though 65% of those recently interviewed say these are an important part of a diet.

Health Objectives for the United States for the Year 2000

Health promotion and disease prevention have been public health strategies in the United States since the late 1970s. One part of this strategy is *Healthy People 2000,* a report issued in 1990 by the U.S. Department of Health and Human Services' Public Health Service. This report consists of national health promotion and disease prevention objectives for the nation for the year 2000 and assigns each of the objectives to appropriate federal agencies to address.

Healthy People 2000's nutrition-related challenges address the following:

- Iron-deficiency **anemia** (progress is evident, especially with infants)
- Stunted growth in infants and children (progress is being made)
- High fat intake (progress is being made, especially by women)
- **Obesity** (we are currently losing this battle)
- Elevated blood lipids (progress is being made)
- High sodium intake (degree of progress currently unclear)
- Low calcium intake (mixed findings on progress to date but doesn't look very promising)
- Low complex carbohydrate and dietary fiber intakes (no data on progress to date)
- The need for more home-delivered meals for elderly people (no data on progress to date)
- A relative lack of breastfeeding, poor general nutrition knowledge, and the lack of nutrition education (mixed findings on progress to date)

The main objective of *Healthy People 2000* is to promote healthful lifestyles and reduce preventable death and disability in all Americans. A new report to set health objectives for the year 2010 is under development.

Anemia
Generally refers to a decreased oxygen-carrying capacity of the blood. This can be caused by many factors.

Obesity
A condition characterized by excess body fat, typically defined as a body mass index greater than or equal to 30 (see Chapter 9).

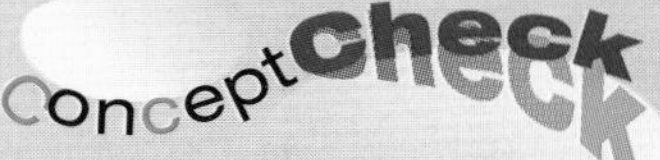

Surveys in the United States show that we generally have a variety of food available to us. However, some of us could improve our diets by focusing on rich food sources of iron, calcium, vitamin A, various B vitamins, vitamin C, zinc, and dietary fiber. In addition, many of us should use more moderation when consuming energy, fat, sodium, and alcoholic beverages. These recommendations are consistent with an overall goal to attain and maintain good health.

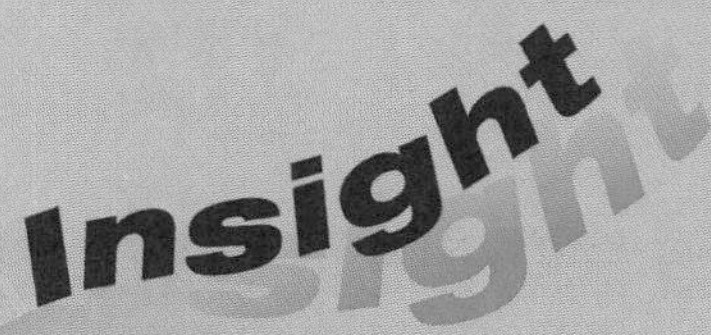

A Fountain of Youth?

Aging is a natural process: your body cells age no matter what health practices you follow. To a considerable extent, however, you can determine how quickly you age throughout your adult years. One's genetic background is important, but so are daily habits. Genetic background can put us at risk for some diseases but does not guarantee these diseases will develop. Obesity is a good example (see Chapter 9 for details).

Overall, how you act now is important to your later health. Successful aging is a result of wise choices. Age quickly or age slowly—you have some choice in the matter (Table 1-4).

The best way to promote your health and prevent chronic diseases in the future is to observe the following guidelines:

- Eat a healthful diet—a varied diet that helps avoid obesity should be a priority. The Food Guide Pyramid and Dietary Guidelines for Americans discussed in Chapter 2 are a great place to start. Choose moderate portion sizes. In addition, do not abuse nutrient supplements, if used. (See Chapter 7 for details.)
- Drink plenty of fluids—because the body is composed mostly of water, which is lost in perspiration and urine, water should continually be replaced. Aim to drink 6 to 8 glasses of water and other fluids daily.
- Physical activity—spend at least 30 minutes almost or all days in a combination of brisk walking, jogging, swimming, stair climbing, and other activities that increase heart rate. Add to that some resistance exercise: sit-ups, push-ups, presses, and curls with dumbbells, etc. See Chapter 10 for other options.
- Don't smoke—lung cancer, caused primarily by smoking cigarettes, is the only major form of cancer for which yearly rates still increase. Currently about 25% of adults smoke; the numbers grow to 28% among college students. The nicotine in tobacco products is the most addictive substance (per milligram) known to man. Most people who smoke wish they could quit.
- Limit alcohol intake—don't drink more than one to two servings of alcohol per day on a regular basis. Women are cautioned to limit intake to one serving because they are more likely than men to develop cirrhosis of the liver with the same intake of alcohol (see Chapter 14).
- Get adequate sleep—establish a regular schedule to allow for an average of 7 to 8 hours of sleep a night.
- Limit stress or adjust to the causes of stress—practice better time management, relax, listen to music, have a massage, and stay physically active. Do what works for you. In addition, maintaining self-esteem, interpersonal relationships, and a positive outlook contributes to limiting stress and reinforces wellness.
- Consult health-care professionals on a regular basis—early diagnosis is especially important for controlling the damaging effects of many diseases.

Proper diet is not the only thing to consider. As just discussed, other behavior is also critical. Taking responsibility for yourself is central to achieving long-term health by establishing appropriate health behavior. This is a goal of Chapters 1 and 2.

TABLE 1-4

What to Expect from Adequate Nutrition and Good Health Habits

DIET

Eating enough essential nutrients and meeting energy needs help prevent
- Birth defects and low birth weight in pregnancy
- Stunted growth and poor resistance to disease in infancy and childhood
- Poor resistance to disease in adulthood
- Deficiency diseases, such as **cretinism** (lack of iodide), scurvy (lack of vitamin C), and anemia (lack of iron, folate, or other nutrients)

Eating enough calcium helps
- Build bone mass in childhood and adolescence
- Prevent some adult bone loss, especially among older individuals

Obtaining adequate intake of fluoride and minimizing sugar intake helps prevent
- Dental caries

Eating enough dietary fiber helps prevent
- Digestive problems such as constipation

Eating enough vitamin A and carotenoids may help reduce
- Susceptibility to some cancers
- Degeneration of the retina in the eye (intake of carotenoids in green and orange vegetables specifically)

Moderating energy intake helps prevent
- Obesity and related diseases, such as the major form of diabetes, high blood pressure, cancer, and heart disease

Limiting intake of sodium helps prevent
- High blood pressure and related diseases of the heart and kidney in susceptible people

Moderating intake of total fat, and especially saturated fat, helps prevent
- Heart disease

Moderating intake of essential nutrients by using vitamin and mineral supplements wisely, if at all, prevents
- Most chances for nutrient toxicities

PHYSICAL ACTIVITY

Adequate, regular physical activity helps prevent
- Obesity
- The major form of diabetes
- Heart disease
- Some adult bone loss
- Loss of muscle tone

LIFESTYLE

Minimizing alcohol intake helps prevent
- Liver disease
- Fetal alcohol syndrome
- Accidents

Not smoking helps prevent
- Lung cancer, other lung disease, and heart disease

In addition, minimum use of medications, no illicit drug use, adequate sleep, adequate fluid intake and a reduction in stress provide a more complete approach to good nutrition and health.

Why Am I So Hungry?

Understanding what drives us to eat and what affects food choice will help put your study of nutrition into greater focus. Specially, this helps you understand the complexity of factors that influence eating, especially the effects of ethnicity and societal change. You can then see why foods may have different meanings to different people and, in turn, allow for greater appreciation of food habits that differ from yours.

Two drives influence our desire to eat and thus take in food energy, **hunger** and **appetite.** These differ dramatically. Hunger, our primarily physical biological drive to eat, is controlled by internal body mechanisms. For example as nutrients are processed by the stomach and small intestine, these organs communicate with the liver and brain, reducing further food intake. The liver then uses its direct nerve pathways to the brain to do the same.

Appetite, our primarily psychological drive to eat, is affected by external food choice mechanisms, such as seeing a tempting dessert. Fulfilling either or both drives by eating sufficient food normally brings a state of **satiety,** temporarily halting our desire to continue eating.

Hunger
The primarily physiological (internal) drive to find and eat food, mostly regulated by innate cues to eating.

Appetite
The primarily psychological (external) influences that encourage us to find and eat food, often in the absence of obvious hunger.

Satiety
State in which there is no longer a desire to eat; a feeling of satisfaction.

The Hypothalamus Contributes to Satiety Regulation

The **hypothalamus,** a portion of the brain, helps regulate satiety. When stimulated, cells in the feeding centers of the hypothalamus signal us to eat. Then as we eat, hunger decreases. Eventually, we stop eating as cells in the satiety centers of the hypothalamus are stimulated. The amount of blood glucose probably stimulates both the feeding and satiety centers. When blood glucose drops, we eat. When it eventually rises after a meal, we no longer have a strong desire to seek food.

Certain chemicals, surgery, and some cancers can destroy both groups of centers in the hypothalamus. Without satiety-center activity, laboratory animals (and humans) eat their way to obesity. Without feeding-center activity, animals eat little and eventually lose weight.

Overall, this entire system depends on the hypothalamus to process the signals generated by nerves responding to the various mediators of food intake. However, this concept of separate satiety and feeding centers is too simplistic to fully describe hunger regulation. We know that the hypothalamus is criss-crossed with a huge amount of nerves that are constantly receiving and passing on information about the body's nutritional state.

Satiety cascade

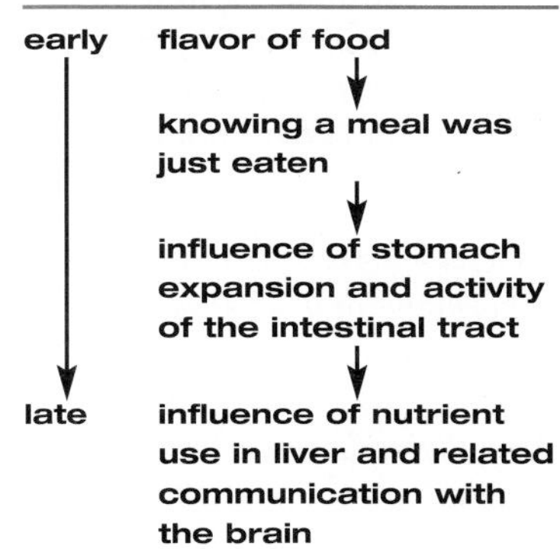

Meal Size Affects Satiety

The effects of stomach expansion and intestinal absorption of nutrients during a meal work to reduce our desire to eat more food. These actions of the **gastrointestinal (GI) tract** contribute to a feeling of satiety. In fact, a meal is generally terminated before significant amounts of nutrients are made available for metabolism and storage. Putting this information into practice, researchers have recently shown that bulky meals produce much more satiety than more concentrated meals. As the dietary fiber and starch content of a meal increases and fat content decreases, humans experience increased satiety and thus do not seek another meal as quickly. Consider how you would feel if you ate five pieces of whole fruit versus one regular serving of French fries (each yielding about 380 kcals).

Gastrointestinal (GI) tract
The main sites in the body used for digestion and absorption of nutrients. It consists of the mouth, esophagus, stomach, small intestine, large intestine, rectum, and anus.

Hormones Affect Satiety

Hormones and hormone-like compounds in our body prod us to eat. Those that increase hunger include **endorphins** and **cortisol.** Those that cause satiety include

Hormone
A compound secreted into the bloodstream by one type of cells that acts to control the function of another type of cells. For example, certain cells in the pancreas produce insulin, which in turn acts on muscle and other types of cells.

Endorphins
Natural body tranquilizers that may be involved in the feeding response.

Cortisol
A hormone made by the adrenal gland that, among other functions, stimulates the production of glucose from amino acids and increases the desire to eat.

Serotonin
A neurotransmitter synthesized from the amino acid typtophan that appears to decrease the desire to eat carbohydrates and to induce sleep.

Cholecystokinin (CCK)
A hormone that stimulates enzyme release from the pancreas, bile release from the gallbladder, and hunger regulation.

Leptin
A hormone made by adipose tissue that influences long-term regulation of fat mass. Leptin also influences reproductive functions, as well as other body processes, such as release of the hormone insulin.

leptin, serotonin, and **cholecystokinin (CCK)**. Researchers are currently trying to produce products that will increase the action of these satiety-inducing hormones. Researchers currently suspect that overweight individuals may have defective leptin utilization, causing satiety to be inhibited. More research is needed in this area. Preliminary studies show that daily leptin injections can contribute to success in weight loss in some overweight people.

Does Appetite Affect What We Eat?

Various feeding and satiety messages from body cells do not single-handedly determine what we eat. Almost everyone has encountered a mouthwatering dessert and devoured it, even on a full stomach. Appetite can be affected by a great variety of external forces, such as environmental and psychological factors as well as social customs (Figure 1–4).

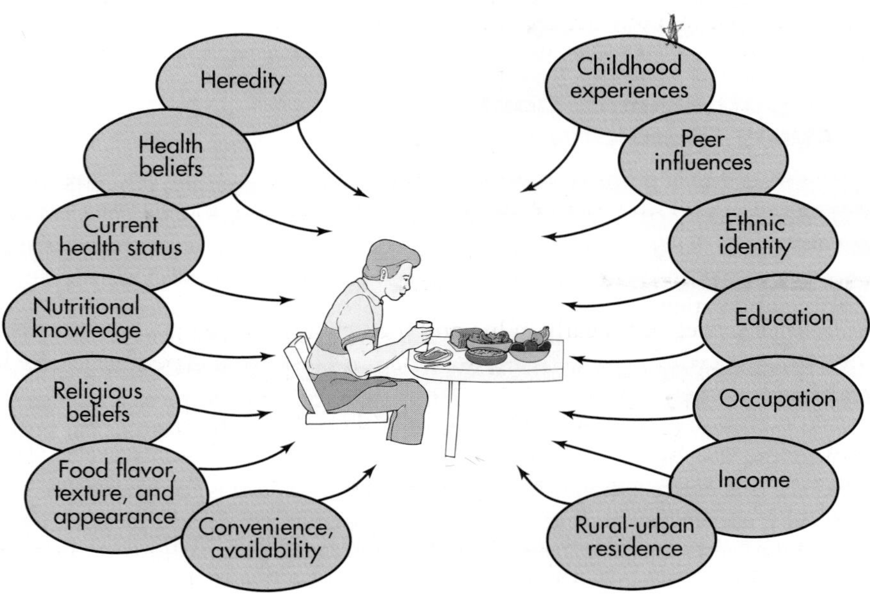

Figure 1–4 *Food behavior is influenced by many sources. Which are important in your life?*

We often eat because food confronts us. It smells good, tastes good, and looks good. We might eat because it is the right time of day, we are celebrating, or we are trying to overcome the blues. After a meal, memories of pleasant tastes and feelings reinforce appetite. If stress or depression sends you to the refrigerator, you are mostly seeking comfort, not food energy. Appetite may not be a biological process, but it does influence food intake.

Putting Hunger and Appetite into Perspective

The next time you pick up a candy bar or ask for second helpings, remember the physical influences on eating behavior. Body cells (brain, stomach, small intestine, liver, and other organs), hormones (like leptin and cortisol), brain chemicals (like serotonin), and social customs all influence food intake. Where food is ample, appetite—not hunger—mostly triggers eating. Keep track of what triggers your eating for a few days. Is it primarily hunger or appetite? Note as well that satiety regulation is not perfect; body weight can fluctuate.

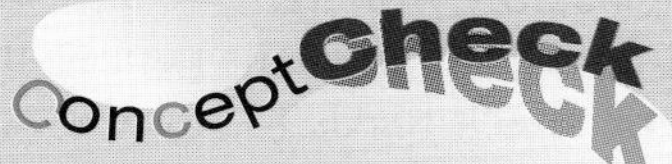

Hunger is the primarily physical or internal desire to find and eat food. Appeasing it creates satiety—no further desire to eat exists. Satiety is influenced by hunger-related (internal) forces in the brain, gastrointestinal tract, liver, and other organs. Various hormones and hormone-like compounds participate. Food intake is also affected by appetite-related (external) forces like social custom, time of day, palatability, and presence of others. Americans probably respond more to external, appetite-related forces than to hunger-related ones in choosing when and what to eat.

What Else Influences Eating?

Flavor and texture are the most important things that influence our actual food choices. After that we consider the cost and convenience of food. What we eat ends up revealing much about who we are—politically, religiously, and socially. Behavior, perception, and environment influence food habits. The Nutrition Issue in Chapter 2 discusses this more fully in the context of ethnic diet pyramids.

Although some people have no concern for nutrition, others will agonize endlessly over the flavor, energy and fat content, and general nutritional value of everything they eat. Where do you fit into the food and nutrition picture?

Social customs, peers, and authority figures can influence the desire to eat. Concern about appearance when on a date can influence the food choices made. A woman concerned about looking "petite" in company may choose a smaller portion of food than when alone. We are also likely to eat more at a meal when with a large group of people than when with a few people or alone, or when someone else is "picking up the check."

Early Experiences with Food Shape Later Choices

Our food preferences begin early in life and then change as we interact with parents, friends, and peers. Unfortunately, as young children our food experiences may have been severely limited by parents or other adults responsible for us. Adults may have introduced us to only a small subset of available foods because some excellent foods are often considered inappropriate for children. For example, at what age did you discover lentils, spinach salad, or salmon? Might now be a good time to become more adventurous?

Just being exposed to a variety of foods can help make us less resistant to try new foods. Preschoolers are usually quite willing to try new things. During school years, children are often strongly influenced by their peers. Adults need to give children under their care a variety of foods to try. It may take time, but children usually come to accept new foods (see Chapter 13).

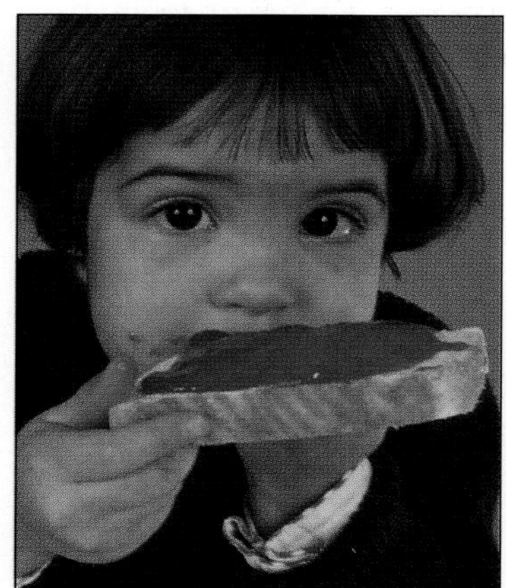

Food likes and dislikes are shaped by early experiences, among other factors. Parents are important "gatekeepers" with regard to the nutritional health of their children. Serving as good role models, parents should strive to instill healthy eating patterns in their children (see Chapter 13 for details).

Some Habits Are Hard to Break

Some food choices are tied to our routines and habits. Only about 100 basic items account for 75% of an individual's total food intake. Narrowing our food choices provides us with security. In this context eating quick-service food (often called "fast food") at a restaurant such as McDonald's provides common expectations, experiences, and behaviors. Some of us are concerned enough about our health that we want to change our diets. Even so, current food habits still strongly influence us.

Health Is a Growing Focus for Some

About half of us consider nutrition, or what we think are good food habits, an important influence on our food purchases. Those Americans who tend to make better food and overall health choices are often well-educated, middle-class professionals. In fact, increased health awareness among minority peoples is a major goal of current federal government health strategies.

Important minority health concerns include drug and alcohol abuse, heart disease, high blood pressure, diabetes, cancer, infant mortality, and AIDS. The Office of Minority Health in Washington, D.C., will answer questions and provide resources regarding these problems (800-444-6472).

Vegetarian
A person who avoids eating animal products to a varying degree ranging from consuming no animal products to simply not consuming four-footed animal products (see Chapter 6).

Sugar used to be the main diet monster; now fat has the limelight. As a result, manufacturers are racing to the market with reduced-fat or nonfat items (many also are lower in cholesterol and sodium), including many snack foods (956 new varieties in 1996 alone), mayonnaise, salad dressings, cheese, dairy spreads, frozen desserts, luncheon meats, sausage, and butter sprinkles (Table 1–5). The consumer must practice caution, though, as many manufacturers may add more sugar or salt to improve the flavor of these fat-reduced foods. Balance in food choice and control of portion size also must not be forgotten.

The American diet does not stand still. If we buy it, the food industry will continue to supply it. The modern supermarket is responding to our health concerns by providing fresh, frozen, ready-to-eat, international, gourmet, ethnic, **vegetarian,** and even not-so-healthful foods. Salad bars in supermarkets have become a big hit, especially for single people. Fruit smoothies and vitamin- and mineral-fortified foods are two other growing trends. For example, orange juice may be fortified with vitamin A, vitamin E, and calcium.

TABLE 1-5

Years When Common American Foods Were Introduced

1875—Chocolate milk
1876—Heinz ketchup
1891—Fig Newtons
1896—Tootsie Roll
1897—Jell-O, Grape-Nuts
1898—Graham crackers
1907—Hershey's Kisses
1912—Life Savers
1912—Oreos
1916—All-Bran
1921—Mounds, Wonder bread
1923—Milky Way
1927—Kool-Aid
1928—Rice Krispies
1930—Birds Eye frozen foods, Snickers
1932—3 Musketeers, Fritos corn chips
1934—Ritz crackers, Bisquick
1941—Cheerios
1944—Hawaiian Punch
1946—Minute Rice, frozen orange juice, instant coffee
1950—Sugar Corn Pops
1952—Kellogg's Sugar Frosted Flakes
1953—Sugar Smacks, frozen pizza
1956—Duncan Hines brownie mix, Jif peanut butter
1958—Tang
1960—Instant potatoes
1963—Tab
1965—Shake 'n Bake
1966—Cool Whip
1968—Pringles, Care Free sugarless gum
1976—Country Time lemonade
1981—TCBY frozen yogurt
1984—Diet Coke (with aspartame)
1986—Pop Secret microwave popcorn
1987—Minute Maid calcium-fortified orange juice
1995—Hellman's (Best Foods) low-fat mayonnaise
1996—Fat-free Pringle's potato chips (with Olestra)

Modified from Staten V: *Can you trust a tomato in January?* New York, 1993, Simon & Schuster, and from other sources.

When people are asked why they don't include foods they know to be healthful in their diets—for instance, green vegetables, low-fat milk, tub margarine, and whole-wheat bread—they say they don't like them. Similarly, people don't want to give up foods such as whole milk, rich cheeses, and fatty meat because they like them too much. This even is the case if they think they should limit fat intake and lower-fat varieties are available. It is clear that although health is a concern for many people, flavor remains a driving force for most of the foods we choose to eat.

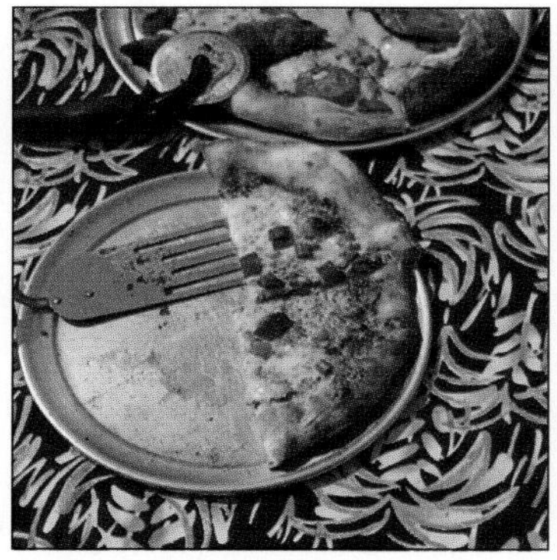

Recently a market research firm surveyed the eating habits of people in 2000 American households. The top meal choice was pizza, followed by ham sandwich, hot dog, peanut butter and jelly sandwich, steak, macaroni and cheese, turkey sandwich, cheese sandwich, hamburger on a bun, and spaghetti.

Advertising Both Helps and Hinders Nutritious Choices

To capture consumers' interest, the food industry spends well over $32 billion per year. The messages we hear influence food choice. Some of this advertising is helpful, as when it promotes the importance of calcium and fiber in our diets. The food industry, however, does not promote all food equally: sellers tend to emphasize brand-name foods, especially highly sweetened cereals, cookies, cakes, and pastries, because they bring higher profits. Food manufacturers often pay for the best place in the supermarkets: at the end of the aisle and, depending on the product, at the child's or adult's eye level. It is important for consumers to be aware of these tactics.

Restaurants and Eating Out Are Growing in Popularity

Restaurants have long been a growth industry in America, reflecting our modern (busy) lifestyles. On weekdays, lunch is eaten out by 30% of all adults and dinner by 24%. Restaurant excursions are no longer a splurge but a real convenience for many people. Some people rely almost entirely on these for nourishment. Traveling sales representatives, students, truck drivers, and others may wolf down 1200 kcal (about half their daily energy needs) via a burger, fries, and shake on a regular basis.

Many restaurants, including quick-service restaurants, offer healthful alternatives to their fat-rich and high-salt foods. Yogurt has replaced ice cream in shakes, and plain hamburgers are offered in some restaurants. Salad bars, grilled chicken, fresh fruit, whole-grain muffins, and fat-reduced milk are widely available as well. Again, consumers must support this healthier fare by buying it, if it is to succeed in a marketplace driven by profit (Figure 1–5).

FOR BETTER OR FOR WORSE / By Lynn Johnston

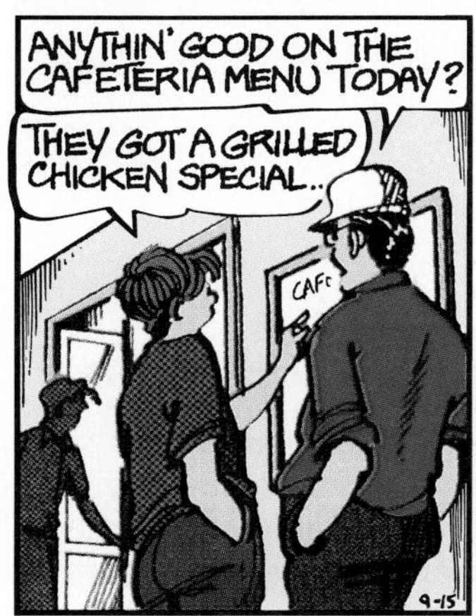

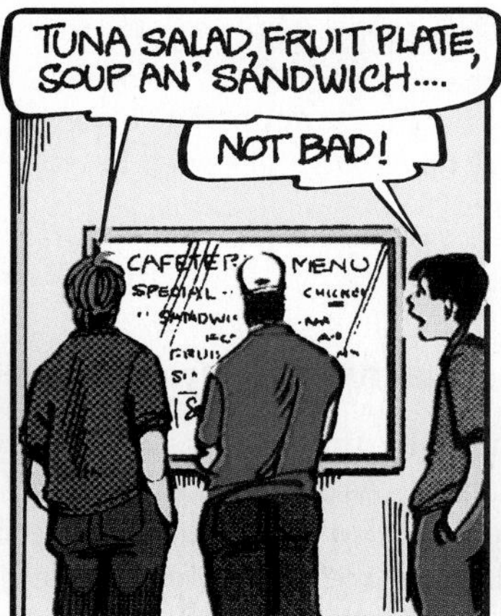

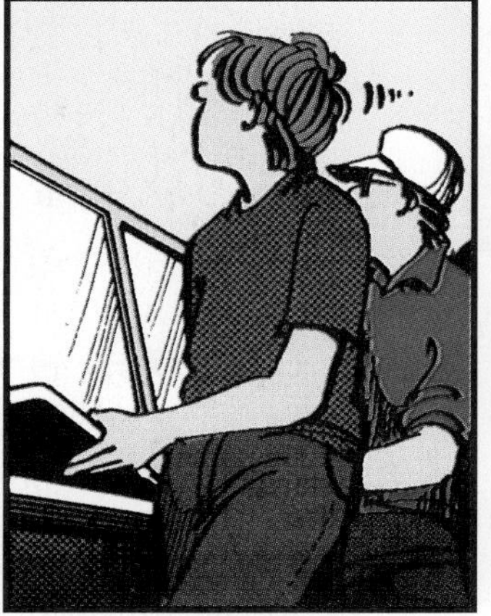

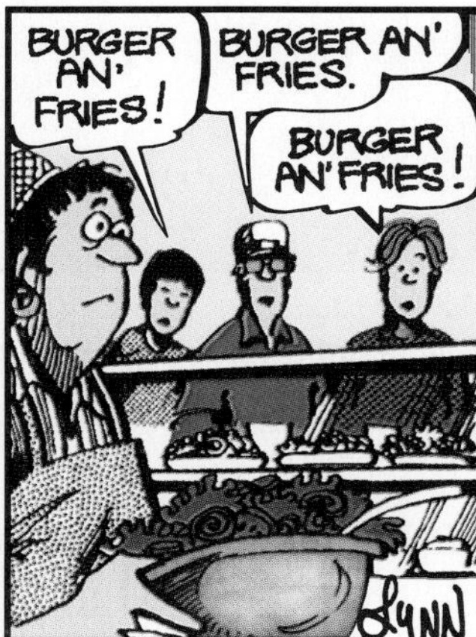

Figure 1–5 *For Better Or For Worse*

Probably the worst trend in the restaurant industry is super-sized meals. Consumers might see these as a bargain, but few need the extra calories supplied by the increased serving sizes.

Still, the temptation to consume foods rich in fat and high in salt is often hard to resist when we eat out. The reality is that a cheeseburger, french fries, and a milk shake are more appealing than a well-stocked salad bar for many of us. Regular visitors to quick-service restaurants must be conscious about the nutritional value of the meals they order if they want to have a healthy diet.

Social Changes Lead to Diet Changes

Many social changes in recent years have strongly affected the food marketplace, especially the large increases in the number of working women and single parents, both young and old. As a result of these and other factors, a general "time-famine" is emerging. Convenience becomes a priority, especially with the well-to-do. Prewashed salad greens in the supermarket is a recent example (see the Rate Your Plate section).

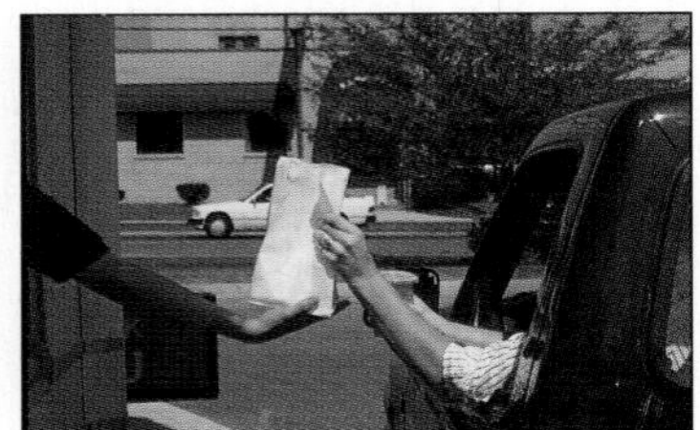

The easy availability of quick-service (fast) food in recent years has made weight control even harder for many people.

Many people now turn to quick-service restaurants for meals on the run. Supermarkets are also competing for these restaurant customers, with already-prepared foods, microwavable entrees, and various other frozen foods being especially popular. Sales for all takeout food business are expected to double in the next 7 years.

Almost 1000 new microwavable products were introduced in a recent year. Sales of ready-to-eat and microwavable products marketed directly to children and weight-conscious adults are among the fastest-growing product segments. Some stores have responded to our "time crunch" by offering grocery shopping on the internet.

Not only do many people eat away from home, they also skip meals. In a recent survey of college students, more than half reported that they ate only two meals a day, eating many snacks to make up the difference. Approximately 25% of adults skip breakfast, which is the appropriate meal to replace the carbohydrate stores used during the night's sleep. Although skipping breakfast might save one a few minutes, the person is likely to be less alert and efficient than if a meal was eaten.

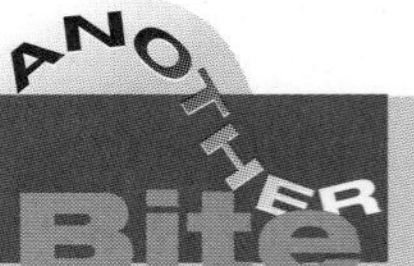

You eat because you see it, you hear it cooking, you smell it, or it's time to eat. All of these stimuli are concentrated in a mall: The food is there, it smells good, and there's so much to choose from. In addition, food may be the most affordable temptation at the mall. After a few hours of trekking through a mall, you would swear you had walked miles. But you would have to walk almost twice around the average mall to chalk up a mile—and that's only 100 kcal worth of physical activity.

The source of shopper's fatigue is psychological—styles, prices, lines, crowds. . .

Tired and frustrated,
the next step is hungry!

Think about that the next time you go shopping. Eat before you go, take a healthful snack, or be on your guard as you sample the smells.

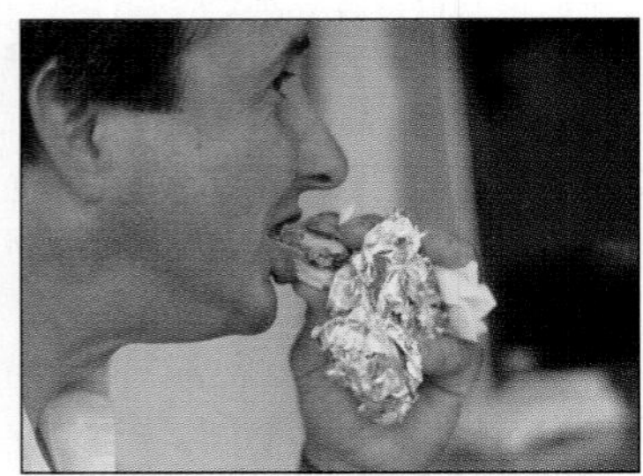

The fast-paced life for some of us requires eating on the run. What we choose should be as important as how fast it is served.

Economics Have a Minor Influence on Food Choice

Food habits are influenced by the amount of money an individual or family has available for food purchases. As income increases, so do meals eaten away from home. More affluent people also tend to consume more vegetables, fruit, cheese, meat, fish, poultry, and fat, while eating fewer dried beans and less rice. However, the average American spends only 13% of after-tax income for food. Compare this to about 50% of income spent on food in China or India. Nevertheless, high meat prices have led to the use of beef as an ingredient rather than as a centerpiece in some households; chicken, turkey, and fish are used as alternatives.

Improving Our Diets

As discussed, while more efforts by the general public are needed to lower fat intake and to improve variety in our diets, our cultural diversity, varied cuisines, and generally high nutritional status should be points of pride for Americans. Today we can choose from a tremendous variety of food products, the result of continual innovation by food manufacturers.

We are eating more breakfast cereals, pizza, pasta entrees, stir-fried meat and vegetables served on rice, salads, tacos, burritos, and fajitas than ever before. Sales of whole milk are down, while in the same time period sales of nonfat and 1% low-fat milk have increased. Consumption of frozen vegetables, rather than canned vegetables, is also on the rise.

A dietary objective that deserves more attention in the United States is to try to eat with others more often. Mealtime is a key social time of the day. The Japanese are ahead of us in recognizing that food's powers go beyond the realm of nutrition. Their national dietary guidelines, which like ours stress the importance of eating a variety of foods, maintaining healthy weight, and moderating fat in the diet, also advise people to make all activities pertaining to food and eating pleasurable.

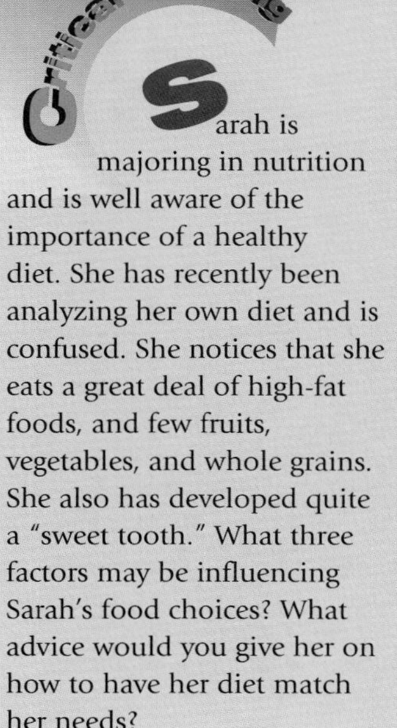

Sarah is majoring in nutrition and is well aware of the importance of a healthy diet. She has recently been analyzing her own diet and is confused. She notices that she eats a great deal of high-fat foods, and few fruits, vegetables, and whole grains. She also has developed quite a "sweet tooth." What three factors may be influencing Sarah's food choices? What advice would you give her on how to have her diet match her needs?

Today, Americans live longer than ever before and enjoy better general health. Many also have more money, more diverse food and lifestyle choices to consider, and more time to relax and enjoy life. The nutritional consequences of these trends are not fully known. Deaths from heart disease and strokes, for example, have dropped dramatically since the late 1960s, partly because of better medical care and diets. Still, if affluence leads to sedentary lifestyles and high intakes of fat, sodium, and alcohol, this lifestyle pattern can lead to problems. Because of better technology and greater choices, we can have a much better diet today than ever before—if we know what choices to make.

The goal of this book is to help you find the best path to good nutrition. There are no good or bad foods, but some foods provide relatively few nutrients in comparison to energy content and thus contribute to less nutritious food behaviors. One's overall diet is the proper focus in a nutritional evaluation. Chapter 2 will emphasize this point and show you how to balance your diet. As you reexamine your nutritional habits, remember your health is partly your responsibility. Your body has a natural ability to heal itself. Offer it what it needs, and it will serve you well. In addition, eating a good diet is one way to affirm that you care about your health.

Confusing and conflicting health messages also hinder diet change. Nutrition science does not have all the answers, but enough is known to (1) help you set a path to good health and (2) put diet-related recommendations you hear in the future into perspective. See Chapter 2 for details.

ConceptCheck

Food choices are influenced mainly by flavor and texture. Recently, factors such as health concerns, economics, convenience, and social changes are also becoming important dietary determinants. Good food habits developed and strengthened early in life can provide many benefits in later years.

Summary

- Nutrition is the study of the food substances vital for health and how the body uses these substances to promote and support growth and maintenance of cells.
- Nutrients in foods fall into six classes: (1) carbohydrates, (2) lipids (mostly fats and oils), (3) proteins, (4) vitamins, (5) minerals, and (6) water. The first three, along with alcohol, provide energy for the body to use.
- The body transforms the energy trapped in carbohydrate, protein, and fat into other forms of energy to allow the body to function. Fat provides on average

9 kcal per gram, while protein and carbohydrates provide 4 kcal per gram. Vitamins, minerals, and water do not supply any energy to the body but are essential for proper body function.

- Public health strategies, such as *Healthy People 2000*, are designed to improve the diets and in turn the health of Americans. Results from large nutrition surveys in the United States suggest that some of us need to concentrate on consuming foods that supply more vitamin A, certain B vitamins, vitamin C, calcium, iron, zinc, and dietary fiber.
- A basic plan for health promotion and disease prevention includes eating a varied diet, performing regular physical activity, not smoking, getting adequate fluid and sleep, limiting alcohol intake (if consumed), and limiting or coping with stress.
- Groups of cells in the hypothalamus and other regions in the brain affect hunger, the primarily internal desire to find and eat food. These cells monitor signals form digestive organs and nutrients and other substances in the blood to control satiety.
- A variety of external (appetite-related) forces affect satiety. Hunger cues combine with appetite cues, such as easy availability of food, to promote food intake.
- The flavor and texture of foods primarily influence our food choices. Several other factors also help determine food habits and choices: our upbringing, various social and cultural factors, the image we want to project to others, economics, and concerns about health.
- There are no good or bad foods. The focus should be on balancing a total diet by choosing many nutritious foods.

Study Questions

1. What are the two types of carbohydrates found in the diet?
2. Describe two types of fats and why the differences are important.
3. Describe the roles of vitamins and minerals in the body.
4. Outline the concept of energy content in foods. List the energy values for a gram of carbohydrate, fat, protein, and alcohol.
5. Name three functions of water in the body.
6. Give four examples of health objectives for the United States for the Year 2000. How could you rate yourself in each area? Why? What additions, if any, would you make to the list of objectives?
7. According to national nutrition surveys, which nutrients tend to be underconsumed by many adult Americans? Why is this the case?
8. Describe the various organs and hormones that control hunger and satiety in the body. List other factors that influence our food patterns.
9. Describe how your own food preferences have been shaped by the following factors:
   - **a.** Exposure to foods at an early age
   - **b.** Advertising (what is the newest food you have tried?)
   - **c.** Eating out
   - **d.** Peer pressure
   - **e.** Economic factors
10. What products in your supermarket reflect the consumer demand for healthier foods? for convenience?

Further Readings

1 Blumenthal SJ: A top woman doctor tells how to get past the hype to the truth, *American Health* p. 36, January/February 1998.
2 Cleveland JD and others: "What we eat in America" survey, *Nutrition Today* 32:37, 1997.
3 Drewnowski A: Energy density, palatability, and satiety: implications for weight control, *Nutrition Reviews* 56:347, 1998.
4 Glanz K and others: Why Americans eat what they do: Taste, nutrition, cost, convenience, and weight control concerns as influences on food consumption, *Journal of the American Dietetic Association* 98:1118, 1998.
5 Hollingsworth P: Lean times for U.S. food companies, *Food Technology* p. 22, July 1995.
6 Kumanyika S: Improving our diet—still a long way to go, *New England Journal of Medicine* 335:738, 1996.
7 Lewis R: Unraveling leptin pathways identifies new drug targets, *The Scientist* p. 4, July 20, 1998.
8 Nemecek S: Unequal health, *Scientific American* p. 40, January 1999.
9 Nestle M and others: Behavioral and social influences on food choice, *Nutrition Reviews* 56:S50, 1998.
10 Pate RR and others: Physical activity and public health: a recommendation from the Centers for Disease Control and Prevention and the American College of Sports Medicine, *Journal of the American Medical Association* 273:402, 1995.
11 Popkin BM, Doak CM: The obesity epidemic is a worldwide phenomenon, *Nutrition Reviews* 56:106, 1998.
12 Porter D and others: Educating consumers regarding choices for fat reduction, *Nutrition Reviews* 56:S75, 1998.
13 Rosenberg IH: Keys to a longer, healthier, more vital life, *Nutrition Reviews* 52:S50, 1994.
14 Schwartz NE, Borra ST: What do consumers really think about dietary fat? *Journal of the American Dietetic Association* 97:S73, 1997.
15 Seven excuses for not eating better, Tufts University Health & Nutrition Letter p. 8, December 1998.
16 Sloan AE: Lunch is no longer traditional, *Food Technology* 53(1):22, 1999.
17 Sloan AE, Stiedemann M: Food fortification, *Food Technology* p. 100, June 1996.
18 Smith GP: Control of food intake, In *Modern Nutrition in Health and Disease,* Shils ME and others, eds, Ninth edition, Baltimore MD, Williams & Wilkins, 1999.
19 Subar AF and others: Dietary sources of nutrients among US adults, 1989 to 1991, *Journal of the American Dietetic Association* 98:537, 1998.
20 Thank you for not smoking, *Journal of the American Medical Association* 280:1968, 1998.
21 The wheat from the chaff: Sorting out nutrition information on the internet, *Journal of the American Dietetic Association* 98:1270, 1998.
22 Woods SC and others: Signals that regulate food intake and energy homeostasis, *Science* 280:1378, 1998.
23 Yet another study—should you pay attention? *Tufts University Health & Nutrition Letter* p. 4, September 1998.
24 Zorilla E: Hunger and satiety, *Journal of the American Dietetic Association* 88:1111, 1998.

RATE

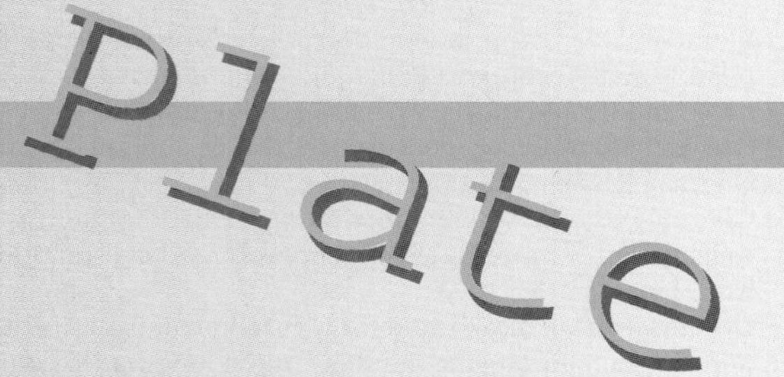

I. Examine the Factors That Affect Your Eating Habits

Choose one day of the week that is typical of your eating pattern. In the first table found in Appendix E, list all foods and drinks you consumed for 1 day. In addition, write down the approximate amounts you ate in units like cups, ounces, teaspoons, and tablespoons. Check the food composition table in Appendix A for examples of appropriate serving units for different types of foods, such as meat, vegetables, etc. After completing this activity, you will use this list of foods for future activities.

After you record each food, drink, and serving size, indicate in the table why you chose to consume each item. Use the following symbols to indicate your reasons. Place the corresponding abbreviation in the space provided, indicating why you picked that particular food or drink.

FLVR	Flavor/texture	HUNG	Hunger
CONV	Convenience	FAM	Family/cultural
EMO	Emotions	PEER	Peers
AVA	Availability	NUTR	Nutritive value
ADV	Advertisement	$	Cost
WTCL	Weight Control	HLTH	Health

There can be more than one reason for choosing a particular food or drink.

APPLICATION

Now ask yourself what your most frequent reason is for eating or drinking. To what degree is health a reason for your food choices?

II. Observe the Supermarket Explosion

Today's supermarkets carry up to 60,000 items, compared to 20,000 items 10 years ago. Think about your last grocery shopping trip and the items you purchased to eat. Below is a list of 20 newer food products added to supermarket shelves. Check the items that you have tried. Then use the Key from Part I of the Rate Your Plate exercise to identify why you might have chosen these products.

_______ **Prepackaged salad greens (variety packs other than iceberg lettuce)** ____________________

_______ **Gourmet salad oils (i.e., walnut, almond, olive, or sesame oil)** ____________________

_______ **Gourmet vinegars (i.e., balsamic or rice)** ____________________

_______ **Prepackaged lunch products (i.e., nacho, pizza, taco, and tortilla Lunchables)** ____________________

_______ **Precooked frozen turkey patties** ____________________

_______ Bean soup mixes (i.e., lentil, black bean, combination bean soups) _______________

_______ Microwaveable sandwiches (i.e., Hotpockets, frozen sandwiches) _______________

_______ Refrigerated, precooked pasta (i.e., tortellini, fettucini) and accompanying sauces (i.e., pesto, tomato basil) _______________

_______ Imported grain products (i.e., riso, farfalline, gnocchi, fusilli) _______________

_______ Frozen dinners (list your favorite of any of the wide variety) _______________

_______ Imported sauces for food preparation (i.e., hoisin or brown bean sauce, mandarin marinade, sesame, curry, or fire oils) _______________

_______ Bottled waters (flavored or unflavored) _______________

_______ Trendy juices (i.e., draft apple cider, hurricane punch) _______________

_______ Roasted and/or flavored coffees (i.e., beans, ground, or instant) _______________

_______ Gourmet jelly beans and candies (i.e., gummi coca-colas or imported chocolates) _______________

_______ Instant hot cereal in a bowl (add water and go!) _______________

_______ "Fast-shake" pancake mix (add water, shake, and ready to cook) _______________

_______ Breakfast bars (i.e., granola or fruit-flavored bars) _______________

_______ Fitness products (i.e., power bars, sports drinks) _______________

Finally, identify three new food products that are not on this list that you have seen in the past year. Discuss the appeal of these products to the American consumer.

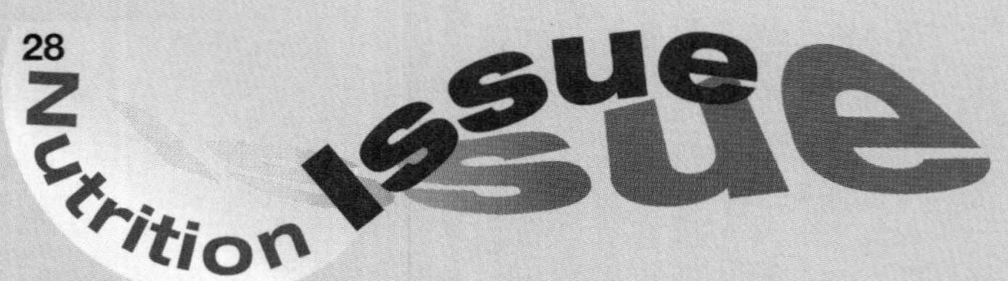

Sorting Fact from Fallacy in Nutrition—the Power of Scientific Research

How do we know what we know about nutrition? How has this knowledge been gained? In a word: research. Like other sciences, the research that underpins nutrition has developed through the use of the *scientific method,* a procedure for testing designed to detect and eliminate error. The first step is observation of a natural phenomenon. Scientists then suggest possible explanations, called **hypotheses,** about its cause. Distinguishing a true cause-and-effect relationship from mere coincidence can be difficult. For instance, earlier in this century many patients in mental hospitals suffered form the disease *pellagra,* which suggested a possible relationship between mental illness and this disease. In time it became clear that this supposed connection was simply coincidental; the real culprit was the poor diet common in mental institutions at that time.

Hypotheses
"Educated guesses" by a scientist to explain a phenomenon.

Experiments
Tests made to examine the validity of a hypothesis.

Theory
An explanation for a phenomenon that has numerous lines of evidence to support it.

To test hypotheses and eliminate coincidental explanations, scientists perform controlled, scientific **experiments.** If the results of many experiments support a hypothesis, the hypothesis becomes generally accepted by scientists and can be called a **theory** (such as the theory of gravity).

The scientific method requires a skeptical attitude. Scientists must not accept proposed hypotheses and theories until they are supported by considerable evidence, and they must reject those that fail to pass critical analyses. Likewise, students should adopt a healthy skepticism and be critical of many current ideas about nutrition (Figure 1–6).

GENERATING HYPOTHESES

Historical events have provided clues to important relationships in nutrition science. In the fifteenth and sixteenth centuries, for example, many European sailors on the long voyages to the Americas developed the disease scurvy. The sailors ate few fruits and vegetables, and eventually British scientists discovered lime juice prevented or cured the scurvy. After this, sailors were given a ration of lime juice, earning them the nickname "limeys." About 200 years later, scientists identified vitamin C, the nutrient present in fruits and vegetables that prevents scurvy.

In a related approach to using historical observation, scientists establish nutritional hypotheses by studying the different dietary and disease patterns among various populations in today's world. If one group tends to develop a certain disease whereas another group does not, scientists can speculate about the role diet plays in this difference. The study of diseases in populations is called **epidmiology.**

An example of this approach occurred in the 1920s, when Dr. Joseph Goldberger noticed that prisoners in jail—but not their jailers—suffered from **pellagra.** He reasoned that if pellagra was an **infectious disease,** both populations would suffer form it. Since this was not the case, he concluded that pellagra was probably caused by a dietary deficiency.

Epidemiology
The study of how disease rates vary among different population groups. For example, the rate of stomach cancer in Japan could be compared with that in Germany.

Pellagra
A disease characterized by inflammation of the skin, diarrhea, and eventual mental incapacity; generally results from an insufficient amount of vitamin niacin in the diet.

Infectious disease
Any disease caused by invasion of the body by microorganism, such as bacteria, fungi, or viruses.

Historical and epidemiological findings can suggest hypotheses about the role of diet in various health problems. To prove the role of particular dietary components, however, requires controlled experiments. For instance, once the high occurrence of pellagra in mental institutions during the 1920s was linked to poor diet, various foods were given to patients who had the disease. These experiments showed that yeast and high-protein foods could cure these patients if the disease was not in its final stage, indicating

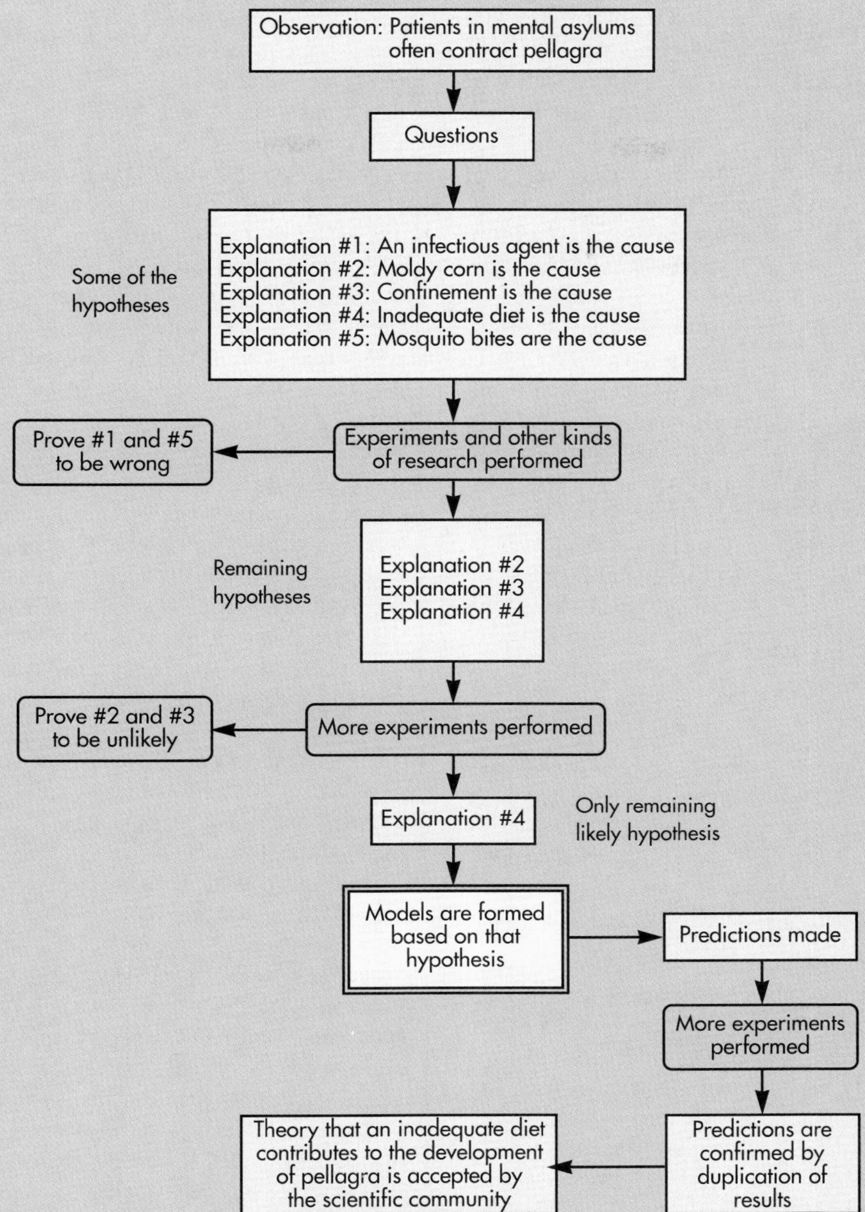

Figure 1-6 *From question to theory—the process of science applied to nutrition. Only after careful and thorough analysis and repeated experimentation should a research finding influence our food choices, such as consuming the vitamin niacin to prevent development of pellagra.*

that pellagra results from a deficiency of some nutrient present in these foods. Eventually this nutrient was found to be the vitamin niacin.

ANIMAL EXPERIMENTS

When scientists cannot test their hypotheses by experiments with humans, they often use animals. Much of what we know about human nutritional needs and functions has been generated from animal experiments. Still, human experiments are the most convincing to scientists. In the 1930s, scientists showed that a pellagra-like disease seen in dogs, called *blacktongue,* was cured by nicotinic acid. Only when nicotinic acid actually cured the disease in humans were scientists convinced that nicotinic acid, later identified as the vitamin niacin, was the critical dietary factor.

Use of humans in certain types of experiments is considered unethical. Although some people argue that

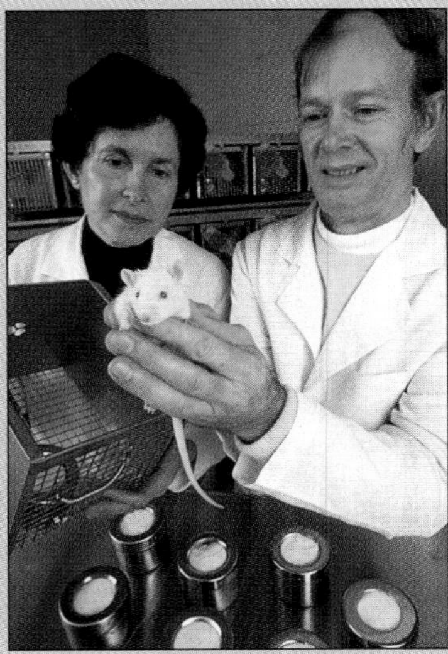

Research using laboratory animals contributes to our nutrition knowledge.

animal experiments are also unethical, most people believe that the careful, humane use of animals is an acceptable alternative to using human subjects. However, use of animal experiments to study the role of nutrition in certain human diseases depends on the availability of an **animal model**—a disease in laboratory animals that closely resembles a particular human disease. If no animal model is available and human experiments are ruled out, scientific knowledge often cannot advance beyond what can be learned from epidemiological studies.

HUMAN EXPERIMENTS

Various experimental approaches are used to test research hypotheses in humans, including case-control and double-blind studies.

Case-Control Study

In a case-control study, individuals who have the condition in question, such as lung cancer,, are compared with individuals who do not have the condition. Comparisons are made only between groups that are matched for other major characteristics (e.g., age and gender) not under study. This type of study may identify factors other than the disease in question, such as fruit and vegetable intake, that differ between the two groups, thus providing researchers with clues about the cause, progression, and prevention of the disease.

Double-blind study
An experimental design in which neither the participants nor the researchers are aware of the participant's assignment (test or placebo) or the outcome of the study until it is completed. An independent third party holds the code and the data until the study has been completed.

Double-Blind Study

An important approach for more definitive testing of hypotheses is the **double-blind study,** in which a group of participants—the experimental group—follows a specific protocol (e.g., consuming a certain food or nutrient), and participants in a corresponding **control group** conform to their normal habits. People are randomly assigned to each group, as by the flip of a coin. Scientists then observe the experimental group over time to see if there is any effect that is not found in the control group.

Control group
Participants in an experiment who are not given the treatment being tested.

Two features of a double-blind study help reduce the introduction of bias (prejudice), which can easily affect the outcome of an experiment. First, neither the participants nor the researchers know which individuals are in the experimental group and which are in the control group. Second, the expected effects of the experimental protocol are not disclosed to the participants or researchers until after the entire study is completed. This approach reduces the possibility that researchers may see the change they want to see in the participants to prove a certain "pet" hypothesis, even though such a change did not actually occur. This approach also reduces the chance that the persons participating may begin to feel better simply because they are involved in a research study or receiving a new treatment, a phenomenon called the *placebo effect.*

Derived from the Latin word **placebo,** meaning "I shall please," the placebo effect cannot be explained by pharmacological or other direct physical action. It may instead be linked to a simple reduction in stress and anxiety. At least one-third of all patients will show improvement after receiving a placebo (generally in the form of a fake medicine). Thus, it is critical to make allowances for the placebo effect in research studies.

Placebo
Generally a fake medicine used to disguise the roles of participants in an experiment.

A recent example illustrates the need to test hypotheses based on epidemiological observations in double-blind studies. Epidemiologists using primarily case-control studies found that smokers who regularly consumed fruits and vegetables had a lower risk for lung cancer than smokers who ate few fruits and vegetables. Some scientists proposed that beta-carotene, a pigment present in many fruits and vegetables, could reduce the damage that tobacco smoke created in the lungs. However, in later double-blind studies involving heavy smokers, the risk of lung cancer was found to be higher for those who took beta-carotene than for those who did not. After these results were reported, the federal agency supporting two other large ongoing studies that employed beta-carotene supplements called a halt to the research, stating that these supplements were ineffective in preventing both lung cancer and heart disease.

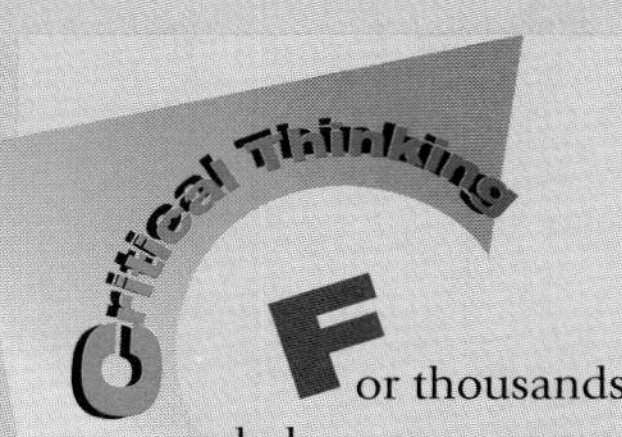

For thousands of years, early humans consumed a diet rich in vegetable products and low in animal products. These diets were generally lower in fat and higher in dietary fiber than modern diets. Do the differences in human diets throughout history necessarily tell us which diet is better—that of early humans or modern humans? If not, what is a more reliable way to pursue this question of potential diet superiority?

Overall, health and nutrition advice provided by grandparents, parents, friends, and other well-meaning individuals can't be verified unless it is put to ultimate scientific scrutiny. Until that is done, we can't be sure that the substance or procedure in question is truly effective. One reason for this is the power of the placebo effect. In addition, many common symptoms, such as sneezing, lower back pain, and headache, are short-lived and go away within a short time without any treatment, reflecting the natural course of the underlying diseases. When people say "I get fewer colds now that I take vitamin C," they overlook the fact that many cold symptoms disappear quickly with no treatment; the apparent curative effective of vitamin C or any other remedy is often coincidental rather than causal to the natural healing process.

PEER REVIEW OF EXPERIMENTAL RESULTS

Once an experiment is complete, scientists summarize the findings and publish the results in a scientific journal. Generally, before articles are published in scientific journals, they are critically reviewed by other scientists familiar with the subject. The objective of this peer review is to ensure that only high-quality research findings are published. This is an important step because most scientific research in this country is funded by the federal government, nonprofit foundations, drug companies, and other private industries. All these funding sources can have strong expectations about the research outcomes. Peer review helps ensure that the researchers are as objective as possible.

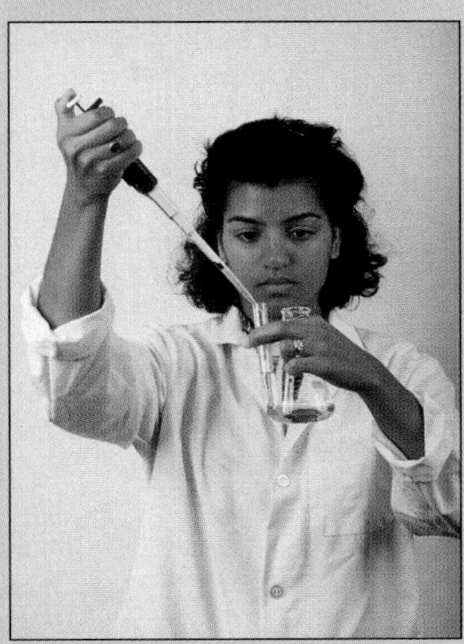

Careful research contributes to nutrition knowledge, more so than personal experience.

Results published in peer-reviewed journals, such as the *American Journal of Clinical Nutrition*, the *New England Journal of Medicine*, and the *Journal of the American Dietetic Association*, are much more reliable than those found in popular magazines or promoted on television talk shows. Unfortunately, reputable journals are not the main sources for the information presented in the popular media.

FOLLOW-UP STUDIES

Finally, even if an acceptable protocol has been followed and the results of a study have been accepted by the scientific community, one experiment is never enough to prove a particular hypothesis or provide a basis for nutritional recommendations. Rather, the results obtained in one laboratory must be confirmed by experiments conducted in other laboratories. Overall, it is important to avoid rushing to accept new ideas as fact or incorporating them into your health habits until they are proved by several lines of evidence.

HOW TO USE THIS KNOWLEDGE TO EVALUATE NUTRITION CLAIMS AND ADVICE

Based on what has been covered so far, the following suggestions should help you make healthful and logical nutrition decisions:

1. Applying the basic principles of nutrition as outlined in this chapter (and the Food Guide Pyramid in Chapter 2) to any nutrition claim. Do you note any inconsistencies? Do reliable references support the claims? Beware of the following:
   - Testimonials about personal experience
   - Disreputable publication sources
   - Dramatic results (rarely true)
   - Lack of evidence from supporting studies made by other scientists
2. Examine the background and scientific credentials of the individual, organizations, or publication making the nutritional claim. Usually, a reputable author is one whose educational background or present affiliation is with a nationally recognized university or medical center that offers programs or courses in the field of nutrition, medicine, or a closely allied specialty.
3. Be wary if the answer is "Yes" to any of the following questions about a health-related nutrition claim:
   - Are only advantages discussed and possible disadvantages ignored?

- Are claims made about "curing" disease? Do they sound too good to be true?
- Is extreme bias against the medical community or traditional medical treatments evident? Physicians as a group strive to cure diseases in their patients, using what proven techniques are available. They do not ignore reliable cures.
- Is the claim touted as a new or secret scientific breakthrough?

4. Note the size and duration of any study cited in support of a nutrition claim. The larger it is and the longer it went on, the more dependable its findings. Also consider the type of study: epidemiology versus case-control versus double-blind. Check out the group studied; a study of men or women in Sweden may be less relevant than one of men or women of Southern European, African, or Hispanic descent, for example. Keep in mind that "contributes to," "is linked to," or "is associated with" does not mean "causes."
5. Beware of press conferences and other hype regarding the latest findings. Much of this will not survive more detailed scientific evaluation.
6. When you meet with a nutrition professional, you should expect that he or she will do the following:
   - Ask questions about your medical history, lifestyle, and current eating habits.
   - Formulate a diet plan tailored to your needs, as opposed to simply tearing a form from a tablet that could apply to almost anyone.
   - Schedule follow-up visits to track your progress, answer any questions, and help keep you motivated.
   - Involve family members in the diet plan, when appropriate.
   - Consult directly with your physician and readily refer you back to your physician for those health problems a nutrition professional is not trained to treat.
7. Avoid practitioners who prescribe large doses of vitamin and mineral supplements for everyone or sell them in connection with their practice.
8. Examine product labels carefully. Be skeptical of any product promotion not clearly stated on the label. A product is not likely to do something that is not specifically claimed on its label or package insert (legally part of the label).

This cautious approach to nutrition-related advice and products is even more important today because of sweeping changes in federal law passed in 1994.

The Dietary Supplement Health and Education Act of 1994 classified vitamins, minerals, amino acids, and herbal remedies as "foods", effectively restraining the U.S. Food and Drug Administration (FDA) from regulating them as heavily as food additives and drugs. According to this act, rather than the manufacturer having to prove a nutritional product is safe, FDA must prove it is unsafe before preventing its sale. In contrast, the safety of food additives and drugs must be demonstrated to FDA's satisfaction before they are marketed.

Currently, a dietary supplement (or herbal product) can be marketed without FDA approval if (1) there is a history of its use or other evidence that it is expected to be reasonably safe when used under the conditions recommended or suggested in its labeling, and (2) the product is labeled as a dietary supplement. It is permissible for the labels on such products to claim a benefit related to a classic nutrient-deficiency disease, describe how a nutrient affects human body structure or function, and claim that general well-being results from consumption of the ingredient(s). However, the label of products bearing such claims also must prominently display in boldface type the following disclaimer: "This statement has not been evaluated by the Food and Drug Administration. This product is not intended to diagnose, treat, cure, or prevent any disease." Despite this warning, when consumers find these products on the shelves of supermarkets, health-food stores, and pharmacies, they may mistakenly assume FDA has carefully evaluated the products.

35 Pounds of Fat.

DR. EDISON'S OBESITY PILLS AND REDUCING TABLETS CURED MRS. MANNING.

No Other Remedies But Dr. Edison's Reduce Obesity—Take No Others.

SAMPLES FREE—USE COUPON.

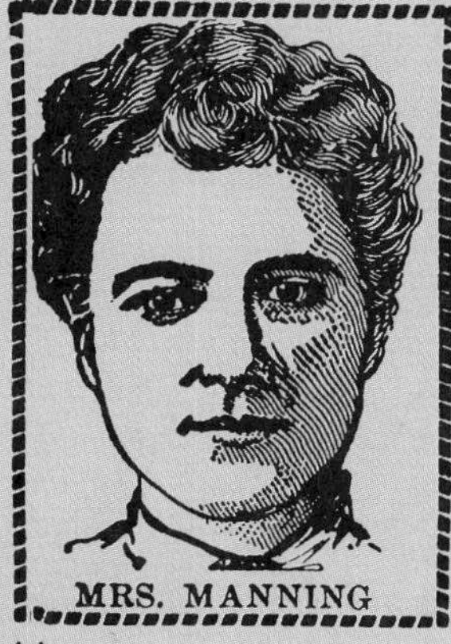

MRS. MANNING

Mary Hyde Manning, one of the best known of Troy's, New York, society women, grew too fleshy, and used Dr. Edison's Obesity Remedies. Read the letter telling of her reduction and restoration to health:—"In six weeks I was reduced 35 pounds, from 171 to 136, by Dr. Edison's Obesity Pills and Reducing Tablets. I recommend these remedies to all fat and sick men and women."

The following well-known men and women have been reduced by DR. EDISON'S OBESITY REMEDIES:
Mrs. H. Mershon, 156 South Jackson St., Lima, O., 148 lbs.
Mrs. Josephine McPherson, 7916 Wright St., Chicago, 42 lbs.
Rev. Edward R. Pierce, 410 Alma St., Chicago, 42 lbs.
C. C. Nichols, 145 Clark St., Aurora, Ill., 36 lbs.
Mrs. W. Davlin, Whitemore, O., 149 lbs.
W. H. Webster, 618 2d Ave., Troy, N. Y., 26 lbs.
J. M. McKinney, 4504 State St., Chicago, 30 lbs.
Mrs. J. M. McKinney, 4504 State St., Chicago, 33 lbs.
Mrs. A. Walker, 1104 Milton Place, Chicago, 20 lbs.

(a)

22% LESS BODY FAT IN SIX WEEKS

University studies have identified CHROMIUM PICOLINATE as a "trigger" for fat loss and lean muscle enhancement. 200 micrograms taken daily caused a 22% fat loss in only 6 weeks.

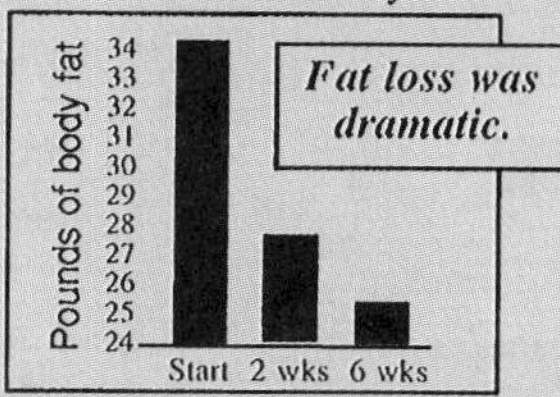

Men and women of every age are talking about the amazing benefits of this safe, essential nutrient:

WEIGHT LOSS • FAT LOSS
MORE ENDURANCE AND STAMINA
MORE LEAN MUSCLE

Our Product is made to the exact specifications of the capsules used in the studies cited above. Each bottle of 60 capsules is a 2-month supply.

SATISFACTION GUARANTEED
(Check or money order only. Canada: U.S. $ m.o.)

(b)

Figure 1–7 *Quackery has been with us for ages.* **A** *Even at the turn of the century, people wanted to believe that fat could be lost without changing habits or without much effort, and* **B** *they still do.*

The fact remains that many Americans are willing to try bogus nutrition products and believe in their miraculous actions (Figure 1–7). Popular products claim to increase muscle growth, enhance sexuality, boost energy, reduce body fat, increase strength, supply missing nutrients, increase longevity, and even improve brain function. Clearly, many nutritional products commonly found in stores are not strictly regulated in terms of effectiveness. Few have been thoroughly evaluated by reputable scientists. If you embark on a self-cure by means of such products, you will probably waste money and possibly risk ill health. A better approach is to consult a physician or registered dietitian first. Appendix J also lists many reputable sources of nutrition advice for your use. Finally, four web sites to help you evaluate ongoing nutrition and health claims are:

http://www.acsh.org
http://www.quackwatch.com
http://www.ncahf.org
http://dietary-supplements.info.nih.gov

The sites are maintained by groups or individuals committed to providing reasoned and authoritative nutrition and health advice to consumers.

The American Dietetic Association has a hotline, staffed by registered dietitians, to answer consumers' food-related questions. Call (900) 225-5267. Cost is $1.95/minute. A toll-free hotline (800) 366-1655 provides dietitian referrals through the Nationwide Nutrition Network and nutrition messages in English and Spanish. You can also find out more about nutrition on their web site http://www.eatright.org.

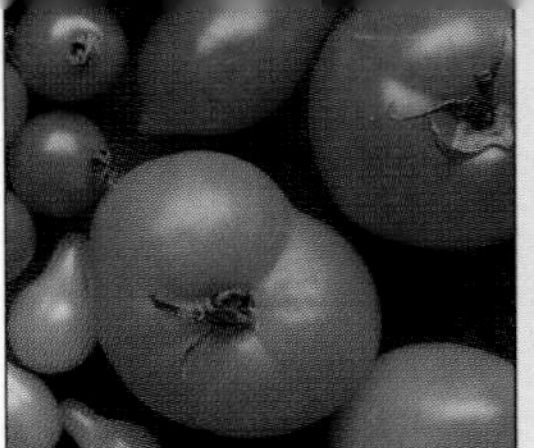

chapter 2

Tools for Diet Design

How many times have you heard wild claims about how healthful certain foods are for you? As consumers focus more and more on diet and disease, food manufacturers are asserting that their products have all sorts of health benefits. Supermarket shelves have begun to look like an 1800s medicine show. "Take aged garlic capsules to avoid a heart attack," "Eat more olive oil and oat bran to lower blood cholesterol." Hearing these claims, you would think that food manufacturers have solutions to all of our health problems.

Advertising aside, nutrient intakes out of balance with nutrient needs—such as energy intake, fat, sodium and sugar—are linked to many of the leading causes of death in the United States, including obesity, high blood pressure, heart disease, cancer, liver disease, and the major form of diabetes. In this chapter you will explore the components of healthy diet plans—those that will minimize your risks of developing nutrition-related diseases. The goal is to provide you with a firm understanding of basic diet-planning concepts before you study the nutrients in detail.

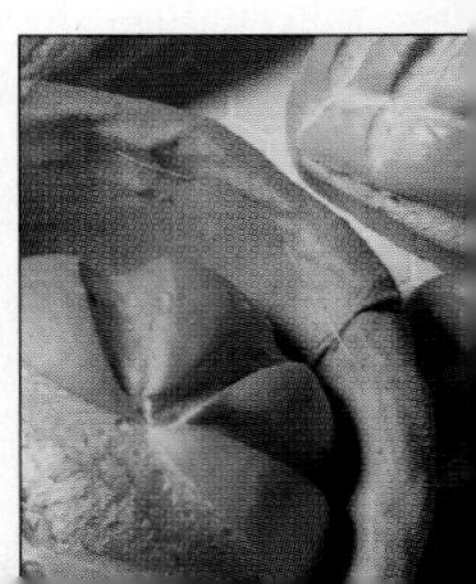

Nutrition Web

Three watchwords of nutrition are variety, balance, and moderation when it comes to designing a diet. Many diet-related tools are available to achieve this combination.

Evaluation of one's nutritional state involves analyzing health background, anthropometric measurements (e.g., weight-for-height), biochemical parameters, clinical symptoms, and diet history. However, it is not always possible to detect existing nutritional inadequacies via such a nutrition assessment since evidence often does not appear for many months or years.

One's nutritional state can be categorized as desirable, in which the body has adequate stores for times of increased needs; undernutrition, which may be present with or without clinical symptoms; and overnutrition, which can lead to vitamin and mineral toxicities, and certain chronic diseases.

The Food Guide Pyramid provides variety, balance, and moderation: sufficient protein, vitamins, and minerals; and a focus on complex carbohydrate sources while moderating fat intake.

Dietary Guidelines have been issued to help fine-tune choices within the Food Guide Pyramid concept. The Guidelines emphasize eating a variety of foods; performing regular physical activity to maintain or improve weight; moderating fat, sodium, and alcohol intake; and other healthful practices.

Recommended Dietary Allowances (RDAs) and related standards are set for many nutrients. The various standards are set to provide enough of each nutrient to meet the needs of healthy Americans.

Daily Values are adapted from the RDAs and other nutrient standards. Daily Values are used to express the nutrient content of foods on the Nutrition Facts panel. These food labels are a valuable tool for tracking nutrient intakes.

Nutrient density compares nutrient content of a food to nutrient needs. A nutrient-dense food is high in one or more nutrients compared to energy content; for example, milk is a nutrient-dense source of calcium.

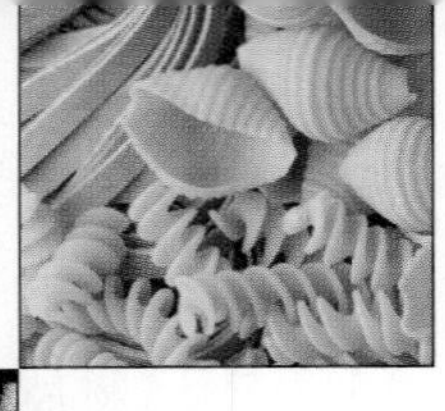

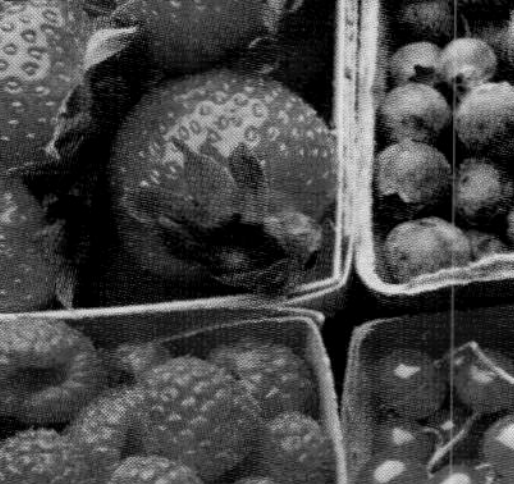

A Food Philosophy That Works

You may be surprised to learn that what you should eat to minimize the risk of developing the common nutrition-related diseases seen in the United States is exactly what you've heard many times before: **Consume a variety of foods balanced by a moderate intake of each food.** A variety of foods is best because no one food meets all your nutrient needs. Human milk comes close to meeting all of an infant's needs, except that it provides only limited amounts of iron, vitamin D, and fluoride. Cow's milk contains very little iron; neither form of milk provides dietary fiber. Meat provides iron but little calcium. Thus, you need variety in your diet because the required nutrients are scattered among many different foods.

It is unfortunate, however, that according to a recent survey conducted by the American Dietetic Association, two of five people in the United States believe that following a healthful diet means giving up foods they enjoy. To the contrary, a healthful diet requires only some simple planning and doesn't have to mean deprivation and misery. Besides, eliminating favorite foods typically doesn't work for "dieters" in the long run.

Variety, balance, and moderation will be continually stressed throughout this book. Let's now fine-tune this advice.

Variety—Choose different types of foods within each food group.
Balance—Choose foods from all five food groups.
Moderation—Control portion size so that balance and variety are possible in your diet.

Variety

For variety in your diet, choose a number of different foods within any given food group rather than the "same old thing" day after day. Variety makes meals more interesting and helps ensure that a diet contains sufficient nutrients. For example, carrots may be your favorite vegetable, but if you choose carrots every day as your only vegetable source, you may miss out on the vitamin folate. Other vegetables, such as broccoli and asparagus, are rich sources of this nutrient. This concept is true of all classes of food: fruits, vegetables, grains, and so on. Different foods within each class vary somewhat in the nutrients they contain, but they generally provide similar types of nutrients.

An added bonus of variety in the diet is the inclusion of a rich supply of what scientists call **phytochemicals**. These substances are not absolutely required parts of the diet. Still, many of these substances probably provide health benefits. Considerable research attention is now focused on various phytochemicals in reducing the risk for certain diseases. Because current vitamin and mineral supplements contain few or none of these potentially beneficial substances, they generally are only available from the diet.

A useful diet/lifestyle acronym is
- **A adequacy of diet**
- **B balance in diet**
- **C calorie control**
- **D diversity in food choice**
- **E exercise on a regular basis**

Numerous epidemiological studies show reduced cancer risk among people who regularly consume fruits and vegetables. This is true for cancer of the gastrointestinal (GI) tract, breast, lung, and bladder. Researchers surmise that some phytochemicals present in the fruits and vegetables block the cancer process. The cancer process is described in the Nutrition Issue in Chapter 7. For now, realize that cancer develops over many years via a multistep process. If an agent such as a phytochemical can block any one of the steps in this process, the chances that cancer will ultimately appear in the body are reduced. Other phytochemicals have been linked to a reduced risk of heart disease. Could it be that because humans evolved on a diet containing a wide variety of plant-based foods, the body developed with a need for these phytochemicals to maintain optimal health?

Phytochemical
A chemical found in plants. Some phytochemicals contribute to a reduced risk of cancer or heart disease in people who consume them regularly.

It will take many years for scientists to unravel the important effects of the myriad of phytochemicals in foods, and it is unlikely that all will ever be available in supplement form. For this reason, leading heart disease and cancer researchers suggest that a diet rich in fruits, vegetables, and whole grains is the most reliable way to obtain the potential benefits of phytochemicals. Table 2–1 lists a variety of phytochemicals under study with their common food sources. Table 2–2 provides a number of suggestions for including more phytochemicals in a diet.

TABLE 2-1

Some of the Phytochemicals Currently Under Study

Phytochemical	Food source
Polyphenols (flavonoids; e.g., quercetin, catechins)	Onions, garlic, red wine, tea* (especially green), dark beer, chocolate, fruits and vegetables
Indoles	Cruciferous vegetables**
Isothiocyanates (e.g., sulforaphane)	Cruciferous vegetables, especially broccoli
Carotenoids (e.g., lycopene)	Orange, yellow, and green vegetables; some fruits
Allyl sulfides	Onions, garlic, leeks, chives
Isoflavones (e.g., genistein)	Legumes (e.g., soybeans)
Monoterpenes (e.g., limonene)	Oils from citrus fruits, cherries; nuts, seeds
Phytic acid	Whole grains, legumes
Lignans	Seeds (e.g., flax); some fruits and vegetables
Phenolic acids (e.g., ellagic acid, ferulic acid)	Seeds (e.g., in strawberries and bananas); fruits and vegetables
p-coumaric acid, chlorogenic acid	Fruits and vegetables
Glutathione	Fruits and vegetables (also freshly prepared meats)
Saponins	Beans and legumes
Curcumin	Tumeric

*Adding milk or cream to tea appears to block absorption of the main phytochemicals present in tea.
**Cruciferous vegetables include bok choy, broccoli, brussels sprouts, cabbage, cauliflower, collards, kale, kohlrabi, mustard greens, rutabaga, turnip greens, and turnips.

A term has been coined to refer to foods rich in phytochemicals—functional foods. This term indicates that the food provides health benefits beyond those supplied by the traditional nutrients it contains. Since a tomato contains the phytochemical lycopene, it can be called a functional food. The food industry especially has begun to use this term.

Finally, a varied diet can make eating fun too. No one ever said that we have to eat the same foods and meals that we've eaten since childhood.

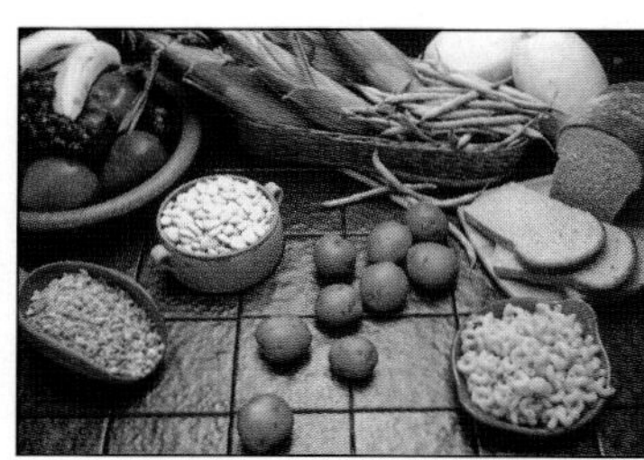

Fruits, vegetables, and whole grains are typically rich in phytochemicals.

Balance

One way to balance your diet as you consume a variety of foods is to select foods from the five major food groups every day:

- Milk, yogurt, and cheese
- Meat, poultry, fish, dry beans, eggs, and nuts
- Vegetable
- Fruit
- Bread, cereal, rice and pasta

A lunch consisting of a bean burrito with tomatoes accompanied by a glass of milk and an apple covers all groups. Fats, oils, and sweets can also be added to a diet in moderation to increase its flavor and help supply certain nutrients, such as vitamin E and essential fatty acids.

Moderation

Some people might like to live on pizza alone. What are pizza's nutrient strengths and inadequacies? Check the food composition table in Appendix A for the vitamin C content of cheese pizza. How many slices would you need to eat to yield the vitamin C RDA of 60 milligrams? (Answer: 25 slices)

Eating moderately requires planning your entire day's diet so that you juggle nutrient sources. For example, if you eat something relatively high in fat, sugar, salt, or energy, such as a bacon cheeseburger with a regular soft drink at a quick-service restaurant, you should eat other foods that are less concentrated sources of the same nutrients, such as fruits and salad greens, the same day.

Although there are no "good" or "bad" foods, many Americans have diets "out-of-balance" because of excessive use of high-fat foods (e.g., whole milk, doughnuts, french fries, hot dogs), white bread and related refined wheat products, and sugared

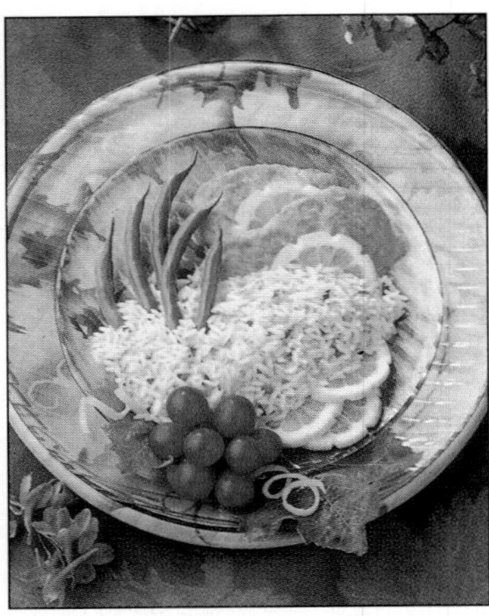

Focus on nutrient-rich foods as you strive to meet your nutrient needs.

TABLE 2-2

Tips for Including Foods Rich in Phytochemicals in a Diet

- Include vegetables in main and side dishes. Add these to rice, omelets, potato salad, tuna salad, and pastas. Try broccoli or cauliflower florets, mushrooms, peas, carrots, corn, or peppers.
- Look for quick-fixing grain side dishes in the supermarket. Pilafs, couscous, rice mixes, and tabbouleh are just a few that you'll find.
- Choose fruit-filled cookies, such as fig bars.
- Use fresh or canned fruit as a topping or direct addition for puddings, hot or cold cereal, pancakes, and frozen desserts.
- Put raisins, grapes, apple chunks, pineapples, grated carrots, zucchini, or cucumber into coleslaw, chicken salad, or tuna salad.
- Be creative at the salad bar: try fresh spinach, leaf lettuce, red cabbage, sprouts, zucchini, yellow squash, cauliflower, peas, mushrooms, or red or yellow peppers.
- Pack fresh or dried fruit for snacks away from home instead of grabbing a candy bar or going hungry.
- On sandwiches, lettuce and tomato are just the beginning. Add slices of cucumber or zucchini, bean sprouts, spinach, carrot slivers, or snow peas.
- Try one or two vegetarian meals per week, such as beans and rice or pasta, vegetable stir fry, or spaghetti, squash, and tomato sauce.
- When daily protein intake more than meets required amounts, reduce the meat, fish, or poultry in casseroles, stews, and soups by one-third to one-half and add more vegetables and legumes.
- In the refrigerator, keep a bowl of fresh vegetables handy for snacks.
- Start the day off with orange or another form of fruit juice.
- Choose 100% fruit or vegetable juices instead of soft drinks.
- Have a bowl of fruit on hand.
- Blend a banana, an orange, orange juice, plain nonfat yogurt and a few ice cubes for a refreshing fruit smoothie. Many fruits and juices can be added to smoothies.
- Switch from iceberg lettuce to leaf lettuce, such as romaine.
- Use salsa as a dip for chips.
- Choose whole-grain breakfast cereals, breads, and crackers.
- Flavor food with plenty of herbs and spices, including ginger, rosemary, basil, thyme, garlic, parsley, and chives.
- Experiment with soy products, such as tofu, soy protein isolate, tempah, soy milk, and roasted soybeans.

soft drinks. Such diets generally lack the foundations of a healthy food plan and in turn pose substantial risks for nutrition-related diseases.

The following sections of the chapter describe various states of nutritional health and provide tools and nutrient guidelines for planning healthy diets to support overall health.

Nutritional state *The nutritional health of a person as determined by anthropometric measurements (height, weight, circumferences, and so on), biochemical measurements of nutrients or their by-products in blood and urine, a clinical (physical) examination, and a dietary analysis; also called nutritional status.*

States of Nutritional Health

The body's nutritional health is determined by the sum of its **nutritional state** with respect to each needed nutrient. Three general categories are recognized: desirable nutrition, undernutrition, and overnutrition. The common term **malnutrition** can refer

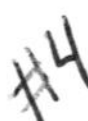

to either **overnutrition** or **undernutrition**. Neither state is conducive to good health.

Desirable Nutrition

The nutritional state for a particular nutrient is desirable when body tissues have enough of the nutrient to support normal metabolic functions as well as surplus stores that can be used in times of increased need. A desirable nutritional state can be achieved by obtaining essential nutrients from a variety of foods.

Undernutrition

Undernutrition occurs when nutrient intake does not meet nutrient needs. Stores are then used up and health declines. Many nutrients are in high demand due to the constant state of cell loss and later regeneration in the body. For this reason, certain nutrient stores are exhausted rapidly, such as for many of the B vitamins. In turn, a regular intake is needed. In addition, some women in the United States do not consume sufficient iron to meet monthly losses and eventually deplete their iron stores (Table 2–3).

Once availability of a nutrient falls sufficiently low, biochemical evidence, in which the body's metabolic processes slow or stop, appears. At this state of deficiency there are no outward symptoms, thus it is termed a **subclinical** deficiency (see Table 2–3). A subclinical deficiency can go on for some time before clinicians are able to detect its effects.

Eventually clinical symptoms will develop, resulting in clinical evidence of a deficiency, perhaps in the skin, hair, nails, tongue, or eyes. Often, clinicians do not detect a problem until a deficiency produces such results, such as in a vitamin C deficiency.

Overnutrition

Prolonged consumption of more nutrients than the body needs can lead to overnutrition. In the short run, for instance a week or two, overnutrition may cause only a few symptoms, such as GI tract distress from excess dietary fiber or iron intake. But if kept up, some nutrients may increase to toxic amounts, which can lead to serious disease. For example, too much vitamin A can have negative effects, particularly in children and pregnant women.

TABLE 2-3

Categories of Nutritional States with Respect to Iron*

General conditions	Condition with respect to iron
Overnutrition: nutrients consumed in excess of body needs (degree of toxicity varies for each nutrient)	Results in toxic damage to liver cells; may contribute to heart disease
Desirable nutrition: nutrients consumed to support body functions and stores of nutrients for times of increased need	Adequate liver stores of iron, adequate blood values for iron-related compounds
Undernutrition: nutrient intake does not meet nutrient needs; biochemical changes then take place.	Many changes in body functions associated with a decline in iron status (e.g., iron-containing proteins and pigments in the blood drop below acceptable amounts and oxygen supply to body tissues is reduced)
Clinical symptoms; these effects eventually are seen.	Pale complexion; greatly increased heart rate during activity; "spooning" of the nails in a severe deficiency; poor body temperature regulation

*This general scheme can apply to all nutrients. Iron was chosen because you are likely to be familiar with this nutrient.

Malnutrition
Failing health that results from long-standing dietary practices that do not coincide with nutritional needs.

Overnutrition
A state in which nutritional intake greatly exceeds the body's needs.

Undernutrition
Failing health that results from a long-standing dietary intake that does not meet nutritional needs.

Subclinical
Disease or disorder that is present but not severe enough to produce symptoms that can be detected or diagnosed.

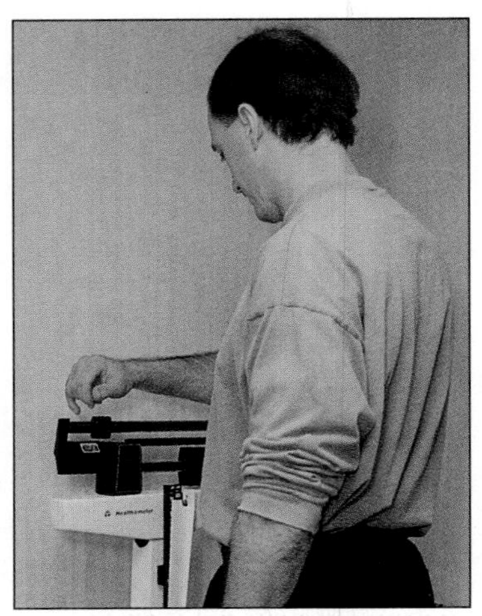

Body weight is a key component of a nutrition assessment.

The most common type of overnutrition in industrialized nations—excess intake of energy-yielding nutrients—often leads to obesity. In the long run, obesity can then lead to other serious diseases, such as certain forms of diabetes and cancer. Use the web site http://www.healthyweight.com to learn more about this problem.

For most vitamins and minerals, the gap between desirable intake and overnutrition is wide. Therefore, even if people take a typical multiple vitamin and mineral supplement daily, they probably won't receive a harmful amount of any nutrient. The gap between optimal intake and overnutrition is narrowest for vitamin A and vitamin D, as well as calcium, iron, copper, and other minerals. Thus, if you take nutrient supplements, keep a close eye on your total vitamin and mineral intake both from food and from supplements to avoid toxicity (see Chapter 7 for further advice on use of nutrient supplements).

How Could Your Nutritional State Be Measured?

To find out how nutritionally fit *you* are, a nutritional assessment—either whole or in part—needs to be performed (Table 2-4).

Analyzing Background Factors

Since family history plays an important role in determining nutritional and health status, it must be carefully recorded and critically analyzed as part of a nutritional assessment. Other related background components include (1) a medical history, especially for any disease states or treatments that could impede nutrient absorptive processes or ultimate use; and (2) socioeconomic history, to determine the ability to purchase and prepare appropriate foods needed to maintain health.

Anthropometric *Pertaining to the measurement of body weight and the lengths, circumferences, and thicknesses of parts of the body.*

Evaluating the ABCDs

Four components in combination further add to the complete nutritional picture. **Anthropometric** measurements of height, weight, body skinfolds, and body circumferences are an excellent first line of attack. They are easy to obtain and

TABLE 2-4

Conducting an Evaluation of Nutritional Health

Component	Example
Background histories	Medical history, including current diseases and past surgeries Medications history Social history (marital status, cooking facilities) Family history Economic status
Nutritional parameters	Anthropometric assessment: height, weight, skinfold thickness, arm muscle circumference, and other parameters Biochemical (laboratory) assessment of blood and urine: enzyme activities, concentrations of nutrients or their by-products Clinical assessment (physical examination): general appearance of skin, eyes, and tongue; rapid hair loss; sense of touch; ability to walk Diet history: usual intake or record or previous days' meals

generally reliable. However, an in-depth examination of nutritional health is impossible without the rather expensive process of biochemical assessment. This involves the measurement of specific blood enzyme activities and of the concentrations of nutrients and nutrient by-products in the blood.

A clinical examination would follow, during which a health professional would search for any physical evidence of diet-related diseases. Last, a diet history, documenting at least the previous few days' intake, is an invaluable took for insight into possible problem areas. Together these activities form the **ABCDs** of nutritional assessment: **a**nthropometric measurements, **b**iochemical assessment, **c**linical examination, and **d**iet history.

Recognizing the Limitations of Nutritional Assessment

As mentioned, a long time may elapse between the initial development of poor nutritional health and the first clinical evidence of a problem. Recall that a diet high in saturated (typically solid) fat often increases blood **cholesterol** concentration, but without producing any clinical evidence for years. However, when the blood vessels become sufficiently blocked by cholesterol and other materials, chest pain during physical activity or a **heart attack** may occur. Much current nutrition research aims to develop better methods for early detection of nutrition-related problems such as this.

Another example in the delay of evidence that serious consequences are occurring is with a calcium deficiency, a particularly relevant issue for adolescent females. Many young women consume well below the needed amount of calcium but often suffer no ill effects in their younger years. However, women whose bone structures do not reach full potential during the years of growth are likely to face an increased risk for osteoporosis later in life.

Furthermore, clinical evidence of nutritional deficiencies is often not very specific, such as diarrhea, an irregular walk, and facial sores. These may have different causes. Long lag times and vague evidence often make it difficult to establish a link between an individual's current diet and nutritional state.

Table 1–4 in Chapter 1 showed the close relationship of nutrition and health. The rest of this current chapter helps you plan a diet to maximize your health and minimize the development of nutrition-related diseases.

Cholesterol
A waxy lipid found in all body cells. It has a structure containing multiple chemical rings that is found only in foods that contain animal products (see Chapter 5).

Heart attack
Rapid fall in heart function caused by reduced blood flow through the heart's blood vessels. Often part of the heart dies in the process (see Chapter 5). Technically called a myocardial infarction.

Concept Check

Variety, balance, and moderation are the foundations of a healthy diet. A desirable nutritional state results when the body has enough nutrients to function fully and contains stores to use in times of increased needs. When nutrient intake fails to meet body needs, undernutrition develops. Symptoms of such an inadequate nutrient intake can take months or years to develop. Overloading the body with nutrients, leading to overnutrition, is another potential problem to avoid. Nutritional state can be assessed by using anthropometric measurements, biochemical evidence, clinical evaluation, and diet history.

Critical Thinking

Tom loves to eat hamburgers, fries, and lots of pizza with double amounts of cheese. He rarely eats any vegetables and fruits, but instead snacks on cookies and ice cream. He insists that he has no problems with his health, is rarely ill, and doesn't see how his diet could cause him any health risks. How would you explain to Tom that despite his current good health, his diet could predispose him to future health problems?

The Food Guide Pyramid—A Menu-Planning Tool

Since the early twentieth century, researchers have worked on various food plans to simplify nutrition science into practical terms so that people with no special training could estimate whether their nutritional needs were being met. In recent years the Food Guide Pyramid has been widely advocated to meet this goal (Figure 2–1). This plan is rich in protein, vitamins, and minerals. An additional intent is to provide the bulk of dietary energy intake from carbohydrate-rich sources while moderating fat intake.

Components of the Food Guide Pyramid

The number of servings to consume from each food group in the Food Guide Pyramid depends on a person's age and energy needs. Service size is also adjusted downward for young children (see Chapter 13). Table 2–5 lists serving sizes and amounts for adults of various ages. The table also lists the major nutrients each food group supplies. Note the similarities and differences among the groups.

Following the Food Guide Pyramid makes it possible to create daily diets containing as few as 1600 to 1800 kcal (Table 2–6), sufficient for a sedentary adult or an older person. Not following this advice can leave a diet of 1600 to 1800 kcal short on the nutrients.

Other food pyramids have been proposed by various nutrition organizations. The Nutrition Issue discusses the Latin American, Asian, Mediterranean, and Soul Food Pyramids.

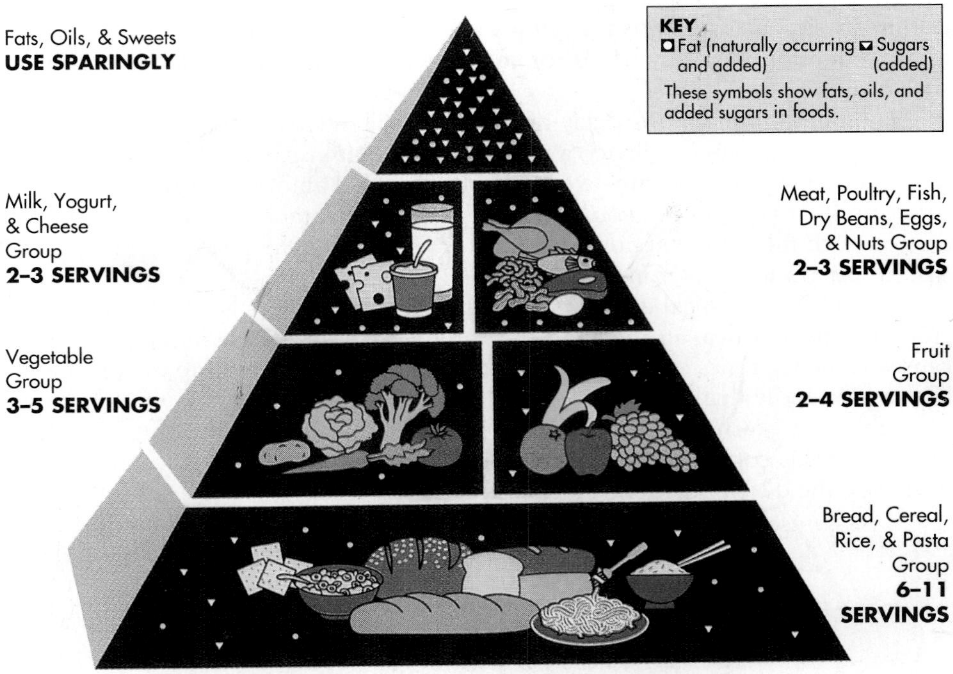

Fats, Oils, & Sweets
USE SPARINGLY

KEY
Fat (naturally occurring and added) Sugars (added)
These symbols show fats, oils, and added sugars in foods.

Milk, Yogurt, & Cheese Group
2–3 SERVINGS

Meat, Poultry, Fish, Dry Beans, Eggs, & Nuts Group
2–3 SERVINGS

Vegetable Group
3–5 SERVINGS

Fruit Group
2–4 SERVINGS

Bread, Cereal, Rice, & Pasta Group
6–11 SERVINGS

Figure 2–1 *USDA's Food Guide Pyramid. You can download the accompanying 17 page pamphlet containing more details from the web (http:\\www.usda.gov:80/fcs/cnpp/using4.htm). The Food Guide Pyramid lists the food groups and the amount to consume from each group. Note that for children, teenagers, and adults under age 25, 3 servings should be chosen from the milk, yogurt, and cheese group. Once you have estimated your energy needs, recommended servings from the other groups with wider ranges are as follows:*

Energy intake	*1600 kcal*	*2200 kcal*	*2800 kcal*
Grain group	*6*	*9*	*11*
Vegetable group	*3*	*4*	*5*
Fruit group	*2*	*3*	*4*
Meat group (ounces)	*5*	*6*	*7*
Total fat (grams)	*53*	*73*	*93*
Total added sugars (teaspoons)	*6*	*12*	*18*

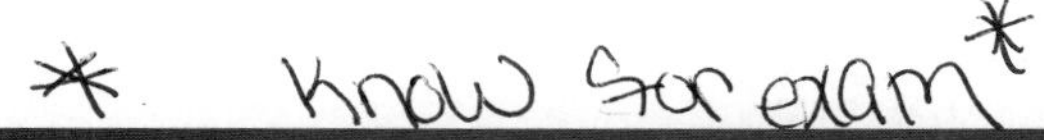

TABLE 2-5

The Food Guide Pyramid—A Summary

Food category	Major contributions	Foods and individual serving sizes*
Milk, yogurt, and cheese	Calcium Phosphorus Carbohydrate Protein Riboflavin Vitamin D Magnesium Zinc	1 cup milk 1½ oz natural cheese 2 oz processed cheese 1 cup yogurt 2 cups cottage cheese
Meat, poultry, fish, dry beans, eggs, and nuts	Protein Thiamin Riboflavin Niacin Vitamin B-6 Folate† Vitamin B-12‡ Phosphorus Magnesium§ Iron Zinc	2–3 oz cooked meat, poultry, or fish 1–1½ cups cooked dry beans 4 tbsp peanut butter 2 eggs ⅔ –1 cup nuts
Fruits	Carbohydrate Vitamin A (few varieties) Vitamin C Folate Magnesium Potassium Dietary fiber	¼ cup dried fruit ½ cup cooked or canned fruit ¾ cup juice 1 whole piece of fruit 1 melon wedge (about ¼) ½ cup berries
Vegetables	Carbohydrate Vitamin A Vitamin C Folate Magnesium Potassium Dietary fiber	½ cup raw or cooked vegetables 1 cup raw leafy vegetables ¾ cup vegetable juice
Bread, cereal, rice, and pasta	Carbohydrate Thiamin Riboflavin§ Niacin Folate‖ Magnesium‖ Iron§ ‖ Zinc‖ Dietary fiber ‖	1 slice of bread 1 oz (about ¾ cup) ready-to-eat cereal ½ cup cooked cereal, rice, or pasta ½ hamburger roll, bagel, or English muffin 3–4 plain crackers 1 small roll, biscuit, or muffin 1 6″ tortilla
Fats, oils, and sweets	Food groups from this category should not replace any from the other groups. Amounts consumed should be determined by individual energy needs.	

*May be reduced for child servings.
†Primarily in plant protein sources.
‡Only in animal foods.
§If enriched.
‖Whole grains and/or enriched products.

To quickly estimate serving size, use the following equivalents:

A thumb = 1 oz. of cheese
4 stacked dice = 1 oz. of cheese
A thumb tip = 1 tsp.
Matchbox = 1 oz. meat
Bar of soap or a pack of cards = 3 oz. meat
Medium Fruit serving = tennis ball
Computer mouse = medium potato
Ping pong ball = 2 tablespoons peanut butter
Yo-Yo = 1 bagel serving
1 ice cream scoop = ½ cup
A fist = 1 cup
A handful = 1 or 2 oz of a snack food

Now test your skills using "Wheel of Portion" (http://www.phys.com)

TABLE 2-6

Putting the Food Guide Pyramid into Practice

Meal	Servings/food group*
BREAKFAST	
1 peeled orange	1 fruit
1½ cups Cheerios	2 bread
with ½ cup low-fat milk	½ milk
1 slice raisin toast	1 bread
with 1 tsp margarine	1 fat/sweet
Optional: coffee or tea	
LUNCH	
Ham sandwich	
2 slices dark rye bread	2 bread
2 oz ham	1 meat
2 tsp mustard	
1 apple	1 fruit
2 oatmeal-raisin cookies (small)	2 fat/sweet
Optional: diet soda or unsweetened iced tea	
3 PM STUDY BREAK	
1 honey whole-wheat bagel	2 bread
1 tbsp peanut butter	¼ meat
½ cup low-fat milk	½ milk
DINNER	
Lettuce salad	
1 cup romaine lettuce	1 vegetable
½ cup sliced tomatoes	1 vegetable
1 tsp regular or reduced fat Thousand Island dressing	1 fat/sweet
½ grated carrot	½ vegetable
3 oz broiled salmon	1 meat
½ cup rice	1 bread
½ cup green beans	1 vegetable
with 1 tsp margarine	1 fat/sweet
Optional: coffee or hot tea	
LATE-NIGHT SNACK	
1 cup low-fat fruit yogurt	1 milk

NUTRIENT BREAKDOWN

1800 kcal	
Carbohydrate	55% of kcal
Protein	20% of kcal
Fat	25% of kcal

Meets estimated nutrient needs for all vitamins and minerals for an average adult. For adolescents, teenagers, and adults under age 25, add 1 additional serving from the milk, yogurt, and cheese group.
*Names of food groups abbreviated as follows: milk = milk, yogurt, and cheese group; meat = meat, poultry, fish, dry beans, eggs, and nuts group; bread = bread, cereal, rice, and pasta group; fat/sweet = fats, oils, and sweets category.

Further fine-tuning then is also recommended to ensure consuming enough vitamin E, vitamin B-6, magnesium, and zinc—nutrients sometimes low in diets based on this plan:

1. Choose primarily low-fat and nonfat items from the milk, yogurt, and cheese group and the meat, poultry, fish, dry beans, eggs, and nuts group. By reducing energy intake in this way, you can select more items from other food groups.

2. Include plant foods that are good sources of proteins, such as beans, at least several times a week because these are rich in minerals, and the dietary fiber present promotes intestinal health.
3. For vegetables and fruits, try to include a dark green vegetable for vitamin A, and a vitamin C–rich fruit, such as an orange, every day. Surveys show that only 25% of adults eat a green vegetable on any given day. Increased consumption of these foods is important because they contribute vitamins, minerals, dietary fiber, and phytochemicals previously mentioned in this chapter.
4. Choose whole-grain varieties of breads, cereals, rice, and pasta often, because they contribute dietary fiber. A daily serving of a whole-grain breakfast cereal with 3 or more grams of fiber per serving is an excellent choice because the vitamins and minerals typically added to it, along with dietary fiber naturally present, help fill in common nutrient gaps.
5. Limit sweets to occasional use in a day. This helps control energy intake.

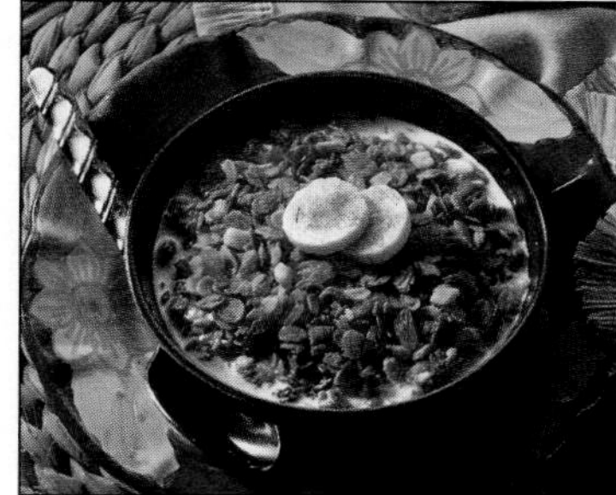

Choosing whole-grain cereals is an excellent way to increase the nutrient value of a diet.

A plate with about two-thirds covered by grains, fruits, and vegetables and one-third or less covered by protein-rich foods promotes this overall fine-tuning. Still, it is also important to observe the serving size for foods when planning and following the Food Guide Pyramid. One can even overconsume nutrient-rich foods when attempting to follow a healthful diet plan.

If 1600 to 1800 kcal represents too much food energy for you, you should first consider becoming more physically active rather than eating less. Obtaining enough nutrients from a diet that supplies fewer than 1600 kcal per day is very difficult. If you can't increase your energy output, you should make a special attempt to choose regularly some nutrient-fortified foods (e.g., breakfast cereals) or take a balanced nutrient supplement (see Chapter 7). In addition, for those whose diets do not include meat or other animal products, the Nutrition Issue on vegetarianism in Chapter 6 provides advice on adapting the Food Guide Pyramid to that dietary practice.

Evaluating the Current American Diet Using the Food Guide Pyramid

The average American diet, based on recent surveys, failed to meet the serving recommendations in the Food Guide Pyramid for many food groups. Fruits and milk products were the most underrepresented groups. Vegetable intake was barely adequate, but half of that came from potatoes, typically french fries. In contrast, the fats, oils, and sweets were well represented.

How Does Your Current Diet Rate?

Regularly comparing your daily food intake with the Food Guide Pyramid recommendations is a relatively simple way to evaluate your overall diet. Strive to meet the recommendations. If that is not possible, identify the nutrients that are low in your diet based on the nutrients found in each food group (see Table 2-5). For example, if you do not consume enough from the milk, yogurt, and cheese group, your calcium intake is most likely too low. After completing the Rate Your Plate activity at the end of this chapter, you will be able to determine more accurately which nutrients are too low in your current diet and by how much. Armed with this knowledge, find foods that you enjoy that supply those nutrients, such as calcium-fortified orange juice. Customizing the Food Guide Pyramid to accommodate your own food preferences may seem a daunting task now, but it is not difficult once you gain some additional nutrition knowledge. To learn more, see the web page sponsored by USDA (http://www.usda.gov/fcs/cnpp.htm).

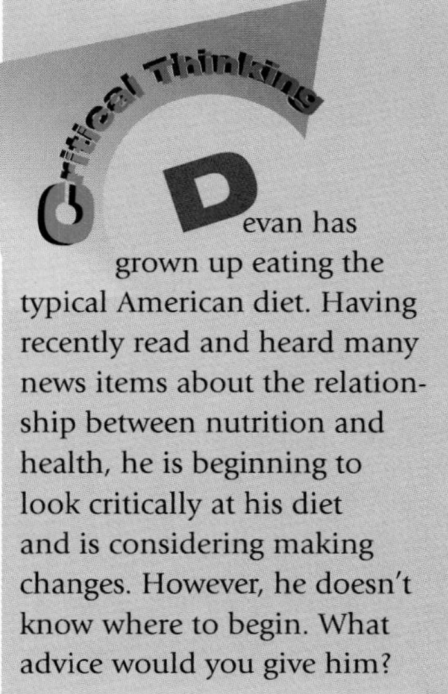

Devan has grown up eating the typical American diet. Having recently read and heard many news items about the relationship between nutrition and health, he is beginning to look critically at his diet and is considering making changes. However, he doesn't know where to begin. What advice would you give him?

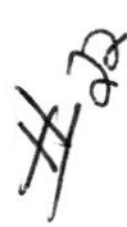

Dietary Guidelines—Another Tool for Menu Planning

The Food Guide Pyramid was designed to mainly help meet nutritional needs for carbohydrate, protein, vitamins, and minerals. However, most of the major chronic "killer" diseases in America, such as heart disease, cancer, and alcoholism, are not primarily associated with deficiencies of these nutrients. For many Americans, the primary dietary culprit is an overconsumption of one or more of the following: energy, saturated and total fat, cholesterol, alcohol, and sodium (salt). Underconsumption of calcium, iron, vitamin A, folate and other B vitamins, vitamin C, zinc, or dietary fiber is also a problem for some people, but easy to fix as the major dietary problems are addressed.

Dietary Guidelines *General goals for nutrient intakes and diet composition set by the USDA and the Department of Health and Human Services (DHHS).*

In response to concerns regarding "killer" disease patterns in the United States, the USDA and Department of Health and Human Services (DHHS) regularly publish **Dietary Guidelines** to aid diet planning. These Dietary Guidelines refer to a total intake over a day or week, not to a single meal or certain food. New guidelines are set to be released in early 2000. The latest version of the guidelines is:

Eat a Variety of Foods. Choose a variety of foods within each group of the Food Guide Pyramid. Many women and adolescent girls need to eat more calcium-rich and iron-rich foods. Supplements do not substitute for proper food choices. Vegetarian diets are consistent with the Dietary Guidelines but must be planned with care (see Chapter 6).

Balance the Food You Eat with Physical Activity—Maintain or Improve Your Weight. Try to do 30 minutes or more of moderate physical activity daily. Devote less time to sedentary activities, such as sitting; spend more time in activities such as walking and climbing stairs. High-fat foods contain more energy per serving than other foods and may increase the likelihood of weight gain. Unless nutritious snacks are part of the daily meal plan, snacking may also lead to weight gain. Most adults should not gain weight. Generally, a gain of more than 10 to 16 pounds after age 21 is not recommended. Excess fat in the abdominal (stomach) area poses a greater health risk than excess fat in the hips and thighs. Slow weight loss is recommended, when needed.

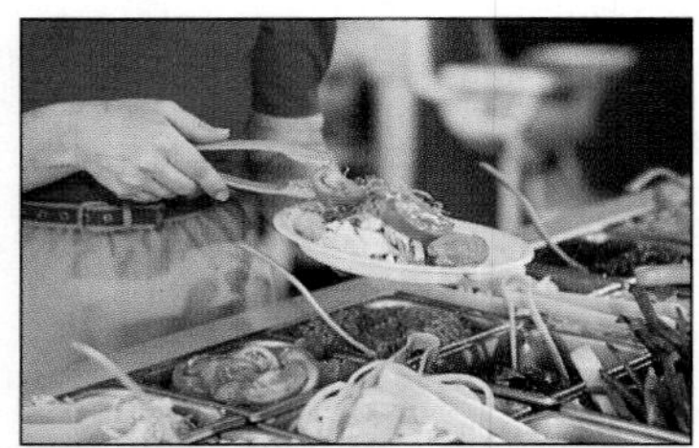

Choose a diet rich in vegetables.

Choose a Diet with Plenty of Grain Products, Vegetables, and Fruits. Most fruits and vegetables are naturally low in fat and provide many essential nutrients. Eat more of these, along with more grain products (breads, cereals, pasta, and rice).

Choose a Diet Low in Fat, Saturated Fat, and Cholesterol. Fats and oils and some types of desserts and snack foods that contain fat provide a great deal of energy but few nutrients. It is often important to choose lower-fat options among these foods to leave room for the recommended servings from the five groups in the Food Guide Pyramid. The fats from meat, milk, and milk products are the main sources of saturated fats in most diets, which is the primary fat that can promote heart disease. Dietary cholesterol comes from animal sources; many cholesterol-rich foods are also high in saturated fat.

Choose a Diet Moderate in Sugars. Because maintaining a nutritious diet and a healthy weight is crucial, sugars should be used in moderation by most healthy people and sparingly by people with low energy needs. Both sugars and starches can also promote tooth decay (see Chapter 4).

Choose a Diet Moderate in Salt and Sodium. Salt and other sodium-containing ingredients are often used in food processing. Most Americans consume more sodium than they need. Many dietary and lifestyle choices influence blood pressure. There is no way at present to tell who might develop high blood pressure from eating too much sodium. However, consuming less salt or sodium is not harmful and is recommended for the healthy normal adult.

If You Drink Alcoholic Beverages, Do So in Moderation. Alcoholic beverages supply energy but few or no nutrients. Although moderate drinking is associated with a reduced risk of certain forms of heart disease and stroke, high amounts of alcohol raise the risk for high blood pressure, heart failure, certain cancers, liver and pancreas disease, accidents, violence, suicides, birth defects, and death by other causes. Those who should not drink are children and adolescents, pregnant women, people who plan to take part in activities that require attention or skill (e.g., driving), and people taking certain medications. A moderate alcohol intake consists of two or fewer servings of 12 ounces of beer, 5 ounces of wine, or 1½ ounces of distilled spirits (80 proof) per day. Women should generally limit alcohol to one serving per day, as they are more vulnerable than men to alcohol-related diseases. People over age 65 should also adhere to the same limit. Any use of alcohol should be with meals.

Practical Use of the Dietary Guidelines

The Dietary Guidelines are designed to promote adequate carbohydrate, protein, vitamin, and mineral intake with the first guideline: Eat a variety of foods. Then the Guidelines emphasize changes that will reduce the risk of obesity, high blood pressure, heart disease, the major type of diabetes, and alcoholism.

The Dietary Guidelines are not difficult to implement (Table 2–7). In addition, this overall diet approach is not especially expensive, as some people suspect. Fruits, vegetables, and low-fat and nonfat milk are no more costly than the chips, cookies, and soft drinks they should in part replace. Note also that the diet recommendations for adults issued by other scientific groups (American Heart Association, U.S. Surgeon General, National Academy of Sciences, American Cancer Society, Canadian Ministries of Health [see Appendix B and the web site http://www.hc-sc.gc.ca/hppb/nutrition] and World Health Organization) are consistent with the spirit of the Dietary Guidelines.

Advice from the American Dietetic Association suggests five basic principles with regard to diet and health. Be realistic, making small changes over time. Be adventurous, trying new foods regularly. Be flexible, balancing some sweet and fatty foods with physical activity. Be sensible, including favorite foods in smaller portions. Finally, be active, including physical activity in daily life.

TABLE 2-7

Advice for Applying the Dietary Guidelines to Practical Situations

You usually eat this	Reconsider and eat this
White bread	Whole-wheat bread (less nutrients lost in refinement processing)
Sugared breakfast cereal	Low-sugar cereal (use the calories you save for a side dish of fruit)
Cheeseburger and french fries	Hamburger (hold the mayonnaise) and baked beans (for less fat and cholesterol, and the benefits of plant proteins)
Potato salad at the salad bar	Three-bean salad
Doughnut, chips, salty snack foods	Bran muffin or bagel (little or no cream cheese)
Soft drinks	Diet soft drinks (save the calories for more nutritious foods)
Boiled vegetables	Steamed vegetables (for more nutrient retention)
Canned vegetables	Frozen vegetables (less nutrients lost in processing)
Fried meats	Broiled meats (watch the fat drain away)
Fatty meats, like ribs	Lean meats, like ground round (also, eat chicken and fish often)
Whole milk and ice cream	1% or nonfat milk and sherbet or frozen yogurt (to reduce saturated fat intake)
Mayonnaise or sour cream salad dressing	Oil and vinegar dressings or diet varieties (to save calories)
Cookies for a snack	Popcorn (air popped with minimal margarine), fruit, raw vegetables (less calories)
Heavily salted foods	Foods flavored primarily with herbs, spices, and lemon juice (lower sodium)
Sour cream dip	Salsa or lite sour cream (less fat)
Sweet and sour pork	Beef with snow peas (less fat)
Cream cheese	Lite cream cheese (less fat)

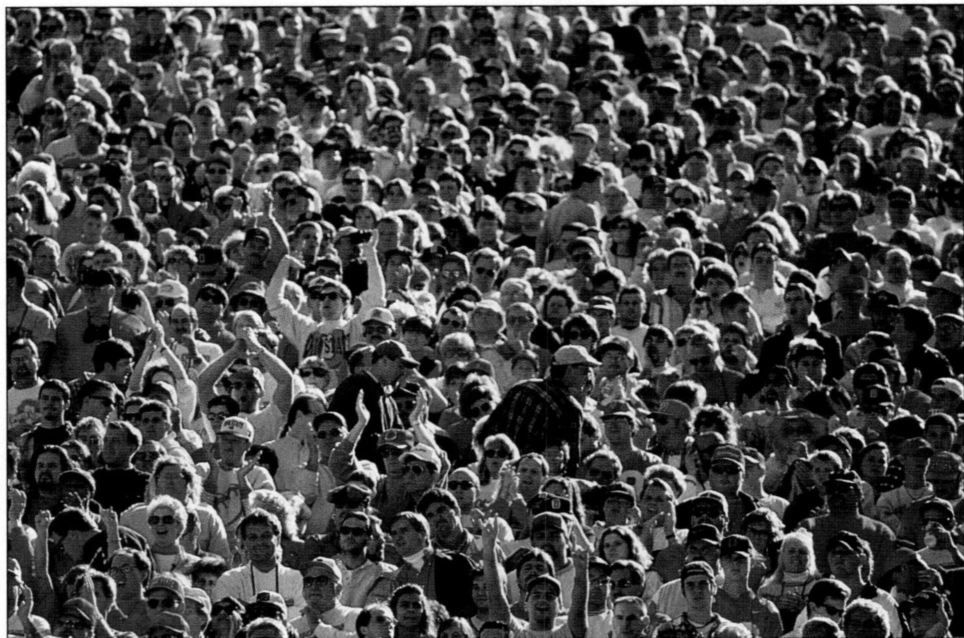

Nutrition recommendations are often made on a population-wide basis. However, in many cases it would be more appropriate if we were evaluated on an individual basis.

The Dietary Guidelines and You

When using the Dietary Guidelines, you should consider your own state of health. Make specific changes and see whether they are effective. Note that results are sometimes disappointing, even when you are following a diet change very closely. Some people can eat a lot of saturated fat and still blood cholesterol remains under control. Other people, unfortunately, have high blood cholesterol even if they eat a diet low in saturated fat. Differences in genetic background can be a key cause in the development of nutrition-related disease. In later chapters, you will see how to tailor diet planning for individuals with various specific needs and characteristics. There is no "optimal" diet. Instead, there are numerous healthful diets. The web page http://www.ificinfo.health.org is a great source to head you in that direction, as is the Nutrition Issue in this chapter.

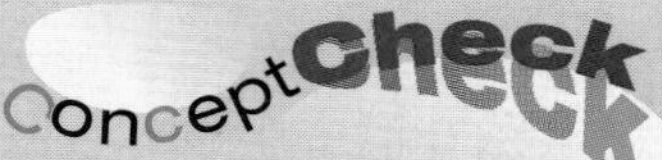

The Food Guide Pyramid is a convenient and valuable tool for planning daily menus that translates general needs for carbohydrate, protein, fat, vitamins, and minerals into the recommended number of daily servings from each of the five major food groups. An added bonus of this diet plan—rich in fruits, vegetables, and whole grains—is an ample intake of phytochemicals and dietary fiber. Dietary Guidelines have been set to fine-tune Food Guide Pyramid choices in order to reduce the risk of developing obesity, high blood pressure, the major type of diabetes, heart disease, and alcoholism. To do so, the Guidelines first recommend eating a variety of foods. They also recommend performing regular physical activity, limiting energy intake to match energy output, and moderating total fat, saturated fat, salt, sugar, and alcohol intake, while focusing more on fruits, vegetables, and grain products—especially whole-grain varieties—in daily menu planning.

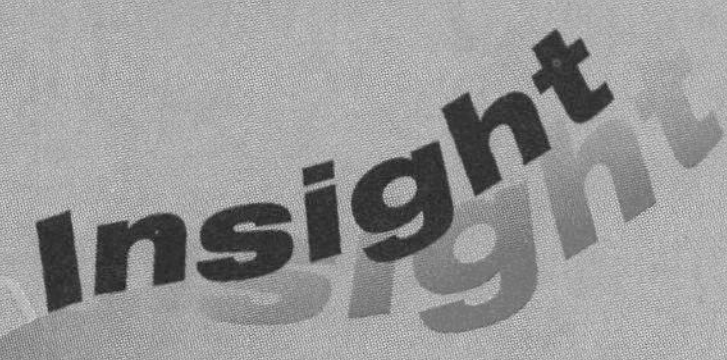

The Alphabet Soup of Specific Nutrient Needs

Before designing a diet plan, such as the Food Guide Pyramid, we must determine what amount of each essential nutrient is needed to maintain health. The standards that have been developed for such nutrient needs, such as DRI, RDA, ESADDI, AI, and UL can often seem like an alphabet soup of abbreviations. However, you can more easily sift through these nutrient standards if you have a base of knowledge concerning their development and use. (Table 2–8).

DRIs: RDAs and Related Standards

Most of the terms that describe nutrient standards, including RDA and AI, fall under one umbrella term—**Dietary Reference Intakes (DRI).** Soon all of the terms mentioned above will fall (or be renamed) under the DRI umbrella as part of ongoing revisions of the DRIs.

You are probably most familiar with the nutrient standard **Recommended Dietary Allowance (RDA).** An RDA represents the nutrient intake that is sufficient to meet the needs of nearly all healthy people (about 97%) in an age and gender group (for specific numbers, see the inside cover of this book). The RDAs are set at about 20% over what is needed by an average person to balance intake with losses; this 20% increase is done in order to accommodate people who may have slightly higher nutrient needs than the average person. A person can compare his or her individual intake of specific nutrients to the RDA and evaluate whether one's diet is inadequate or ample in that nutrient. An intake slightly above or below the RDA is not of great concern since your needs do not likely fall directly on the RDA number. However, a significant deviation below (about ½) or above (about 2 times for some nutrients) the RDA for a considerable length of time can eventually result in a deficiency or toxicity of nutrients.

TABLE 2-8

Putting the Alphabet Soup of Specific Nutrient Needs to Use

Recommended Dietary Allowance (RDA)—use this to evaluate your current intake for a specific nutrient. The further you stray above or below this value, the greater the chance of developing nutritional problems.

Adequate Intake (AI)—use this to evaluate your current intake of nutrients, but realize that an AI designation means that much more research is needed before scientists can establish a more definitive number.

Estimated Safe and Adequate Dietary Intake (ESADDI)—use this the same as you would an AI.

Minimum Requirement for Health—use this as a guide for the lowest intake of sodium, chloride, and potassium that allows for health. Note that our typical intakes greatly exceed the minimum requirements for sodium and chloride.

Upper Limit (UL)—use this as a maximum daily intake of a nutrient. An intake below this is unlikely to cause adverse health effects in almost all people (97% to 98%) in a population. This number applies to chronic daily use and is set to protect even very susceptible people in the healthy general population.

Daily Value (DV)—use this as a rough guide for comparing the nutrient content of a food to approximate human needs. Typically the Daily Value used on food labels refers to ages 4 years old through adulthood. It is based on a 2000 kcal diet; Daily Values for fat, saturated fat, protein, carbohydrate, and fiber increase slightly with higher energy intakes (see Figure 2–2).

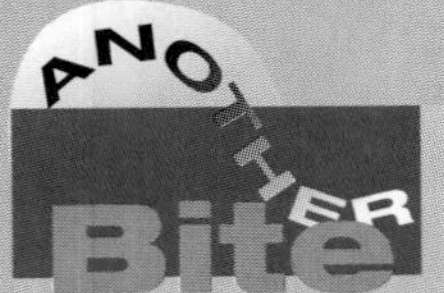

The RDAs for energy are set at the average needs for various age groups (see the inside cover). These are not increased by 20% to reflect the higher needs of some people—as is done for most vitamins and minerals—because excess energy consumed is not excreted. Thus, to promote weight maintenance, a more conservative standard is used for energy needs compared to that used for nutrient needs. The energy RDA should be viewed as only a rough estimate, because energy needs depend on energy use. For most adults, the ability to obtain and maintain a healthy weight is the best yardstick for assessing one's current energy intake.

An RDA for a nutrient can be set only if there is much information on the human needs for that particular nutrient. Today there is not enough information on nutrients such as calcium, vitamin D, copper, and biotin to set such a precise standard as an RDA. For these and other nutrients, the DRIs include a category called **Adequate Intake (AI).** The AIs are similar in context to the older term **Estimated Safe and Adequate Daily Dietary Intake (ESADDI).** These standards (AI and ESADDI) are based on observing dietary intakes of people that appear to be maintaining nutritional health. That amount of intake is assumed to be adequate, as no evidence of a nutritional deficiency is apparent. Both of the AI and ESADDI terms are now being used, but the ESADDI term is being phased out as the DRIs are being revised. Finally, minimum requirements to maintain health are set for sodium, chloride, and potassium, and **Tolerable Upper Intake Levels (UL)** have been set for some vitamins and minerals (see Chapters 7 and 8).

How Should These Nutrient Standards Be Used?

RDAs and related standards are intended mainly for diet planning. Specifically, a diet plan should aim to meet the RDA, AI (or ESADDI), and minimum requirements, as appropriate, and not exceed the UL if one has been set. However, the AI or ESADDI should not be used alone, as the RDA can be, to evaluate individual nutrient intake and needs. For these standards, individual characteristics from person to person should be more carefully considered. For example, it is recommended that the AI and ESADDI estimates be used in combination with the clinical, biochemical, and anthropometric measures of one's nutritional state, discussed earlier in this chapter. To learn more about these nutrient standards use the web page http://www.nas.edu.

Daily Values: The Standards Used for Food Labeling

Though it is worthwhile to understand the intent behind the terms discussed in this Nutrition Insight, a nutrition standard more relevant to everyday life is **Daily Values.** These are generic standards used on food labels. The actual version used on foods labels is applicable to ages 4 years old through adulthood. No gender categories are used with the Daily Values, and age categories are wide, as just noted. This condensed system is essential for food labeling, since the RDAs and other nutrient standards are highly age and gender specific; there are too many categories for each nutrient for RDA and related standards to be used on food labels.

Daily Values exist for vitamins, minerals, and protein. These are mostly set at or close to the highest RDA value or related nutrient standard seen in the various age and gender categories for a specific nutrient (Table 2–9). Daily Values are also set for dietary components that are not part of the DRIs, such as cholesterol, carbohydrate, fiber, and others. The values are based on current dietary advice from federal agencies.

Overall, Daily Values are designed to allow consumers to compare their intake to desirable (or maximum) intakes. It is nevertheless important to understand that the nutrient standards expressed on food labels are not the same as the RDAs. Food labels will be discussed further in the following section.

TABLE 2-9

Comparison of Daily Values with the Latest RDAs and Other Nutrient Standards*

Dietary constituent	Unit of measure	Current daily values for people over 4 years of age	RDA or other current dietary standard: Males 19 years old	RDA or other current dietary standard: Females 19 years old
Fat‡	g	<65	—	—
Saturated fatty acids‡	"	<20	—	—
Protein‡	"	50	58	46
Cholesterol§	mg	<300	—	—
Carbohydrate‡	g	300	—	—
Fiber	"	25	—	—
Vitamin A	Retinol Equivalents	1000	1000	800
Vitamin D	International Units	400	200	200
Vitamin E	"	30	10	8
Vitamin K	μg	80	70	60
Vitamin C	mg	60	60	60
Folate	μg	400	400	400
Thiamin	mg	1.5	1.2	1.1
Riboflavin	"	1.7	1.3	1.1
Niacin	"	20	16	14
Vitamin B-6	"	2	1.3	1.3
Vitamin B-12	μg	6	2.4	2.4
Biotin	mg	0.3	0.03	0.03
Pantothenic acid	"	10	5	5
Calcium	g	1	1	1
Phosphorus	"	1	0.7	0.7
Iodide	μg	150	150	150
Iron	mg	18	10	15
Magnesium	"	400	400	310
Copper	"	2	1.5–3.0	1.5–3.0
Zinc	"	15	15	12
Sodium†	"	<2400	500	500
Potassium†	"	3500	2000	2000
Chloride†	"	3400	750	750
Manganese	"	2	2–5	2–5
Selenium	μg	70	70	55
Chromium	"	120	50–200	50–200
Molybdenum	"	75	75–250	75–250

Abbreviations: g = gram, mg = milligram, μg = microgram.

*Daily Values are generally set at the highest RDA in a specific age and gender category. Many Daily Values exceed current nutrient standards. This is in part because aspects of the Daily Values were originally developed in the early 1970s using estimates of nutrient needs published in 1968. The Daily Values have yet to be updated to reflect our current state of knowledge.

†Sodium, potassium, and chloride values are based on the minimum requirement for health. The considerably higher Daily Values you see for sodium and chloride are there to allow for more diet flexibility, but the extra amounts are not needed to maintain health.

‡No RDA has been set for these nutrients. These values are based on a 2000 kcal diet, with a caloric distribution of 30% from fat (and ⅓ of this total from saturated fat), 60% from carbohydrate, and 10% from protein.

§Based on recommendations of federal agencies.

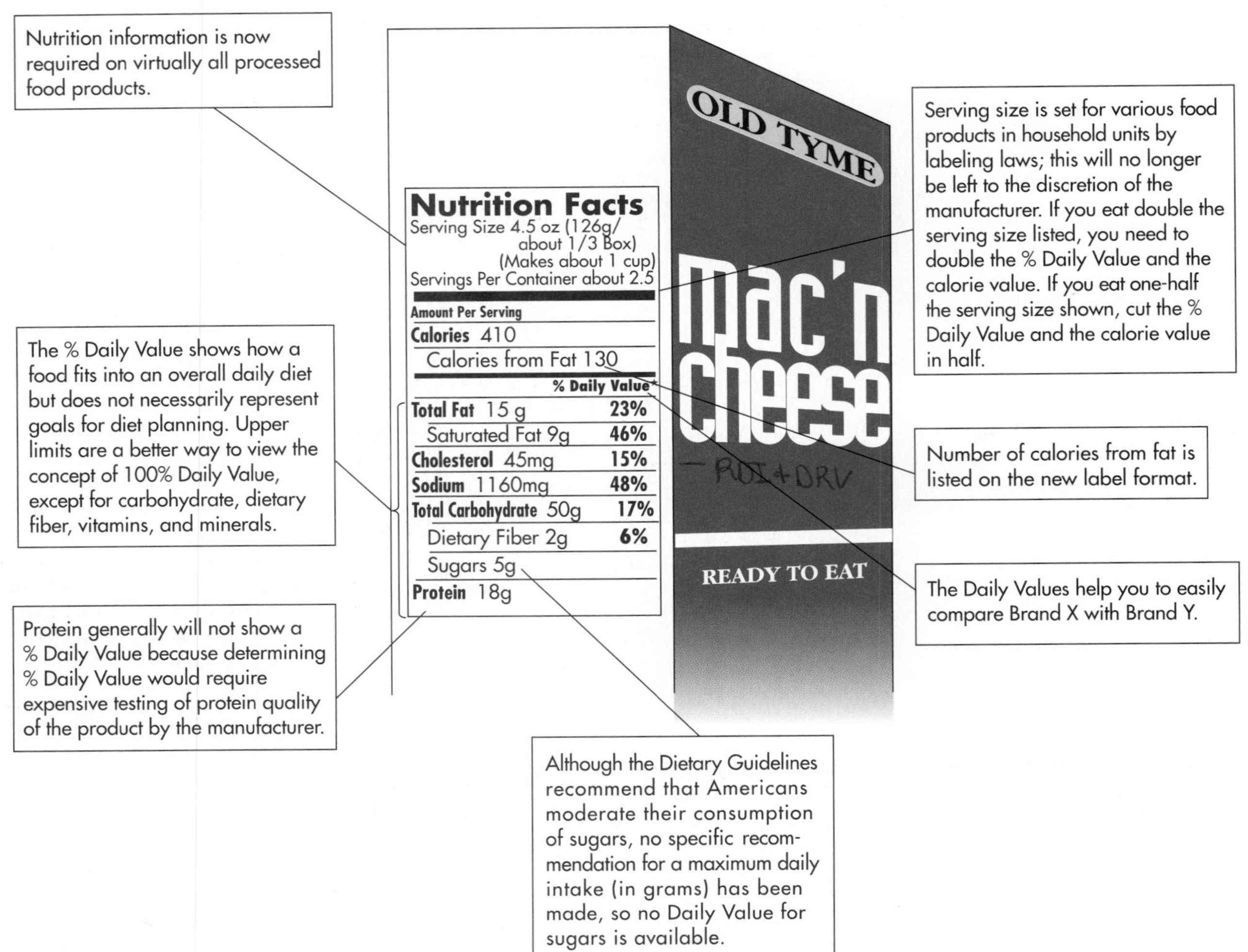

Figure 2-2 *The Nutrition Facts panel on a current food label. The box is broken into two parts: A is the top, and B is the bottom. The % Daily Value listed on the label is the percentage of the generally accepted amount of a nutrient needed daily that is present in 1 serving of the product. You can use the % Daily Values to compare your diet with current nutrition recommendations for certain diet components. Let's consider dietary fiber. Assume that you consume 2000 kcal per day, which is the energy intake corresponding to the % Daily Values listed on labels. If the total % Daily Value for dietary fiber in all the foods you eat in one day adds up to 100%, your diet meets the recommendations for dietary fiber.*

What Does the Food Label Have to Offer as a Tool in Diet Planning?

As mentioned in Chapter 1, health is becoming a driving force in the food purchasing practices of Americans. For this reason, food manufacturers have jumped on the "healthy foods" bandwagon, and government agencies in response have raised the bar on related labeling standards.

Today nearly all foods sold in the grocery store must be labeled with the product name, name and address of the manufacturer, amount of product in the package, and ingredients listed in descending order by weight. This was not the case just 10 years ago. This food and beverage labeling is monitored by government agencies such as the Food and Drug Administration (FDA).

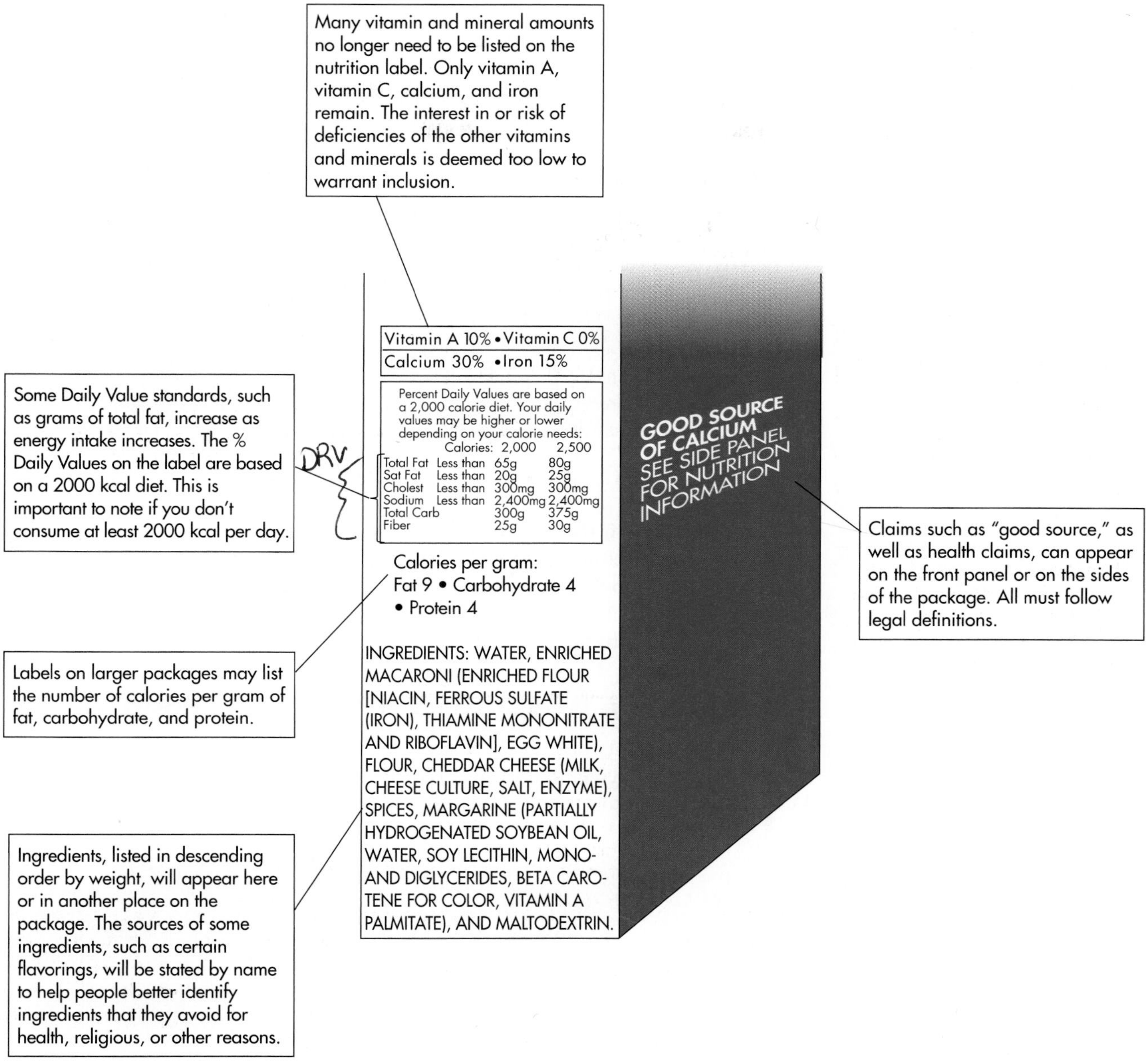

Many vitamin and mineral amounts no longer need to be listed on the nutrition label. Only vitamin A, vitamin C, calcium, and iron remain. The interest in or risk of deficiencies of the other vitamins and minerals is deemed too low to warrant inclusion.

Some Daily Value standards, such as grams of total fat, increase as energy intake increases. The % Daily Values on the label are based on a 2000 kcal diet. This is important to note if you don't consume at least 2000 kcal per day.

Labels on larger packages may list the number of calories per gram of fat, carbohydrate, and protein.

Ingredients, listed in descending order by weight, will appear here or in another place on the package. The sources of some ingredients, such as certain flavorings, will be stated by name to help people better identify ingredients that they avoid for health, religious, or other reasons.

Claims such as "good source," as well as health claims, can appear on the front panel or on the sides of the package. All must follow legal definitions.

Vitamin A 10% • Vitamin C 0%
Calcium 30% • Iron 15%

Percent Daily Values are based on a 2,000 calorie diet. Your daily values may be higher or lower depending on your calorie needs:

		Calories: 2,000	2,500
Total Fat	Less than	65g	80g
Sat Fat	Less than	20g	25g
Cholest	Less than	300mg	300mg
Sodium	Less than	2,400mg	2,400mg
Total Carb		300g	375g
Fiber		25g	30g

Calories per gram:
Fat 9 • Carbohydrate 4 • Protein 4

INGREDIENTS: WATER, ENRICHED MACARONI (ENRICHED FLOUR [NIACIN, FERROUS SULFATE (IRON), THIAMINE MONONITRATE AND RIBOFLAVIN], EGG WHITE), FLOUR, CHEDDAR CHEESE (MILK, CHEESE CULTURE, SALT, ENZYME), SPICES, MARGARINE (PARTIALLY HYDROGENATED SOYBEAN OIL, WATER, SOY LECITHIN, MONO- AND DIGLYCERIDES, BETA CAROTENE FOR COLOR, VITAMIN A PALMITATE), AND MALTODEXTRIN.

GOOD SOURCE OF CALCIUM
SEE SIDE PANEL FOR NUTRITION INFORMATION

Figure 2–2 *For legend see opposite page.*

The listing of certain food constituents also is required on the Nutrition Facts panel (Figure 2–2). The following components must be listed: total kcal, kcal from fat, total fat, saturated fat, cholesterol, sodium, total carbohydrate, dietary fiber, sugars, protein, vitamin A, vitamin C, calcium, and iron. In addition to these required components, manufacturers can choose to list polyunsaturated and monounsaturated fat, potassium, dietary fiber, and others. Listing these components is *required* however, if a claim is made about the health benefits of the specific nutrient (see the second Nutrition Insight in this chapter), or if the food is fortified with that nutrient.

The percentage of the Daily Value (% Daily Value) is usually given for each nutrient per serving (recall that Daily Values were discussed in the first Nutrition Insight in this chapter). It is important for the consumer to understand that these percentages are based on a 2000 kcal diet. In other words, they are not as applicable to people who require considerably more or less than 2000 kcal per day with respect to fat and carbohydrate intake.

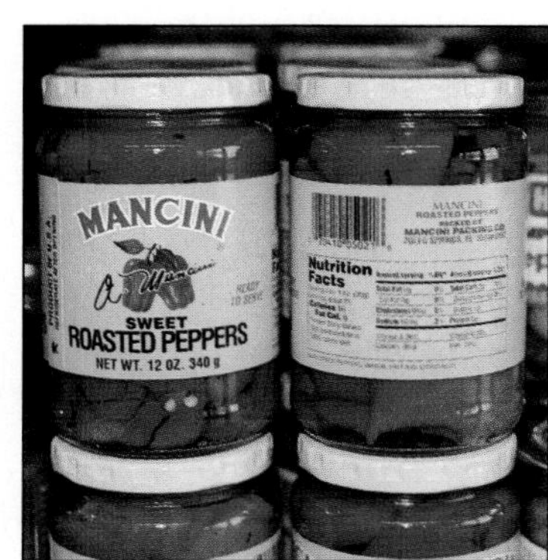

Use the Nutrition Facts label to learn more about the nutrient content of the foods you eat.

Recall from Chapter 1 that the nutrition label uses the term *calorie* for energy values, but *kilocalorie* (kcal) values are actually listed.

Many manufacturers list the actual Daily Values for dietary components such as fat, cholesterol, and carbohydrate on the Nutrition Facts panel. This can be useful as a reference point. They are based on 2000 kcals; if the label is large enough amounts based on 2500 kcal are listed as well.

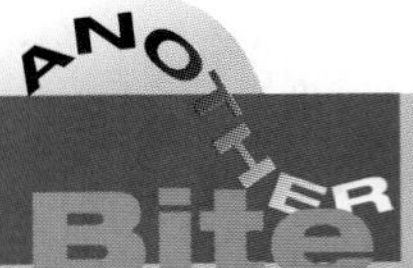

Because protein deficiency is not a public health concern in the United States, declaration of the % Daily Value for protein is not mandatory on foods for people over 4 years of age. If the % Daily Value is given on a label, FDA requires that the product be analyzed for protein quality. Because this procedure is expensive and time consuming, many companies opt not to list a % Daily Value for protein rather than undergo the expense. However, labels on food for infants or children under 4 years of age must include the % Daily Value for protein, as must the labels on any food carrying a claim about protein content (see Chapter 13).

Serving sizes on the Nutrition Facts panel must be consistent between similar foods. This means that all brands of ice cream, for example, must use the same serving size on their labels. In addition, food claims made on packages now follow legal definitions (Table 2–10). For example, if a product claims to be "low sodium," it must have 140 milligrams of sodium or less per serving.

What Are the Benefits of the Current Food Labels?

Though the current food label requirements are meant to make the labels more user-friendly for the general public, consumers must have a basic knowledge of the label components in order to take full advantage of the information provided. With

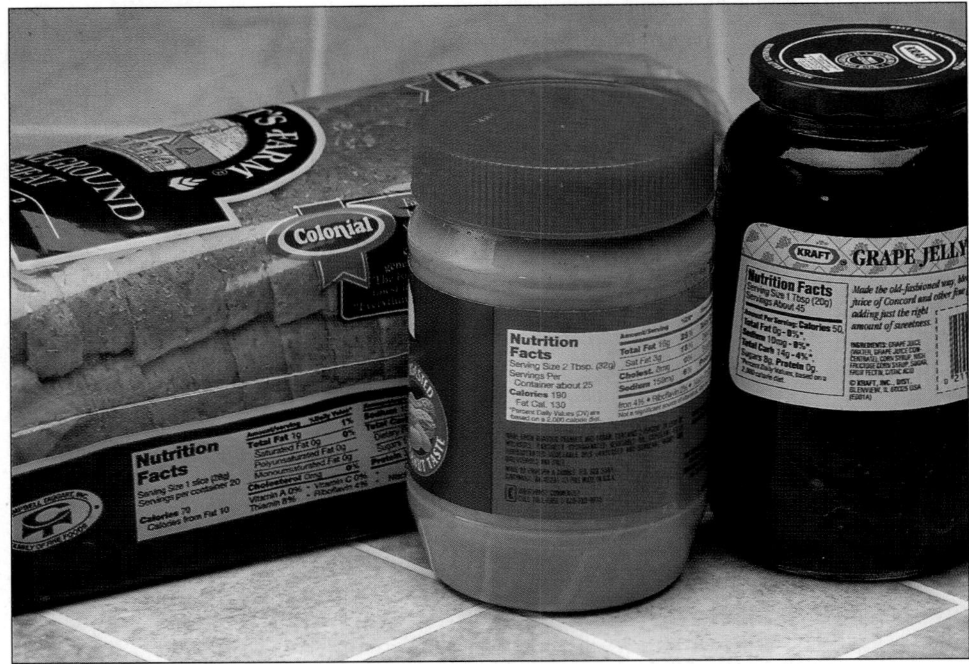

The food labels on these three products can be combined to indicate nutrient intake for a meal—a peanut butter and jelly sandwich.

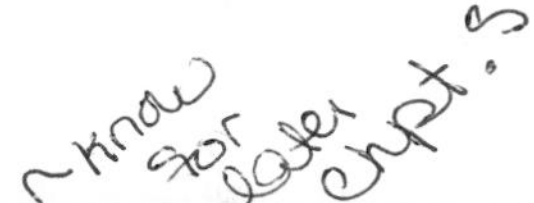

TABLE 2-10

Definitions for Nutrient Claims on Food Labels

SUGAR

- *Sugar free:* less than 0.5 g per serving.
- *No added sugar; Without added sugar; No sugar added:*
  - No sugars added during processing or packing, including ingredients that contain sugars (e.g., fruit juices, applesauce, or jam).
  - Processing does not increase the sugar content above the amount naturally present in the ingredients. (A functionally insignificant increase in sugars is acceptable for processes used for purposes other than increasing sugar content.)
  - The food that it resembles and for which it substitutes normally contains added sugars.
  - If the food doesn't meet the requirements for a low- or reduced-calorie food, the product bears a statement that the food is not low-calorie or calorie-reduced and directs consumers' attention to the nutrition panel for further information on sugars and calorie content.
- *Reduced sugar:* At least 25% less sugar per serving than reference food.

CALORIES

- *Calorie free:* Fewer than 5 kcal per serving.
- *Low calorie:* 40 kcal or less per serving and, if the serving is 30 g or less, or 2 tbsp or less, per 50 g of the food.
- *Reduced or fewer calories:* At least 25% fewer kcal per serving than reference food.

FIBER

- *High fiber:* 5 g or more per serving. (Foods making high-fiber claims must meet the definition for low fat, or the level of total fat must appear next to the high-fiber claim.)
- *Food source of fiber:* 2.5 to 4.9 g per serving.
- *More or added fiber:* At least 2.5 g more per serving than reference food.

FAT

- *Fat free:* Less than 0.5 g of fat per serving.
- *Saturated fat free:* Less than 0.5 g per serving, and the level of trans fatty acids does not exceed 0.5 g per serving.
- *Low fat:* 3 g or less per serving and, if the serving is 30 g or less, or 2 tbsp or less, per 50 g of the food. 2% milk can no longer be labeled low-fat as it exceeds 3 g per serving. Reduced fat will be the term used instead.
- *Low saturated fat:* 1 g or less per serving and not more than 15% of kcal from saturated fatty acids.
- *Reduced or less fat:* At least 25% less per serving than reference food.
- *Reduced or less saturated fat:* At least 25% less per serving than reference food.

CHOLESTEROL

- *Cholesterol free:* Less than 2 mg of cholesterol and 2 g or less of saturated fat per serving.
- *Low cholesterol:* 20 mg or less cholesterol and 2 g or less of saturated fat per serving, and if the serving is 30 g or less, or 2 tbsp or less, per 50 g of the food.
- *Reduced or less cholesterol:* At least 25% less cholesterol and 2 g or less of saturated fat per serving than reference food.

SODIUM

- *Sodium free:* Less than 5 mg per serving.
- *Very low sodium:* 35 mg or less per serving and, if the serving is 30 g or less, or 2 tbsp or less, per 50 g of the food.
- *Low sodium:* 140 mg or less per serving and, if the serving is 30 g or less, or 2 tbsp or less, per 50 g of the food.
- *Light in sodium:* At least 50% less per serving than reference food.
- *Reduced or less sodium:* At least 25% less per serving than reference food.

OTHER TERMS

- *Fortified/Enriched:* Vitamins and/or minerals have been added to the product in amounts in excess of at least 10% of that normally present in the usual product.
- *Healthy:* An individual food that is low fat and low saturated fat and has no more than 360 to 480 mg of sodium or 60 mg of cholesterol per serving can be labeled "healthy" if it provides at least 10% of vitamin A, vitamin C, protein, calcium, iron, or dietary fiber. Fruits and vegetables have recently been granted exceptions to this rule. All can be labeled healthy.
- *Light or lite:* The description "light" or "lite" can mean two things; first, that a nutritionally altered product contains one-third fewer kilocalories or half the fat of the reference food (if the food derives 50% or more of its calories from fat, the reduction must be 50% of the fat); and second, that the sodium content of a low-calorie low-fat food has been reduced by 50%.

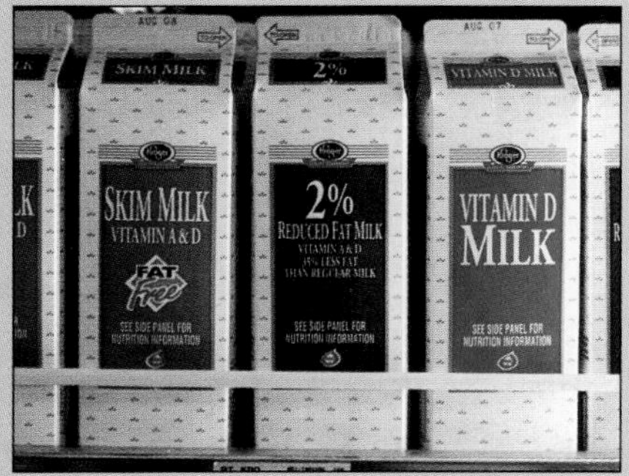

2% milk can no longer be labeled low fat because it has more that 3 grams of fat per serving.

In addition, "light in sodium" may be used for foods in which the sodium content has been reduced by at least 50%. The term "light" may still be used to describe such properties as texture and color, as long as the label explains the intent; for example, "light brown sugar" and "light and fluffy".

- *Diet:* A food may be labeled with terms such as "diet," "dietetic," "artificially sweetened," or "sweetened with nonnutritive sweetener" only if the claim is not false or misleading. The food can also be labeled "low calorie" or "reduced calorie."
- *Good source:* "Good source" means that a food contains 10% to 19% of the Daily Value for a particular nutrient.
- *High:* "High" means that a food contains 20% or more of the Daily Value for a particular nutrient.
- *Organic:* FDA has deferred rulemaking regarding the use of the term "organic" until USDA has adopted appropriate regulations. At that time, FDA will determine whether any regulations governing the term "organic" are necessary.
- *Natural:* The food must be free of food colors, synthetic flavors, or any other synthetic substance.

THE FOLLOWING TERMS APPLY ONLY TO MEAT AND POULTRY PRODUCTS REGULATED BY USDA.

- *Extra lean:* The product has less than 5 g of fat, 2 g of saturated fat, and 95 mg of cholesterol per serving (or 100 g of an individual food).
- *Lean:* The product contains less than 10 g of fat, 4.5 g of saturated fat, and 95 mg of cholesterol per serving (or 100 g of an individual food).

Many definitions are from FDA's *Dictionary of Terms,* as established in conjunction with the 1990 NLEA; g = gram, mg = milligram.

Nutrition Insight

Health Claims on Foods—What Is Currently Allowed and What Isn't

As a marketing tool directed toward the health-conscious consumer, food manufacturers are asserting that their products have all sorts of health benefits. This campaign began in earnest in 1984, when the Kellogg Company, in conjunction with The National Cancer Institute, printed a health claim on its "high-fiber" cereals stating that fiber may help prevent certain forms of cancer. This type of label message was not allowed at the time and caused a heated debate among nutrition scientists.

Currently, FDA limits the use of health messages to specific diseases in which there is significant scientific agreement concerning the relationship between a nutrient, food, or food constituent and the disease. The currently allowed claims may show a link between the following:

- A diet with enough calcium and a reduced risk of osteoporosis
- A diet low in total fat and a reduced risk of some cancers
- A diet low in saturated fat and cholesterol and a reduced risk of heart disease
- A diet rich in dietary fiber–containing grain products, fruits, and vegetables and a reduced risk of some cancers
- A diet low in sodium and a reduced risk of high blood pressure
- A diet rich in fruits and vegetables and a reduced risk of some cancers
- A diet adequate in the vitamin folate and a reduced risk of neural tube defects (a type of birth defect)
- Use of sugarless gum and a reduced risk of tooth decay, especially when compared with foods high in sugars and starches
- A diet rich in fruits, vegetables, and grain products that contain fiber and a reduced risk of heart disease. Oats (oatmeal, oat bran, and oat flour) and psyllium are two fiber-rich ingredients that can be singled out in reducing the risk of heart disease, as long as the statement also says the diet should also be low in saturated fat and cholesterol.

A "may" or "might" qualifier must be used in any statement.

In addition, before a health claim can be made for a food product, it must meet two general requirements. First, the food must be a "good source" (before fortification) of dietary fiber, protein, vitamin A, vitamin C, calcium, or iron. The legal definition of "good source" appears in Table 2–10 (on page 55 in this chapter).

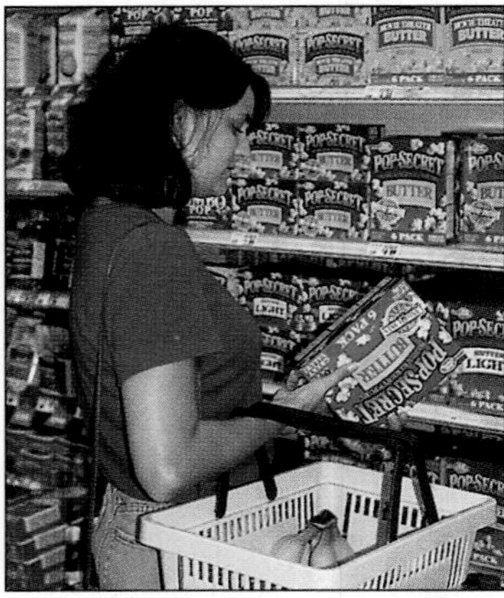

Nutrient content in foods is expressed on the nutrition label in terms of Daily Values.

a little bit of practice, the labels can allow consumers to compare products and choose the one that is more appropriate for one's dietary needs (see the Rate Your Plate section in this chapter). Furthermore, the uniformity of serving sizes is beneficial because these serving sizes are in common household units and are realistic. In addition, product claims are now more credible since the definition of each is regulated. Finally, a detailed list of ingredients is required, making it easier for those who need to avoid certain substances for health or religious reasons.

Overall, the current food label, particularly the Nutrition Facts panel, is a useful tool in planning a healthful diet. It is worthwhile to invest the small amount of time required to understand the components of the food label.

Exceptions to Food Labeling

Foods such as fresh fruits and vegetables, fish, meats, and poultry are not required to have Nutrition Facts labels. However, many grocers have voluntarily chosen to

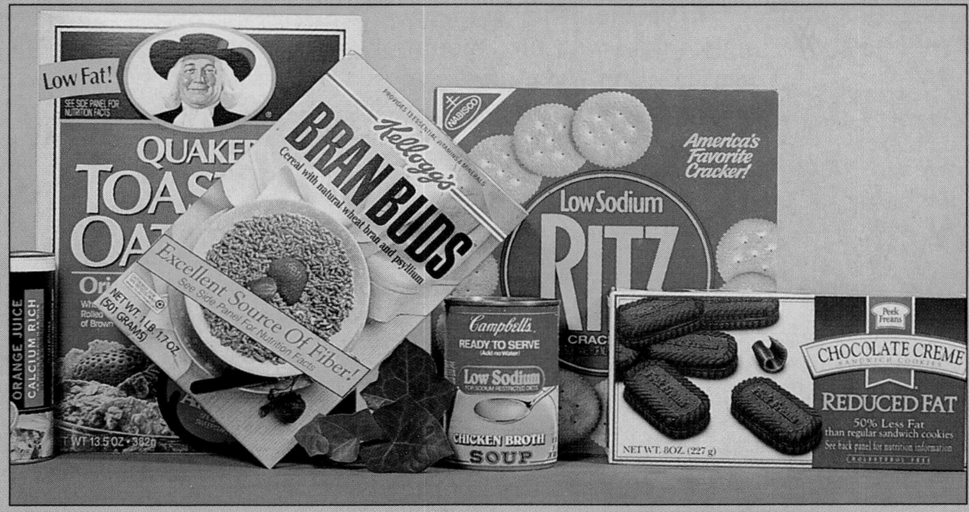

Many food packages prominently feature health claims.

Second, a single serving of the food product cannot contain more than 13 grams of fat, 4 grams of saturated fat, 60 milligrams of cholesterol, or 480 milligrams of sodium. If a food exceeds any one of these amounts, no health claim can be made for it despite its other nutritional qualities. For example, even though whole milk is high in calcium, its label can't make the health claim about calcium and osteoporosis because whole milk contains 5 grams of saturated fat per serving.

In addition, the product must meet criteria specific to the health claim being made. For example, a health claim regarding fat and cancer can be made only if the product contains 3 grams or less of fat per serving, which is the standard for low-fat food.

The primary danger with health claims is that not all the facts may be presented in some cases. For example, claims about dietary fiber often omit the negative information, such as the fact that too much wheat-bran fiber can lead to decreased absorption of iron, zinc, and calcium, as well as to intestinal problems, such as gas (see Chapter 4). A more complete statement is that too much—as well as too little—fiber can be harmful.

The bottom line for health claims is honesty. FDA is vigilant in controlling the claims made about foods on supermarket shelves.

provide their customers with information on these products. The next time you are at the grocery store, ask where you might find information on these fresh products. You will likely find some type of poster or pamphlet near the product; often these pamphlets contain recipes in which to use your favorite fruit, vegetable, or cut of meat. It is important to utilize these tools so that they continue to be made available; they may even assist you in your endeavor to improve your diet.

Nutrient Density Can Help Guide Food Choice

As you've seen already, the RDAs and related nutrient standards are used for planning diets. However, these nutrient standards aren't necessarily useful for assessing the nutritional quality of an individual food. For this purpose the concept of **nutrient density** has gained acceptance.

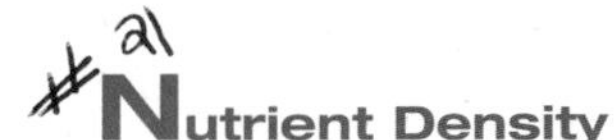

Nutrient Density *The ratio formed by dividing a food's contribution to nutrient needs by its contribution to energy needs. When its contribution to nutrient needs exceeds its energy contribution, the food is considered to have a favorable nutrient density.*

Energy density is another way to evaluate foods. These foods are rich calorie sources compared to their relatively small serving size. Nuts, avocados, and ice cream are three examples. Energy-dense food choices can be helpful for people with problems maintaining weight, such as some elderly or ill people, but should be used sparingly by people with weight problems.

To determine the nutrient density of a food, simply compare its vitamin or mineral content with the amount of energy it provides. A food is said to be nutrient dense if it provides a high amount of a nutrient for a relatively small amount of kcals (compared with other food sources). The higher a food's nutrient density, the better it is as a nutrient source in comparison to an energy source.

Generally, nutrient density is assessed with respect to individual nutrients. For example, many fruits and vegetables have a high content of vitamin C compared with their modest energy content: that is, they are nutrient-dense foods for vitamin C. Moreover, as Figure 2–3 shows, nonfat milk is much more nutrient dense than sugared soft drinks for many nutrients.

Searching for nutrient-dense foods such as the ones mentioned above is important in some cases. For example, this strategy can aid diet planning for people who tend to consume little food energy, including some older people and those following weight-loss diets.

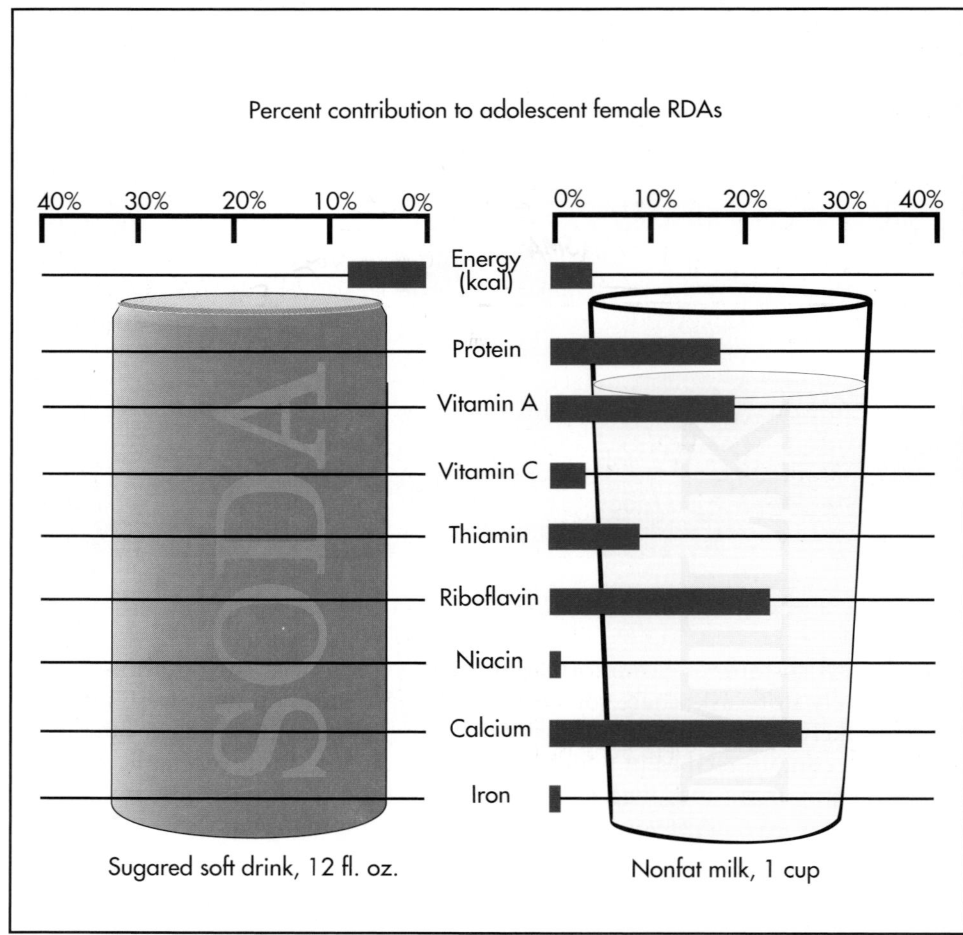

Figure 2–3 *Comparison of the nutrient density of a sugared soft drink with that of nonfat milk. Choosing a glass of nonfat milk makes a significantly greater contribution to nutrient intake in comparison with a sugared soft drink. An easy way to determine nutrient density is to see how many of the nutrient bars are longer than the kcal bar. The soft drink has no longer nutrient bars. Nonfat milk has longer nutrient bars for protein, vitamin A, thiamin, riboflavin, and calcium. Including many nutrient-dense foods in your diet aids in meeting nutrient needs.*

Epilogue

The tools discussed in this chapter greatly aid in menu planning. Menu planning can start with the Food Guide Pyramid. The totality of choices made within the groups can then be evaluated using the Dietary Guidelines. Individual foods that make up a diet can be examined more closely using the comparison to the Daily Values listed on the Nutrition Facts panel of the product. For the most part, these Daily Values are in line with the Recommended Dietary Allowances and related nutrient standards, as well as the Dietary Guidelines. The Nutrition Facts panel is especially useful in identifying nutrient-dense foods—foods that are high in a specific nutrient, such as vitamin C, but low in comparison to the relative amount of energy provided. Generally speaking, the more you learn about and use these and other nutrition tools, the more they will benefit your diet (Figure 2–4).

A final menu-planning tool is the Exchange System. This tool organizes foods based on energy, protein, carbohydrate, and fat content. A manageable framework for designing diets is the result. For more information on the Exchange System see Appendixes C and D.

FRANK & ERNEST ® by Bob Thaves

BOOKS
NEW! "EAT SMART"
EAT SMART
EAT SMART
EAT SMART
WHAT DOES IT SAY?
"GET SOMEBODY ELSE TO PICK UP THE CHECK"
THAVES 12-28
© 1991 by NEA, Inc.

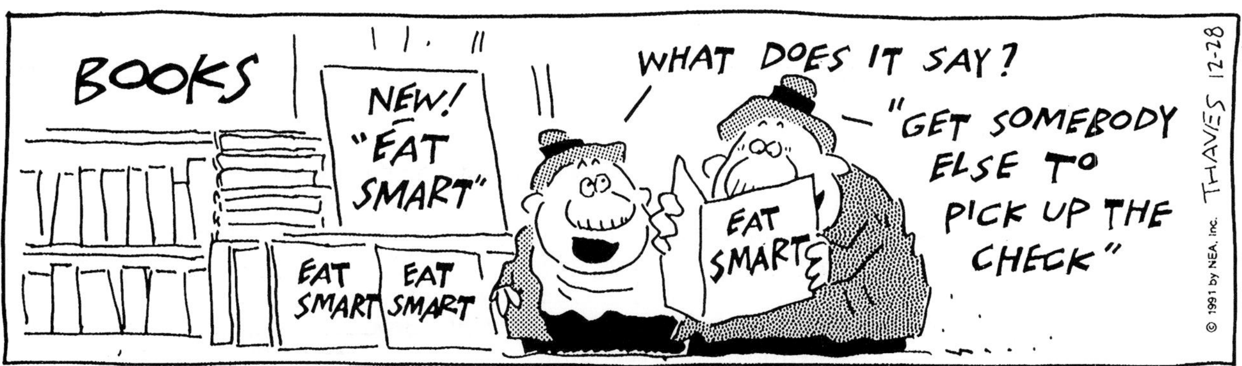

Figure 2–4 FRANK AND ERNEST © United Feature Syndicated. Reprinted by Permission.

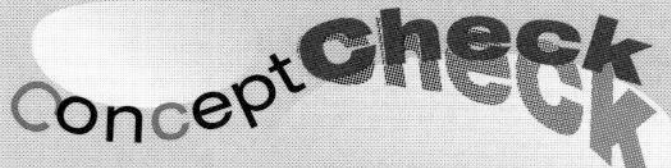

Daily Values are currently used as a benchmark for representing the nutrient content of foods on nutrition labels. Nutrient content is expressed as percentages of the Daily Values, which in turn are based roughly on RDAs and related nutrient standards and various Dietary Guidelines. Nutrient density is a measure of the nutrient contributions made by each food compared with its total energy content. Nutrient-dense foods supply much of one or many nutrients while providing a modest amount of energy. Current food labels are a valuable tool for diet planning. The nutrition information required is both accurate and extensive, and undergoes continuing scrutiny by FDA.

Summary

- The watchwords of nutrition are variety, balance, and moderation when it comes to designing a diet.
- A person's nutritional state can be categorized as desirable nutrition, in which the body has adequate stores for times of increased needs; undernutrition, which may be present with or without clinical symptons; and overnutrition, which can lead to vitamin and mineral toxicities and various chronic diseases.

- ➤ Evaluation of nutritional state involves analyzing background factors, anthropometric measurements, biochemical parameters, clinical evidence, and diet history. It is not always possible to detect nutritional inadequacies via nutrition assessment since such evidence often does not appear for many years.
- ➤ The Food Guide Pyramid is designed to translate nutrient recommendations into a food plan that exhibits variety, balance, and moderation. The best results are obtained by using low-fat or nonfat milk products; including some vegetable proteins in addition to animal-protein foods; including citrus fruits and dark green vegetables; and emphasizing whole-grain breads and cereals.
- ➤ Dietary Guidelines have been issued to help reduce chronic diseases in our population. The Guidelines emphasize eating a variety of foods; performing regular physical activity; maintaining or improving weight; moderating consumption of fats, cholesterol, sugar, salt, and alcohol; and eating plenty of grain products (especially whole grain), fruits, and vegetables.
- ➤ Recommended Dietary Allowances (RDAs) are set for many nutrients. These amounts yield enough of each nutrient to meet the needs of healthy people within specific gender and age categories. The Adequate Intake (AI) standards are similar to the RDAs, but use of an AI indicates not enough is known about these nutrients. Upper Limits (UL) for nutrient intake have been set for some vitamins and minerals. All fall under the umbrella term Dietary Reference Intakes (DRIs).
- ➤ Daily Values are used as a basis for expressing the nutrient content of foods on the Nutrition Facts panel. These are based roughly on RDAs and related nutrient standards. Daily Values also are set for food components not covered by the RDAs, such as fat and dietary fiber.
- ➤ Food labels are a powerful tool to use to track your nutritional intake and learn more about the nutritional characteristics of the foods you eat.
- ➤ Nutrient density reflects the nutrient content of a food in relation to its energy (kcal) content. Nutrient-dense foods are relatively rich in nutrients, in comparison with energy content.

Study Questions

1. Describe the philosophy underlying the creation of the Food Guide Pyramid. What dietary changes would you need to make to meet the Pyramid guidelines on a regular basis?
2. Trace the progression, in terms of physical results, of a person who went from an overnourished to an undernourished state.
3. How could the nutritional state of the person at each state in question 2 be evaluated?
4. Describe the intent of the Dietary Guidelines. Point out one criticism for its general application to all American adults.
5. Based on surveys of current food patterns of adults, suggest two key dietary changes the typical American adult should consider making.
6. What three key points should you make when explaining the significance of the RDAs to a friend?
7. How do RDAs and AIs differ from Daily Values in intention and application?
8. Nutritionists encourage all people to read labels on food packages to learn more about what they eat. What four nutrients could easily be tracked in your diet if you regularly read the Nutrition Facts panels on food products?
9. Explain why consumers can have more confidence in health claims on food packages today than in years past.
10. How would you explain the concept of nutrient density to a fourth-grade class?

Further Readings

1 ADA Reports: Position of the American Dietetic Association: Phytochemicals and functional foods, *Journal of the American Dietetic Association* 95: 493, 1995.
2 Bialostosky K, St Jeor ST: The 1995 Dietary Guidelines for Americans, *Nutrition Today* 31:6, 1996.
3 Craig WJ: Phytochemicals: guardians of our health, *Journal of the American Dietetic Association* 97(suppl 2): S199, 1997.
4 FDA's final regulations of health claims for foods, *Nutrition Reviews* 51:90, 1993.
5 Food servings, *Mayo Clinic Health Letter* p. 7, April 1997.
6 Hahn NJ: Variety is still the spice of a healthful diet, *Journal of the American Dietetic Association* 95:1096, 1995.
7 Hasler CM: Functional foods: Their role in disease, prevention and health promotion, *Food Technology* 52(11):63, 1998.
8 Jaret P: Only 5 a day, *Health* p. 78, May–June 1998.
9 Katz F: USDA surveys show what Americans eat, *Food Technology* 52(11):50, 1998.
10 Kurtzweil P: Staking a claim to good health, *FDA Consumer* p. 16, November–December 1998.
11 Lycopene, *Mayo Clinic Health Letter* p. 7, September 1998.
12 Marwick C: Learning how phytochemicals help fight disease, *Journal of the American Medical Association* 274:1328, 1995.
13 McBean L: The Dietary Guidelines: change and implications, *Dairy Council Digest* 67:7, 1996.
14 Most frequently asked questions about 1997 Dietary Reference Intakes (DRIs), *Nutrition Today* 32:189, 1997.
15 Porter DV: Health claims on food products; NLEA, *Nutrition Today* 31:35, 1996.
16 Schweitzer CM and others: How do Americans eat (and think they eat) today? *Food & Nutrition News* 67(2):11, 1995.
17 Sloan AE: Way beyond burritos, *Food Technology* 52(7):24, 1998.
18 Translating the science behind the Dietary Reference Intakes, *Journal of the American Dietetic Association* 98:756, 1998.
19 Truswell AS: Dietary goals and guidelines: national and international perspectives in *Modern Nutrition in Health and Disease,* Shils ME and others, eds, Ninth edition, Baltimore MD, Williams & Wilkins, 1999.
20 Voelker R: Ames agrees with mom's advice: eat your fruits and vegetables, *Journal of the American Medical Association* 273:1077, 1995.
21 Welsh S and others: Development of the Food Guide Pyramid, *Nutrition Today,* November–December 1992.
22 Willet WC: The dietary pyramid: does the foundation need repair? *American Journal of Clinical Nutrition* 68:218, 1998.
23 Yates AA and others: Dietary reference intakes, *Journal of the American Dietetic Association* 98:699, 1998.

RATE Your Plate

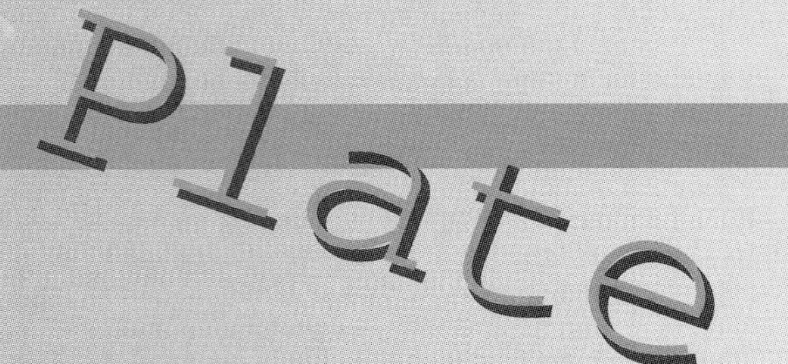

I. Does Your Diet Meet Nutrient Needs and Food Guide Pyramid Recommendations?

Complete either Part I or Part II. Then complete Parts III, IV, and V. (For help in following the instructions for this activity, see the sample assessment in Appendix E.)

PART I

Manual RDA analysis

A. Take the information from the 1-day food-intake record you completed in Chapter 1 and record it on the blank form provided in Appendix E or by your instructor. Be sure to record the food or drink ingested and the amount (e.g., weight) consumed. NOTE: Your instructor may require you to keep the food record for more than 1 day. A still longer period increases the accuracy of the assessment.

B. Review the RDAs or related nutrient standards (in the inside cover of this book) and choose the appropriate recommendations for your gender and age. Write the appropriate value for each nutrient on the line on the form labeled "RDA or related nutrient standard." Note that the values for sodium and potassium from the table on the inside cover of the book are labeled "Estimated Sodium, Chloride, and Potassium Requirements of Healthy Persons."

C. Look up the foods and drinks that you listed on the form in the food composition table, Appendix A. Record on the form the amounts of each nutrient and the kcal present in them, based on the serving size and the number of servings you ate. For example, if you drank 2 cups of milk and the serving size listed in Appendix A is 1 cup, double all nutrient values as you record them. If the food is not listed, choose a substitute, such as cola for root beer.

D. For each food and drink, add the amounts in each column and record the results on the line labeled "Totals."

E. Compare the totals to your estimated needs. Divide the total for each nutrient by the specific number and multiply that by 100. Record the result on the line labeled "% of Nutrient Needs."

F. Keep this assessment for use in subsequent activities in other chapters.

PART II

Computer diet analysis

A. Obtain copies of the computer software from your instructor. Load the software into the computer.

B. Choose RDAs and related nutrient standards based on your age and gender.

C. Enter the information from the 1-day food intake record you kept in Chapter 1. Be sure to enter each food and drink and the specific amount you ate.

D. This software program will give you the following results:
   1. The appropriate RDA or related nutrient standard for each nutrient
   2. The total amount of each nutrient and the kcal consumed for the day
   3. The percentage of intake compared to needs for each nutrient that you consumed

E. Keep this assessment for use in subsequent activities in other chapters.

PART III

Evaluation of nutrient intakes

Remember that you don't necessarily need to consume 100% of estimated nutrient needs. A general standard is meeting needs averaged over 5 to 8 days. It is best not to generally exceed 200% (2 times) to avoid potential toxic effects for some nutrients.

A. **For which nutrients did your intakes fall below the RDAs or related nutrient standards?**
B. **Did you exceed the minimum needs for sodium? To what degree?**
C. **For which nutrients did you exceed estimated needs by greater than 200%? (2 times greater)?**
D. **What dietary changes could you make to correct or improve your dietary profile? If you're not sure, future chapters will help guide your decisions.**

PART IV

Food Guide Pyramid

Using the same food-intake record used in Part I or II, place each food item in the appropriate group of the Food Guide Pyramid in Appendix E. That is, for each food item indicate how many servings it contributres to each group based on the amount you ate (see Table 2-5 for serving sizes). Note that many of your food choices may contribute to more than one group. For example, toast with margarine contributes to two categories: (1) the breads, cereals, rice, and pasta group; and (2) fats, oils, and sweets. After entering all the values, add the number of servings consumed in each group. Finally, compare your total in each food group with the recommended number of servings shown in Figure 2-1. Enter a − if your total falls below the recommendation or a + if it equals or exceeds the recommendations.

PART V

Further diet evaluation

Do the weaknesses, if any, suggested in your nutrient analysis (see Part III) correspond to missing servings in the Food Guide Pyramid chart? If so, consider changing your food choices based on the Food Guide Pyramid to help improve your nutrient profile. Finally, indicate whether your day's diet did or did not conform to the following items in the Dietary Guidelines:

	Yes	No
• Eat a variety of foods.	________	________
• Choose a diet with plenty of grain products, vegetables, and fruits.	________	________
• Choose a diet low in fat, saturated fat, and cholesterol.	________	________
• Choose a diet moderate in sugars.	________	________
• Choose a diet moderate in salt and sodium.	________	________
• Drink alcoholic beverages in moderation, if at all.	________	________

If your diet comes up short on any of these evaluations, take appropriate action to improve your eating patterns.

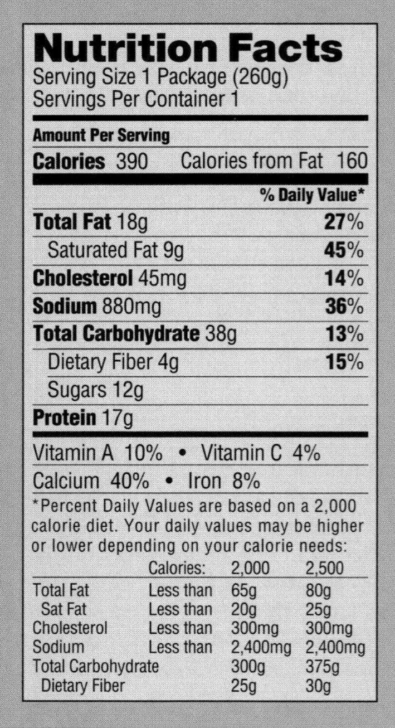

Nutrition Facts
Serving Size 1 Package (260g)
Servings Per Container 1

Amount Per Serving
Calories 390 Calories from Fat 160

	% Daily Value*
Total Fat 18g	**27**%
Saturated Fat 9g	**45**%
Cholesterol 45mg	**14**%
Sodium 880mg	**36**%
Total Carbohydrate 38g	**13**%
Dietary Fiber 4g	**15**%
Sugars 12g	
Protein 17g	

Vitamin A 10% • Vitamin C 4%
Calcium 40% • Iron 8%

*Percent Daily Values are based on a 2,000 calorie diet. Your daily values may be higher or lower depending on your calorie needs:

	Calories:	2,000	2,500
Total Fat	Less than	65g	80g
Sat Fat	Less than	20g	25g
Cholesterol	Less than	300mg	300mg
Sodium	Less than	2,400mg	2,400mg
Total Carbohydrate		300g	375g
Dietary Fiber		25g	30g

Nutrition Facts
Serving Size 1 Package (260g)
Servings Per Container 1

Amount Per Serving
Calories 230 Calories from Fat 35

	% Daily Value*
Total Fat 4g	**6**%
Saturated Fat 2g	**10**%
Cholesterol 15mg	**4**%
Sodium 590mg	**24**%
Total Carbohydrate 28g	**9**%
Dietary Fiber 3g	**12**%
Sugars 10g	
Protein 19g	

Vitamin A 10% • Vitamin C 10%
Calcium 35% • Iron 4%

*Percent Daily Values are based on a 2,000 calorie diet. Your daily values may be higher or lower depending on your calorie needs:

	Calories:	2,000	2,500
Total Fat	Less than	65g	80g
Sat Fat	Less than	20g	25g
Cholesterol	Less than	300mg	300mg
Sodium	Less than	2,400mg	2,400mg
Potassium		3,500mg	3,500mg
Total Carbohydrate		300g	375g
Dietary Fiber		25g	30g

II. Applying the Nutrition Facts Label to Your Daily Food Choices

Imagine that you are at the grocery store looking for a quick meal before a busy evening. In the frozen food section you find two different brands of frozen cheese manicotti (see labels A and B). Which of the two brands would you choose? What information on the Nutrition Facts label contributed to this decision?

____

____

____

____

____

____

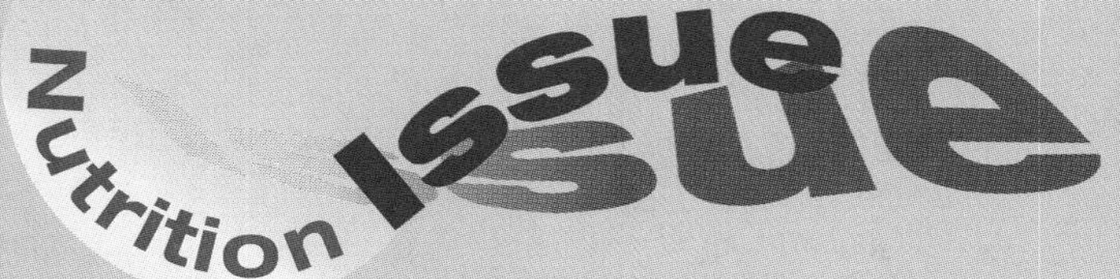

Ethnic Influences on the American Diet

Over the centuries, people of various cultures have migrated to new locations. Typically, migrants keep some traditional dietary habits, or *foodways,* change some habits, and abandon others. As people migrate and mingle with those of other cultures their cuisines tend to mingle as well. Note that about 25% of all restaurants in the United States have an ethnic theme. Changes in affluence and technology also affect dietary habits, some for better and some for worse.

This Nutrition Issue examines how the cuisines of various cultures have affected the American diet. Examining the nutrition attributes of a number of ethnic diets will help you to understand that no single cuisine is either completely healthful or unhealthful. The trick to finding healthful food is to evaluate individual dishes carefully. Let's look at several cuisines that contribute to food "American style." Note that almost all Americans sample at least one of these on a regular basis.

NATIVE AMERICANS

The size and varied geography of the American continent meant that different foods were available to people living in different locations. Some of these people were hunter-gatherers, relying on wild vegetation and wild game, such as bison, for subsistence. Others learned to grow vegetable crops. Depending on where they lived, Native American groups cultivated early forms of such plant foods as tomatoes, corn, squash, beans, sweet potatoes, vanilla, and cocoa, all of which are important contributors to American cuisine today. Their diets tended to be low in sodium and fat and high in dietary fiber. In the far North, native populations subsisted on fish, sea mammals, other game, and a few plants, such as seaweed, willow leaves, and berries.

In contrast, today many Native Americans have food patterns that are very similar to other Americans. Recent studies also have shown that the diseases that affected traditional Native American societies differed significantly from the diseases common in American society today. For example, Alaskan natives following the traditional diet had heart disease rates lower than those in the general United States population. Younger generations of Alaskan natives, however, who usually do not eat the traditional diet, have developed heart disease at rates

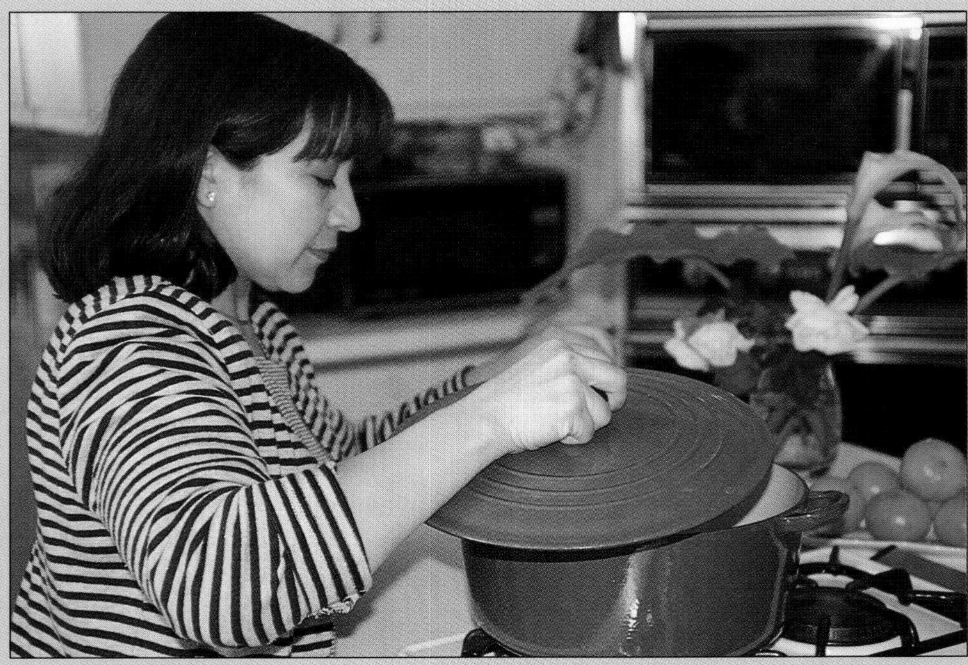

Our cooking habits often reflect our ethnic heritage.

similar to those in the U.S. population in general. These and other studies indicate that as societies become more uniform in dietary choices, so too do disease patterns.

HISPANIC AMERICANS

When Spanish colonists arrived in what is now called Latin America, they brought foods, flavors, and cooking techniques that they combined with locally available foods. Several cuisines developed from those combinations, influenced also by the arrival of other groups. Thus, the Cuban cuisine combined native foods with those of both Spanish and Chinese immigrants, whereas the Puerto Rican cuisine combined native foods with Spanish and African contributions. In Mexico, the Spanish influence mingled with that of local Native American cuisines.

The Mayans, Aztecs, and other populations in Mexico grew corn, beans, squash, and chili peppers; these were the basis of Mexican cuisine. They also grew such fruits as avocados, papayas, and pineapples. By the end of the fifteenth century, wheat, chickpeas, melons, radishes, grapes, and sugarcane had been brought to the New World. Rice, citrus fruits, and some kinds of nuts came soon afterward. The Spanish also introduced beef, lamb, and chicken. Native inhabitants had previously eaten mostly fish and wild game. Spices such as cinnamon, black pepper, cloves, thyme, marjoram, and bay leaves were introduced and also became part of the cuisine.

Mexican cuisine today shows regional variety. In southern Mexico, savory sauces and stews and corn tortillas reflect the native heritage. The Gulf states are renowned for delicious seafood dishes prepared with tomatoes, herbs, and olives, whereas Yucatán cuisine follows Mayan tradition, with such specialties as wild turkey and fish flavored with lime juice. Fresh produce adds color, flavor, and nutrients to authentic Mexican dining. Markets in the United States are now beginning to offer some of these plant foods, such as chayote, squash, jicama root, plantains, and cactus leaves and fruit. Traditional Mexican cooking is healthful in that it is high in complex carbohydrates, beans, and fruits and vegetables, particularly those rich in vitamins A and C. This pattern is reflected in the Latin American Diet Pyramid issued by Oldways Preservation & Exchange Trust in 1996 (Figure 2–5). For more information on this and other ethnic diet Pyramids, see the web site http://www.oldwayspt.org.

Today, true Mexican cooking bears little resemblance to the dishes usually found in "Mexican" restaurants. Restaurant Mexican food tends to use larger portions of meat, as well as adding portions of high-fat sour cream, guacamole, and cheese to many dishes. To lower your fat intake in such a restaurant, order a bean burrito without cheese. Or have a bean or meat taco with a soft (unfried) shell. Fajitas can also be constructed with low-fat ingredients. Consume such fried dishes as tortilla chips, chimichangas, or enchiladas infrequently.

NORTHERN EUROPEAN-AMERICANS

Immigrants from Northern Europe are responsible for the "meat-and-potatoes" presentation of traditional American home cooking. The first large group of settlers from Europe—the English, French, and Germans—adapted to the foods available in the regions in which they settled. Native Americans shared new foods that are now staples of the American diet: corn and corn products such as popcorn and hominy, some kinds of squash, and tomatoes.

However, because the new immigrants often settled in regions of the "new land" that most closely resembled their homes in Europe, they were able to grow many familiar foods and retain many of their traditional foodways. One of these foodways involved the way food is presented.

A sizable portion of meat arranged with vegetables and potatoes in separate portions on a plate in the European pattern, compared with other cuisines in which a mixture of starch, vegetables, and a much smaller portion of protein (such as a stir-fry) is more typical. The meat on the "American" dinner plate may be, for example, sausage or roast beef, the potatoes may be boiled or mashed, and the vegetable may be sauerkraut or green peas. Whatever the choices, the Northern European pattern is still followed by many in this country.

This traditional pattern provides abundant protein and nutrients from dairy and meat products. However, the protein also contains saturated fat, and the large portions of protein and starch may mean that insufficient amounts of whole grains, vegetables, and fruits are eaten. In response, try a smaller portion of skinless chicken breast, accompanied by a romaine lettuce salad, plain baked potato with the skin, and a hearty portion of green beens or broccoli as one example. This combination of foods follows the traditional pattern while allowing for more healthful food choices.

AFRICAN-AMERICANS

Involuntary immigrants to the New World, people from West Africa struggled to survive under harsh conditions. Their ability to adapt familiar foodways to new conditions became a lasting influence on today's American cuisine.

The "soul food" of African-Americans is the basis of the regional cuisines of the American South. Many understand "soul food" to consist mainly of barbecued meat, fried chicken, sweet potatoes, and chitterlings. In fact, true soul food includes a wide range of dishes

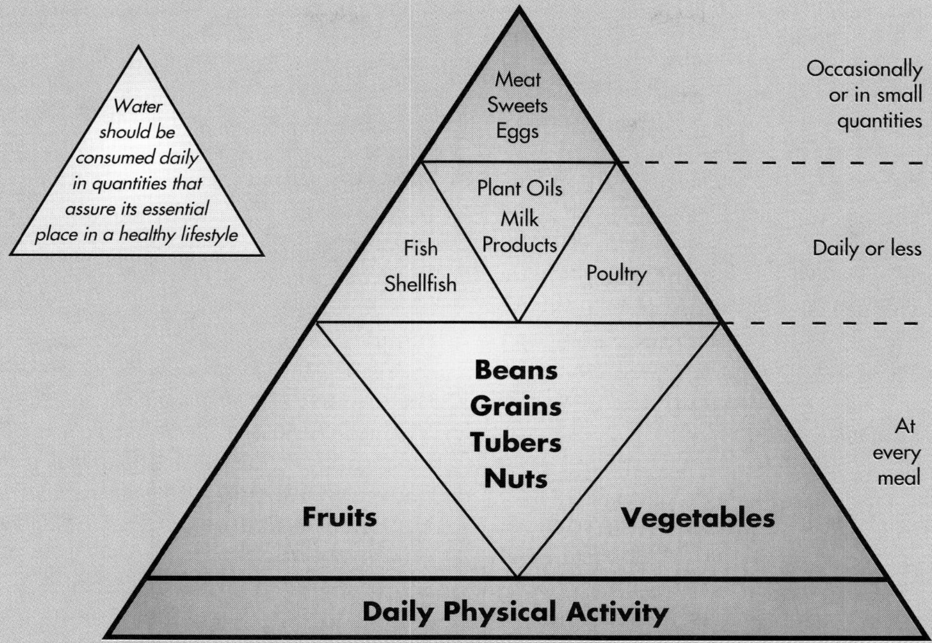

Figure 2-5 *The traditional healthy Latin American Diet Pyramid. A variety of diet Pyramids have been developed by Oldways Preservation & Exchange Trust. These pyramids reflect the typical diets of rural peoples in the region, in this case Latin America. Text accompanying the Latin American Pyramid, as is true for the other Oldways ethnic pyramids, states that alcohol may be consumed with meals, but consumption should be avoided during pregnancy and whenever it would put the individual or others at risk. As you will notice throughout this Nutrition Issue, all pyramids developed by governmental or private organizations always have fruits, vegetables, and grains at the base. The Latin American Diet Pyramid then adds nuts and beans to this base; other pyramids also slightly alter the base.*

created by African-American cooks. They used traditional methods and foods brought from Africa, such as yams, okra, and peanuts, as well as what was available in the New World. African-American women, cooking for their families, created dishes that they often adapted for the plantation owner's table as well, creating the basis of Southern cuisine. The combination of these African-American foodways with Native American, Spanish, and French traditions produced the Cajun and Creole cuisines enjoyed today in Louisiana and throughout the nation.

Pork and corn products were the basis of soul food. The plantation owner ate the better parts of the pig. As with other foods, slaves learned to make the less desirable parts of the pig, such as entrails, feet, ears, and head, palatable. Corn was ground for corn bread. Unrefined yellow cornmeal was mixed with water and lard to make "hoecake," baked on a hoe blade by cooks who had neither ovens nor cooking utensils for their own use. The plantation owner probably ate white cornbread made from refined cornmeal.

Among other dishes still considered soul food staples are greens, usually cooked with a small portion of smoked pork. The greens used include collards, mustard, turnip, or dandelion greens, and kale. Black-eyed peas, first brought to the New World by slaves, are also cooked with pork. Sweet potatoes and yams were and remain basic soul foods; sweet potato pie is the soul food equivalent of pumpkin pie.

Today's traditional African-American cuisine has both nutritional benefits and deficits. The variety of fruits, vegetables, and grain products used provides ample vitamins, minerals, and dietary fiber. For instance, African-Americans in general consume more cruciferous vegetables, and fruits and vegetables containing vitamins

A and C than do Caucasian Americans. However, cured pork products contribute undesirable levels of sodium as well as saturated fat. Traditional reliance on frying, especially with lard, also adds much fat to the diet. Boiling vegetables for long periods depletes water-soluble vitamins. Dairy products may not be used enough, especially by older people who follow traditional dietary customs. This avoidance is based in part on the difficulty many African-American adults experience in digesting lactose; see Chapter 4 for details.

To help guide African-Americans toward a healthy food plan, Hebni Nutrition Consultants has developed a Soul Food Pyramid. It differs from the Food Guide Pyramid primarily by emphasizing lactose-reduced dairy products in the Milk, Yogurt, and Cheese group and placing very high-fat meats such as bacon and sausage in the Fats, Oils, and Sweets category. To obtain a copy of the Soul Food Pyramid, call/fax 407-345-7999.

ASIAN-AMERICANS

Okinawa, an island southwest of Japan, boasts some of the oldest, healthiest people in the world. Their diet of fresh vegetables, minimal amounts of meat (mainly pork and fish), and moderate fat (lower than American diets, but higher than traditional Japanese fare), has influenced the eating habits of Japan and the United States alike. Studies prove that the Okinawan diet of more fresh versus pickled vegetables, more fiber, less salt, and a little more fat than traditional Japanese cuisine has protected them from premature death from problems such as stroke. Since this discovery, the Japanese diet has become more like that of the Okinawans.

Two issues addressed by various ethnic Diet Pyramids developed by Oldways Preservation & Exchange Trust but not specifically included as part of the Food Guide Pyramid diagram are physical activity and alcohol intake. The ethnic Diet Pyramids recommend daily physical activity. Alcohol may be consumed by adults in moderation with meals, but consumption should be avoided during pregnancy and whenever it would put the individual or others at risk. The booklet accompanying the Food Guide Pyramid does address alcohol intake, suggesting adults have no more than 1 to 2 drinks per day.

This idea of large portions of vegetables and grains, and small portions of meat is becoming known in the United States as well, but people are having difficulty complying with this more disciplined way of eating. Also influenced by Japanese cuisine is the growing popularity of soy products, such as tofu, soy milk, and miso; as well as use of flavors such as soy sauce, cilantro, and ginger.

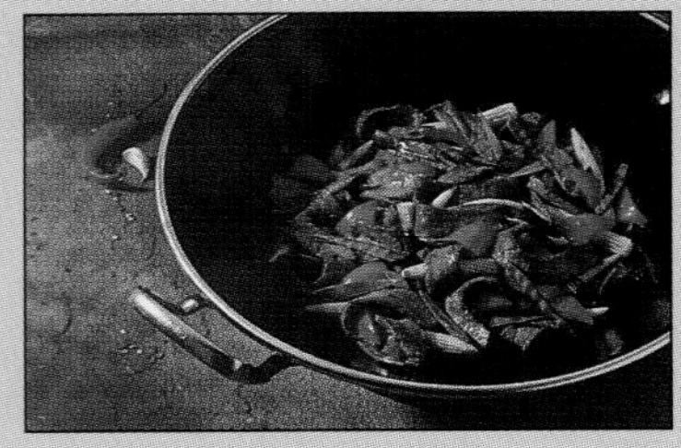

Stir-fry is commonly used in Chinese cooking.

More than 200 different vegetables are used in Chinese cuisine; bok choy and other forms of Chinese cabbage are perhaps the most widely eaten vegetables in the world. In the southeastern coastal region of China, home of the Cantonese cuisine, the number of dishes may be as high as 50,000. Southern Chinese cuisine is the least greasy, with seafood, fish and stir-fried vegetables making up the majority of meals. This is the most popular Chinese style in the United States. In the temperate North however, wheat is used in noodles (China is the original home of pasta), bread, and dumplings. Garlic, leeks, and scallions are commonly used to flavor a meal. Popular dishes include hot pots (stews containing many ingredients) and stir-fried mixtures of vegetables and small amounts of meat or fish cooked in a lightly oiled, very hot pan.

An Asian Pyramid has recently been developed to reflect the Asian dietary pattern (Figure 2–6). Like the Latin American Diet Pyramid the bulk of the diet consists of grains, fruits, vegetables, and plant sources of protein, such as legumes, nuts, and seeds.

Chinese immigration to America began with the California gold rush in the middle of the nineteenth century. Chinese workers brought with them food preparation methods that tend to preserve nutrients, as well as a variety of sauces and seasonings, such as ginger root, garlic, rice wine, scallions, and sesame seeds and oil. Although many of the traditional foodways have been preserved, North American restaurant versions of Chinese cuisine, whether Cantonese, Szechuan, or Mandarin, are usually not authentic. Chinese-American restaurant food is often prepared with far more fat than in true Chinese cooking, which tends to use flavorful but fat-free sauces and seasoning. The restaurant versions of Chinese dishes also contain much larger portions of protein.

However, choosing a healthful meal in an Asian-American restaurant is still possible. Select dishes that are not deep-fat fried (such as egg rolls or batter-coated meats or seafood). Choose at least one vegetable dish instead of just meat entrées. Leave most of the sauce behind by lifting the food from the sauce and placing it on top of a mouthful of rice, which in Asia is the basis of the meal. Limit the amount of soy sauce you sprinkle on the rice. (Even in Asia, health authorities are now calling for a cut in salt intake and a switch from saturated to unsaturated fats, particularly as diets in these areas are becoming more Westernized.)

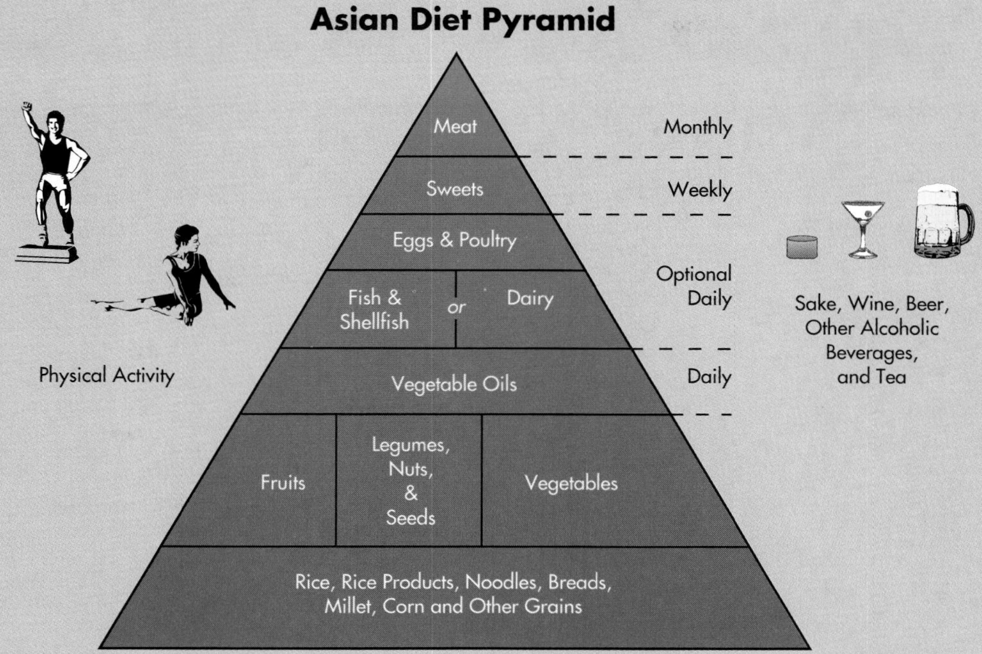

Figure 2-6 *The Asian Diet Pyramid. This pyramid was inspired by the cuisines of South and East Asia, including such countries as China, Japan, South Korea, India, Thailand, Vietnam, Cambodia, Indonesia, Malaysia, Philippines, and other related Pacific Rim areas. If meat is consumed more often than monthly it should be in small amounts. If dairy foods are consumed on a daily basis, they should be used in low to moderate amounts, and preferably low in fat. Grain products chosen should be minimally refined whenever possible.*

ITALIAN-AMERICANS

Authentic Italian cuisine, like Asian cuisine, is more diverse than most Americans realize. Foods of different regions reflect Italy's varied geography and climate. Northern Italy, the more affluent part of the country, is the principal producer of meat and dairy products, such as butter and cheese. Rice dishes such as risotto are popular there. Fish is more important in regions near the sea, and lighter foods, such as fresh vegetables prepared with herbs, garlic, and olive oil, are characteristic. The poorer regions south of Rome, as well as the island of Sicily, have a diet rich in grains, vegetables, dried beans, and fish, with little meat or oil. Compared with northern Italians of the same class, southern Italians eat less beef, veal, chicken, and butter, and more bread, pasta, vegetables, fruit and fish.

Pasta is the heart of the Italian diet. Italians eat six times more of this simple wheat and water product than do North Americans, although Americans have also learned to love this nutritious dish. Pasta in America, however, often means spaghetti, with a tomato-based sauce that includes meatballs or sausage. In contrast, Italians eat pasta in a variety of shapes and with a variety of sauces, often excluding meat.

Most of the Italian-American cuisine found in restaurants offers foods more common to the north of Italy, including veal, cheese, and cream and pesto sauces for pasta. Pizza, a southern Italian dish, is the exception, and it is fast becoming the most frequently consumed food in the United States. Pizza in this country is served on a variety of flour crusts topped with anything from high-fat meats, such as pepperoni, to vegetables or even fruit, combined with a variety of cheeses, tomatoes, and oregano for seasoning. Purists in Naples, however, insist that classic pizza consists only of a thin crust, tomato, basil, and mozzarella cheese.

Although some components of the Italian diet contain substantial amounts of saturated fat, nutritionists now know that other components, such as pasta, olive oil, and vegetables, contribute to healthy diets. One approach to American-Italian cuisine could be the Mediterranean Diet Pyramid (Figure 2–7). This is a plan based on food choices like those traditionally found in the simple cuisines of Greece and southern Italy. The Mediterranean Diet Pyramid allows up to 35% of total calories as fat in the diet, compared with the typical recommendation of not more than 30%. However, it recommends consuming the type of fat consumed in the Mediterranean region: olive oil.

Overall, healthy choices in an Italian-American restaurant might include a pasta dish with fresh tomato sauce, rather than cheese-laden Alfredo sauce, and an entrée of fish and vegetables cooked with wine, olive oil, and herbs. Limiting the cheeses and meats offered on the

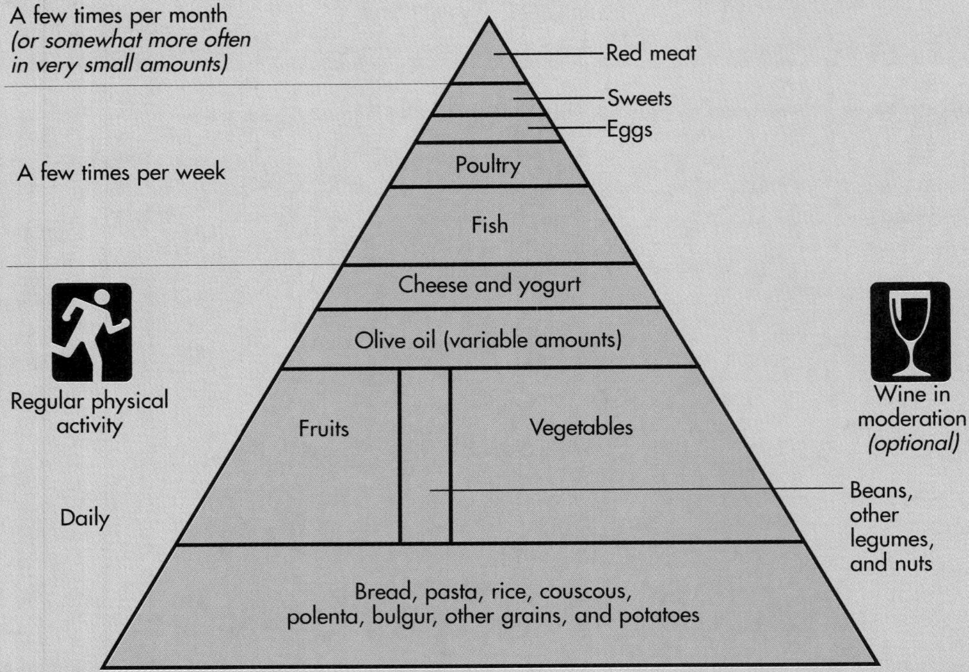

Figure 2-7 *The traditional healthy Mediterranean Diet Pyramid. This plan is based on long-standing eating habits in southern Italy, Crete, and Greece. The base of the diet is bread and grains, fruits and vegetables, and beans and potatoes. Red meat is consumed sparingly—moderate amounts of fish and poultry are preferred. Most of the fat in this plan comes from olive oil. Cheese and yogurt supply some calcium, other low-fat and nonfat milk products also can be included.*

antipasto tray and limiting fried foods such as veal parmigiana, are also wise moves.

JEWISH-AMERICANS

Though Jewish immigrants arrive from all over the world, the two predominant groups are the Ashkenazic Jews, from Eastern European countries such as Russia, Germany, Poland, and Romania and from South Africa; and the Sephardic Jews from Spain, Portugal, and North Africa. Religious laws and the consumption of only kosher foods influence the dietary practices of some Jews, but many discontinue such practices, especially as they become more integrated into the United States.

Common foods for Ashkenazic Jews include dark rye bread, borscht, and herring. The Sephardic Jews eat foods that are also common in the Middle East, such as eggplant, humus, tahini, and couscous. Many of these foods have become popular in American cuisine, including rye bread, bagels with cream cheese, corned beef, and pastrami. In Israel the food practices are similar to that of the Sephardic Jews, who traditionally ate only small amounts of meat due to economic constraints. The Ashkenazic diet is traditionally higher in fat and sodium due to the consumption of foods such as high-fat meats, chicken fat, chopped liver, cream cheese, corned beef, smoked fish, sauerkraut, and pickles. Clearly, foodways of each group of Jewish immigrants have been preserved. Some are beneficial to health, while others should be practiced only occasionally.

ETHNIC DIETS AND PRESENT TRENDS

Only several ethnic diets have been described here; see Table 2–11 for a summary of their advantages and disad-

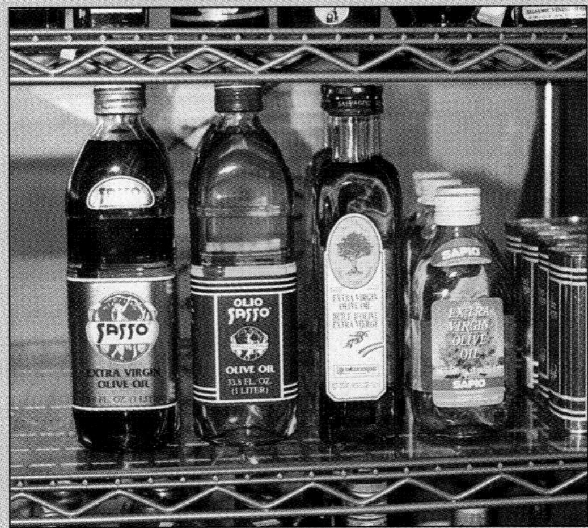

Olive oil is a principal fat source in the Mediterranean diet. Canola oil offers a similar monounsaturated fat composition at a lower price.

vantages. Many other cuisines have also influenced the American diet and new arrivals continue to bring their traditions and foodways to this country. For example, recent social upheavals have increased the immigration of Russians and other Eastern European peoples to the United States. On the other side of the world, continuing unrest in southeast Asia has brought peoples from that area here. Restaurants serving traditional Russian or Thai fare, for instance, are now offering new foodways to those willing to experiment.

Using research also begun many years ago, still other scientists suggest that a healthful diet consists of the inexpensive traditional dishes based on grains, fruits, and vegetables that form the backbone of a number of ethnic cuisines. These are precisely the dishes that people abandon as they become affluent and seek convenience. Simple foods prepared in simple ways have fed most of humanity for virtually its entire existence. As we turn toward a new century, some Americans are rediscovering the simple foods of their respective pasts, learning to enjoy a variety of cuisines, and finding how the positive aspects of each cuisine can contribute to a healthier American diet.

TABLE 2-11

The World's Fare Has Influenced the American Diet

	Advantages	Shortcomings
Native American: Alaskan Native	Variety of seafood, lean wild game; early Native Americans ate variety of vegetables, berries, leaves	High fat content of some meat/seafood; low in calcium
Hispanic-American	Excellent variety of vegetables, legumes, fruits; high in dietary fiber	Traditional Hispanic diet may fall short in calcium; Mexican-American restaurants serve much high-fat fare, rich in sour cream, cheese, and guacamole
Northern European-American	Abundant sources of protein, iron, and calcium from meat and milk groups	Less variety from vegetables, fruits, and legumes; high in fat
African-American	Good variety of carotenoid-containing vegetables; high in dietary fiber. Many variations including Cajun, Creole dishes	Traditional meals high in fat; may fall short in calcium
Asian-American	Excellent variety of vegetables, grains; cooking methods retain nutrients in foods	Some sauces are high in salt and fat; may fall short in calcium
Italian-American	Varies regionally—some regions provide excellent variety of seafood; overall high grain intake, good vegetable and fruit variety	Italian-American restaurants often serve many foods made with high-fat cheese, sauces, and meats; may fall short in calcium
Jewish-American	Good variety of whole-grain products, legumes, and some types of seafood. Many traditions regarding food as an important part of Jewish culture have been retained	Traditional Jewish foods often high in saturated fat and sodium. Limited variety from vegetables and fruits; may fall short on calcium

This is a brief summary of healthful attributes and shortcomings of the ethnic diet influences covered in this Nutrition Issue.

Certain Jewish laws dictate the separation of meat and milk products in a meal as well as in pots and pans used for cooking. In addition, it is important for meat to be completely drained of blood. To be sure that food laws are followed in processing, foods are labeled "kosher," meaning that a rabbi has approved food handling.

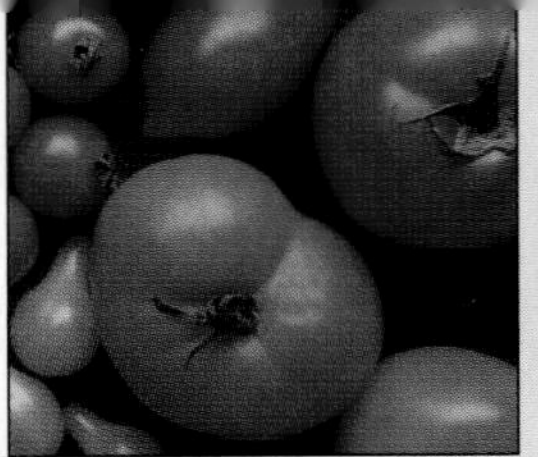

chapter

3

The Human Body
A Nutrition Perspective

Merely eating food won't nourish you. You must first digest the food—in other words, break it down into usable forms of the essential nutrients that can be absorbed into the bloodstream. Once nutrients are taken up by the bloodstream, they can be distributed to body cells.

We rarely think about, let alone control, the digesting and absorbing of foods. Except for a few voluntary responses—such as deciding what and when to eat, how well to chew food, and when to eliminate the remains—most digestion and absorption processes control themselves. We don't consciously decide when the pancreas will secrete digestive substances into the small intestine or how quickly to propel foodstuffs down the intestinal tract. Various hormones and the nervous system mostly control these functions. Your only awareness of these involuntary responses may be a hunger pang right before lunch or a "full" feeling after eating that last slice of pizza.

Let's examine digestion and absorption as part of the study of the human physiology that supports nutritional health. In the process you will become acquainted with the basic anatomy (structure) and physiology (function) that contribute to circulatory, regulatory (control), digestive, excretory, storage, and immune functions of the body.

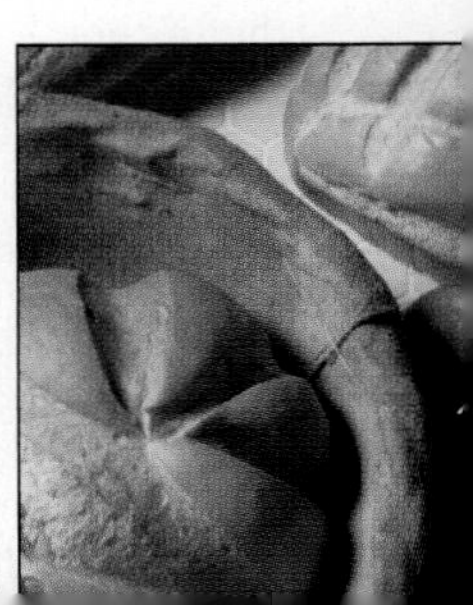

Nutrition Web

The cell is the basic building block of body tissues. Cells combine to form tissues, organs, and organ systems.

The circulatory system carries blood, nutrients, and water to cells.

Blood travels to the lungs to pick up oxygen. It then delivers nutrients, oxygen, and water to cells. These nutrients are exchanged for waste products in the capillaries.

Cells can store only a short-term supply of most nutrients. When the body suffers a nutrient deficiency due to poor diet, it can break down vital tissues to release needed nutrients in many cases. This can lead to poor health, as can an excess intake of any nutrient.

The gastrointestinal (GI) tract is a sort of tube consisting of the mouth, esophagus, stomach, small intestine, large intestine, rectum, and anus.

The liver, gallbladder, and pancreas also contribute to GI tract digestion and absorption by supplying enzymes and bile.

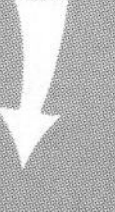

The majority of digestion and absorption of nutrients occur in the small intestine. Some protein digestion (and alcohol absorption) takes place in the stomach, and some plant fiber and remaining starch digestion takes place in the large intestine. Final water and mineral absorption also takes place in the large intestine.

Water-soluble compounds travel from the small intestine to the liver via the portal vein, while fat-soluble compounds travel directly to the bloodstream via the lymphatic system.

Waste products, such as undigested plant fibers and bacteria, are excreted through the rectum. The presence of feces in the rectum encourages elimination.

Other areas for body excretion include the kidneys, skin, and lungs.

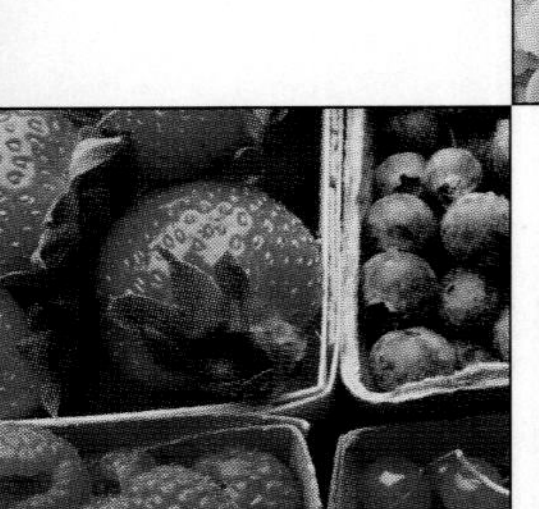

Overview of Body Systems Used in Digestion and Absorption

Many aspects of human anatomy and physiology contribute to nutritional health. In this context the stomach and intestinal tract, part of the gastrointestinal (GI) tract, should quickly come to mind. However, other systems, such as the circulatory system, excretory system, endocrine system, and nervous system, also play key roles. Use of carbohydrate, protein, fat, vitamins, minerals, and water requires input from all these systems (Table 3–1).

From Cells to Organ Systems

Tissue
A group of cells designed to perform a specific function; muscle tissue is an example.

Organ
A group of tissues designed to perform a specific function—for example, the heart. It contains muscle tissue, nerve tissue, and so on.

The various body systems are composed of millions of cells. (See Appendix F for a review of the parts and structure of a cell if you do not recall this from previous course work.) Cells represent the basic building blocks of the body and ultimately form all body structures.

When cells of the same type work together for a common purpose—bound together by intercellular substances—they form **tissues,** such as bone, cartilage, muscle, and nerve. Often two or more tissues combine in a particular way to form more complex **organs,** such as skin, kidneys, and liver. At still higher levels of coordination, several organs can cooperate to achieve a common purpose and form an organ system, such as the respiratory system or the digestive system. The human body is a coordinated unit of many such organ systems and is called an **organism** (Figure 3–1).

TABLE 3-1

Organ Systems of the Body

System	Major Components	Key Functions
Integumentary	Skin, hair, nails, and sweat glands	Protects, regulates temperature, prevents water loss, and produces a substance that converts to vitamin D
Skeletal	Bones, associated cartilage, and joints	Protects, supports, and allows body movement, produces blood cells, and stores minerals
Muscular	Muscles attached to the skeleton	Produces body movement
Nervous	Brain, spinal cord, nerves, and sensory units	Detects sensation, controls movements, controls physiological and intellectual functions
Endocrine	Endocrine glands such as the thyroid gland	Participates in the regulation of metabolism, reproduction, and many other functions
Cardiovascular	Heart, blood vessels, and blood	Transports nutrients, waste products, gases, and hormones throughout the body; plays a role in the immune response and the regulation of body temperature
Lymphatic	Lymph vessels, lymph nodes, and other lymph organs	Removes foreign substances from the blood and lymph, maintains tissue fluid balance, and aids in fat absorption
Respiratory	Lungs and respiratory passages	Exchanges gases (oxygen and carbon dioxide) between the blood and the air and regulates blood acidity
Digestive	Mouth, esophagus, stomach, intestines, and accessory structures	Performs digestion and absorption of nutrients, and elimination of wastes
Urinary	Kidneys, urinary bladder, and the ducts that carry urine	Removes waste products from the circulatory system; helps regulate overall chemical balance and water balance in the body
Reproductive	Gonads, accessory structures, and genitals of males and females	Allows for reproduction

The cardiovascular and lymphatic organ systems contribute to the circulatory functions. The endocrine and nervous organ systems contribute to the regulatory functions. The digestive, urinary, integumentary, and respiratory organ systems contribute to the excretory functions, while the muscular and skeletal organ systems contribute to storage functions in the body. Note, however, that excessive or long-term use of these nutrient stores harms health, such as release of much calcium from bones.

Every cell in the human body performs a specialized job. A cell's master plan for its work is encoded into the cell's genetic material, the **deoxyribonucleic acid (DNA).** The DNA acts as a blueprint for constructing specific proteins required to perform specific tasks in the body. Although most cells in our bodies contain the same DNA information, each cell is programmed to use only the parts of the DNA instructions that apply to its own tasks, depending on the type of tissue it is part of. For example, stomach cells and bone marrow cells receive the same master plan. However, stomach cells use only a subset of the DNA code to make **mucus,** while cells in the bone marrow do not use that part of the DNA code.

Chemical processes occur all the time in every living cell: the chemical synthesis of new substances is balanced by the chemical breakdown of other materials into smaller units. For these reactions to occur, the cell requires a continuous supply of energy and oxygen. Cells also need water, the medium in which they live. Furthermore, they need their own building blocks, especially the materials they can't make themselves—the essential nutrients supplied by food.

Healthful nutrition can supply an adequate amount of nutrients to all body cells. Still, to ensure the best use of these nutrients by cells, the following organ systems must also be healthy and working efficiently.

Deoxyribonucleic acid (DNA)
The site of hereditary information in cells; DNA directs the synthesis of cell proteins.

Mucus
A thick fluid secreted by glands throughout the body. It contains a compound that is both carbohydrate and protein in nature. Mucus acts as both a lubricant and protectant for cells.

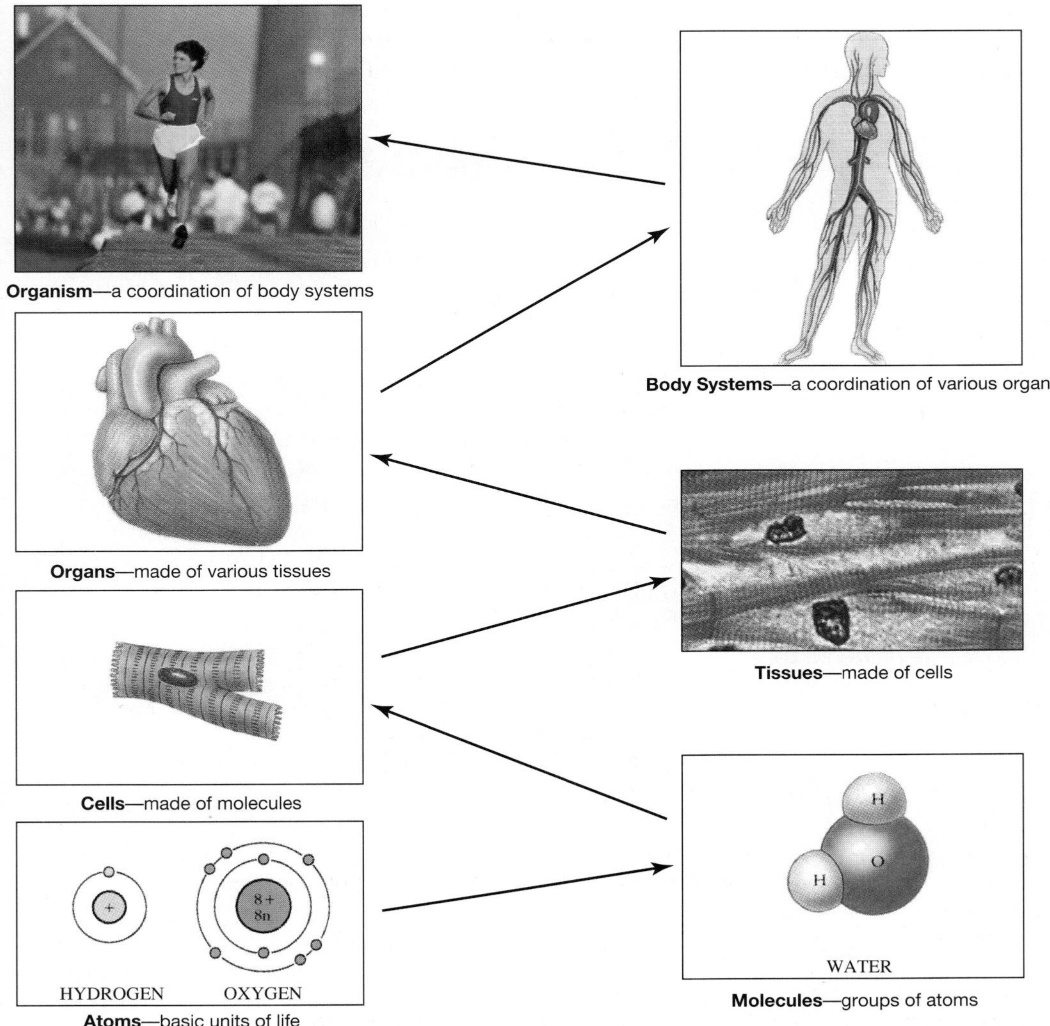

Figure 3-1 *The levels of human biological organization. We are as simple as a collection of atoms and as complex as a whole organism.*

Nutrition Insight

Genetics and Nutrition

The growth, development, and maintenance of cells, and ultimately of the entire organism, are directed by genes present in the cells. The genes contain the codes that control expression of individual traits, such as height, eye color, and susceptibility to many diseases. An individual's genetic risk for a given disease is an important factor, although often not the only factor, in determining whether he or she develops that disease.

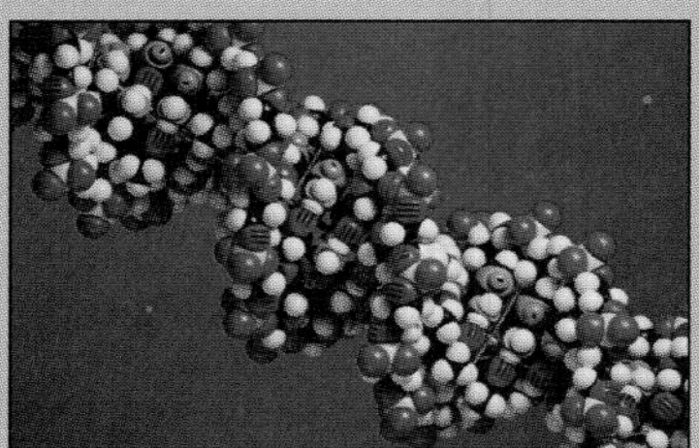

Genes are present on DNA—a double helix. The cell nucleus contains most of the DNA in the body.

Nutritional Diseases with a Genetic Link

Most chronic diseases in which nutrition plays a role are also influenced by genetics. Such diseases include:

- Heart disease (see Chapter 5)
- High blood pressure (see Chapter 8)
- Obesity (see Chapter 9)
- Diabetes (see Chapter 4)
- Cancer (see Chapter 7)
- Osteoporosis (see Chapter 8)
- Metabolic diseases, such as phenylketonuria (PKU; see Chapter 6)

Studies of families, including those with twins and adoptees, provide strong support for the effect of genetics in these disorders. In fact, family history is considered to be one of the important factors in the development of many serious diseases.

Your Genetic Profile

From this brief introduction you can see that a family history of certain diseases raises your risk of developing those diseases. By recognizing your potential for developing a particular disease, you can avoid behavior that contributes to it. For example, women with a family history of breast cancer could take action by not becoming obese, minimizing alcohol use, and obtaining regular mammograms. In general, the more of your relatives who had a genetically transmitted disease and the closer they are related to you, the greater your risk. One way to assess your risk is to put together a family tree of illnesses and deaths by compiling a few key facts on your primary relatives: siblings, parents, aunts and uncles, and grandparents.

Figure 3–2 shows an example of a family tree (also called a genogram). In this family, prostate cancer killed the man's father. This means that the son should be tested regularly for prostate cancer. Because heart disease and stroke are also common in the family, all the children should adopt a lifestyle that minimizes the risk of developing these diseases. Other genetic risk factors should be identified and precautions taken in order to maximize health outcomes.

Genetic Testing

In recent years, human genetics has become a major area of research. With the information gained, scientists have developed ways of testing a person's genes for the likelihood of developing certain diseases. For cases such as Huntington's disease, a degenerative brain disorder, a positive gene test guarantees the eventual development of the disease. However, with diseases such as cancer and Alzheimer's disease, a positive gene test simply indicates a greater risk for developing the disease. In addition to the diseases mentioned, risk factors for birth defects, cystic fibrosis, certain forms of muscular dystrophy, and a host of other diseases can be detected through genetic testing.

Benefits of genetic testing include the potential for more individualized nutrition and health advice, more informed decisions by couples attempting to have children (i.e., alternatives such as adoption or therapeutic abortion), and the ability to appropriately plan for the future. However, it is not possible, given the resources presently allocated to medical care in America, to identify all people at genetic risk for the major chronic diseases and other health problems. And, in almost all cases, there is no way to cure a specific gene alteration—only the health problems that result can be treated. Thus, the wisdom of genetic testing in many cases is an open question. Perhaps preventive measures and careful scrutiny for the specific genetically linked diseases in one's family would suffice.

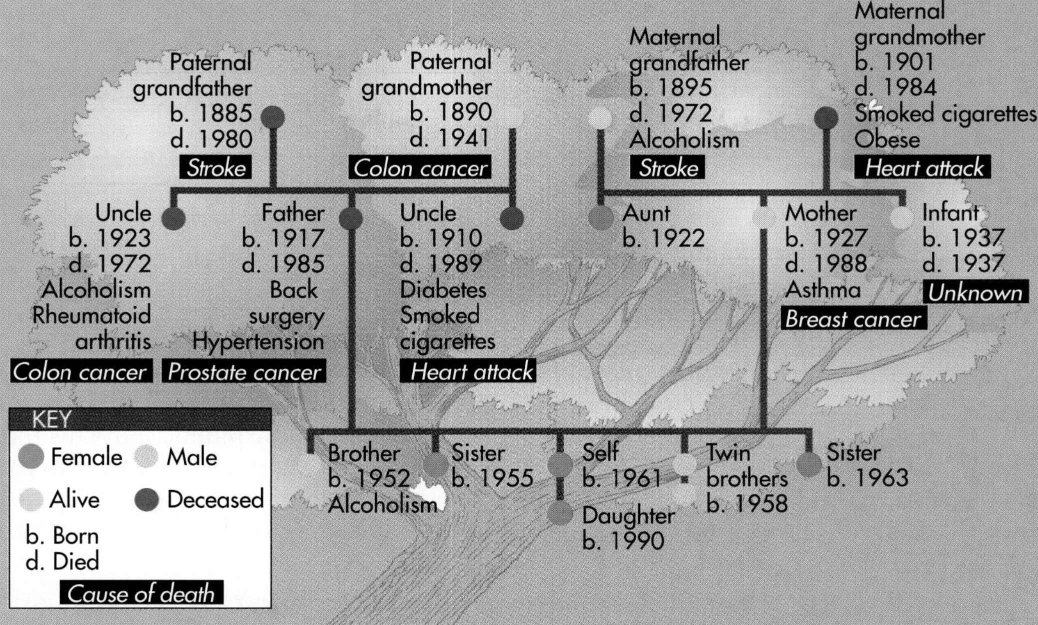

Figure 3–2 *Example of a family tree. Create your family tree of frequent diseases, age, and cause of death, using the example here as a guide. Then show your tree to your physician to get a full picture of what the information means for your health.*

Researchers also worry that people who are found to have genetic alterations that increase disease risk may face job and insurance discrimination. This also is a concern of many who contemplate being tested. Testing positive could also lead to unnecessary radical treatment. As well, a seemingly hopeless diagnosis could result in depression or withdrawal from life when a cure is out of reach.

Consider the following situations with regard to genetic testing.

- Using the family tree such as in Figure 3–2, you realize that colon cancer runs in your family. Knowing that the mortality rate for colon cancer is quite high, would you be tested for the colon cancer gene (note: this gene does not guarantee colon cancer, but does indicate greater risk)? What implications would affect your decision?
- You as a female (or your female partner, if you are a male) carry the breast cancer genes BRAC1 or BRAC2, or have a family history of breast cancer. Would you consider mastectomies to try to make sure the disease does not develop? This has been shown to be effective therapy, reducing risk of breast cancer and death by 90%. However, even many high risk women never actually develop the disease.
- You and your (future) spouse would like to have children. You know that cystic fibrosis runs in your family and would like to be tested as a carrier. It turns out that both you and your spouse carry the gene for cystic fibrosis. Any offspring have a 1 in 4 chance of having the fatal disease. How would this affect your decision to have a child? How would your decision change if you (or your spouse) were already pregnant?

In the final analysis, would you rather know if you were at high risk for a specific disease that a genetic test could point out? If so, ask your physician about the possibility and wisdom of testing you for the genetically linked diseases in your family tree. You may be referred to a genetic counselor who can help you make your decision. Also, be aware that throughout this book discussions will point out how you can personalize nutrition advice based on your genetic background. In this way, you can identify and avoid the "controllable" risk factors that would contribute to development of genetically linked diseases present in your family.

The following web links will help you gather more information about genetic conditions and testing:

Alliance of Genetic Support Groups
http://medhlp.netusa.net/www/agsg.htm
Genetic Conditions and Rare Conditions Information
http://www.kumc.edu/gec/support/groups.html
March of Dimes Genetics Site
http://www.modimes.org/pub/genetics.htm
Genetics information from the National Cancer Institute
http://cancernet.nci.nih.gov/p_genetics.html
Understanding Gene Testing
http://www.gene.com/ae/AE/AEPC/NIH/index.html
Human Genome Project Information
http://www.ornl.gov/techresources/human_genome/publicat/publications.html

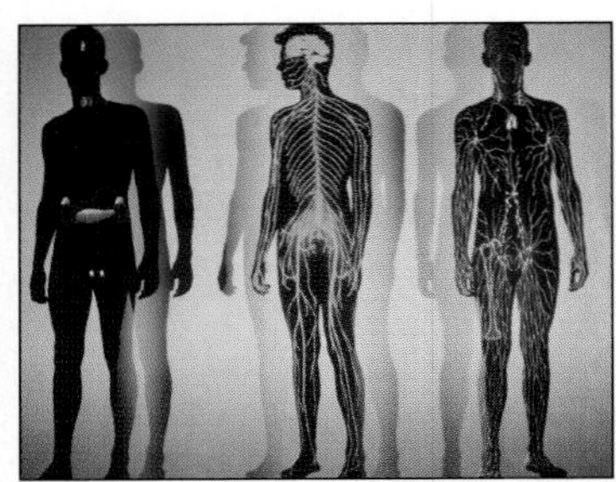

The body is made up of numerous organ systems.

Circulatory System

Blood travels two basic routes. In the first route it circulates from the right side of the heart, through the lungs, and then back to the heart (the pulmonary circuit). Then, in the second route the blood later circulates between the left side of the heart and all other body parts, eventually returning back to the right side of the heart (the systemic circuit) (Figure 3–3). The heart is a muscular pump that normally contracts and relaxes 50 to 90 times per minute while the body is at rest. This continuous pumping keeps blood moving through the circuits.

The circulatory system distributes nutrients yielded from digestion and absorption, along with oxygen from the air, to all body cells. All blood goes to the lungs to pick up oxygen and release carbon dioxide. The oxygenated blood then returns to the heart to be pumped to all other body tissues. In the capillaries, which are made up of a network of tiny blood vessels, cells exchange nutrients and wastes with the blood. That is, cells empty their waste products into the blood and take nutrients from it. Capillaries service every region of the body via individual capillary beds that are only one cell layer thick. Nutrients, gases, and other substances can pass through capillary cells to both enter into and exit out of other body cells.

Portal and Lymphatic Circulation Plays an Important Role in Nutrient Absorption

Fluids and particles, once absorbed through the intestinal wall, travel one of two different routes. One pathway is the bloodstream. As just noted, the blood—laden with oxygen and nutrients—leaves the heart and enters the arteries. Some of this blood travels to the intestine and ends up in capillary beds inside the intestine. From there, some nutrients are taken up by intestinal cells for nourishment, whereas much of the nutrients from recently eaten foods transfers into the bloodstream. The actual transfer points are the capillary beds. The blood then passes into veins and eventually collects in a very large vein, called the **portal vein** (see Figure 3–3). This vein leads directly to the liver. Note that most veins in the body double back directly to the heart. However, by going first to the liver, the portal vein enables the liver to process absorbed nutrients before they enter the general circulation of the bloodstream. Water-soluble nutrients—such as glucose and amino acids—enter the bloodstream through this portal vein.

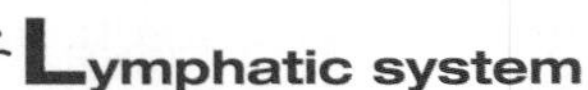

Lymphatic system
A system of vessels that can accept fluid surrounding cells and large particles, such as products of fat absorption. This lymph fluid eventually passes into the bloodstream via the lymphatic system.

The **lymphatic system** is the other system of circulatory vessels that serves the body. It carries lymph, which is mostly composed of a clear fluid that forms between cells (see Figure 3–3). This fluid filters into tiny lymphatic vessels composing a one-way network that funnels lymph from all over the body into large lymphatic vessels. From these vessels, the lymph fluid empties into major veins returning to the heart. The lymphatic system thereby serves as a second route to return fluids that emanate from the capillaries to the circulatory system.

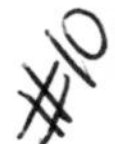

Lymphatic vessels that serve the small intestine play an important role in nutrition. These vessels pick up and transport the majority of products yielded from fat absorption. These products are too large to enter the bloodstream directly. The lymphatic vessels from the intestine drain into a large duct that connects with the bloodstream through a vein near the neck. Most of the absorbed fat products eventually enter the bloodstream in this way.

Regulatory (Control) Systems

The hormonal and nervous systems have regulatory functions that greatly influence nutrient use in the body. The term *hormone* comes from the Greek word for "to stir or excite." To be a true hormone, a regulatory compound must have a specific synthesis site from which it enters the bloodstream to reach target cells.

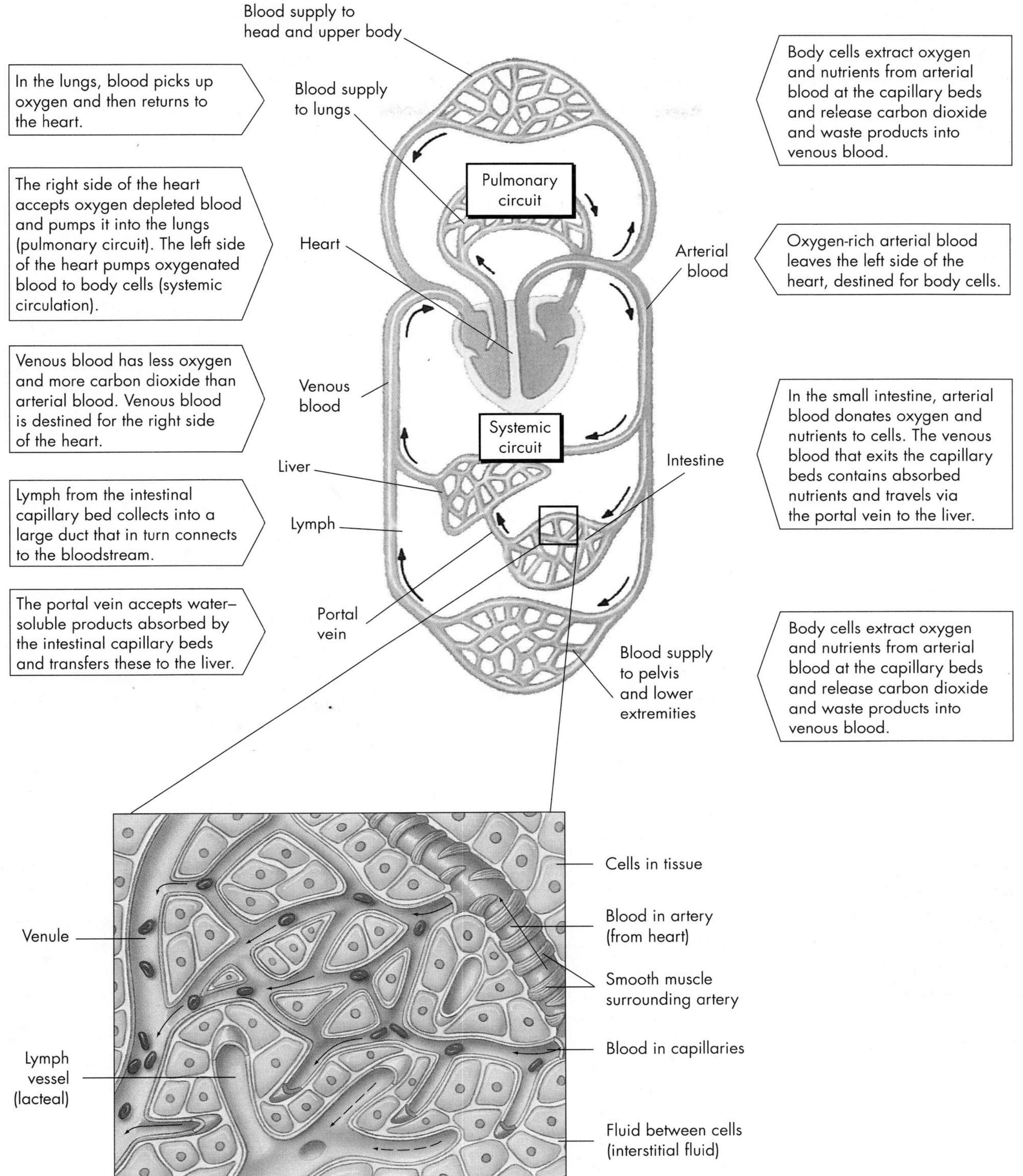

Figure 3–3 *Blood circulation throughout the body. This represents the route blood takes through the two circuits that begin and end at the heart. For proper orientation, temporarily place this figure across your chest. The red color indicates blood that is richer in oxygen; blue is for blood carrying more carbon dioxide. Oxygen and nutrients are exchanged for carbon dioxide and waste products in the capillaries, the points at which the arteries and veins merge. The bottom box shows a close up of a capillary bed in the small intestine, including the location of the lymphatic vessels. This second set of circulatory vessels—part of the lymphatic system—picks up fluid that builds up between cells (interstitial fluid) and large particles, such as some fats and some cells. This becomes lymph, which travels through further lymph vessels to reach the bloodstream. Lymph vessels in the intestine are also called* lacteals.

TABLE 3-2

Important Secretions and Products of the Digestive Tract

Secretion	Site of production	Purpose
Saliva	Mouth	Contributes to starch digestion, lubrication
Mucus	Mouth, stomach, small intestine, large intestine	Protects cells, lubricates
Enzymes	Mouth, stomach, small intestine, pancreas	Promote digestion of foodstuffs into particles small enough for absorption
Acid	Stomach	Promotes digestion of protein among other functions
Bile	Liver (stored in gallbladder)	Suspends fat in water to aid fat digestion in the small intestine
Bicarbonate	Pancreas and small intestine	Neutralizes stomach acid when it reaches the small intestine
Hormones	Stomach, small intestine	Stimulate production and/or release of acid, enzymes, bile, and bicarbonate; help regulate peristalsis and overall GI tract flow

The hormone insulin helps control the amount of glucose in the blood, and thyroid hormones help control the body's metabolic rate. Other hormones are especially important in regulating digestive processes, such as the hormone gastrin, which is produced in the stomach (Table 3–2).

Many hormone-like compounds also control important aspects of GI tract function. These compounds diffuse from GI tract cells or nerve endings to act on nearby cells. Many of these hormone-like compounds are found in both the intestine and the brain. When a person thinks about eating or prepares to eat, the whole GI tract begins to prime itself for action. Hormone-like substances participate in this process.

Secrete
To produce and then release a substance, generally called a secretion, from a cell into the body.

Nervous system input is also important for the GI tract. Nerves influence acid **secretion** in the stomach and regulate intestinal muscle action. The senses of sight, hearing, touch, smell, and taste all use nerve pathways to communicate information—such as the availability of food or the need for it—to the brain. Some nutrients are important in nerve functioning, especially the vitamins thiamin and niacin.

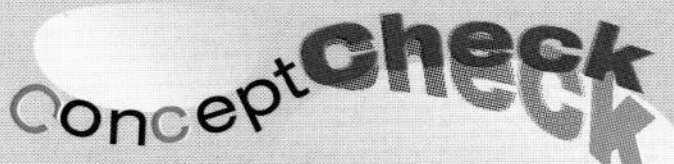

Digestion and absorption require the coordinated efforts of many body systems. These processes aid in supplying energy, oxygen, water, and essential nutrients to all body cells. The circulatory and lymphatic systems transport nutrients throughout the body. The hormonal and nervous systems have regulatory (control) functions that help direct nutrient use and the digestive process.

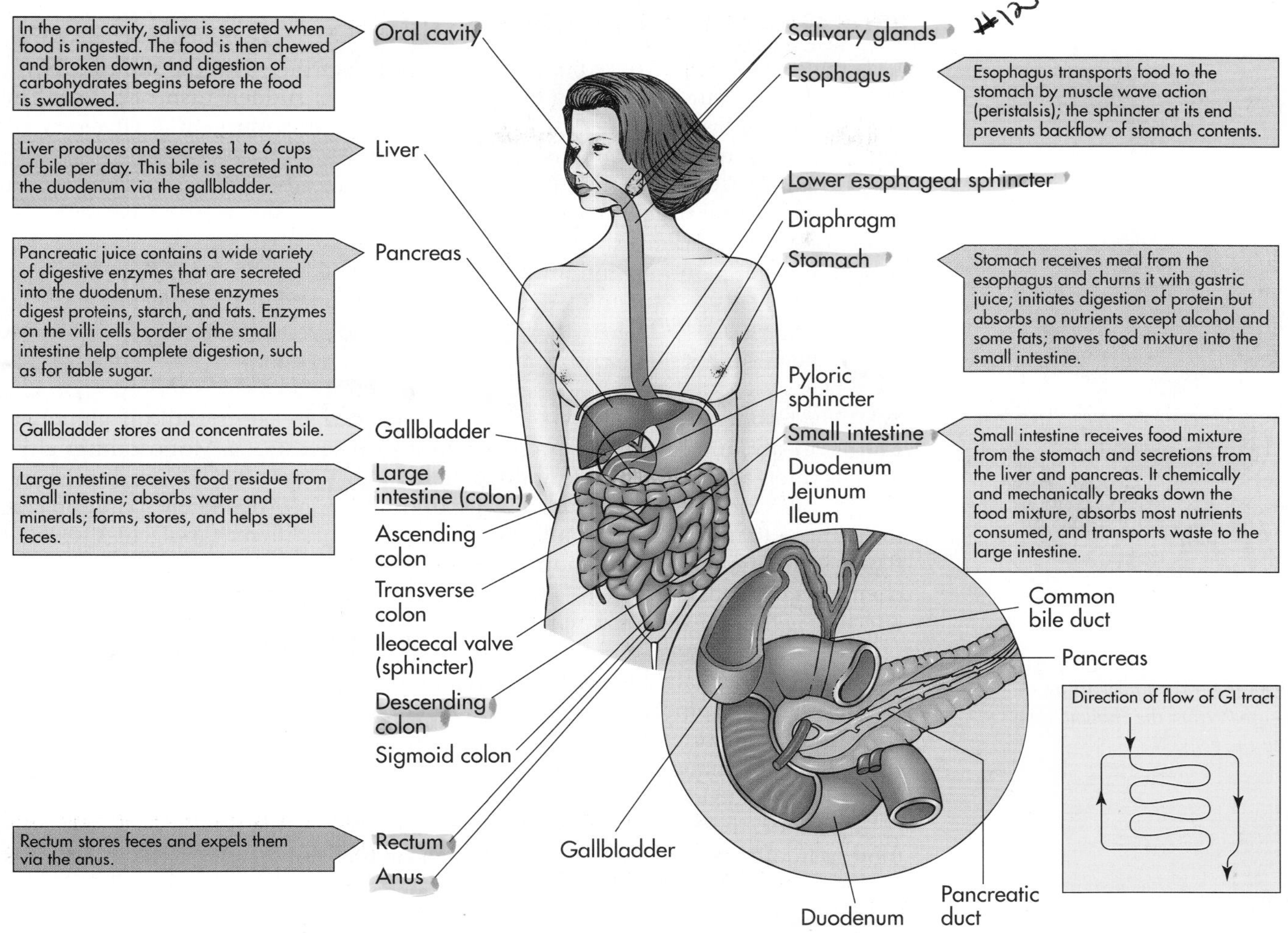

Figure 3–4 *Physiology of the GI tract. Many organs cooperate in a regulated fashion to allow digestion and subsequent absorption of nutrients in foods.*

The Anatomy and Physiology of Digestion

The gastrointestinal (GI) tract is the site of nutrient **digestion** and later of absorption. This long hollow tube stretches from the mouth to the anus (Figure 3–4). Nutrients from the food we eat must pass through the walls of this tube—from the inside to the outside—to be absorbed into the bloodstream. The GI tract promotes digestion and absorption through a variety of functions: it simultaneously moves and mixes foods (as part of a process called *motility*). The GI tract also secretes chemical substances to promote the breakdown of foods. Finally, the GI tract eliminates wastes. Adding to this, the GI tract promotes nutrient production; the bacteria living in the intestine make vitamin K and the vitamin biotin, which we can then use. Most of these processes are under autonomic control; that is, they are involuntary. Almost all functions involved in digestion and absorption are controlled by hormones, hormone-like compounds, and nerves.

Digestion
The process whereby food is broken down into forms that can be taken up by the GI tract.

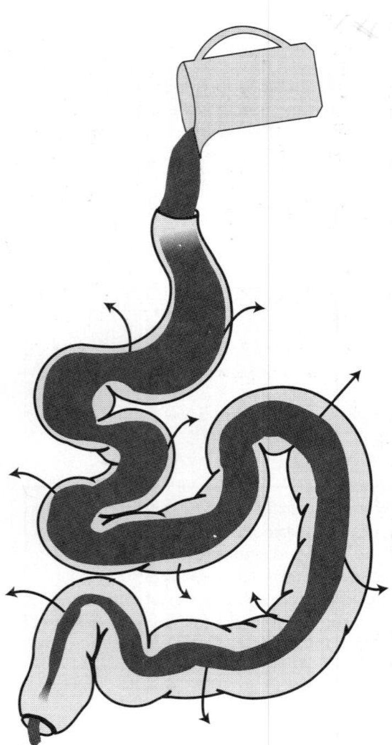

As the intestinal contents pass down the tract, nutrients are absorbed from the "hollow tube" into the body.

The Flow of Digestion

Let's review the major body parts of the GI tract, starting with the mouth. As you put food into your mouth, the typical response is a sudden rush of **saliva.** This saliva, secreted by special glands in the mouth, contains mucus that envelops and lubricates each morsel, easing its passage down the GI tract (see Table 3–2). Saliva also contains specific enzymes that break down large carbohydrates into small units (see Figure 3–7 on page 85). Chewing then breaks food into small pieces, exposing more food surface to digestive action. The more surface exposed, the more efficient digestion is in the mouth and throughout the entire GI tract as well. This shows the importance of also maintaining dental health, as it contributes to nutritional health.

The tongue aids chewing and also contains taste sensors for sweet, salt, sour and bitter. The sweet and salt sensors are near the tip of the tongue; the sour are along the edges; and bitter sensors are near the back. A fifth taste sensation called ***umami*** has been proposed. This taste sensation is elicited by monosodium glutamate. Brothy, meaty, and savory are examples of umami sensations. Monosodium glutamate is often added to Chinese and Japanese foods to enhance the umami flavor.

Umami
A brothy, meaty, savory flavor in some foods. Monosodium glutamate enhances this flavor when added to foods.

The sensation of flavor is aided by input from the approximately 6 million **cells** in the nose that can detect hundreds of thousands of different molecules. Overall, flavor is a complex combination of taste, smell, physical sensations from certain chemicals in foods (such as in chili peppers), and textural sensations. Flavor is also affected by human genetic variability in both taste and nasal sensations.

The mouth and stomach are connected by a tube called the *esophagus*. At its top is a flap of tissue (called the *epiglottis*) that prevents food from being swallowed into the trachea (windpipe). During swallowing, food lands on the flap, folding it down to cover the opening of the trachea. Breathing also automatically stops. These responses ensure that swallowed food will only travel down the esophagus. This uses muscular contractions by the esophagus, as well as lubricating mucus and gravity.

The food then enters the stomach, which can hold approximately 4 cups of food or liquid. Note that a child has a much smaller stomach capacity, and so must eat more frequently than an adult.

Only proteins are significantly digested in the stomach. This protein digestion proceeds as the stomach secretes acid and enzymes to help break down the food and slowly churns these into the food. (Later sections discuss the role of acid and enzymes in the digestive process in detail.) A meal usually leaves the stomach within 2 to 4 hours after eating. The stomach performs the important duty of slowly releasing or "squirting" small amounts of food into the small intestine. In this way, the body prevents too much food from reaching the small intestine at one time. Solids take longer than liquids to leave the stomach, and a fat meal usually leaves later than a meal containing mostly protein or carbohydrate.

The considerable length of the small intestine (about 10 feet) provides ample opportunity for digestion to occur. The small intestine is then divided into three sections: the first part, the duodenum, is about 10 inches long; the middle segment, the jejunum, is about 4 feet long; and the last section, the ileum, is about 5 feet long. The small intestine is considered small because of its narrow (1 inch) diameter. Most digestion is completed in the duodenum and upper jejunum, with the help of enzymes made by intestinal cells and the pancreas.

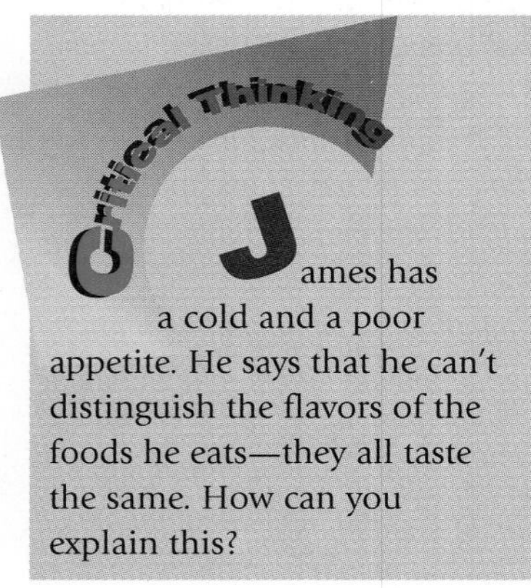

James has a cold and a poor appetite. He says that he can't distinguish the flavors of the foods he eats—they all taste the same. How can you explain this?

Muscular contractions constantly mix the food in the small intestine. This churning enhances digestive action because it exposes more food surface to enzyme action. A meal remains in the small intestine about 3 to 10 hours. About 95% of a total meal has been digested by the time it leaves.

From the small intestine, food is moved into the large intestine, also called the ***colon.*** This organ is about 3½ feet long and is separated into five sections: the cecum, ascending colon, transverse colon, descending colon, and sigmoid colon. Bacteria in the large intestine digest mostly leftover plant fibers. Little else remains to be digested. The food remnants and wastes stay in the large intestine for about 24 to 72 hours before being eliminated.

The large intestine ends in a cavity called the *rectum,* which connects to the anus, the end of the GI tube. These final sections work with the large intestine to prepare the feces for elimination.

As mentioned before, other organs associated with the GI tract aid digestion in the small intestine (see Figure 3–4 and Table 3–1). The liver secretes **bile** needed to digest fat. The body stores bile in the gallbladder until it is needed. Bile helps suspend fat in the watery digestive mixture, making the fat more available to the digestive processes. This process is analogous to the way dishwashing liquid breaks up oil spots in dishwater.

The pancreas secretes enzymes that aid digestion, and bicarbonate (the chemical in baking soda) to neutralize the acid produced earlier in the stomach. Ducts leading from the pancreas and gallbladder merge, allowing the pancreatic juices and bile to blend as they are released into the upper small intestine for digestion. In this way the liver, pancreas, and gallbladder work with the GI tract.

Most foods we eat consist of carbohydrates, protein, and fat. Our bodies break down each of these nutrients in a different way.

GI Tract Control Valves: Sphincters

A variety of ringlike muscles form valves, called ***sphincters,*** are spaced at various points along the GI tract (Figure 3–5). Sphincters retard or prevent backflow of partially digested food. These sphincters respond to various stimuli, such as signals from the nervous system, hormones, acid versus alkaline conditions, and the pressure that builds up around sphincters. A sphincter in the lower esophagus (lower esophageal sphincter) is critical in preventing backflow of stomach contents up into the esophagus. If highly acidic stomach contents come in contact with the esophagus, they can cause pain, known as **heartburn.** Another sphincter (pyloric sphincter), located at the base of the stomach, controls the flow of processed foodstuffs from the stomach into the small intestine, as described earlier.

At the end of the small intestine, another sphincter (typically called the *ileocecal sphincter*) prevents the contents of the large intestine from reentering the small intestine. At the end of the large intestine are two final anal sphincters, one of which is under voluntary control. Once children are toilet trained, they can generally determine when the outer anal sphincter will relax and when it will stay rigid, in turn affecting whether elimination occurs. Relaxation of the sphincter allows for elimination.

GI Tract Propulsion: Peristalsis

Food is moved down the GI tract mainly by a wavelike process called ***peristalsis.*** A snake swallowing its prey illustrates the process. Groups of muscles encircle the GI tract, whereas other groups run along its length (see Figure 3–5). When food is swallowed, coordinated squeezing and shortening by the muscle groups in the esophagus create the first waves. In the stomach, the same muscle action creates a mixing and grinding motion. The most active peristaltic waves occur in the small intestine, about every 4 to 5 seconds (Figure 3–6). In contrast, the large intestine has very sluggish peristalsis, using occasional large contractions to help eliminate the feces.

Enzymes Play a Vital Role in Digestion

As noted earlier, enzymes are critical to digestion. These substances bring specific chemicals close together and then create an environment that allows these to

Bile
A substance secreted by the liver and stored in the gallbladder; it is released into the small intestine to aid fat absorption by suspending fat in tiny droplets within a watery fluid.

Sphincter
A muscular valve; these valves help control the flow of foodstuffs in the GI tract.

Heartburn
A pain arising from the esophagus caused by stomach acid backing up into the esophagus and irritating its tissue.

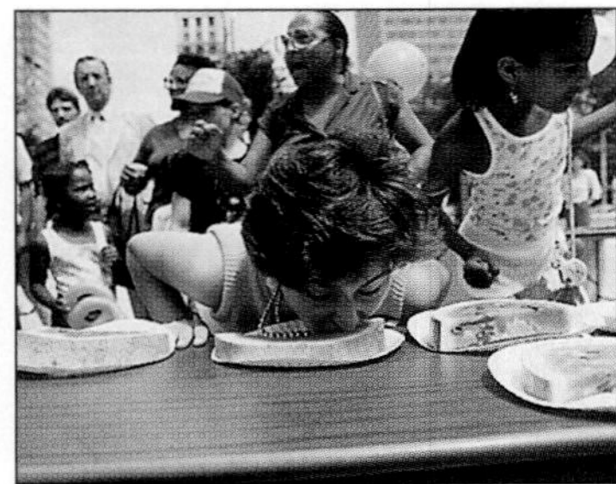

The GI tract is ready for what we call on it to do—snack or gorge.

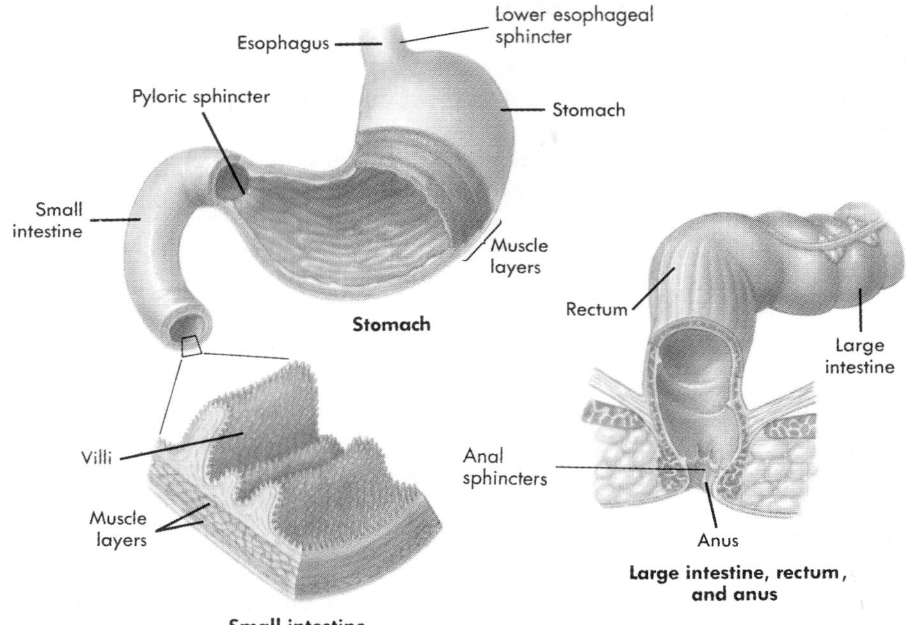

Figure 3–5 *A close-up view of the intestinal tract—muscles, sphincters, and villi. These features of the GI tract perform key roles in digestion, absorption, and elimination.*

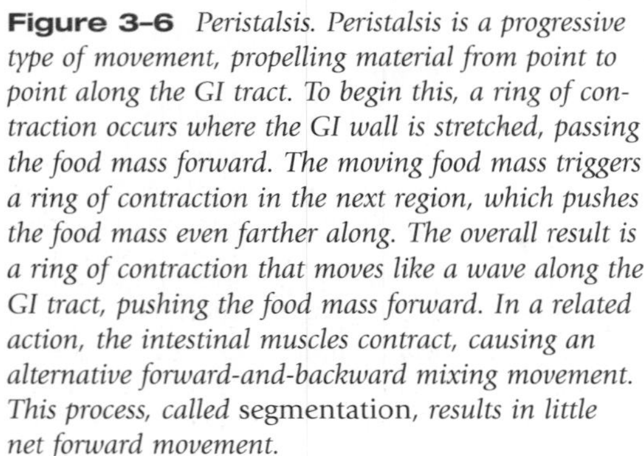

Figure 3–6 *Peristalsis. Peristalsis is a progressive type of movement, propelling material from point to point along the GI tract. To begin this, a ring of contraction occurs where the GI wall is stretched, passing the food mass forward. The moving food mass triggers a ring of contraction in the next region, which pushes the food mass even farther along. The overall result is a ring of contraction that moves like a wave along the GI tract, pushing the food mass forward. In a related action, the intestinal muscles contract, causing an alternative forward-and-backward mixing movement. This process, called* segmentation, *results in little net forward movement.*

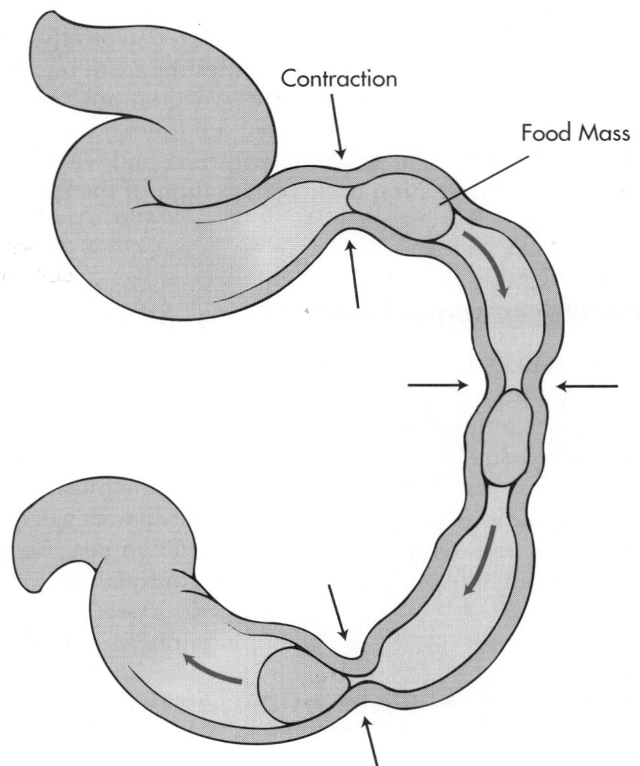

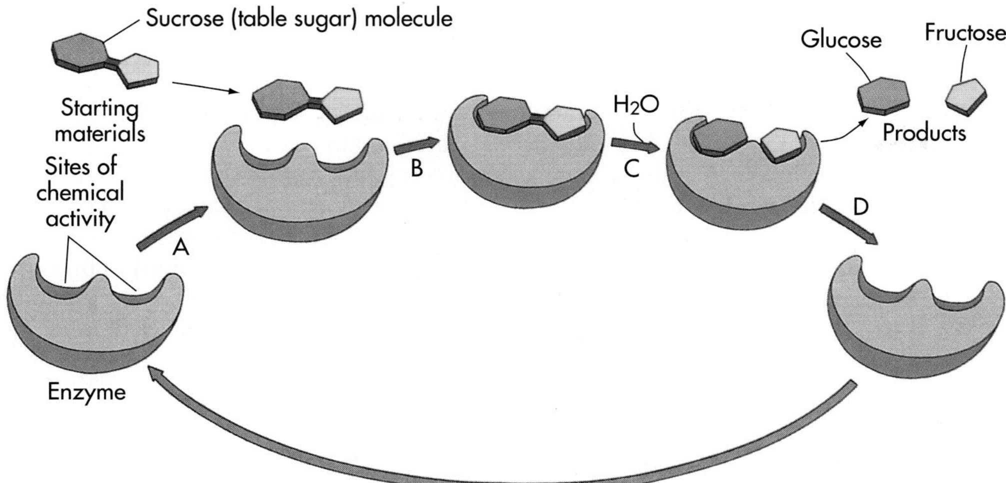

Figure 3-7 *A model of enzyme action. Enzymes act as catalysts to speed chemical reactions, including those that contribute to the digestion of foodstuffs. In this example an enzyme is contributing to the breakdown of sucrose (from* **A** *to* **D***) into the smaller sugar forms glucose and fructose. Only these smaller sugar forms are absorbed from the small intestine to enter the bloodstream. Note that with some enzymes the action can go both ways. In addition, sometimes energy input is needed to allow the enzyme to push the reaction along.*

change in structure (Figure 3–7). Almost every chemical process in the body, including the digestion of food, requires an enzyme to hasten the event. Figure 3–7 shows how an enzyme contributes to the breakdown of table sugar (sucrose) into the smaller sugars glucose and fructose. Only the latter sugars are absorbed from the GI tract. The pancreas and small intestine produce most digestive enzymes. A few are secreted by the mouth and stomach.

Each type of enzyme can speed only one specific type of chemical process. For example, enzymes that recognize and digest table sugar ignore milk sugar (lactose). The body can even increase the synthesis of certain digestive enzymes in response to the type of diet consumed—for example, producing more fat-digesting enzymes in response to a high-fat diet. Besides working only on particular types of chemicals, enzymes are sensitive to acid and alkaline conditions, temperature, and the types of vitamins (acting **coenzymes**) and minerals they require. Digestive enzymes that work in the acid environment of the stomach do not work well in the alkaline (basic) environment of the small intestine.

Coenzyme
The active form of many vitamins; the coenzyme aids enzyme function.

ConceptCheck

The gastrointestinal (GI) tract consists of the mouth, esophagus, stomach, small intestine, large intestine (colon), rectum, and anus. Organs that assist in digestion and absorption are the liver, gallbladder, and pancreas. Together these organs perform the digestion needed to extract nutrients from food and funnel them into the bloodstream. In the GI tract, peristalsis propels food from the esophagus to the anus. During this journey, digestion is aided by enzymes produced by the mouth, stomach, pancreas, and small intestine cells. The transit time between eating food and eventually eliminating the indigestible remains is usually about 1 to 3 days.

In cystic fibrosis—an inherited disease of infants, children, and sometimes adults—the pancreas often develops thick mucus that blocks its ducts, and active cells then die. As a result, the pancreas is not able to effectively deliver its digestive enzymes into the small intestine. Digestion of carbohydrate, protein, and—most notably—fat then is impaired. Often the missing enzymes must be ingested in capsule form with meals to aid in digestion.

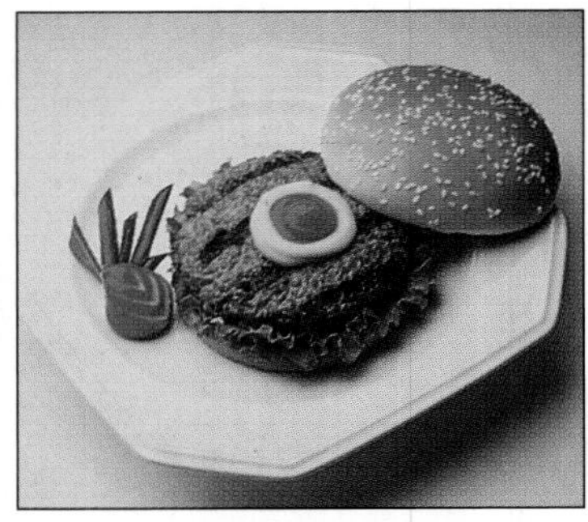

The body digests the foods presented—the order in which foods are eaten plays no role. You can eat the bun and then the burger, or both at the same time.

A Closer Look at the Digestive Process

Even before we eat a morsel of many foods, the work of digestion—the breakdown of foods into usable forms we can absorb—is often already partially accomplished. Cooking or other preparations, such as marinating, pounding, or dicing, have probably begun the process. Starch granules in foods swell as they soak up water during cooking, making them much easier to digest. Cooking also softens the tough connective tissues in meats and the fibrous tissue of plants, such as is found in broccoli stalks. As a result, the food is easier to chew, swallow, and break down during later digestion. As you will see in Chapter 15 cooking also makes many foods, such as eggs, meats, fish, and poultry, much safer to eat.

Key Digestive Processes in the Stomach

The key digestive process that takes place in the stomach is protein digestion. The stomach secretes an enzyme used for protein digestion. Hormones and stimulus from the brain control this enzyme's release.

You might wonder how the stomach protects itself from the enzymes (and acid) it produces. First the stomach has a thick layer of mucus that lines and insulates it from the acid and enzymes produced for digestion. The production of acid and enzymes is also tied to the release of a specific hormone, and this release happens primarily when we are thinking about eating or actually in the process of eating. Lastly, as the concentration of acid in the stomach increases, acid production tapers off, also because of hormonal control.

Chyme
A mixture of stomach secretions and partially digested food.

Ulcer
Erosion of the tissue lining in either the stomach or upper small intestine; generally referred to as a peptic ulcer.

Key Digestive Processes in the Small Intestine

All liquids consumed with a meal combine with stomach acid to form a very watery food mixture called ***chyme.*** As chyme squirts into the upper small intestine (the *duodenum*), the acid in the chyme triggers the release of another hormone that stimulates the pancreas to release bicarbonate. This neutralizes the acid. If the chyme is not neutralized, it corrodes the wall of the duodenum, and could quickly lead to an **ulcer,** because, unlike the stomach, the small intestine lacks a protective layer of mucus. This form of protection is not possible because it would impede nutrient absorption. A second hormone causes the pancreas and gallbladder to release their products—enzymes from the pancreas and bile from the gallbladder.

Another Bite

In part because of hormonal fine-tuning, the digestive tract responds to the nutritional makeup and amount of the food consumed. Foods generally contain a mixture of macronutrients and vitamins and minerals; therefore a multiple enzymatic attack on the contents of the small intestine is the rule. The contention of the authors of some fad diet books that ingestion of certain combinations of foods, such as meats and fruits together, hinders the digestive process does not make sense in light of both our knowledge about gastrointestinal physiology and our collective experience.

FRANK & ERNEST® by Bob Thaves

M.D.
I DON'T SEEM TO BE DIGESTING MY FOOD.
THEN WHO IS?
THAVES 7-29
© 1991 by NEA, Inc.

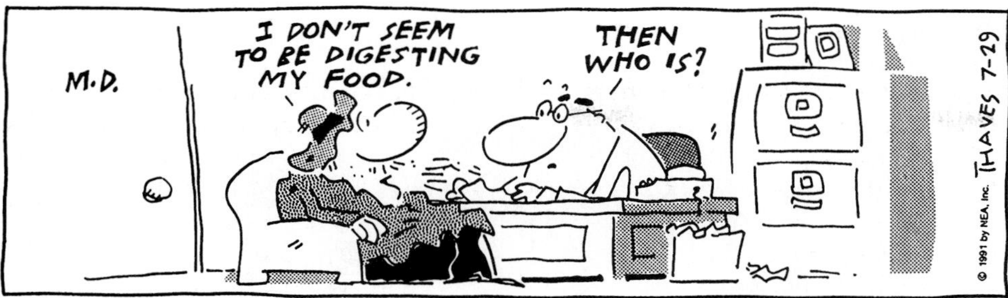

Figure 3-8 *Frank and Ernest.*

Small Intestine: Site for Most Nutrient Absorption

Most nutrient absorption—that is, the transfer of nutrients from the intestine and to the bloodstream—occurs in the small intestine; little occurs in the stomach and large intestine. The small intestine can absorb about 95% of the energy it receives in the form of protein, carbohydrate, fat, and alcohol (see Figure 3–8). This list does not include dietary fiber since it can't be digested by the stomach or small intestine.

The mouth and stomach absorb only water, some alcohol, certain types of minor fats, and some glucose. (Many medications are designed to allow for absorption in the stomach as well.) The large intestine absorbs some minerals, water, and some fat and carbohydrate by-products (produced by bacterial action).

The enormous surface area of the small intestine promotes efficient nutrient absorption. The wall of the small intestine is folded, and within the folds are fingerlike projections called ***villi*** (see Figure 3–5). These "fingers" are in constant movement, which helps trap foodstuffs between them to enhance absorption. Each villus "finger" is made up of numerous absorptive cells, and each of these cells has a highly folded cap. The combined folds, fingers, and folded caps in the small intestine increase its surface area 600 times beyond that of a simple tube.

Villi
Fingerlike protrusions in the small intestine that participate in digestion and absorption of foodstuffs.

New absorptive cells are constantly produced and appear daily along the surface of each villus "finger," probably because absorptive cells are subjected to a harsh environment. This environment demands constant renewal of the intestinal lining, and it leads to a high nutrient demand from the small intestine. The health of these cells is further enhanced by the various hormones and other substances that participate in or are produced as part of the digestive process.

ANOTHER Bite

Cancer treatments often involve the use of medications (chemotherapy) to prevent rapid cell growth. Cancer cell growth is the intended target. However, although the medications can slow the growth of rapidly dividing cancer cells, they also affect other body cells that normally reproduce rapidly, such as the absorptive cells in the small intestine. This is the reason that diarrhea is a common side effect of chemotherapy.

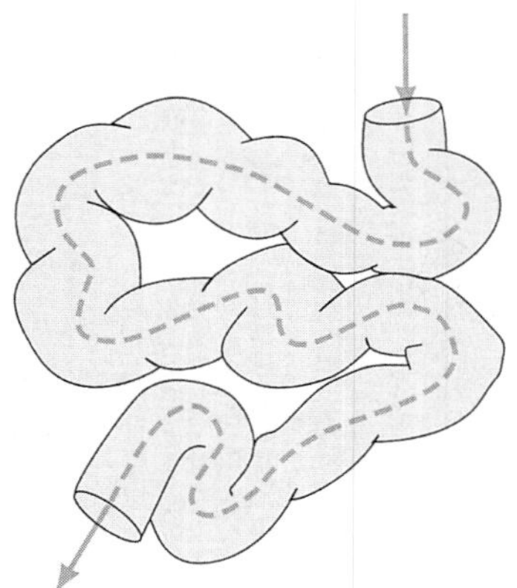

Lumen: The inside of a tube, such as the inside cavity of the GI tract.

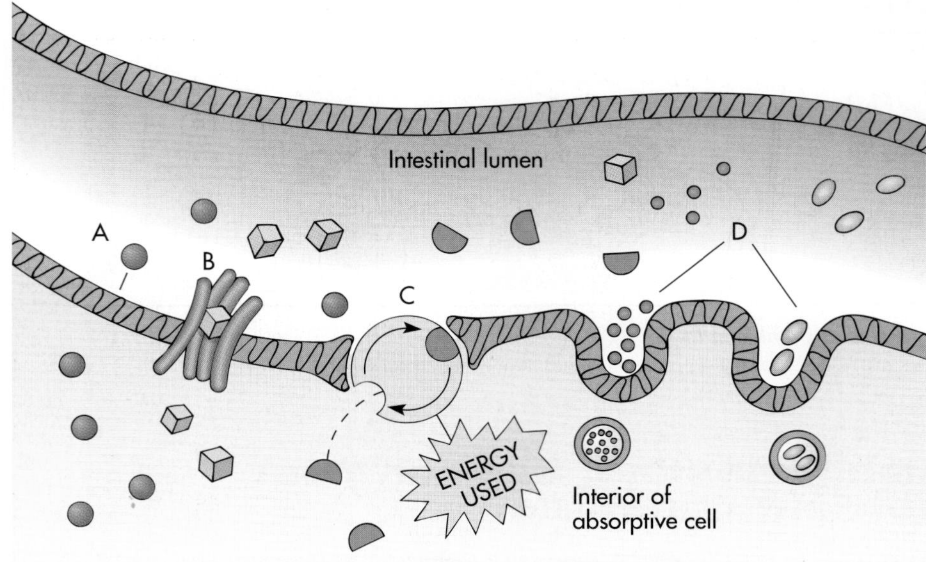

Figure 3-9 *Nutrient absorption relies on these major forms of absorptive processes.* **A,** *Passive absorption involves simple diffusion of substances across the cell membrane of absorptive cells. No energy is expended because the substances follow a favorable concentration gradient (from high to low concentrations). Water and fats are absorbed in this manner.* (**B,** *Facilitated absorption [not described in the chapter] uses a carrier protein or other process to aid in absorption of specific substances, such as fructose, but no energy is expended; the process is simply aided by the carrier.)* **C,** *Active absorption uses a carrier protein and expends energy in the process. The use of energy allows the absorptive cells to absorb nutrients against their concentration gradient (from low to high concentrations). Glucose undergoes active absorption.* **D,** *Phagocytsis—"cell eating" involves cells taking in substances, including whole particles, by forming an indentation in the cell membrane and then surrounding the particle, with eventual incorporation into the cell. This is an active form of transport of substances. Pinocytosis—"cell drinking" involves cellular uptake of liquids in a manner analogous to phagocytosis.*

Types and Means of Absorption

The small intestine absorbs nutrients into the intestinal cells through various means and processes. When the nutrient concentration is higher in the inside cavity **(lumen)** of the small intestine than in the **absorptive cells,** the difference in nutrient concentration drives absorption because nutrients naturally move from higher to lower concentrations. Fats and other nutrients now enter the absorptive cells from the lumen of the small intestine via a **passive absorption** route with the concentration difference driving the process. Water and some minerals are also absorbed in this way (Figure 3-9).

Absorptive cells
A class of cells that line the villi (fingerlike projections in the small intestine) and participate in nutrient absorption.

Active absorption
Absorption using a carrier protein and expending energy. In this way the absorptive cell absorbs nutrients, such as glucose, when a high concentration of the nutrient is already present in the absorptive cells.

Another absorption mechanism uses both a carrier protein and energy input to actively pump nutrients from the lumen of the small intestine into the absorptive cells. This makes it possible for the body to take up nutrients even when they are not present in great concentrations in the diet. Some sugars, such as glucose, follow this route, called **active absorption.**

A further means of active absorption entails the absorptive cells literally engulfing compounds (phagocytosis) or liquids (pinocytosis). A cell membrane can form an indentation itself so that when particles or fluids move into the indentation, the cell membrane surrounds and engulfs them. This process is used when an infant absorbs immune substances from human milk (see Chapter 12).

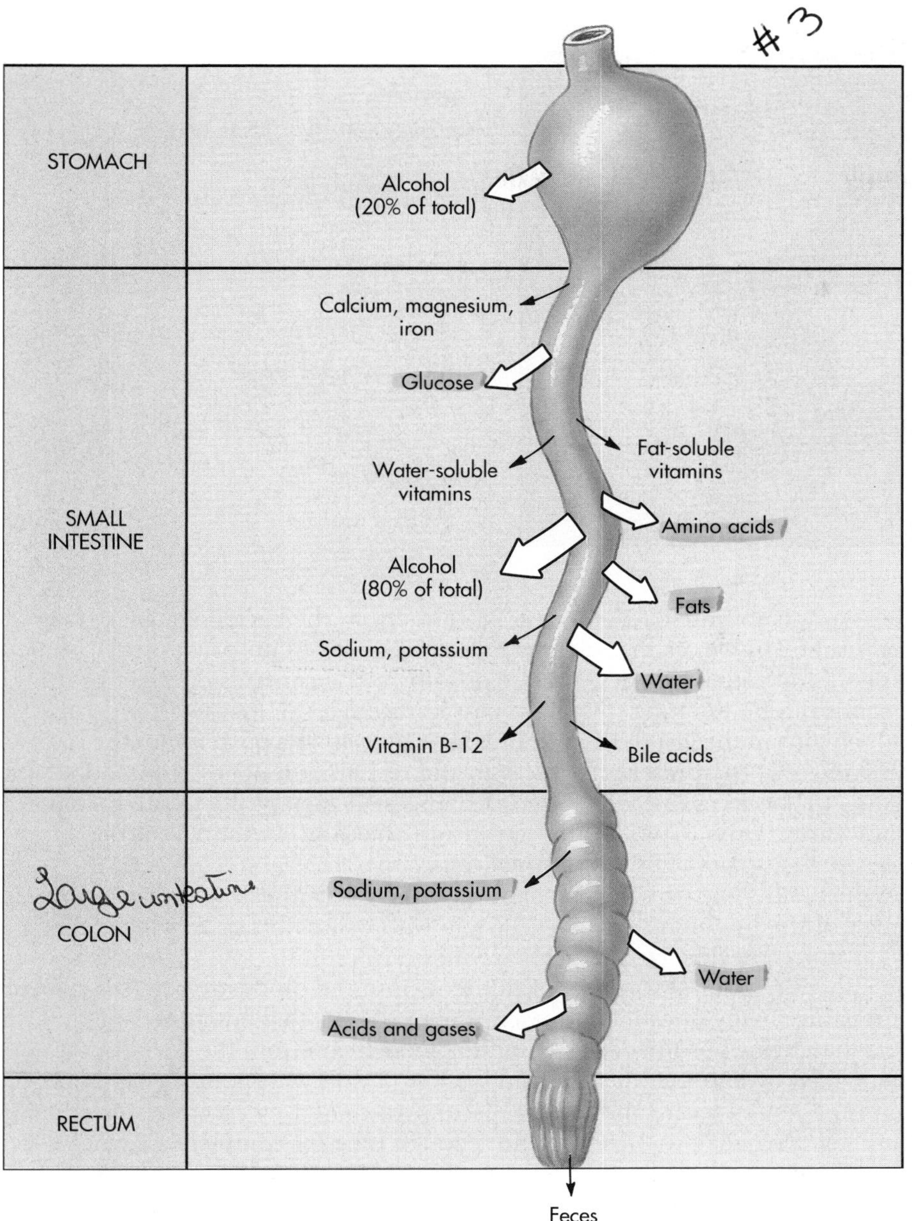

Figure 3-10 *Major sites of absorption along the GI tract. The size of the arrow indicates the relative amount of absorption at that site.*

Critical Thinking

The medical history of a young girl who is greatly underweight shows that she had three quarters of her small intestine removed after she was injured in a car accident. Explain how this accounts for her underweight condition, even though her medical chart shows that she eats well.

The Large Intestine Completes Absorption

When the intestinal contents enter the large intestine, little of the original foodstuff eaten still remains. Only a minor amount (5%) of carbohydrate, protein, and fat has escaped absorption (Figure 3-10). Some water is still present because the small intestine absorbs only 85% to 90% of the fluid it receives, which includes large amounts of GI-tract secretions produced during digestion. The remnants of the meal also include some minerals and what we call dietary fiber.

In the upper half of the large intestine, much of the remaining water and the minerals—mostly sodium and potassium—are absorbed. The unabsorbed water

Nutrient intake also directly influences nutrient absorption. For example, vitamin C in a meal modestly increases iron absorption in the same meal because it changes iron into a more absorbable state.

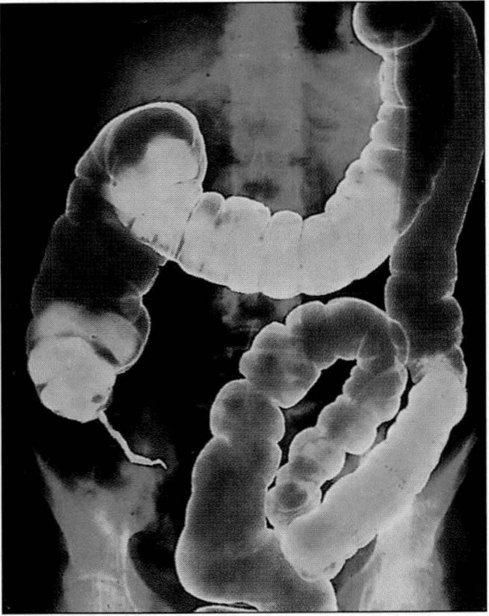

The large intestine (colon) has a large diameter and no villi.

now amounts to only a few ounces. Products from the bacterial activity that takes place in the large intestine, such as by-products of certain constituents of dietary fiber and undigested starches, are also absorbed. The contents of the large intestine are semisolid by the time they have passed through the first two-thirds of it. The stool remains in the last third until muscular movements push it into the rectum to be eliminated. The presence of feces in the rectum stimulates elimination. What remains in the feces, besides water, is undigested dietary fiber, tough connective tissues (from animal foods), bacteria from the large intestine, and some body wastes, such as parts of dead intestinal cells.

When either the small intestine or the pancreas is diseased, it may not produce enough of the important enzymes. People with cystic fibrosis may have this problem, as noted previously. A lack of enzymes can result in poor digestion and, consequently, very poor absorption of nutrients into the bloodstream. This condition accompanies many intestinal diseases. Any foodstuffs that enter the large intestine, rather than being absorbed mostly in the bloodstream from the small intestine, are metabolized by bacteria into acids and gas. A person with poor intestinal function often experiences severe abdominal discomfort caused by excessive intestinal gas. Insufficient enzyme production or not enough time for complete enzyme action is often the source of these problems.

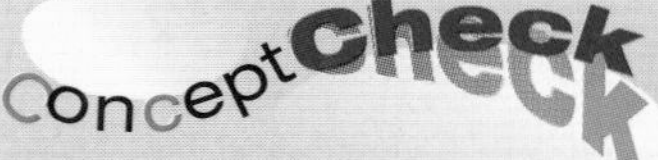

A variety of factors—such as hormones, nerves, muscles, and sphincters—help regulate the rate of digestion. Stomach acid and enzymes contribute to digestion of some foodstuffs. The small intestine is the major site for nutrient digestion and absorption, which are aided by enzymes and bile. Numerous folds and fingerlike projections in the small intestine create a large amount of absorptive surface for nutrient absorption. Because absorptive cells have a life span of only a few days, the lining of the small intestine is constantly renewed. Absorptive cells can perform passive types of absorption promoted by a concentration difference that is greater in the lumen of the intestine than in the absorptive cell. They also perform more active forms of absorption by either overcoming the resistance of high concentrations through the use of a carrier protein and energy input or physically engulfing compounds.

Excretory System

The kidneys, digestive tract, skin, and lungs all remove wastes from the body. For example, as blood passes through the kidneys, body wastes such as **urea** are removed and shunted into the urine to be excreted via the bladder. Excess intakes of water-soluble nutrients and other substances are also filtered and excreted in that manner. So, if the body already has enough vitamin C, for example, the kidneys screen the extra amount out of the blood and redirect it into the urine. The skin excretes body wastes, along with perspiration, through the pores. The lungs remove the carbon dioxide produced during the metabolism of energy-yielding nutrients, including carbohydrates, fats, and proteins. The carbon dioxide is then exhaled into the air.

Urea
Nitrogen-containing waste product found in urine. Most nitrogen excreted from the body leaves in this form.

Storage Systems

The human body must maintain reserves of nutrients. Otherwise, we would need to eat continuously. Storage capacity varies for each different nutrient. Most fat is stored at sites designed specifically for this—**adipose (fat) tissue.** Short-term storage of carbohydrate occurs in muscle and liver, and the blood maintains a small reserve of glucose and amino acids. Many vitamins and minerals are stored in the liver, while other nutrient stores are found in other sites in the body.

Adipose (fat) tissue
A grouping of fat-storing cells.

When people do not meet their nutrient needs, some nutrients are obtained by breaking down a tissue that contains high concentrations of the nutrient. Calcium is taken from bone, and protein is taken from muscle. These nutrient losses in cases of long-term deficiency harm these tissues.

Many people believe that if too much of a nutrient is obtained—for example, from a vitamin or mineral supplement—only what is needed is stored and the rest is excreted by the body. Though partially true, as with vitamin C, the large dosages found frequently in supplements such as vitamins A and D can cause harmful side effects because these are not readily excreted. This is one reason that obtaining your nutrients primarily (or exclusively) from a balanced diet is the safest means to acquire the building blocks you need to maintain the good health of all body systems.

This review of human anatomy and physiology from a nutrition perspective sets the stage for developing a more detailed understanding of the nutrients. The next three chapters will build on this information.

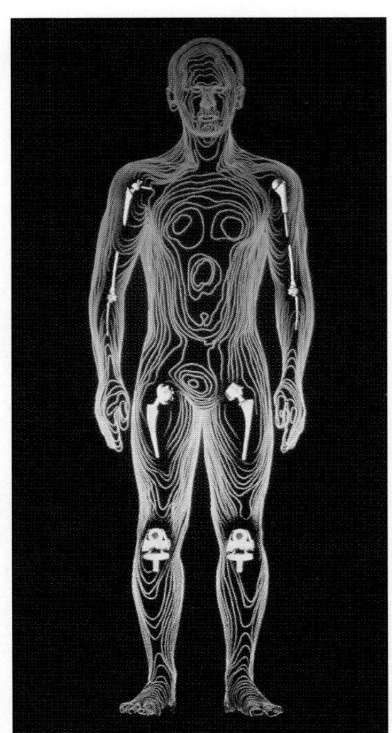

The skeletal system provides a reserve of calcium and phosphorus for day-to-day needs when dietary intake is inadequate. Long-term use of this reserve, however, reduces bone strength.

ConceptCheck

Besides the digestive tract, the kidneys, skin, and lungs all perform excretory functions of the body. The health of these organ systems depends on a sufficient and appropriate supply of nutrients. Nutrients are constantly present in the blood for immediate use and are stored to a greater or lesser extent in the body tissues for later use when sufficient food is unavailable. However, when the body suffers a nutrient deficiency caused by an inadequate diet, it breaks down vital tissues for their nutrients, which can lead to ill health. Additionally, too much of any nutrient can be detrimental. It's best to focus on obtaining all essential nutrients from a balanced diet.

Nutrition Insight

The Immune System—with a Nutrition Focus

Many types of body cells work in cooperation to maintain a defense against infection. It is easy to demonstrate the importance of good nutrition for immune function. Early humans were plagued by famine, infections, and death. Today, because of better nutrition, many of us avoid that cycle. In striving to eat healthfully, however, we may easily go too far. Although a proper nutrient intake is needed to maintain immune function, excess quantities can in fact jeopardize it. In reviewing some major components of the immune system—the skin, intestinal cells, and white blood cells—let's also consider how nutrient intake affects each component (Figure 3-11).

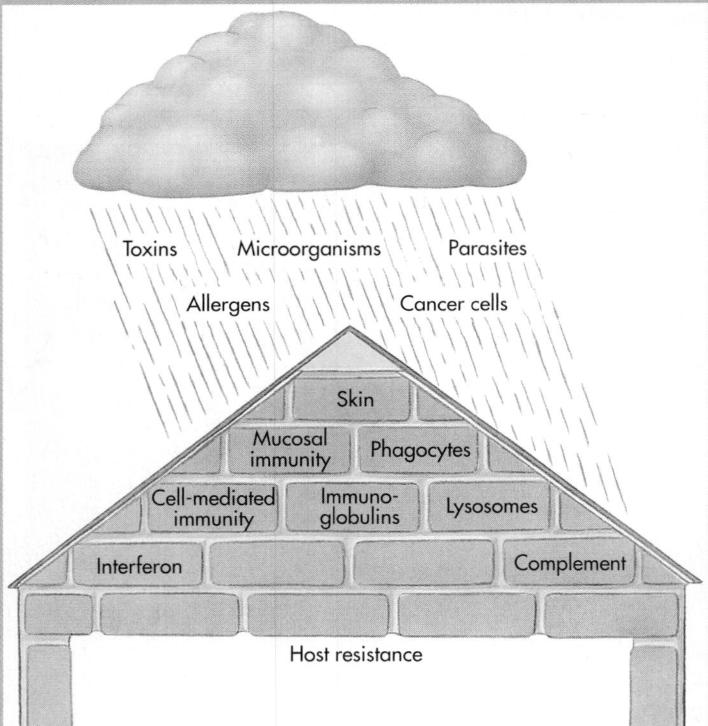

Skin

The skin forms an almost continuous barrier surrounding the body. Invading microbes have difficulty penetrating the skin. However, if the skin is split by lesions, bacteria can easily penetrate this barrier. Skin health is hampered by deficiencies of such nutrients as essential fatty acids, vitamin A, niacin, and zinc. Vitamin A deficiency also decreases gland secretions in the skin—necessary secretions that contain enzymes capable of killing bacteria. Bacterial eye infections in citizens of poorer countries are often due to vitamin A deficiency.

Intestinal Cells

The cells of the intestines form an important barrier to invading microbes. Not only are the cells closely packed together, but specialized cells that produce immune bodies—such as immunoglobulins—are also scattered throughout the intestinal tract. These immune bodies bind to the invading microbes, preventing them from entering the bloodstream. This process is called "mucosal immunity."

For a person in a nutritionally deficient state, the intestinal cells break down so that microbes more easily enter the body and cause infections. Two common results

Figure 3-11 *Host protective factors. The immune system has many components, all of which are affected by nutrient intake.*

of undernutrition are diarrhea and bacterial infections of the bloodstream. To protect the health of the intestinal tract, an adequate nutrient intake is necessary—especially of protein; vitamins A, B-6, B-12, and C; the vitamin folate; and zinc.

White Blood Cells

Once a microbe enters the bloodstream, white blood cells move in to attack it. A variety of types of white blood cells participate in this response and function in unique ways. For example, a class called *phagocytes* circulates throughout the circulatory system and ingests and sometimes digests microbes and foreign particles. Other white blood cells participate in cell-mediated immunity, achieved when certain immune cells recognize foreign cells and directly attack and destroy them. White blood cells, along with proteins in the blood called *immunoglobulins* and *complement*, contribute to an antibody response that binds microorganisms, engulfs and digests them, and then creates a template (memory) that allows future recognition of the microbe. Recognition allows more rapid attacks in the future.

Some white blood cells live only a few days. Their constant resynthesis requires a steady nutrient input. The immune system needs (1) iron to produce an important killing factor (2) copper for the synthesis of a specific type of white blood cell, and (3) adequate amounts of protein; vitamins B-6, B-12, and C; and folate for general cell synthesis and, later, cell activity. Zinc and vitamin A are also needed for the overall growth and development of the immune cells.

One proof that nutrition is important to immune status is the body's response to microbes: microbes normally present in the body usually cause disease only in severely undernourished people. A good example is measles. Your parents probably had this viral infection and survived. (You were probably vaccinated against measles.) However, many undernourished children who contract it die. Thus, the presence of a virus or microbe in the body does not guarantee its triumph over the immune system in a healthy person. However, if a person's health status is compromised through undernutrition, the chances that a destructive microbe will win are greater.

A Note of Caution

Many studies show that good nutritional status is associated with good immune status. However, other studies also show that an overabundance of certain nutrients can actually harm the immune system. Excess intake of total fat and polyunsaturated fatty acids has been implicated in a decreased immune response. Taking too much zinc also decreases immune function, as does excess vitamin E when administered to preterm infants.

The message here is that eating a balanced diet will help us maintain the health of all components of our immune systems. Our bodies need this system to continuously defend us from harmful microbes in the environment. The diets of some older people are a concern in this context because their energy intakes may be too low to meet all nutrient needs. Careful nutrient supplementation, especially with folate vitamin B-6 and vitamin B-12, then deserves consideration (see Chapter 14 for more details). However, keep in mind that consuming megadoses of nutrients is not going to boost the immune system to even higher abilities. In fact, it can harm certain aspects of immune function.

Summary

- The cell is the basic building block of body tissues. DNA is the blueprint found in all cells. This determines the cell type, its function and structure, and the types of proteins each type of cell will produce.
- Blood travels the pulmonary circuit, picking up oxygen at the lungs. Then, via the systemic circuit, the blood delivers essential nutrients, oxygen, and water to all body cells. Nutrients and wastes are exchanged between the blood and cells across the cell membrane. This exchange occurs in the capillaries.
- Water-soluble compounds in the villi enter the portal vein and travel to the liver. Fat-soluble compounds enter the lymphatic system, which eventually connects to the bloodstream.
- The gastrointestinal (GI) tract consists of the mouth, esophagus, stomach, small intestine, large intestine (colon), rectum, and anus. The majority of digestion and absorption of nutrients occur in the small intestine.
- The liver, gallbladder, and pancreas participate in digestion and absorption. Products from these organs, such as enzymes and bile, enter the small intestine and play important roles in digesting protein, fat, and carbohydrate.
- Spaced along the GI tract are ringlike valves (sphincters) that regulate the flow of foodstuffs. Muscular contractions, called *peristalsis,* move the foodstuffs down the GI tract. A variety of nerves, hormones, and other substances control the activity of sphincters and peristaltic muscles.
- Digestive enzymes are secreted by the mouth, stomach, wall of the small intestine, and pancreas. The presence of food in the small intestine stimulates the release of pancreatic enzymes. Bile needed for fat digestion is synthesized by the liver, stored in the gallbladder, and released in digestion, as directed by hormonal action.
- The major absorptive sites consist of fingerlike projections called *villi,* located in the small intestine. Absorptive cells cover the villi. This intestinal lining is continually renewed. Absorptive cells can perform various passive and active forms of absorption.
- Little digestion and absorption occur in the stomach or large intestine, but some protein is digested in the stomach. Some constituents of dietary fiber and undigested starch are digested by bacteria in the large intestine; undigested dietary fiber that remains is eliminated in the feces.
- Final water and mineral absorption takes place in the large intestine. Products from bacterial breakdown of some dietary fibers and other substances are also absorbed here. The presence of feces in the rectum provides a strong impetus for elimination.
- The kidneys, skin, and lungs all perform excretory functions for the body. Limited stores of nutrients are present in the blood for immediate use and stored to a greater or lesser extent in body tissues for later use when sufficient food is unavailable. When the body suffers a nutrient deficiency caused by a poor diet, it breaks down vital tissues for their nutrients, which can lead to ill health. Additionally, too much of any nutrient can be detrimental.

Study Questions

1. Explain how the nerves and hormones interact in "priming" the digestive tract.
2. Describe the physiological mechanisms by which the health and absorptive abilities of the cells of the small intestine are protected.
3. Describe the role of the portal and lymphatic systems in the digestive process.
4. What is the difference between nature and nuture? Relate these terms to the attempt to prevent three chronic diseases.
5. Contrast the processes of active and passive absorption of nutrients.
6. Describe the process of peristalsis in physiological terms.
7. Explain why the small intestine is better suited than the other GI tract organs to carry out the absorptive process.
8. Explain where and how each of the following nutrients is absorbed:
   a. Glucose
   b. Fats
   c. Amino acids
   d. Water
9. Show where acid is secreted and how its production is controlled. What are its roles in digestion?
10. Indicate how blood is routed through the digestive system. Which nutrients enter the bloodstream directly? Which nutrients are first absorbed into the lymph?

Further Readings

1 Axel R: The molecular logic of smell, *Scientific American* p. 154, October 1995.
2 Chandra RK: Nutrition and the immune system: an introduction, *American Journal of Clinical Nutrition* 66:460s, 1997.
3 Constipation becomes more common with age, *Tufts University Health & Nutrition Letter* p. 7, February 1999.
4 Eisen A, Weber B: Prophylactic mastectomy—the price of fear, *New England Journal of Medicine* 340:137, 1999.
5 Fass R and others: Contemporary medical therapy for gastroesophageal reflux disease, *American Family Physician* 55:205, 1997.
6 Feinberg A: Treating troubled stomachs, *Health News* p. 4, May 6, 1997.
7 Hahn NI: The flavor of food? It's all in your head, *Journal of the American Dietetic Association* 96:655, 1996.
8 Heartburn relief: the acid test, *UC Berkeley Wellness Letter* p. 1, October 1997.
9 Huston DP: The biology of the immune system, *Journal of the American Medical Association* 278:1804, 1997.
10 Kelly OS, Bendich A: Essential nutrients and immunity, *American Journal of Clinical Nutrition* 63:994S, 1996.
11 Laine L, Fendrick AM: *Helicobacter pylori* and peptic ulcer disease, *Postgraduate Medicine* 103:231, 1998.
12 Laxatives and constipation, *Mayo Clinic Health Letter* p. 7, February 1998.
13 Leland JV: Flavor interactions: the greater whole, *Food Technology* 51:75, 1997.
14 Lowdown on hemorrhoids, *UC Berkeley Wellness Letter* p. 5, May 1997.
15 Lynch HT, Lynch JF: Pros and cons of genetic screening for breast cancer, *American Family Physician* 59(1):43, 1999.
16 Mattes RD: Physiologic responses to sensory stimulation by food: nutritional implications, *Journal of the American Dietetic Association* 97:406, 1997.
17 Mayes PA: Nutrition, digestion, and absorption. In Murray RK and others editors: *Harper's biochemistry,* Norwalk, CT, 1996, Appleton & Lange.
18 Neumann DA and others: Conference on nutrition and immunity, *Nutrition Today* 32:240, 1997.
19 Rosenthal TC, Puck SM: Screening for genetic risk of breast cancer, *American Family Physician* 59(1):99, 1999.
20 Schardt D: Building immunity—what can help? *Nutrition Action Health Letter* 24(7):1, 1997.
21 Scrimshaw NS, San Giovanni JP: Synergism of nutrition, infection and immunity: an overview, *American Journal of Clinical Nutrition* 66:464S, 1997.
22 Titus K: Benefit is bottom line in genetic testing, *Journal of the American Medical Association* 276:1016, 1996.

RATE

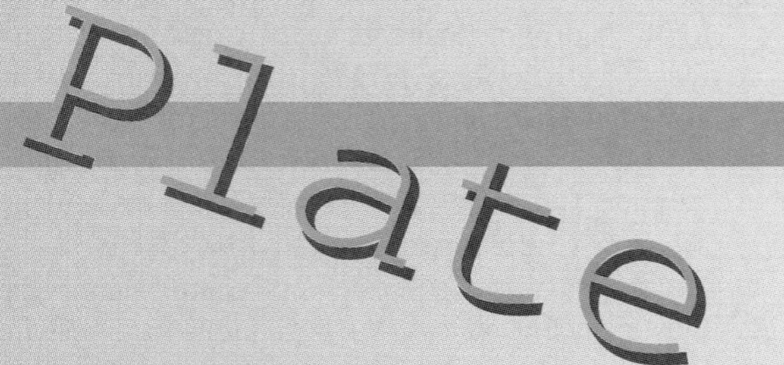

I. Are You Taking Care of Your Digestive Tract?

People need to think about the health of their digestive tracts. There are symptoms we need to notice as well as habits we need to practice in order to protect it. The following assessment is designed to help you examine your habits and symptoms associated with the health of your digestive tract. The Nutrition Issue explains why these habits are important to examine. Put a Y in the blank to the left of the question to indicate yes and an N to indicate no.

____ **1. Are you currently experiencing greater-than-normal stress and tension?**

____ **2. Do you have a family history of digestive tract problems (ulcers, hemorrhoids, diverticulosis, constipation, lactose intolerance)?**

____ **3. Do you experience pain in your stomach region about 2 hours after you eat?**

____ **4. Do you smoke cigarettes?**

____ **5. Do you take aspirin frequently?**

____ **6. Do you have heartburn at least once per week?**

____ **7. Do you commonly lie down after eating a large meal?**

____ **8. Do you drink alcoholic beverages more than two or three times per day?**

____ **9. Do you experience abdominal pain, bloating, and gas about 30 minutes to 2 hours after consuming milk products?**

____ **10. Do you often have to strain while having a bowel movement?**

____ **11. Do you consume less than 6 to 8 cups of a combination of water and other fluids per day?**

____ **12. Do you perform physical activity (e.g., jog, swim, walk briskly, row, stair climb) less than 20 to 30 minutes on most days?**

____ **13. Do you eat a diet relatively low in dietary fiber (recall that significant dietary fiber is found in whole and dried fruits, vegetables, legumes, nuts and seeds, whole-grain breads, and whole-grain cereals)?**

____ **14. Do you frequently have diarrhea?**

____ **15. Do you frequently use laxatives or antacids?**

INTERPRETATION

Add up the number of "yes" answers you gave and record the total in the blank to the right.

If your score is from 8 to 15, your habits and symptoms put you at risk for experiencing future digestive tract problems. Take particular note of the habits to which you answered yes. Consider trying to cooperate more with your digestive tract, based on what is discussed in the Nutrition Issue.

II. Take A Closer Look at Heartburn

As discussed as well in the Nutrition Issue, heartburn is a major problem for some people. Generally, people assume that their only option for treatment is medication. Below are some popular heartburn medications and their method of action:

Medication	Method of Action
Pepcid AC, Tagamet HB 200, Zantac 75, Axid AR	Reduce stomach acid production
Tums, Rolaids, Alka-Seltzer Mylanta, Maalox	Antigas, antacids, and pain relievers
Pepto-Bismol	Protective stomach-coating action

Note, however, that Table 3–3 provides suggestions for some dietary and lifestyle changes that could be tried instead of the medication. Additional changes that may help reduce heartburn include the following: eat smaller meals that are lower in fat; limit foods that may contribute to heartburn such as onions, garlic, peppermint, caffeine, alcohol, chocolate, orange juice, tomato products, and fried foods. Remember also that self-medication of heartburn for longer than a week is not advised. If heartburn remains after both dietary and lifestyle changes and medications have been tried, it is best to consult with a physician. Chronic heartburn may be due to a treatable cause, and if left untreated, can lead to serious health problems.

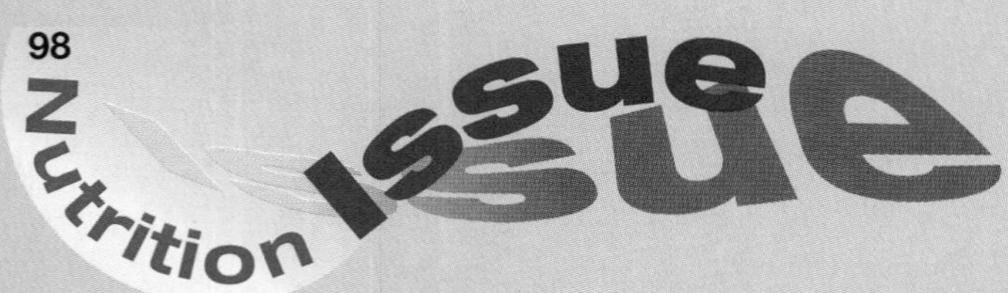

When the Digestive Processes Go Awry

The fine-tuned organ system we call the *GI tract* can develop problems. Knowing about these common problems can help you avoid them.

ULCERS

Many adults develop ulcers each year. An estimated 25 million Americans develop this during their lifetimes. The principal causes are a specific bacterial infection of *Helicobacter pylori* (*H. pylori*), heavy use of aspirin and related medications, and disorders that cause excessive acid production in the stomach. As the stomach lining deteriorates and loses its mucus layer protection, the acid erodes the stomach tissue. This specific chain of events will result in a gastric ulcer. Acid can also erode the tissue lining of the initial part of the small intestine, the duodenum, and result in a duodenal ulcer. *Peptic ulcer* is the general term for both of these two cases.

Most ulcers in young people occur in the duodenum; in older people they occur primarily in the stomach. The typical symptom of an ulcer is pain about 2 hours after eating. Digestive acids acting on a meal irritate the ulcer after most of the meal has moved to the jejunum area of the small intestine.

The primary risk associated with an ulcer is the possibility that is will penetrate entirely through the stomach or intestinal wall. The GI contents could then spill into the body cavities, causing a massive infection. In addition, an ulcer may erode a blood vessel, leading to massive blood loss. For these reasons it is important not to ignore the early warning signs of ulcer development.

In the past, milk and cream therapy—the Sippy diet—was used to help cure ulcers. Clinicians now know that milk and cream are two of the worst foods for an ulcer. The calcium in these foods stimulates stomach acid secretion and actually inhibits ulcer healing.

Today a combination of approaches is used for ulcer therapy. People infected with *H. pylori* are given antibiotics with antacid or bismuth therapy to eradicate that agent. In many cases, there is a 90% cure rate of *H. pylori* in the first week of this treatment. Recurrence is unlikely if the infection is cured.

Other medications may also be a part of ulcer care, all of which reduce acid secretion in the stomach. Some of these medications are now available over the counter in nonprescription doses for cases of indigestion and heartburn. Medications that coat the ulcer are also commonly used today.

People with ulcers should also refrain from smoking and minimize the use of aspirin and related products. These practices reduce the mucus secreted by the stomach. Overall, this combination of lifestyle therapy and modern medical treatment has so revolutionized ulcer therapy that dietary changes are of minor importance today (Table 3–3). Current diet-therapy approaches recommend simply avoiding foods that increase ulcer symptoms.

Note also that stomach acid is not a problem for those not prone to or currently experiencing ulcers. The

TABLE 3-3

Recommendations to Prevent Ulcers and Heartburn from Occurring or Recurring

ULCERS

1. See your physician, as *H. pylori* may be the cause.
2. Stop smoking, if you are now a smoker.
3. Avoid regular/heavy use of aspirin, ibuprofen, and other aspirin-like compounds unless a physician advises otherwise.
4. Limit coffee, tea, and alcohol (especially wine), if this helps.
5. Limit pepper, chili powder, and other strong spices, if this helps.
6. Eat nutritious meals on a regular schedule.
7. Chew foods well.
8. Lose weight if you are currently overweight.

HEARTBURN

1. Wait about 3 hours after a meal before lying down.
2. Don't overeat at mealtime. Smaller meals that are low in fat are advised.
3. Try elevating the head of the bed (6" blocks).
4. Observe the recommendations for ulcer prevention.

acid in the stomach enhances absorption of iron, calcium, and vitamin B-12. Acid also minimizes bacterial growth in the stomach; the stomach is essentially bacteria free because of its high acid content. Bacteria in food are quickly destroyed, which reduces the risk of cancer-causing agents or food-borne illness formed by these bacteria. Thus, acid production by the stomach is an important part of the physiology of digestion and absorption. This means that despite their usual presence alongside the breath mints in a convenience store, antacids should not be used excessively. If an antacid contains magnesium (and many do), magnesium toxicity is another possible result of antacid abuse.

HEARTBURN

Many adults regularly have heartburn. This gnawing pain in the upper chest is caused by the movement of acid from the stomach into the esophagus and so the problem is more formally called **gastroesophageal reflux disease (GERD).** Unlike the stomach, the esophagus has no mucus lining to protect it, so acid quickly erodes the lining of the esophagus, causing pain.

Gastroesophageal reflux disease (GERD)
Disease that results from stomach acid backing up into the esophagus. The acid irritates the lining of the esophagus, causing pain.

An important dietary measure for avoiding heartburn is to eat smaller meals, especially meals that are low in fat (see Table 3–3). Fatty meals remain in the stomach longer than low-fat meals. The large volume of food and secretions that remains in the stomach creates pressure that can force the stomach contents up into the esophagus.

Several other steps may be taken to prevent heartburn. Cigarette smokers should quit smoking. In addition, it is best not to lie down after eating and to limit foods and other substances that can specifically contribute to heartburn, mostly by irritating the esophagus, such as chili powder, onions, garlic, peppermint, caffeine, alcohol, and chocolate. Individuals should discover irritants and tailor their diets accordingly.

Certain physical conditions can lead to heartburn. For example, both pregnancy and obesity result in increased production of estrogen and progesterone. These hormones relax the lower esophageal (cardiac) sphincter, making heartburn more likely. A pregnant woman may find it helpful to eat smaller, more frequent meals. An obese person should slim down to a more healthy weight so that blood concentrations of these hormones decrease.

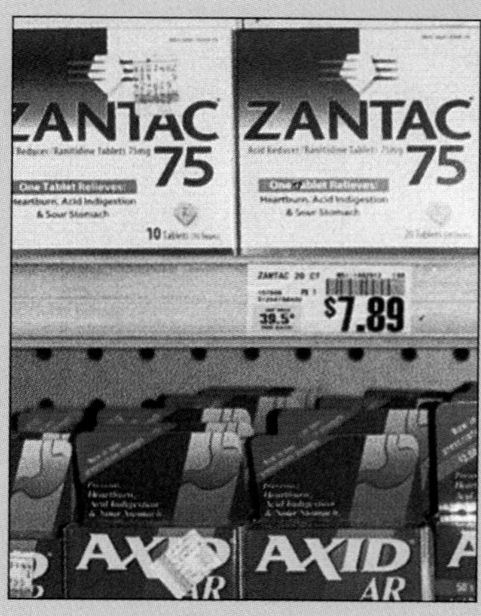

A number of over-the-counter medications are marketed for heartburn. However, attention to diet and lifestyle, such as not overeating, are more important measures to take.

Occasional heartburn can be treated with dietary lifestyle changes and medications. The action and proper use of these medications are summarized in the Rate Your Plate exercise of this chapter. Attention to diet and lifestyle, however, are two healthful measures that can provide longer-lasting relief from heartburn. And though it is true that many people suffer occasional heartburn, it is important that this problem not be accepted as a normal part of daily life or self-treated for an extended time. Heartburn that recurs several times a week for at least a month should be investigated by a physician. This heartburn may require aggressive medical therapy because it can lead to alteration in the cells of the esophagus, which increases the risk of a rare form of cancer.

CONSTIPATION

Constipation, which is difficult or infrequent evacuation of the bowels, is commonly reported by adults. Slow movement of fecal material through the large intestine causes constipation. As fluid is increasingly absorbed during the extended time the feces stay in the large intestine, they become dry and hard.

Constipation
A condition characterized by infrequent bowel movements.

Constipation can result when people regularly inhibit their normal bowel reflexes for long periods. In addition, muscle spasms of an irritated large intestine can slow the movement of feces and contribute to constipation. Medications such as antacids and calcium and iron supplements can also cause constipation.

Constipation is difficult to diagnose. The normal frequency of bowel movements is 3 to 12 times per week, varying from person to person. The best indication of constipation is unusually hard, dry feces at infrequent intervals, rather than failure to meet a general prescription of "once a day." Sudden, prolonged changes in the frequency of bowel movements should be evaluated by a physician. This may be a warning that a more serious intestinal disorder is developing.

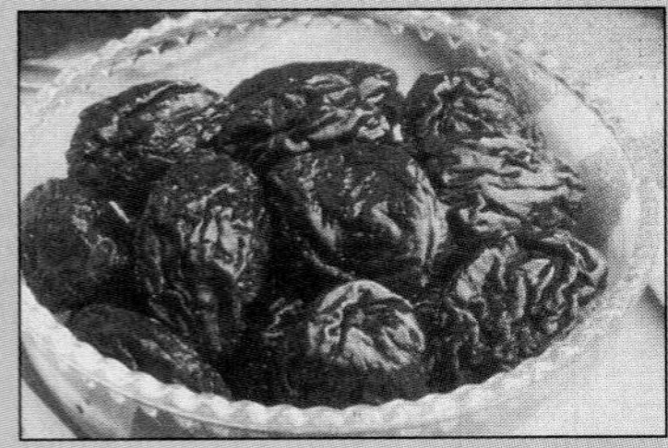

Dried fruits, like prunes, aid in treating constipation.

Eating foods with plenty of dietary fiber, such as whole-grain breads and cereals and dried fruits, is the best alternative for treating typical cases of constipation. Dietary fibers stimulate peristalsis by drawing water into the large intestine and helping form a bulky, soft fecal output. People with constipation should also drink more fluids. In addition, people with constipation may need to develop more regular bowel habits. Finally, relaxation facilitates regular bowel movements, as does regular physical activity.

Laxative

A medication or other substance that stimulates evacuation of the intestinal tract.

Laxatives can also lessen constipation. These work by irritating the intestinal nerve junctions to stimulate the peristaltic muscles, or by drawing water into the intestine to enlarge fecal output. The larger output stretches the peristaltic muscles, making them rebound and then constrict. Regular use of laxatives, especially irritating ones, however, can decrease muscle action in the large intestine, in time causing more constipation. The GI tract can then actually become dependent on laxatives. Thus it is unwise for anyone to use laxatives routinely, although people in certain circumstances—for example, those who are bedridden or quite elderly—may need periodic help from laxatives to relieve constipation.

HEMORRHOIDS

Hemorrhoids, also called *piles,* are swollen veins of the rectum and anus. The blood vessels in this area are subject to intense pressure, especially during bowel movements. Added stress to the vessels from pregnancy, obesity, prolonged sitting, violent coughing or sneezing, or straining during bowel movements, particularly with constipation, can lead to a hemorrhoid. Symptoms may include pain, itching, and bleeding. If you think you have a hemorrhoid, you should consult your physician. Rectal bleeding, although usually caused by hemorrhoids, may also indicate other problems, such as cancer.

A physician may suggest a variety of self-care measures for hemorrhoids. Pain can be lessened by applying warm, soft compresses or sitting in a tub of warm water for 15 to 20 minutes. Dietary recommendations are the same as those for treating constipation, emphasizing the need to consume adequate dietary fiber and fluid. Over-the-counter remedies can also offer relief of symptoms.

Perhaps you have heard that taking laxatives after overeating prevents deposition of body fat from the excess energy intake. This erroneous and dangerous premise has gained popularity among followers of numerous fad diets. You may temporarily feel less full after using a laxative because laxatives hasten emptying of the large intestine and increase fluid loss. Most laxatives, however, do not speed the passage of food through the small intestine, where digestion and most nutrient absorption take place. As a result, you can't count on laxatives to prevent fat gain from excess energy intake.

Diarrhea, a GI tract disease that generally lasts only a few days, is defined as increased fluidity, frequency, or amount of bowel movements compared to a person's usual pattern. Most cases of diarrhea result from infections in the intestines, with bacteria and viruses the usual offending agents. They produce substances that cause the intestinal cells to primarily secrete fluid rather than absorb fluid. Another form of diarrhea can be caused by consumption of substances that are not readily absorbed, such as the sugar alcohol sorbitol found in sugarless gum (see Chapter 4). When consumed in large amounts the unabsorbed substance draws much water into the intestines, in turn leading to diarrhea. Treatment of diarrhea generally requires drinking lots of fluid during the affected stage; reduced intake of the poorly absorbed substance also is important if that is a cause. Prompt treatment—within 24 to 48 hours—is especially important for infants and elderly people, as they are more susceptible to the effects of dehydration associated with diarrhea (see Chapters 13 and 14). Diarrhea that lasts more than seven days in adults should be investigated by a physician as it can be a symptom of more serious intestinal disease, especially if there is also blood in the stool.

part 2

Nutrients: The Heart of Nutrition

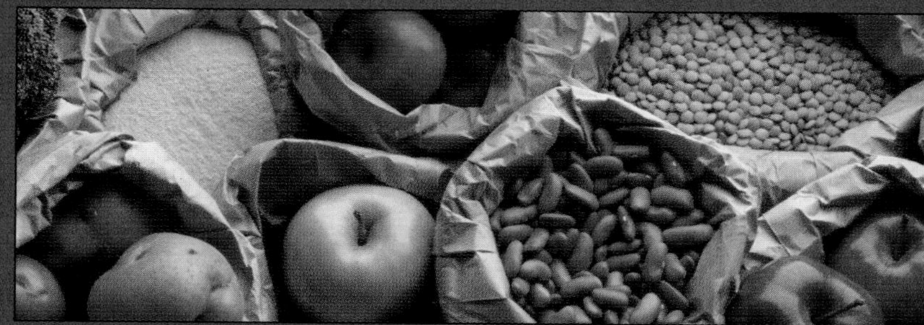

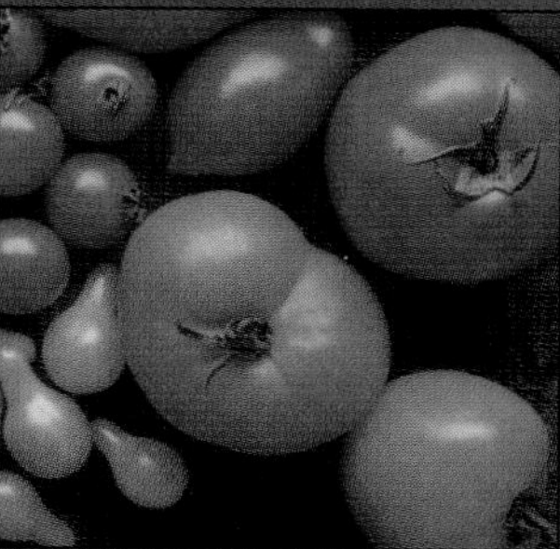

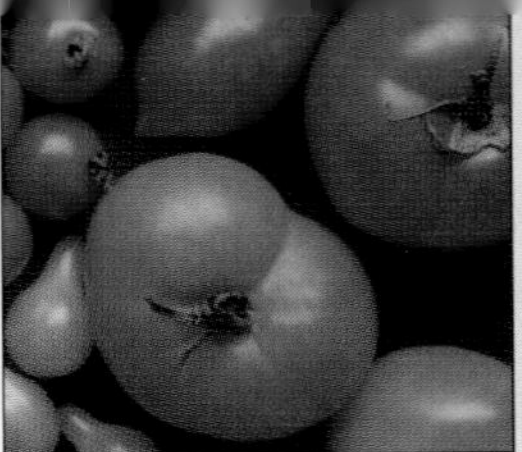

chapter

4 Carbohydrates

What did you eat to obtain the energy you are using right now? The next three chapters will examine this question by focusing on the nutrients the human body uses for fuel. These energy-yielding nutrients are mainly carbohydrates (on average 4 kcal per gram) and fats and oils (on average 9 kcal per gram). Not much protein (on average 4 kcal per gram) is used to fuel the body. Most people know that potatoes have carbohydrates and steak has fat and protein, but few people know what those terms mean. Knowing more about them helps you choose appropriate foods for your needs.

You have likely consumed fruits, vegetables, dairy products, cereals, breads, or pasta in the past 24 hours. All these foods supply carbohydrates. Unfortunately, the benefits of these foods are often misunderstood. Many people think carbohydrate-rich foods are necessarily fattening—they are not. In fact, they are much less fattening than fats and oils, pound for pound. Some people think sugars cause hyperactivity—this is highly unlikely. If you see carbohydrates as being unhealthful, it is unfortunate. In fact, carbohydrates, especially when naturally part of beans, fruits, vegetables, and whole grains, have been the class of nutrients most promoted by diet recommendations in recent years. These should generally constitute about 60% of your daily energy intake. The link between fat—especially animal fat—and heart disease should prompt us all to switch our focus away from high-fat foods and toward more high-carbohydrate foods. It is unfortunate that affluence tends to drive us the other way.

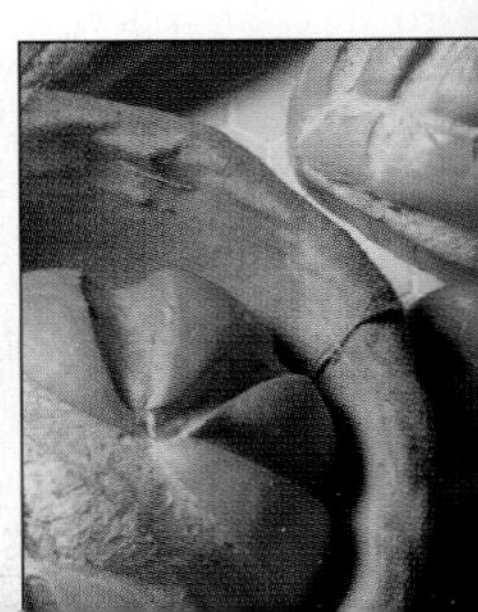

Nutrition Web

The forms of carbohydrates include monosaccharides and disaccharides (simple sugars), polysaccharides (starches), and dietary fiber.

The bulk of carbohydrate digestion takes place in the small intestine. Some plant fibers are digested by bacteria in the large intestine, and undigested plant fibers exit in the feces.

In some people the intestinal cells do not produce sufficient lactase, the enzyme needed to digest lactose. This condition is called *lactose intolerance,* and results in abdominal discomfort when large servings of milk products are consumed. Most sufferers can tolerate moderate amounts of milk, cheese, and yogurt.

Carbohydrates should generally form the bulk of energy in the diet, approximately 60% of total calorie intake.

Carbohydrates are found in grain products, fruits, vegetables, legumes, milk products, and sweets, such as jelly, table sugar, and syrup.

Sugar should be consumed in moderation; rich starch and dietary fiber choices should be the focus of the diet. Moderate use of alternative sweeteners such as aspartame can help in controlling sugar and overall energy intake.

Carbohydrates supply energy for cells, contribute to fat metabolism, and spare protein as an energy source. Dietary fiber provides mass to the stool, thus easing elimination.

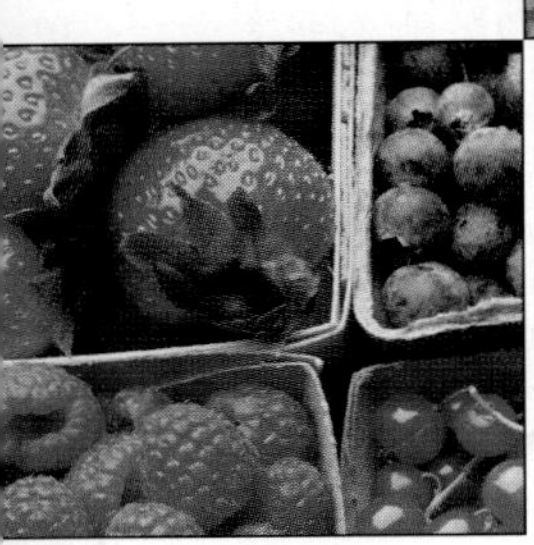

Photosynthesis
Process by which plants use solar energy from the sun to synthesize energy-yielding compounds, such as glucose.

Sugar
A simple carbohydrate, generally with the chemical composition $(CH_2O)_n$.

Monosaccharide
A simple sugar, such as glucose, that is not broken down further during digestion.

Carbohydrates are a primary fuel source for some cells, such as those in the brain and in the bloodstream. Muscles also rely on a dependable supply of carbohydrate in order to support intense physical activity. Yielding on average 4 kcal per gram, carbohydrates are a readily available fuel for all cells in the form of blood glucose, and stored in the liver and muscles as **glycogen.** That stored in the liver can be used to maintain blood glucose availability in times when the diet does not supply enough. Regular intake of carbohydrate is important as the liver glycogen is used up in only about 18 hours when no carbohydrate is consumed. After that point the body is forced to produce its own carbohydrate from body protein; this eventually leads to health problems.

We obtain about 50% of our energy intake from carbohydrate; this percentage is higher in the developing world. We have sensors on our tongue that recognize sweet carbohydrates. Researchers surmise that this sweetness indicated a safe energy source to early man, and so it became an important energy source. The returning Crusaders brought sugar from the Holy Land to Europe. Columbus introduced sugarcane to the Americas. The French later exploited sugar beets as a source of sugar.

Primarily choosing the healthiest carbohydrate sources, while moderating intake of those that are less healthful, contributes to well-planned diet. It is difficult to eat so little carbohydrate that body needs are not met, but it is easy to over consume the carbohydrates that can contribute to health problems. Let's explore this concept further as we look at carbohydrates in detail.

Forms of Simple Carbohydrates

Green plants create the carbohydrates in our foods. Leaves capture the sun's solar energy in their cells and transform it to chemical energy. This energy is then used to produce the carbohydrate glucose from carbon dioxide and water. This complex process is called ***photosynthesis.***

$$\text{6 Carbon dioxide } (CO_2) + \text{6 Water } (H_2O) \rightarrow \text{Glucose } (C_6H_{12}O_6) + \text{6 Oxygen } (O_2)$$

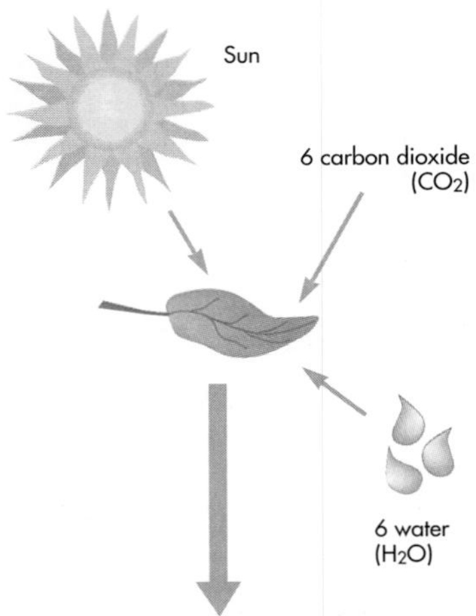

Glucose is stored in the leaf, but can also undergo further metabolism.

As the name suggests, most carbohydrate molecules are composed of carbon, hydrogen, and oxygen atoms. Simple forms of carbohydrates are called ***sugars.*** Larger, more complex forms are primarily called either *starches* or *dietary fibers,* depending on their digestibility by human GI tract enzymes. Starches are the digestible form.

Monosaccharides—Glucose, Fructose, and Galactose

Monosaccharides are the single sugar forms (*mono* means one) that serve as the basic unit of all sugar structures. Glucose is the major monosaccharide found in the body (Figure 4–1). Glucose is also known as *dextrose,* and that found in the bloodstream may be called blood sugar. Glucose is a primary source of energy for human cells, although foods contain little in this form. Most glucose comes from starches and **sucrose** (common table sugar). The latter is made up of the monosaccharides glucose and fructose. For the most part, sugars in foods are eventually converted to glucose in the liver and this goes on to serve as a source of cellular energy.

Fructose, also called *levulose* or *fruit sugar,* is another common sugar. After it is consumed, fructose is absorbed by the small intestine and then transported to the liver, where it is quickly metabolized. Much is converted to glucose, and the rest goes on to form other compounds. Most of the fructose as such in our diets comes from the use of **high-fructose corn syrup** in food production (see later discussion). Fructose also forms half of sucrose, as previously noted, and is found in fruits.

The sugar **galactose** has nearly the same structure as glucose. Large quantities of pure galactose do not exist in nature. Instead, galactose is usually found attached to glucose in **lactose,** a sugar found in milk and other milk products. After it is ab-

Monosaccharides

Glucose Fructose Galactose

Disaccharides

Sucrose: glucose + fructose
Lactose: glucose + galactose
Maltose: glucose + glucose

Sucrose

Figure 4-1 *Some common sugars. Sucrose and fructose are the most common sugars in our diets.*

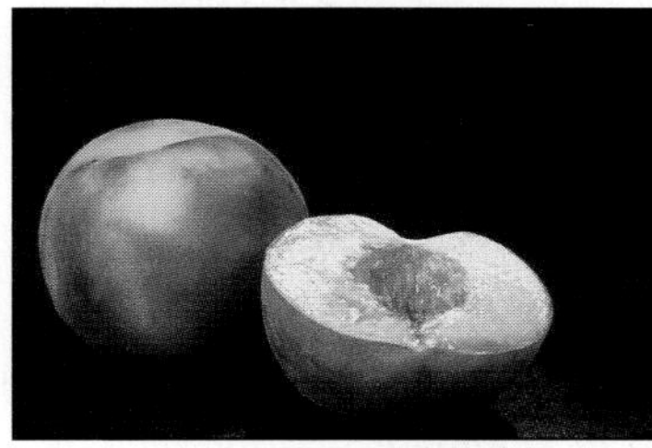

Fruits contain sugars, such as fructose.

sorbed, galactose arrives in the liver. There it is either transformed into glucose per se or further metabolized. One product of this metabolism is glycogen, a special storage form of glucose found in liver and muscle.

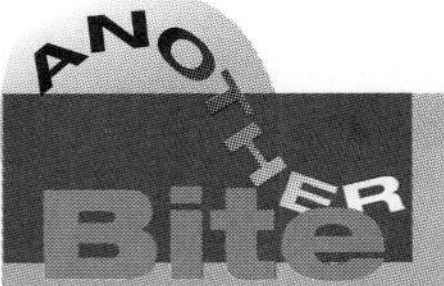

Now is a good time to begin emphasizing a key concept in nutrition: the difference between intake of a substance and the body's use of that substance. The body often does not use all nutrients in their original states. Some of these substances are broken down and later reassembled into the same or a different substance when and where necessary. For example, much of the galactose in the diet is metabolized to glucose. When later required, as in the mammary gland of the lactating female, galactose is resynthesized.

Disaccharides—Sucrose, Lactose, and Maltose

Disaccharides are formed when two monosaccharides combine (*di* means two). The most common disaccharides in food are sucrose, lactose, and maltose.

Disaccharides *Class of sugars formed by chemically linking two monosaccharides.*

Sucrose forms when the two sugars glucose and fructose join together. Sucrose is found in sugarcane, sugar beets, honey, and maple sugar. These products are processed to varying degrees to make brown, white, and powdered sugars. Animals do not produce sucrose, or typically any appreciable amount of carbohydrate for that matter.

Lactose forms when glucose joins with galactose. Again, our major food source for lactose is milk products. The second Nutrition Insight discusses the problems that result when a person can't readily digest lactose.

Maltose forms when two glucose molecules combine. Maltose is of nutritional interest primarily because of its role in alcohol production in the beer and liquor

Fermentation
The conversion, without the use of oxygen, of carbohydrates to alcohols, acids, and carbon dioxide.

Polysaccharides
Large carbohydrates containing from hundreds to 3000 or more glucose units; also known as complex carbohydrates.

Amylose
A straight-chain digestible polysaccharide made of glucose units; primary component of starch in foods.

industry. In the production of alcoholic beverages, starches in various cereal grains are first converted to simpler carbohydrates by enzymes present in the grains. The end products of this step—maltose, glucose, and other sugars—are then mixed with yeast cells in the absence of oxygen. The yeast cells convert most of the sugars to alcohol (ethanol) and carbon dioxide, a process termed ***fermentation.*** Little maltose remains in the final product. Few other food products and beverages contain maltose. In fact, most maltose that we ultimately digest in the small intestine is produced during the digestion of starch.

Monosaccharides and disaccharides are often referred to as *simple sugars* because they contain few sugar units. Food labels lump all these sugars under one category, listing them as "sugars."

Forms of the More Complex Carbohydrates

The scientific name for the large, complex carbohydrates is **polysaccharides.** They are often referred to as complex carbohydrates for this reason. Polysaccharides are very long carbohydrate chains composed of many monosaccharide units, mainly glucose (*poly* means many). Some polysaccharides have 3000 or more glucose units, and are found primarily in grains, vegetables, and fruits. When food labels on breakfast cereals list "Other Carbohydrates," this primarily refers to starch content.

Amylose, a long, straight chain of glucoses (Figure 4–2), forms much of the starch found in vegetables, beans, breads, pasta, and rice. In corn, for example, glucose is converted to starch as the corn ages. This reflects the function of starch as a carbohydrate storage form in plants.

Dietary fiber is an indigestible form of polysaccharide. This means that dietary fiber passes through the small intestine without being digested. Detailed information about the forms, recommendations, and benefits of dietary fiber can be found in the first Nutrition Insight in this chapter.

Glycogen (animal starch) is made by humans and is a storage form for glucose. This polysaccharide consists of a chain of glucoses with many branches. Enzymes that break down starches to glucose and other simple sugars can start digestion only at the ends of the molecules. The numerous branches of glycogen provide many sites (ends) for enzyme action. Glycogen is thus an ideal form for carbohydrate storage in the body because it can be quickly broken down.

The liver and muscles are the major storage sites for glycogen. Because only about 120 kcal of glucose are available as such in body fluids, these storage sites for carbohydrate energy—amounting to about 1800 kcal—are extremely important. As noted in the introduction, the 400 kcal of liver glycogen can be turned into blood glucose, but the 1400 kcal of muscle glycogen cannot. Still, glycogen in muscles can supply glucose for muscle use, especially during high-intensity and endurance exercise. (See Chapter 10 for a detailed discussion of carbohydrate use in exercise.)

Though animals contain carbohydrate in the form of glycogen, meat, fish, and poultry are not good sources of this (or any other) carbohydrate. This is because glycogen stores are quickly used up in the process of death.

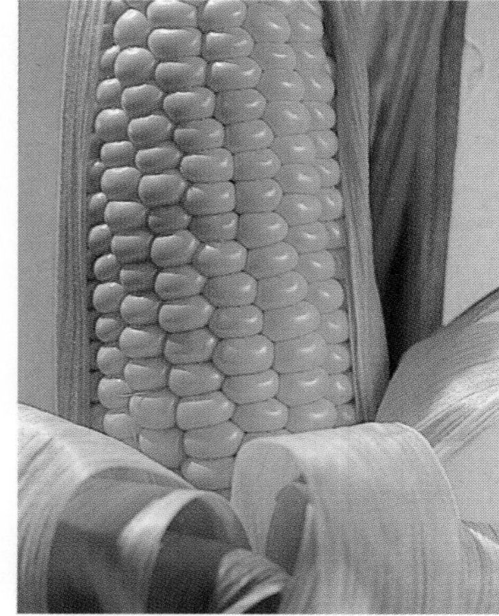

As plants mature, some sugars are turned into starch.

ConceptCheck

Important monosaccharides in nutrition are glucose, fructose, and galactose. Glucose is a primary energy source for body cells. Disaccharides form when two monosaccharides combine. Important disaccharides in nutrition are the table sugar sucrose (glucose joined with fructose), maltose (glucose joined with glucose), and the milk sugar lactose (glucose joined with galactose). Once digested into monosaccharide forms and absorbed, most carbohydrates are transformed into glucose in the liver.

The major digestible polysaccharides—starches—contain multiple glucose units linked together. Glycogen is animal starch and acts as a storage form of glucose in the liver and muscles.

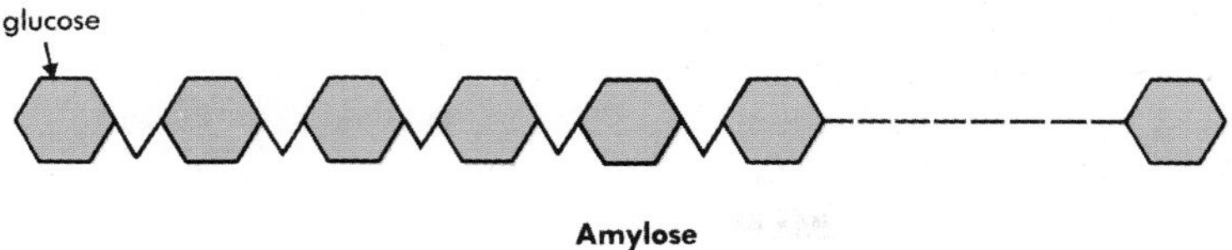

Simple → Complex

Monosaccharides
Glucose, fructose, galactose

Disaccharides
Sucrose, lactose, maltose

Polysaccharides
Starches (amylose), glycogen, most dietary fiber

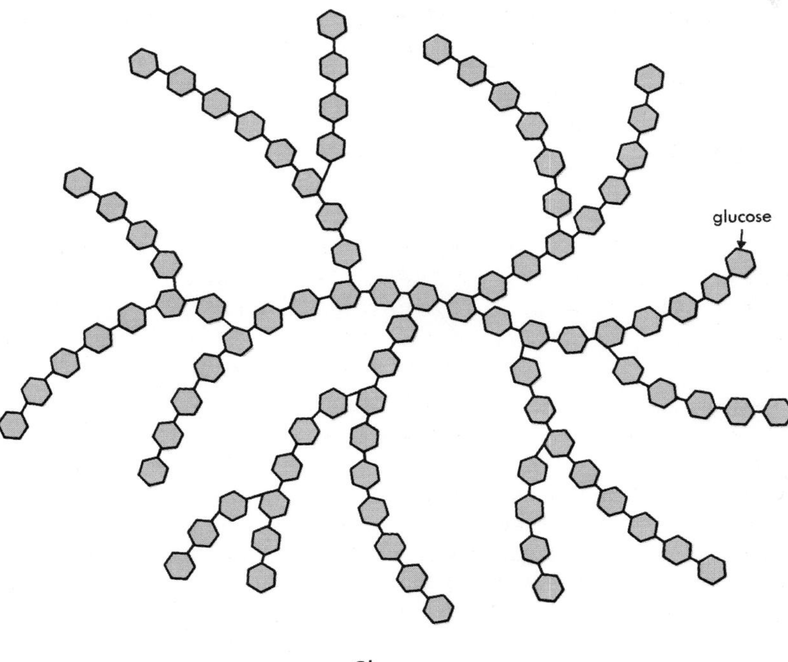

Figure 4–2 *Some common starches. We consume essentially no glycogen. All glycogen found in the body is made by our cells, primarily in the liver and muscles.*

Carbohydrates in Foods

The foods that yield the highest percentage of energy from carbohydrates are table sugar, honey, jam, jelly, fruit, and plain baked potatoes. These foods are nutrient dense for carbohydrate; that is, carbohydrates deliver much of their food energy. Corn flakes, rice, bread, and noodles all contain at least 75% of energy as carbohydrates. Foods less rich in carbohydrate energy are vegetables in general, oatmeal, dry beans and other legumes, cream pies, french fries, and nonfat milk. In many of these foods the carbohydrate content is diluted either by protein, as in the case of nonfat milk, or by fat, as in the case of a cream pie.

Chocolate, potato chips, and whole milk contain 30% to 40% of energy as carbohydrates. Again, the energy supplied from the carbohydrate content of these foods is overwhelmed by either their fat content or their protein content. Foods with essentially no carbohydrates include beef, chicken, fish (as mentioned above), and vegetable oils, butter, and margarine.

Figure 4–3 shows that, in planning a high-carbohydrate diet, you should emphasize potatoes, grains, pasta, beans, fruits, and vegetables. Sugar-rich sources then are secondary considerations. Note also that you can't create a diet high in carbohydrate energy from mostly chocolate, potato chips, and french fries because these foods contain too much fat. The percentage of energy from carbohydrate, and the type of carbohydrate, is more important than the total amount of carbohydrate in a food when planning a high-carbohydrate diet. Currently the top five carbohydrate

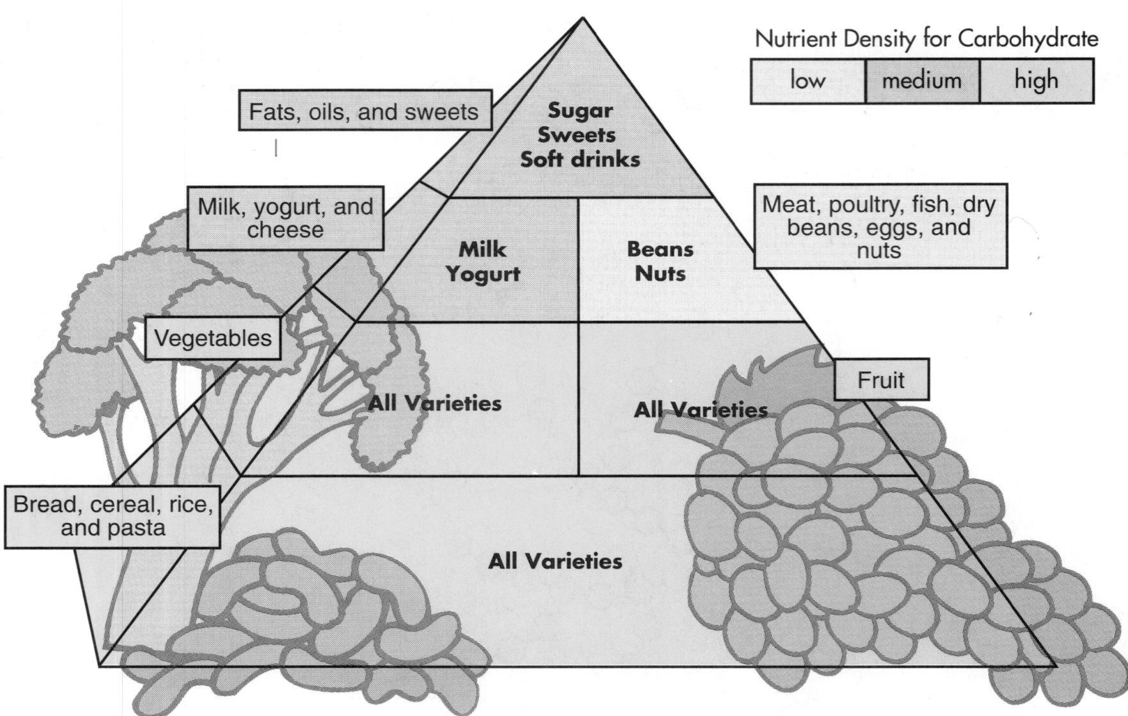

Figure 4–3 *Sources of carbohydrates from the Food Guide Pyramid. The bread, cereal, rice, and pasta group, fruit group, vegetable group, and milk, yogurt, and cheese group contain many foods rich in carbohydrate. Based on serving sizes for the Food Guide Pyramid, milk and yogurt contain about 12 grams, beans about 40 grams, nuts about 20 grams, fruits and grain products about 15 grams, and vegetables about 5 grams of carbohydrates. The background color of each group indicates the average nutrient density for carbohydrate in that group.*

Names of sugars used in foods:
Sugar
Sucrose
Brown sugar
Confectioners' sugar (powdered sugar)
Fruit juice concentrate
Syrup
Turbinado sugar
Invert sugar
Glucose
Levulose
Polydextrose
Lactose
Honey
Corn syrup or sweeteners
High-fructose corn syrup
Molasses
Caramel
Maple syrup
Dextrose
Fructose
Maltose

sources for U.S. adults are white bread, soft drinks, cookies and cakes (including doughnuts), sugars/syrups/jams, and potatoes. Clearly many Americans (teenagers included) should take a closer look at their main carbohydrate sources and strive to improve these from a nutritional standpoint.

A Closer Look at Nutritive Sweeteners in Foods

Sucrose is the tried-and-true sweetener. A relatively new sweetener in food is high-fructose corn syrup, which contains 40% to 90% fructose. It is made by treating corn starch with acid and enzymes. Much of the starch is broken down into glucose and then changed into fructose. The syrup is usually as sweet as sucrose (Table 4–1). Its major advantage is that it is cheaper and can be shipped in a more concentrated form than sucrose. Also, it has better freezing properties because it doesn't encourage the formation of ice crystals. High-fructose corn syrups are used in soft drinks, candies, jams, jellies, other fruit products, and desserts.

In addition to sucrose and high-fructose corn syrup, brown sugar, honey, maple syrup, and other sugars are added to foods. A partially refined version of raw sugar that can be sold is turbinado sugar. This has a slight molasses flavor. Brown sugar is basically sucrose containing some molasses; either the molasses is not totally removed from the sucrose during processing or it is added back to the sucrose crystals. Maple syrup is made by boiling down the sap from sugar maple trees. Pancake syrup sold in supermarkets is sweetened mostly with corn syrup—not maple syrup.

To make honey, bees alter nectar from plants, breaking down the sucrose into fructose and glucose. Honey offers the same nutritional value as other simple sugar sources. A common misconception is that honey contains vitamins and minerals. It

TABLE 4-1

The Sweetness of Sugars and Alternative Sweeteners

Type of sweetener	Relative sweetness* (sucrose = 1)	Typical sources
SUGARS		
Lactose	0.2	Dairy products
Maltose	0.4	Sprouted seeds
Glucose	0.7	Corn syrup
Sucrose	1	Table sugar, most sweets
Invert sugar†	1.3	Some candies, honey
Fructose	1.2–1.8	Fruit, honey, some soft drinks
SUGAR ALCOHOLS		
Sorbitol	0.6	Dietetic candies, sugarless gum
Mannitol	0.7	Dietetic candies
Xylitol	0.9	Sugarless gum
ALTERNATIVE SWEETENERS		
Cyclamate	30	Not currently in use in the United States
Aspartame	200	Diet soft drinks, diet fruit drinks, sugarless gum, tabletop use
Acesulfame-K	200	Sugarless gum, diet drink mixes, powdered diet sweeteners, puddings, gelatin desserts
Saccharin (sodium salt)	200–700	Diet soft drinks, tabletop use
Sucralose	600	Soft drinks, sugarless gum, jams, frozen desserts, tabletop use

*On a per gram basis.
†Sucrose broken down into glucose and fructose.
Adapted from the American Dietetic Association, 1993, and other sources.

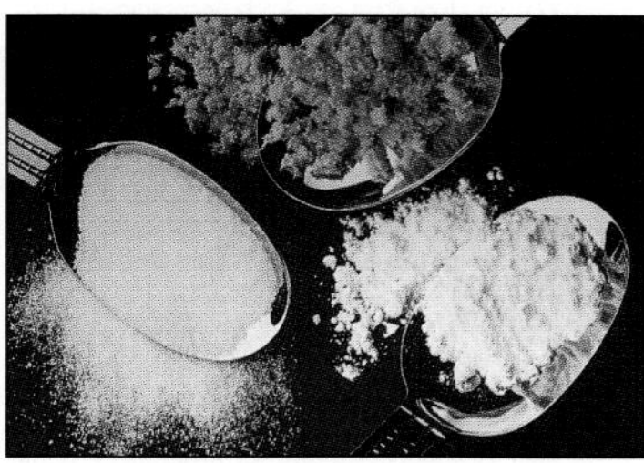

There are many forms of sugar on the market. Used in many foods, together they contribute to our daily intake of approximately 20 teaspoons (85 grams) of added sugars.

is a source of energy but little else (see Appendix A). Only the sweetener black strap molasses, a by-product of sugar production, contains any appreciable amounts of minerals. However, our consumption of molasses in foods is very low.

Alternative Sweeteners in Foods

People who want to limit sugar have two sets of alternative sweeteners to consider. One set is the sugar alcohols: this includes **sorbitol,** mannitol, and xylitol. Although sugar alcohols contribute energy (about 1.5 to 3 kcal per gram), they are absorbed and metabolized to glucose more slowly than simple sugars. Still, these substances do not provide a significant advantage for people with diabetes because large amounts can cause diarrhea (due to slow absorption), and they are usually found primarily in diabetic candy and gum. Nonetheless, products containing these sugar alcohols are marketed to people with diabetes. Sorbitol and xylitol also are used in sugarless gum, breath mints, and candy. These are not readily metabolized by bacteria in the mouth and thus do not promote **dental caries** as readily as simple sugars, such as sucrose (see later section.).

The other major class of alternative sweeteners currently available in the United States includes saccharin, aspartame, acesulfame-K, and sucralose.

Saccharin. Although widely used in soft drinks and table sweeteners, **saccharin** has been linked with cancer. Laboratory animals have developed bladder cancer when given high doses of saccharin. Arguments continue concerning the interpretation of data from these experiments, mostly because of saccharin's weak carcinogenic nature. In 1977 FDA attempted to ban saccharin because of this association with

Sorbitol
An alcohol derivative of glucose that yields about 3 kcal per gram but is slowly absorbed from the small intestine. It is used in some sugarless gums and dietetic foods.

Dental caries (KARE-ees)
Erosions in the surface of a tooth caused by acids made by bacteria as they metabolize sugars.

Saccharin
An alternative sweetener that yields no energy to the body; it is 300 times sweeter than sucrose.

INGREDIENTS: SORBITOL, GUM BASE, MANNITOL, GLYCEROL, HYDROGENATED GLUCOSE SYRUP, XYLITOL, ARTIFICIAL AND NATURAL FLAVORS, ASPARTAME, RED 40, YELLOW 6 AND BHT (TO MAINTAIN FRESHNESS). PHENYLKETONURICS: CONTAINS PHENYLALANINE. *NUTRASWEET IS A REGISTERED TRADEMARK OF THE NUTRASWEET CO.

Sugarless Gum

Sugar alcohols can be found in sugarless gum. Note that aspartame is also used to sweeten this product.

cancer. Many saccharin users protested a ban because it left them with no low-calorie sweetener (the others were not available in 1977). Public pressure persuaded Congress to prevent FDA from banning saccharin; however, products containing saccharin are currently required to contain a label warning of the cancer risk.

Aspartame. The trade name of **aspartame** is NutraSweet when added to foods and Equal when sold as powder. Aspartame is composed of the amino acids phenylalanine and aspartic acid, with the addition of methanol. Because amino acids are the building blocks of proteins, aspartame belongs more in the protein class than in the carbohydrate class. Aspartame yields energy—about 4 kcal per gram—but is much sweeter than sucrose. This means that much less aspartame yields the same sweetening potency as sucrose. Today aspartame is used mostly in beverages, gelatin desserts, chewing gum, and toppings and fillings for precooked bakery goods and cookies. Aspartame does not cause tooth decay. Like other proteins, however, aspartame is damaged when heated for a long time and thus cannot be widely used in products that require cooking.

Although aspartame has never been linked with cancer, some individuals have filed complaints with FDA claiming adverse reactions to aspartame—headaches, dizziness, seizures, nausea, allergic reactions, and other side effects. People who are sensitive to aspartame should avoid it. However, the percentage of sensitive people is extremely small. Considering its wide use, the relatively small numbers of complaints made against aspartame to date suggests most people can use it. In addition, careful research casts doubt on whether it causes headaches and mood swings or stimulates later food intake. FDA also does not consider the recent concern over it causing brain tumors credible.

An acceptable daily intake set by FDA is equivalent to about 14 cans of diet soft drinks a day for an adult or about 80 packets of Equal. Aspartame is safe for children and pregnant women to consume, but some scientists suggest cautious use by these groups.

One final note about aspartame: a rare disease called ***phenylketonuria (PKU)*** lessens a person's ability to metabolize phenylalanine. PKU is discussed in Chapter 6. For now, note that labels on products containing aspartame (such as diet soft drinks) warn people with PKU against using the product. (Babies are tested for this disease at birth.)

Aspartame
An alternative sweetener made of two amino acids (part of proteins) and methanol; it is about 200 times sweeter than sucrose.

Phenylketonuria (PKU)
A disease in which the liver cannot readily metabolize the amino acid phenylalanine. Toxic by-products of phenylalanine can then build up in the body and lead to mental retardation.

Acesulfame-K
An alternative sweetener that yields no energy to the body; it is 200 times sweeter than sucrose.

Sucralose
An alternative sweetener that has chlorines in place of some hydroxyl (–OH) groups on sucrose. It is 600 times sweeter than sucrose.

Acesulfame-K. **Acesulfame-K** (Sunette) is much sweeter than sucrose. Presently, it can be used in chewing gum, powdered drink mixes, gelatins, puddings, nondairy creamers, baked goods, yogurt, frozen desserts, syrups, and toppings. It contributes no energy to the diet because it is not broken down by the body. Acesulfame-K is used as a sweetener in foods and beverages in at least 60 countries including Canada. Acesulfame-K can be used in baking, whereas the current form of aspartame cannot because it breaks down when heated. Acesulfame-K may therefore become more widely used. There is also a trend to blend it with aspartame, such as in soft drinks.

Sucralose. **Sucralose**, which is made by substituting three chlorines for three hydroxyl groups (−OH) on sucrose, is much sweeter than sucrose. FDA approved sucralose's use in 1998 as an additive to foods such as soda, gum, baked goods, syrups, gelatins, frozen dairy desserts such as ice cream, jams, processed fruits and fruit juices, and for tabletop use. Sucralose doesn't break down under high heat conditions and can be used in cooking and baking. It is also excreted as such in the feces, or in the urine for the little that ends up being absorbed. Because of such recent introduction, it is not clear whether the public will embrace this new product. Canadians have had access to sucralose before its U.S. introduction.

Overall, alternative sweeteners enable people with diabetes to enjoy the flavor of sweetness while controlling calories and simple sugars in their diets; they also provide noncaloric or very low-calorie sugar substitutes for persons trying to lose or control weight.

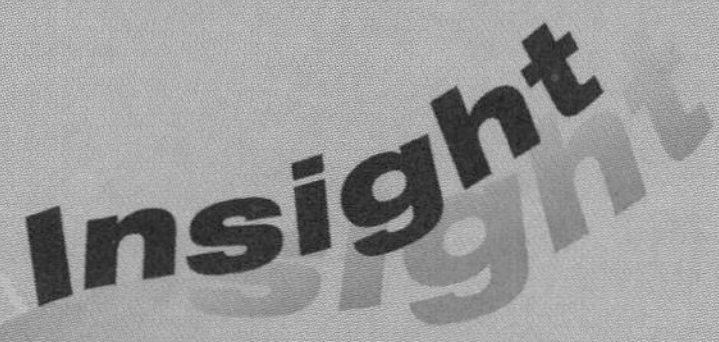

Dietary Fiber: An Often Underappreciated Class of Carbohydrates

Dietary fibers as a class are mostly made up of polysaccharides, but they differ from starches insofar as the chemical links that join individual sugar units cannot be digested by human enzymes in the GI tract. This prevents the small intestine from absorbing the sugars that make up dietary fibers. Dietary fiber is not a single substance but a group of substances with similar characteristics (Table 4–2). The group comprises the carbohydrates cellulose, hemicelluloses, pectins, gums, and mucilages, as well as the noncarbohydrate lignin. In total these constitute all the nonstarch polysaccharides in foods.

Cellulose, hemicelluloses, and lignin form the structural parts of plants. A cotton ball is pure cellulose. Bran fiber is rich in hemicelluloses. The woody fibers in broccoli are partly lignin. Because the majority of these compounds neither readily dissolve in water nor are readily metabolized by intestinal bacteria, they are called ***insoluble fibers*** (Figure 4–4).

Pectins, gums, and mucilages are contained around and inside plant cells. These compounds either dissolve or swell when put into water and are therefore called ***soluble fibers.*** They also are readily metabolized by bacteria in the large intestine. These exist as gum arabic, guar gum, locust bean gum, and various pectin forms and are found in several foods, especially in salad dressings, some frozen desserts, jams, and jellies. Some forms of hemicelluloses also fall into the soluble category.

Most foods contain mixtures of soluble and insoluble fibers, but food labels do not distinguish between the two types. Still, if food is listed as a good source of one type of fiber, it usually contains some of the other type of dietary fiber as well.

Dietary Fiber Provides Health Benefits

As mentioned, many types of dietary fiber absorb water and hold on to it in the intestine. When enough fiber is consumed, its water-retaining property helps enlarge and soften the stool, easing elimination. Basically the larger stool size stimulates the intestinal muscles that promote peristalsis (see Chapter 3). Consequently, less pressure is needed to expel the stool.

When too little dietary fiber is eaten, the opposite can occur: the stool may be small and hard. Constipation may result, requiring strong pressures to move the stool in the large intestine during elimination. Hemorrhoids may then result from excessive straining. Also, the high pressures can force parts of the large intestine wall to pop

TABLE 4-2

Classification of Dietary Fibers

Type	Component(s)	Examples	Physiological effects	Major food sources
INSOLUBLE				
Noncarbohydrate	Lignin	Wheat bran	Under study	All plants
Carbohydrate	Cellulose	Wheat products	Increases fecal bulk	All plants
	Hemicelluloses	Brown rice	Decreases intestinal transit time	Wheat, rye, rice, vegetables
SOLUBLE				
Carbohydrate	Pectins, gums, mucilages, some hemicelluloses	Apples Bananas Oranges Carrots Barley Oats Kidney beans	Delays gastric emptying; slows glucose absorption; can lower blood cholesterol	Citrus fruits, oat products, beans

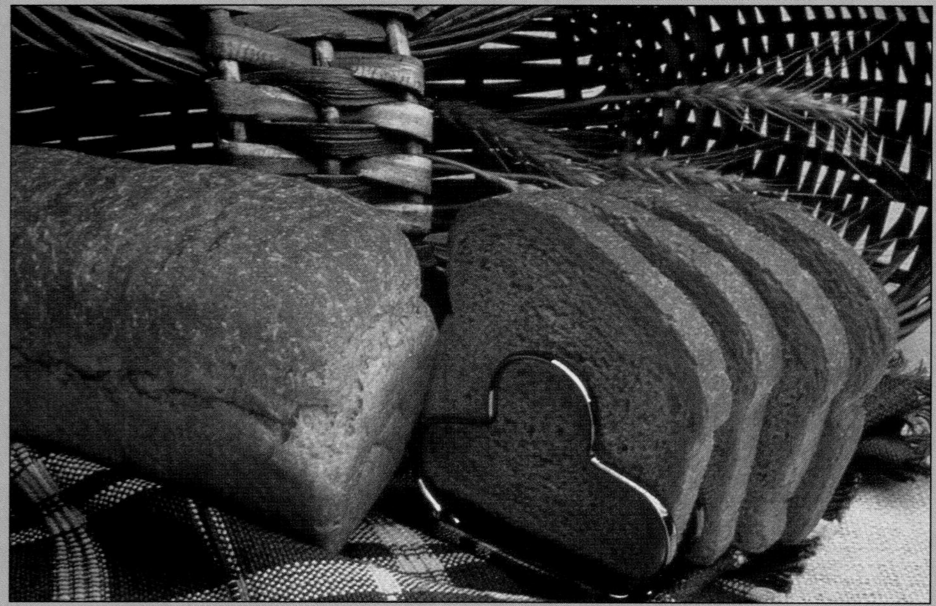

Whole grains are an excellent source of dietary fiber.

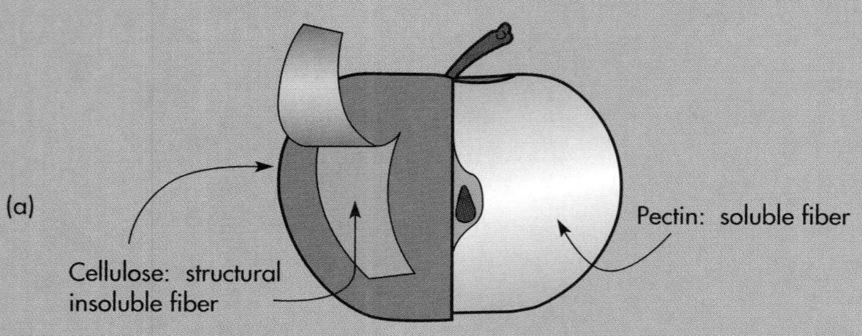

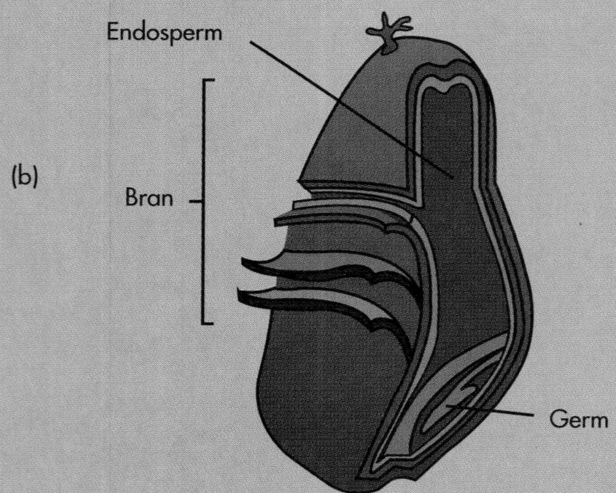

Figure 4-4 *Soluble and insoluble fiber.* ***A,*** *The skin of an apple consists of the insoluble fiber cellulose, which provides structure for the fruit. The soluble fiber pectin "glues" the fruit cells together.* ***B,*** *The outside layer of a wheat kernel is made of layers of bran—insoluble fiber—making this whole grain a good source of fiber. Overall, fruits, vegetables, whole grains and legumes are rich in dietary fiber.*

out from between the surrounding bands of muscle. This forms small pouches, called ***diverticula,*** leading to a condition called *diverticulosis.* About 50% of older people have many of these pouches (Figure 4-5). Diverticula rarely occur in people in developing countries, probably because of their high dietary fiber intakes. In contrast, people in Western countries often ingest much less dietary fiber in their diets.

Diverticulosis is normally not noticeable. But if the diverticula become filled with food particles, especially hulls or seeds, bacteria can metabolize them into acids and gases. This irritates the diverticula and may eventually cause inflammation, a condition known as ***diverticulitis.*** Treatment includes taking antibiotics to counter the bacterial action and eating a limited amount of dietary fiber to reduce the food source for bacterial activity. Once the inflammation subsides, a high fiber intake (but free of seeds) and increased fluid intake is recommended to ease elimination and reduce the risk of a future attack. Performing regular physical activity to stimulate peristalsis and maintaining regular bowel movements are also helpful in these cases.

Can Dietary Fiber Play Other Roles in Preserving Health?

Dietary fiber may also play a role in preventing colon cancer, but the research findings are mixed at this time. Epidemiological studies have linked its occurrence to diets low in **whole grains** (grains containing the entire seed of the plant, including the bran, germ, and starchy interior), fruits, and vegetables—all good sources of dietary fiber—and high in fat, meat, and excess energy intake. Many other factors, however, are also involved in the development of the disease, such as

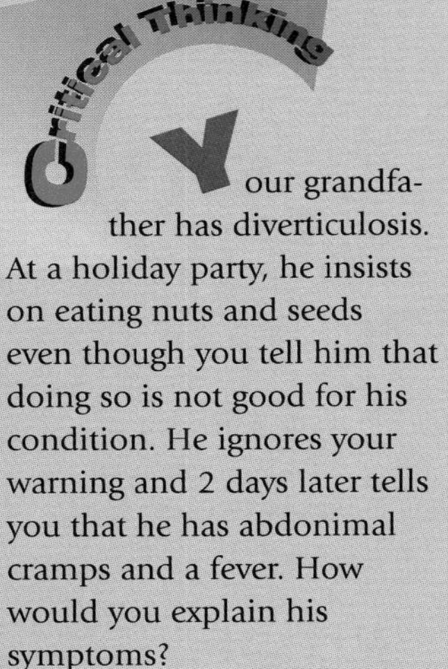

Your grandfather has diverticulosis. At a holiday party, he insists on eating nuts and seeds even though you tell him that doing so is not good for his condition. He ignores your warning and 2 days later tells you that he has abdonimal cramps and a fever. How would you explain his symptoms?

genetic background. Weaker but intriguing evidence implicates obesity; smoking; a generous alcohol intake (more that two drinks per day); lack of regular physical activity; inadequate intakes of the vitamins C, D, and folate and the mineral calcium; and low starch intakes.

Researchers are not sure how dietary fiber might reduce colon cancer development. However, they have proposed that potential cancer-causing compounds in the intestinal contents are diluted by fluid attracted to the fibers, bound to the fibers, and more rapidly excreted as fibers speed passage of feces through the intestinal tract.

In human studies, dietary fiber from fruits and vegetables has tended to be most protective against colon and rectal cancers. This finding suggests that increased consumption of vitamin C and phytochemicals from fruits and vegetables, or simply the reduction in meat and fat intake when a high-fiber diet is instituted, may exert the main protective effect, rather than dietary fiber alone. In other words, the presence of a high fiber diet might simply be a marker for an otherwise healthy diet (and related healthy lifestyle).

Adequate dietary fiber intake promotes cardiovascular health. Soluble fibers taken in high amounts in the diet can decrease blood cholesterol. The dose, if oat bran is used, needs to be about 80 to 100 grams (about ¾ of a cup uncooked) per day. With cooked beans, about 150 grams (1½ cups) is needed. The effect is partly caused by inhibiting bile recycling in the intestinal tract. Bile, which is formed from cholesterol, is then pulled into the feces for elimination. Additional mechanisms may be at work as well. Other rich sources of soluble fibers include fruits and vegetables in general, soybean fiber, rice bran, and **psyllium** seeds (found in many commercial fiber laxatives).

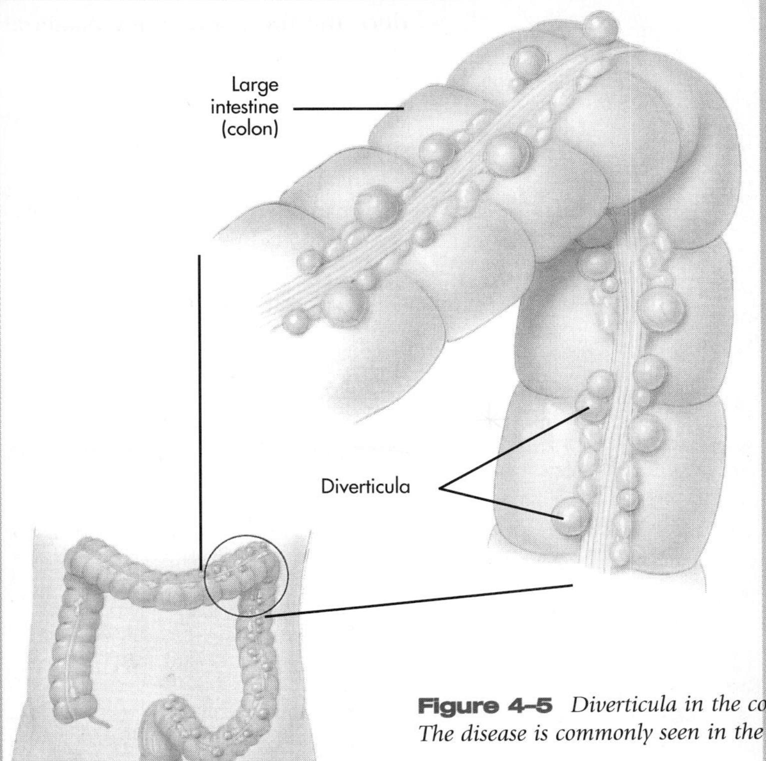

Figure 4–5 *Diverticula in the colon. A low-fiber diet increases the risk for their development. The disease is commonly seen in the elderly in Western societies.*

A recent study showed that men who ate more than 25 grams of fiber per day had a 36% lower risk of developing heart disease, and those eating 29 grams of fiber per day decreased their risk of a heart attack by 41%. For this reason, experts are recommending a 10 gram per day increase in fiber above our typical 14 to 15 gram per day intake, especially from grain sources, to prevent heart disease in the average American. Overall, a fiber-rich diet containing fruits, vegetables, beans, and whole grains (including whole-grain breakfast cereals) is advocated as part of a strategy to reduce heart disease risk.

A diet high in fiber may also aid weight control and reduce the risk of developing obesity. As noted in Chapter 1, the bulky nature of high-fiber foods fills us up without yielding much energy. High-fat foods tend to do just the opposite, contributing to obesity. Increasing intake of foods rich in dietary fiber is one strategy for remaining satisfied after a meal even if the fat content in a diet is low.

Finally, when consumed in large amounts, soluble dietary fiber slows glucose absorption from the small intestine. This effect can be helpful in treatment of diabetes (see the Nutrition Issue).

How Much Dietary Fiber Do We Need?

A reasonable goal for dietary fiber intake is 20 to 35 grams per day. As just mentioned, the average intake for Americans is closer to 14 to 15 grams per day. (For children over the age of 2, experts recommend a fiber intake of their age plus 5 grams per day.) Men eat more dietary fiber on average than do women, partly because they eat more food. Increasing dietary fiber intake to 20 to 35 grams is not difficult to achieve (Table 4–3). For example, eating a high-fiber cereal for breakfast is one easy way to increase dietary fiber intake.

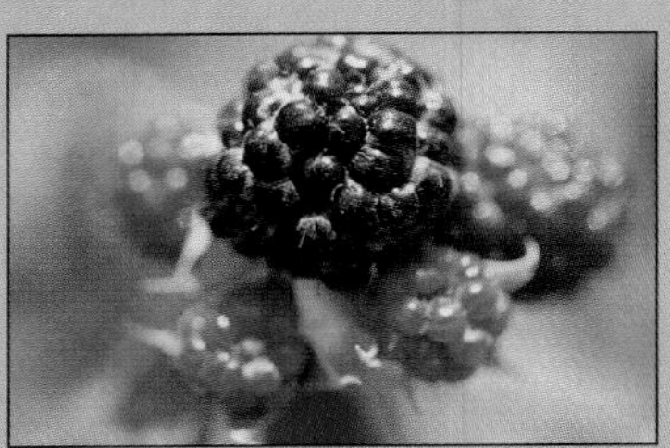

In the search for dietary fiber sources, berries may be overlooked. Just 1 cup of blackberries contains up to 6 grams of fiber.

Whole-food sources such as cereals, not bran supplements, are preferable because foods provide a broader variety of nutrients, particularly many natural high-fiber foods—whole grains, fruits, vegetables, and beans. Note also that drinking fluids with fiber-containing foods is recommended because fibers tend to bind water. Recall from Chapter 2 that the Food Guide Pyramid suggests we consume 5 to 9 servings of fruits/vegetables and 6 to 11 serving of breads/cereals each day. In addition, consuming legumes 1 to 2 times per week further increases fiber content in the diet. All these food choices can provide dietary fiber.

Read the Label

To check for whole grains, read the label on the food package (Figure 4–6). Note that manufacturers often list enriched white flour as wheat flour on food labels. Many people think that if a product is labeled *wheat,* they are getting a whole-wheat product. However, if the label does not say *whole-wheat* flour in the ingredient list, it is not a whole-wheat product. Bread made from white (refined) flour lacks the bran that forms a protective coating around the wheat kernel. Bran makes flour coarser but contains important parts, including dietary fiber.

Problems with High-Fiber Diets

Very high dietary fiber intakes—for example, 60 grams per day—can pose some health risks. Again, a high dietary fiber intake such as this also requires a high fluid intake. Not consuming enough fluid with the dietary fiber can leave the stool very hard, making elimination difficult and painful. Intestinal blockage has occurred in elderly people who consume great amounts of wheat bran and oat bran. Large amounts of dietary fiber can also bind important minerals, especially calcium, zinc, and iron, making them less available to the body. High-fiber diets also contribute to intestinal gas. Finally, great amounts of dietary fiber can make children feel full before they eat enough foot to meet energy needs. As with many practices, moderation with dietary fiber is the best approach.

TABLE 4-3

What's Your Fiber Score?

Although the foods below are particularly good sources of dietary fiber, many other foods—including all fruits and vegetables—contain smaller amounts that add up each day. What would it take to have your typical intake meet the recommended amount of 20 to 35 grams of fiber per day?

About 2 grams per serving	About 3 grams per serving	About 4 grams per serving
Banana	Apple with skin	Baked beans
Broccoli	Blueberries	Bran cereals
Carrot	Corn	Dried figs
Cauliflower	Orange	Kidney beans
Mango	Potato with skin	Lentils
Mixed vegetables	Raisins	Navy beans
Nectarine	Strawberries	Pear with skin
Pear, canned	Whole-grain cereals	Raspberries
Peas		Whole-wheat spaghetti
Oatmeal		
Peach		
Pineapple		
Rye crisp		
Whole-wheat bread		

Data from Pennington JAT: *Bowes and Church's food values of portions commonly used,* 17th ed. Philadelphia: J. B. Lippincott, 1998.

Nutrition Facts

Serving Size 1 cup (55g/2.0 oz.)
Servings Per Container 10

Amount Per Serving	Cereal	Cereal with ½ Cup Vitamins A & D Skim Milk
Calories	170	210
Calories from Fat	10	10
		% Daily Value**
Total Fat 1.0g*	**2%**	**2%**
Sat. Fat 0g	**0%**	**0%**
Cholesterol 0mg	**0%**	**0%**
Sodium 300mg	**13%**	**15%**
Potassium 340mg	**10%**	**16%**
Total Carbohydrate 43g	**14%**	**16%**
Dietary Fiber 7g	**28%**	**28%**
Sugars 16g		
Other Carbohydrate 20g		
Protein 4g		
Vitamin A	15%	20%
Vitamin C	20%	22%
Calcium	2%	15%
Iron	65%	65%
Vitamin D	10%	25%
Thiamin	25%	30%
Riboflavin	25%	35%
Niacin	25%	25%
Vitamin B_6	25%	25%
Folate	30%	30%
Vitamin B_{12}	25%	35%
Phosphorus	20%	30%
Magnesium	20%	25%
Zinc	25%	25%
Copper	10%	10%

*Amount in cereal. One half cup skim milk contributes an additional 40 calories, 65mg sodium, 6g total carbohydrate (6g sugars), and 4g protein.
**Percent Daily Values are based on a 2,000 calorie diet. Your daily values may be higher or lower depending on your calorie needs:

	Calories:	2,000	2,500
Total Fat	Less than	65g	80g
Sat Fat	Less than	20g	25g
Cholesterol	Less than	300mg	300mg
Sodium	Less than	2,400mg	2,400mg
Potassium		3,500mg	3,500mg
Total Carbohydrate		300g	375g
Dietary Fiber		25g	30g

Calories per gram:
Fat 9 • Carbohydrate 4 • Protein 4

Ingredients: Wheat bran with other parts of wheat, raisins, sugar, corn syrup, salt, malt flavoring, glycerin, iron,niacinamide, zinc oxide, pyridoxine hydrochloride (vitamin B_6), riboflavin (vitamin B_2), vitamin A palmitate, thiamin hydrochloride (vitamin B_1), folic acid, vitamin B_{12}, and vitamin D.

Nutrition Facts

Serving Size: ¾ Cup (30g)
Servings Per Package: About 17

Amount Per Serving	¾ Cup Cereal	Cereal With ½ Cup Skim Milk
Calories	120	160
Calories from Fat	0	5
	%Daily Value**	
Total Fat 0g*	**0%**	**1%**
Saturated Fat 0g	**0%**	**1%**
Cholesterol 0mg	**0%**	**1%**
Sodium 40mg	**2%**	**4%**
Potassium 60mg	**2%**	**8%**
Total Carbohydrate 26g	**9%**	**11%**
Dietary Fiber 1g	**4%**	**4%**
Sugars 15g		
Other Carbohydrate 10g		
Protein 2g		
Vitamin A	25%	30%
Vitamin C	0%	2%
Calcium	0%	15%
Iron	10%	10%
Vitamin D	10%	20%
Thiamin	25%	25%
Riboflavin	25%	35%
Niacin	25%	25%
Vitamin B6	25%	25%
Folate	25%	25%
Vitamin B12	25%	30%
Phosphorus	4%	15%
Magnesium	4%	8%
Zinc	10%	10%
Copper	2%	2%

*Amount in Cereal. One-half cup skim milk contributes an additional 65mg sodium, 6g total carbohydrate (6g sugars), and 4g protein.
**Percent Daily Values are based on a 2000 calorie diet. Your daily values may be higher or lower depending on your calorie needs:

	Calories:	2,000	2,500
Total Fat	Less than	65g	80g
Sat. Fat	Less than	20g	25g
Cholesterol	Less than	300mg	300mg
Sodium	Less than	2,400mg	2,400mg
Potassium		3,500mg	3,500mg
Total Carbohydrate		300g	375g
Dietary Fiber		25g	30g

Calories per gram:
Fat 9 • Carbohydrate 4 • Protein 4

Ingredients: Wheat, Sugar, Corn Syrup, Honey, Caramel Color, Partially Hydrogenated Soybean Oil, Salt, Ferric Phosphate, Niacinamide (Niacin), Zinc Oxide, Vitamin A (Palmitate), Pyridoxine Hydrochloride (Vitamin B6), Riboflavin, Thiamin Mononitrate, Folic Acid (Folate),Vitamin B12 and Vitamin D.

Figure 4-6 *Reading the NUTRITION FACTS on food labels helps us choose more nutritious foods. Based on the information from these nutrition labels, which cereal is the better choice for breakfast? Consider the amount of dietary fiber in each cereal, based on the amount per 100 kcal. Did the ingredient lists give you any clues? (Note: Ingredients are always listed in descending order by weight on a label.) When choosing a breakfast cereal, it is generally wise to focus on those that are rich sources of dietary fiber and low in fat. Sugar content can also be used for evaluation. However, sometimes this number does not reflect added sugar but simply the addition of fruits such as raisins, complicating the evaluation.*

ConceptCheck

Table sugar, honey, jam, fruit, and plain baked potatoes contain the highest percentage of energy from carbohydrates. Foods such as cream pies, potato chips, whole milk, and oatmeal contain moderate amounts of carbohydrate. Common nutritive sweeteners added to foods include sucrose, maple sugar, honey, brown sugar, and high-fructose corn syrup. For people who want to limit sugar intake, alternative sweeteners are available and include the sugar alcohols, saccharin, aspartame, acesulfame-K, and sucralose. Of these, aspartame is the most common alternative sweetener in use.

Making Carbohydrates Available for Body Use

As discussed in Chapter 3, simply eating a food does not supply nutrients to body cells. Digestion and absorption must occur first.

Carbohydrate Digestion

Carbohydrate digestion actually begins before we start eating. Preparing food can be viewed as the first step in digestion. Cooking softens tough connective tissues in the fibrous tissue of plants, such as broccoli stalks. When starches are heated, the starch granules swell as they soak up water, making them much easier to digest. All these effects of cooking generally make food easier to chew, swallow, and break down during digestion.

Digestion of starches begins as these mix with saliva during the chewing of food. Saliva contains an enzyme called *salivary amylase*. This enzyme breaks down starch into many smaller sugar units (disaccharides, such as maltose) (Figure 4–7). You can observe this conversion while chewing a saltine cracker. Prolonged chewing of the cracker causes it to taste sweeter as some starch breaks down into the sweeter sugars.

Salivary amylase does not work in an acidic environment. Once food moves down the esophagus into the stomach, the stomach's acidity soon halts further salivary amylase action and subsequently any starch digestion. However, this halting of salivary amylase is not very important because other enzymes including pancreatic amylase finish in the small intestine what salivary amylase begins in the mouth.

After the carbohydrates are in the intestine and pancreatic amylase and other enzymes have had time to act, the original carbohydrates in a food will be present as monosaccharides (mostly any glucose and fructose present as such in food), as well as disaccharides (maltose from starch breakdown, lactose mainly from dairy products, and sucrose from food preparation and that added at the table). Eventually all the disaccharide forms are digested to their monosaccharide forms by specialized enzymes attached to the cells of the small intestine. The enzyme maltase acts on maltose to produce two glucose molecules. Sucrase acts on sucrose to produce glucose and fructose. Lactase acts on lactose to produce glucose and galactose.

When considering carbohydrate digestion, you should remember that key digestive enzymes come from both the pancreas and the cells of the intestinal wall. Intestinal diseases can interfere with the production of the intestinal wall enzymes. Such conditions may interfere with the efficient digestion of the sugars maltose, lactose, and sucrose. The portion of these carbohydrates that is not fully digested will not be absorbed. When these unabsorbed carbohydrates eventually end up in the large intestine, the bacteria there will use the sugars to produce acid and gas. If produced in large amounts, these can cause abdominal discomfort. People recovering from intestinal disorders, such as diarrhea or bacterial infections, may need to avoid

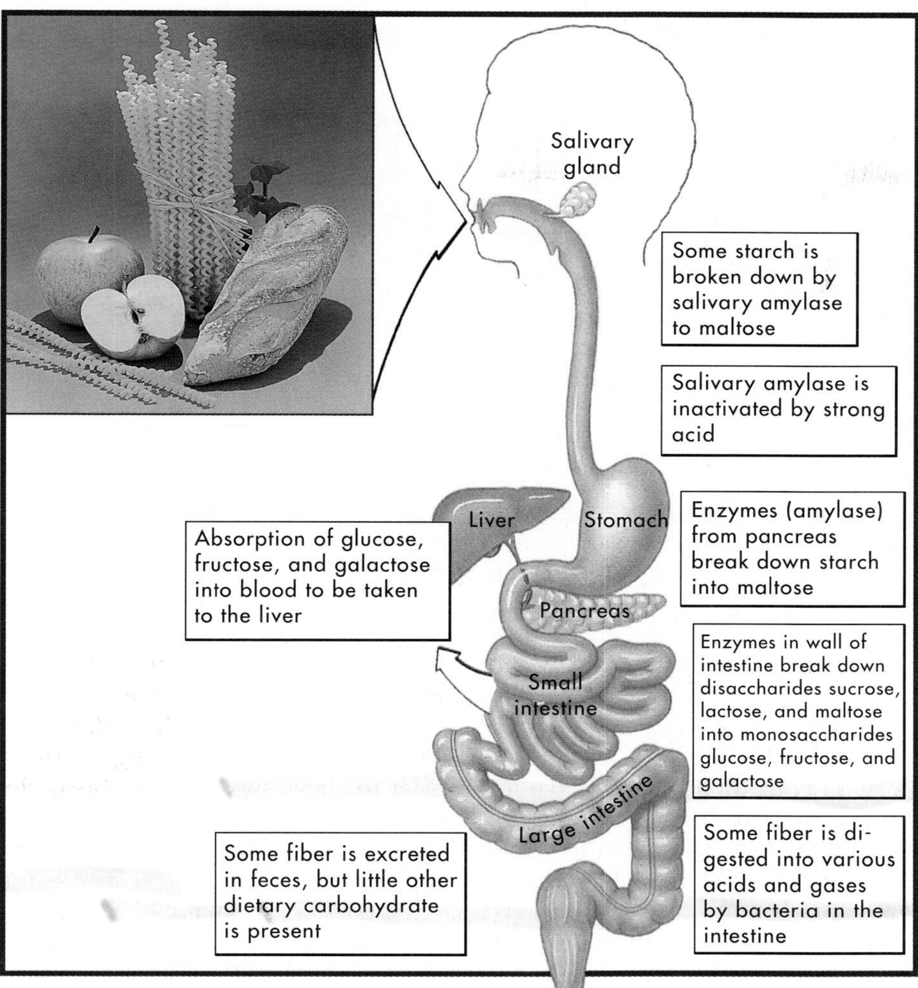

Figure 4-7 *Carbohydrate digestion and absorption. Enzymes made by the mouth, pancreas, and small intestine participate in the process of digestion. Most carbohydrate digestion and absorption take place in the small intestine.*

lactose for a few weeks if temporary lactose intolerance is experienced. Two weeks will be sufficient time for the small intestine to resume producing enough lactase enzyme to allow for lactose digestion (see the next Nutrition Insight).

Carbohydrate Absorption

Single sugars found naturally in foods and those formed as by-products of earlier starch digestion in the mouth and small intestine generally follow an active absorption process (one that requires energy input) when they are taken up by the absorptive cells in the small intestine. Once glucose, galactose, and fructose enter the intestinal cells, they are transported via the portal vein to the liver. The liver then exercises its metabolic options—transforming monosaccharides into glucose and releasing them directly into the bloodstream, producing the storage form of the carbohydrate, glycogen, or producing fat. Of these three options, producing fat is the least likely. Only a minor amount of starch (about 5%) escapes absorption. This travels down to the large intestine and is digested there by bacteria. Then some is absorbed in the form of acids and gases produced by bacterial metabolism, as is true for undigested lactose. Scientists suspect that some of these products actually promote health of the large intestine by providing a source of energy.

As bacteria in the large intestine metabolize soluble fibers into such products as acids and gases, these in turn can cause intestinal gas (flatulence). Gas is not harmful but can be inconvenient. However, the body tends to adapt over time to a high fiber intake and produce less gas.

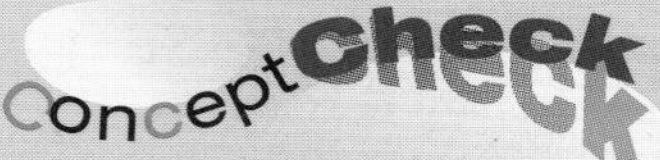

Carbohydrate digestion is the process of breaking down larger carbohydrates into their absorbable components. Digestion of starches begins in the mouth with salivary amylase. Enzymes made by the pancreas and small intestine complete the digestion of carbohydrates to single sugars in the small intestine. Primarily following an active absorption process, the single sugars (monosaccharides)—either resulting from the digestive process or present in the meal—are taken up by absorptive cells in the intestine and ultimately transported via the portal vein to the liver. Then the liver exercises its metabolic options, primarily producing glucose and glycogen.

Putting Simple Carbohydrates to Work in the Body

The functions of glucose in the body start with supplying energy, but that is only the beginning. Because the other sugars can generally be converted to glucose and starches are broken down to yield glucose, the functions described here apply to most carbohydrates.

Yielding Energy

The main function of glucose is to supply energy for the body. Certain tissues in the body, such as red blood cells, can use only glucose and other simple carbohydrate forms for energy. Most parts of the brain also derive energy only from simple carbohydrates, unless the diet contains almost none. In that case, much of the brain can use partial breakdown products of fat—called ***ketones***—for energy (see below). Simple carbohydrates can also fuel muscle cells and other body cells, but many of these cells can also use fat for energy needs (see Chapter 10 for details on muscle metabolism).

Ketone
Incomplete breakdown products of fat containing three or four carbons.

Sparing Protein from Use as an Energy Source and Preventing Ketosis

The importance of carbohydrate fuel for the body cannot be overstated. As a fuel for the brain and red blood cells, carbohydrate is critical. If you don't eat enough carbohydrates, your body is forced to make glucose from other nutrients, mainly certain amino acids that make up proteins. When this occurs, some of the proteins from your diet can't be used to make body tissues and perform other vital functions. Under normal circumstances, digestible carbohydrates in the diet mostly end up as blood glucose to be used by the brain, red blood cells, and most other body cells for fuel. This allows proteins to be saved for their normal functions, like building and maintaining muscles. Therefore digestible carbohydrates are considered protein sparing.

During long-term starvation, proteins in the muscles, heart, liver, kidneys, and other vital organs break down into amino acids, and certain forms are turned into needed glucose. If the process occurs over weeks at a time, these organs become partially weakened. (See Chapters 6 and 16 for discussions of the specific effects of starvation.)

When you don't eat enough carbohydrates, an additional result is that fats don't break down completely in metabolism. In other words, without enough carbohydrate present, fat metabolism is hampered. Partial breakdown products of fats, called *ketones*, then form. This condition, known as ***ketosis***, should be avoided because it disturbs the body's normal acid-base balance and leads to other health problems.

For now, keep in mind that eating at least 50 to 100 grams of carbohydrates per day ensures complete metabolism of fats. It also prevents the body weakness that usually results from having to use protein to compensate for an insufficient carbohydrate intake. Still, typical adults in the United States need not worry. Our daily carbohydrate intakes usually exceed 100 grams, averaging closer to 200 to 300 grams per day.

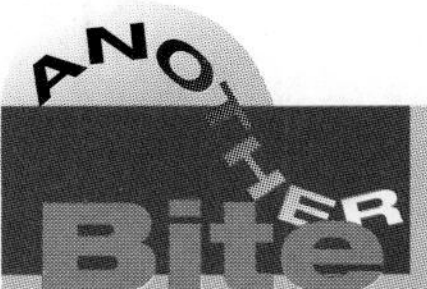

The life-threatening wasting of protein that occurs during long-term fasting has prompted companies that produce medical products for rapid weight loss to include 30 to 120 grams of carbohydrate in the formulation. This significantly decreases protein breakdown and thereby helps protect vital tissues and organs, including the heart (see Chapter 9 for details).*

*Most of these products are powders that can be mixed with different kinds of fluids, are consumed five or six times per day, and are very low in calories.

Regulating This Energy Source

Under normal circumstances a person's blood glucose concentration is regulated within a very narrow range.

Recall from Chapter 3 that when carbohydrates are digested and taken up by the absorptive cells of the small intestine, the portal vein then transports the resulting monosaccharides to the liver. The liver is the first organ to screen the absorbed sugars. One of its roles is to guard against excess glucose entering the bloodstream after a meal.

The pancreas works with the liver to control blood glucose. As soon as eating begins, the pancreas releases small amounts of the hormone **insulin**. Once much glucose enters the bloodstream, the pancreas releases more insulin. This insulin stimulates the liver to synthesize glycogen—the storage form of glucose in the body—and stimulates muscle cells, adipose (fat) cells, and other cells to increase glucose uptake. By triggering both glucose storage in the liver and glucose movement out of the bloodstream into certain cells, insulin keeps glucose from rising too high in the blood (Figure 4–8).

Other hormones have the opposite effect of insulin. When a person has not eaten for a few hours and blood glucose begins to fall, the pancreas releases the hormone **glucagon**. This hormone prompts the breakdown of glycogen into glucose, which is then released from the liver into the bloodstream. In this way glucagon keeps blood glucose from falling too low.

A different mechanism increases blood glucose during times of stress. **Epinephrine** (adrenaline) is the hormone responsible for the "flight or fight" reaction. Epinephrine and a related compound are released in large amounts from the adrenal gland (located on each kidney) and various nerve endings in response to a perceived threat, such as a car approaching head-on. These cause glycogen in the liver to break down into glucose. The resulting rapid flood of glucose from the liver into the bloodstream helps promote quick mental and physical reactions.

In essence, the actions of insulin on blood glucose are balanced by the actions of glucagon, epinephrine, and other hormones. If hormonal balance is not maintained, such as during over- or under-production of insulin or glucagon, major changes in blood glucose concentrations occur.

Before we move on, let's step back and look at one of the intricacies of our body's metabolism. To maintain blood glucose within an acceptable range, the

Insulin
A hormone produced by the beta cells of the pancreas. Among other processes, insulin increases the synthesis of glycogen in the liver and the movement of glucose from the bloodstream into body cells.

Glucagon
A hormone made by the pancreas that stimulates the breakdown of glycogen in the liver into glucose; this ends up increasing blood glucose. Glucagon also performs other functions.

Epinephrine
A hormone also known as adrenaline; *it is released by the adrenal gland (located on each kidney) and various nerve endings in the body. It acts to increase glycogen breakdown in the liver, among other functions.*

Nutrition Insight

Lactose Intolerance

The ability to digest lactose depends on the activity of the enzyme lactase. This enzyme, which is embedded within the surface of intestinal cells, splits lactose into glucose and galactose. These monosaccharides are absorbed from the small intestine into the bloodstream, but lactose is not. When lactase activity is low, lactose travels unaltered into the large intestine, where resident bacteria metabolize it into acids and gases, causing intestinal gas, bloating, cramping, and discomfort.

Primary lactose intolerance is common in Asians, Hispanics, Native Americans, people of Mediterranean descent, African-Americans, and some other ethnic races. In this case, the loss of lactase activity is not due to another disease per se—hence its designation as a **primary disease.** Some individuals may be born with little or no lactase, but more commonly the lactase activity declines with age, starting at about 2 years of age. Even though lactose intolerance is more common in some ethnic groups than others, between 30 and 60 million Americans and up to 70% of adults worldwide experience a large decrease in their ability to synthesize lactase as they age.

Secondary lactose intolerance by definition develops as a result of another disease, as is true of **secondary diseases.** Most cases are caused by intestinal bacterial infections. The inability to digest lactose may also result from the use of certain medications, especially anticancer drugs. Both infection and some drugs can inhibit the growth of the rapidly reproducing cells that line the GI tract and produce lactase.

Clinically, lactose intolerance can be diagnosed from a history of gas and bloating after milk consumption. This history can then be confirmed by having the person consume lactose. If blood glucose does not rise much after consuming the lactose, lactose maldigestion is the likely cause. Other, more technical procedures are available to confirm the diagnosis of lactose intolerance.

An individual who is sensitive to even small amounts of lactose must become an avid label reader in order to avoid products with ingredients such as milk, milk solids, casein, and whey. Some medications contain lactose as binders or fillers. Moderate lactose intolerance, however, is much more common than nearly complete intolerance. Most people who are moderately intolerant quickly learn by trial and error how much lactose they can tolerate and easily adjust the amount of dairy products in their diet. Such people need not avoid all milk and milk products; nor is this recommended, because these foods are very good sources of calcium, riboflavin,

body relies on a complex regulatory system. This provides a safeguard against extremely high or low blood glucose if one control mechanism fails. Suppose instead there were only one mechanism for controlling blood glucose, such as a nerve connection between the brain and pancreas that when appropriately stimulated caused release of insulin. Damage to this nerve would prevent insulin release, causing extreme fluctuations in blood glucose, with dire physiological consequences. In fact, a disturbance in one of the body's control mechanisms—such as insulin release from the pancreas—can greatly influence blood glucose, but it doesn't knock out all of the other regulatory systems. The liver and adrenal glands still act to provide moderate regulation of blood glucose. This example of checks and balances is typical of how the body maintains blood and other tissue concentrations of its key constituents within fairly narrow ranges.

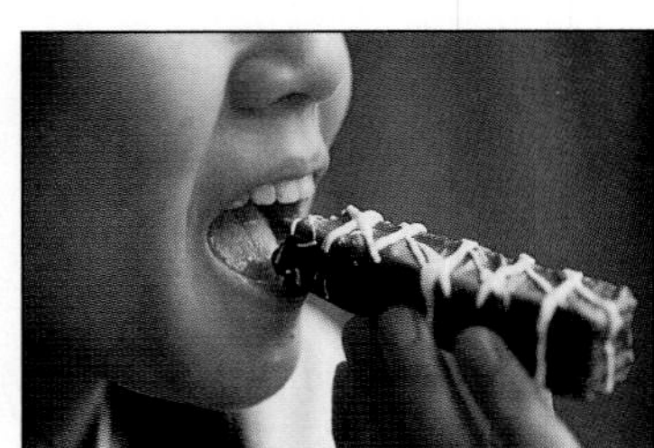

Many foods we enjoy are sweet. These should be eaten in moderation.

Flavoring and Sweetening Foods

Even a baby responds to sugars with a smile. Sensors on the tip of the tongue recognize a variety of sugars and even some noncarbohydrate substances. Sugars improve the palatability of many foods and thus enhance diets in general. For example, a small amount of sucrose on a grapefruit improves the taste of this sour fruit. Moderation in using sugars is recommended, but there is no need to avoid sugars altogether.

potassium, and magnesium. Although these four nutrients are present in other food groups, many people don't eat much of these alternative sources. Obtaining enough of these nutrients is much easier if milk and milk products are included in the diet.

Recent studies show that nearly all lactose-intolerant individuals can tolerate ½ to 1 cup of milk with breakfast and 1 cup with dinner. In addition, this portion of milk product is often better tolerated when taken with other foods because fat in a meal slows digestion, allowing more time for lactase action. Also, individuals with lactose intolerance can eat cheese. Much lactose is lost when milk is made into cheese. Yogurt can be tolerated as well.

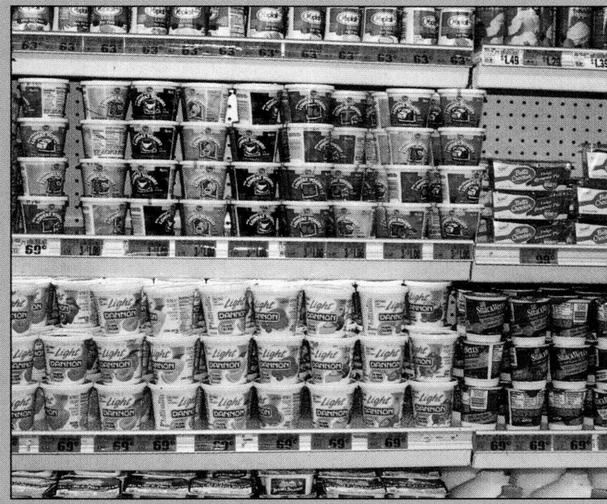

Use of yogurt helps moderately lactose intolerant individuals to meet calcium needs.

The bacteria that make yogurt provide their own lactase activity. Thus, if the yogurt contains active bacteria cultures, the lactose present is essentially digested by the yogurt. Freezing destroys the bacteria's activity, so frozen yogurt—as currently manufactured—may have little remaining lactase activity. In general, the foods tolerated best by lactose-intolerant individuals are hard cheeses and regular yogurt.

During the past few years, manufacturers have been producing low-lactose milk by treating regular milk with lactase isolated from yeast. The added lactase breaks down most of the lactose into glucose and galactose, yielding a milk that causes few symptoms in most moderately intolerant people. Compared with regular milk, low-lactose milk tastes sweeter because of its higher concentration of glucose, which is three to four times sweeter than lactose. Low-lactose milk can be made at home by adding a commercially available lactase preparation to regular milk. Lactase pills are also available and can be used at mealtimes. Few people actually need to use enzyme-treated milk or lactase pills, because their intolerance is moderate. Minor changes in diet suffice, even for people who feel they are quite sensitive to lactose. Researchers also suggest that lactose-intolerant individuals who continue to drink milk for 4 to 6 months may adapt to intestinal gas production. For those who nevertheless wish to consume less lactose, low-lactose products allow greater versatility in the diet. Thus, several options are available to lactose-intolerant people, only one of which is abandoning milk products. People with severe lactase deficiency who avoid all dairy products should seek other sources of calcium (see Chapter 8).

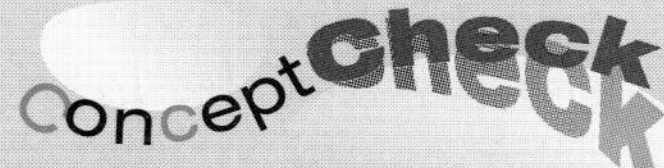

In addition to providing sweetness to food, carbohydrates provide glucose for the energy needs of red blood cells and parts of the brain. Eating less than 50 to 100 grams of carbohydrates per day forces the body to make glucose using primarily amino acids from proteins found in vital organs. A low glucose supply in cells also inhibits efficient metabolism of fats. Ketosis can then result.

Blood glucose concentration is maintained within a very narrow range. When blood glucose rises after a meal, the hormone insulin is released in great amounts from the pancreas. Insulin acts to lower blood glucose by increasing glucose storage in the liver and glucose uptake by many body cells. If blood glucose falls during fasting, then glucagon and other hormones increase the liver's release of glucose into the bloodstream to restore normal blood glucose values. In a similar way the hormone epinephrine can make more glucose available in response to stress. This balance in hormone activity helps maintain blood glucose within a healthy range.

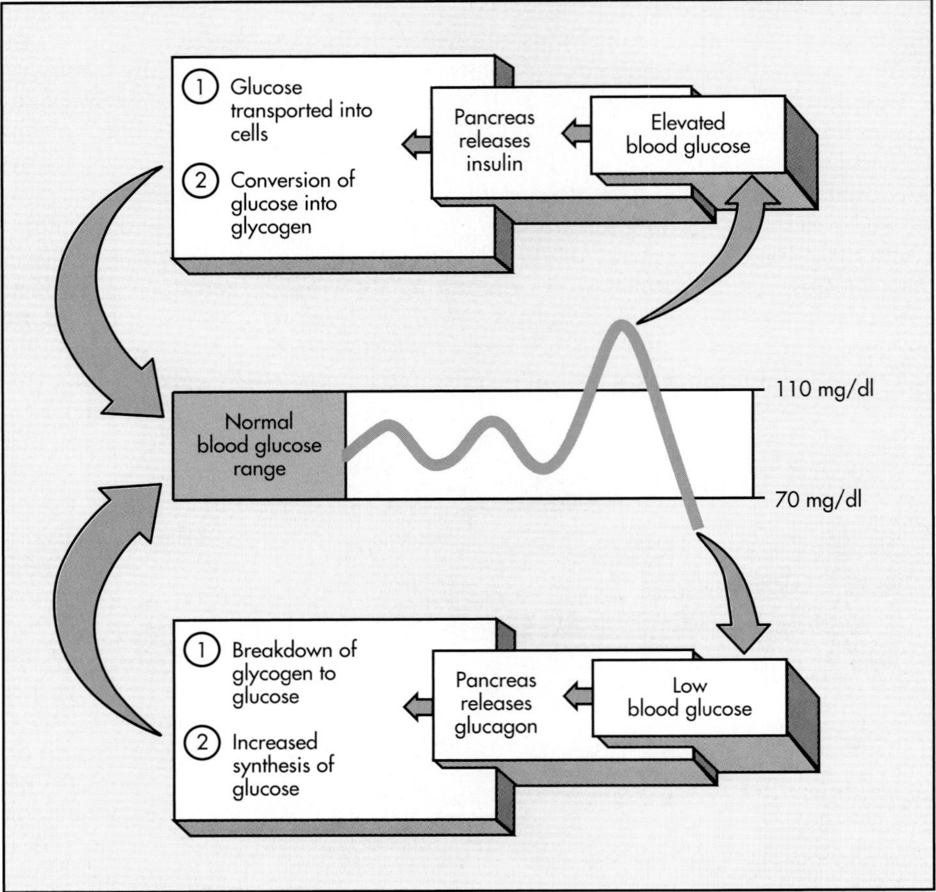

Figure 4-8 *Regulation of blood glucose. Insulin and glucagon are key hormones in controlling blood glucose. Other hormones, such as epinephrine, norepinephrine, cortisol, and growth hormone, also contribute to blood glucose regulation. When we eat a meal insulin is released to promote glucose uptake by cells, thus lowering high blood glucose. When fasting, glucagon is released to promote glucose release from liver stores (those are present in the form of glycogen). This raises blood glucose.* Illustration by William Ober.

Recommendations for Carbohydrate Intake

No RDA for carbohydrate intake has been established. As previously discussed, consuming at least 50 to 100 grams of carbohydrate per day is critical to prevent ketosis. The diet must also contain enough total energy to meet needs.

Consuming 50 grams of carbohydrate is easy. Just 3 pieces of fruit, 3 slices of bread, or a little more than 3 cups of milk suffice. In fact, eating so little carbohydrate that ketosis results is rare.

The average adult American eats more than 200 grams of a combination of all digestible carbohydrates—sugars and starches—per day. This adds up to about 50% of energy intake. As noted in Chapter 2, many health authorities recommend boosting carbohydrate intake to about 60% of energy intake and reducing fat intake, with an emphasis on whole grains, fruits, and vegetables. As carbohydrate intake increases—by eating more foods from the bottom part of the Food Guide

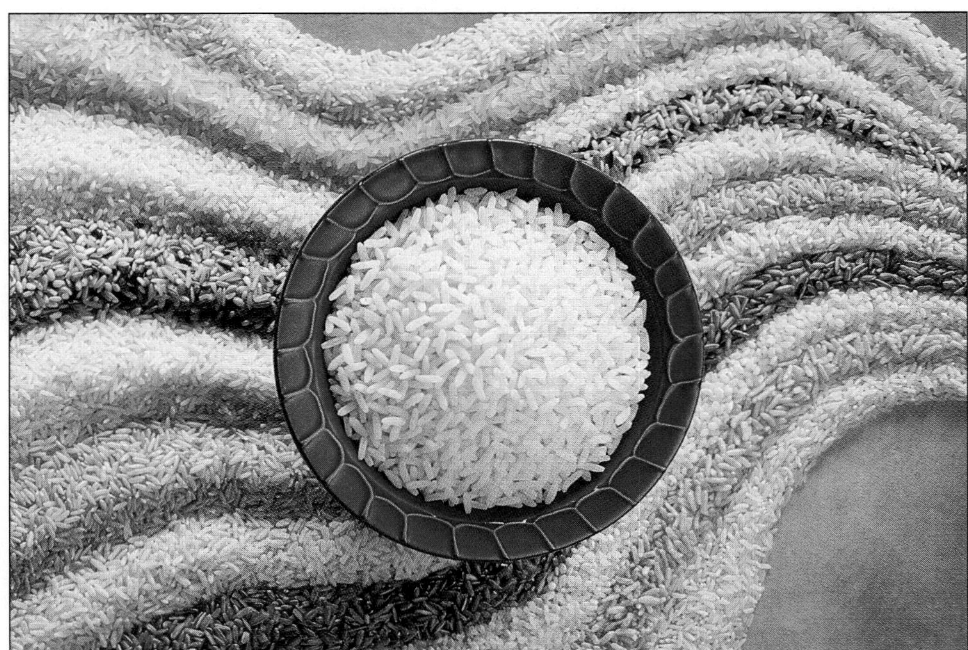

Rice is a rich source of carbohydrates.

Pyramid—fat intake should automatically decrease, as long as added fat is kept to a minimum and foods are prepared and served without additional fat.

Only in cases where a person's blood triglycerides are high is a carbohydrate-rich diet not recommended. (This will be covered further in Chapter 5.) Actually the chief culprits in this case are excessively large meals full of foods both rich in simple sugars and low in dietary fiber, and these aren't practices that should form the basis of a diet. But unfortunately, they often do.

Keep in mind, however, that any nutrient can lead to health problems when consumed in excess, including complex carbohydrate and dietary fiber. The contribution of high-carbohydrate foods to total energy intake still needs to be watched. Generally speaking, though, Americans are becoming fatter not because they are eating too much bread and pasta but because they are physically inactive and their diets are high in fat and simple sugars. In fact, added sugars, such as those in soft drinks, comprise about 16% of energy intake of adults. That corresponds to about 20 teaspoons (85 grams) per day. Recall from Chapter 2 that the Food Guide Pyramid suggests considerably lower intakes for many of us: 1600 kcal, 8 teaspoons; 2200 kcal, 12 teaspoons; 2800 kcal, 18 teaspoons. These allotments work out to 10% or less of total calories, a typical recommendation made by many health authorities. Overall, most adults are not active enough to warrant current use of added sugars (Figure 4–9).

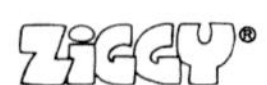

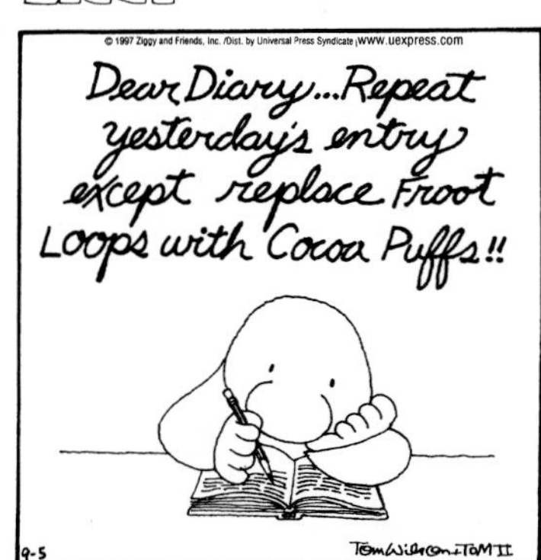

ZIGGY®

Dear Diary...Repeat yesterday's entry except replace Froot Loops with Cocoa Puffs!!

Figure 4–9
Ziggy.

ANOTHER
Bite

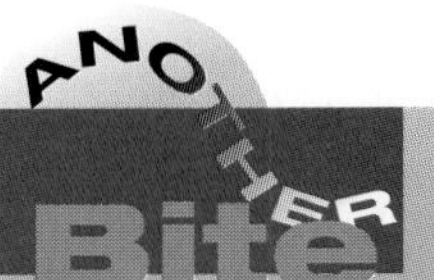

During food processing, the sugar content is often increased. Usually, the more processed the food, the higher the sugar content. An apple has 0 grams of added sugar, canned apples in heavy syrup have 10 to 15 grams, and one sixth of a 9-inch apple pie has 30 grams of added sugar. For comparison purposes, 1 teaspoon of sugar is 4 grams.

Is Sugar Actually Harmful?

Some people think that any consumption of sugar is unhealthy. Certainly, foods high in simple sugars may supply few, if any, vitamins, minerals, or proteins compared with the number of calories they supply. However, if you can afford to consume some extra calories, moderate amounts of sugar are not harmful. Sugar is mostly a problem when it is eaten at the expense of more nutritious foods. When this happens, a person could become deficient in vitamins and other important nutrients, especially if restricting energy intake from other sources.

Many reputable scientific groups have reviewed the current research concerning the health effects of the typical sugars in American diets. In general, these groups have given consumption of a moderate amount of simple sugars a clean bill of health except for the tendency of many sugars to cause dental caries. Caries are formed when sugars and other carbohydrates are metabolized into acids by bacteria that live in the mouth (Figure 4–10). The acid produced dissolves the tooth enamel and underlying structure. These bacteria lodge themselves in fissures in the teeth. Bacteria also use the sugars to make plaque, a sticky substance that both adheres bacteria to teeth and diminishes the acid-neutralizing effect of saliva.

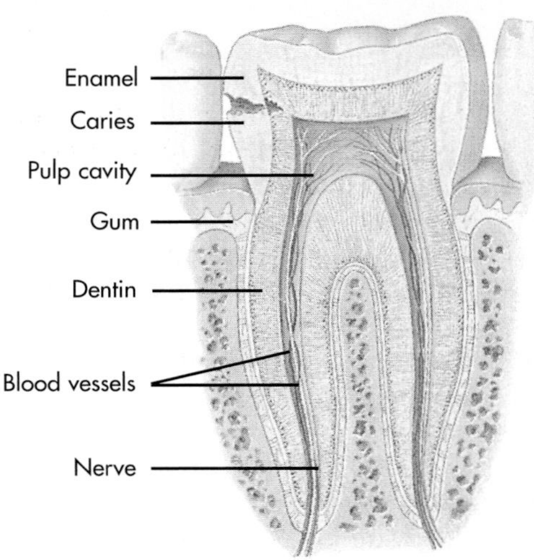

Figure 4–10 *Dental caries. Bacteria can collect in various areas on a tooth. Using simple sugars, bacteria then create acids that can dissolve tooth enamel, leading to caries. If the caries process progresses and enters the pulp cavity, damage to the nerve and resulting pain are likely. The bacteria also produce plaque whereby they adhere to the tooth surface.*

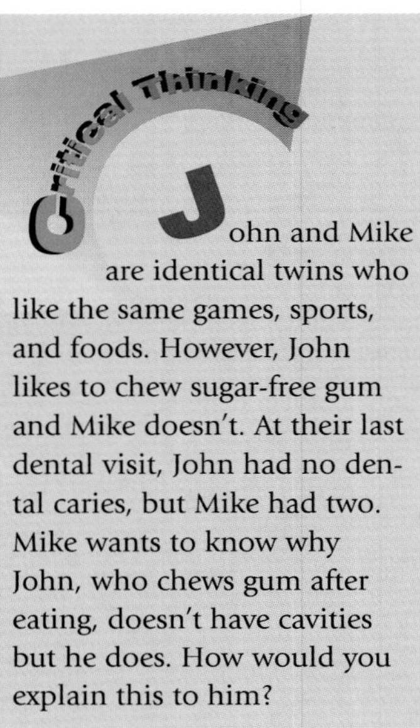

John and Mike are identical twins who like the same games, sports, and foods. However, John likes to chew sugar-free gum and Mike doesn't. At their last dental visit, John had no dental caries, but Mike had two. Mike wants to know why John, who chews gum after eating, doesn't have cavities but he does. How would you explain this to him?

The worst offenders in terms of sugars and dental caries are sticky or gummy foods high in sugars, such as caramel, because they stick to the teeth and supply the bacteria with a long-lived carbohydrate source. Although liquid sugar sources (e.g., fruit juices) are not as potent at causing dental caries as sticky or gummy foods, they still warrant consideration. Some experts caution that sports drinks may also lead to dental caries due to their acid content.

In the last few decades, dental caries rates have decreased in the United States, even though simple-sugar consumption has remained about constant. This decline is primarily due to the addition of flouride to water. When teeth develop in the presence of this mineral, they become much more resistant to acid (see Chapter 8). Flouride in toothpaste also contributes to dental health because it promotes remineralization of damaged teeth and inhibits the metabolism and growth of bacteria on the teeth. Research has also indicated that certain foods—such as cheese, peanuts, and sugar-free chewing gum—can actually help reduce the amount of acid on teeth. In addition, rinsing the mouth after meals and snacks reduces the acidity in the mouth. Certainly, good nutrition, habits that do not present an overwhelming challenge to oral health, and routine visits to the dentist all contribute to improved dental health.

It has been mentioned several times that milk and some milk products contain the sugar lactose. This should in no way be construed to mean that milk is a food to avoid when limiting simple-sugar consumption. In fact, lowfat and nonfat dairy products have an overall high nutrient density and would be one of the last sources of sugars to limit.

Are There Risks from Sugar Use Besides Dental Caries?

Some people claim that simple sugars by their nature cause diabetes, juvenile delinquency, obesity, and other problems. Little or no credible research supports these allegations. A cause-and-effect relationship between these conditions and moderate consumption of sugars—specifically sucrose—has not been established. As noted earlier, a sugar-rich, low-fiber diet can cause blood triglycerides to go too high in some people, and does cause higher spikes in blood insulin as the body utilizes this sugar load. For about 25% of Americans these effects can increase the risk for heart disease (see the discussion of Syndrome X in Chapter 5). For many adults, however, this is only a secondary concern when it comes to evaluating the risk for heart disease.

There is a widespread notion that high sugar intake by children causes hyperactivity, typically part of the syndrome called *attention deficit hyperactive disorder (ADHD)*. Some people claim that sucrose creates an excited—even antisocial—state, which may lead to violence and disruptive behavior. However, most research shows that sucrose itself is not the villain and indeed may have the opposite effect. A high-carbohydrate meal, for example, calms many children and induces sleep. Negative behavioral changes probably result from the excitement or tension in situations in which high-sucrose foods are served, such as birthday parties and on Halloween. Any improvement in behavior observed in children on relatively sugar-free diets is probably due to the extra attention they receive, not the reduction in the intake of sugars.

In the final analysis, by regularly visiting the dentist, practicing good dental hygiene, and following the Food Guide Pyramid while keeping weight under control, you can consume sugar in reasonable amounts without risking your health. Table 4–4 lists ways to reduce sugar intake if you think you eat too much of it.

ConceptCheck

There is no RDA for carbohydrate; the general advice is an intake of more than 50 to 100 grams, emphasizing grains, vegetables, and fruits, to about 60% of total energy intake. We should limit total consumption of simple sugars to about 10% of total calories. Most simple sugars are added to foods and beverages during manufacturing or at the table. To reduce simple sugar consumption, one must eat fewer items that have had a lot of sugar added, such as some baked goods, certain beverages, and some breakfast cereals. Simple sugars contribute to dental caries and provide few vitamins and minerals, if any.

TABLE 4-4

Suggestions for Reducing Simple-Sugar Intake

AT THE SUPERMARKET

- Read ingredient labels. Identify all the added sugars in a product. Select items lower in total sugar when possible.
- Buy fresh fruits or fruits packed in water, juice, or light syrup rather than those packed in heavy syrup.
- Buy fewer foods that are high in sugar, such as prepared baked goods, candies, sugared cereals, sweet desserts, soft drinks, and fruit-flavored punches. Substitute vanilla wafers, graham crackers, bagels, English muffins, and diet soft drinks, for example.
- Buy reduced-fat microwave popcorn to replace candy for snacks.

IN THE KITCHEN

- Reduce the sugar in foods prepared at home. Try new recipes or adjust your own. Start by reducing the sugar gradually until you've decreased it by one-third or more.
- Experiment with spices such as cinnamon, cardamom, coriander, nutmeg, ginger, and mace to enhance the flavor of foods.
- Use home-prepared items (with less sugar) instead of commercially prepared ones that are higher in sugar.

AT THE TABLE

- Use less of all sugars. This includes white and brown sugars, honey, molasses, and syrups.
- Choose fewer foods high in sugar, such as prepared baked goods, candies, and sweet desserts.
- Reach for fresh fruit instead of a sweet for dessert or between-meal snacks.
- Add less sugar to foods—coffee, tea, cereal, and fruit. Get used to using half as much; then see if you can cut back even more.
- Cut back on the number of sugared soft drinks and punches you drink. Substitute water, fruit juice, and diet soft drinks.

Modified from USDA *Home and Garden Bulletin* No. 232–5, 1986.

Summary

- The monosaccharides in our diet include glucose, fructose, and galactose (the latter as part of lactose). Once absorbed via the small intestine and transported through the portal vein into the liver, much of the fructose and galactose is turned into glucose.
- The major disaccharides are sucrose (glucose plus fructose), maltose (glucose plus glucose), and lactose (glucose plus galactose). When digested, these yield monosaccharide forms. Both monosaccharides and disaccharides are classified as simple sugars.
- The major digestible polysaccharides—starches—contain multiple glucose units linked together. Glycogen is an animal starch that acts as a storage form of glucose in the liver and muscles.
- Table sugar, honey, jelly, fruit, and plain baked potatoes are some of the most concentrated sources of carbohydrates. Other high-carbohydrate foods, such as pie and nonfat milk, are diluted by either fat or protein. Nutritive sweeteners in food include sucrose, high-fructose corn syrup, brown sugar, and maple syrup.
- Dietary fibers include the indigestible polysaccharides cellulose, hemicelluloses, pectins, gums, and mucilages, as well as the noncarbohydrate lignin. Dietary fiber, especially insoluble varieties, provides mass to the stool, thus easing elimination. It may also decrease the risk for colon cancer. In high doses,

soluble fibers can help control blood glucose in diabetic people and also lower blood cholesterol.

- Some starch digestion occurs in the mouth. Carbohydrate digestion is finished in the small intestine. Some plant fibers are digested by the bacteria present in the large intestine; undigested plant fibers end up in the feces. Single sugars mostly follow an active absorption process in the small intestine. They are then transported to the liver.
- Carbohydrates provide energy (on average 4 kcal per gram), protect against needless metabolism of protein for energy, and add flavor and sweetness to foods. They are not necessarily fattening. Many types of carbohydrates can be matabolized to acids by bacteria on teeth. The acid can erode the tooth surface, leading to dental caries.
- Lactose is the sugar found in milk. Lactose intolerance is a condition that results when cells of the intestine wall do not make sufficient or any lactase, the enzyme necessary to digest lactose. Undigested lactose travels to the large intestine, resulting in such symptoms as abdominal gas, pain, and diarrhea. Most people with lactose intolerance can tolerate cheese and yogurt, although tolerance to dairy products as a whole varies among affected individuals.
- There is no RDA for carbohydrate. A minimal intake of 50 to 100 grams is needed; about 60% of total energy intake is generally recommended. If carbohydrate consumption is inadequate, the body can make what sugars it needs to support cell metabolism. However, if inadequate carbohydrate intake continues for weeks at a time, the price is a loss of body protein, ketosis, and a general weakening of the body.
- Diets high in complex forms of carbohydrates are encouraged as a replacement for high-fat diets, with an emphasis on starch- and fiber-rich foods. The foods to emphasize would be whole grains, pastas, fruits, and vegetables. Sugar intake should be limited to 10% of energy intake. Moderating sugar intake, especially between meals, reduces the risk of dental caries. Use of alternative sweeteners, such as aspartame, can help in limiting sugar intake.

Study Questions

1. Outline the basic steps in blood glucose regulation, including the roles of insulin and glucagon.
2. What are the three major monosaccharides and the three major disaccharides? Describe how each plays a part in the human diet.
3. Why are some foods that are high in carbohydrates, such as cookies and nonfat milk, not considered to be concentrated sources of carbohydrates?
4. Describe the digestion of the various types of carbohydrates in the body.
5. Describe the reason why some people are unable to tolerate high intakes of milk.
6. What are the important roles that dietary fiber plays in the diet?
7. What, if any, are the proven ill effects of sugar in the diet?
8. Why do we need carbohydrates in the diet? How does the body regulate the blood concentration of these carbohydrates?
9. Summarize current carbohydrate intake recommendations.
10. List three alternatives to simple sugars for adding sweetness to the diet.

Further Readings

1 Amazing grain. *Harvard Health Letter* p. 6, March 1997.
2 American Dietetic Association Reports: Health implications of dietary fiber, *Journal of the American Dietetic Association* 97:1158, 1997.
3 American Dietetic Association Reports: Position of the American Dietetic Association: Use of nutritive and nonnutritive sweeteners, *Journal of the American Dietetic Association* 98:580, 1998.
4 American Dietetic Association Reports: Position of The American Dietetic Association: oral health and nutrition, *Journal of the American Dietetic Association* 96:184, 1996.
5 Bennett WG, Cerda JJ: Benefits of dietary fiber, *Postgraduate Medicine* 99(2):153, 1996.
6 Carroccio A and others: Lactose intolerance and self-reported milk intolerance, *Journal of the American College of Nutrition* 17:631, 1998.
7 Conner WE, Conner SL with reply by Katan MB and others: Should a low-fat, high-carbohydrate diet be recommended for everyone? *New England Journal of Medicine* 337:562, 1997.
8 Diabetes Control and Complications Trial Research Group: Lifetime benefits and costs of intensive therapy as practiced in the Diabetes Control and Complications Trial, *Journal of the American Medical Association* 276:1409, 1996.
9 Fishman L: About diabetes, *Nutrition Today* 32:46, 1997.
10 Hingley A: Diabetes demands a triad of treatments, *FDA Consumer* p. 33, May–June 1997.
11 Jacobs DR and others: Whole-grain intake may reduce the risk of ischemic heart disease death in post-menopausal women, *American Journal of Clinical Nutrition* 68:248, 1998.
12 Kirby J: Beyond bran: overlooked fiber options, *American Health* p. 84, July–August 1997.
13 Levin RJ: Carbohydrates in *Modern Nutrition in Health and Disease,* Shils ME and others, eds, Ninth edition, Baltimore MD, Williams & Wilkins, 1999.
14 Liebman B: The whole grain guide, *Nutrition Action Healthletter* p. 1, March 1997.
15 Liebman B: Sugar: the sweetening of the American diet, *Nutrition Action Health Letter* p. 1, November 1998.
16 Papazian R: Bulking up fiber's healthful reputation, *FDA Consumer* p. 23, July–August 1997.
17 Suarez FL and others: Lactose maldigestion is not an impediment to the intake of 1500 mg calcium daily as dairy products. *American Journal of Clinical Nutrition* 68:111, 1998.
18 Tillotson JL: Relation of dietary fiber to blood lipids in the special intervention and usual care groups in the Multiple Risk Factor Intervention Trial. *American Journal of Clinical Nutrition* 65:327S, 1997.
19 Wolraich ML and others: Effects of diets high in sucrose or aspartame on the behavior and cognitive performance of children, *New England Journal of Medicine* 330:301, 1994.
20 Wynder EL and others: High fiber intake—indicator of a healthy lifestyle, *Journal of the American Medical Association* 275:486, 1996.

RATE Your Plate

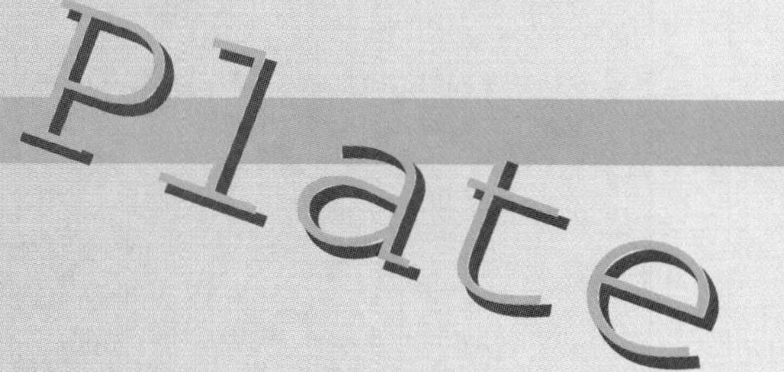

I. How Does Your Diet Rate for Carbohydrate and Dietary Fiber?

Let's reevaluate the nutritional assessment you completed at the end of Chapter 2. Here are your tasks:

1. Look at your analysis and find the total number of grams of carbohydrate you ate.

   TOTAL GRAMS OF CARBOHYDRATE ________

   A. Did you consume more than the minimum amount to avoid ketosis, 50 to 100 grams?

   B. Now calculate the percentage of energy in your diet from carbohydrate. You will need the total grams of carbohydrate from your assessment as well as the total kcals you ate. Use this formula to calculate it:

$$\frac{\text{Total grams of carbohydrate} \times 4}{\text{Total kcals consumed}} \times 100 = \text{\% of energy intake from carbohydrate}$$

   ANSWER: ________

   Was about 60% of your total energy intake from carbohydrate? YES________ NO ________
   If not, list several ways you could increase your carbohydrate intake.

____

____

____

2. Look again at the list of foods you ate, including the amounts, and determine the total amount of dietary fiber you consumed. If you have a computer analysis of your diet, your dietary fiber intake is listed in the printout. Otherwise, look up the dietary fiber content of each food you ate in the food composition table in Appendix A, then calculate your total intake, taking into account the amount of each food you ate.

TOTAL AMOUNT OF DIETARY FIBER CONSUMED ________ grams

   A. Did you eat the 20 to 35 grams suggested in this chapter?

   B. If not, what could you do to increase your dietary fiber intake? What foods could you substitute for some of the foods you ate?

____

____

____

3. Finally, use Table 4-4 to see if you can reduce your intake of sugars, especially if you need to watch your total energy intake to maintain a healthy weight. What three foods might you limit in the future?

____

____

____

II. Can You Choose the Best Source of Dietary Fiber?

Assume the sandwiches on the blackboard below are available at your local deli and sandwich shop. All of the sandwiches provide about 350 kcal. The dietary fiber content ranges from about 1 gram to about 7.5 grams. Rank the sandwiches from highest amount of dietary fiber to lowest amount, then check your answers at the bottom of the page.

Deli Specials
Turkey & Swiss on Rye
Served with tomato slices, alfalfa sprouts, romaine lettuce, and mustard
Ham & Swiss on Sourdough
Extra-lean ham served with mayonnaise
Tuna Salad on Whole Wheat
Our tuna salad contains tuna, grated carrots, onions, and mayonnaise, and is served with alfalfa sprouts, romaine lettuce, and cucumber slices
Hot Dog
Served on a white bun with relish, mustard, and catsup
Soyburger
Served on a whole-wheat English muffin with tomato and pickle slices, romaine lettuce, and mayonnaise
PB & J
Soft white bread with strawberry jelly and smooth peanut butter

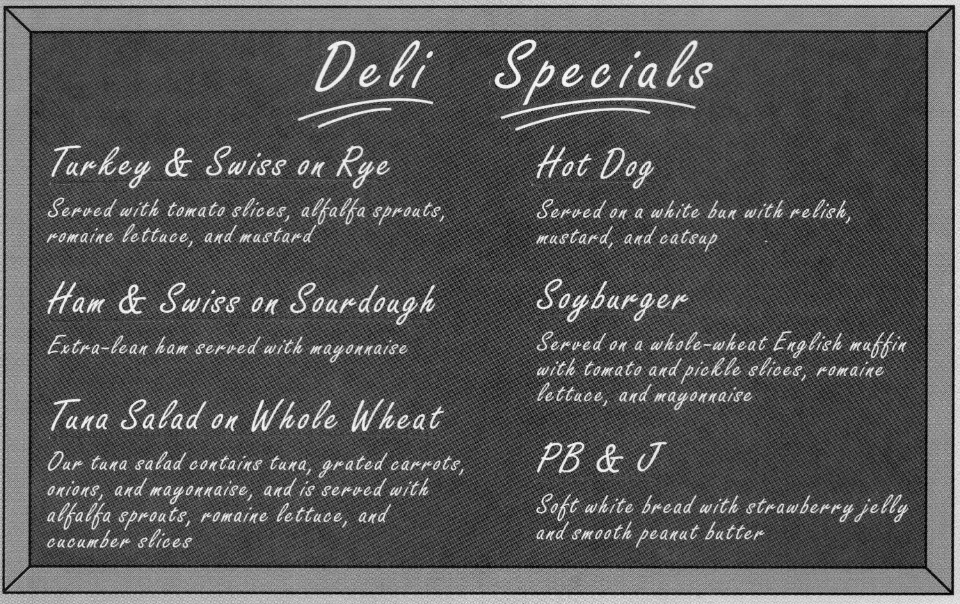

Answer Key: 1. Soyburger: 7.5 grams, 2. Tuna Salad on Whole Wheat: 7 grams, 3. Turkey and Swiss on Rye: 4 grams, 4. PB & J: 3 grams, 5. Ham and Swiss on Sourdough: 1.5 grams, 6. Hot dog: 1 gram.

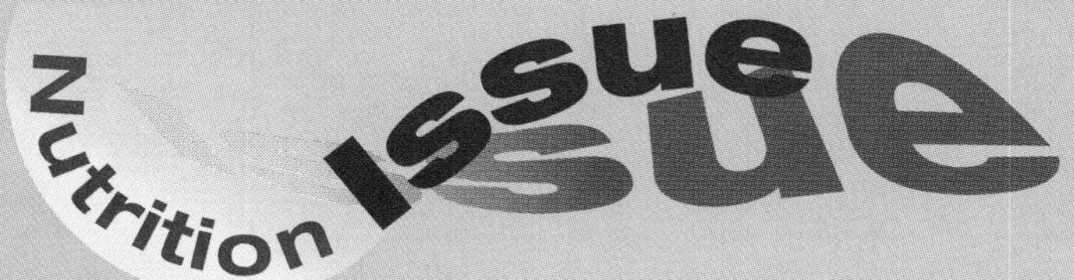

When Blood Glucose Regulation Fails

Improper regulation of blood glucose results in either **hyperglycemia** (high blood glucose) or **hypoglycemia** (low blood glucose). High blood glucose is most commonly associated with diabetes (technically *diabetes mellitus)*, a disease that affects about 16 million Americans. Of these, it is estimated that up to 5 to 8 million do not know that they have the disease. New recommendations promote testing fasting blood glucose in adults over age 45 every 3 years to help diagnose these missed cases. In contrast, low blood glucose is a much rarer condition.

Hyperglycemia
High blood glucose; above 125 milligrams per 100 milliliters of blood.

Hypoglycemia
Low blood glucose; below 40 to 50 milligrams per 100 milliliters of blood.

DIABETES MELLITUS

There are two major forms of diabetes: **Type 1** (formerly called insulin-dependent or juvenile-onset diabetes), and **Type 2** (formerly called non–insulin-dependent or adult-onset) **diabetes.** The change in names to Type 1 and Type 2 diabetes stems from the fact that many "non–insulin-dependent diabetics" eventually have to also rely on insulin injections as a part of their treatment.

Type 1 diabetes
A form of diabetes prone to ketosis and that requires insulin therapy.

Type 2 diabetes
A form of diabetes in which ketosis is not commonly seen. Insulin therapy can be used but is often not required. This form of the disease is often associated with obesity.

Type 1 Diabetes

Type 1 diabetes often begins in late childhood, around the age of 8 to 12 years, but can occur at any age. The disease runs in certain families, indicating a clear genetic link. The symptoms of the disease are abnormally high blood glucose after eating and the tendency to develop ketosis.

The onset of Type 1 diabetes is generally associated with decreased release of insulin from the pancreas. As insulin in the blood declines, blood glucose increases, especially after eating. When blood glucose exceeds the kidney's threshold, excess glucose spills over into the urine.

An exciting new finding regarding the cause of Type 1 diabetes may help physicians to treat this disease, or even prevent its onset in the future. At least some cases of Type 1 diabetes begin with an immune system disorder that causes destruction of the insulin-producing (beta) cells in the pancreas. Most likely a virus or protein foreign to the body sets off the destruction. Cow's milk is suspected of supplying such a protein, so its introduction before 1 year of age is not advised (see Chapter 13). In response to the destruction, the affected beta cells release other proteins that stimulate a more furious attack. Eventually the pancreas loses its ability to synthesize insulin, and the clinical stage of the disease begins. Because of this immune process that destroys beta cells, pancreas

TAKE CHARGE of Your Diabetes, updated guidelines for persons with diabetes, is available on the web site of the CDC, at http://www.cdc.gov/nccdphp/ddt/tcoyd.htm. This document provides information about steps to help promote health and prevent complications in people with diabetes. More information on diabetes also is listed at http://www.diabetes.org.

transplants have proven very difficult in these patients as this same process may destroy the new beta cells. Consequently, early treatment to stop the immune-linked destruction in children may be important. Research on this is continuing.

Currently, Type 1 diabetes is treated primarily by insulin therapy. In addition, dietary measures include three regular meals and one or more snacks (including one at bedtime) having a regulated carbohydrate:protein:fat ratio to maximize insulin action and minimize swings in blood glucose. If one does not eat often enough, the injected insulin can cause severe hypoglycemia, since it acts on whatever little glucose is available. The diet should be ample in complex carbohydrates, include ample dietary fiber at each meal, and supply an amount of energy in balance with energy needs.

Traditional symptoms of diabetes, known as the three poly's, are polyuria (excessive urination), polydipsia (excessive thirst), and polyphagia (excessive hunger). No one symptom is diagnostic of diabetes, and other symptoms such as unusual weight loss, exhaustion, blurred vision, tingling in hands and feet, frequent infections, and impotence often accompany traditional symptoms.

The hormone imbalances that occur in people with untreated diabetes lead to mobilization of body fat, which floods into liver cells. Ketosis is the result because the fat is mostly converted to ketones. Ketone concentration can rise excessively in the blood, eventually forcing ketones into the urine. These ketones pull sodium and potassium ions with them. This series of events can contribute to a chain reaction that eventually leads to dehydration, ion imbalance, coma, and even death, especially in patients with poorly controlled Type 1 diabetes.

Other complications of Type 1 diabetes can be degenerative conditions, such as blindness, heart disease, kidney disease, and numbness from nerve damage; all are caused by poor blood glucose regulation. Because of nerve deterioration in the extremities, many people with diabetes lose the sensation of pain associated with injuries or infections. Not having as much pain, they often delay treatment of hand or foot problems. This delay, combined with a rich environment for bacterial growth (bacteria thrive on glucose) sets the stage for complications in the extremities. High blood glucose also contributes to a rapid buildup of fats on blood vessel walls, which eventually chokes off the blood supply to nearby organs. See Chapter 5 for details on this latter process, called **atherosclerosis.**

Atherosclerosis *A buildup of mostly fatty material (plaque) in the arteries, including those surrounding the heart.*

Diabetic complications such as those mentioned can be slowed with aggressive treatment directed at keeping blood glucose within the normal range. The therapy poses some risks of its own, such as hypoglycemia, so it must be implemented under close supervision of a physician. Also, exercise can aid the control of blood glucose if it is performed under the same supervision.

Type 2 Diabetes

Type 2 diabetes usually begins after age 20. This is the most common type of diabetes, accounting for about 90% of the cases diagnosed in the United States. The number of people affected is on the rise, primarily because of widespread inactivity and obesity in our population. This type of diabetes is also genetically linked, but the initial problem is not with the insulin-producing cells of the pancreas. Instead it arises with the insulin receptors on the cell surfaces of certain body tissues, especially muscle tissue. Insulin needs to bind to these receptors if it is to promote glucose uptake in the tissues. If limited binding is instead the case, blood glucose is not readily transferred into cells, so the patient develops hyperglycemia as a result of the glucose's remaining in the bloodstream. The pancreas attempts to increase insulin output to compensate, but its ability to do so is limited. Rather than insufficient insulin production, there is an abundance of insulin, particularly during the onset of the disease. Thus Type 2 diabetes can be viewed as a state in which the pancreas is unable to compensate for the insulin resistance present in body tissues. As the disease develops, pancreatic function can fail, leading to reduced insulin output. Because of the genetic link for Type 2 diabetes, those who have a family history should be careful to avoid risk factors such as obesity and inactivity and be tested regularly.

Many cases of Type 2 diabetes are associated with obesity (especially that located in the abdominal region), but the hyperglycemia is not directly caused by the obesity. In fact, some lean people also develop this type of diabetes, while some obese people do not. Obesity associated with oversized fat cells simply increases the risk for insulin resistance by the body.

Type 2 diabetes linked to obesity often disappears if the obesity is corrected. Achieving a healthy weight should be a primary goal of treatment, but even limited weight loss can lead to better blood glucose regulation. Oral medications that can reduce glucose production by the liver, increase the ability of the pancreas to release insulin, and increase the body's response to its own insulin, are often prescribed. Another class of oral agents used works by delaying carbohydrate digestion and glucose absorption.

Sometimes it may be necessary to provide insulin injections in Type 2 diabetes because nothing else is able to control the disease. Regular physical activity also helps the muscles to take up more glucose. And regular meal patterns, with an emphasis on control of energy intake, consumption of complex carbohydrates, and ample dietary fiber, is important therapy. Distributing carbohydrates throughout the day is also important, as this helps minimize the high and low swings in blood glucose concentrations. Moderate intake of sugars is fine with meals in both forms of diabetes, but again these must be substituted for other carbohydrates, not simply added to the meal plan.

Diabetes that develops in pregnancy is called gestational diabetes. Management of it is reviewed in Chapter 12.

Although many cases of Type 2 diabetes can be relieved by reducing excess fat stores, many people are not able to lose weight. They remain affected with diabetes and may experience the degenerative complications seen in the Type I form of the disease. Ketosis, however, is not usually seen in Type 2 diabetes.

Hypoglycemia

As noted earlier, diabetic people who are taking insulin sometimes have hypoglycemia if they don't eat frequently enough. Hypoglycemia can also develop in nondiabetic individuals, though it occurs rarely if at all according to some scientists. Symptoms of hypoglycemia are described as irritability, nervousness, headache, sweating, and confusion. These symptoms may result due to excessive insulin output by the pancreas in otherwise healthy individuals and occasionally in people with pancreatic cancer.

It is normal for healthy people to have some hypoglycemic symptoms, such as irritability, headache, and shakiness, if they have not eaten for a prolonged period of time. Although not diagnostic of hypoglycemia, if you sometimes have symptoms of hypoglycemia, the standard nutrition therapy is to eat regular meals, make sure you have some protein and fat in each meal, and eat complex carbohydrates with ample soluble fiber. In addition, avoid meals or snacks that contain little more than simple sugars. If symptoms continue, try small protein-containing snacks between meals. Fat, protein, and soluble fiber in the diet tend to moderate swings in blood glucose. Last, moderate caffeine and alcohol intake.

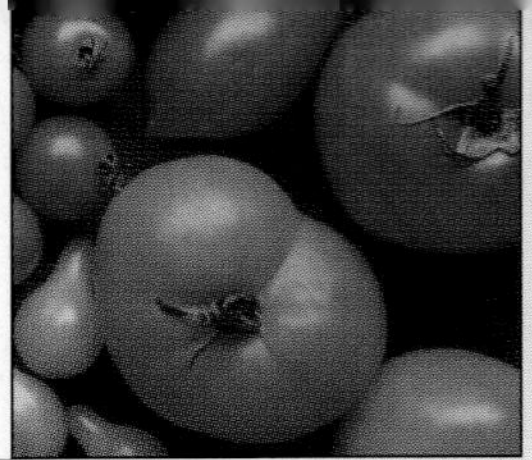

chapter

5

Lipids

Your doctor informs you that your "triglycerides are up." Your bill from a medical laboratory reads, "Blood lipid profile—$55." A health food advertisement suggests using omega-3 fatty acids from fish oil capsules to lower blood cholesterol. Advertisers plug foods "lowest in saturated fat." All of these substances—triglycerides, omega-3 fatty acids, saturated fat, and cholesterol—are lipids, a collective term referring to fats and oils.

Lipids contain more than twice the energy per gram (on average 9 kcal) as proteins and carbohydrates. Consumption of certain saturated fatty acids also is linked to the risk of heart disease. For this reason, some concern about lipids is warranted, but lipids also play vital roles both in the body and in foods. Their presence in at least small amounts in the diet is essential to good health.

Let's look at lipids in detail—their forms, functions, metabolism, and food sources. This chapter will then conclude with a look at the link between lipid intake and the major "killer" disease in the United States, heart disease.

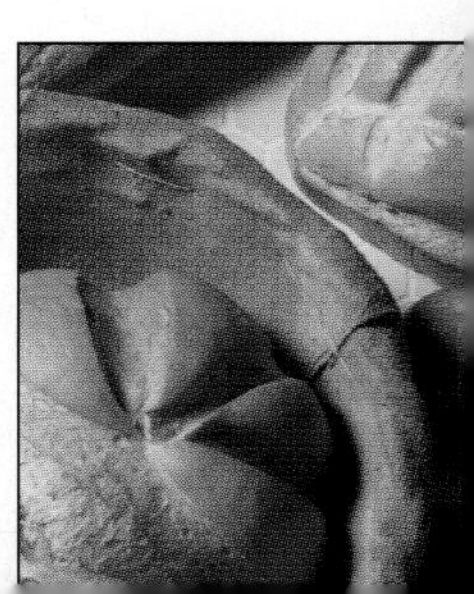

Nutrition Web

Lipids are a group of compounds that don't readily dissolve in water and include fatty acids, triglycerides, glycerol, phospholipids, and sterols (e.g., cholesterol). Most forms fall into the category of fats and oils.

Fatty acids are part of most lipids and can be grouped according to the type of bonds between the carbons: saturated fatty acids contain no double bonds, monounsaturated fatty acids contain one double bond, and polyunsaturated fatty acids contain two or more double bonds.

Lipids composed of saturated fatty acids, such as in animal fat, tend to be solid at room temperature. Those with polyunsaturated fatty acids, such as in vegetable oils, are usually liquid at room temperature.

Turning liquid oils into solid fats (e.g., shortenings) creates an alteration in the shape of the fatty acids, among other changes. This causes the fatty acids to increase the risk of heart disease, rather than decrease it.

Certain polyunsaturated fatty acids are essential parts of our diet because our bodies need them but don't produce them. We can obtain these essential fatty acids by consuming small amounts of vegetable oils and some fish on a regular basis.

Besides supplying certain essential polyunsaturated fatty acids to the body, triglycerides supply energy, allow efficient energy storage, insulate and protect the body, and transport fat-soluble vitamins.

Fats are carried in the bloodstream by various lipoproteins: chylomicrons, very low-density lipoproteins (VLDLs), low-density lipoproteins (LDLs), and high-density lipoproteins (HDLs). Both elevated LDL and low HDL in the blood speed the development of heart disease.

Major contributors of fat to our diets include animal foods, whole milk and cheese, and salad dressings. Eggs are the major source of dietary cholesterol. Fat in food is not always obvious. Careful label reading helps monitor total fat and cholesterol intake.

Fat free does not mean *calorie free.* As with other foods, the calorie content of fat-free products must be considered when evaluating a diet.

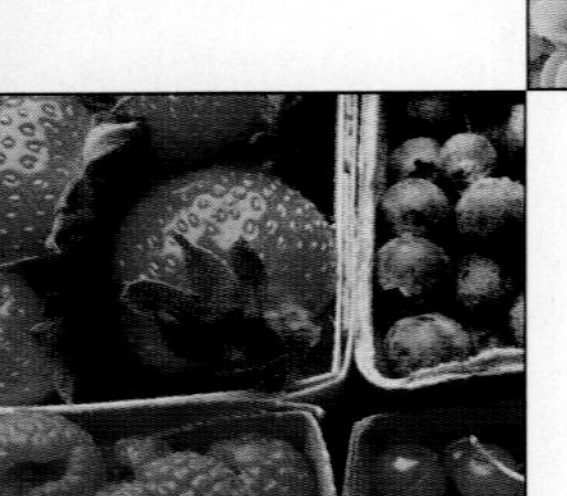

Current recommendations for fat intake range from about 10% of calories if you want to follow the Dr. Dean Ornish plan to reverse cholesterol-laden blockages in the arteries to about 35% of calories if you follow the Mediterranean Diet Pyramid. For the last 25 years health authorities have generally recommended that a diet contain no more than 30% of calories from fat. The U.S. diet yields about 33%. As noted in the Nutrition Web, some fat must be consumed, as certain types are necessary for specific body functions. However, the amount of fat needed is negligible, such that one could follow a Dr. Dean Ornish type plan (which is considered very low in fat) and typically not harm health. After learning more about the various lipids in this chapter you can decide for yourself how much fat you want to consume and where that fat should come from in the diet, and as well how to track your fat intake.

Lipids in General

Lipids are a diverse group of chemical compounds, but they share one main characteristic: they do not readily dissolve in water. Think of an oil and vinegar salad dressing. The oil does not dissolve in the water-based vinegar; upon standing, the two separate into distinct layers, with oil on top and vinegar on the bottom.

The diversity of lipids is evident when you compare the structures of two of the many types: a fatty acid shown in Figure 5–1 and cholesterol in Figure 5–2.

As noted in Chapter 1, lipids that are solid at room temperature are called *fats,* and lipids that are liquid are called *oils.* People often use the word *fat* to refer to all lipids because they don't know any differences exist. As already noted, however, *lipid* is a generic term that includes triglycerides and many other substances. To simplify our discussion, this chapter primarily uses the term *fat;* but as you will see later, not all the substances we call *fats* truly are fats. When necessary for clarity, the name of a specific lipid, such as cholesterol, will be used. This word usage is consistent with the way many people use these terms today.

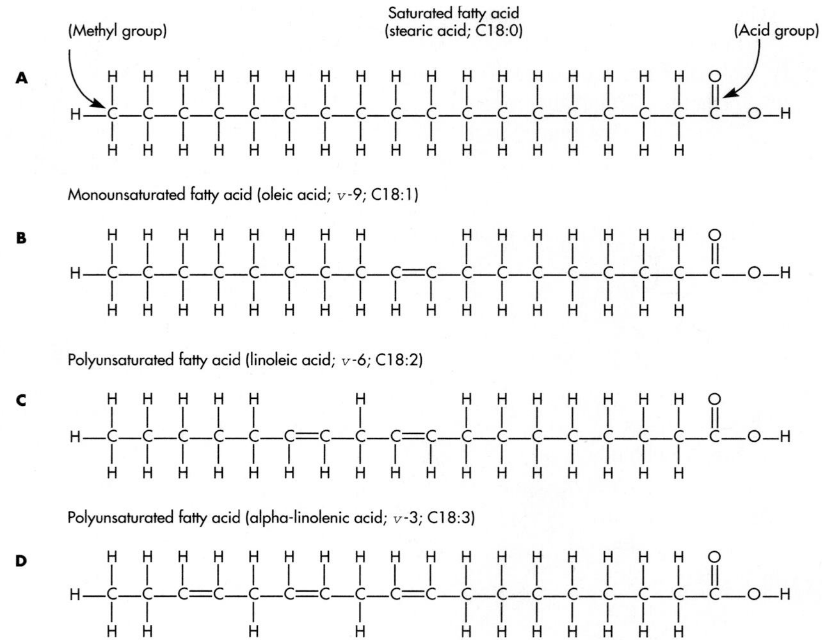

Figure 5–1 *Chemical forms of saturated, monounsaturated, and polyunsaturated fatty acids.*

Fatty Acids: The Simplest Form of Lipids

The **fatty acid** is common to most lipids, both in the body and in foods. It is basically a long chain of carbons linked together and flanked by hydrogen (see Figure 5–1). Fats in foods are not composed of a single type or category of fatty acid. Rather, each dietary fat is a complex mixture of different fatty acids.

If all the links (technically referred to as ***chemical bonds***) between the carbons are single connections and the carbons are filled with hydrogen, a fatty acid is said to be **saturated** (see Figure 5–1, A). To understand this concept, picture a sponge saturated (full) with water.

As noted earlier, most fats high in saturated fatty acids, such as animal fats, remain solid at room temperature. A good example is the solid fat surrounding a piece of uncooked steak at room temperature. Chicken fat, semisolid at room temperature, contains less saturated fat. In some foods, like whole milk, saturated fats are suspended in liquid along with the more liquid oils, so the solid nature of these fats at room temperature is less apparent.

If a fatty acid is unsaturated, hydrogens are missing from the carbon chain, specifically at the area of the carbon-carbon double bonds. If a fatty acid has one double bond between the carbons, it is **monounsaturated** (see Figure 5–1, B). Canola and olive oils contain a high percentage of monounsaturated fatty acids. If two or more bonds between the carbons are double bonds, the fatty acid is **polyunsaturated** and thus even less saturated with hydrogens (see Figure 5–1, C and D). Corn, soybean, and safflower oils are rich in polyunsaturated fatty acids.

Note, however, that dietary fats and oils contain a mixture of various saturated and unsaturated fatty acids. A fat or oil is classified as saturated, monounsaturated, or polyunsaturated based on the nature of the fatty acids present in the greatest concentration.

Fatty acid
Acids found in fats. These are composed of a chain of carbons linked together. The chain is flanked by hydrogens and has an acidic chemical group at one end.

Saturated fatty acid
A fatty acid with no carbon-carbon double bonds.

Monounsaturated fatty acid
A fatty acid containing one carbon-carbon double bond.

Polyunsaturated fatty acid
A fatty acid containing two or more carbon-carbon double bonds.

Triglyceride

Lecithin

Cholesterol

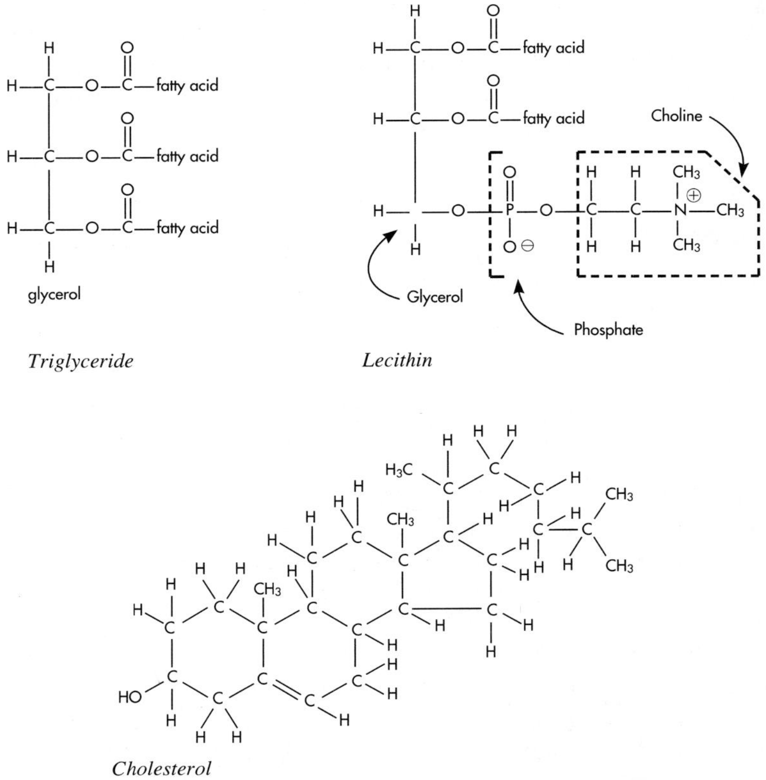

Figure 5-2 *Chemical forms of triglycerides, a phospholipid (lecithin), and cholesterol.*

Saturated fatty acids are linear, allowing them to pack tightly together. In contrast, unsaturated fatty acids have a kinked shape and thus pack together only loosely (this is depicted later in Figure 5-8). The loose organization of unsaturated fats is more easily disrupted by heat than is the more ordered organization of saturated fats. Thus fats high in unsaturated fatty acids melt at a lower temperature than fats high in typical saturated fatty acids.

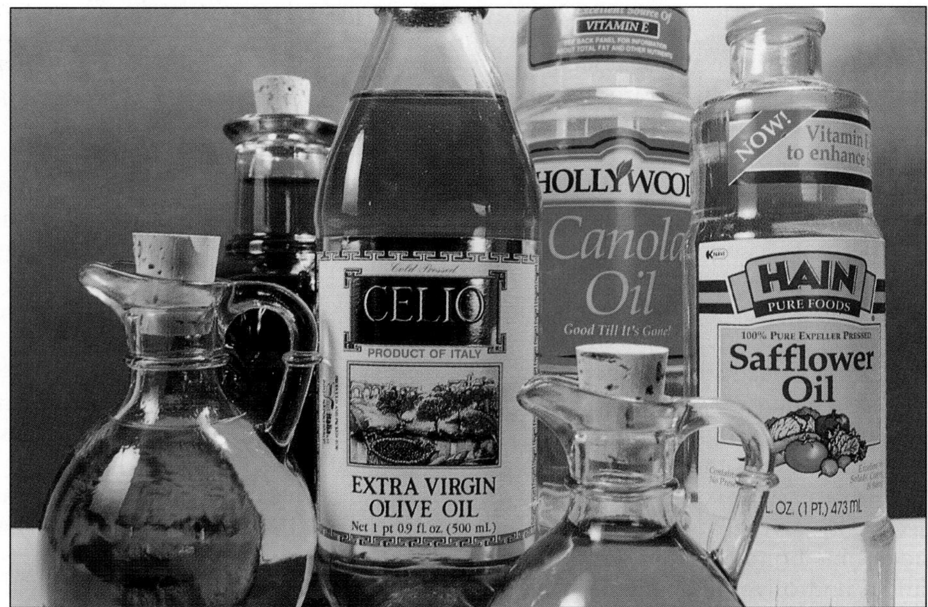

Olive and canola oil are rich in monounsaturated fats, while safflower oil is rich in polyunsaturated fat. Olive oil has been awarded much attention in recent years.

Chain Length Affects Fatty Acid Characteristics

Fats in foods that contain primarily saturated fatty acids are solid at room temperature, especially if the fatty acids have a **long chain** (12 carbons or longer). **Medium-chain** saturated fatty acids (6 to 10 carbons long), such as those in coconut oil, produce liquid oils at room temperature. The shorter chain length overrides the effect of saturation. **Short-chain** saturated fatty acids (less than 6 carbons long) also form liquid oils at room temperature. Fats in milk products are sources of these short-chain fatty acids. Fats containing primarily polyunsaturated or monounsaturated fatty acids are also usually liquid at room temperature. These are not affected by chain length to any major extent.

Triglycerides

Glycerol
A three-carbon alcohol used to form triglycerides.

Monoglyceride
A breakdown product of a triglyceride consisting of one fatty acid attached to a glycerol backbone.

Phospholipid
Any of a class of fat-related substances that contain phosphorus, fatty acids, and a nitrogen-containing base. Phospholipids are an essential part of every cell.

Fats and oils in foods are mostly in the form of triglycerides. The same is true for fats found in body structures. Some fatty acids are found attached to proteins in the bloodstream as they are being transported, but fatty acids usually do not exist in the body as such. Instead they form into triglycerides.

Triglycerides contain a simple three-carbon alcohol, **glycerol,** which serves as a backbone for the three attached fatty acids (Figure 5–2). Removing one fatty acid from a triglyceride forms a diglyceride. Removing two fatty acids from a triglyceride forms a **monoglyceride.** Later you see that before most dietary fats are absorbed in the small intestine, the upper and lower fatty acids are typically removed from the triglyceride. This produces fatty acids and monoglycerides, which are absorbed into the intestinal cells. After absorption the fatty acids and monoglycerides are mostly re-formed into triglycerides.

Phospholipids

Phospholipids are another class of lipid. Like triglycerides, they are built on a backbone of glycerol. However, at least one fatty acid is replaced with a compound containing phosphorus (and often other chemicals, such as nitrogen) (see Figure 5–2).

Many types of phospholipids exist in the body, especially in the brain. They form important parts of the membrane that surrounds body cells. The various forms of **lecithin** are common examples of phospholipids. These are found in body cells, and they participate in fat digestion in the intestine. We produce these lipids; there is no reason to seek a dietary source.

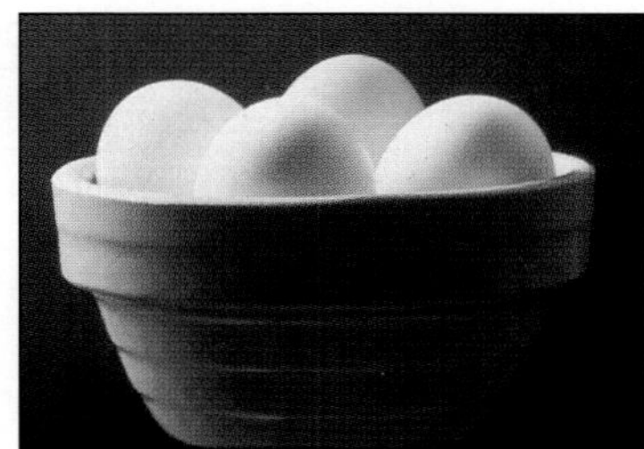

Lecithins are found in abundance in egg yolks. This phospholipid acts as an emulsifier.

Sterols

Sterols are the last class of lipids this chapter covers. Their characteristic multi-ringed structure makes them different from the other lipids already discussed (see Figure 5–2). Consider the sterol cholesterol. This waxy substance doesn't look like a triglyceride—it doesn't have a glycerol backbone or any fatty acids. Still, because it doesn't really dissolve in water, it is a lipid. Among other functions, cholesterol is used to form certain hormones and bile acids, and is incorporated into cell structures. The body can make all the cholesterol it needs.

Sterol
A compound containing a multi-ring (steroid) structure and a hydroxyl group (−OH).

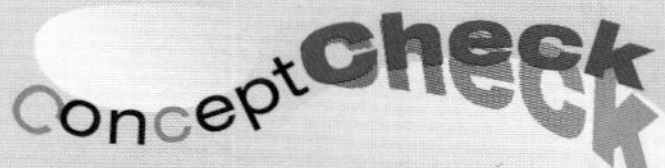

Lipids are a group of compounds that do not dissolve readily in water. They include fatty acids, triglycerides, phospholipids, and sterols. Fatty acids can differ from each other in the number of the double bonds between carbons in the carbon chain. Saturated fatty acids contain no carbon-carbon double bonds; that is, they are fully saturated with hydrogens. Monounsaturated fatty acids contain one carbon-carbon double bond, and polyunsaturated fatty acids contain two or more carbon-carbon double bonds.

Triglyceride is the major form of fat in the body and in food. It is formed by attaching three fatty acids to a glycerol backbone. Phospholipids differ from triglycerides: their glycerol backbone has fatty acids attached, but at least one fatty acid is replaced by another type of compound. Many phospholipids are present in cells, and some act as emulsifiers. Sterols, another class of lipids, are constructed quite differently from either triglycerides or phospholipids. Cholesterol, a sterol, forms parts of cells, some hormones, and bile acids.

Lipids in Food

The foods with the highest energy density for fat are salad oils, butter, margarine, and mayonnaise (Figure 5–3). All contain close to 100% of energy as fat. Many fat-reduced margarines have been introduced, with water replacing some of the fat. Typical margarines are 80% fat by weight (11 grams per tablespoon). Some fat-reduced margarines are as low as 30% fat by weight (4 grams per tablespoon). The extra water added to these margarines can cause texture and volume changes when used in recipes. Cookbooks can provide guidance for appropriate use for these products by suggesting alterations in recipes to compensate.

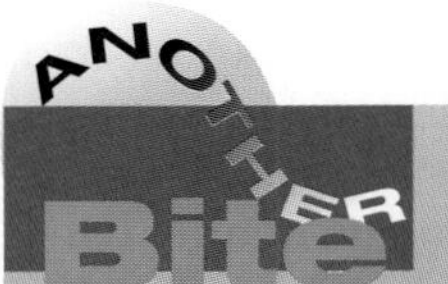

You may be surprised to note that some margarines are even advertised as being fat-free. Close inspection of the label shows that these products are made up of monoglycerides and diglycerides. These are not considered to be fats for labeling purposes, as they are not triglycerides, but of course they are still fats and energy dense.

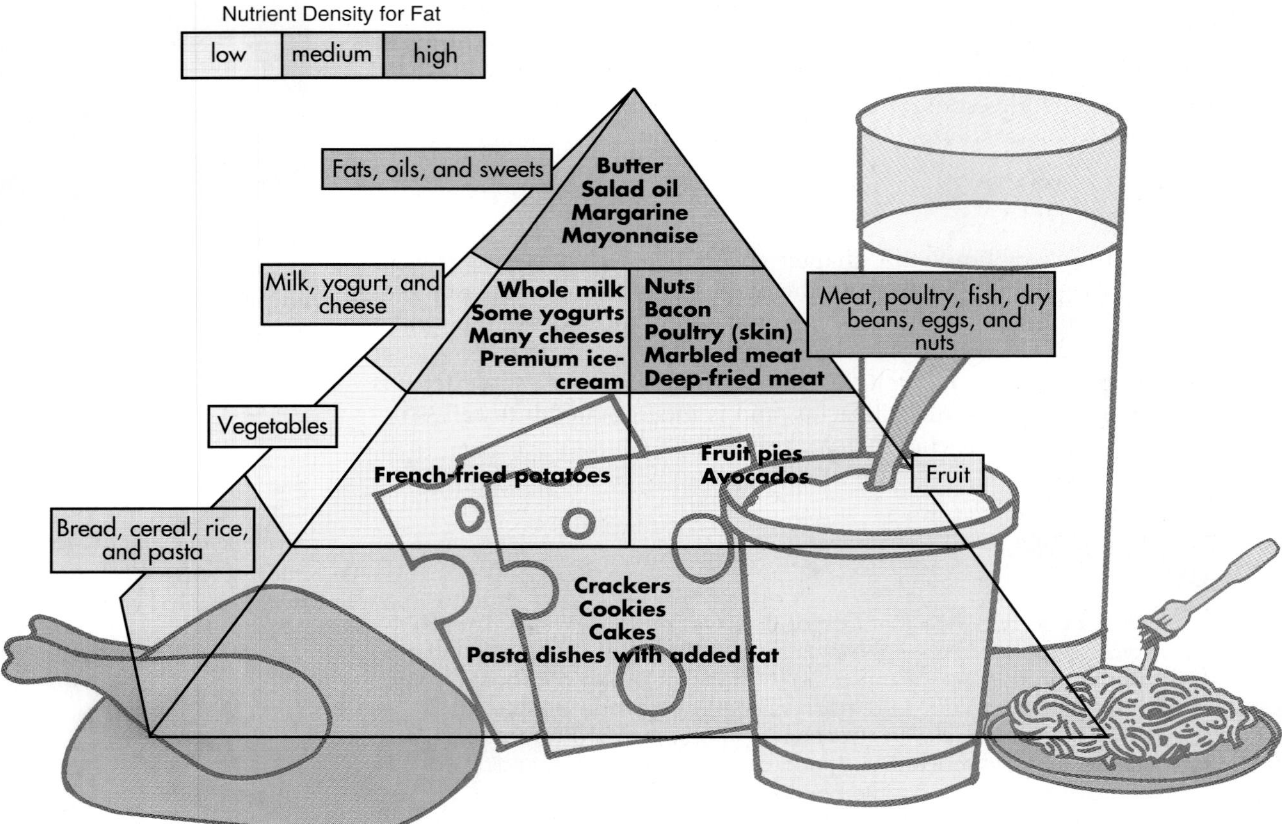

Figure 5-3 *Sources of fats in foods from the Food Guide Pyramid. The background color of each group indicates the average nutrient density for fat in that food group. The fruit group and vegetable group are generally very low in fat. In the other groups both low-fat and fat-rich choices are available. In general, any type of frying adds significant amounts of fat to a product, as with french-fried potatoes and fried chicken. Use Nutrition Labels to assess actual fat content.*

Walnuts, bologna, avocados, and bacon have about 80% of energy as fat. Peanut butter and cheddar cheese have about 75%. Marbled steak and hamburgers (ground chuck) have about 60%, and chocolate bars, ice cream, doughnuts, and whole milk have about 50% of energy as fat. Eggs, pumpkin pie, and cupcakes have 35%, as do lean cuts of meat, such as top round (and ground round) and sirloin. Bread contains about 15%. Cornflakes, sugar, and nonfat milk have essentially no fat. Careful label reading is necessary to determine the true fat content of a food—these are only rough guidelines.

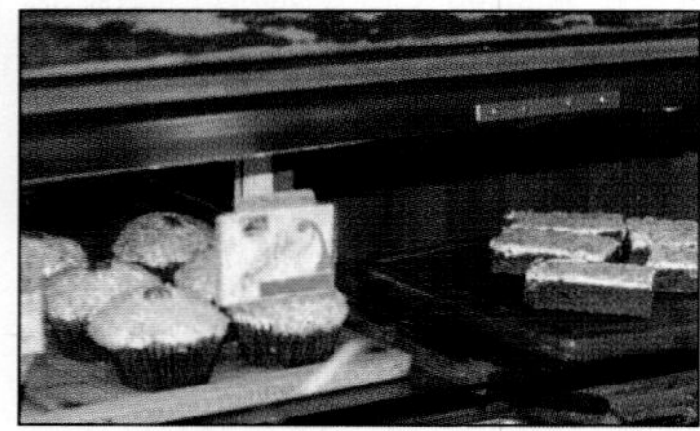

The American diet contains many high-fat foods—including typical cookie and cake choices.

Animal fats, which contain about 40% to 60% of total fat as saturated fatty acids, are the chief contributor of saturated fatty acids to the American diet (Figure 5-4). In some plant oils, these saturated fatty acids also make up a notable percentage of the total fat: for example, cottonseed oil (27%) and coconut oil (89%). Saturated fatty acids with 12, 14, and 16 carbons (lauric acid, myristic acid, and palmitic acid, respectively) are the primary contributors to elevated blood cholesterol in humans. Of these, the 14-carbon myristic acid is mainly responsible. Fats in milk products are rich in myristic acid. The 16-carbon palmitic acid does the same primarily when there is much cholesterol in the diet (more than 200 to 300 milligrams per day) and blood cholesterol is elevated. In contrast, stearic acid, the saturated fatty acid with 18 carbons, does not raise blood cholesterol; it constitutes about 20% of the

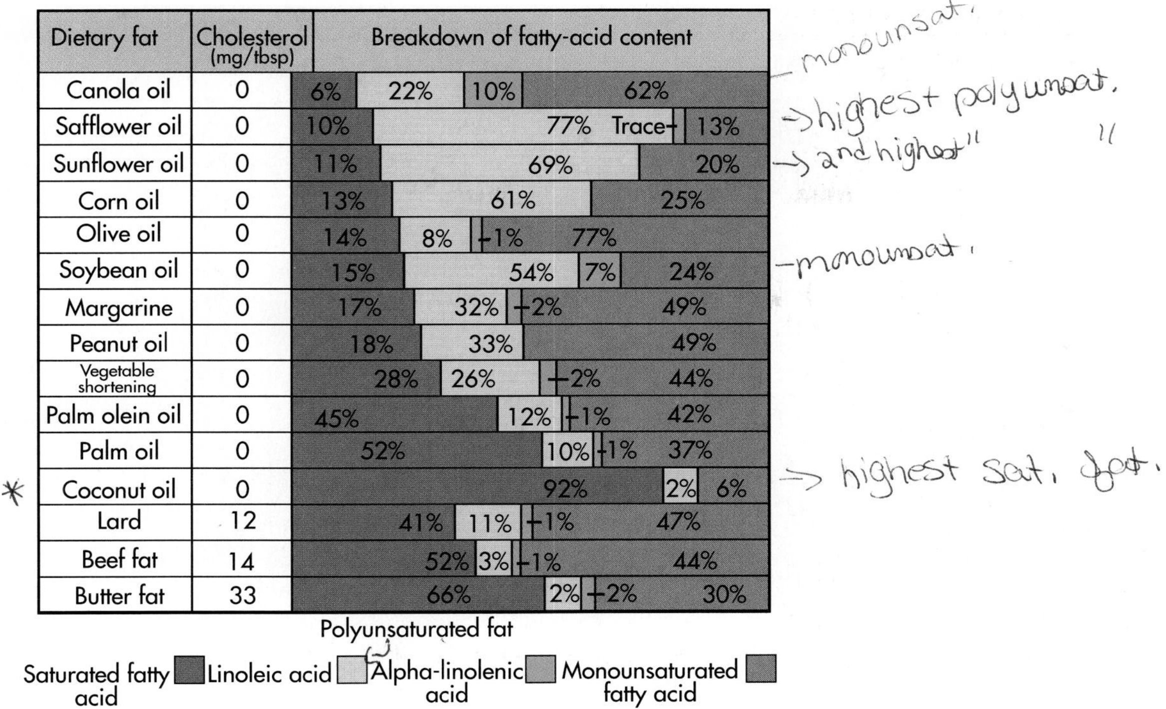

Figure 5–4 *Comparison of dietary fats in terms of saturated fatty acids, the most common unsaturated fatty acids, and cholesterol content.*

saturated fat in meats. The saturated fatty acids with 12, 14, or 16 carbons generally constitute about 25% to 50% of the total fat in animal foods. As you will see later, the fatty acids found in vegetable shortenings can also increase blood cholesterol.

Plant oils contain mostly unsaturated fatty acids, ranging from 73% to 94% of total fat. Canola oil, olive oil, and peanut oil contain moderate to high amounts of total fat as monounsaturated fatty acids. Some animal fats are also good sources of monounsaturated fatty acids. Corn, cottonseed, sunflower, soybean, and safflower oils contain mostly polyunsaturated fatty acids in terms of total fat. Note that plant oils vary in their content of polyunsaturated fatty acids; oils that are similar in appearance still may vary significantly in fatty acid composition.

Egg yolks, wheat germ, peanuts, and organ meats are rich sources of phospholipids. Cholesterol is found only in the animal foods we eat (Table 5–1). An egg yolk contains about 210 milligrams of cholesterol. This is our main dietary source of cholesterol, along with meats and whole milk. Some plants contain related sterols, but none we typically eat contains cholesterol. Manufacturers who advertise peanut butter, vegetable shortening, margarines, and vegetable oils as containing "no cholesterol" are taking advantage of uninformed consumers. Peanut butter and margarine never contain cholesterol—it's not part of their nature!

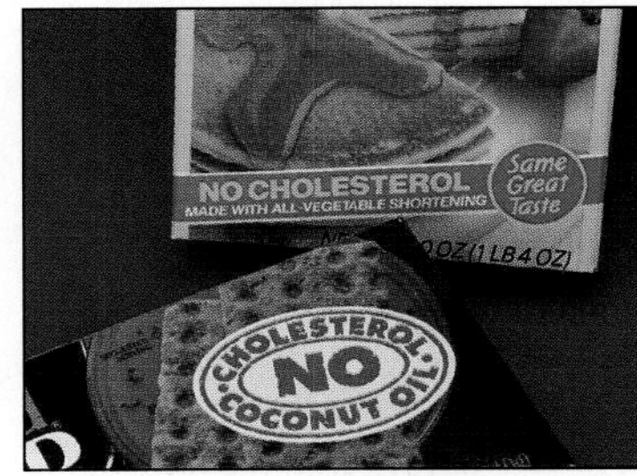

Manufacturers now offer a variety of low-cholesterol foods.

Recall from Chapter 2 that "low fat" signifies in most cases that a product contains no more than 3 grams of fat per serving. Products claimed to be fat free must have less than ½ gram of fat per serving. A claim of "reduced fat" means the product has at least 25% less fat than is usually found in that food.

When there is no food label to inspect, moderating portion size is a good way to control fat intake. Table 5–2 lists many ways you can avoid eating too much fat. Whether or not to choose a fat-rich food should depend on how you intend to use it: as a staple item, as an occasional treat, or as a garnish for other foods.

TABLE 5-1

Cholesterol Content of Common Measurements of Selected Foods (in ascending order)

Food	Amount	Cholesterol (milligrams)	Food	Amount	Cholesterol (milligrams)
Skim milk	1 cup	4	Cheeseburger	1	52
Snack cake w/cream filling	1	6	Clams, halibut, tuna	3 oz	55
Mayonnaise, lard	1 tbsp	10	Crab, lobster	3 oz	65
Butter	1 pat	11	Chicken, turkey (white meat)	3 oz	70
Cottage cheese	½ cup	15	Beef,* pork	3 oz	75
Low-fat milk (2%)*	1 cup	22	Oysters, salmon	3 oz	90
Half and half	¼ cup	23	Lamb	3 oz	85
Hot dog	1	29	Shrimp	3 oz	165
Ice cream, ≈10% fat	½ cup	30	Heart, beef	3 oz	165
Cheese, cheddar*	1 oz	30	Egg (egg yolk)*	1 each	210
Whole milk*	1 cup	34	Kidney	3 oz	330
Cheese pizza	2 slices	36	Liver, beef	3 oz	425
Hamburger sandwich	1	42	Brains	3 oz	1700
Chocolate milkshake	12 fl oz	44			

*One of 5 leading contributors of cholesterol to the U.S. diet (milk in all of its forms is one category).

Using Reduced Fat Foods Wisely

In recent years, manufacturers have introduced reduced-fat versions of numerous food products (Figure 5–5). The fat content of these alternatives ranges from 0% in fat-free Fig Newtons to about 75% of the original fat content in other products. However, the total energy content of most fat-reduced products is not substantially lower than that of their conventional versions. Generally, when fat is removed from a product, something must be added, commonly sugars, in its place. It is very difficult to reduce both the fat and sugar content of a product at the same time. For this reason, most fat-reduced products (e.g., cakes, cookies, and sugared yogurt) are still very energy dense. Similarly, some cookbooks are modifying recipes to make them lower in fat. This is accomplished by replacing the fat with applesauce or other fruit purees. Keep in mind that these carbohydrate replacements still contain calories, but not as much as the fat that is left out. Overall, don't be fooled into thinking you can eat *substantially* more of such foods just because some or all of the fat has been removed. "Reduced fat" is not a license to overeat. Use the Nutrition Facts label to guide the portion size you choose.

GRIN & BEAR IT By Wagner

"Figby Foods has reduced its fat content by another gram! This is war, gentlemen!"

Figure 5–5 *Grin & Bear It.* Reprinted with special permission of North America Syndicate.

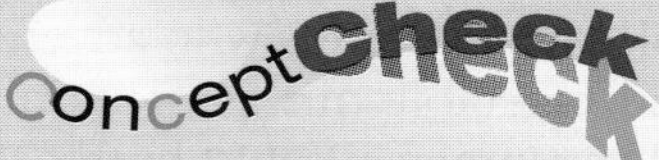

Fat-dense foods—those with more than 60% of total energy as fat—include plant oils, butter, margarine, mayonnaise, walnuts, bacon, avocados, peanut butter, cheddar cheese, steak, and hamburger. Of the foods we typically eat, cholesterol is found naturally only in those of animal origin, with eggs being a primary source. Fat free doesn't mean calorie free; moderation in the use of fat-reduced products is still important.

TABLE 5-2

Tips for Avoiding too Much Fat

1. Steam, boil, or bake vegetables. For a change, stir-fry in a small amount of vegetable oil. Consider buying an insert for a pot so you can easily steam your vegetables.
2. Season vegetables with herbs and spices rather than with sauces, butter, or margarine.
3. Try lemon juice on salad or use limited amounts of oil-based salad dressing.
4. To reduce saturated fat, use tub margarine instead of butter or stick margarine in baked products. When possible, use vegetable oil instead of either of these solid fats or hydrogenated shortenings.
5. Limit baked goods made with large amounts of fat: croissants, doughnuts, muffins, biscuits, and butter rolls.
6. Try whole-grain flours to enhance flavors when baking goods with less fat. Use applesauce and other fruit purees in place of fat.
7. Replace whole milk with nonfat or reduced-fat milk in puddings, soups, and baked products and for use as a beverage.
8. Substitute plain low-fat yogurt, blender-whipped low-fat cottage cheese, or buttermilk in recipes that call for sour cream or mayonnaise.
9. Choose lean cuts of meat. Look for 'round' or 'loin' in the name. Limit bacon, ribs, and meatloaf.
10. Trim fat from meat before and after cooking.
11. Roast, bake, or broil meat, poultry, and fish so that fat drains away as the food cooks.
12. Remove skin from poultry before cooking. This eliminates the temptation to eat it along with the meat.
13. Use a nonstick pan for cooking so that added fat will be unnecessary; use a vegetable spray for frying.
14. Chill meat or poultry broth until the fat solidifies. Spoon off the fat before using the broth.
15. Eat a vegetarian main dish at lease once a week. Include fish (cooked without much added fat) in the diet about two times a week.
16. Choose fat-reduced ice cream, low-fat frozen yogurt, sorbet, and Popsicles as substitutes for regular ice cream.
17. Try angel food cake, fig bars, and gingersnaps as substitutes for commercial baked goods high in fat.
18. Limit high-fat cheese intake.
19. Read labels on commercially prepared foods to find out how much fat they contain.
20. Use mostly jam, jelly, or marmalade on bread and toast instead of mostly butter or margarine.
21. Buy whole-grain breads and rolls. They have more flavor and do not need butter or margarine to taste good. The dietary fiber present is an added bonus.
22. Watch portion size, especially in restaurants (see the second Nutrition Insight).

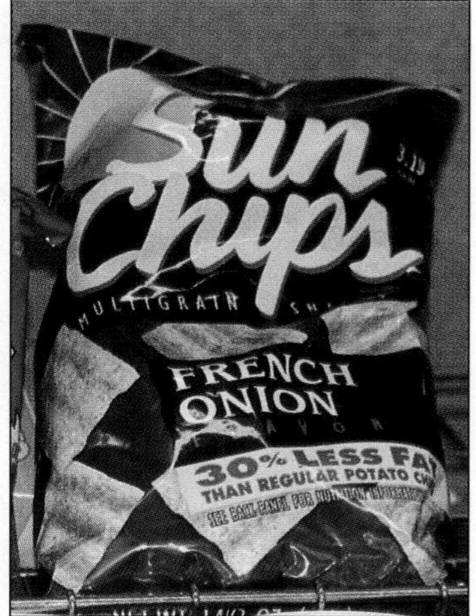

Many manufacturers offer products that are lower in fat than the traditional product.

When many Americans think of a low-fat diet, they include generous amounts of reduced-fat versions of pastries, cookies, and cakes. Consequently, reduced-fat food sales are projected to soar to nearly $32 billion by the year 2001. When health professionals refer to a low-fat diet, they have a very different plan in mind: replacing high-fat snacks primarily with fruits, vegetables, and whole grains. Most Americans could benefit from this paradigm shift.

Nutrition Insight

Fat Replacement Strategies

Currently five different types of fat replacements are available in the United States. Addition of these substances during manufacture yields products that to varying degrees satisfy consumers desire for fat-reduced products that are still tasty. About 90% of adults consume fat-reduced foods on a regular basis.

Water, Starch Derivatives, and Gums

The simplest fat replacement is water. Addition of water yields a product, such as diet margarine, with less fat per serving than the normal product. Starch derivatives that bind water form another type of fat replacement. The resulting gel replaces some of the mouth feel lost by the removal of fat. Starch derivatives commonly used by food manufacturers include Z-trim, cellulose, Maltrin, Stellar, and Oatrim. These substances are used in a variety of foods, including luncheon meats, salad dressings, frozen desserts, table spreads, dips, baked goods, and candies. Most starch derivatives contain some calories, though they have at least less than half the amount that is in fat. Note that these starch derivatives cannot be used in fried foods.

Gums extracted from plants can also be used to replace fat. They thicken a product and replace some of the body that fat provided. Diet salad dressings have gums added for this reason.

Protein-Derived Fat Replacements

A new type of fat replacement on the market consists of proteins that have been treated to produce microscopic, mistlike protein globules. Both egg and milk proteins can be used. When these substances replace fat in a food product, they feel like fat in the mouth, although the product does not contain any fatty acids. Simplesse is a currently used fat replacement of this type. Since it contains protein, Simplesse yields some energy—but only about 1 to 2 kcal per gram. Simplesse has this low energy value primarily for two reasons: proteins contain only about 4 kcal per gram, and the product has a high water content.

Simplesse is used primarily in frozen desserts. It reduces the energy content of these products by about one-half and fat content to a negligible amount. Because high temperatures alter the structure of Simplesse so much that it no longer resembles fat, it cannot be used for cooking or frying. Note also that people who are allergic to milk or egg proteins should not consume Simplesse.

Engineered Fats

The final form of fat replacement is the engineered fat. This type of product is synthesized in the laboratory

Making Lipids Available for Body Use

Dietary fat is digested and absorbed primarily in the small intestine.

Fat Digestion

In the first phase of fat digestion the stomach secretes an enzyme that acts primarily on triglycerides with fatty acids of short-chain and medium-chain lengths, such as those found in butterfat. The action of this enzyme, however, is usually dwarfed by that of an enzyme released from the pancreas and active in the small intestine. In addition, triglycerides and other lipids found in common vegetable oils and meats are generally not digested until they reach the small intestine (Figure 5–6).

from various food constituents. The recently introduced product olestra (Olean) is a good example. It is made by chemically linking fatty acids to sucrose (table sugar), similar to the way fatty acids attach to glycerol to form a triglyceride. The resulting product cannot be digested by either human digestive enzymes or bacteria that live in the intestine. Therefore olestra yields no energy to the body.

Olestra can replace much of the fat in salad dressings and cakes and is also the first fat replacement that can be used for frying. Use is currently limited by FDA to fried snack foods.

Some problems are associated with the use of olestra. It binds the fat-soluble vitamins A, D, E, and K, thus reducing absorption. To compensate, the manufacturer adds these vitamins to olestra. Olestra also may cause abdominal cramping and loose stools in some people, because even though it is not absorbed in the small intestine, it still may influence intestinal function. The problem is mostly seen with intakes of 20 grams at a meal. In comparison, a 1-ounce bag of chips will have about 10 grams of olestra.

One final problem linked to olestra is its ability to bind carotenoids, the yellow, orange, or red pigments found in many fruits and vegetables. Recall from Chapter 2 the discussion of phytochemicals and their proposed contribution to overall health; one class of phytochemicals is **carotenoids.** There is no planned attempt to add carotenoids to olestra. This effect of olestra will be most important when it is consumed in large amounts with meals rich in carotenoids. Typical projected intakes of 10 to 20 grams don't have much of an effect. Nevertheless, this ability to bind carotenoids has caused some experts to recommend that we not consume olestra. At the very least, organizations such as the American Heart Association recommend moderate intake until we know more about its long-term effects.

Food manufacturers are working on still other types of engineered fats that either wholly or partially escape absorption by the body. One example is Salatrim, which is marketed under the name Benefat and yields only about 5 kcal per gram. It is generally composed of stearic acid, a long-chain fatty acid that the body absorbs poorly, and short-chain fatty acids (two to three carbons long in this case). Benefat is currently used in reduced-fat chocolate products.

Fat Replacement in Perspective

So far, fat replacements have had little impact on the American diet, partly because the currently approved forms either are not very versatile or have not been used extensively by manufacturers. In addition, fat replacements are of little use in many foods that contribute the most fat to our diets—beef, margarine, salad dressings/mayonnaise, cheese, milk, and pastries—to name some key players. We consumers must decide to limit our intake of these fat sources; the replacements currently can't help us much.

The main benefit of fat replacements will be in helping people cut some fat from their diets. The reduction in overall energy intake will probably be less impressive because people tend to make up the lost energy by increasing their intake of other foods or by eating more of fat-reduced foods than the corresponding conventional foods.

In the small intestine, triglycerides break down into smaller products, namely monoglycerides (glycerol backbones with single fatty acids attached) and fatty acids. In the right circumstances, digestion is very rapid and thorough. The "right" circumstances include the presence of bile from the gallbladder. Bile acids help emulsify the digestive products of enzyme action, in effect acting like dishwashing detergent when it breaks up oil spots in dishwater. This improves digestion and absorption because as large fat globules are broken down into smaller ones, the total surface area for enzyme action increases.

During meals, bile circulates in a path that begins in the liver, goes on to the gallbladder, and then moves to the small intestine. After participating in fat digestion, the bile constituents are absorbed and end up back at the liver. Approximately 98% of the bile constituents are recycled. Only 1% to 2% ends up in the large

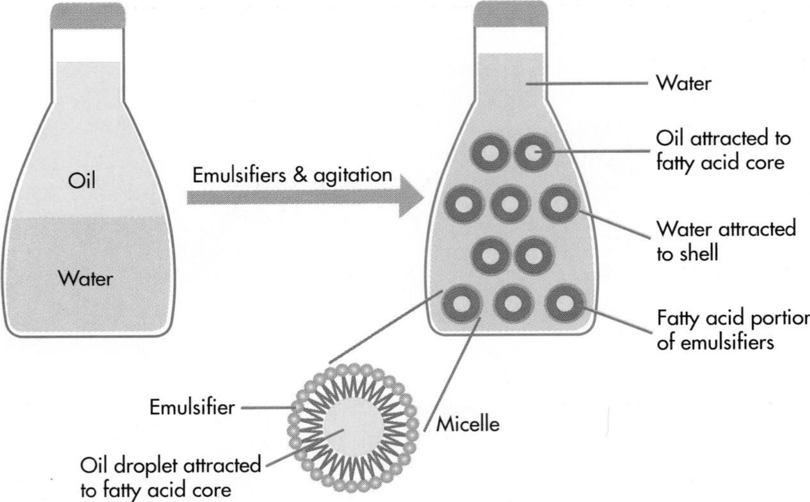

Figure 5-6 *Emulsifiers in action. Emulsifiers are what keep many brands of salad dressings and other condiments from separating into layers of water and fat. Emulsifiers attract fatty acids inside, and have a water-attracting group on the outside. Add them to salad dressing, shake well, and they hold the oil in the dressing away from the water. Emulsification is important in both food production and fat digestion/absorption.*

intestine to be eliminated in the feces. Using medicines to block some of this reabsorption of bile acids is a way physicians can treat high blood cholesterol. The liver takes cholesterol from the bloodstream to form replacement bile acids. Soluble fiber in the diet can produce the same effect as these medicines (see the Nutrition Issue for details).

Fat Absorption

Most products of fat digestion have by now been reduced to mere fatty acids and monoglycerides in the small intestine. These diffuse as such into the absorptive cells of the small intestine. One key characteristic of fatty acids and monoglycerides affects their ultimate fate after absorption. If the chain length of a fatty acid is less than 12 carbon atoms (a short-chain or medium-chain variety), it is water soluble and will therefore probably travel as such through the portal vein to the liver. If the fatty acid is long-chain variety (especially 14 or more carbon atoms), it must eventually be re-formed into a triglyceride and eventually enter circulation via the lymphatic system (see Chapter 3 for a review of this process).

ConceptCheck

In the small intestine an enzyme released from the pancreas digests dietary triglycerides into smaller breakdown products, namely monoglycerides (glycerol backbones with single fatty acids attached) and fatty acids. The breakdown products then diffuse into the absorptive cells of the small intestine. These products are mostly resynthesized into triglycerides, using the lymphatic system to enter the bloodstream.

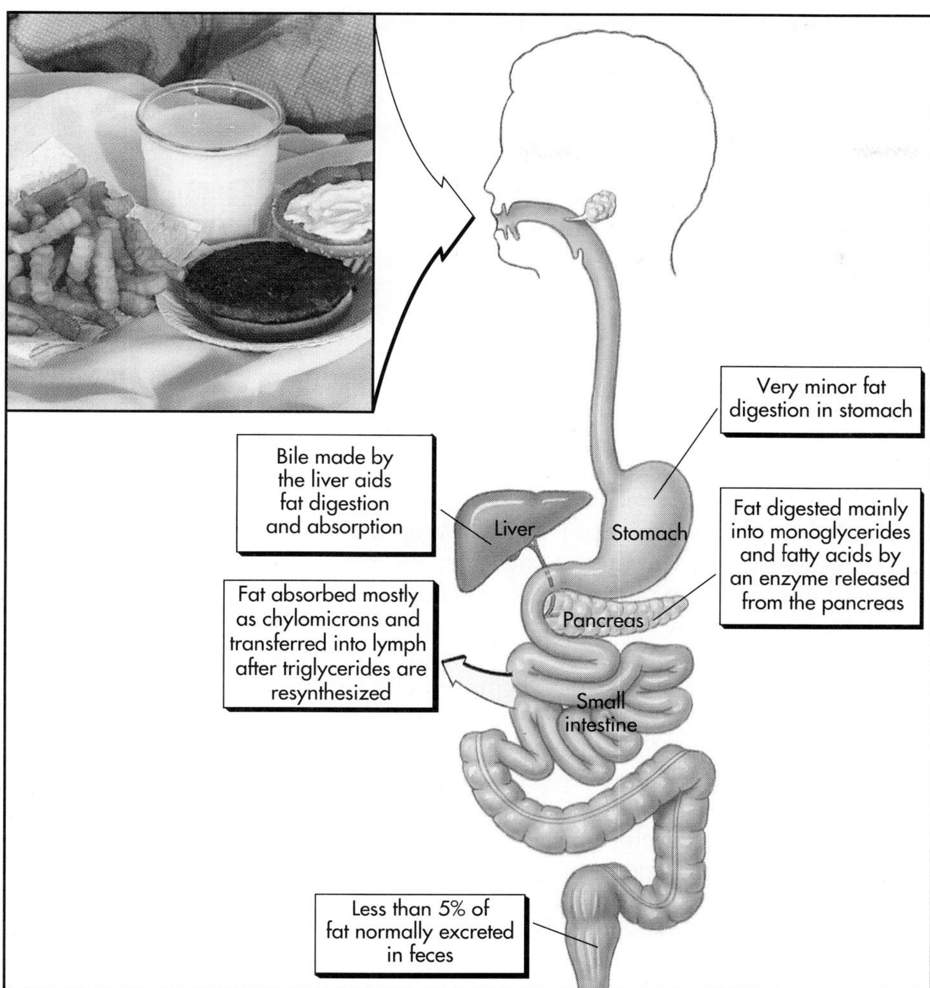

Figure 5-7 *A summary of fat digestion and absorption. Chapter 3 covered general aspects of this process.* Illustration by William Ober.

Carrying Lipids in the Bloodstream

As noted earlier, fat and water don't easily mix. This incompatibility presents a challenge in transporting fats through the watery mediums of the blood and lymph systems.

Carrying Dietary Fats

The various dietary fats absorbed into the small intestine cells and re-formed into triglycerides combine with phospholipids, protein, and cholesterol to form a chylomicron. This is one of many types of blood **lipoproteins.** This lipoprotein structure allows fats to float freely in the water-based bloodstream (Figure 5-7).

Lipoprotein
A compound found in the bloodstream containing a core of lipids with a shell of protein, phospholipid, and cholesterol.

Chylomicrons enter the lymphatic system and travel into the bloodstream. Once there, the triglycerides in the chylomicrons are broken down into fatty acids and glycerol by an enzyme on the inside wall of the blood vessel. Muscle cells, adipose cells, and other cells in the vicinity then absorb most of the fatty acids. Cells can immediately use absorbed fatty acids for fuel, or they can re-form them into triglycerides and store them as such. Muscle cells tend to burn the fatty acids, whereas adipose cells tend to store them.

Lipoprotein	*Key role*
Chylomicron	**Carries dietary fat to cells**
VLDL	**Carries lipids made by liver to cells**
LDL	**Carries cholesterol made by liver and other sources to cells**
HDL	**Contributes to cholesterol removal from cells, and in turn excretion of it from the body**

Transporting Various Lipids Made by the Body

The liver produces more fat and cholesterol than does any other body organ. The source of the needed carbons, hydrogens, and energy to make such substances as triglycerides and cholesterol includes the carbohydrate and protein the liver takes up from the bloodstream. Any alcohol consumed can also be used as a source. The liver coats the cholesterol and triglycerides it makes with a shell of protein and lipids. This process produces what is called a **very low-density lipoprotein (VLDL).**

When the VLDLs leave the liver, enzymes on the blood vessels break down the triglyceride in the VLDLs into fatty acids and glycerol. Again fatty acids and glycerol are released into the bloodstream, and are taken up by the body cells. Because fats are less dense than water, VLDLs become denser as triglyceride is released. Much of what eventually remains of these VLDLs becomes particles called **low-density lipoprotein (LDL).** LDL is composed primarily of cholesterol.

LDL particles are absorbed from the bloodstream by cells and broken down. Most LDL is taken up by liver cells. Diets low in saturated fat and cholesterol encourage this process, whereas diets high in those lipids can reduce LDL uptake by the liver (see the Nutrition Issue). The cholesterol and protein parts then are transported throughout the cell. In this way, liver and other body cells absorb the building blocks used to make bile acids, certain hormones, and other compounds.

If LDL is not rapidly taken up by this route, scavenger cells buried in blood vessels detect, alter **(oxidize),** engulf, and digest the extra circulating LDL. Once within the scavenger cells the altered LDL is prevented from reentering the bloodstream. Over time, cholesterol builds up in the scavenger cells, especially when the amount of LDL in the bloodstream is excessive.

When scavenger cells have collected and deposited cholesterol for many years at a heavy pace, cholesterol builds up on the inner blood vessel walls—especially in arteries—and **plaque** develops (see Figure 5–12 in the Nutrition Issue). The plaque eventually mixes with protein and is then covered with a cap of muscle cells and calcium. Atherosclerosis, also referred to as *hardening of the arteries,* develops as plaque grows in the vessel. This eventually chokes off the blood supply to organs, setting the stage for heart problems. Plaque is probably first deposited to repair injuries in a vessel lining. The injuries that start plaque formation can be caused by smoking, diabetes, high blood pressure, and LDL itself. Viral and bacterial infections also are implicated and related vessel inflammation.

Oxidize
In the most basic sense this means a chemical substance has either lost an electron or gained an oxygen. This change typically alters the shape and/or function of the substance. An oxidizing agent then is a substance capable of capturing an electron from another source. That source is then "oxidized" when it loses the electron.

Plaque
In terms of heart disease, a cholesterol-rich substance deposited in the blood vessels. It also contains various white blood cells and smooth muscle cells, cholesterol and other lipids, and eventually calcium.

Antioxidant
Generally, a compound that can donate electrons to electron-seeking (oxidizing) compounds. This reduces the destructive nature of oxidizing compounds. Some compounds have antioxidant capabilities (i.e., they stop oxidation) but are not electron donors per se.

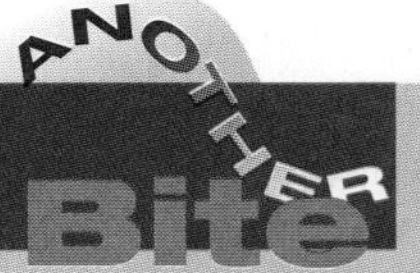

*Some nutrients have **antioxidant** properties. These likely reduce LDL oxidation in the bloodstream and thus slow LDL uptake into scavenger cells. Fruits and vegetables are rich in such antioxidants, including carotenoids and vitamin C. Eating fruits and vegetables regularly is one positive step we can take to reduce cholesterol buildup and slow the progression of heart disease. Consuming vitamin E supplements may also accomplish this, but it should only be done with a physician's approval (see Chapter 7). On the other hand, an excessive intake of iron probably speeds LDL oxidation, making it wise not to take an iron supplement unless a physician prescribes it (see Chapter 8).*

A final critical participant in this extensive process of fat transport is the **high-density lipoprotein (HDL).** Its high proportion of protein makes it the heaviest (densest) lipoprotein. The liver and intestine produce most of the HDL in the blood. It roams the bloodstream, picking up cholesterol from dying cells and other sources. HDL donates the cholesterol to other lipoproteins for transport back to the liver; some HDL travels directly back to the liver. Another beneficial function of HDL is that it may block oxidation of LDL.

The amount of HDL in the bloodstream helps predict the risk for heart disease. The risk increases with low HDL because little blood cholesterol is transported back to the liver and excreted. Women tend to have high HDL, especially before **menopause,** whereas low values are more common in men.

Menopause
The cessation of menses in women, usually beginning at about age 50.

Because high HDL slows the development of heart disease, any cholesterol carried by HDL can be considered "good" cholesterol. By convention, then, cholesterol carried by LDL would be "bad" cholesterol because high LDL speeds the development of heart disease. Still, LDL is only a problem when it is too high in the bloodstream; low amounts are needed as part of routine body functions.

Note that in the clinical laboratory the amount of cholesterol in the HDL fraction of blood lipids is what is determined, rather than the amount of HDL itself. The same generally holds true for LDL. Thus it is more correct to refer to HDL cholesterol and LDL cholesterol. To simplify the discussion, the shorthand terms LDL and HDL will be used.

ConceptCheck

The bloodstream carries absorbed dietary fat as chylomicrons. Lipid synthesized by the liver is carried in the bloodstream as very low-density lipoprotein (VLDL). Once a VLDL has most triglycerides removed, it eventually becomes low-density lipoprotein (LDL), which is rich in cholesterol. LDL is picked up by body cells, especially liver cells. High-density lipoprotein (HDL) picks up cholesterol from cells and transports it primarily to other lipoproteins for eventual transport back to the liver. HDL may also decrease LDL oxidation, thereby reducing LDL uptake into atherosclerotic plaque. Elevated LDL is one major risk factor associated with heart disease, as is low HDL.

Critical Thinking

As part of his annual health checkup, Juan has a blood sample drawn for measurement of cholesterol values. The results of the test indicate that his total blood cholesterol is a bit too high, but his HDL is high as well. Juan has read that high total blood cholesterol is linked to cardiovascular problems. However, his physician is happy with the results of the blood test. How would Juan explain his physician's satisfaction to his parents?

Putting Lipids to Work in the Body

The various classes of lipids have diverse functions in the body. All are necessary for health, but, as mentioned earlier, not all are needed in our diet. Of all the classes of lipids, only certain polyunsaturated fatty acids are essential parts of a diet.

Essential Fatty Acids

This essentiality of certain polyunsaturated fatty acids in the diet is based on the location of the carbon-carbon double bonds in the fatty acids. Greek letters are used to signify this location. For example, if the double bonds start directly after the third carbon (counting from the end with a $-CH_3$ group), the fatty acid is an **omega-3 (ω-3) fatty acid.** If these bonds start directly after the sixth carbon, it is an **omega-6 (ω-6) fatty acid,** and so on. **Alpha-linolenic acid** is the major omega-3 fatty acid found in food; **linoleic acid** is the major omega-6 fatty acid.

Humans can't produce omega-3 and omega-6 fatty acids; we get them only by ingesting them. That is why this structural uniqueness is important. These fatty acids are essential for us to eat because they participate in immune processes and vision, help form cell structures, and aid in the production of hormone-like compounds. Because we must get linoleic acid (omega-6) and alpha-linolenic acid (omega-3) from foods, they are called ***essential fatty acids.***

In the Greek alphabet, *alpha* is the first letter and *omega* is the last.

We need to get about 1% to 2% of our total energy intake from linoleic acid. On a 2500-kcal diet, that corresponds to 1 tablespoon of plant oil each day. We easily get that much—via mayonnaise, salad dressings, margarine, and other foods—without even noticing. Barring these foods, regular consumption of whole grains and vegetables can also supply enough essential fatty acids.

Our diets should include a regular supply of either alpha-linolenic acid or its related omega-3 forms, such as **eicosapentaenoic acid (EPA).** To get this supply, we

Alpha-linolenic acid
An essential fatty acid with 18 carbons and three carbon-carbon double bonds (omega-3).

Linoleic acid
An essential fatty acid with 18 carbons and two carbon-carbon double bonds; omega-6.

Essential fatty acids
Fatty acids that must be present in the diet to maintain health; these consist of linoleic acid and alpha-linolenic acid.

Stroke
Damage to part of the brain caused by interruption of its blood supply or leakage of blood outside vessel walls. Sensation, movement, or function controlled by the damaged area is then impaired.

should eat fish—such as salmon, halibut, trout, tuna, and sardines—about twice a week. Regular use of canola or soybean oil or nuts also supplies omega-3 fatty acids. It is interesting to note that fatty fish do not produce these omega-3 fatty acids. They obtain these acids as part of their diet via algae—a plant source.

This recommendation for consuming omega-3 fatty acids stems from the observation that compounds made from omega-3 fatty acids tend to decrease blood clotting and inflammatory processes in the body, whereas the omega-6 fatty acids generally increase these processes. People who eat fish about twice a week (total weekly intake: 8 ounces or 240 grams) run lower risks for heart attacks than do people who rarely eat fish. In these cases, the omega-3 fatty acids in fish oil are probably acting to reduce blood clotting. (Blood clots are part of the heart attack process.) Consequently the risk of heart attack decreases, especially for people already at high risk (see the Nutrition Issue at the end of this chapter to learn about the link between blood clots and heart attacks). Better heart rhythm is also induced by eating omega-3 fatty acids, as are other heart-healthy benefits.

We need to remember, however, that blood clotting is a normal body process. Certain groups of people, such as Eskimos in Greenland, eat so much seafood that their blood-clotting ability can be impaired. An excess of omega-3 fatty acid intake can allow uncontrolled bleeding and may cause one form of **stroke.**

Overall, excessive consumption of omega-3 fatty acids can be as problematic as inadequate consumption. Thus, health experts do not recommend that healthy people use megadose fish oil supplements, suggesting instead that people stick to eating fish about two times a week. People with heart disease should strive for the full two servings per week.

If regular fish intake is not acceptable to a person, experts recommend seeking plant sources of omega-3 fatty acids. Use of low doses of fish oil capsules is also appropriate (2 to 3 grams per day).

Effects of a Deficiency of Essential Fatty Acids

If humans don't receive enough essential fatty acids, one's skin will become flaky and itchy, and diarrhea and other symptoms such as infections often are seen. Growth and wound healing also may be retarded, and anemia can develop. These signs of deficiency have been seen in people fed **intravenous nutrition** solutions containing little or no fat for 2 to 3 weeks, and in infants receiving formulas low in fat. However, because our bodies need the equivalent of only about 1 tablespoon of polyunsaturated plant oil a day, even a very low-fat diet will provide enough EFAs if it follows the Food Guide Pyramid and includes some fish.

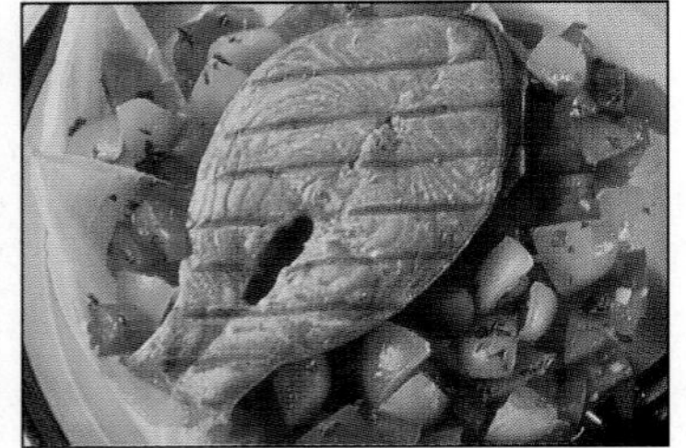

Eating fish about twice a week makes a healthy addition to a diet as it contributes to omega-3 fatty acid intake.

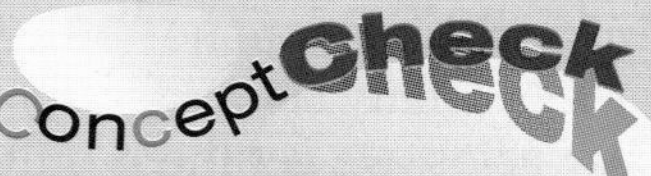

Because humans can't make either omega-3 or omega-6 fatty acids, which perform vital functions in the body, they are essential parts of a diet and therefore called essential fatty acids. Plant oils are generally rich in omega-6 fatty acids. Eating fish about twice a week is a good way to meet omega-3 fatty acid needs. Essential fatty acid deficiency can occur after 2 to 3 weeks if fat is left out of intravenous nutrition solutions, which in turn can lead to skin disorders, diarrhea, and other problems.

Broader Roles for Fatty Acids and Triglycerides

Many key functions of fat in the body require the use of fatty acids in the form of triglycerides. Triglycerides are used for energy storage, insulation, and transportation of fat-soluble vitamins. As well, triglycerides contribute to the sensation of satiety (fullness) after eating.

Intravenous nutrition *Nutrition that is supplied directly into the veins, rather than via the GI tract.*

Providing Energy for the Body

The fatty acids supplied by triglycerides both contained in the diet and stored in adipose (fat) tissue are the main fuel for muscles while at rest and during light activity. Only in endurance exercise, such as long-distance running and cycling, or short bursts of intense activity, such as a 200-meter run, do muscles burn much of carbohydrate in addition to fatty acids. Other body tissues also use fatty acids for energy. Overall, about half of the energy used by the entire body at rest and during light activity comes from fatty acids. On a whole-body basis the use of fatty acids by muscles is balanced by the use of glucose by the brain and red blood cells. Recall from Chapter 4 that all cells also need carbohydrate to efficiently process fatty acids for fuel.

Storing Energy

Humans store energy mainly in the form of triglycerides. The body's ability to store fat is essentially limitless. Its fat storage sites, adipose (fat) cells, can increase about 50 times in weight. If the amount of fat to be stored exceeds the ability of the cells to expand, the body can form new adipose cells. (This is discussed further in Chapter 9.)

An important advantage of using triglycerides to store energy in the body is that they are energy dense. In addition, when the body stores triglycerides in adipose cells, little else is included; adipose cells contain about 80% lipid and only 20% water and protein. In contrast, imagine if humans stored energy as muscle tissue, which is about 73% water. Body weight linked to energy storage would increase dramatically.

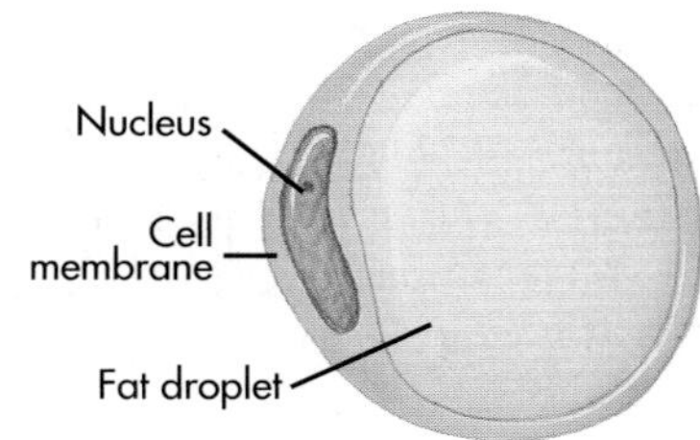

Adipose cell.

Insulating the Body and Protecting Organs

The layer of fat just beneath our skin is made mostly of triglycerides. This fat tissue insulates and protects some organs—kidneys, for example—from injury. We usually don't notice the important insulating function of fat tissue, because we wear clothes and add more as needed. But a layer of insulating fat is quite apparent in animals, particularly in those cold climates. Polar bears, walruses, and whales all build a thick layer of fat tissue around themselves to insulate against cold-weather environments. The extra fat also provides energy storage for times when food is scarce.

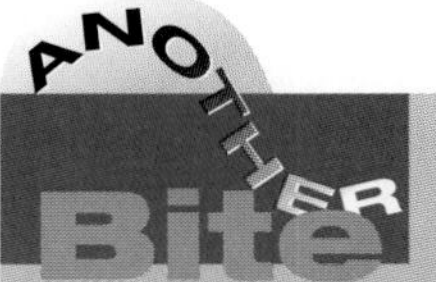

We can never be totally fat free because fat is an essential part of all cells. However, people with ***anorexia nervosa*** *often lose 25% or more of body weight and end up about as fat free as biologically possible. This poses many health risks, such as a loss of menstrual periods and related bone loss (see Chapter 11). In addition, in place of the layer of fat tissue under the skin, people with anorexia nervosa often develop downy hair called* ***lanugo*** *all over the body. These hairs insulate the body by standing up and trapping air.*

Transporting Fat-Soluble Vitamins

Triglycerides and other fats in foods carry fat-soluble vitamins to the small intestine and aid their absorption. If the small intestine is diseased, however, it may not be able to adequately digest and absorb fat from foods. When this happens, the

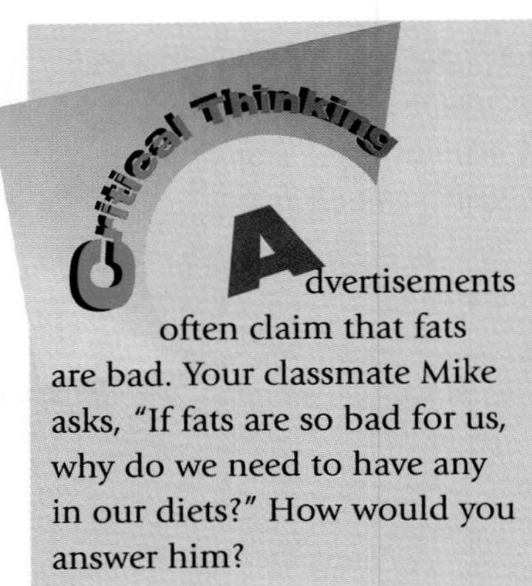

Advertisements often claim that fats are bad. Your classmate Mike asks, "If fats are so bad for us, why do we need to have any in our diets?" How would you answer him?

unabsorbed fat carries the fat-soluble vitamins—A, D, E, and K—into the large intestine. From there they are eliminated with the feces, and the body loses the benefits of the vitamins. If the disease doesn't resolve quickly, medical attention is necessary.

People who absorb fat poorly, such as those with the disease cystic fibrosis, are also at risk for deficiencies of fat-soluble vitamins. Supplements are used in these cases. A similar risk accrues from taking mineral oil, the undigested oil carries the fat-soluble vitamins from the meal into the large intestine, where they are eliminated.

Contributing to Satiety

If you are fond of cheesecake, you know that a little goes a long way. This is because triglycerides in foods help give us a full and contented feeling after a meal. The fat we eat triggers hormones that cause the stomach to retain foods longer than when we eat mostly carbohydrate or protein. This is why a high-fat meal allows us to feel full longer.

Many people who want to lose weight cut much of the fat from their diet. However, if dieters cut too much fat, they lose its *satiety* value and get hungry more quickly. Thus reducing fat intake below about 20% of total energy intake can actually be self-defeating, unless high-fiber foods are added to contribute bulk, which also makes us feel full. Having some low-fat snacks around to respond to intense hunger in this instance is also a good idea. Fruit is an excellent choice.

Phospholipids in the Body

Many types of phospholipids exist in the body, such as in the brain and other nerve tissue. Although phospholipids are necessary components of body tissues, however, we don't have to consume phospholipids as such because the body can make them when and where they are needed.

Emulsifier
A compound that can suspend fat in water by isolating individual fat droplets using a shell of water molecules or other substances to prevent the fat from coalescing.

Some phospholipids, such as the family of compounds mentioned earlier called *lecithins,* function as **emulsifiers.** These allow fat and water to mix. By breaking fat globules into small droplets, emulsifiers enable a fat to be suspended in water. For example, when lecithins are added to an oil and water mixture, they act as bridges between the oil and water that in turn lead to the formation of tiny oil droplets surrounded by thin shells of water. In an emulsified solution, millions of tiny oil droplets are separated by shells of water (Figure 5–8).

The body's main emulsifiers are the lecithins and bile acids which are produced by the liver and released into the small intestine via the gallbladder during digestion. By breaking up the fat globules, the emulsifiers create more fat surface for fat-digesting enzymes to act on.

Cholesterol in the Body

Cholesterol forms part of some important hormones, such as estrogen, testosterone, and a form of the active vitamin D hormone. Cholesterol is also the building block of bile acids, which are needed for fat digestion. Finally, cholesterol is an essential structural component of cells and the outer layer of particles that transport lipids in the blood, as discussed in the next section. The cholesterol content of the heart, liver, kidney, and brain is quite high, reflecting its critical role in these organs.

Each day your liver makes about 1000 milligrams of cholesterol. About one third is made into bile acids; the rest circulates through the bloodstream to function as the body needs it. In comparison, we eat about 200 to 400 milligrams of cholesterol per day. About half of this cholesterol is absorbed. There is interest in using plant sterols (these look much like cholesterol) to reduce cholesterol absorption.

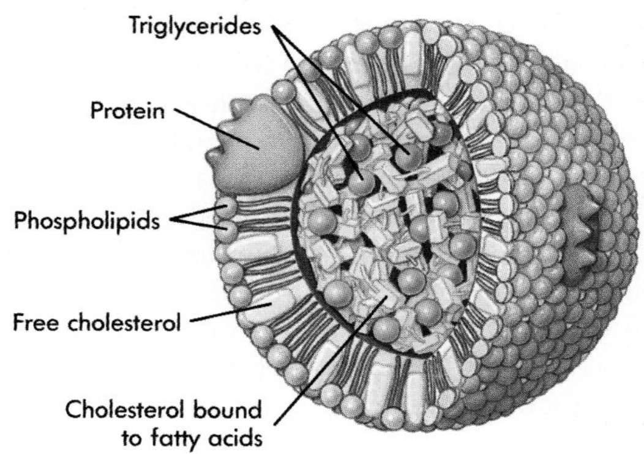

Figure 5-8 *The structure of a lipoprotein, in this case an LDL. This structure allows fats to circulate in the water-based bloodstream. Various lipoproteins are found in the bloodstream. Chylomicrons carry fats absorbed from foods through the bloodstream to body cells. VLDLs do the same but mostly carry various lipids made by the liver. LDLs carry cholesterol to the body cells and result from breakdown of VLDLs. HDLs carry cholesterol primarily back to other lipoproteins that in turn are mostly taken up by the liver. HDLs also take their cholesterol load directly back to the liver.*

These are added to margarine in Finland, and have been shown to reduce cholesterol absorption to about 5% of intake. This in turn leads to a fall in LDL. FDA is currently reviewing the request to allow this use of plant sterols (Benechol) in the United States.

When a diet doesn't contain enough cholesterol, the liver makes what the body needs. Medication to reduce liver synthesis of cholesterol are commonly used by physicians to lower elevated blood cholesterol (see the Nutrition Insight).

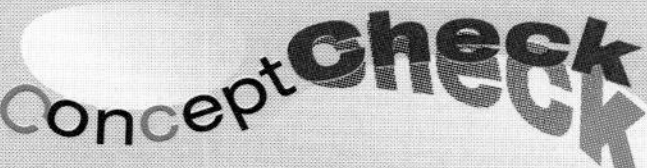

Triglycerides are the major form of fat in the body. Used for and stored as energy, they also insulate and protect body organs, transport fat-soluble vitamins, and promote satiety. Many phospholipids act as emulsifiers, compounds that suspend fat as small droplets in water. Phospholipids also form parts of cells and various other compounds in the body. Cells produce the phospholipids the body needs. Cholesterol, a sterol, forms parts of cells, hormones, and bile acids; it is essential to the body. Cholesterol is manufactured in the liver, and if sufficient amounts are not ingested, the body makes what it needs.

Exploring Another Dimension of Fat—Roles in Food

Various fats play important roles in foods.

Fat Provides Flavor and Texture to Foods

Many flavorings dissolve in fat. Heating spices in oil intensifies the flavors of an Indian curry or Mexican dish far more than simply adding them at the table. The oil then carries these flavors to the sensory cells that discriminate taste and smell in the mouth. We quickly associate flavor with fatty foods.

If you've ever eaten a high-fat yellow cheese or cream cheese, you probably agree that fat melting on the tongue feels good. The fat in whole milk also gives body that nonfat milk lacks. This love of fat is universal. Western, Eskimo, and Mediterranean diets are all rich in fat. Immigrants to Western cultures, such as many Japanese, quickly embrace the high-fat diet found in the United States. A person who has been following a typical American diet will probably need some time to adjust to a lower-fat diet. For example, if one changes from regular use of whole milk to 1% low-fat milk, after a few weeks switching back to the whole milk will have it taste more like cream than milk. One has thus adjusted to the flavor of the low-fat milk and will likely now find the whole milk to be not as palatable. Emphasizing flavorful fruits, vegetables, and whole grains also helps to adapt to a low-fat diet. Thus, it is certainly possible to make the change from a higher-fat diet to a lower-fat diet, but it takes some effort.

Hydrogenation of Fatty Acids Is Used for Some Types of Food Production

In some kinds of food production, such as pastry making, solid fats work better than liquid oils. In pie crust, for example, solid fats yield a flaky product, whereas crusts made with liquid oils tend to be greasy. The polyunsaturated fatty acids must become more saturated to solidify vegetable oils into shortenings and margarines for use in pastries and other products. In other words, more hydrogen must be added to turn double bonds between the carbons into single bonds. In the **hydrogenation** process the hydrogens are added by bubbling hydrogen gas into liquid vegetable oils (Figure 5–9).

Hydrogenation
Addition of hydrogen to a carbon-carbon double bond, producing a single bond. Because hydrogenation of unsaturated fatty acids in a vegetable oil increases its hardness, this process is used to convert liquid oils into more solid fats, which are used in making margarine and shortening.

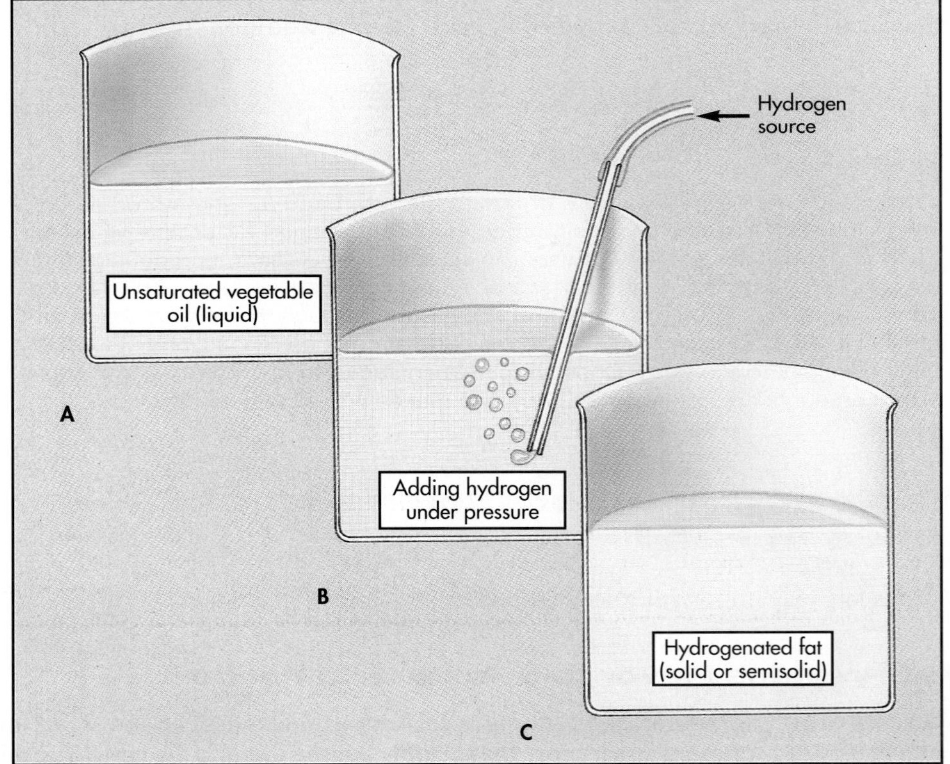

Figure 5–9 *How liquid oils become solid fats.* **A,** *Unsaturated fatty acids are present in liquid form.* **B,** *Hydrogens are added (hydrogenation) changing some carbon-carbon double bonds to single bonds and producing some trans fatty acids.* **C,** *The completed hydrogenated product, which is likely to be used in margarine, shortening, or deep-fat frying.*

During hydrogenation, changes also occur in the fatty acid, casting it in a so-called trans shape from its more typical *cis* form. The resulting substance is called a ***trans* fatty acid** (Figure 5–10). This structural change also causes the *trans* fats to raise blood cholesterol, just as many saturated fatty acids do. Thus people with elevated LDL should minimize intake of hydrogenated fat. It is less clear that this is important for the average person, as long as total fat intake is not excessive. However, since these fatty acids serve no particular role in maintaining body health, many experts now recommend this practice.

***Trans* fatty acid**
A form of an unsaturated fatty acid, usually a monounsaturated one when found in food, in which the hydrogens on both carbons forming the double bond lie on opposite sides of that bond. A cis *fatty acid has the hydrogens lying on the same side of the carbon-carbon double bond.* Trans *fatty acids are a by-product of hydrogenation of vegetable oils.*

Generally the more hydrogenation that occurs, the harder the product is; for example, stick margarine is more hydrogenated (saturated) than tub margarine. If a liquid oil is listed before any hydrogenated oil on food labels, the food probably contains a greater amount of unsaturated than saturated fat. Note that food labels don't currently list the amount of *trans* fatty acids present. Consumers have to look for the words 'hydrogenated' or 'hardened' to see if *trans* fatty acids are present. During the next few days, study food labels and notice how many chips, snack products, and crackers contain a "partially hydrogenated vegetable oil."

It's easy to avoid eating much hydrogenated fat and in turn taking in high amount of *trans* fatty acids. First, use little or no stick margarine or shortening; instead, substitute softer, tub margarine (whose labels list vegetable oil or water as the first ingredient) and vegetable oils. Second, minimize consumption of deep fat-fried foods in restaurants, which tend to use hydrogenated fat in the fryer. Foods to eat sparingly include french fries, doughnuts, fried potato skins, and any deep fat-fried meat, fish, or poultry. As an alternative a typical hamburger sandwich, bowl of chili, and soft drink or milk in a quick-service restaurant contain minimal hydrogenated fat. Finally, limit intake of high-fat baked foods, such as pastries, and nondairy coffee creamers.

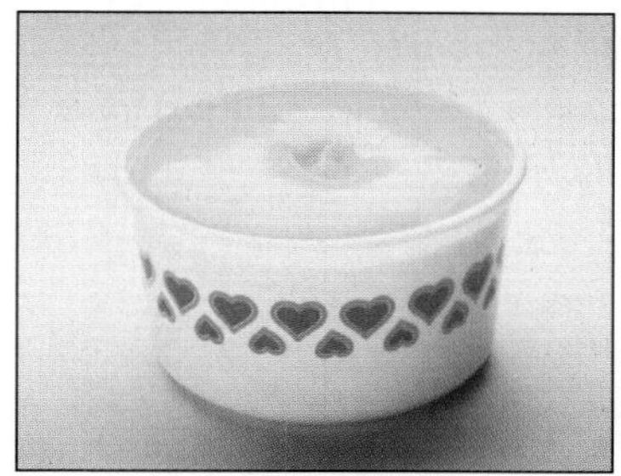

Tub margarine is much lower in trans *fatty acids than stick margarine or shortenings.*

Oleic acid

Elaidic acid

Cis form (causes backbone of molecule to bend)

Trans form

Figure 5-10 Cis *and* trans *fatty acids. In the* cis *form at double carbon-carbon bonds in a fatty acid, the hydrogens (in blue) lie on the same side of the double bond. This causes a "kink" at that point in the fatty acid, which is typical of unsaturated fatty acids in nature. In contrast, in the* trans *form at double carbon-carbon bonds in a fatty acid, the hydrogens lie across from each other at the double bond. This causes the fatty acid to exist in a linear form, like a saturated fatty acid.* Cis *fatty acids are much more common in foods than* trans *fatty acids. The latter are primarily found in foods containing hydrogenated fats, notably stick margarine, shortening, and deep fat-fried foods.* Trans *fatty acids raise LDL and lower HDL.* Illustration by William Ober..

Fat Rancidity Limits Shelf Life of Foods

Decomposing oils emit a disagreeable odor and also taste sour and stale. Stale potato chips are a good example. As double bonds in fatty acids break down, the

Rancid
Containing products of decomposed fatty acids; they yield unpleasant flavors and odors.

BHA and BHT
Butylated hydroxyanisol and butylated hydroxytoluene—two common synthetic antioxidants added to foods.

by-products are said to be **rancid.** Ultraviolet rays of light, oxygen, and certain other procedures can break double bonds, break them, and in turn destroy the structure of polyunsaturated fatty acids. Saturated fats can much more readily resist these effects. Why?

Rancidity is not a major problem for consumers because although eating rancid oils can cause sickness, the odor and taste generally discourage us from eating enough to become sick. However, rancidity is a problem for manufacturers because it reduces a product's shelf life. For this reason, manufacturers often add hydrogenated plant oils to products to increase shelf life. Foods most likely to become rancid are deep-fried foods and foods with a large amount of exposed surface (such as powdered eggs or powdered milk). The fat in fish is also very susceptible to rancidity because it is highly polyunsaturated, and so refrigeration is very important.

Vitamin E helps protect foods against rancidity because it acts as an antioxidant. It guards against fat breakdown caused by various agents, such as metals found as impurities in vegetable oils. The vitamin E in plant oils reduces the breakdown of double bonds in fatty acids. In Chapter 7 the role of vitamin E is explained more fully. When food manufacturers want to prevent rancidity in polyunsaturated fats, they often add **BHA** and **BHT.** (Chapter 15 discusses these additives.) Look for BHA and BHT in salad dressings, cake mixes, and other products that contain fat. Vitamin C also may be added for the same reason. Manufacturers also tightly seal products and use other methods to reduce the amount of oxygen inside packages.

Emulsifiers Improve Many Food Products

Food manufacturers add emulsifiers in the preparation of many food products, primarily to improve texture. For example, lecithins, polysorbate 60, monoglycerides, and other emulsifiers are added to salad dressings to keep the vegetable oil suspended in water. Eggs added to cake batters likewise emulsify the fat with the milk. Over the next few days, examine the labels of salad dressings and cake mixes, and see how many emulsifiers are listed.

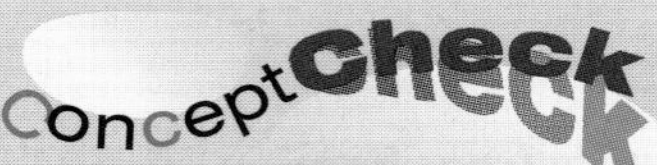

At room temperature, fats rich is saturated fatty acids tend to form solid fats, and fats rich in polyunsaturated and monounsaturated fatty acids tend to form liquid oils. During hydrogenation of unsaturated fatty acids, hydrogen is added to carbon-carbon double bonds to produce single bonds; some *trans* fatty acids are also created. Hydrogenation changes vegetable oil to solid fat. The carbon-carbon double bonds in polyunsaturated fatty acids are easily broken, yielding products responsible for rancidity. The presence of antioxidants, such as vitamin E in oils, naturally protects unsaturated fatty acids against oxidative destruction. Manufacturers can use hydrogenated fats and add various antioxidants to reduce the likelihood of rancidity.

Commercial salad dressings find practical use for emulsification. Emulsifiers such as lecithins, polysorbate 60, and monoglycerides are added to salad dressings and other fat-rich products to keep the vegetable oils and other fats suspended in water.

Recommendations for Fat Intake

No specific recommendation for fat intake has yet been set as part of development of the Dietary Reference Intakes. This will be considered by the Committee, but at a later date. As noted before, to obtain the essential fatty acids, adults should consume about 4% of total energy intake from plant oils incorporated into foods and eat fish about twice a week. Recall that it takes only about 1 tablespoon of oil per day to meet linoleic acid needs. The typical American diet derives about 7% of energy content from polyunsaturated fatty acids. An upper limit of 10% of energy intake as polyunsaturated fatty acids is often recommended, in part because the breakdown (oxidation) of those present in lipoproteins is linked to increased cholesterol deposition in the arteries, as just discussed. This breakdown may also increase the risk of cancer. Reduction in immune function also is suspected to be caused by an excessive intake of polyunsaturated fats.

Dietary fat supplies about 33% of Americans' total energy intake. Vegetable and animal foods each supply about half of the fat. Major sources of total fat in the U.S. diet include animal flesh, milk, pastries, cheese, margarine, mayonnaise, and salad dressing. Careful label reading helps one find which foods are rich in fat, especially those in which the fat content is not readily apparent (Figure 5-11).

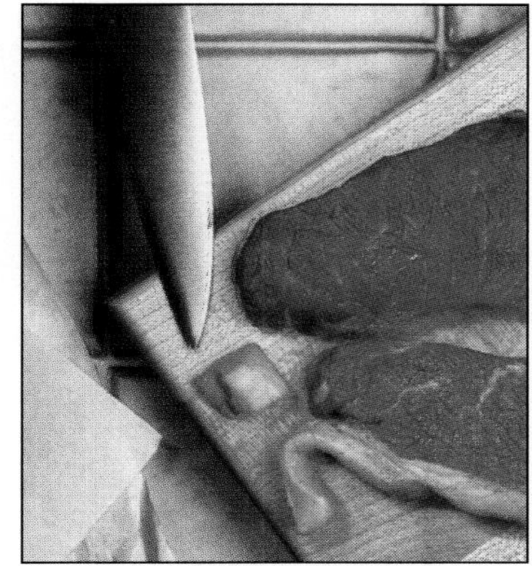

Trim meats before cooking to help reduce your saturated fat intake.

Wiley's
Our BEST
WIENERS
INGREDIENTS: PORK, WATER, BEEF, SALT, FLAVORINGS, CORN SYRUP SOLIDS, DEXTROSE, HYDROLYZED SOY AND POTATO PROTEIN, SODIUM PHOSPHATES, EXTRACT OF PAPRIKA, SODIUM ERYTHORBATE, SODIUM NITRITE.
KEEP REFRIGERATED
U.S. INSPECTED AND PASSED BY DEPARTMENT OF AGRICULTURE EST. 575
NET WT. 16 OZ. (1 LB.) 454g.
0 73593 11212 2
Nutrition Facts
Serving Size 1 Link (45g)
Servings Per Container 10
Amount Per Serving
Calories 140 Calories from Fat 120
% Daily Value*
Total Fat 13g 20%
Saturated Fat 5g 23%
Cholesterol 20mg 7%
Sodium 420mg 17%
Total Carbohydrate 2g 1%
Dietary Fiber 0g 0%
Sugars 1g
Protein 5g
Vitamin A 0% • Vitamin C 0%
Calcium 0% • Iron 2%
*Percent Daily Values are based on a 2,000 calorie diet.

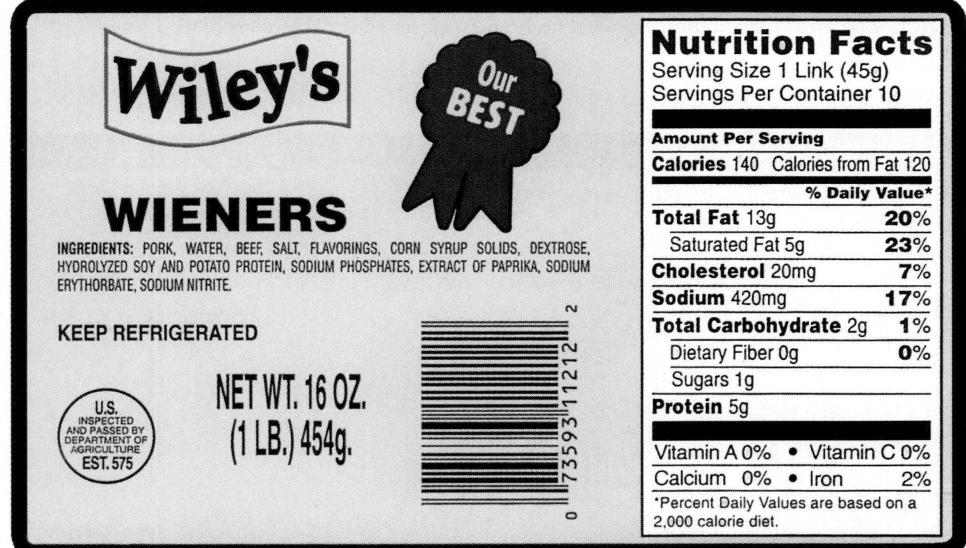

Figure 5-11 *Reading labels helps locate hidden fat. Who would think that wieners (hot dogs) can contain 85% of food energy as fat? Looking at the hot dog itself does not suggest that almost all of its food energy comes from fat, but the label shows otherwise.*

Because many Americans are at risk for developing heart disease, the American Heart Association (AHA) promotes dietary changes aimed at reducing this risk (Table 5-3). Many health agencies agree with the AHA recommendation that total fat intake averaged over a day or so should not exceed 30% of total energy intake, with no more than 8% to 10% of total energy intake from saturated fat. The intake of saturated fats currently averages about 12% of energy intake. Table 5-4 shows a diet that follows the basic AHA guidelines. Other experts suggest that fat can exceed 30% to 35% of energy intake, but in that case the diet should emphasize monounsaturated fat, as is in canola oil, or follow a pattern similar to the Mediterranean Diet Pyramid, which emphasizes olive oil (see the Nutrition Issue in Chapter 2).

For people who have elevated LDL even when following the guidelines of 30% or less of energy intake from fat, the AHA recommends a more stringent diet that includes no more than 20% of total energy from fat. Some cancer researchers

TABLE 5-3

Dietary Guidelines for Healthy American Adults: A Statement for Physicians and Health Professionals by the Nutrition Committee, American Heart Association (AHA)

- Elimination of cigarette smoking
- Appropriate levels of caloric intake and physical activity to prevent obesity and reduce weight in those who are overweight
- Consumption of 30% or less of the day's total calories from fat
- Consumption of 8% to 10% of total calories from saturated fatty acids
- Consumption of up to 10% of total calories from polyunsaturated fatty acids
- Consumption of up to 15% of total calories from monounsaturated fatty acids
- Consumption of less than 300 milligrams per day of cholesterol
- Consumption of no more than 2.4 grams per day of sodium
- Consumption of 55% to 60% of calories as complex carbohydrates
- For those who drink and those for whom alcohol (ethanol) is not contraindicated, consumption should not exceed 2 drinks (1 to 2 oz of ethanol) per day

These guidelines apply to one's diet over a few days to a week, rather than to a specific food or meal. "Moderate fat intake" is a common general health message for adults, regardless of who issues the report.

TABLE 5-4

Daily Menus Containing 2000 kcal and Various Percentages of Fat

30% OF ENERGY AS FAT	Teaspoons of fat	20% OF ENERGY AS FAT	Teaspoons of fat
BREAKFAST			
Orange juice, 1 cup	0	Same	0
Shredded wheat, ¾ cup	⅕	Shredded wheat, 1 cup	⅕
Bagel, toasted	⅕	Same	⅕
Margarine, 2 tsp	1¾	Margarine, 1 tsp	⅞
1% low-fat milk, 1 cup	½	Nonfat milk, 1 cup	⅒
LUNCH			
Whole-wheat bread, 2 slices	½	Same	½
Roast beef, 2 oz	2	Ham, extra lean, 3 oz	1
Mayonnaise, 2 tsp	1½	Mayonnaise, 1 tsp	¾
Lettuce	0	Same	0
Tomato, sliced	0	Same	0
Animal crackers, 8	½	Animal crackers, 10	⅔
SNACK			
Apple	⅙	Same	⅙
DINNER			
Chicken Parmigiana frozen dinner	4	Healthy Choice Chicken Parmigiana frozen dinner	⅔
Dinner roll, 1	½	Dinner roll, 2	1
Banana, 1	⅒	Margarine, 2 tsp	1¾
1% low-fat milk, 1 cup	½	Nonfat milk, 1 cup	⅒
SNACK			
Raisins, 2 tbsp	0	Raisins, ¼ cup	0
Popcorn, air-popped, 6 cups	½	Same	½
with 2 tsp margarine	1¾	with 1 tsp margarine	⅞
TOTALS	14⅔		9⅓

also advocate such a diet for adults in general (see Chapter 7). To achieve this goal, fat intake must be strictly limited (see Table 5–4). The advice and counsel of a registered dietitian are helpful in planning such diets. In addition, physician monitoring is important, as this degree of fat restriction can greatly increase blood triglycerides in some people, which is not a healthful change.

The National Cholesterol Education Program of the Federal government recommends reducing saturated fatty acids to 7% of total energy intake if elevated LDL does not respond to the reduction in saturated fat intake of closer to 10% of energy intake. Cholesterol intake in this regard should be limited to 300 milligrams per day, with a reduction to 200 milligrams per day if LDL remains elevated when following a fat-restricted diet containing the higher amount of cholesterol. Recall that adults consume an average of about 200 to 400 milligrams of cholesterol per day, with men generally consuming the higher amount. By encouraging a reduction in total fat, saturated fat, and cholesterol intake, all of these suggestions are in line with the Dietary Guidelines discussed in Chapter 2. Keep in mind, however, that the latter two suggestions are most important for people with elevated LDL.

Unfortunately, exceeding 30% of energy intake of fat is all too easy. For example, a bologna and cheese sandwich with mayonnaise contains about 39 grams of fat, or about 60% of the fat allowance for a 2000-kcal diet. A half-cup of premium ice cream contains about 18 grams, and a slice of apple pie contains about 19 grams, almost all of which is in the crust. A large (super-sized) order of fries has 26 to 30 grams, and much of it is *trans* fat.

Most people have no idea how much of the energy in their diets comes from fat. You've already tracked your food intake for one day. The Rate Your Plate exercise asks you to compare your food intake to current guidelines. Using the information on food labels and occasionally recording and analyzing daily food intake allow you to track your fat intake.

A final note: The advice to consume 20% to 30% of energy as fat does not apply to infants and toddlers below the age of 2 years. These youngsters are forming much new tissue, especially in the brain, so their intake of fat and cholesterol should not be greatly restricted. After that age, children should gradually adopt a diet that contains no more than 30% of energy from fat and 300 milligrams of cholesterol per day (see Chapter 13 for details). As children begin to consume less fat, they should replace the missing calories with more grain products, fruits, vegetables, and reduced-fat milk products.

Recommendations for fat intake are stated as a percentage of total energy intake—usually 20% to 30%. This chart shows how many grams of fat per day would be allowed with diets ranging from 1000 to 3900 kcal.

Energy intake (kcal)	*Fat intake grams 30% of energy*	*20% of energy*
1000	33	22
1200	40	27
1500	50	33
1800	60	40
2100	70	47
2400	80	53
2700	90	60
3000	100	67
3600	120	80
3900	130	87

ConceptCheck

We need about 4% of total energy intake from plant oils to obtain the needed essential fatty acids. (Eating fish about twice a week is also advised to supply omega-3 fatty acids.) Many health-related agencies recommend a diet containing no more than 30% of energy intake as fat, with no more than 7% to 10% of energy intake as saturated fat. Limiting *trans* fat intake is also advocated by many experts. The current American diet contains about 33% of energy content as fat, with about 12% of energy content as saturated fat. If fat intake exceeds 30% of total calories, a diet emphasizing monounsaturated fat is advised.

Nutrition Insight

Eating on the Run, with a Focus on Fat

Choosing healthful foods is becoming easier in many of today's quick-service (also called "fast-food") restaurants. Some restaurants have evolved beyond hamburgers, french fries, and milk shakes to include a variety of vegetables, salad bars, and ethnic foods. In addition, some restaurants are trying to cater to their more health-conscious clientele. If we buy more healthful foods, these restaurants will continue to meet this market demand. Still, between 40% and 50% of the energy in most quick-service choices come from fat. See Appendix A to evaluate your typical choices (100 × (grams of fat × 9)/total kcal). Overall, many of these meal selections are high-calorie options when compared with the amounts of other nutrients provided.

People who eat regularly at quick-service restaurants should choose meals carefully to meet their nutrient needs without exceeding their energy needs. Because these food outlets serve a need in our fast-paced society, they are probably a permanent part of the lifestyle of many Americans. What follows is a list of suggestions for making good nutritional choices in quick-service restaurants. Keep in mind that when no nutrition information is provided by the restaurant, moderating portion size is a good way to keep calorie and fat intake under control with foods you suspect are rich in fat, such as fried foods, potato and macaroni salads, desserts, and salad dressings.

Breakfast

Before entering a local quick-service restaurant for breakfast, decide whether you can fix this meal at home. Can breakfast be prepared the night before so it's ready for the next morning? The effort might be as simple as stocking the refrigerator with yogurt, putting bread next to the toaster, placing cereal on the counter with a bowl. Breakfast can be a relaxing time, and many of us need time away from the fast pace of daily life. If you've abandoned breakfast at home, think again. Breakfast at home is usually faster than a visit to a quick-service restaurant.

If you still prefer breakfast out, consider hot or cold cereal with milk. Another option is a plain scrambled egg or an English muffin with no more than 1 teaspoon of margarine. Add orange juice to round out a tasty breakfast. Substitute pancakes without the butter and minimal syrup instead of the egg and English muffin. Either way, you consume a lot less fat and calories than if you choose the typical meat, egg, and cheese-laden muffin or croissant. Be especially wary of croissants: they are loaded with fat. If you still want meat, consider Canadian bacon, a leaner breakfast meat than regular bacon.

Lunch and Dinner

A good choice for lunch or dinner is a sandwich made of whole-wheat bread and some lean meat or tuna. Pizza is a good idea once or twice a week. If ordered with vegetable toppings—mushrooms, green peppers, and onions—pizza provides a very nutritious meal for a moderate number of calories. The cheese most commonly used in pizza is a low-fat variety. The next best choice is probably a hamburger, but not the king-size model. Consider buying the basic hamburger. Be especially wary of mayonnaise, sauces, melted cheese, fried onions, and other sources of added fat. Chili is another alternative. It's lower in fat than a king-size hamburger, and the beans supply dietary fiber. Finally, ordering soup and a salad is another lower-fat option. Burritos with beans or chicken also are often moderate in fat, if added cheese is kept to a minimum.

Bite-size pieces of chicken should be made from chicken breast only and not from processed chicken that can include ground chicken skin. Ask the restaurant manager from which parts of the chicken the entrée is made. Let him or her know your nutrition and health interests and see to what extent your needs can be accommodated. Broiled or baked chicken is the most healthful. If the chicken is fried, remove the coating. The same applies to fish: remove the coating. Actually, chicken and fish start out as low-fat protein sources, but by the time they're deep-fat fried, their protein:fat ratio resembles that of a typical hamburger sandwich.

For side dishes, consider portion sizes. Order a small rather than a large portion of french fries. Order a baked potato, and to spice it up, put on plenty of chives but not more than a pat of margarine. Minimize sour cream, cheese, and other toppings—you can save 300 kcal. Also watch the fats you add to vegetables.

At the salad bar, pay particular attention to the addition of cheese, bacon bits, and dressing. Mayonnaise-based salads, such as macaroni and potato salad, are relatively high in calories. To minimize saturated fat intake, try the oil and vinegar and French dressings rather than the creamy types such as bleu cheese dressing. Some people find fresh-squeezed lemon juice is a satisfying alternative to dressing. Some restaurants do supply low-calorie dressings. Try these, or otherwise add as little regular dressing as possible. Salad bars also offer fresh fruits and vegetables, which can contribute to a healthful meal.

For beverages, consider 1% low-fat or nonfat milk, water, diet soft drinks, or iced tea. A typical milk shake contains about 350 to 400 kcal. In contrast, a cup of 1% milk has only 100 kcal.

Above all, focus on fat in the overall meal you choose. By all means, however, enjoy eating out. Look at your total diet, not at whether one food or another is going to ruin your health. For example, if you know you're going to have a high-fat lunch, plan to have a leaner dinner to compensate. We should think of eating as a pleasurable experience. There are some hurdles to clear, but once you learn these tips for eating on the run, you can make choices that fit into a healthful diet even at quick-service restaurants.

Summary

- Lipids are a group of compounds that don't readily dissolve in water. Fatty acids can be grouped according to the type of bonds between the carbons: saturated fatty acids contain no double bonds, monounsaturated fatty acids contain one double bond, and polyunsaturated fatty acids contain two or more double bonds.
- Fats composed of saturated fatty acids tend to be solid at room temperature. Those with polyunsaturated fatty acids are usually liquid at room temperature.
- Triglycerides are the major form of fat in our bodies. Besides supplying essential fatty acids to the body, triglycerides supply energy, allow efficient energy storage, insulate and protect the body, transport fat-soluble vitamins, and promote satiety, or a feeling of fullness.
- Phospholipids are derived from triglycerides. They form parts of cell membranes. Some act as efficient emulsifiers, allowing fats to disperse in water.
- Cholesterol is in the class of lipids called sterols. It forms part of vital compounds, such as hormones and bile acids. Cells in the body can make all the cholesterol we need; there is no dietary requirement. Fat-rich foods include plant oils, butter, margarine, mayonnaise, walnuts, bacon, avocados, peanut butter, cheddar cheese, steak, and hamburger. Cholesterol is present in those of animal origin, with eggs being a primary source. Fat free doesn't mean calorie free; moderation in the use of fat-reduced products is still important.
- If the double bonds in a fatty acid begin at the third carbon from the $-CH_3$ end of the chain, the fatty acid is an omega-3 fatty acid. In omega-6 fatty acids the double bonds begin at the sixth carbon. Both omega-3 and omega-6 fatty acids are essential parts of a diet because our bodies need them but don't produce them.
- Body cells use omega-3 fatty acids to synthesize compounds that tend to reduce blood clotting and inflammatory responses. Because many types of fish contain ample amounts of the omega-3 fatty acids, eating fish about twice a week is a recommended dietary practice.
- Fat digestion takes place primarily in the small intestine. An enzyme released from the pancreas digests the triglycerides into smaller breakdown products, namely monoglycerides (glycerol backbones with single fatty acids attached) and fatty acids. The breakdown products then are absorbed by the small intestine. These products are mostly resynthesized into triglycerides and combined with cholesterol, protein, and other substances to yield a chylomicron. Chylomicrons enter the lymphatic system, in turn passing into the bloodstream.
- Fats are carried in the bloodstream by various lipoproteins: chylomicrons, very low-density lipoproteins (VLDLs), low-density lipoproteins (LDLs), and high-density lipoproteins (HDLs). The greater the amount of triglycerides in the lipoproteins, the less their density. Both elevated LDL and low HDL speed the development of heart disease.

- Fats add flavor and texture to foods. Hydrogenation is the process of adding hydrogens to fatty acids to turn many double bonds into single bonds. This process also forms *trans* fatty acids. Manufacturers hydrogenate (increase saturation of) fats to solidify vegetable oils for making shortenings and margarine. This practice also reduces the breakdown of polyunsaturated fatty acids, which lessens rancidity.
- We need to eat at least the equivalent of about 1 tablespoon of plant oils daily in foods to get the needed omega-6 essential fatty acids. Fish is a rich source of needed omega-3 fatty acids.
- The typical American diet contains about 33% of total energy as fat. Many health agencies and scientific groups suggest reducing fat intake to no more than 30% of energy intake and cholesterol intake to between 200 and 300 milligrams. Some health experts advocate an even greater reduction to 20% of energy intake, but such a diet is generally difficult to plan and requires physician monitoring. Limiting *trans* fat intake is also encouraged by many experts. If fat intake exceeds 30% of total calories, the diet should emphasize monounsaturated fat.

Study Questions

1. Describe the chemical structures of saturated and polyunsaturated fatty acids and their different effects in both food and the human body.
2. Relate the need for omega-3 fatty acids in the diet to the recommendation to consume fish about two times per week.
3. Describe the structures, origins, and roles of the four major blood lipoproteins.
4. What are the various recommendations of health-care professionals regarding fat intake? What does this mean in terms of actual food choices?
5. What are two important attributes of fat in food? How are these different from two general functions of lipids in the human body?
6. What are the significance of and possible uses for the new reduced-fat foods?
7. Why is there growing concern over *trans* fats in the diet? How would one limit *trans* fat intake?
8. Does the total cholesterol concentration in the bloodstream tell the whole story with respect to coronary heart disease risk?

Read the Nutrition Issue before answering the following questions:

9. List five risk factors for the development of heart disease.
10. What actually brings on a myocardial infarction? What practices are thought to precipitate this event?

Further Readings

1 ADA Reports: Position of the American Dietetic Association: fat replacers, *Journal of the American Dietetic Association* 98:463, 1998.
2 AHA Medical/Scientific Statement: Dietary guidelines for healthy American adults, *Circulation* 94:1795–1800, 1996.
3 Byers T: Hardened fats: hardened arteries, *New England Journal of Medicine* 337:1544, 1997.
4 Conner SL, Conner WE: Are fish oils beneficial in the prevention and treatment of coronary heart disease? *American Journal of Clinical Nutrition* 66(suppl):1020S, 1997.
5 Drewnowski A: Why do we like fat? *Journal of the American Dietetic Association* 97(suppl):S58, 1997.
6 Folsom AR and others: Physical activity and incidence of coronary heart disease in middle-aged women and men, *Medicine & Science in Sports & Exercise* 29:901, 1997.
7 Grundy SM: Cholesterol management in high-risk patients without heart disease, *Postgraduate Medicine* 104(5):117, 1998.
8 Grundy SM: What is the desirable ratio of saturated, polyunsaturated, and monounsaturated fatty acids in the diet? *American Journal of Clinical Nutrition* 66(suppl):988S, 1997.
9 Hayes KC: Designing a cholesterol-removed fat blend for frying and baking, *Food Technology* p. 92, April 1996.
10 Henkel J: Keeping cholesterol under control, *FDA Consumer* p. 23, January–February 1999.
11 Katan MB: Effect of low-fat diets on plasma high-density lipoprotein concentrations, *American Journal of Clinical Nutrition* 67(suppl):573S, 1998.
12 Kris-Etherton P, Yu S: Individual fatty acid effects on plasma lipids and lipoproteins: human studies, *American Journal of Clinical Nutrition* 65(suppl):1628S, 1997.
13 Kromhout D: Fish consumption and sudden cardiac death, *Journal of the American Medical Association* 279:65, 1998.
14 Lichtenstein AH and others: Dietary fat and health, *Nutrition Reviews* 56(11):S3, 1998.
15 Liebman B: Fat: fine-tuning the message, *Nutrition Action Health Letter* 25(2):1, 1998 (March).
16 Masley SC: Dietary therapy for preventing and treating coronary artery disease, *American Family Physician* 57:1299, 1998.
17 McBean LD: Coronary Heart Disease, *Dairy Council Digest* 69(2):7, 1998.
18 McCully KS: Homocysteine, folate, vitamin B-6, and cardiovascular disease, *Journal of the American Medical Association* 279:392, 1998.
19 Miller GJ: Effects of diet composition on coagulation pathways, *American Journal of Clinical Nutrition* 67(suppl):542S, 1998.
20 Ornish D and others: Intensive lifestyle changes for reversal of coronary heart disease, *Journal of the American Medical Association* 280:2001, 1998.
21 Pearson TA: Alcohol and heart disease, *American Journal of Clinical Nutrition* 65:1567, 1997.
22 Pierre C: Are you getting enough fat? *American Health* p. 68, March 1998.

RATE

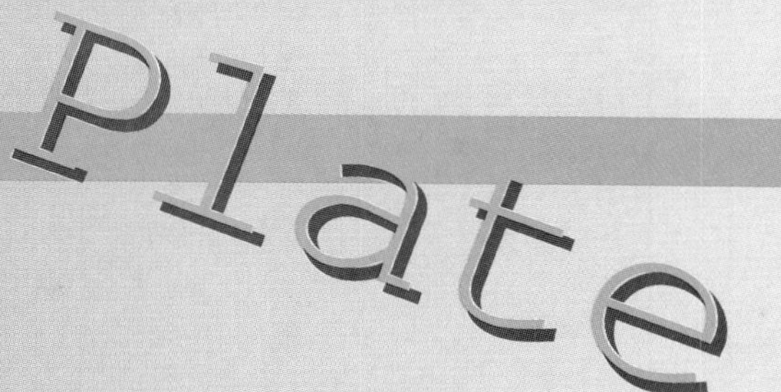

I. Are You Eating A Diet That Includes Many Saturated-Fat Sources?

Instructions:

Check the food you would typically select from the two choices given.

1.	____ **Bacon and eggs**	____ **Ready-to-eat whole-grain breakfast cereal**
2.	____ **Doughnut or sweet roll**	____ **White or whole-wheat roll, bagel, or bread, no margarine**
3.	____ **Breakfast sausage**	____ **Fruit**
4.	____ **Whole milk**	____ **Low-fat or nonfat milk**
5.	____ **Cheeseburger**	____ **Turkey sandwich, no cheese**
6.	____ **French fries**	____ **Plain baked potato with minimal added fat or salad with low-cal or fat-free dressing**
7.	____ **Meal including fried hamburger or fatty beef**	____ **Meal including broiled lean hamburger (ground round), chicken, or fish**
8.	____ **Creamed soup**	____ **Clear soup (could have meat or vegetables in it)**
9.	____ **Potato salad**	____ **Baked potato, limited added fat**
10.	____ **Cream/fruit pie**	____ **Graham crackers**
11.	____ **Ice cream**	____ **Frozen yogurt, sherbet, or fat-reduced ice cream**
12.	____ **Butter or stick margarine**	____ **Soft margarine in a tub**

INTERPRETATION

The foods listed on the left tend to be high in saturated fat, *trans* fat, cholesterol, and total fat. Those on the right generally are low. If you want to help reduce the risk of heart disease, choose the foods on the right more often than the foods on the left.

II. What Is Your Fat and Cholesterol Intake?

How do your food practices actually compare with general guidelines suggested for fat, saturated fat, and cholesterol intake? Refer to the nutritional assessment you completed at the end of Chapter 2, and compare it with the guidelines listed below, issued by the American Heart Association and the National Cholesterol Education Program:

- **Limit or reduce total fat intake to 30% or less of total energy intake.**
- **Reduce saturated fat intake to 7% to 10% of energy intake or less.**
- **Limit cholesterol to 200 to 300 milligrams per day.**

To compare your nutritional assessment with these guidelines, first fill in the values for your intakes of the following:

Total Energy: ________ Total Fat:________ Saturated Fat:________ Cholesterol: ________

Now complete the following steps:

1. **Multiply your total grams of fat by 9 (kcal per gram of fat). Then divide the result by your total energy intake. Next multiply this number by 100. This will give you the percentage of energy you consumed from fat.**

   % OF ENERGY FROM FAT ____ IS IT 30% OR LESS OF TOTAL ENERGY? YES ____ NO ____

2. **Multiply your grams of saturated fat by 9 (kcal per gram of fat). Divide the result by your total energy intake. Now multiply this number by 100. This will give you the percentage of energy you consumed from saturated fat.**
   % OF ENERGY FROM SATURATED FAT ____
   IS IT 10% OF ENERGY OR LESS? YES ____ NO ____
3. **Look at your milligrams of cholesterol.**
   IS YOUR INTAKE LESS THAN 300 MILLIGRAMS? YES ____ NO ____
4. **Look back at the foods you ate and notice the foods that contributed the most fat, saturated fat, and cholesterol. If you didn't meet one or more of the guidelines and had elevated LDL, how could you change what you ate that day to improve your diet?**
5. **Now take the next step. Do you know your LDL, HDL, and triglyceride values? If not, have them checked soon. All adults should know whether these values are in the abnormal ranges.**
6. **Finally, fill in the following assessment of your risk for developing heart disease. Decide today how you could modify your diet and lifestyle, if necessary, to reduce your risk.**

Do you have . . .	Yes	No		Yes	No
a history of smoking?	____	____	diabetes?	____	____
high blood pressure?	____	____	a history of physical inactivity?	____	____
high LDL?	____	____	a family history of premature heart disease (before age 60 years)?	____	____
low HDL?	____	____	a history of obesity?	____	____
high triglycerides?	____	____	a diet that lacks sufficient B vitamins, such as B-6, folate, and B-12?	____	____

Other factors also could be considered, as discussed in the Nutrition Issue, but this provides a good start for assessing your risk.

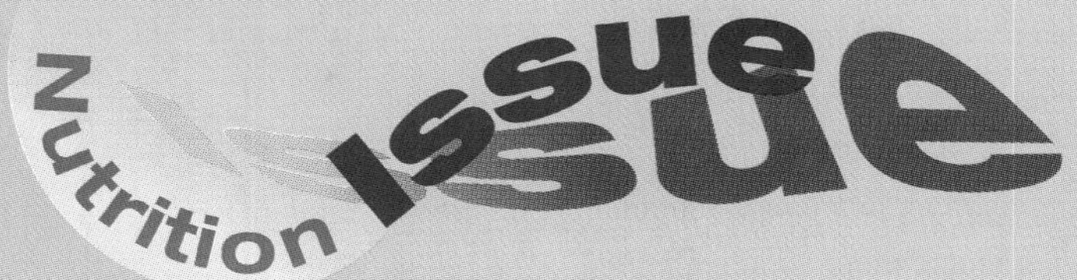

Heart Disease

A heart attack can strike with the sudden force of a sledgehammer, with pain radiating up the neck or down the arm. It can also sneak up at night, masquerading as indigestion, with slight pain or pressure in the chest. Typical warning signs are:

If a person senses a heart attack is beginning, one should chew an aspirin (325 milligrams). Chewing the medicine allows it to act more quickly than simply swallowing it. This aspirin use decreases blood clotting, and especially formation of large clots, in turn greatly decreasing the chance of related death. For the same reason, low dose aspirin therapy (80 to 160 milligrams per day) is commonly prescribed for people with evidence of heart disease or who otherwise are at high risk of a heart attack.

- Intense, prolonged chest pain or pressure, sometimes radiating to other parts of the upper body (men and women)
- Shortness of breath (men and women)
- Sweating (men and women)
- Nausea and vomiting (especially women)
- Dizziness (especially women)
- Weakness (men and women)
- Jaw, neck, and shoulder pain (especially women)

Heart disease—more precisely termed coronary heart disease or **cardiovascular disease**—is the major killer of Americans. Each year about 500,000 people die of heart disease in the United States, about 60% more than die of cancer. The figure rises to almost 1 million if strokes and other circulatory diseases are included in the more global term cardiovascular disease. About 1.5 million people each year have a heart attack. The overall male-to-female ratio for heart disease is about 2:1. Women generally lag about 10 years behind men in developing the disease. Still, heart disease eventually kills more women than any other disease—twice as many as cancer. Women also fare worse than men after a heart attack, partly because these come later in life.

Cardiovascular disease
Disease of the heart and blood vessels.

DEVELOPMENT OF HEART DISEASE

The symptoms of heart disease develop over many years and generally do not become obvious until old age. Nonetheless, autopsies of young adults under 20 years of age have shown that many of them have atherosclerotic plaque in their arteries. This finding indicates that plaque buildup can begin in childhood and continue throughout life, although it usually goes undetected for quite some time.

Preventing premature heart disease—that which appears before age 60 years—deserves everyone's consideration. Although we all die, one key to a better life is to prevent premature death and live in good health until essentially the entire body wears out, the heart included. Heart attacks at ages 40 through 60 are closely linked to the risk factors discussed later. Most people at risk can greatly improve their chance to avoid premature heart disease by making some long-term lifestyle changes.

Heart disease and strokes are associated with inadequate blood circulation in the heart and brain. Blood supplies the heart muscle and brain—and other body organs—with oxygen and nutrients. When blood flow via the coronary arteries surrounding the heart is interrupted, the heart muscle can be damaged. A heart attack, or **myocardial infarction,** may result (Figure 5-12). This may cause the heart to beat irregularly or to stop altogether. About 25% of people do not survive their first heart attack. If blood flow to parts of the brain is interrupted long enough, part of the brain dies, causing a stroke. When a stroke causes loss of muscle control, death may occur.

Myocardial infarction
Death of part of the heart muscle.

Almost all heart attacks are caused by blood clots that stop blood flow to the heart or brain. Clots form more readily where atherosclerotic plaque has built up in the arteries that serve the heart (coronary arteries) or brain (carotid arteries). Actually, the most dangerous lesions aren't the large, advanced ones, but smaller, unstable lesions

Heart disease involves the coronary arteries and thus is frequently termed coronary heart disease (CHD) or coronary artery disease (CAD).

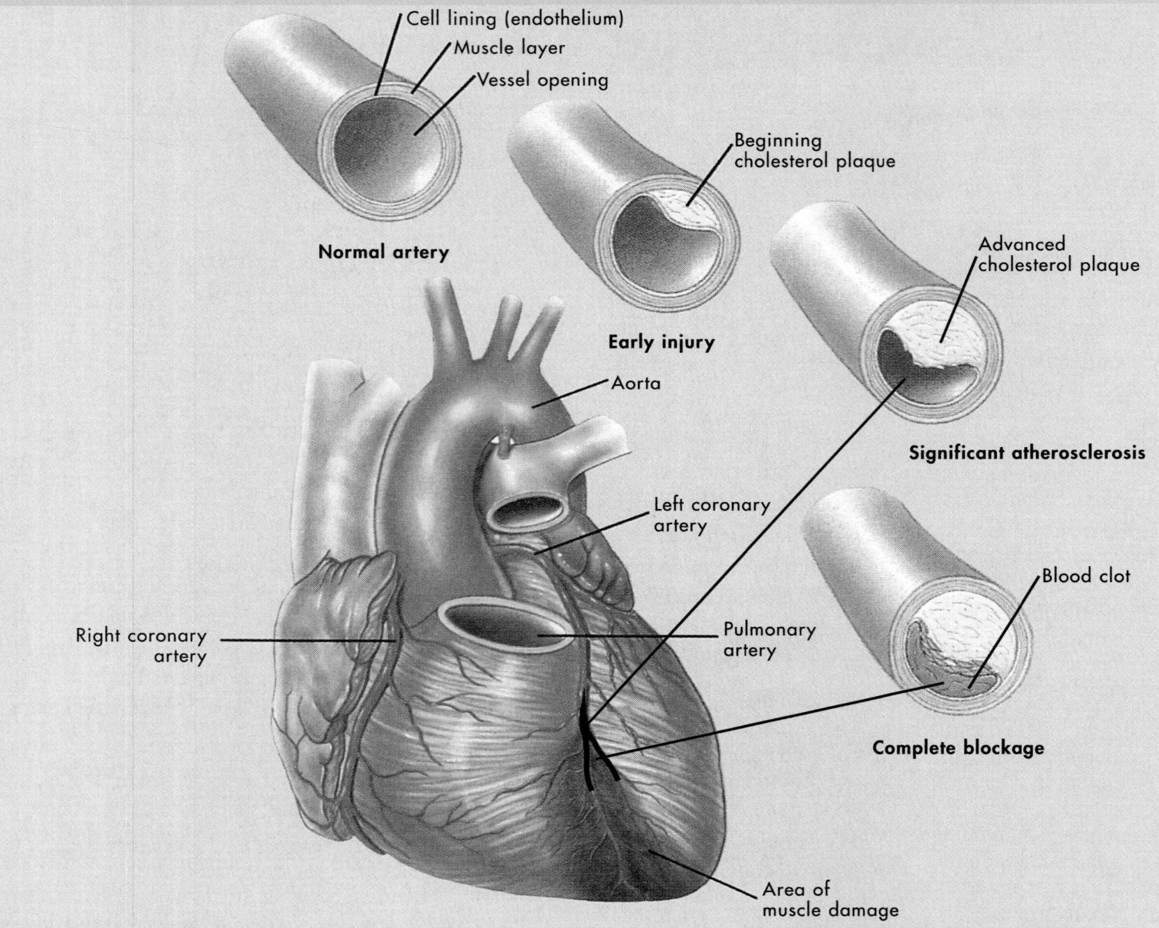

Figure 5-12 *The road to a heart attack. Injury to an artery wall begins the process. This is followed by a progressive buildup of plaque in the artery walls. The heart attack represents the final phase of the process. Blockage of the left coronary artery by a blood clot is evident. The point where arteries such as these branch into small arteries is the typical site of major blockage. The heart muscle that is served by the portion of the coronary artery beyond the point of blockage lacks oxygen and nutrients; it is damaged and may die. This can lead to a significant drop in heart function and often total heart failure. Current research suggests that the smaller, early plaques cause most heart attacks as they break up and in turn stimulate blood clotting.*

covered by a small fibrous cap. In essence, heart attacks are caused not by total blockage of the coronary arteries by plaque, but by disruption of a partial blockage, leading to eventual clot formation.

As mentioned earlier in this chapter, plaque is probably first deposited to repair injuries in a vessel lining. The *athero* in "atherosclerosis" comes from the Greek and means "gruel or paste." This process of damage repair is part of the initial phase of atherosclerosis. The rate of further plaque deposition in the next phase, called the progression phase, partly depends on the amount of LDL in the blood. The plaque thickens as layers of cholesterol (part of LDL), protein, smooth muscle, and calcium are deposited. Arteries harden and narrow as plaque builds up, making them less elastic. They are thus unable to expand to accommodate alterations in blood pressure.

Affected arteries become further damaged as blood pumps through them and pressure increases. Then, in the final phase, a clot or spasm in a plaque-laden artery leads to a myocardial infarction.

Factors that typically bring on a heart attack in a person at risk include dehydration, acute emotional stress (such as firing an employee), strenuous physical activity when not otherwise physically fit (shoveling snow and deer hunting in the fall, for example), waking during the night or the process of getting up in the morning (linked to an abrupt increase in stress), and consuming high-fat meals (increases blood clotting).

RISK FACTORS FOR HEART DISEASE

Many of us are free of the risk factors that contribute to rapid development of atherosclerosis and premature heart disease. If so, the advice of health experts is to simply consume a balanced diet, perform regular physical activity, and reevaluate risk factors every 5 years.

When 28-year-old gold medallist Sergei Grinkov died suddenly of a heart attack while ice skating, researchers investigated the case and discovered a protein abnormality in his blood. This abnormal protein caused Grinkov's blood to clot easier than normal. Grinkov was otherwise healthy. The only heart disease risk factor he had was that his father died of heart disease at the age of 52. It is thought that up to 25% of Americans may have this same protein abnormality, and that the only sign is a family history of heart-related death under age 60. For this reason, it is wise for all adult Americans to have a careful evaluation of heart disease risks conducted by a physician.

People who face the highest risk for premature heart disease have one or another rare genetic defect that substantially blocks clearance of chylomicrons and triglycerides from the blood, greatly reduces LDL uptake by the liver, limits synthesis of HDL, or enhances blood clotting. Other medical conditions, such as certain forms of liver and kidney disease and use of certain medications, can increase LDL and thus increase the risk for heart disease.

For most people, however, the most likely risk factors for premature heart disease are:

- Total cholesterol over 200 milligrams per 100 milliliters of blood (mg/dl, as dl is short for 100 milliliters), especially when it is at or over 240 mg/dl and coupled with LDL over 130 to 160 mg/dl
- HDL under 35 mg/dl, especially when the ratio of total cholesterol to HDL is greater than 4:1
- Age: men over 45 years; women over 55 years who are not receiving estrogen replacement therapy
- Family history of premature heart disease
- Smoking. Note that this generally negates the female advantage of later presentation of the disease, and is the main cause of about 20% of heart disease deaths. A combination of smoking and oral contraceptive use worsens matters even more.
- High blood pressure
- Diabetes. This disease also negates the female advantage.

Elevated triglyceride in the blood is also thought to be a risk factor for heart disease. The typcial cutoff is currently below 150 to 200 mg/dl, but some studies have shown that values over 100 mg/dl can increase the risk of heart attack.

In addition, elevated triglycerides (over 200 mg/dl) are often accompanied by other lipoprotein abnormalities. Thus, experts recommend that such people should be screened carefully to find other possible risk factors.

Lack of physical activity and obesity (especially fat accumulation around the waist) are also significant risk factors for premature heart disease. Typical weight gain in adults is a chief contributor to increased LDL seen with aging. Regular exercise helps prevent this, and also improves insulin action. The corresponding reduction in insulin output leads to a reduction in lipoprotein synthesis in the liver. Researchers are currently trying to unravel and quantify numerous other factors that may be linked to premature heart disease, such as loneliness and stress, and the connection between inadequate intake of vitamin B-6, folate, and vitamin B-12 and increased homocysteine in the blood. Homocysteine damages the cells lining the blood vessels, in turn promoting atherosclerosis. Elevated homocysteine may one day be included as a known risk factor for heart disease, but until then, it is wise to meet fruit and vegetable intake recommendations of the Food Guide Pyramid, particularly those rich in the vitamin folate or find a supplemental source (see Chapter 7).

The term "risk factor" is not intended to mean causality, nevertheless, the more of these risk factors one has, the greater the chances of ultimately developing heart disease. An example of this is the pattern of symptoms called Syndrome X. These people have high blood triglycerides and low HDL, high blood pressure, and excessive insulin output. This combination greatly increases heart disease risk, more so than each individual risk factor. In addition premature heart disease is rare in populations who have low LDL, normal blood pressure, and do not smoke.

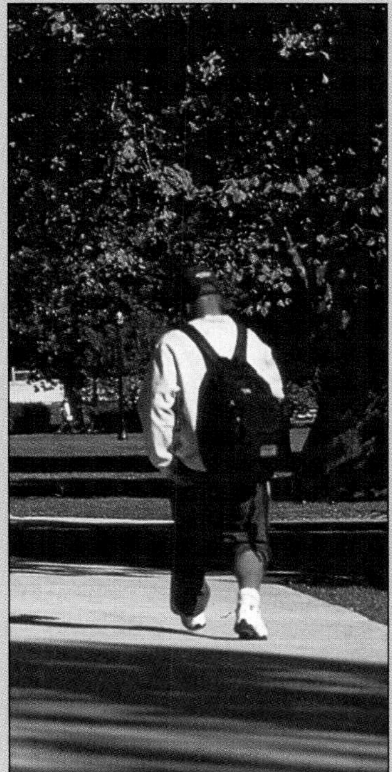

Regular physical activity contributes to heart health.

Minimizing risk factors as possible, along with following a varied diet and staying physically active, constitutes a total lifestyle plan. In addition, heart disease expert Dr. Richard Havel recommends that if a person has a history of premature heart disease in the family, but the usual risk factors aren't typically present, some rarer defect might be the cause. In this case he advises having a detailed physical examination for other rarer causes of heart disease.

Smoking

Substances in smoke alter blood vessels, enabling plaque to build up faster. Smoking greatly contributes to the ultimate expression of a person's genetically linked risk for heart disease. Smoking also makes blood more likely to clot.

Systolic blood pressure
The pressure in the bloodstream associated with pumping blood from the heart.

Diastolic blood pressure
The pressure in the bloodstream when the heart is between beats.

High Blood Pressure

If **systolic blood pressure** is over 140 (milliliters of mercury) or your **diastolic blood pressure** is 90 or more, high blood pressure is the diagnosis. (Treatment is reviewed in Chapter 8.)

High HDL

Total cholesterol greater than 200 mg/dl is widely touted in the popular press as the key value for predicting heart disease risk. In fact, much more important are LDL (over 130 to 160 mg/dl), HDL (under 35 mg/dl), and the ratio of total cholesterol to HDL (above 4:1). As explained in the chapter, LDL is the main contributor to plaque formation, whereas HDL helps dispose of cholesterol and may decrease oxidation of LDL as well.

If total cholesterol is greater than 200 mg/dl but HDL is high (especially above 60 mg/dl), the risk of heart disease is not increased and may even be lower than average. Thus in assessing heart disease risk, both total cholesterol and HDL must be considered, along with family history and other contributing factors. It is not uncommon for premenopausal women to have a relatively high total cholesterol because of high HDL. Unfortunately, men with elevated total cholesterol usually also have elevated LDL, and the ratio of total cholesterol to HDL is above 4:1.

All people over age 20 should have their total cholesterol and HDL measured. Children over 2 years of age with a family history of heart disease deserve similar scrutiny. Heart disease experts also recommend having blood triglycerides measured, as this is likely a risk factor in and of itself.

LOWERING LDL BY DIET CHANGES

If you discover that your LDL is high, the first step is to consult a physician. Some diseases (for example, a form of kidney disease) raise LDL, and treating the disease may remedy the LDL problem as well. If no such disease is present, diet change is advised. In fact, diet and related lifestyle modification is the primary therapy for those at increased risk for heart disease.

Nutrition experts recommend several approaches for lowering LDL. Because changes that work for one person may be ineffective for another, LDL and HDL values should be rechecked a month or so after any of the changes discussed here are implemented.

Reducing Dietary Saturated Fat and Cholesterol Intake

Reducing saturated-fat intake can lower elevated LDL. Although high cholesterol in the blood indicates that an individual is at risk for heart disease, the most potent dietary factor associated with high LDL is overconsumption of saturated fat, not of cholesterol.

Almost everyone who minimizes saturated-fat intake can lower elevated LDL by about 15% to 20%, especially if the person has been eating lots of foods that are high in saturated fats. About 10% of the population has trouble decreasing LDL by dietary means. Genetic defects are one reason. On the other hand, about 10% can expect an even bigger drop in LDL.

About 30% of the population who eat a diet low in saturated fat finds that reducing dietary cholesterol lowers LDL even more. Some people can eat six eggs a day for a month without having fasting LDL values increase, most likely because of a genetic propensity of the liver to compensate by making less cholesterol. Still, most authorities encourage limiting cholesterol intake to less than 200 to 300 milligrams per day, partly to minimize the cholesterol content of the chylomicrons that arise right after eating. Deposition of cholesterol from circulating chylomicrons probably contributes to atherosclerosis. In addition, as noted in this chapter, the tendency for palmitic acid—one of the main saturated fatty acids in our diets—to raise LDL is especially prominent when dietary cholesterol intake exceeds 200 to 300 milligrams per day and total cholesterol is elevated.

High intakes of saturated fat affect the liver's ability to clear LDL from the bloodstream, in turn leading to increased LDL. It appears that saturated fatty acids promote an increase in the amount of free cholesterol (not attached to fatty acids) in the liver, while unsaturated fatty acids do the opposite. As free cholesterol in the liver increases, it causes the liver to reduce cholesterol uptake from the bloodstream, contributing to elevated LDL.

The contribution of dietary saturated fat to elevated LDL can be minimized by eating no more than 7% to 10% of total energy as saturated fats. Finding substitutes for foods rich in animal fat, such as butter, as well as shortening and hydrogenated (solid) fats is a must. Only animal and fish products contain cholesterol (see Table 5–1). Although egg whites contain no cholesterol, a single egg yolk contains about 210 mg of cholesterol. Thus to meet the general recommendation for cholesterol intake, intake of egg yolks must be limited to four per week. A reduction to 200 would essentially mean not consuming egg yolks as such except occasionally. Many egg-containing foods (for example, pancakes, French toast, cookies, and cakes) can be prepared using egg whites rather than whole eggs. Cholesterol-free egg substitutes are also available in the grocery store. Most of these are egg whites colored yellow, to which a small amount of fat has been added to improve the flavor. Trimming the fat before and after cooking a 3- to 4-ounce serving of chicken, beef, or pork leaves roughly one-third to one-half the cholesterol content of an egg. A 10-ounce portion of meat contains about 260 milligrams of cholesterol, slightly more than the amount of one egg. If meats have a reputation for being high in cholesterol, it is mainly because of an overly generous portion size.

Increasing Monounsaturated and Polyunsaturated Fats in the Diet

Until recently, polyunsaturated fatty acids, but not monounsaturated fatty acids, were recommended as a substitute for saturated fatty acids in the diet to lower LDL. However, recent studies show that both monounsaturated and polyunsaturated fatty acids have this effect. In fact, monounsaturated fatty acids may be more beneficial, since LDLs containing these fatty acids are less likely to be oxidized. Recall that oxidized LDL probably contributes more to plaque formation in the arteries than does LDL itself. The key here is to replace saturated fat with monounsaturated fat, not simply to add it to the diet. This may also be beneficial for both blood triglycerides and HDL, because diets that are very low in fat and very high in carbohydrate can raise triglycerides and decrease HDL in some people. However, many people eventually adapt to a very low-fat diet, and in turn this effect is not that great.

Most fruits and vegetables are low in fat; however, avocados are an exception. Most of this fat is monounsaturated.

Increasing intake of monounsaturated fat would be difficult for the typical American. Foods and meals rich in monounsaturated fats are not widely available in the United States, nor are they a big part of our cuisine. If you do much of your own cooking, using canola oil, olive oil, or canola oil blended with other vegetable oils on a regular basis will increase your intake of monounsaturated fats. A further emphasis on monounsaturated fat would probably require the counsel of a registered dietitian to design a specific weekly meal pattern.

Increasing Dietary Fiber

Another dietary means of reducing LDL is increasing intake of soluble fibers, as discussed in Chapter 4. Although large amounts of fiber must be eaten to have a significant effect on LDL, any amount helps—and has other health benefits. Diets with an overall fiber content of 25 to 50 grams per day, especially those that emphasize soluble fiber, such as in oatmeal, are most effective in lowering LDL. Most people would have to change their diets extensively to achieve high intakes of soluble fiber. Instead, the focus could simply be on high-fiber foods—fruits, vegetables, dry beans, and whole grains. Moreover, dietary fiber intake above 35 grams per day may cause binding of dietary minerals and other potentially deleterious side effects. Consultation with a physician is recommended before beginning a very high-fiber diet.

LOWERING BLOOD TRIGLYCERIDES

Blood triglycerides are the most diet-responsive blood lipid. Not overeating, watching alcohol and simple-sugar intake, spreading meals throughout the day (not just one or two), and including some fish in the diet all help. Controlling diabetes if present also is important, as is losing excess weight and performing regular physical activity.

RAISING HDL: A MORE DIFFICULT TASK

Physical activity is one way to raise HDL. Exercising for at least 45 minutes four times a week can raise HDL by about 5 mg/dl. It also contributes to lowering LDL when a typical heart-healthy diet is instituted. Losing excess weight (especially around the waist) and avoiding smoking also help to raise HDL. Estrogen replacement in postmenopausal women also is effective.

In addition, eating regularly (three or more balanced meals daily), watching the amount of energy eaten with that expended, and eating less total fat often raise HDL because these practices lower blood triglycerides. This in turn, as just reviewed, is associated with higher HDL. Certain medications also act to lower blood triglycerides, thereby indirectly increasing HDL.

Consumption of alcohol is also associated with higher HDL and reduced blood clotting—two factors that reduce the risk of heart attack. However, excessive consumption of alcohol has many negative effects. The Dietary Guidelines indicate that most people can consume 1 (women) to 2 (men) drinks daily (no more) without negative health consequences. But for people at risk for alcoholism, any alcohol may be too much (see discussion in Chapter 14).

MEDICAL INTERVENTION

Some people need even more aggressive therapy added to their regimen of a diet and lifestyle overhaul. The clearest indication for this more aggressive approach is in people who already have had a heart attack or have heart disease symptoms.

Medications are the cornerstone of this more aggressive therapy. Currently, medications work to lower LDL in one of two ways. Some reduce cholesterol synthesis in the liver. The cost of being on one of these drugs ranges from $300 to $1000 per year, depending on the dose needed. The other group of medications binds bile acids in the small intestine and leads to their elimination in the feces. This requires the liver to synthesize new bile acids. The liver removes LDL from the blood to do this. These medications taste gritty and therefore are not very popular. Use of one or both of these classes of medications should ideally drive LDL down to about 100 mg/dl—the current therapeutic goal for people with heart disease.

A third group of drugs can be used to lower triglyceride production by the liver, and so lower blood triglycerides. An added benefit of this triglyceride lowering is an accompanying increase in HDL. Use can result in pesky side effects, but these are typically manageable. All these medications work better when coupled with a heart-healthy diet and lifestyle.

For postmenopausal women, estrogen replacement also deserves consideration, in part because this lowers LDL and raises HDL. As noted in Chapter 8, estrogen replacement therapy does pose some risks, but for women at risk for heart disease and osteoporosis, the benefits can outweigh concerns. Experts recommend that such women discuss the appropriateness of estrogen therapy with their physician.

Overall, death from heart disease is reduced when treatment to lower elevated LDL in people at high risk for heart disease or who have had a heart attack is followed for a few years or more. Furthermore, new research shows that plaque even regresses with aggressive use of medications. A total vegetarian (vegan) diet also has been shown to have the same effect, when combined with exercise, stress reduction, and group interactive therapy (i.e. the Dr. Dean Ornish Diet plan; the Nutrition Issue in Chapter 6 discusses vegan diets). It is suspected that aggressive therapies to lower LDL stabilize the development of atherosclerotic plaque, thereby lowering the risk of rupture and in turn reducing the chance of a heart attack caused by clot formation.

In summary, individuals with elevated LDL, in consultation with their physicians, are best suited to determine their desire and ability to make lifestyle changes, supplemented by medications (if necessary) to lower heart disease risk. Some physicians also recommend caution about initiating aggressive LDL-lowering treatment in persons over 65 to 70 years of age because of concern about the safety and cost-effectiveness of such interventions in older people (see Chapter 14).

For more information on heart disease, see the web site of the American Heart Association at http://www.amhrt.org or the heart disease section of Healthfinder at http://www.healthfinder.gov/tours/heart.htm. This is a site created by the U.S. government for consumers. In addition, visit the web site http://www.nhlbi.nih.gov/chd.

GENERAL STRATEGY FOR REDUCING HEART DISEASE RISK

Table 5–5 outlines a general strategy for lowering LDL. The bottom line for diet changes is actually quite simple: Remove as much saturated fat from the diet as possible while moderating total fat, *trans* fat, and cholesterol intake. To do this, select foods that are lower in total fat and especially in saturated fat. That means eating fewer high-fat foods of animal origin, such as marbled meat, eggs, and whole-milk dairy products, while eating more plant foods, such as fruits, vegetables, some nuts, and whole grains. Minimizing fried foods and hydrogenated fats helps as well.

TABLE 5-5

General Diet-Related Strategy for Reducing the Risk of Heart Disease and Heart Attack, Especially for People at Risk

Action	Rationale
Follow the Food Guide Pyramid, consuming less total fat, especially saturated fat and *trans* fat, and less cholesterol. Some researchers advocate a switch to a primarily vegetarian diet to help meet this goal (see Chapter 6).	In particular, the bottom half of the pyramid supplies vitamins associated with reduced risk of heart disease. The key focus is on reducing intake of animal fat and hydrogenated (*trans*) fat (especially deep fat-fried foods) as choices from the top half are made. Use of a balanced vitamin and mineral supplement to complement a healthy diet such as this is appropriate. Use of megadose Vitamin E therapy is also recommended by some experts, but one should be under physician scrutiny (see Chapter 7).
Meet calcium needs (AI).	One study has shown that this approach can lower LDL, probably by binding saturated fatty acids in the GI tract and so reducing their absorption.
Eat plenty of fruits, vegetables, and whole grains. Include some nuts, soy, and garlic on a regular basis.	The dietary fiber, antioxidants, and other phytochemical substances present in these foods can contribute to lower risk of heart disease.
Eat regularly spaced meals, not one or two large ones.	The frequency of meals affects blood triglycerides. Studies show that increasing meal frequency (from three to nine meals per day or so) can even help reduce LDL and reduce blood glucose swings. This effect on blood glucose is beneficial for the body in many ways, including heart health.
Minimize fat-rich meals, especially those high in saturated fat.	These meals cause the blood to clot more than is regularly seen.
Lose weight if needed, ideally to attain a healthy body weight (see Chapter 9).	This especially helps reduce blood triglycerides (if elevated), lowers blood pressure, and can increase HDL, especially if the fat is lost from the abdominal region.
Eat fish about twice a week. If this is not agreeable, consider fish oil capsules (2 to 3 grams per day).	This provides omega-3 fatty acids to reduce blood clotting and thus lessens the risk of heart attack. Regular use of aspirin for people at high risk of a heart attack (under a physician's scrutiny) is promoted for the same reason.
Consume moderate amounts of alcohol with meals if you can control this practice, your physician gives approval, and you are of legal age.	Consumption of red wine in particular has been noted to reduce heart disease risk in some studies, but it is speculated that small doses of any form of alcohol may do the same. A reduction in blood clotting is one mechanism.
Avoid unfiltered coffee intake.	Unfiltered coffee (Espresso and French press types) increases LDL. Moderate use of filtered coffee appears to be fine for most people.
Use iron supplements with caution.	Although this point is still being debated, some experts recommend that iron-containing supplements not be consumed unless medically needed because this may increase LDL oxidation. This message is especially important for adult men. With regard to dietary iron intake, the iron found in animal products is most highly linked to the risk of heart attack, rather than the iron found in plants or added to enriched grains (see Chapter 8).

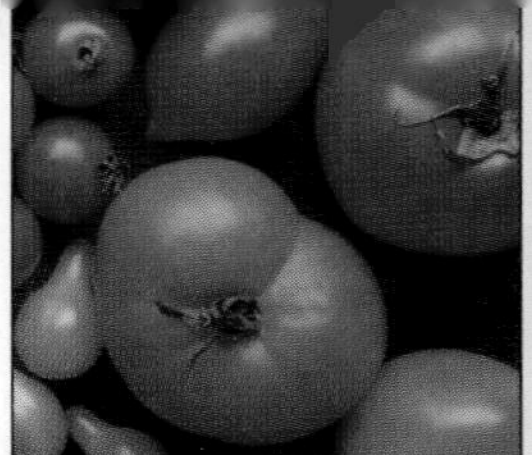

chapter 6

Proteins

Eating enough protein is vital for maintaining health. Proteins form important structures in the body, make up a key part of the blood, help regulate many body functions, and can fuel body cells.

Americans generally eat more protein than is needed to maintain health. For many of us, protein translates into meat, poultry, fish, and eggs. Turkey, hamburger, cheese, and T-bone steak are some favorite animal protein foods in America. In contrast, many other countries obtain a greater percentage of their protein from vegetables. It is only the more affluent countries that can afford to consume most of their protein from animal products. As we will explore, diets that consist primarily of vegetable proteins can be very adequate with just a small amount of planning.

Few of us wish to exchange our comfortable modern lifestyles with those of our less affluent world citizens, and yet we could benefit from eating more plant sources of proteins. It is possible—and desirable—to incorporate the most nutritious practices of both ways of life and enjoy the benefits of *both* animal and plant protein. Let's see why this is worth your attention.

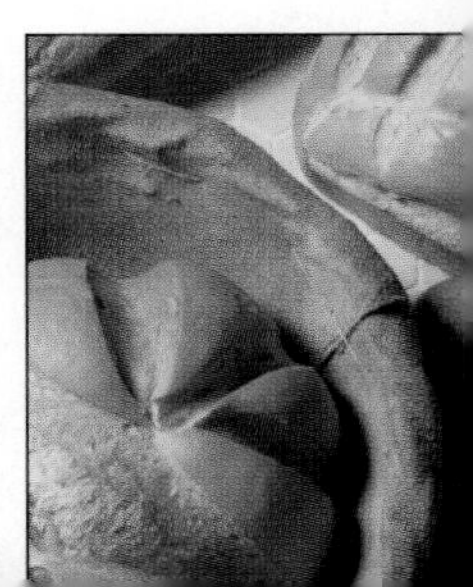

Nutrition Web

About 15% of total energy intake as protein is desirable.

Amino acids are the building blocks of proteins and contain a usable form of nitrogen for humans. There are 9 essential amino acids that must be supplied by the diet and 11 nonessential amino acids. The body can make the nonessential forms.

High-quality protein sources provide all of the essential amino acids, while lower-quality protein sources are low in one or more of the essential amino acids. Animal foods in general and soybeans provide high-quality protein sources, and plant foods in general provide lower-quality protein sources.

Many protein sources are a regular part of our diets. Animal products are the most nutrient-dense sources of protein in the diet. However, plant foods such as legumes are an excellent source of protein.

By eating a variety of plant sources, an overall high-quality protein diet can be achieved. Two plant proteins that result in a high-quality protein source when eaten together are said to be complementary with respect to the essential amino acids donated to the meal.

Proteins are part of body constituents such as blood-clotting factors, enzymes, immune factors, and more. In addition, proteins help regulate fluid balance, contribute to acid-base balance, and provide energy to the body when necessary.

The protein RDA for adults is 0.8 grams per kilogram of healthy body weight. Americans generally consume much more than the RDA for protein.

Inadequate intakes of energy and protein can result in protein-energy malnutrition. Marginal energy intake with little protein results in kwashiorkor, a disease characterized by edema with some subcutaneous fat. Starvation, with poor energy and protein intake, results in marasmus, in which little or no subcutaneous fat remains.

Protein recommendations for athletes range from 1.2 to 1.6 grams per kilogram. However, even this higher need can be met easily through the diet. It is not advised for anyone to take supplements of individual amino acids as they can compete with each other for absorption when taken in excess.

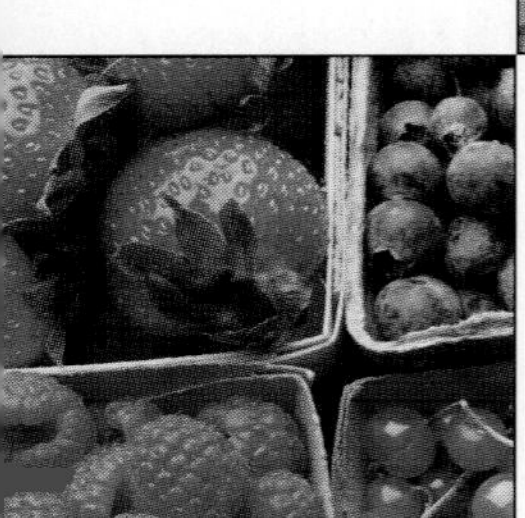

Proteins—Vital to Life

Thousands of various substances in the body are made of **proteins.** Aside from water, proteins form the major part of a lean human body, about 16% of body weight. Amino acids—the building blocks for these proteins—contain a special form of nitrogen. This form of nitrogen, essentially carbon linked to nitrogen, is generated by plants. By combining nitrogen from soil and air with carbon and other elements, plants form amino acids. They then link these amino acids together to make proteins. We ordinarily must get the nitrogen we need by consuming it in proteins. This form of nitrogen is something carbohydrates and fats can't provide us. Proteins are thus very important because they supply nitrogen in a form we can readily use—namely, amino acids. Directly using simpler forms of nitrogen is, for the most part, impossible for humans.

Proteins
Food components made of amino acids. Proteins contain the form of nitrogen used by the human body.

Proteins are crucial to the minute-by-minute regulation and maintenance of our bodies. Body functions such as blood clotting, fluid balance, hormone and enzyme production, visual processes, and cell repair require specific proteins. Your body generates proteins in many configurations and sizes so that they can serve these greatly varied functions. All these proteins use the amino acids in protein-containing foods we eat. Proteins can also supply energy for the body—on average 4 kcal per gram.

If you don't regularly eat enough protein, many of your metabolic processes slow down. This is because the body does not have enough amino acids available to build the proteins it needs. For example, the immune system no longer functions efficiently when it lacks key proteins, thereby increasing the risk of infections, disease, and eventually death. Therefore proteins deserve their name, which comes form the Greek word *protos,* meaning "to come first."

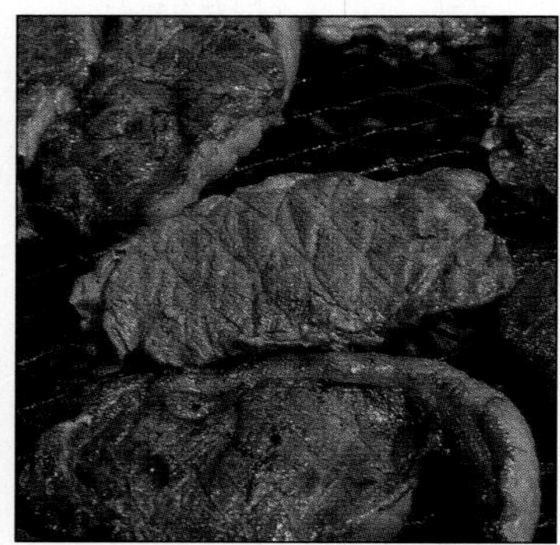

Animal protein foods are typically our favorite sources of amino acids.

Amino Acids

Amino acids—the building blocks of proteins—are formed mostly of carbon, hydrogen, oxygen, and nitrogen. Note that the key part of an amino acid is nitrogen. The diagram below shows the general form of an amino acid and what a typical amino acid looks like. The amino acids used to make protein have different chemical makeups, but all are slight variations of the glutamic acid pictured.

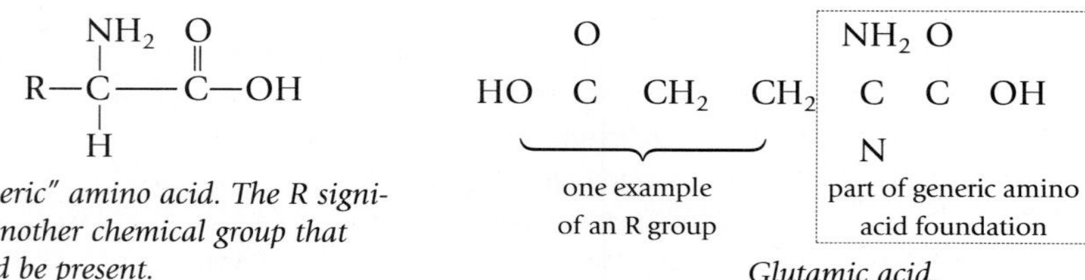

"Generic" amino acid. The R signifies another chemical group that would be present.

Glutamic acid.

Your body needs to use 20 different types of amino acids to function. Although they are all important, 11 of these amino acids are considered **nonessential** (also called ***dispensable***) with respect to our diets. Human cells can produce these certain amino acids as long as the right ingredients are present—the key factor being nitrogen that is already part of another amino acid (Table 6–1).

Nonessential amino acids
Amino acids that can be synthesized by a healthy body in sufficient amounts; there are 11 nonessential amino acids. These are also termed dispensable amino acids.

The nine amino acids the body cannot make are known as ***essential*** (also called ***indispensable***)—they must be obtained from foods. This is because body cells either cannot make the needed carbon-based foundation of the amino acid, cannot put a nitrogen group on the needed carbon-based foundation, or just cannot do the whole process fast enough to meet body needs.

Both nonessential and essential amino acids are present in foods that contain protein. If you don't eat enough essential amino acids, your body first struggles to conserve what essential amino acids it can. However, eventually your body progressively slows production of new proteins until at some point you will break protein down faster than you can make it. When that happens, as noted, health deteriorates.

TABLE 6-1

Classification of Amino Acids

Essential (indispensable) amino acids	Nonessential (dispensable) amino acids
Histidine	Alanine
Isoleucine	Arginine
Leucine	Asparagine
Lysine	Aspartic acid
Methionine	Cysteine*
Phenylalanine	(Cystine)
Threonine	Glutamic acid
Tryptophan	Glutamine
Valine	Glycine
	Proline
	Serine
	Tyrosine*

*These amino acids are also classed as semiessential. This means they must be made from essential amino acids if insufficient amounts are eaten. When that occurs, the body's supply of certain essential amino acids is depleted. Researchers now suggest that some other nonessential amino acids assume a more essential status when the body cannot readily generate them. This occurs during some illnesses. Glutamine may assume an essential status in traumatic injury, especially in the period after intestinal surgery, and arginine is essential for children born preterm.

Essential amino acids *The amino acids that cannot be synthesized by humans in sufficient amounts and therefore must be included in the diet; there are nine essential amino acids. These are also called* indispensable amino acids.

Because two cysteine molecules can bind to form a new amino acid called cystine, the number of nonessential amino acids is sometimes listed as 12. If this form of cysteine is not counted as a unique form, then there are 11 nonessential amino acids. This discussion will not count cystine, and will thus use the figure of 20 amino acids in foods—9 essential and 11 nonessential.

Putting Essential and Nonessential Amino Acids into Perspective

Eating a balanced diet can supply us with both the essential and nonessential amino acids (or building blocks needed) to maintain good health. Let's now take a more detailed look at this concept of essential amino acids, especially in relationship to nonessential amino acids.

Physiological Aspects. The disease phenylketonuria (PKU) illustrates the importance of one essential amino acid. Recall from Chapter 4 that the person with PKU has a limited ability to metabolize the essential amino acid phenylalanine. Normally the body converts much of this essential amino acid consumed in the diet into the nonessential amino acid tyrosine, because the body's need for phenylalanine is easily exceeded by our typical diets. However, in PKU, liver enzyme activity may be mildly or grossly insufficient in processing phenylalanine to the amino acid tyrosine. When the enzymes cannot synthesize enough tyrosine, both amino acids must then be derived from foods. The key point here is that both amino acids now end up to be *essential* in terms of dietary needs. In the treatment of PKU, consumption of phenylalanine must also be controlled because it can rise to toxic amounts in the body. This then hampers growth and development of the infant.

Dietary Considerations. Animal and plant proteins can differ greatly in proportions of essential and nonessential amino acids. Animal proteins contain ample amounts of all nine essential amino acids. (Gelatin—made from the animal protein collagen—is an exception because it loses one essential amino acid during processing and is also low in other essential amino acids.) With the exception of soybeans, plant proteins don't match our needs for essential amino acids as precisely as animal proteins. Many plant proteins, especially those found in grains, are low in one or more of the nine essential amino acids.

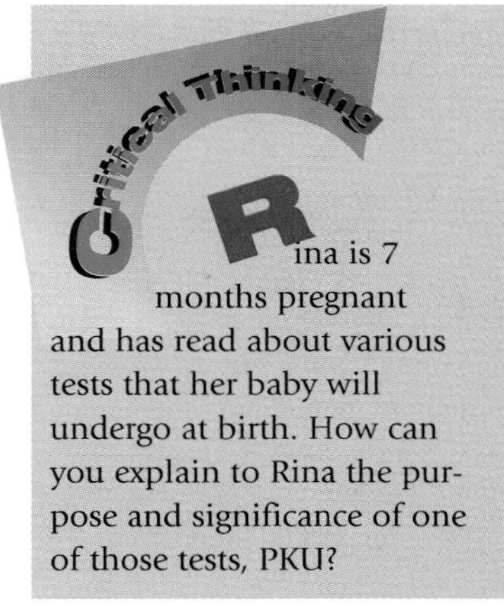

Rina is 7 months pregnant and has read about various tests that her baby will undergo at birth. How can you explain to Rina the purpose and significance of one of those tests, PKU?

High-quality (complete) proteins
Dietary proteins that contain ample amounts of all nine essential amino acids.

Lower-quality (incomplete) proteins
Dietary proteins that are low in or lack one or more essential amino acids.

Complementary proteins
Two food protein sources that make up for each other's inadequate supply of specific essential amino acids; together they yield a sufficient amount of all nine and so provide high-quality (complete) protein for the diet.

As you might expect, human tissue composition resembles animal tissue more than it does plant tissue. The similarities enable us to use proteins from single animal sources more efficiently to support human growth and maintenance than we do those from single plant sources. For this reason, animal proteins, except gelatin, are considered **high-quality** (or ***complete***) **proteins**—they contain all the amino acids we need in sufficient amounts. Individual plant sources of proteins for the most part are considered **lower-quality** (or ***incomplete***) **proteins** because their amino acid patterns can be quite different from ours. A single plant protein, such as wheat alone, cannot support needs, especially in times of growth.

Because the depletion of just one of the essential amino acids prevents protein synthesis, the process illustrates the *all or none principle:* either all essential amino acids are available or none can be used. The essential amino acid in smallest supply in a food or diet becomes the limiting factor (called the ***limiting amino acid***) because it limits the amount of protein the body can synthesize. For example, assume the letters of the alphabet represent the 20 different amino acids we eat. If A represents an essential amino acid, we would need four of these to spell the hypothetical protein ALABAMA. If the body had an L, B, and M, but only 3 As, the "synthesis" of ALABAMA would not be possible. "A" would then be seen as the limiting amino acid because it is the limiting factor with respect to the body's ability to synthesize ALABAMA.

Most of us eat large enough amounts and such an assortment of protein-rich foods that we easily get a sufficient amount of all nine essential amino acids. That is, Americans in general eat a diet in which overall protein quality is high. Even worldwide, most adults who eat sufficient protein get enough essential amino acids to yield a high-quality protein diet, even if the various protein sources in the diet are of lower quality. This is because the various lower-quality protein sources eaten can make up for deficiencies in essential amino acids that each individual protein presents.

When two or more proteins combine to compensate for deficiencies in essential amino acid content in each individual protein, the proteins are called ***complementary proteins*** (Table 6–2). Mixed diets generally provide high-quality protein because a complementary protein pattern results. In addition, these complementing proteins need not be consumed at the same meal by adults. Meeting amino acid needs over the course of a day is a reasonable goal for adults because muscles are able to create a pool of essential amino acids for later use.

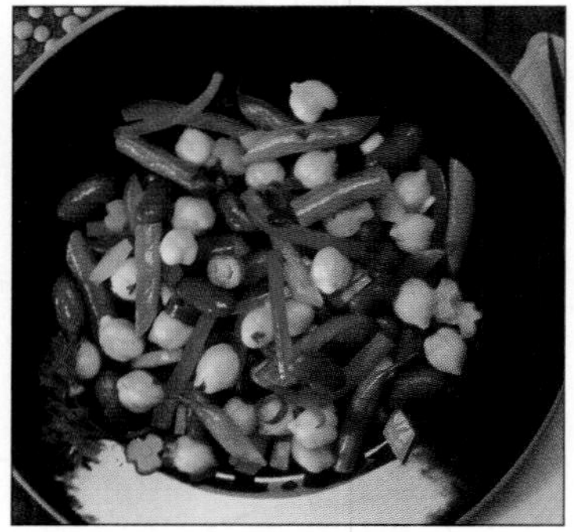

Amino acids in vegetables are best used when a combination of sources is consumed.

Infants and preschool children, on the other hand, need much of their protein supplied by essential amino acids. As noted earlier, diets for young children must be carefully planned to make sure enough proteins are present to yield high-quality protein intake. Including some animal products in the diet, such as human milk, infant formula, or cow's milk, helps ensure this. Otherwise, complementary amino acids from plant proteins should be consumed in each individual meal or within two subsequent meals. A major health risk for children occurs in famine situations in which only one type of grain is available, increasing the probability that one or more of the nine essential amino acids may be lacking in the total diet. This is discussed further in a later section in the chapter.

TABLE 6-2

Limiting Amino Acids in Plant Foods

Food	Limiting amino acids	Good plant source of the limiting amino acids*	Traditional uses where the proteins complement each other
Beans (legumes)	Methionine	Grains, nuts, and seeds	Red beans and rice
Grains	Lysine, threonine	Legumes	Rice and red beans; lentils, curry, and rice
Nuts and seeds	Lysine	Legumes	Soybeans and ground sesame seeds (miso); peanuts, rice, and black-eyed and green peas
Vegetables	Methionine	Grains, nuts, and seeds	Green beans and almonds
Corn	Tryptophan, lysine	Legumes	Corn tortillas and pinto beans

As you might suspect from the information in this table, the amino acids most likely to be low in a diet are lysine, methionine, threonine, and tryptophan. If a diet is low in an amino acid, nutrition experts recommend finding a good food source to supply it. Forget about amino acid supplements—they can lead to problems, as discussed later in this chapter.

*Animal products in the diet serve the same purpose, such as when fish is consumed with rice.

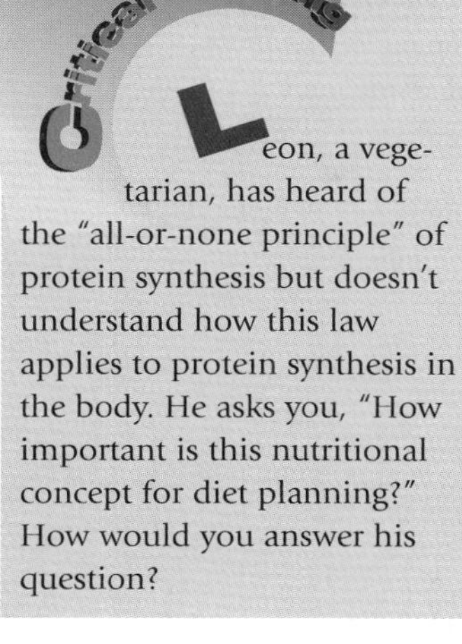

Leon, a vegetarian, has heard of the "all-or-none principle" of protein synthesis but doesn't understand how this law applies to protein synthesis in the body. He asks you, "How important is this nutritional concept for diet planning?" How would you answer his question?

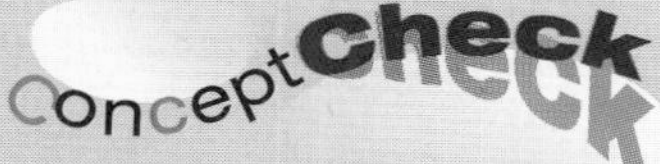

The human body uses 20 different forms of amino acids from foods. Because a healthy body can synthesize 11 or so of the different amino acids, it is not necessary to get all amino acids from foods—only the building blocks for protein synthesis of these amino acids are needed. Nine of the various amino acids used by the body must be consumed and are therefore termed *essential (indispensable) amino acids*. Foods that contain all 9 essential amino acids in about the proportions we need are considered high-quality (complete) protein foods. Those low in one or more essential amino acids are lower-quality (incomplete) protein foods. When different lower-quality protein foods are eaten together, the total intake of amino acids generally makes up for the individual foods' shortcomings to yield a high-quality protein meal.

Proteins—Amino Acids Joined Together

Peptide bond
A chemical bond formed to link amino acids in a protein.

Amino acids are joined by chemical links—technically called ***peptide bonds***—to form proteins. Although these links are difficult to break, acids, enzymes, and other agents are able to do so, as occurs, for example during digestion.

Protein Organization

By linking various combinations of the 20 types of amino acids, the body synthesizes thousands of different proteins. This process is comparable to using the alphabet to create a dictionary full of words. Amino acids are joined together in specific sequences to form distinct proteins, just as various sequences of letters form specific words. The DNA in a cell directs this ordering during protein synthesis, as noted in Chapter 3. The sequential order of the amino acids determines a protein's shape. The key point is that only correctly positioned amino acids can interact and fold properly to form the intended shape for the protein. The resulting unique three-dimensional form dictates the function of each particular protein. If it lacks the appropriate configuration, a protein cannot function (Figure 6–1).

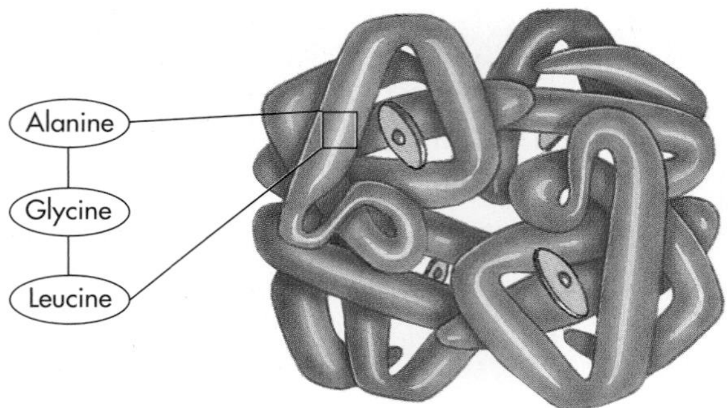

Figure 6–1 *Protein organization. Proteins often form a coiled shape, as shown by this drawing of the blood protein hemoglobin. This shape is dictated by the order of the amino acids in the protein chain. To get an idea of its size, note that each teaspoon (5 milliliters) of blood contains about 10^{18} hemoglobin molecules. Note that one billion is 10^9.*

Sickle cell disease (also called ***sickle cell anemia***) illustrates what happens when amino acids are out of order on a protein. African-Americans are especially prone to this genetic disease. It originates in defective production of the protein chains of hemoglobin, a compound found in red blood cells. In two of its four protein chains, a slight error in the amino acid order occurs. This small error produces a profound change in hemoglobin structure: it can no longer form the shape needed to carry oxygen efficiently inside the red blood cell. Instead of forming normal circular disks, the red blood cells collapse into crescent shapes. Health deteriorates, and eventually episodes of severe bone and joint pain, abdominal pain, headache, convulsions, and paralysis may occur.

These life-threatening symptoms are caused by a minute but critical error in the hemoglobin amino acid order. Why does this error happen? It results from a defect in a person's genetic blueprint, DNA, which is inherited through one's parents. A defect in the DNA can dictate that a wrong amino acid will be built into the sequence of the body proteins. Many diseases stem from incorrect DNA information passed on in the body. Cancer, which is discussed in Chapter 7, is an example.

Denature
Alteration of a protein's three-dimensional structure, usually because of treatment by heat, enzymes, acid or alkaline solutions, or agitation.

Denaturation of Proteins

Treatment with acid or alkaline substances, heat, or agitation can severely alter a protein's folded structure, leaving it unfolded and in a **denatured** state. The protein now can no longer perform its function. For example, once the bacteria in yogurt have synthesized enough acid and enzymes to precipitate some of the milk protein, the product solidifies irreversibly.

Unraveling a protein's shape often destroys its normal functioning. The characteristic is useful for some body processes, such as digestion. The secretion of stomach acid denatures some bacteria, plant hormones, many active enzymes, and other forms of proteins in foods. The heat produced during cooking likewise denatures these proteins. Both processes make foods safer to eat. Digestion is also enhanced because the unraveling increases exposure of the food to digestive enzymes. Denaturing proteins in some foods can also reduce their tendencies to cause allergic reactions.

Recall that we need proteins in the diet to supply essential amino acids—not the active proteins themselves. We dismantle the proteins we get from foods and use the amino acids to assemble proteins we need.

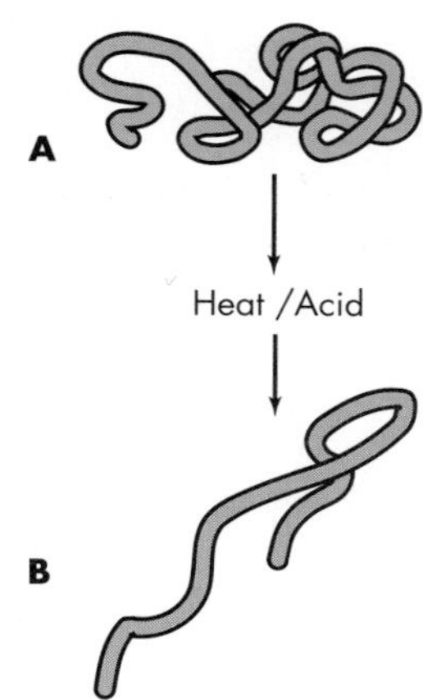

A, Protein showing typical coiled state. B, Protein is now partly uncoiled. This uncoiling can reduce protein function.

Protein in Foods

The most nutrient-dense source of protein is water-packed tuna, which has over 80% of energy as protein. Of the typical foods we eat, over 65% of our protein comes from animal sources (Figure 6–2). The top 5 contributors of protein to the U.S. diet are beef, poultry, milk, white bread and cheese. In the United States, meat, poultry, and fish consumption amounts to about 145 pounds (weight without bones) per person per year. Worldwide, 35% of protein comes from animal sources. In Africa and East Asia, about 20% of the protein eaten comes from animals.

Primarily vegetarian diets are typical among rural peoples throughout the world.

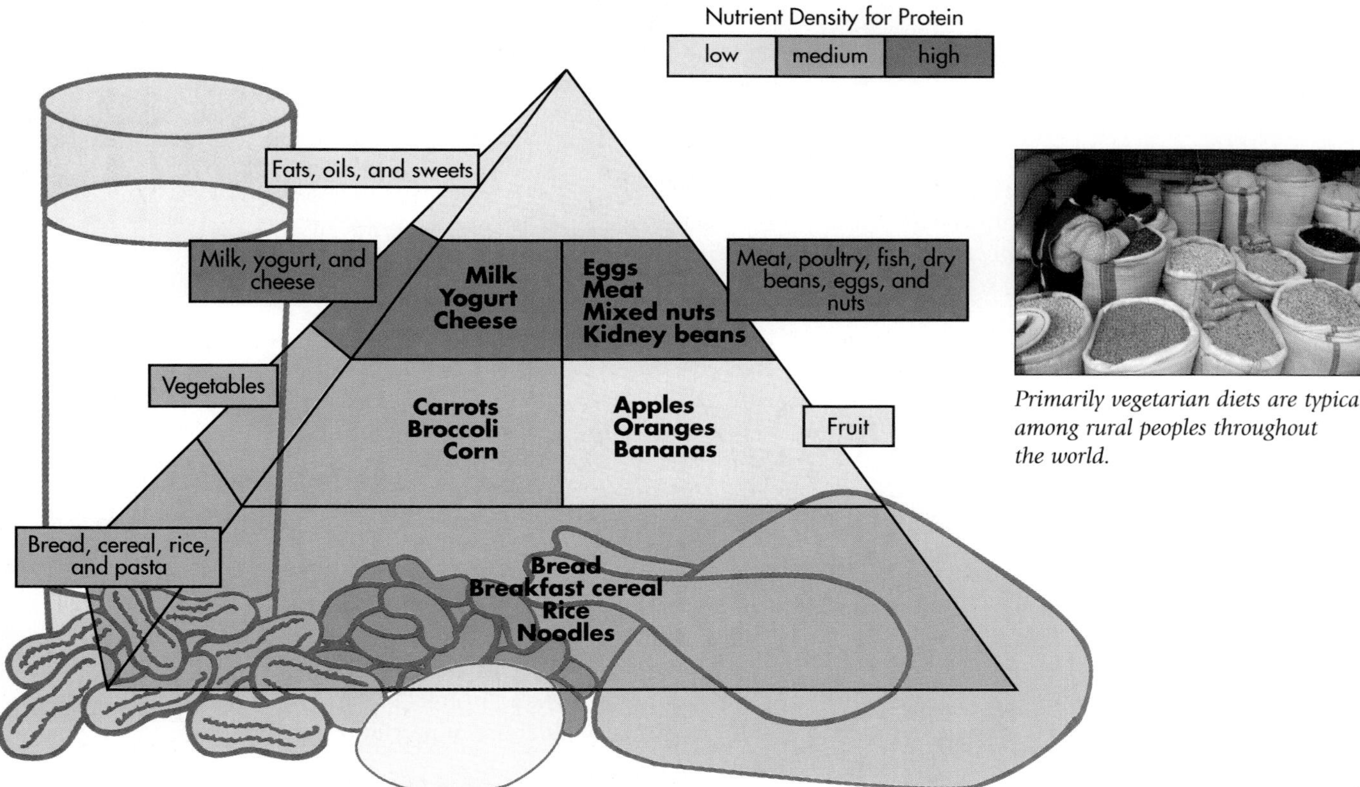

Figure 6–2 *Sources of protein in foods from the Food Guide Pyramid (FGP). The fruit group, vegetable group, and fats, oils, and sweet category generally contain little protein (about 0.1 to 3 grams per FGP serving), whereas the other groups contain moderate to high amounts (about 8 to 10 grams per FGP serving for milk products, 12 grams per FGP serving for nuts and beans, and 7 grams per ounce for meat, fish, and poultry). The background color of each group indicates the average nutrient density for protein in that group.*

Nutrition Insight

Legumes: They Deserve a Closer Look

Legumes are a plant family with pods that contain a single row of seeds: garden and black-eyed peas; green, black, red, great northern, lima, kidney, pinto, and garbanzo beans; lentils; and soybeans. Dried varieties of the mature seeds—what we know as beans—make an impressive contribution to the protein, vitamin, mineral, and dietary fiber content of a meal. Moreover, as discussed in earlier chapters, the soluble fiber in them can help lower blood cholesterol and moderate the swings in blood glucose that occur after eating. In addition, these plant proteins contain no cholesterol and little saturated fat, unless these are added during food processing, cooking, or from additions at the table.

Many people dismiss beans. This unfortunate oversight may be rooted in the Depression of the 1930s, when people could afford little else. Beans, however, are a versatile food: they can anchor or blend into soups, salads, casseroles, sandwich spreads, and cracker dips; they can be added in small quantities wherever extra body, texture, and nutritional value are desired. Because legumes tend to soak up flavors during the cooking process, it is possible to incorporate delicate flavors from combinations of herbs, spices, and broths. Incorporating legumes into your weekly menu can add variety and new flavors.

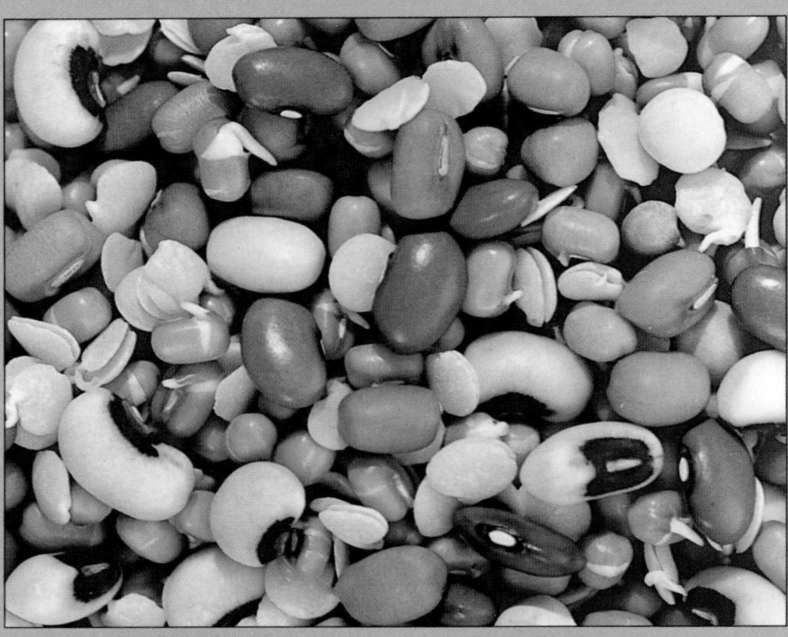

Legumes add color and many nutrients to meals.

Another Bite

Nuts are often overlooked as a source of plant protein. Recent studies have linked consumption of nuts to decreased blood cholesterol and so heart disease. The protective action of nuts probably stems from their lack of cholesterol and abundance of unsaturated fatty acids. These unsaturated fats do not raise total cholesterol like saturated fat. Of course, this benefit occurs only if nuts are used to replace saturated fats in the diet. Phytochemicals in nuts, such as flavonoids, also provide health benefits. For these reasons, a 30 gram (1 ounce) serving of nuts per day makes a nice addition to one's diet. Regular use of peanut butter is one way to put this recommendation into action.

When you initially add legumes to your diet, they may cause intestinal gas. Split peas, limas, and lentils are less likely to cause this problem than the others, so start with them. Eat small servings at first, and give your GI tract a few weeks to adjust.

You can also reduce your risk of getting intestinal gas by cooking dry beans in boiling water for 3 minutes to soften them. Then turn off the heat and let the covered beans soak for a few hours. Much of the indigestible sugars that cause the gas (recall that this happens when certain sugars in beans escape digestion in the small intestine and are broken down by the bacteria in the large intestine) will leach into the water. The water should be poured off and the beans further cooked in fresh water as desired. This practice will lead to some vitamin loss but will not affect protein or dietary fiber content. For canned beans, draining and rinsing with water is an excellent way to lower the content of gas-forming sugars.

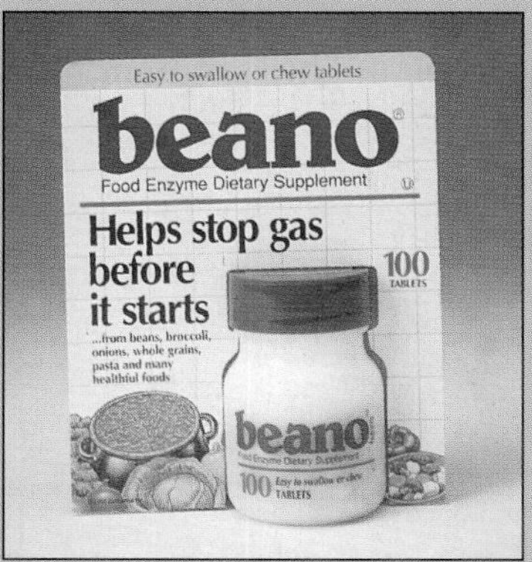

Beano® reduces intestinal gas produced by bacterial metabolism in the large intestine of the undigestible sugars in legumes. It does so by breaking down these sugars so the breakdown products (monosaccharides) can be absorbed in the small intestine.

Many people have no trouble with beans and other legumes, but it's best to be cautious. An enzyme preparation called *Beano* is also available to ease gas symptoms. Taken right before a meal in tablet or liquid form and according to directions, it helps digest the beans' undigestible carbohydrates in the small intestine and thereby lessens the intestinal gas production in the large intestine. Because Beano is made from mold, people sensitive to molds may have allergic reactions and should avoid this product or use it with care. For more information and/or free samples, contact the manufacturer at 1-800-257-8650.

Like all foods, though, legumes do not offer every nutrient and cannot serve as a complete diet by themselves. They contain no vitamin A, vitamin C, or vitamin B-12. The protein in beans is somewhat deficient in methionine, one of the essential amino acids. Serving beans with a food high in methionine, such as meat, eggs, or cheese in typical diets or rice, corn, or other grains in vegetarian diets compensates for this deficiency (see Table 6–2). Many traditional ethnic dishes combine legumes with grains and vegetables to yield a high-quality protein in the meal: lentil curry on rice, pinto beans and corn tortillas, and corn and lima beans (succotash). Try these combinations or create your own.

As you prepare foods or order them in a restaurant, look for beans—salad bars usually provide a few choices. Black bean and other bean soups, baked beans, chili, red beans and rice, and soy burgers are other possibilities.

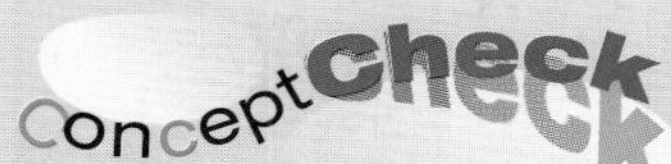

Amino acids are linked together in specific sequences to form distinct proteins. The amino acid order within a protein determines its ultimate shape. Destroying the shape of a protein denatures it. Acid and alkaline conditions present during the body's digestive processes, heat, and other factors can denature proteins, causing them to lose their biological activity.

In the United States most of our protein comes from animal sources. However, in other countries plants supply the majority of protein in the diet.

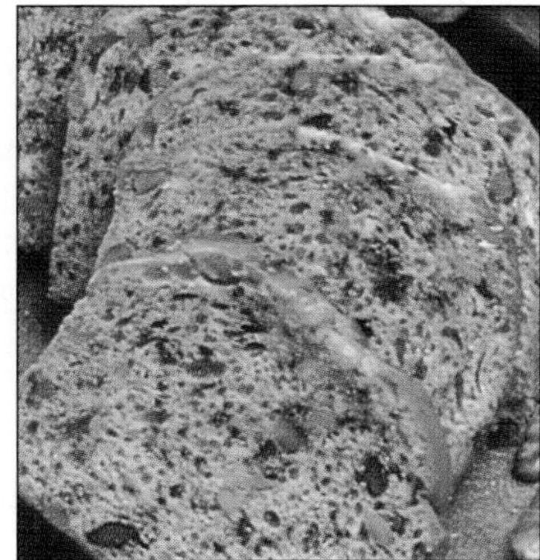

Nuts, like walnuts, can be incorporated into one's diet in numerous ways, such as adding it to banana bread.

Protein Digestion and Absorption—Supplying Amino Acids to Body Cells

As discussed in Chapter 3, digestion of protein begins in the stomach (Figure 6–3). Certain cells of the stomach secrete pepsin, a major enzyme used for this digestion. Pepsin attacks all proteins and breaks them down into shorter amino acid units, called *peptones.* Pepsin does not completely separate the protein into amino acids because it can break only a few of the chemical bonds found in protein molecules. The release of pepsin is controlled by the hormone gastrin. Just thinking about or chewing food stimulates gastrin release. Gastrin also stimulates other cells in the stomach to produce acid. This acid, in turn, activates pepsin and enhances protein digestion. The partially digested proteins now move with the rest of the nutrients from the stomach into the small intestine.

One in the small intestine the peptones (and any fats accompanying the incoming peptones produced from a meal) trigger the release of another hormone. This hormone causes the pancreas to release enzyme-rich juice into the small intestine.

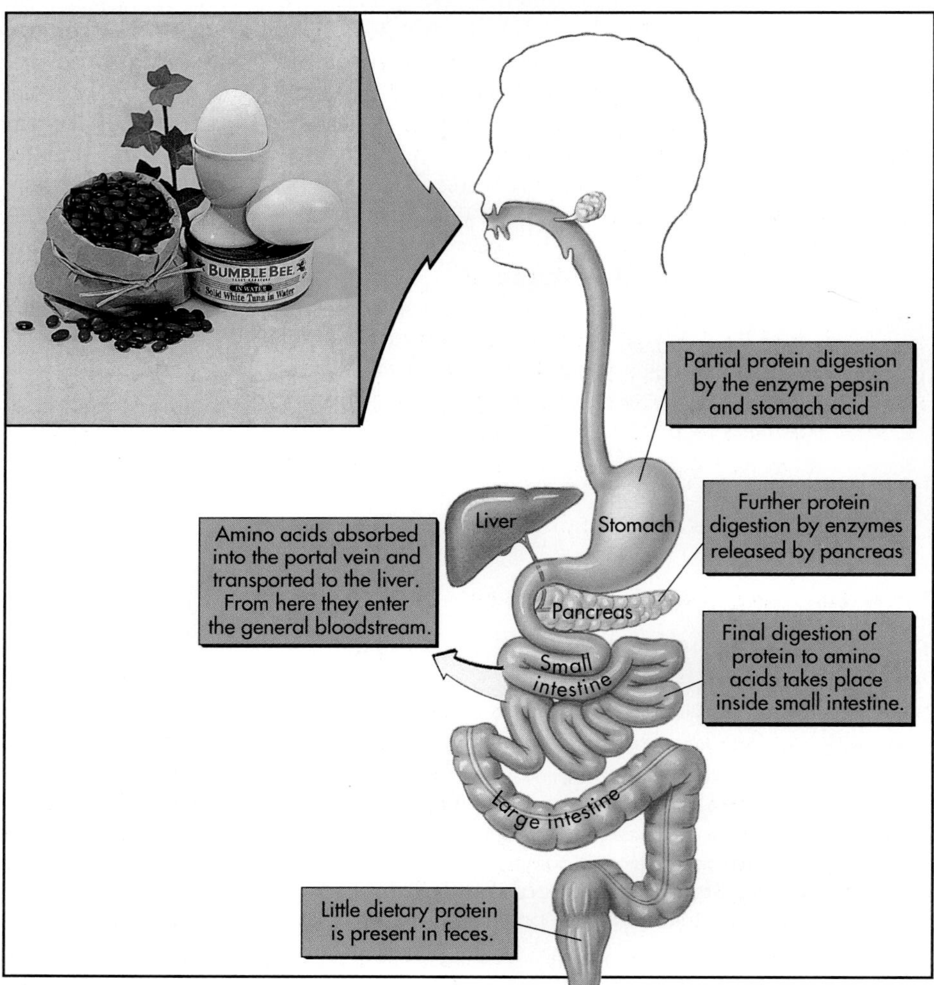

Figure 6–3 *Protein digestion and absorption. Protein digestion begins in the stomach and ends in the absorptive cells of the small intestine, where it is finally broken down into single amino acids. Stomach acid and enzymes from the stomach and pancreas also contribute to protein digestion.*

Enzymes from the digestive juice and other digestive enzymes from the small intestine divide the peptones into shorter products. The eventual digestion of these divided peptones into amino acids occurs inside the absorptive cells of the small intestine. The amino acids then travel to the liver via the portal vein, where they are either combined into protein, converted into glucose or fat, used for energy needs, or released into the bloodstream.

Putting Proteins to Work in the Body

As you have learned, proteins function in many crucial ways in human metabolism and the formation of body structures. Note, however, that only when we also eat enough carbohydrate and fat can food proteins be used most efficiently. If we don't consume enough energy to meet energy needs, some amino acids from proteins are broken down to produce needed energy, rather than being used to make needed body proteins.

Producing Vital Body Constituents

Every cell contains protein. Muscles, connective tissue, blood-clotting factors, blood-transport proteins, lipoproteins, enzymes, immune bodies, some hormones, visual pigments, and the support structure inside bones are mainly made of protein. Measurements of the amounts of certain body proteins, particularly some of those in the blood, are used as indicators of health or disease. Excess protein in the diet doesn't enhance the synthesis of body components, but eating too little can impede it.

Most vital body proteins are in a constant state of breakdown, rebuilding, and repair. The GI tract lining, for example, is constantly **sloughed** off. The digestive tract treats sloughed cells just like food particles and absorbs the amino acids released during their digestion. In fact, most protein breakdown products—amino acids—released throughout the body can be recycled and are added to the pool of amino acids available for future protein synthesis.

Slough
To shed or cast off.

However, some protein breakdown products, such as the nitrogen that ends up as **urea,** are lost rather than recycled (Figure 6–4). If a person habitually doesn't eat enough protein to replace this loss, the protein rebuilding and repairing process slows. Eventually, skeletal muscles, heart, liver, blood proteins, and other organs decrease in size or amount. Only the brain resists breakdown. To ensure good health, a person must eat enough protein.

Maintaining Fluid Balance

Blood proteins—albumins and globulins—help maintain body fluid balance. Blood pressure in the arteries forces blood through blood vessels into capillary beds. The blood fluid then enters from the capillary beds into the spaces between nearby cells to provide nutrients to those cells (Figure 6–5). Proteins in the bloodstream are too large to move out of the capillary beds into the tissues. The presence of these proteins in the capillary beds attracts the fluid back to them, partially counteracting the force of blood pressure. This is especially true of the areas of the capillary beds right next to their venous connections.

Unless enough protein is eaten, the concentration of proteins eventually decreases in the bloodstream. Excessive fluid then builds up in the tissues because the counteracting force produced by the smaller amount of blood proteins is too weak to pull much of the fluid back from the tissues into the bloodstream. As fluids pool in the tissues, the tissues swell. Clinical **edema** results. Because edema sometimes leads to serious medical problems, the cause must be identified. An important step in diagnosing the cause is to measure the concentration of blood proteins.

Edema
The buildup of excess fluid outside body cells (technically called extracellular spaces).

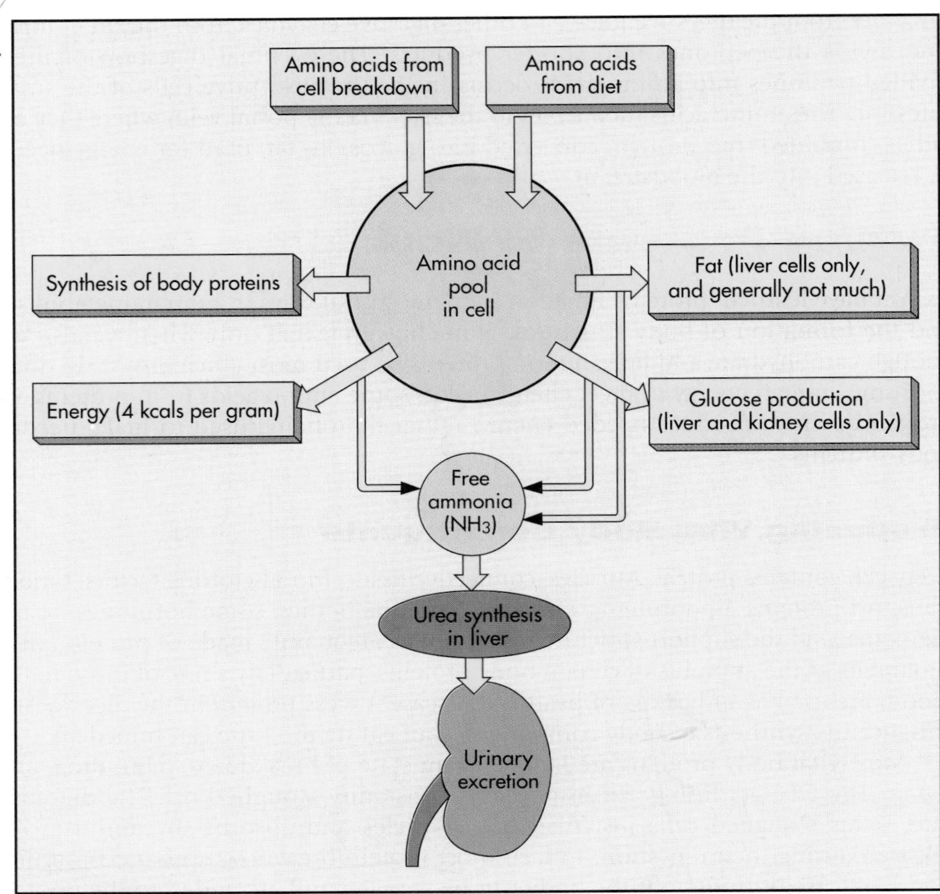

Figure 6-4 *Amino acid metabolism. The amino acid pool in a cell can be used to form body proteins, as well as a variety of other possible products—from fat and glucose to urea. The urea is a waste product made from the nitrogen-containing ammonia (NH_3) released during amino acid breakdown.*

Contributing to Acid-Base Balance

Proteins help regulate the **pH**—the acid-base balance—in the blood. Special proteins located in cell membranes act to pump chemical ions in and out of cells. The pumping action, among other factors, works to keep the blood slightly alkaline. **Buffers**—compounds that maintain acid-base conditions within a narrow range—are another means to regulate acid-base balance in the blood. Some blood proteins are especially good buffers for the body.

Buffer
A compound that helps a solution resist changes in acid-base balance. This is generally done by either having the compound take up or release hydrogens.

Forming Hormones and Enzymes

Protein is required for the synthesis of many hormones—our internal body messengers. Some hormones, such as the thyroid hormones, are made from only one or a few amino acids. Insulin, on the other hand, is composed of 48 amino acids. These and other hormones classified as proteins perform important regulatory functions in the body, such as controlling the metabolic rate (thyroid hormone) and amount of glucose taken up from the bloodstream (primarily insulin and glucagon).

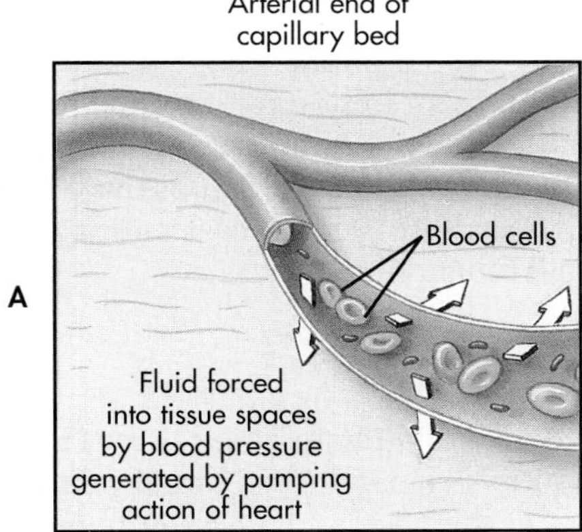

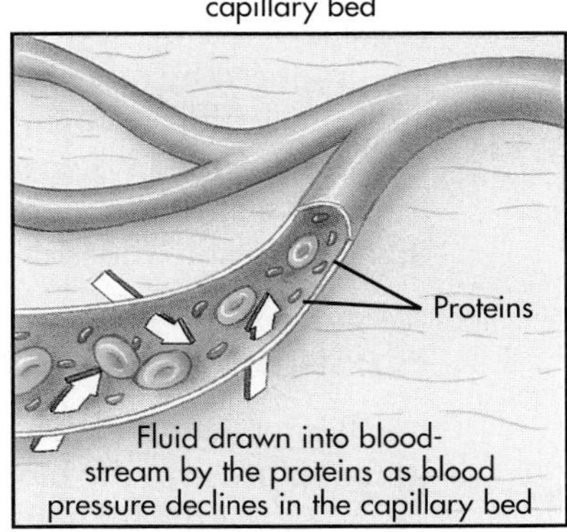

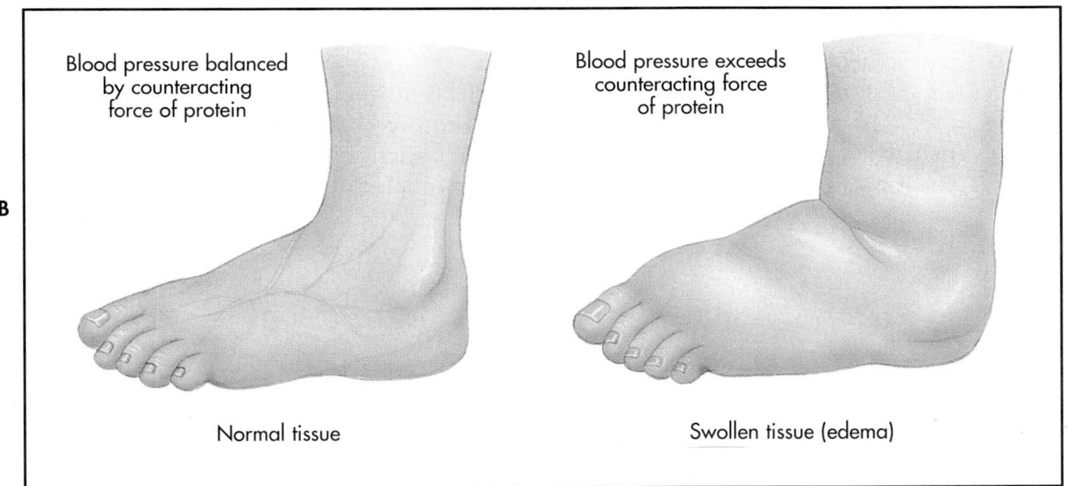

Figure 6-5 *Blood proteins in relation to protein balance. A, Blood proteins are important for maintaining the body's fluid balance. B, Without sufficient protein in the bloodstream, edema develops.*

Another Bite

Some hormone medicines from the protein class, such as the insulin used to treat some cases of diabetes, must be injected. If taken orally, insulin would be destroyed: the stomach and small intestine would digest the hormone, dismantling it into amino acids.

Almost all enzymes are proteins. Recall that enzymes are compounds that speed chemical reactions. Occasionally a cell lacks the correct genetic information to make needed enzymes. For example, an infant who has the disease **galactosemia** can't make an enzyme needed to metabolize the single sugar galactose. If the infant is not put on a galactose-free diet soon after birth—which in practical terms means no cow's milk, human milk, liver, and certain other foods—its growth and mental development will be depressed. A special infant formula must be used. The galactose-free diet is then continued, ideally throughout life. This example demonstrates the crucial roles that enzymes, and thus proteins, play in cell function.

Galactosemia
A disease characterized by the buildup of the sugar galactose in the bloodstream; the buildup occurs because the liver is unable to metabolize galactose. If present at birth and left untreated, this condition results in severe mental and growth retardation.

Antibodies
Blood proteins that inactivate foreign proteins found in the body. This helps to prevent and control infections.

Contributing to the Immune Function

Proteins make up key parts of cells used by the immune system. Protein **antibodies** are produced by one type of immune cell. In an important immune response these antibodies bind to foreign proteins in the body. Without enough protein from the diet the immune system will eventually not produce enough of the cells and other tools needed to function properly and resist disease. However, eating more protein than is necessary doesn't boost immune function.

Forming Glucose

Neurotransmitters, made by nerve endings, are often derivatives of amino acids. This is true for dopamine (synthesized from tyrosine), epinephrine (synthesized from tyrosine), and serotonin (synthesized from tryptophan). The way in which diet influences the synthesis of some of these neurotransmitters is currently under study. For example, high-carbohydrate meals can induce sleepiness as a result of increased serotonin synthesis in the brain.

In Chapter 4 you learned that the body must maintain a fairly constant concentration of glucose in the bloodstream to supply energy for red blood cells and nervous tissue. At rest the brain uses about 19% of the body's energy requirements, which is supplied by glucose. If you don't eat enough carbohydrate to supply the glucose, your liver (and kidneys to a lesser extent) will be forced to make glucose from amino acids (see Figure 6–5).

Making some glucose from amino acids is normal. For example, when you skip breakfast and haven't eaten since 7 P.M. the preceding evening, glucose must be manufactured. Taken to an extreme, however, such as occurs in starvation, the conversion of amino acids into glucose wastes much muscle tissue and consequently impairs health.

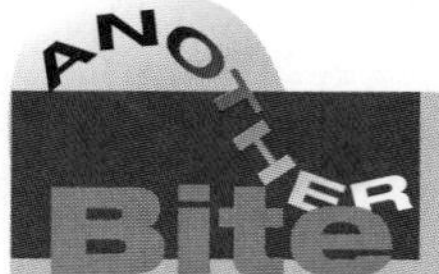

Research over the last few years suggests that soybeans have many unique properties. The protein in soy can lower blood cholesterol, even beyond the degree that would be expected from its low-fat and high dietary fiber content. To reap the benefits a person must consume about 25 grams or more of soy protein per day—10 grams is provided by ½ cup tofu, 1 to 2 cups soy milk, or 1 ounce soy flour (read the label, in any case, to be sure).

A compound in soy called genistein*—one of the many phytochemicals mentioned in Chapter 2—can reduce cancer risk, most notably breast cancer. Genistein can block cancer development and prevent tumors from creating blood vessels, thus preventing the cells from growing by depriving them of the means to obtain nourishment. The effective dose of soy products is one serving per day (1 cup soy milk, ½ cup tofu or soybeans). Researchers are investigating still other benefits. Including some soy milk, tofu, soy protein powder, tempeh or soybeans in your diet is worth considering. In the near future, food manufacturers will probably make it easier to incorporate soy protein in our diets, as they have with the recent introduction of soy nut butter to be used like peanut butter.*

Peanuts are rich in protein.

Providing Energy

Proteins generally directly supply little of the energy the body uses (see the next Nutrition Insight for information about the use of amino acids for energy during exercise). Most cells use primarily carbohydrates and fats for energy. Excess amino acids in the body generally undergo metabolism to form these products rather than being used directly as an energy source. It is only after this metabolism that we typically use most of the energy content of proteins. Proteins and carbohydrates contain the same amount of usable energy. However, proteins are a very costly source of energy, considering the amount of metabolism and processing the liver and kidneys must perform to use this energy source.

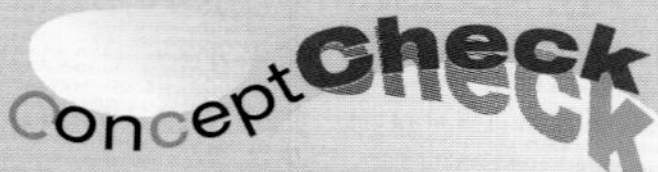

Protein digestion begins in the stomach, producing breakdown products called *peptones.* In the small intestine, peptones separate eventually into amino acids and enter the portal vein en route to the liver.

Vital body constituents—such as muscle, connective tissue, blood transport proteins, enzymes, hormones, buffers, and immune factors—are mainly proteins. Proteins can also provide fuel for the body and be used for glucose production.

The Recommended Dietary Allowance for Protein

How much protein (actually, amino acids) do we need to eat each day? People who aren't growing need to eat only enough protein to match whatever they lose daily in urine, feces, skin, hair, nails, and so on. This maintains a state of protein equilibrium (Figure 6–6).

When a body is growing or recovering from an illness, it needs a positive protein balance to supply raw materials required to build new tissues. To achieve this, a person must eat more protein daily than he or she loses. In addition, the hormones insulin, growth hormone, and testosterone all stimulate positive protein balance. Merely eating more protein does not guarantee a positive balance; building extra body tissues requires the right hormonal condition as well. Resistance exercise (weight training) also enhances positive balance.

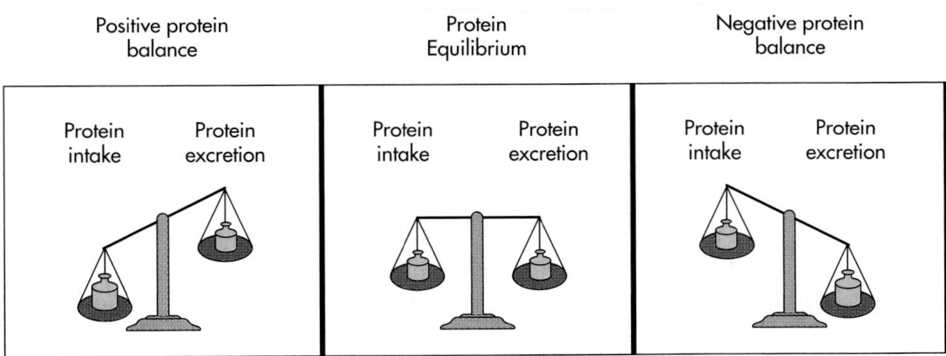

Figure 6–6 *Protein balance in practical terms.*

Situations in which protein balance is positive:

Growth
Pregnancy
Recovery stage after illness
Athletic training*
Increased secretion of hormones, such as insulin, growth hormone, and testosterone

Situations in which protein balance is negative:

Inadequate intake of protein (fasting, intestinal tract diseases)
Inadequate energy intake
Conditions such as fevers, burns, and infections
Bed rest (for several days)
Deficiency of essential amino acids
Increased protein loss (as in some forms of kidney disease)
Increased secretion of certain hormones, such as thyroid hormone and cortisol

*Only when additional lean body mass is being gained. Nevertheless, the athlete is probably already eating enough protein to support this extra protein synthesis; protein supplements are not needed.

Frequently during semistarvation or illness the body loses much more protein than is replaced. The body then falls into a negative protein balance—not enough nitrogen is being obtained from protein foods to maintain normal protein status.

For healthy people the amount of dietary protein needed to maintain nitrogen equilibrium (where intake equals output) can be determined by increasing protein intake until it just equals losses. Energy needs must be met so that amino acids are not diverted for energy use. Any protein intake above equilibrium also maintains a balance between intake and output. To estimate the requirement, we need to determine the least amount of protein intake necessary to balance intake with output.

Today the best estimate for the amount of protein required for nearly all adults is 0.8 grams of protein per kilogram (kg) of healthy body weight. This amount at least doubles during infancy. (Specific values for infants and children are discussed in Chapter 13 and the concept of healthy weight in Chapter 9.) Healthy weight is used as a baseline because excess fat storage doesn't contribute much to protein needs. This recommended amount works out to about 56 grams of protein daily for a typical 70-kilogram (154-pound) man and about 44 grams of protein daily for a typical 55-kilogram (120-pound) woman.

$$\textbf{Put weight into kilograms: } \frac{\text{154 pounds}}{\text{2.2 pounds/kg}} = \text{70 kg}$$

$$\textbf{Calculate RDA: 70 kg} \times \frac{\text{0.8 gram protein}}{\text{kg healthy body weight}} = \text{56 grams protein}$$

$$\textbf{Put weight into kilograms: } \frac{\text{120 pounds}}{\text{2.2 pounds/kg}} = \text{55 kg}$$

$$\textbf{Calculate RDA: 55 kg} \times \frac{\text{0.8 gram protein}}{\text{kg healthy body weight}} = \text{44 grams protein}$$

To estimate a recommendation for you, just substitute your body weight in kilograms in the formula listed above. Approximate protein needs are listed in the inside cover of this textbook. Using either method, it is easy to eat the amount of protein suggested each day to meet body needs (Table 6–3). American men typically consume about 95 grams of protein daily, whereas women typically consume about 65 grams daily.

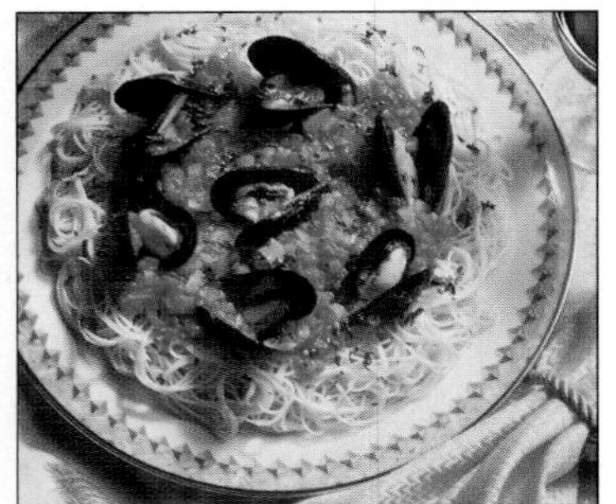

Small amounts of animal protein in a meal easily add up to meet daily protein needs.

Recall that an RDA is an allowance, not a requirement. Some people need less than that amount of protein. Most of us, however, get much more because we like many high-protein foods and can afford to buy them. Pregnancy raises protein needs by about 10 to 15 grams per day averaged over the 9 months, totaling 60 grams per day for the diet. However, mental stress, physical labor, and routine weekend sports activities do not require an increase in the protein RDA. Also, protein intakes above usual adult intakes are rarely needed, even for athletes (see the next Nutrition Insight), as our intakes are typically 1.5 to 2 times body needs.

Surveys show that only older women as a group fail to eat enough protein to meet the RDA, and the discrepancy is very slight. Older adults may also have slightly higher protein needs than those set by the RDA. Some researchers advocate up to 1.2 grams of protein per kilogram of healthy body weight. If older people eat inadequate amounts of protein, which may happen because their energy intake is so low, health can suffer.

Does Eating a Mainly High-Protein Diet Harm You?

People frequently ask whether the high protein intake of adults in America is harmful. (Getting too much protein can be very harmful to infants. This is discussed in detail in Chapter 13.) The extra vitamin B-6, iron, and zinc that accompany protein foods are often beneficial, but the extra fat—especially saturated fat—found in

TABLE 6-3

The Protein Content of a 1400-Kcal Diet and a 2400-Kcal Diet*

1200 kcal diet	Protein (grams)	2400 kcal diet	Protein (grams)
BREAKFAST			
Nonfat milk, 1 cup	8	2% milk, 1 cup	8
Cheerios, ¾ cup	3	Cheerios, ¾ cup	3
Orange	1	Eggs, soft-boiled, 2	13
		Orange	1
LUNCH			
Whole-wheat bread, 2 slices	7	Whole-wheat bread, 2 slices	7
Chicken breast, 2 oz	18	Chicken breast, 2 oz	18
Mayonnaise, 1 tsp	—	Provolone cheese, 2 oz	15
Tomato slices, 2	—	Tomato slices, 2	—
Carrot sticks, 1 cup	1	Mayonnaise, 1 tsp	—
Fig	0.5	Oatmeal-raisin cookies, 2	2
Diet soda	—	Figs, 2	1
		Diet soda	—
DINNER			
Mixed green salad, ½ cup	—	Mixed green salad, ½ cup	—
Italian dressing, 2 tsp	—	Italian dressing, 2 tsp	—
Beef tenderloin, 2 oz	17	Beef tenderloin, 4 oz	35
Spinach pasta, 1 cup with garlic butter, 1 tsp	6	Spinach pasta, 1 cup with garlic butter, 1 tsp	6
Zucchini, ½ cup, sautéed in oil, 1 tsp	0.5	Zucchini, ½ cup, sautéed in oil, 1 tsp	0.5
Nonfat milk, 1 cup	8	Carrot sticks, ½ cup	1
SNACK			
Multigrain bagel, toasted, ½	3	2% milk, 1 cup	8
Jam, 2 tsp	—	Multigrain bagel, toasted	6
		Jam, 2 tsp	—
		Fruited yogurt, 1 cup	11
TOTAL	73		133

*This table illustrates how little energy need be consumed while still meeting the RDA for protein. It also shows how much protein we eat when we consume typical energy intakes.

many high-protein animal foods is not. As a consequence, consumption of animal protein has been linked to heart disease in humans, likely due to this saturated fat content.

High-protein diets increase calcium loss in urine. Certain types of amino acids—especially some of those rich in animal proteins—cause this effect. Populations noted for high animal protein consumption tend to experience more osteoporosis, but other factors such as inadequate calcium intakes and little physical activity, excessive alcohol intakes, and smoking need to be considered (see Chapter 8 for more information on the risk factors for osteoporosis). Based on the research to date, it is reasonable to assume that individuals who have inadequate calcium intakes are further compromising bone health by consuming excessive amounts of protein. People meeting their calcium needs likely need not be concerned about this effect of dietary protein.

Excessive intake of red meat is linked to colon cancer in population studies. This link could be attributable to the protein or fat in the food products or to substances that form during cooking of red meat at high temperatures. Excessive fat intake associated with diets rich in red meat, or low dietary fiber intake, may also be contributing factors. More research on this topic is needed before red meat can be singled out as a causative factor in colon cancer.

Insight

Protein and the Athlete

Contrary to popular belief, fat and carbohydrate are more important fuels for exercising muscles than the amino acids in protein. Endurance exercise is the only case in which proteins contribute significantly to energy needs, perhaps as much as 10% to 15% of needs. Thus, promotion of high-protein products to weight lifters is misleading, as protein is not the major fuel for these athletes.

Though protein is not the major fuel for exercise, typical recommendations for athletes range from 1.2 to 1.6 grams of protein per kilogram of body weight, considerably higher than the RDA of 0.8 of body weight. Endurance athletes should aim for the higher end of this range, but the vast majority of athletes can meet protein needs without having to exceed twice the RDA. Furthermore, benefits with intakes above twice the RDA have not been supported by sufficient research.

Table 6–4 shows the actual amount of protein that people of different body weights need to consume to meet the RDA and twice the RDA. Any athlete can easily have a protein intake twice the RDA simply by eating a variety of foods. For example, a 123-pound (53-kilogram) woman can consume 82 grams of her upper range of 85 grams of protein (twice the RDA) by eating 4 ounces of chicken (one chicken breast), 3 ounces of beef (a small lean hamburger), and ½ cup of cooked beans, and drinking 2 glasses of milk during a single day. A 180-pound (77-kilogram) man needs to consume only 6 ounces of chicken (a large chicken breast), ½ cup of cooked beans, a 6–ounce can of tuna, and 2 glasses of milk during a day to consume 122 grams of his upper range of 123 grams of protein (twice the RDA). And for both athletes this does not even include the protein in the grains or vegetables they will also eat. In meeting their energy needs, many athletes consume even more protein.

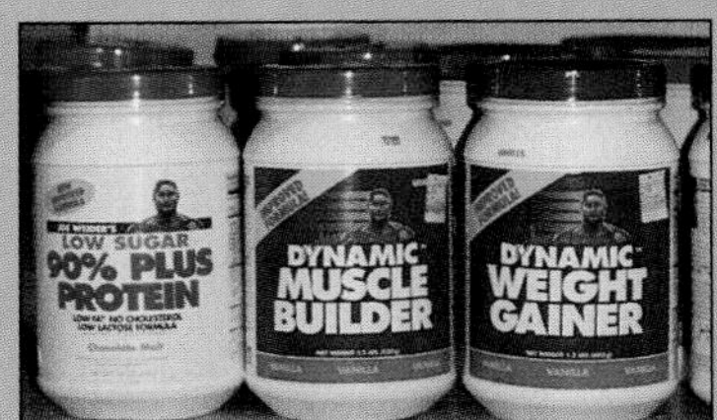

High-protein products, which are marketed to athletes, are unnecessary.

High protein diets have recently been promoted as a weight-loss strategy. However, as noted in Chapter 9, total energy intake is the focus—no source of calories is immune from scrutiny. Promotion of high-protein diets for weight loss are just another gimmick being sold to adults. Watching one's total calorie intake and performing regular physical activity are the most important habits to keep in mind for weight control.

Some researchers have also expressed the concern that a high protein intake may unduly burden the kidneys to excrete the resulting excess nitrogen (mostly as urea) into the urine. Low-protein diets marginally slow the decline in kidney function in humans if begun early in the course of developing kidney disease, and laboratory animal studies show that protein intakes that just meet nutritional needs preserve kidney function over time better than high-protein diets. Preserving kidney function is especially important for people with diabetes and for people who show signs of kidney disease, such as excess urea in the blood, or who have only one functioning kidney. High-protein diets are discouraged in these cases (especially when coupled with high blood pressure). For people without diabetes or kidney disease the risk of suffering kidney failure is very low, and thus the risk of a high-protein diet contributing to kidney disease in later life is also low.

High-protein diets increase fluid needs, as the excretion of the extra urea produced from protein metabolism increases urine output. This is primarily a concern for athletes, as they already experience increased fluid losses from sweat. Fluid intake is very important to monitor for athletes; dehydration can produce deleterious effects on performance (see Chapter 10). For nonathletes, fluid needs are easy to meet (about 1 milliliter per calorie expended by the body; [see Chapter 8]), and so this effect of protein is not a concern.

Because protein needs are so easily met, amino acid supplements are not necessary. No significant amount of free amino acids are present in our food. Nor is there any dietary need for or unique dietary value from eating free amino acids. In fact, when individual amino acid supplements are taken, they can overwhelm the absorptive mechanism, triggering amino acid imbalances in the body. These imbalances occur because groups of chemically similar amino acids compete for absorption into the bloodstream. Overall, every amino acid taken in excess can be harmful. Stick to whole foods as your source for amino acids.

Athletes who either feel they must significantly limit their energy intake or are vegetarians should specifically determine how much protein they eat. They should make sure to choose foods that provide at least 1.2 grams of protein per kilogram of body weight. Skimping on protein is not a good idea.

TABLE 6-4

Grams of Protein That Meet Recommendations for Individuals of Different Weights

Body Weight		Protein Allotment (Grams)	
Pounds	Kilograms	RDA (0.8 gram per kilogram)	2 × RDA (1.6 grams per kilogram)
110	50	40	80
130	60	48	96
155	70	56	112
175	80	64	128
200	90	72	144
220	100	80	160

Compare these quantities with protein intake from the diets listed in Table 10-4 in Chapter 10. Note that diets supplying enough total energy for athletes yield plenty of protein, even for those who make no special attempt to consume high-protein foods.

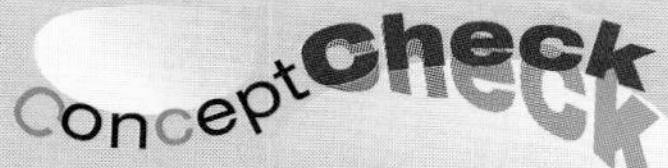

The Recommended Dietary Allowance (RDA) for adults is 0.8 gram of protein per kilogram of healthy body weight. This adds up to 56 grams of protein daily for a 70-kilogram (156-pound) person. Typically, we eat more than enough protein to meet our needs. Current research has not firmly established that this excess poses a major health risk for most of us, aside from the fat present in most high-protein diets, but it is also not necessary.

Protein-Energy Malnutrition

Rarely an isolated condition, protein deficiency worldwide usually accompanies a deficiency of dietary energy and other nutrients resulting from insufficient food intake. In developing areas of the world, this state of undernutrition stunts growth in childhood and causes more susceptibility to disease throughout life. (Note that undernutrition is a main focus of Chapter 16.) In the United States, certain populations also are at risk such as the elderly, the homeless, individuals who undertake severe prolonged dieting, people with certain disease states, and those who experience long-term hospitalization.

Protein-energy malnutrition (PEM)
A condition resulting from regularly consuming insufficient amounts of energy and protein. The deficiency eventually results in body wasting and an increased susceptibility to infections.

Marasmus
A disease that results from consuming a grossly insufficient amount of protein and energy; one of the diseases classed as protein-energy malnutrition. Victims will have little or no fat stores, little muscle mass, and poor strength. Death from infections is common.

Kwashiorkor
A disease occurring primarily in young children who have an existing disease and consume a marginal amount of energy and considerably insufficient protein despite high needs. The child generally suffers from infections and exhibits edema, poor growth, weakness, and an increased susceptibility to further illness.

People who eat too little protein and energy food can develop **protein-energy malnutrition (PEM),** also referred to as ***protein-calorie malnutrition (PCM).*** If the nutrient deficiency—especially for energy and protein—is quite severe, a deficiency disease called ***marasmus*** can result. On the other hand, when a poor nutrient intake—protein included—is added to other problems from concurrent diseases and infections, a disease called ***kwashiorkor*** can develop. These two diseases form the tip of the iceberg with respect to all states of undernutrition, and symptoms of these two diseases even can be present in the same person (Figure 6–7).

Kwashiorkor

Kwashiorkor often occurs in developing countries when the diet of a young child (approximately 1 to 1.5 years of age) is abruptly changed due to the arrival of another child. The diet changes from nutritious human milk to native starchy roots and gruels that are low in protein. The filling nature of these foods also makes it difficult to meet the child's energy requirements.

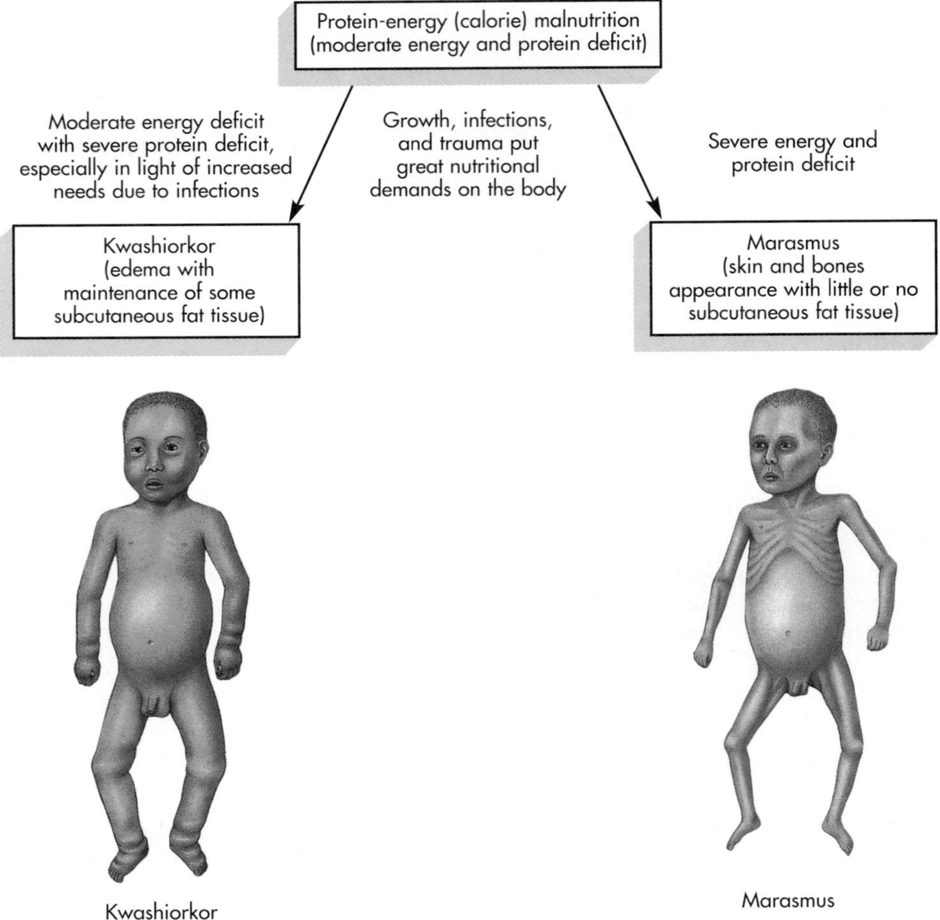

Figure 6–7 *A schema for classifying undernutrition. The presence of subcutaneous fat (directly underneath the skin) is a diagnostic key for distinguishing kwashiorkor from marasmus.*

Symptoms that result from this inadequate diet reflect protein deficiency and include apathy, growth and weight gain failure, poor immune function, and others. The presence of edema with some subcutaneous fat still present is the hallmark of this disease (see Figure 6–7). These symptoms can be reversed if adequate protein and energy are given in time. Unfortunately, by the time many of these children are treated, they already have severe infections that lead to death. Or, if they survive, they return home only to repeat the cycle.

Marasmus

Marasmus typically occurs as a person slowly starves to death. It is caused by diets containing greatly insufficient amounts of protein, energy, and other nutrients. The word *marasmus* means "to waste away." Victims have the "skin and bones" appearance you see on posters from relief agencies (see Figure 6–7). Little or no subcutaneous fat is present.

Marasmus commonly develops in infants when the weaning formula used is improperly prepared because of unsafe water and/or when parents cannot afford sufficient infant formula for the child's needs. The latter problem may lead the parents to dilute the formula to provide more feedings, not realizing that this provides only more water for the infant. An infant with marasmus requires large amounts of energy and protein—like a preterm infant—and unless the child receives them, full recovery from the disease is not likely to occur.

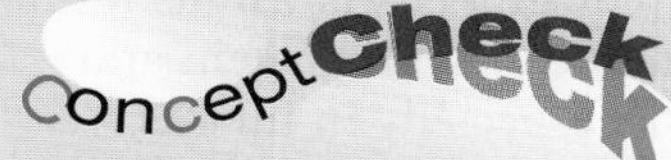

Multiple dietary deficiencies often exist in developing countries. Together the deficiencies in energy and protein are called protein-energy malnutrition. Specifically, ill children who also receive marginal food energy and little protein often develop kwashiorkor, a disease characterized by edema with some subcutaneous fat. People who are starving to death, with severely inadequate protein and energy intake, develop marasmus. In this case, little or no subcutaneous fat remains. If treated in the early stages, protein-energy malnutrition can be reversed, but often victims of this type of deficiency receive treatment too late.

Summary

- The building blocks of proteins, amino acids contain a very usable form of nitrogen for humans. Of the 20 types of amino acids found in food, 9 must be consumed as food and the rest can be synthesized by the body.
- High-quality, also called *complete,* protein foods contain ample amounts of all nine essential amino acids. Animal foods and soybeans typically supply all of them in approximately the right amounts. Lower-quality, also called *incomplete,* protein foods lack sufficient amounts of one or more essential amino acids. This is typical of plant foods, especially cereal grains. Plant foods eaten together often complement each other's amino acid deficits, thereby providing high-quality protein in the diet.
- Individual amino acids are linked together to form proteins. The sequential order of amino acids determines the protein's ultimate shape and function. Diseases such as sickle cell disease can occur if the amino acids are out of order in a protein. And if the three-dimensional shape of the protein is unfolded—denatured—by treatment with heat, acid or alkaline solutions, or other processes, the protein loses also its biological activity.

- Animal products are the most nutrient-dense sources of protein. For example, water-packed tuna contains over 80% of its energy content as protein. The high quality of these proteins means we can easily convert them into body proteins. Plant foods generally contain less than 20% of their energy content as protein; however, legumes are an excellent source of high-quality protein if eaten with grain proteins or animal products.
- Protein digestion begins in the stomach, producing breakdown products called *peptones*. In the small intestine, peptones eventually separate into amino acids. These travel via the portal vein to the liver.
- Body components, such as muscles, connective tissue, transport proteins, visual pigments, enzymes, some hormones, and immune bodies, are made of proteins. Proteins also can be used to synthesize glucose when necessary.
- The protein RDA for adults is 0.8 gram per kilogram of healthy body weight. For a typical 70-kilogram (156–pound) person, this corresponds to 56 grams of protein daily. The American diet generally supplies plenty of protein. The combined protein intake is also of sufficient quality to support body functions.
- Evidence suggests that high-protein diets should be avoided by some people, such as those with diabetes or kidney problems. However, more information is needed before significantly decreasing protein intake is recommended for other groups.
- Though athletes require a higher amount of protein (1.2 to 1.6 grams per kilogram) than the RDA suggests, most can easily meet their needs through the diet.
- Undernutrition occasionally leads to kwashiorkor and marasmus. Kwashiorkor results in otherwise ill children, primarily from an inadequate energy and protein intake in comparison to body needs. Kwashiorkor often occurs when a child is weaned from human milk to mostly starchy gruels. Marasmus results primarily from extreme starvation—a negligible intake of both protein and energy. Marasmus commonly occurs during famine, especially in infants.

Study Questions

1. Discuss the relative importance of essential and nonessential amino acids in the diet. Why is it important for essential amino acids lost from the body to be replaced in the diet?
2. Describe the concept of complementary proteins.
3. What amino acids may be low in the diet of a vegan (one who eats no animal foods)? List some suggestions for appropriate diet planning for these individuals.
4. Why is protein organization so important to protein function in the body?
5. What are four of the functions of protein?
6. Describe how the functions of protein break down in protein-energy malnutrition.
7. Briefly outline protein digestion and absorption, emphasizing the location in the body and the enzyme(s) and hormone(s) involved.
8. How does the concept of protein balance affect setting the RDA for an infant? A healthy adult? Someone recovering from an extended illness with extreme weight loss?
9. Several health problems may be associated with high-protein diets. What are they? Why don't more health professionals encourage average Americans to significantly cut down on protein intake?
10. If your grandmother was eating little more than tea and toast for meals, what consequences could this have to her health, based on what you now know about proteins?

Further Readings

1 ADA reports: Position of the American Dietetic Association: vegetarian diets, *Journal of the American Dietetic Association* 97:1317, 1997.
2 Americans and red meat: a love-hate relationship, *Harvard Health Letter* p. 1, May 1998.
3 Dwyer JT: Vegetarianism for women. In Krummel DA, Kris-Etherton PM, (editors): *Nutrition in women's health.* Gaithersburg, Md., 1996, Aspen.
4 Farley D: More people trying vegetarian diets, *FDA Consumer* p. 10, October 1995.
5 Geil PB, Anderson JW: Nutrition and health implications of dry beans: a review, *Journal of the American College of Nutrition* 13:549, 1994.
6 Giovannuci E and others: Intake of fat, meat, and fiber in relation to colon cancer in men, *Cancer Research* 54:2390, 1994.
7 Haddad E: Health implications of vegetarian diets, *Nutrition & the MD* 22(8):1, 1996.
8 Jeret P: The new vegetarians, *Health* p. 82, May–June 1996.
9 Lemon PWR: Is increased dietary protein intake necessary or beneficial for individuals with a physically-active lifestyle, *Nutrition Reviews* 54(II):S169, 1996 (April).
10 Liebman B: Plants for supper? 10 reasons to eat more like a vegetarian, *Nutrition Action Healthletter* p. 10, October 1996.
11 Mestel R: Soy wonder, *Health* p. 82, January–February 1998.
12 Rainey C, Nyquist L: Nuts—nutrition and health benefits of daily use, *Nutrition Today* 32:157, 1997.
13 Raloff J: High fat and healthful: scientists offer a nutty recipe for hale hearts and slim physiques, *Science News* 154:328, 1998.
14 Raloff J: Soya-nara, heart disease, *Science News* 153:348, 1998.
15 Russell RM: The impact of disease states as a modifying factor nutrition toxicity, *Nutrition Reviews* 55:50, 1997.
16 Sanders TA: Vegetarian diets and children, *Pediatric Clinics of North America* 42:955, 1995.
17 Spiller GA, Bruce B: Vegan diets and cardiovascular health, *Journal of the American College of Nutrition* 17:407, 1998.
18 Walter P: Effects of vegetarian diets on aging and longevity, *Nutrition Reviews* 55(II):S61, 1997.

RATE Your Plate

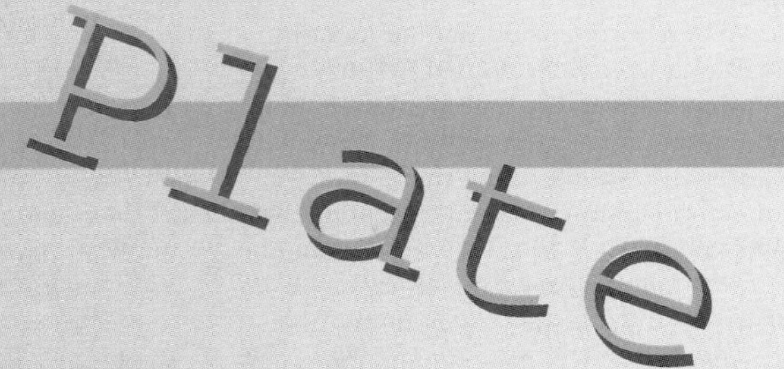

I. How Much Protein Are You Eating?

How much protein do you eat in a typical day? Look at the nutrition assessment you completed at the end of Chapter 2. Review it closely. Find the figure indicating the amount of protein you consumed on that day, and write it in the space below:

TOTAL PROTEIN ________

Compare your protein intake with your RDA for protein. Find your healthy weight for height in pounds using Table 9–1 in Chapter 9. Choose a midrange value. Divide this number by 2.2 to reveal your healthy weight in kilograms. Next, multiply by 0.8 grams per kilogram of this weight (or your current body weight if the two numbers are close). This will indicate the RDA for protein for your age and gender. Write it in the space below:

RDA FOR PROTEIN ________

How does your consumption compare with your RDA?

____

____

____

If you consumed either more or less than the RDA, what foods could you add, subtract, or eat more or less of? (Look at the foods you ate.)

____

____

____

____

Was most of your protein from animal or plant sources?

____

____

If your protein intake was primarily from plants, did this come from a wide variety to encourage protein complementarity for the day?

____

____

II. Evaluating protein intake—a case study

Marcus is a college student who has been lifting weights at the student recreation center. The trainer at the center recommended a protein drink to help Marcus build muscle mass. Evaluate Marcus' current food intake, and determine whether a protein drink is needed to supplement Marcus' diet.

1. The following is a tally of yesterday's intake.

Breakfast	**Frosted Mini-Wheats cereal, 2 oz**
	1% milk, 1½ cups
	Orange juice, chilled, 6 oz
	Glazed yeast doughnut, 1
	Brewed coffee, 1 cup
Lunch	**Double hamburger w/condiments, 1**
	French fries, 30
	Cola, 12 oz
	Medium apple, 1
Dinner	**Frozen lasagna w/meat, 2 pieces**
	1% milk, 1 cup
	Looseleaf lettuce, chopped, 1 cup
	Creamy Italian salad dressing, 2 tsp
	Medium tomato, ½
	Whole carrot, raw, 1
Evening snack	**Vanilla ice milk, 1 cup**
	Hot fudge chocolate topping, 2 tsp
	Soft chocolate chip cookies, 2

a. Evaluate Marcus' diet—is he meeting the minimum recommendations of the Food Guide Pyramid?____________________

2. Marcus' weight has been stable at 80 kilograms (176 pounds). Determine his protein needs based on the RDA (0.8 grams per kilogram).

a. Marcus' estimated protein RDA. ____________________

b. What are the maximum recommendations for protein intake for athletes? (see p. 193) ________

c. Apply this maximum recommendation to Marcus. ____________________

____

3. An analysis of the total kcal and protein content of Marcus' current diet is: 3470 kcals, 125 grams of protein (14% of total calories supplied by protein). This diet is representative of the food choices and amounts of food that Marcus chooses on a regular basis.

a. What is the difference between Marcus' estimated protein needs if an athlete (from exercise 2) and the amount of protein that his current diet provides?____________________

b. Is his current protein intake inadequate, adequate, or excessive? ____________________

4. Marcus takes his trainer's advice and goes to the grocery store to purchase a protein drink to add to his diet. Four products are available; they contain the following label information.

	Amino Fuel	Joe Weider's Sugar-Free 90% Plus Protein	Joe Weider's Dynamic Muscle Builder	Victory Super Mega Mass 2000
Serving size	3 tbsp	3 tbsp	3 tbsp	¼ scoop
Kcal	104	110	103	104
Protein (grams)	15	24	10	5

The trainer recommends adding the supplement to Marcus' diet two times a day. Marcus chooses Joe Weider's Dynamic Muscle Builder.

a. **How much protein would be added to Marcus' diet daily from two servings of the supplement alone (prior to mixing it with a beverage)?**____________________

b. **Marcus mixes the powder with 8 ounces of milk at lunch and dinner. How much protein total would Marcus now consume in one day? ________ (Add the protein amount from the nutrition analysis to the value from the previous question.)**

c. **What is the difference between Marcus' estimated protein needs as an athlete and this total value?**____________________

5. What is your conclusion—does Marcus need the protein supplement? ________________

____

ANSWERS TO CALCULATIONS

2a Marcus' estimated protein RDA: 80 kilograms × 0.8 grams/kg = 64 grams
2b Maximum recommendation for protein intake for athletes = 2 × RDA
2c Applied to Marcus: 2 × 64 = 128 grams
3a Difference between Marcus' estimated maximum protein needs if an athlete and the amount of protein provided by his current diet: 128 − 125 = 3 grams protein
3b Marcus' current diet is adequate to excessive
4a Two servings of protein supplement alone = 20 grams of protein
4b Marcus' total protein consumption: 125 grams + 20 grams = 145 grams protein
4c Difference between Marcus' estimated maximum protein needs as an athlete and total value (from above): 145 grams − 128 grams = 17 grams protein

Nutrition Issue

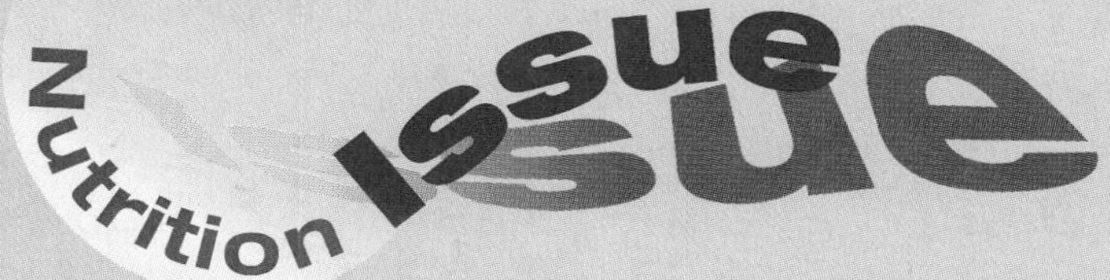

Vegetarianism

Today there are about 12 million vegetarians in the United States, about double the number in 1985. Over the past two decades vegetarian diets have gone from dull to delicious, with the inclusion of such new products as soy-based sloppy joes, chili, tacos, burgers, and more. In addition, cookbooks that feature use of a variety of fruits, vegetables, and seasonings are enhancing food selection for vegetarians of all degrees.

Vegetarianism is popular among college students. Fifteen percent of college students in one survey said they select vegetarian options at lunch or dinner on any given day. In response, dining services offer vegetarian options at every meal, the most common being pastas with meatless sauce and pizza. And a recent survey by the National Restaurant Association found that 20% of their customers want a vegetarian option when they eat out.

As nutrition science has grown, new information has enabled the design of adequate vegetarian diets. It is important for vegetarians to take advantage of this information because a diet with a limited variety of only plants can lead to various nutrient deficiencies and a substantial growth retardation in infants and children. People who choose a vegetarian diet can meet their nutritional needs by following a few basic rules and knowledgeably planning their diets (Figure 6–8).

Recent studies show that death rates from some chronic diseases such as certain forms of heart disease, cancer, and Type 2 diabetes, are lower for vegetarians than for nonvegetarians. Healthful lifestyles (not smoking, abstinence from alcohol and drugs, and increased physical activity) and social class bias probably partially account for these findings.

WHY DO PEOPLE PRACTICE VEGETARIANISM?

People choose vegetarianism for a variety of reasons. Some believe that killing animals for food is unethical. Hindus and Trappist monks eat vegetarian meals as a practice of their religion. In the United States, many Seventh Day Adventists base their practice of vegetarianism on biblical texts and believe it is a more healthful way to live. Some people might pursue vegetarianism because meat is expensive. Others cite health and flavor as reasons for choosing vegetarian fare.

People might choose vegetarianism after realizing that animals are not efficient protein factories. Animals actually use much of the protein they eat just to maintain themselves rather than to synthesize new muscle tissue. Note that 40% of the world's grain production is used to breed meat-producing animals. Animals that humans eat sometimes eat grasses that humans cannot digest. Many, however, also eat grains humans can eat.

People might also practice vegetarianism because it encourages a high intake of carbohydrates, vitamins A, E and C, carotenoids, magnesium, and dietary fiber, while limiting saturated fat and cholesterol intake. This produces a diet closely resembling that suggested in the Dietary Guidelines for Americans covered in Chapter 2.

FRANK & ERNEST® by Bob Thaves
Sid's Diner
TODAY'S MENU INCLUDES ELBOW MACARONI, EARS OF CORN, HEAD LETTUCE, BLACK-EYED PEAS, KIDNEY BEANS, HEARTS OF ARTICHOKE, AND LADYFINGERS.
SORRY -- I'M A VEGETARIAN.
© 1990 by NEA, Inc. THAVES 10-5

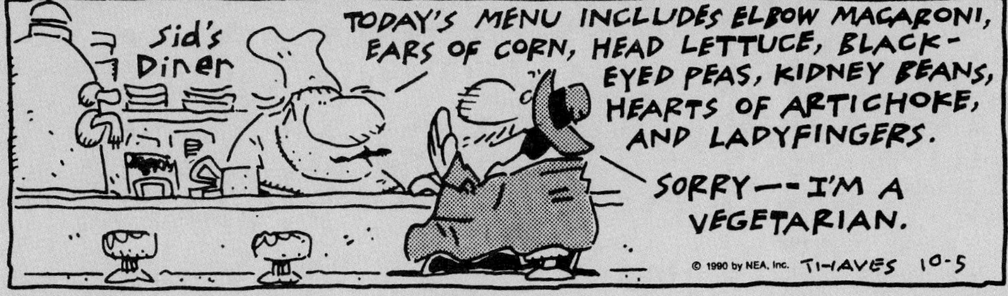

Figure 6–8 *Frank & Ernest.*

Vegan
A person who eats only plant foods.

Fruitarian
A person who primarily eats fruits, nuts, honey, and vegetable oils.

Lacto-vegetarian
A person who consumes plant products and dairy products.

Lacto-ovo-vegetarian
A person who consumes plant products, dairy products, and eggs.

FOOD PLANNING FOR VEGETARIANS

There are a variety of vegetarian styles. **Vegans** eat only plant foods. **Fruitarians** primarily eat fruits, nuts, honey, and vegetable oils. This plan is not recommended because it can lead to nutrient deficiencies in people of all ages. **Lacto-vegetarians** modify vegetarianism a bit—they include dairy products and plant foods. **Lacto-ovo-vegetarians** modify the diet even further and eat dairy products and eggs, as well as plant foods. Including these animal products makes food planning easier because they are rich in some nutrients missing or present in low amounts in plants. Overall, the wider the variety of foods eaten, the easier it is to meet nutritional needs. Thus, the practice of eating no animal sources of food significantly separates the vegans and fruitarians from all other semivegetarian styles.

Oldways Preservation & Exchange Trust has published a Vegetarian Pyramid. The base consists of fruits, vegetables, whole grains, and legumes (at every meal). The middle tier is nuts, seeds, egg whites, soy milks, dairy products, and plant oils (daily). Eggs and sweets form the tip (small quantities). Alcohol intake is optional, and daily physical activity is recommended. See their site for further information (htpp://www.oldwayspt.org).

It has been suggested that "almost vegetarians" (those who allow dairy, eggs, and occasional fish or chicken) are the healthiest group of all vegetarians. Perhaps this is due to the health benefits of a high fruit and vegetable diet, rather than the complete exclusion of all animal products.

Most people who call themselves vegetarians consume at least some dairy products, if not all dairy products and eggs. A Food Guide Pyramid plan has been developed for lacto-vegetarians. This plan includes servings of nuts, grains, legumes, and seeds to help meet protein needs. There is also a vegetable group, a fruit group, and a milk group.

This plan differs a little from the Food Guide Pyramid for **omnivores.** Figure 6–9 shows how the Food Guide Pyramid could be adapted for lacto- or lacto-ovo-vegetarians. The key to this plan is seeking foods other than meat that supply the nutrients contained in meat. It's not nutritionally sound simply to stop eating meat without making sure the body's needs are still met. Good-quality plant sources of nutrients, such as nuts, grains, legumes, and seeds, should be eaten to supply nutrients that normally come from meat in the diet. By following such a food plan, a lacto-vegetarian should be able to have an adequate diet.

Omnivore
A person who consumes both plant and animal food sources.

THE VEGAN—SPECIAL CONSIDERATIONS

A vegan diet requires some creative planning. A real effort must be made to use grains and legumes to yield high-quality protein and other key nutrients in meals, especially when used in pregnancy or with infants and children. Then, if energy needs are satisfied, protein needs should also be met. Including a wide variety of protein sources should provide all amino acids needed for a high-quality protein diet. The essential amino acids deficient from one food protein are supplied by those of another protein in the same meal or in the next. For example, many legumes do not provide enough of the essential amino acid methionine, while cereal grains are limited in lysine. When a combination of these two foods is eaten, the body is supplied with adequate amounts of both amino acids. So cereal grains and legumes complement each other.

Table 6–2 lists traditional dishes in which vegetable proteins combine to provide high-quality (complete) protein in the meal.

Purchasing some vegetarian cookbooks will simplify the task of menu planning. They provide numerous ideas for imaginative and nutritious ways to use plant foods.

The vegan diet must also include good sources of riboflavin, vitamins D and B-12, calcium, iron, and zinc (Table 6–5). A fortified breakfast cereal provides a good start in meeting those needs. Riboflavin can be obtained from green leafy vegetables, whole grains, yeast, and legumes, part of most vegan diets. Vitamin D can be obtained through regular sun exposure and fortified margarine. Otherwise, a supplement containing vitamin D should be considered (see Chapter 7).

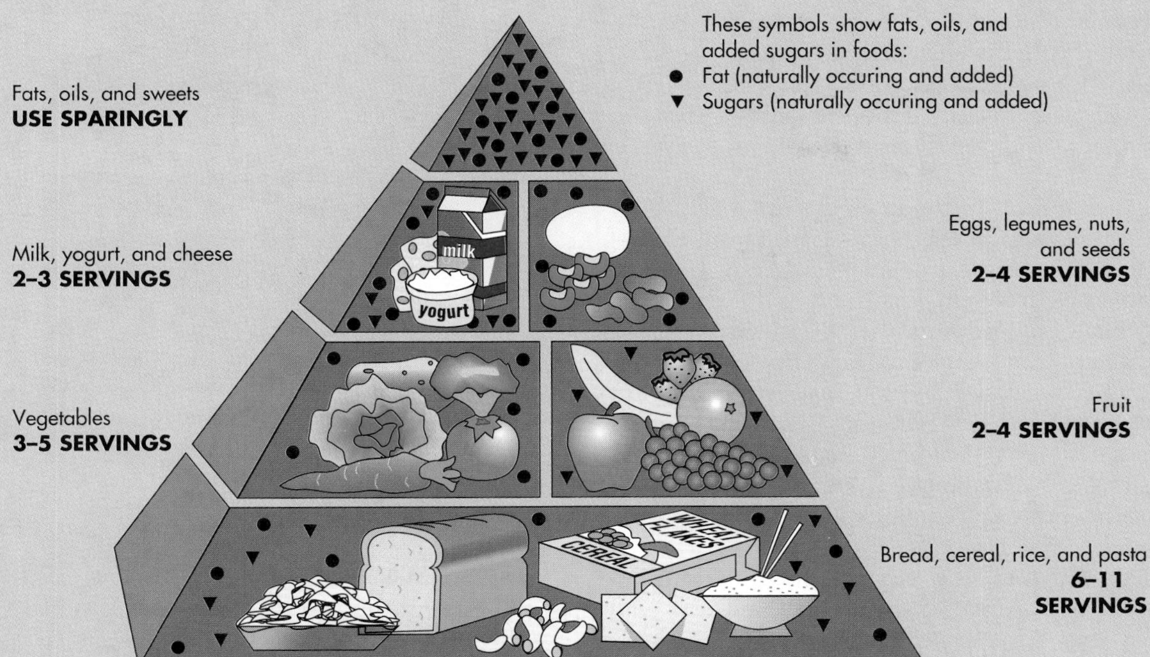

Figure 6–9 *Food Guide Pyramid for lacto-ovo-vegetarian (lacto-vegetarians would omit eggs as a choice). Base serving size on Food Guide Pyramid in Chapter 2. This plan yields about 1800 kcal and about 75 grams of protein. One should increase the number of servings, or add other foods to meet higher energy needs. To adapt this Pyramid to a vegan plan, one should aim for the higher range of servings in the fruits, vegetables, and bread, cereal, rice, and pasta groups. In addition, servings from the protein-rich group should include 2 from legumes and 2 from nuts. These changes keep total calorie and protein content about the same as shown for the lacto-ovo-vegetarian plan.*

TABLE 6-5

Nutrients Likely to be Marginal in the Vegan Diet

Nutrient	Plant sources
Vitamin D	Fortified margarine, fortified breakfast cereal
Riboflavin	Whole and enriched grains, leafy vegetables, mushrooms, beans, nuts, seeds
Vitamin B-12	Fortified breakfast cereal, fortified yeast, fortified soy milk
Iron	Whole grains, prune juice, dried fruits, beans, nuts, seeds, leafy vegetables
Calcium	Fortified soy milk, tofu, almonds, dry beans, leafy vegetables, some fortified breakfast cereals, flour, certain brands of orange juice, and certain snacks
Zinc	Whole grains, wheat germ, beans, nuts, seeds

The vegan should find a reliable source of vitamin B-12, such as fortified soybean milk and special yeast grown on media rich in vitamin B-12. Vitamin B-12 occurs naturally only in animal foods; plants can contain soil or microbial contamination that provides at most a trace amount of vitamin B-12. Because the body can store enough vitamin B-12 for about 4 years, a deficiency can take a long time to develop after animal foods are removed from the diet. If a deficiency develops, nerves can be damaged irreversibly and brain function can decrease. Evidence of a vitamin B-12 deficiency has been noted in vegetarian mothers and their infants. The milk produced by the vegetarian mothers was low in vitamin B-12 The earliest sign of a vitamin B-12 deficiency is mental dysfunction; a prolonged deficiency can lead to irreversible nerve damage. Therefore vegans need to be careful to prevent a vitamin B-12 deficiency (see Chapter 7).

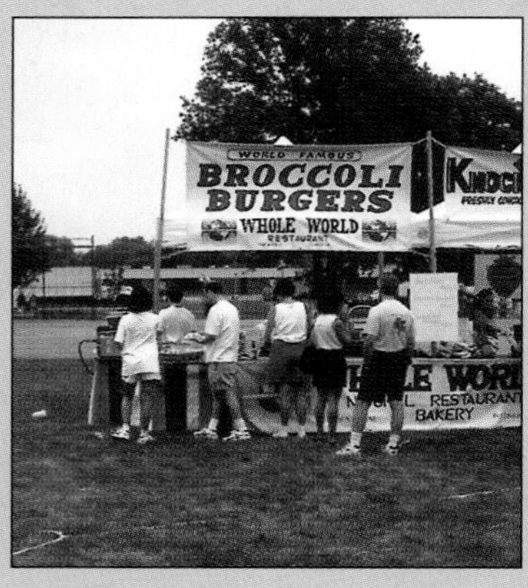

Vegetarian adaptations of traditional foods is a growing trend in our society.

To obtain calcium, the vegan can drink fortified soybean milk or fortified orange juice and consume calcium-rich tofu (check the label) or other calcium-fortified foods, such as certain breakfast cereals and snacks. Green leafy vegetables and nuts also contain calcium, but the calcium is either not well absorbed or not very plentiful. Calcium supplements are another option (see Chapter 8).

For iron the vegan can consume whole grains, dried fruits and nuts, and legumes. The iron in these foods is not absorbed as well as that found in animal foods, but a good source of vitamin C taken with these foods modestly enhances iron absorption. Thus a recommended strategy is to consume vitamin C with every meal that contains adequate iron-rich plant foods. Cooking in iron pots and skillets can also add iron to the diet (see Chapter 8).

The vegan can find zinc in whole grains, nuts, and legumes, but phytic acid and other substances in these foods limit zinc absorption. Grains are most nutritious when leavened, as in bread, because this process reduces the influence of phytic acid.

Of all these nutrients, calcium and iron are the most difficult to consume in sufficient quantities. Special diet planning is required.

Veganism during childhood can pose problems. The sheer bulk of a plant-based diet may make it difficult for a child to eat foods that supply enough energy to permit dietary protein to be used for synthesis of body proteins rather than for energy needs. Vegan children need concentrated sources of energy to avoid this problem. Examples include fortified soybean milk, nuts, dried fruits, avocados, cookies made with vegetable oils or tub margarine, and fruit juices. Soy milk, soy yogurt and soy cheese are excellent choices for vegan children (and vegan adults). When fortified with calcium and vitamin B-12, these substitutes can provide many of the key nutrients found in milk. Finding excellent iron and zinc sources is important in planning vegan diets for infants and children.

For a web site that provides much information on vegetarianism, see http://www.veg.org/veg/.

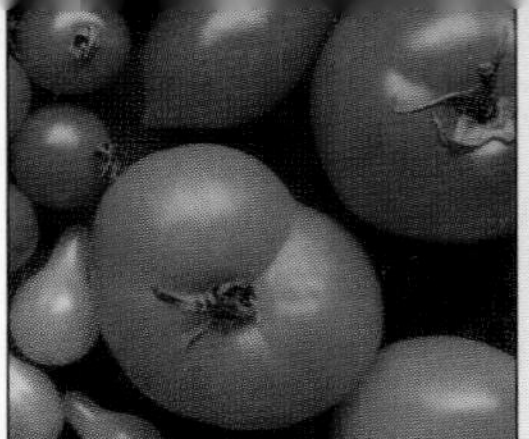

chapter 7

Vitamins

When it comes to vitamins, we often hear, "If a little is good, then more must be better." Some people believe that consuming vitamins far in excess of their needs provides them with extra energy, protection from disease, and prolonged youth. About 70% of adults in the United States take vitamin and mineral supplements on at least an occasional basis, with about half of those people taking a vitamin and mineral supplement daily. This helps fuel what has become a $13 billion industry.

Our total vitamin needs to prevent deficiency symptoms are actually quite small. In general, humans require a total of about 1 ounce (28 grams) of vitamins for every 150 pounds (70 kilograms) of food consumed. Vitamins are found in plants and animals. Plants synthesize all the vitamins they need. Animals vary in their ability to synthesize vitamins. For example, guinea pigs and humans are two of the very few organisms that are unable to synthesize their own supply of vitamin C.

This chapter first briefly reviews some general properties of the vitamins. Attention then focuses on the functions and sources of, and the need for, these vitamins and finishes with a look at their role in cancer prevention. In the process, the need for supplement use is explored.

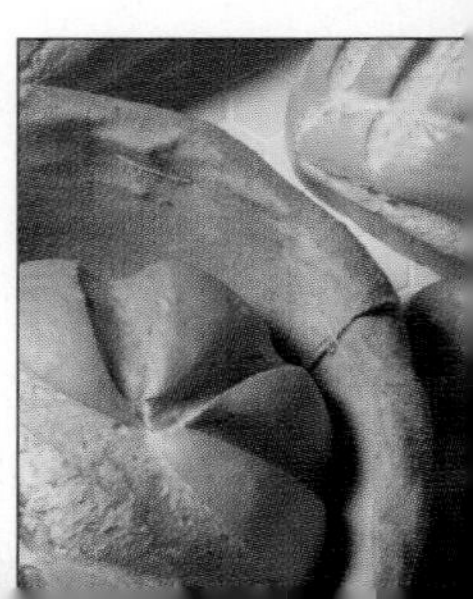

Nutrition Web

Vitamins are compounds we generally need daily or so in small amounts from food. They yield no energy directly, but many contribute to energy-yielding chemical reactions in the body and promote growth and development.

Vitamins A, D, E, and K are fat soluble. Vitamins A and D have a notable potential for toxicity since they are not readily excreted by the body.

The key roles of vitamin A include aiding in vision, immune function, and cell development. Vitamin A is found in fortified milk and breakfast cereals, eggs, and fish. The provitamin form of vitamin A is found in dark green and orange vegetables.

Vitamin D primarily acts to regulate calcium and bone metabolism. The body can synthesize vitamin D with adequate sun exposure, but needs can also be met by consuming fish and fortified milk.

The primary role of vitamin E is as an antioxidant, and it is found in plant oils and foods made with these oils.

Vitamin K is vital for blood clotting and is found in green and leafy vegetables. Some vitamin K used by the body comes from bacterial synthesis in the intestines.

Some segments of the population—such as pregnant women, strict vegans, and those on low-calorie diets—generally benefit from nutrient supplementation. Supplements are very loosely regulated by FDA. Any supplement use should be made known to one's physician.

The B vitamins and vitamin C are water soluble. These vitamins are more readily excreted by the body than the fat-soluble vitamins, making toxicity less likely. However, if very large amounts are consumed, toxicity can still result in some cases.

Thiamin, riboflavin, niacin, biotin, and pantothenic acid all aid in energy-yielding reactions and related nutrient metabolism. Food sources of one or more of these vitamins include whole- and enriched grain products, breakfast cereals, eggs, meats, and milk products.

Folate and vitamin B-12 are involved in cell development and homocysteine metabolism. Excellent sources include leafy vegetables and orange juice for folate, and animal foods for vitamin B-12. Grain products are generally fortified with folate.

The key function of vitamin B-6 is its role in protein and homocysteine metabolism. It is found in animal foods and some fruits and vegetables.

Vitamin C is crucial for synthesizing protein for connective tissue and other body tissues. Fruits and vegetables, especially citrus fruits, are rich sources of vitamin C.

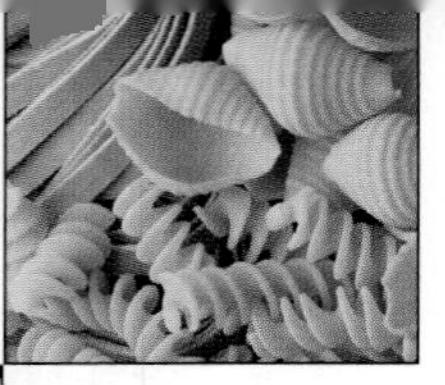

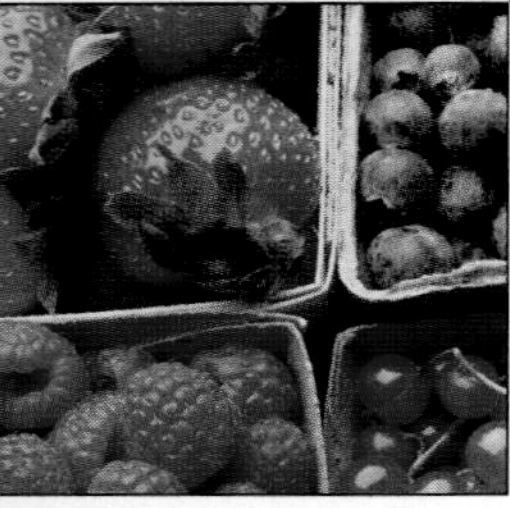

Vitamins: Vital Dietary Components

By definition, **vitamins** are essential organic (carbon-containing) substances needed in small amounts in the diet for normal function, growth, and maintenance of the body. Although vitamins themselves yield no energy to the body, they often participate in energy-yielding reactions. Vitamins A, D, E, and K are **fat soluble,** whereas the B vitamins and vitamin C are **water soluble.** In addition, the B vitamins and vitamin K function as parts of **coenzymes** (that is, compounds that help enzymes function) (Figure 7–1).

Vitamins are generally indispensable in human diets because they can't be synthesized in the human body, or because their synthesis can be curtailed by environmental factors. Notable exceptions to a strict dietary need are vitamin D, which is synthesized by the skin in the presence of sunlight; niacin, which is synthesized from an amino acid; and vitamin K and biotin, which are synthesized to some extent by bacteria in the intestinal tract.

For a substance to be classified as a vitamin, not only must the body be unable to synthesize enough of it, but its absence from the diet for a defined period of time also must produce deficiency symptoms that, if caught in time, are quickly cured when the substance is resupplied. A substance does not qualify as a vitamin merely because the body can't make it. Evidence must suggest that health declines when the substance is not consumed.

As scientists began to identify various vitamins, related deficiency diseases such as scurvy, beriberi, pellagra, and rickets were dramatically cured. For the most part, as the vitamins were discovered, they were named alphabetically: A, B, C, D, E, and so on. Later many substances originally classified as vitamins were found not to be essential for humans and were dropped from the list. This explains the many gaps in the alphabetical listing. Other vitamins, thought at first to have only one chemical form, turned out to take many forms, so the alphabetical name had to be broken down by numbers (B-6, B-12, and so on).

In addition to their use in correcting deficiency diseases, a few vitamins have also proved useful in treating several nondeficiency diseases. These medical applications require administration of **megadoses,** well above typical human needs for the vitamins. For example, megadoses of niacin can be employed as part of blood cholesterol–lowering treatment for appropriately selected individuals. Other examples of medical use include forms of vitamin D in the treatment of psoriasis. This chapter will mention others as well. Still, any claimed benefits from use of vitamin supplements, especially intakes in excess of 100% of the Daily Value listed on a supplement label, should be viewed critically because many unproven claims have been and are continually made.

Vitamins
Carbon-containing compounds that are needed in very small amounts in the diet to help promote and regulate chemical reactions and processes in the body. Absence from the diet must result in a disease that timely replacement of the vitamin will cure.

Fat-soluble vitamins
Vitamins that dissolve in such substances as ether and benzene but not readily in water. These vitamins are A, D, E, and K.

Water-soluble vitamins
Vitamins that dissolve in water. These vitamins are the B vitamins and vitamin C.

Have Scientists Found All the Vitamins?

You may wonder whether still more vitamins are lurking in foods that have not been discovered. After all, the first chemical formula of a vitamin (thiamin) was not determined until 1937, and the last structure was characterized in 1948 (vitamin B-12). Though some optimistic researchers hope to discover one or more additional vitamins such as choline (see p. 244), most scientists are confident that all vitamins needed by humans that are otherwise healthy have been discovered. Evidence supports this assumption. For example, people have lived well for years on intravenous solutions that consist of protein, carbohydrate, fat, all the known vitamins, and the essential minerals. With appropriate medical monitoring, these people not only continue to live but also build new body tissues, have babies, heal wounds, and fight existing diseases.

Storage of Vitamins in the Body

The fat-soluble vitamins, especially A and D, are not readily excreted from the body. In contrast, the water-soluble vitamins are generally lost from the body quite rapidly, partly because the water in cells dissolves these vitamins and excretes them out of the body via the kidneys. An exception is water-soluble vitamin B-12, which is stored much more readily than the other water-soluble vitamins.

Because of the limited storage of many vitamins, they should be consumed in the diet daily, although an occasional lapse in the intake of even water-soluble vitamins generally causes no harm. An average person, for example, must consume no thiamin for 10 days or no vitamin C for 20 to 40 days before developing the first symptoms of deficiency of these vitamins.

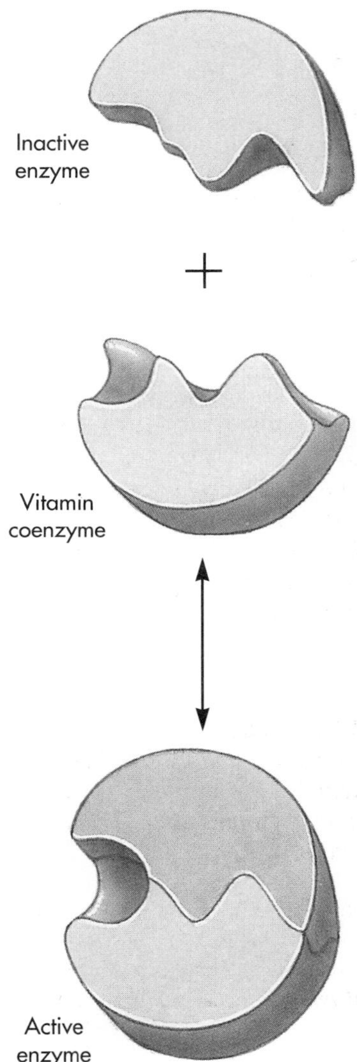

Figure 7-1
Coenzymes, such as those formed from B vitamins, aid in the function of various enzymes. Without the coenzyme, the enzyme cannot function, and deficiency symptoms associated with the missing vitamin eventually appear.

Vitamin Toxicity

Because the fat-soluble vitamins A and D are not readily excreted, they can easily accumulate in the body and cause toxic effects. Although a toxic effect from an excessive intake of any vitamin is theoretically possible, toxicities of these fat-soluble vitamins are the most frequently observed. Fat-soluble vitamin E and the water-soluble vitamins niacin, vitamin B-6, and vitamin C can also cause toxic effects but only when consumed in very large amounts. These four vitamins are unlikely to cause toxic effects unless taken in supplement (pill) form. In comparison, vitamins A and D generally are toxic with long-term intake at just three to five times human needs, with the lowest value referring to vitamin A intake during early stages of pregnancy.

Because regular use of a "once-a-day" type of multivitamin and mineral supplement usually yields less than two times the Daily Values for the components, this practice is unlikely to cause toxic effects. Consuming many vitamin pills, however, especially highly potent sources of vitamin A and vitamin D, can cause problems. The first Nutrition Insight will help you determine whether to take a vitamin and mineral supplement and, if so, how to do it safely. Most nutrition scientists agree that a well-chosen diet including some animal products can supply the vitamin needs of almost all people. In addition, any supplement use by you or others in your care—especially beyond 100% of the Daily Values—should be made known to one's physician. Note that some vitamins and minerals counteract the effect of certain medications. Professional advice, which includes evaluation of your current diet, can help you evaluate whether supplementation is in your best interest.

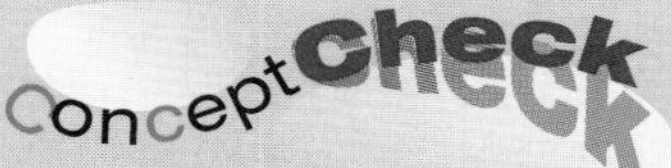

Vitamins are compounds needed in small amounts by the body; their absence from the diet results in a disease that timely replacement of the vitamin cures. Vitamins do not directly yield energy, but many are needed for energy-yielding processes in the body. Vitamins A, D, E, and K are fat soluble, whereas the B vitamins and vitamin C are water soluble. The fat-soluble vitamins A and D are not readily excreted from the body and so have the potential to build up rapidly to toxic amounts. Water-soluble vitamins are much more readily excreted.

THE FAT-SOLUBLE VITAMINS—A, D, E, AND K

First, let's look at what we know about the fat-soluble vitamins—vitamins A, D, E, and K (Table 7–1).

Absorption of Fat-Soluble Vitamins

Vitamins A, D, E, and K are absorbed along with dietary fat. These vitamins travel with dietary fats through the bloodstream to reach body cells. Special carriers in the bloodstream help distribute some of these vitamins. Fat-soluble vitamins are stored mostly in the liver and fatty tissues.

TABLE 7-1

Summary of the Fat-Soluble Vitamins, Their Functions, Deficiency Conditions, and Food Sources

Vitamin	Major functions	Deficiency symptoms	People most at risk	Dietary sources	RDA or AI	Toxicity symptoms
Vitamin A (retinoids) and provitamin A (carotenoids)	Promote vision: light and color Promote growth Prevent drying of skin and eyes Promote resistance to bacterial infection	Night blindness Xerophthalmia Poor growth Dry skin	People in poverty, especially preschool children (still very rare in the United States) Alcoholism People with AIDS	Vitamin A Liver Fortified milk Fortified breakfast cereals Provitamin A Sweet potatoes Spinach Greens Carrots Cantaloupe Apricots Broccoli	Females: 800 RE (4000 IU) Males: 1000 RE (5000 IU)	Fetal malformations, hair loss, skin changes, pain in bones (beyond 3000 RE per day)
D (chole- and ergocalciferol)	Facilitate absorption of calcium and phosphorus Maintain optimal calcification of bone	Rickets Osteomalacia	Breastfed infants not exposed to sunlight, elderly	Vitamin D–fortified milk Fortified breakfast cereals Fish oils Sardines Salmon	5–15 micrograms (200–600 IU)	Growth retardation, kidney damage, calcium deposits in soft tissue (beyond 2000 IU per day)
E (tocopherols)	Act as an antioxidant: prevent breakdown of vitamin A and unsaturated fatty acids	Hemolysis of red blood cells Nerve destruction	People with poor fat absorption, smokers (still rare as far as we know)	Vegetable oils Some greens Some fruits Fortified breakfast cereals	Females: 8 milligrams (alpha-tocopherol equivalents) Males: 10 milligrams (alpha-tocopherol equivalents)	Muscle weakness, headaches, fatigue, nausea, inhibition of vitamin K metabolism (beyond 1200 IU per day)
K (phyllo- and menaquinone)	Help form prothrombin and other factors for blood clotting and contribute to bone metabolism	Hemorrhage	People taking antibiotics for months at a time (still quite rare)	Green vegetables Liver	60–80 micrograms	Anemia and jaundice (medicinal forms only)

Abbreviations: RE = retinol equivalents, IU = international units.

When fat absorption is efficient, about 40% to 90% of the fat-soluble vitamins are absorbed. Anything that interferes with normal digestion and absorption of fats also interferes with fat-soluble vitamin absorption. People who use mineral oil as a laxative at mealtimes risk fat-soluble vitamin deficiencies because the intestine does not absorb mineral oil. Fat-soluble vitamins are simply eliminated with the mineral oil in the feces.

Vitamin A

The amount of vitamin A you consume is very important. Either too much or too little vitamin A can cause severe problems. Vitamin A is found in foods in a variety of forms. Retinol is one example. As a family, the various forms are called *preformed vitamin A* or ***retinoids*** (and found naturally only in animal foods). Vitamin A activity in the diet also occurs in the form of common plant pigments—**carotenoids**—such as the yellow-orange, beta-carotene pigment in carrots. Thus, carotenoids can be termed provitamin A because parts can be turned into vitamin A as needed. Over 600 carotenoids are found in nature; about 50 of them serve as provitamin A. The most potent form of provitamin A is beta-carotene. The preformed vitamin A and the provitamin A carotenoids both make up what is generically referred to as *vitamin A*.

Retinoids
Chemical forms of preformed vitamin A; one source is animal foods.

Carotenoids
Pigment substances in plants that can often form vitamin A. Beta-carotene is the most active form in terms of vitamin A activity.

Functions of Vitamin A

Vitamin A performs many important functions in the body, though its exact roles in the cell are still under study. Its importance to vision is perhaps its best-known role and the only role clearly understood. Body changes that occur when vitamin A is lacking provide clues to its function.

Vision

The link between vitamin A and night vision has been known since ancient Egyptian times, when juice extracted from liver was used as a cure for night blindness. Vitamin A performs important functions in light-dark and color vision. For a person to see in dim light, one form of vitamin A is required to start the chemical process that signals the brain that light is striking the eye. This allows the eye to adjust from bright to dim light (such as after seeing the headlights of an oncoming car). Without sufficient dietary vitamin A, eventually the eye cannot quickly readjust to dim light. The condition is known as **night blindness.**

Night blindness
A vitamin deficiency condition in which the retina (in the eye) cannot adjust to low amounts of light.

Xerophthalmia
Literally "dry eye." This is a cause of blindness that results from a vitamin A deficiency. The specific cause is linked to a lack of mucus production by the eye, which then leaves it at a greater risk of damage from surface dirt and bacteria.

If night blindness is not corrected and vitamin A deficiency progresses, the cells that line the cornea of the eye (the clear window of the eye) also lose their ability to produce mucus. The eye then becomes dry. Eventually, when dirt particles scratch the dry surface of the eye, bacteria infect it. The infection soon spreads to the entire surface of the eye and leads to blindness. This disease process is called ***xerophthalmia***, which means *dry eye.*

Vitamin A deficiency is second only to accidents as a worldwide cause of blindness. Americans are at little risk because of generally good diets. However, people—especially children—in less-developed nations are very susceptible to vitamin A deficiency. Poor dietary intakes and low stores of vitamin A fail to meet the children's high needs during rapid childhood growth. Millions of children in Asia become blind each year because of vitamin A deficiency and die soon after from infections (see the next section). As covered in more detail in Chapter 16, worldwide attempts to reduce this problem have included giving large doses of vitamin A twice yearly and supplementing sugar, margarine, and monosodium glutamate with vitamin A. These food vehicles are used because they are commonly consumed by the populations of less-developed nations. In some countries this effort has proved effective.

In the United States the leading cause of blindness in adults is diabetes; in children, it is accidents.

Epithelial cells
The cells that line the outside of the body and the inside of all external passages within it, such as the GI tract.

Health of Cells

Vitamin A maintains the health of cells that line internal and external "skin" surfaces in the lungs, intestines, stomach, vagina, urinary tract, and bladder, as well as those of the eyes and skin. These cells (called ***epithelial cells***) serve as important barriers to bacterial infection. As just noted for the eye, some epithelial cells secrete mucus, a needed lubricant. Without vitamin A, mucus-forming cells deteriorate and no longer synthesize mucus. Vitamin A deficiency also causes insufficient mucus production in the intestines and lung cells and poor health of cells in general. All of this increases the risk of body infections. Vitamin A deficiency also reduces the activity of certain immune system cells. Together, these effects leave the vitamin A–deficient person at great risk for infections.

Growth, Development, and Reproduction

Vitamin A is necessary for cell growth and development. Vitamin A causes a cell to increase its synthesis of proteins that stimulate proper growth and development. One consequence of vitamin A deficiency in laboratory animals is that they cannot reproduce. Resorbing old bone, which must occur before new bone can be deposited, requires bone cells that also use vitamin A. In addition, producing some components of bone requires vitamin A.

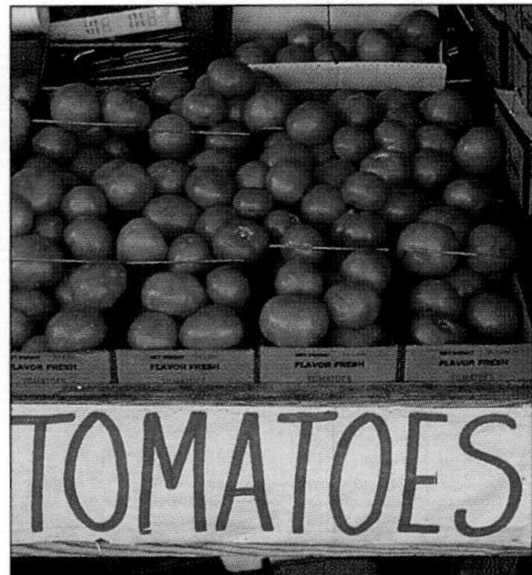

When the word carotenoids is mentioned, most people think of carrots. Perhaps their minds should jump first to tomatoes. This juicy vegetable contains 14 carotenoids (including lycopene), compared with 3 found in carrots.

Cancer Prevention

Most forms of cancer arise from cells that are influenced by vitamin A. Coupled with its ability to aid immune system activity, vitamin A may be a valuable tool in the fight against cancer. This is especially true for skin, lung, bladder, and breast cancers. The results to date indicate that use of vitamin A supplements can lower the risk of breast cancer among women with very low intakes of dietary vitamin A. However, studies on prostate and colon cancers indicate no protective effect from dietary vitamin A. Because of the potential for toxicity, unsupervised use of megadose vitamin A supplements to reduce cancer risk is not advised.

Carotenoids by themselves also may help prevent cancer. The many double bonds present in some carotenoids make them effective traps for the energy in certain **free radical** compounds that can probably initiate the cancer process (see the discussion on vitamin E for details). Epidemiological evidence shows that regular consumption of foods rich in carotenoids decreases the risk of lung and oral cancer and possibly prostate cancer in men. However, recall from Chapter 1 that recent studies from here and in Finland failed to show a reduction in lung cancer or heart disease in male smokers and nonsmokers who were given supplements of beta-carotene for 5 or more years. In fact, beta-carotene use increased the lung cancer cases compared with the control groups. No comparable studies have been done with women. Though further research continues, most researchers are now convinced that beta-carotene supplementation offers no protection against cancer or heart disease. The overwhelming advice is to rely on food sources of this or any other carotenoids. The best related advice is to eat a combination of at least five fruits and vegetables a day (and not smoke).

Analog
A chemical compound that differs slightly from another, usually natural, compound. Analogs generally contain extra or altered chemical groups and may have similar or opposite metabolic effects compared with the native compound.

Vitamin A Analogs for Acne

The acne medication tretinoin (Retin-A) is made of one **analog** form of vitamin A. It has been used as a topical treatment (applied to the skin) for acne for more than 10 years. It appears to work by altering cell activity in the skin. Another derivative of vitamin A, 13-*cis* retinoic acid (Accutane), is an oral drug used to treat serious acne. Note that taking high doses of vitamin A itself would not be safe. Even Accutane, a less potentially toxic form, can induce toxicity symptoms, as well as birth defects in the offspring of women using it during pregnancy.

Vitamin A in Foods and Needs

Preformed vitamin A is found in liver, fish oils, vitamin A–fortified milk and breakfast cereals, and eggs. Butter and margarine are also sources because they are fortified with vitamin A. Provitamin A is found mainly in dark green and orange vegetables and some fruits. Carrots, spinach, winter squash, broccoli, papayas, and apricots are examples of sources. Consuming a varied diet rich in green vegetables and carrots ensures sufficient sources for meeting vitamin A needs (Figure 7–2). About half of the vitamin A in the American diet comes from animal sources, the other half from plants.

Recently, derivatives of vitamin A have been put into creams (Renova) that reduce some effects of aging on the skin. Note that if the skin is already deeply wrinkled, these creams are ineffective.

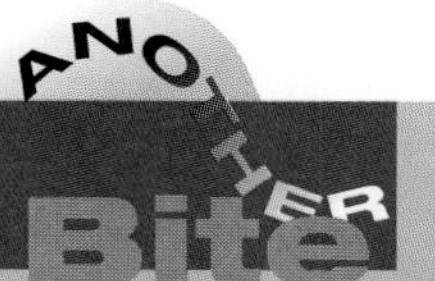

Most nutrient amounts in foods, including vitamin A, were formerly expressed in less precise ***international units (IU).*** *Some supplement labels still show the older IU values for vitamin A. For vitamin A the current unit of measurement is the retinol equivalent (RE). In this system, all potential forms of vitamin A are scaled based on their activity. Based on a mixture of preformed and provitamin A, 1 RE of vitamin A is equivalent to 5 IU of vitamin A.*

International unit (IU) *A crude measure of vitamin activity, often based on the growth rate of animals. Today these units have largely been replaced by more precise milligram and microgram measures.*

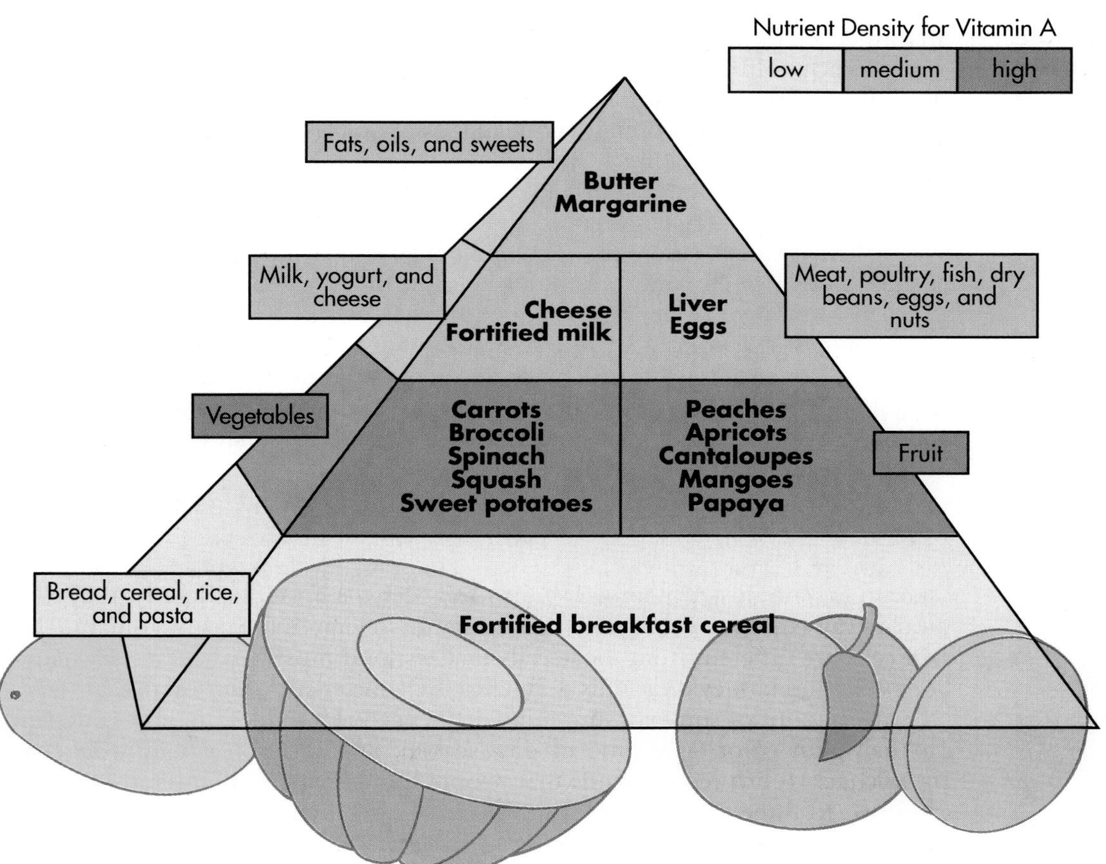

Figure 7–2 *Food sources of vitamin A from the Food Guide Pyramid. The fruit and vegetable groups supply abundant carotenoids if they have an intense yellow-orange or green color. Some of these carotenoids yield vitamin A. Liver is the richest source of preformed vitamin A, because that is the major site of vitamin A storage in animals. Milk is often fortified with vitamin A. The background color of each food group indicates the average nutrient density (RE per kcal) for vitamin A in that group.*

Dietary sources of vitamin A

Food item and amount	Vitamin A (RE)	Vitamin A (IU)
Fried beef liver, 1 oz	**3,042**	**10,236**
Baked sweet potato, 1	**2,487**	**24,877**
Carrot, 1	**2,025**	**20,253**
Cooked squash, ¾ cup	**1,286**	**12,864**
Mango, 1	**805**	**8,061**
Cooked spinach, ½ cup	**739**	**7,395**
Cantaloupe, 1 cup	**515**	**5,158**
Apricots, 3	**274**	**2,743**
Tomato juice, 8 oz	**136**	**1,351**
Cooked broccoli, ½ cup	**108**	**1,083**

Fetus
The developing human life form from 8 weeks after conception until birth.

The RDA for vitamin A is 1000 RE for men and 800 RE for women. (Throughout this and the next chapter, refer to the inside cover for nutrient recommendations for other ages and to Appendix B for Canadian recommendations.) The Daily Value is expressed in the IU form (5000 IU). The average intake for adult men and women in the United States is slightly above these values.

In America, poor vitamin A status has been noted among preschool children who do not eat enough vegetables. The urban poor, older people, and people who are alcoholics or who have liver disease (which limits vitamin A storage) can also show poor vitamin A status. Finally, children with severe fat malabsorption, as in cases of cystic fibrosis, may also show a vitamin A deficiency, as can adults with AIDS or severe intestinal disease.

Toxicity of Vitamin A

An intake of just three times the RDA for vitamin A can cause problems if taken for a prolonged time, especially during pregnancy and in the elderly years. A high preformed vitamin A intake is especially dangerous during the early months of pregnancy because it may cause **fetal** malformations, birth defects and spontaneous abortions. In nonpregnant adults, skin, hair, internal organs, and the central nervous system are most affected. These adverse effects in adults generally disappear after the doses stop. Permanent damage to the liver, bones, and eyes and recurrent joint and muscle pain, however, can occur.

FDA recommends that women in childbearing years limit their overall intake of preformed vitamin A to about 100% of the Daily Value and consume rich food sources, such as liver and highly fortified breakfast cereals, in moderation. This also applies to women who may become pregnant. Because vitamin A is stored in the body for long periods, women who take large amounts during the months before pregnancy place their babies at risk.

The ingestion of large amounts of vitamin A–yielding carotenoids does not cause toxic effects. If someone consumes large amounts of carrots or takes pills containing beta-carotene (more than 30 milligrams daily), or if infants eat a great deal of squash, high carotenoid concentration in the blood can occur. This can turn the skin yellow-orange. The palms of the hand and soles of the feet in particular become colored. This condition does not appear to cause harm and disappears when the excess carotenoids decrease. Dietary carotenoids do not produce toxic effects because (1) their rate of conversion into vitamin A is relatively slow and regulated, and (2) the efficiency of carotenoid absorption from the small intestine decreases markedly as oral intake increases.

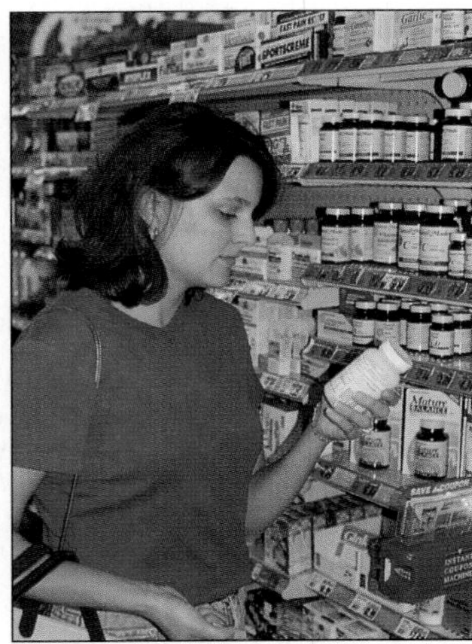

Long-term intake of just three or more times the RDA for some fat-soluble vitamins—particularly vitamin A during pregnancy—can cause toxic effects. Read supplement labels carefully for excess amounts of vitamins (> 100% of the Daily Value).

Vitamin D

Vitamin D is not just a vitamin. It is also considered a hormone because the cells in the skin can convert a cholesterol-like substance to vitamin D, using sunlight. These skin cells are different from those cells that respond mostly to vitamin D, namely bone cells and kidney cells. This difference is characteristic of hormones.

The amount of sun exposure individuals need to produce vitamin D depends on their skin color, age, time of day, season, and location. Vitamin D expert Dr. Michael Holick recommends that people should expose their hands, face, and arms two to three times a week to 30% to 50% of the amount of sun needed to cause a sunburn. In other words, for a person who would sunburn in just a half hour, 10 to 15 minutes of exposure is recommended. Persons with dark skin would need additional exposure, but the amount is not known. This sun exposure is only effective for vitamin D synthesis if sunscreen over SPF 8 is not used during this time, and it is done between about eight A.M. and four P.M. Still, this practice is not effective at all in the winter in northern climates. Some people may be able to use vitamin D stored from summer months in their fat cells, but most people in northern climates should find alternate vitamin D sources in the winter months. Overall, anyone who does not receive enough sunshine to synthesize an adequate amount of vitamin D must have a dietary source of the vitamin.

Functions of Vitamin D

To become the active hormone, vitamin D must be acted on by the liver and then the kidneys. The main function of this vitamin D hormone (called ***calcitriol***) is to help regulate calcium and bone metabolism. In concert with other hormones, especially **parathyroid hormone (PTH),** vitamin D closely regulates blood calcium to supply appropriate amounts of it to all cells. This task entails a variety of processes: the vitamin D hormone helps regulate absorption of calcium and phosphorus from the intestine, it reduces kidney excretion of calcium, and it helps regulate the deposition of calcium in the bones.

Even tissues in the brain, pancreas, and pituitary gland appear to be influenced by the vitamin D hormone. More interestingly, vitamin D is capable of influencing development in some cancer cells, such as skin, bone, and breast cancer cells. Vitamin D hormone also controls the growth of the parathyroid gland, aids in the function of the immune system, and contributes to skin cell development.

The most obvious result of vitamin D hormone action is increased calcium and phosphorus deposition in bones. Without adequate calcium and phosphorus, bones weaken and bow under pressure. A child with these symptoms has the disease **rickets.** Symptoms also include enlarged head, joints, and rib cage and a deformed pelvis.

For the prevention of rickets, infant diets, especially those of breastfed infants after their first 9 months of life, should contain a food source or supplement of vitamin D (the latter under a physician's guidance) if sufficient exposure to sunlight is not possible. Keep in mind that supplements should be used very carefully to avoid vitamin D toxicity. Vitamin D fortification of milk has greatly reduced the risk of rickets in children. Today, rickets is most commonly associated with fat malabsorption, such as occurs in children with cystic fibrosis.

An adult disease comparable to rickets is **osteomalacia,** which means *soft bones.* It results when calcium is withdrawn from the bones to make up for inefficient absorption in the intestine or poor conservation by the kidneys. Both of these calcium-rated problems can be caused by vitamin D deficiency. Bones then lose their minerals and become porous and weak and break easily. This leads to fractures in the hip and other bones. A recent study showed that treatment with 10 to 20 micrograms per day (400 to 800 IU per day) of vitamin D (in conjunction with adequate dietary calcium) greatly decreased fracture risk in the elderly in nursing homes.

Osteomalacia in adults occurs most commonly in people with kidney, stomach, gallbladder, or intestinal disease (especially when most of the intestine has been removed) and in people with cirrhosis of the liver. These diseases affect both vitamin D activation and calcium absorption. Adults with limited sun exposure may also develop the disease. Combinations of sun exposure, vitamin D intake, or both can prevent this problem.

Calcitriol
The active hormone form of vitamin D (1,25-dihydroxy-vitamin D).

Vitamin D

↓ action by the liver

25-hydroxy vitamin D

↓ action by kidney

1,25 dihydroxy vitamin D (active hormone form, called calcitriol)

Rickets
A disease characterized by softening of the bones because of low calcium content. This deficiency disease arises from insufficient vitamin D activity in the body.

Osteomalacia
Adult form of rickets. The weakening of the bones that is seen in this disease is caused by low calcium content. A reduction in the amount of the vitamin D hormone activity in the body is the cause.

Dietary Sources of Vitamin D and Needs

Few foods contain appreciable amounts of vitamin D. Rich sources are fatty fish (e.g., sardines and salmon), fortified milk, and some fortified breakfast cereals. In the United States, milk usually is fortified with 10 micrograms (400 IU) per quart. Although eggs, butter, liver, and a few brands of margarine contain some vitamin D, large servings must be eaten to obtain an appreciable amount of the vitamin; thus these foods are not considered significant sources.

Be careful not to confuse osteomalacia with osteoporosis, another type of bone disorder discussed in Chapter 8.

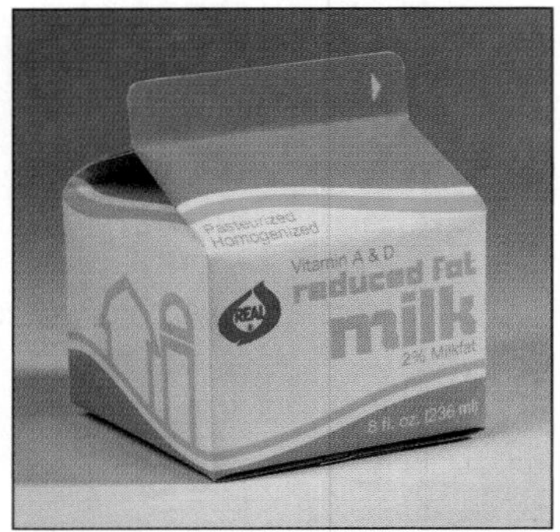

Milk is usually fortified with vitamin D.

The adequate intake (AI) set for vitamin D is 5 micrograms per day (200 IU per day) for people under age 51 and increases two to three times for older Americans. Experts suggest an upper limit of 50 micrograms per day (2000 IU per day). As mentioned, young, light-skinned people can synthesize all the vitamin D needed from casual sun exposure on just the face and hands.

As little as 5 to 10 times vitamin D needs taken regularly can create an overdose, especially in children. Toxicity results in overabsorption of calcium and eventual calcium deposits in the kidneys and other organs. The person also suffers the typical symptoms of high blood calcium: weakness, loss of appetite, diarrhea, vomiting, mental confusion, and increased urine output. Calcium deposits in organs cause metabolic disturbances and cell death. However, vitamin D toxicity does not result from tanning in the sun too long because the body regulates the amount made in the skin.

Dietary sources of vitamin D

Food item and amount	*Vitamin D (IU)*	*Vitamin D (micrograms)*
Baked herring, 3 oz	**1,775**	**44**
Smoked eel, 1 oz	**1,021**	**26**
Baked salmon, 3 oz	**238**	**6**
Canned tuna, 3 oz	**136**	**3.5**
Skim milk, 8 oz	**98**	**2.5**
Sardines, 1 oz	**77**	**2**
Raisin bran cereal, ¾ cup	**42**	**1**
Pork sausage, 1 oz	**31**	**0.75**
Egg yolk, 1	**25**	**0.66**

ConceptCheck

Vitamin A is found in foods as preformed vitamin A and as provitamin A carotenoids. The most fully understood function of vitamin A is its importance in vision. Blindness caused by vitamin A deficiency is a major problem in many parts of the world. Vitamin A is also needed to maintain the health of many types of cells, support the immune system, and promote proper growth and development. Vitamin A may be important in preventing cancer. However, because taking supplements of preformed vitamin A can be toxic, especially in pregnancy, the best recommendation is to focus primarily on eating plenty of provitamin A–rich foods, such as fruits and vegetables.

Vitamin D is a true vitamin only for people who fail to produce enough from sunlight, such as some older people. Using a cholesterol-like substance, people synthesize vitamin D by the action of sunlight on their skin. The vitamin D is later acted on by the liver and kidneys to form the hormone calcitriol. This hormone increases calcium absorption in the intestine and works with another hormone to maintain calcium metabolism in bones and other organs in the body. Rich food sources of vitamin D are fish oils and fortified milk. Megadose vitamin D intake can be quite toxic.

Vitamin E

Health-food literature attests to many benefits of vitamin E, including prevention of arthritis, cataracts, stroke, diabetes, cancer, and heart disease; increased immune function; delayed symptoms of Alzheimer's disease; relief of asthma; and protection of the skin from pollution. Though only some of these benefits are actually supported by reliable studies, American are spending more than $300 million on vitamin E supplements each year. The following section attempts to sort out fact from fiction in the debate over this high-profile vitamin.

Functions of Vitamin E

Acting as a fat-soluble antioxidant, vitamin E resides mostly in cell membranes. As discussed earlier in the book, an antioxidant can form a barrier between a target molecule—an unsaturated fatty acid in a cell membrane, for example—and a compound seeking its electrons (Figure 7–3). The antioxidant donates electrons of hydrogens or both to the electron-seeking compound (called an ***oxidizing compound***) to neutralize it. This protects other molecules or parts of a cell from having electrons nabbed. Note that vitamin C is a water-soluble antioxidant.

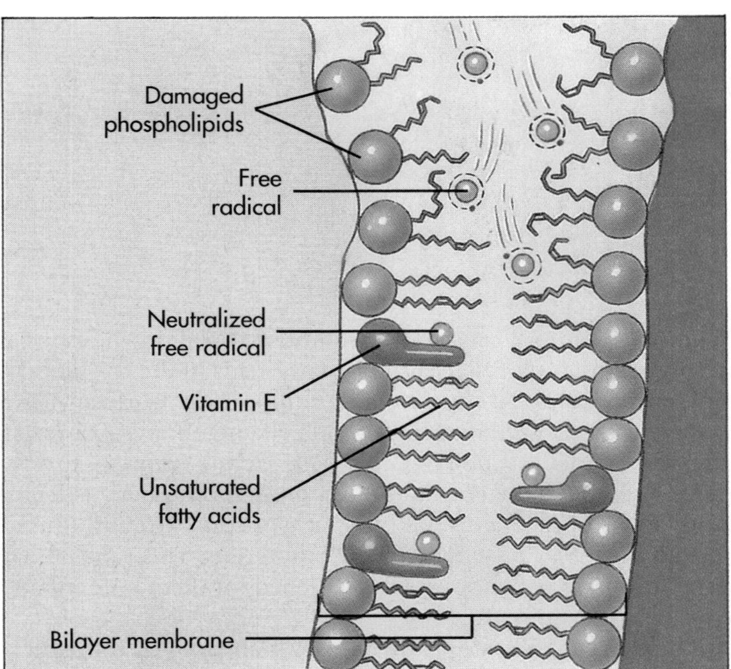

Figure 7–3 *Fat-soluble vitamin E can insert itself into cell membranes, where it helps stop free-radical chain reactions. If not interrupted, these reactions cause extensive oxidative damage to cells and ultimately cell death.*

If vitamin E is not available to do its job, an electron-seeking compound, such as a free radical, can pull electrons from cell membranes, DNA, and other electron-dense cell components. This either alters the cell's DNA, which may increase the risk for cancer, or injures cell membranes, possibly causing the cell to die. Recall that free radicals are highly reactive compounds containing an unpaired electron. This free-radical production is a normal result of cell metabolism and immune-system function. For example, white blood cells generate free radicals as part of their action to stop infection. Some exposure to free radicals, then, is part of life. Overall, however, the body needs to carefully regulate this exposure to avoid their undesirable effects. Once vitamin E acts on free radicals and related compounds, some of it is excreted and some of it is recycled by the addition of an electron from other antioxidants (e.g., vitamin C).

Many other antioxidant systems exist in cells as well. Cells do not rely exclusively on vitamin E for protection from free radicals. Systems also exist in cells to repair molecules (such as DNA) that have been damaged by free radicals.

This discussion raises the question of the relative role of vitamin E in oxidant protection in the body. Experts do not know whether taking vitamin E supplements by otherwise healthy people confers any additional protection against heart disease and cancer than that achieved by improving diet (especially fruit, vegetable and whole-grain intake), performing regular physical activity, not smoking, and maintaining a healthy body weight. This advice has the widest scientific support in the battle against these diseases. Furthermore, the proven benefits of these lifestyle changes are far greater than the postulated benefits of supplemental antioxidants, including vitamin E. Thus, as reviewed in the first Nutrition Insight, even if antioxidant supplements eventually are determined to be effective in preventing heart disease and cancer, they should be used (even in people at high risk) only as an adjunct—not as an alternative—to a healthful lifestyle.

People who have had a heart attack are often prescribed megadose vitamin E therapy (about 400–800 IU per day). One study from England supports this practice, as it found a reduction in further heart attacks with this use. Other studies are in progress to verify the effectiveness of this therapy.

Hemolysis
Destruction of red blood cells. The red blood cell membrane breaks down, allowing cell contents to leak into the fluid portion of the blood.

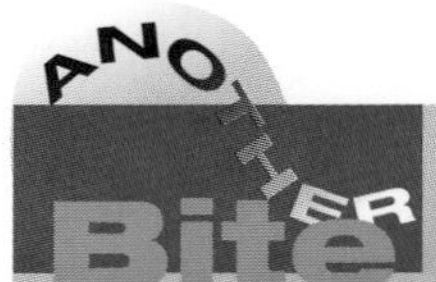

The mineral selenium can spare some of the body's need for vitamin E. Selenium enables an enzyme in cells to decrease the formation of certain oxidizing compounds. Thus an adequate dietary intake of selenium (from cereals, meats, and seafood) reduces the need for vitamin E, whereas low selenium intake in the diet increases it.

Dietary sources of vitamin E

Food item and amount	Vitamin E (α–TE)	Vitamin E (IU)
Sunflower seeds, 1 oz	14	21
Sunflower oil, 1 tbsp	7	10
Almonds, 1 oz	7	10
Safflower oil, 1 tbsp	6	9
Wheat germ, ¼ cup	5	8
Peanut butter, 2 tbsp	3	5
Italian dressing, 2 tbsp	3	5
Avocado, 1	2.7	4
Mango, 1	2	3.5
Mayonnaise, 1 tbsp	0.5	1

A deficiency of vitamin E causes cell membrane breakdown, especially in red blood cells of premature infants. Unsaturated fatty acids in the red blood cell membrane are very sensitive to attack by oxidizing compounds. Because vitamin E neutralizes these agents, it protects the red blood cell membrane from damage. Red blood cell breakage, called ***hemolysis,*** commonly occurs in premature infants because they did not receive sufficient vitamin E from their mothers. The rapid growth of premature infants, coupled with the high oxygen concentration found in infant incubators, greatly increases the stress on red blood cells. This raises the risk of cell damage. Special formulas and supplements designed for premature infants can help compensate for lack of vitamin E.

Finally, vitamin E can help improve vitamin A absorption if the dietary intake of vitamin A is low. In addition, vitamin E is used to metabolize iron in the cell and help maintain nervous tissue, immune, and insulin function.

Vitamin E in Foods and Needs

Major sources of vitamin E are plant oils and foods rich in these; fortified breakfast cereals; some fruits and vegetables, such as asparagus, tomatoes, and green leafy vegetables; eggs; and margarine. The vitamin E in plant oils is used to protect the unsaturated fats present in plant oils. Animal fats and fish oils, on the other hand, have practically no vitamin E (Figure 7–4). The actual vitamin E content of a food depends on how it was harvested, processed, stored, and cooked because vitamin E is very susceptible to destruction by oxygen, metals, light, and especially repeated use of oils in deep-fat frying.

Tocopherols
The chemical name for some forms of vitamin E. The alpha form is the most potent.

Isomers
Different chemical structures for compounds that share the same chemical formula.

The RDA of vitamin E for adults is 8 to 10 milligrams per day of **alpha-tocopherol**, the most active form of what is called vitamin E. This is about the amount we eat each day. To convert from the older IU system, 10 milligrams equals about 10 IU, based on the synthetic (dl **isomer**) form of vitamin E found in most supplements. If vitamin E is from a food source (d isomer) 10 milligrams equals 15 IU, as the food forms of vitamin E are more potent than the synthetic forms.

The likelihood of finding signs of a vitamin E deficiency in the United States among healthy nonsmokers is very low. (For smokers, the most reliable way to improve vitamin E status is to stop smoking. Smoking readily destroys vitamin E, especially in the lungs.) However, the beneficial effects of vitamin E and other antioxidants in counteracting free radical damage in biological systems will be most apparent when viewed on a long-term basis because free radical–related damage to cells occurs over time. Thus current research can't rule out that some benefit may occur from intakes of vitamin E in excess of the RDA. Studies in otherwise healthy people are under way using megadoses from 100 to 800 milligrams (IU) per day.

Excessive amounts of vitamin E can antagonize vitamin K's role in the clotting mechanism. The risk of insufficient blood clotting is especially high if vitamin E is taken in conjunction with anticoagulant medications (this will be discussed in the next section). Otherwise, daily intakes of vitamin E of up to 1200 milligrams (IU) are probably safe for people who are not taking anticoagulant medicines.

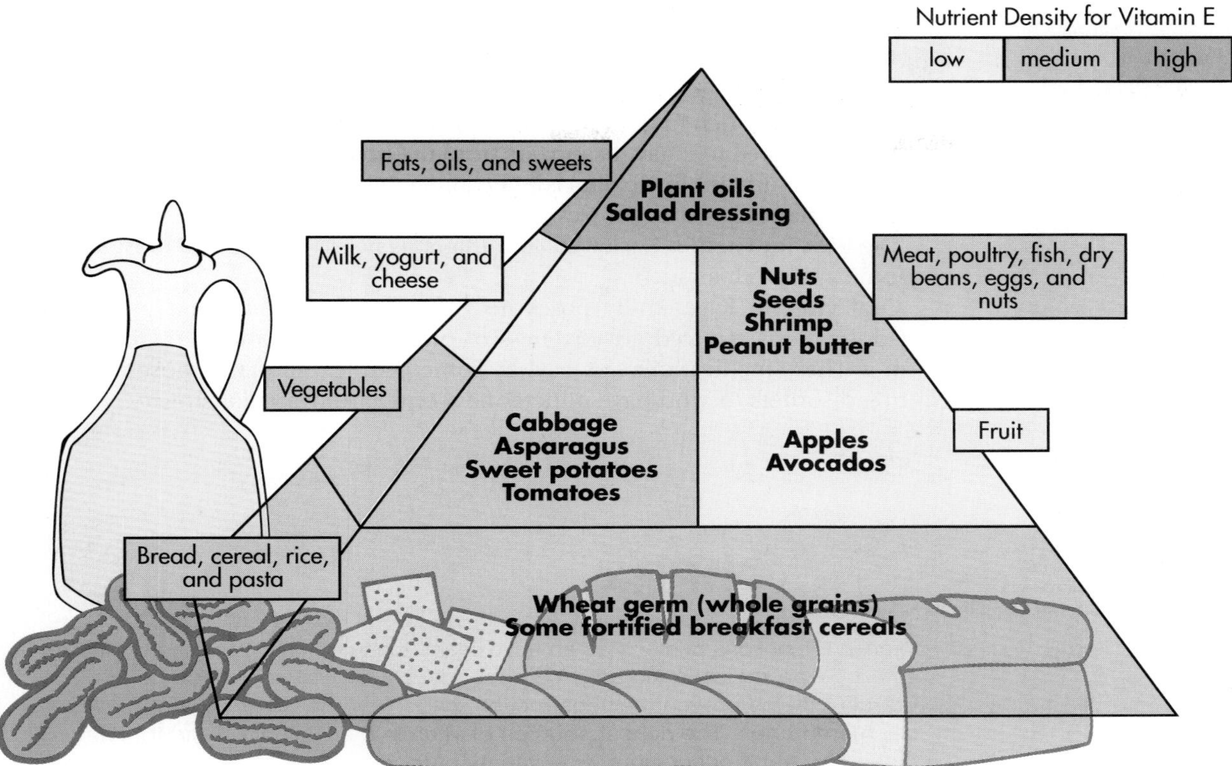

Figure 7–4 *Food sources of vitamin E from the Food Guide Pyramid. Vitamin E is concentrated in plant oils, nuts, seeds, and some vegetables. The background color of each food group indicates the average nutrient density (milligram [or IU] per kcal) for vitamin E in that group.*

Vitamin K

A family of compounds known collectively as vitamin K is found in plants, fish oils, and meats. One form is synthesized by bacteria in the human intestine. These bacteria supply us with some of the vitamin K we absorb every day. Most, however, comes from diet.

Vitamin K is vital for blood clotting. The *K* stands for *koagulation,* as it is spelled in Denmark. This spelling is used because a Danish researcher first noted the relationship between vitamin K and blood clotting. Vitamin K contributes to the synthesis of several blood-clotting factors. Vitamin K also helps form proteins present in bone, muscle, and kidneys, thereby imparting calcium-binding potential to these organs.

Inactive blood-clotting factors

↓ Action of vitamin K

Active blood-clotting factors

A newborn's intestinal tract lacks sufficient vitamin K–producing bacteria to allow for blood to clot effectively if the infant is injured. Therefore vitamin K also is routinely given by injection shortly after birth to bridge the gap until enough bacteria are present to synthesize the vitamin K needed by the infant. In adult, deficiencies of vitamin K have occurred when a person takes antibiotics for a long period and in the presence of severe long-standing fat malabsorption. Long-term antibiotic use also can lead to this problem because it destroys many of the intestinal bacteria that normally account for some of the vitamin K absorbed.

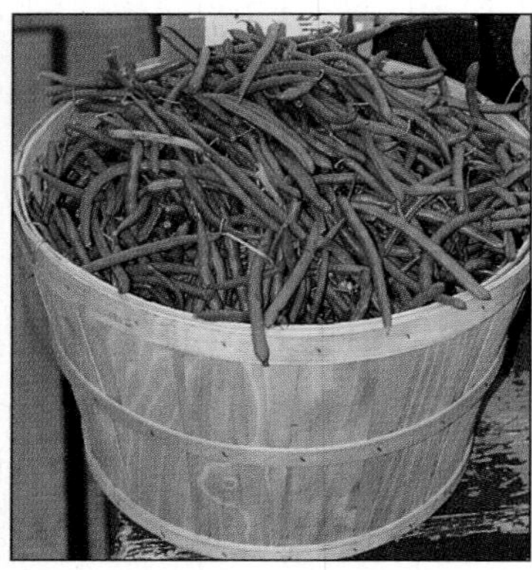

Green beans are a good source of vitamin K.

Dietary sources of vitamin K

Food item and amount	Vitamin K (micro-grams)
Raw cauliflower, 1 cup	**300**
Dried seaweed, .5 oz	**243**
Cooked broccoli, ½ cup	**211**
Raw spinach, 1 cup	**120**
Raw turnip greens, 1 cup	**182**
Fried beef liver, 1 oz	**30**
Egg, 1	**27**
Cooked green beans, ½ cup	**24**
Strawberries, 1 cup	**21**
Skim milk, 1 cup	**9**

Vitamin K in Foods and Needs

Major food sources of vitamin K are liver, green leafy vegetables (for example, kale, turnip greens, cabbage, and spinach), broccoli, peas, and green beans. One reason to consume a diet rich in green vegetables is to obtain sufficient vitamin K. Most vitamin K consumed in a day disappears from the body by the next day. Nevertheless, vitamin K is abundant in a balanced diet, and a deficiency is uncommon. Vitamin K is quite resistant to cooking losses.

The RDA for vitamin K is 60 to 80 milligrams per day for adults. Most Americans consume at least this much.

Oral vitamin K generally poses no risk of toxicity. The main problem with megadose use is reduced effectiveness of oral medications used to reduce blood clotting. These medications are used by some people, especially those with blood-clotting disorders or who have undergone recent cardiovascular surgery.

ConceptCheck

Vitamin E functions primarily as an antioxidant. It can donate electrons to electron-seeking free radical (oxidizing) compounds. By neutralizing these compounds, vitamin E helps prevent cell destruction, especially the destruction of red blood cell membranes. The richest sources of vitamin E are plant oil and foods rich in these oils, but it occurs in a wide variety of foods.

Vitamin K plays a key role in efficient blood clotting; it contributes to the synthesis of certain blood-clotting proteins. In addition, vitamin K increases the calcium-binding potential of some organs. Some of the vitamin K we absorb every day is synthesized by intestinal bacteria; most comes from our diets. The amount in the diet alone generally meets our daily needs. Thus, except for newborns, a deficiency of vitamin K is unlikely when one consumes vegetables on a regular basis.

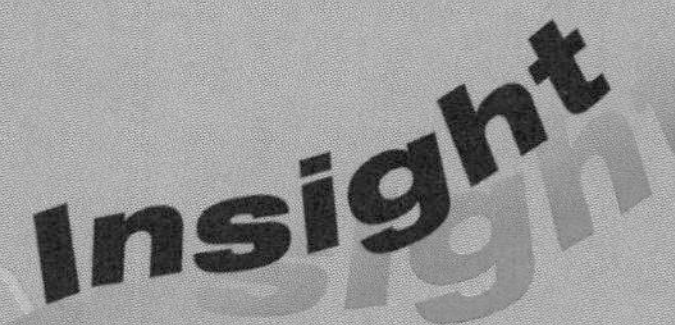

Vitamin Supplements: Who Needs Them?

The question of whether you should take vitamin and/or mineral supplements is not that simple. Typically, nutrition scientists have recommended that supplement use is needed only by a few groups of our population at large. However, over the last few years some reputable nutrition scientists have recommended supplementation for all adults.

This change in philosophy has arisen primarily because Americans have been unwilling to change their food habits, such as include ample fruits and vegetables. This gap leaves many diets low in the vitamin folate—adequate folate status when a woman is pregnant reduces the risk of certain birth defects in her offspring, and as well limits homocysteine in the blood, a likely risk factor for heart disease that can affect all of us. In addition, the committee that set current nutrient needs suggested that adults over age 50 consume vitamin B-12 in a synthetic form, such as that added to breakfast cereals or present in supplements. Synthetic vitamin B-12 is more easily absorbed than that found in food; this helps compensate for the fall in vitamin B-12 absorption typically seen as we age into our later years (see p. 239).

An example of this change in philosophy is a recent editorial in the *New England Journal of Medicine* entitled "Eat Right and Take a Multivitamin." Note that "eat right" is part of the recommendation. All the health-promoting effects of foods cannot be found in a bottle; recall the discussion of phytochemicals in Chapter 2. Few or no phytochemicals are present in supplements.

Overall, supplement use cannot fix a poor diet in all respects. As well, uninformed megadose supplement use can lead to harm and even death. Thus, we are advised to first take a good look at our dietary habits (Table 7–2), and then improve them as possible, as outlined in Chapter 2. Finally, find out which nutrient gaps remain, and identify food sources that can help. Examples could be breakfast cereals to increase folate and vitamin B-6 intake and provide highly absorbable forms of vitamin B-12, calcium-fortified orange juice to increase calcium intake, or milk to increase vitamin D and calcium intake. Only after that should we worry about the need to take supplements (Figure 7–5).

If supplement use is desired, one should discuss this practice with a physician, as some supplements can

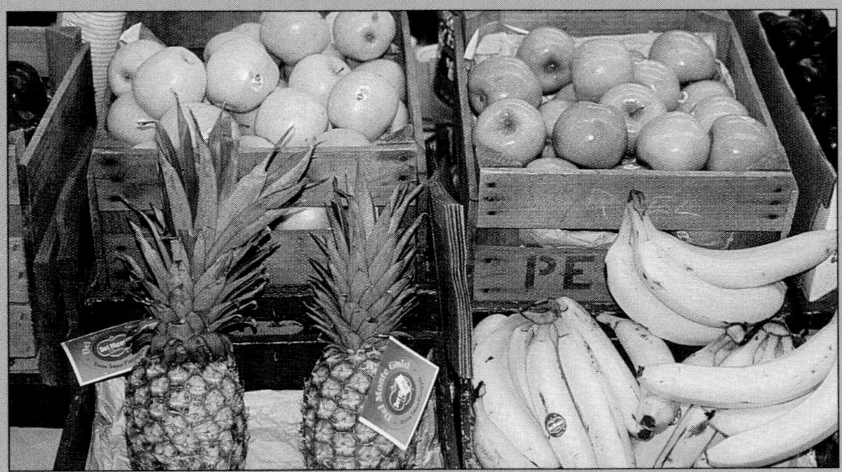

Focus first on foods for meeting nutrient needs.

interfere with certain medicines. For example, vitamin B-6 can offset the action of L-dopa (used in treating Parkinsons's disease), and high intakes of vitamin K or vitamin E alter the action of oral anticoagulants. Remember, you can get too much of a good thing.

Some research is also pointing to the advantages for some of us of taking specific supplements in amounts not possible to achieve by diet alone. Two examples are vitamin E and vitamin B-12. To meet the recommendations arising from this research, one would need to take supplements (Table 7–3). Vitamin B-12 supplement use has a low potential for toxicity and is inexpensive. Some multivitamins sold in grocery stores and drugstores (costing about $0.10 per day) already contain the intended amounts. Vitamin E supplement use is fairly nontoxic for most adults and inexpensive (again about $0.10 per day). Still, we do not have solid information that supports widespread megadose vitamin E supplementation. The intent is to reduce the risk of heart disease and possibly certain forms of cancer and age-related mental decline.

TABLE 7-2

Two Dietary Paths of Adulthood—Which One Looks More Like Your Typical Choices?

Unhealthful	Healthful
BREAKFAST	**BREAKFAST**
Glazed doughnut, 1 Coffee or tea (if desired)	Grapefruit juice, 1 cup Healthy choice cereal, 1 cup 1% milk, ½ cup Coffee or tea (if desired)
SNACK	**SNACK**
	Granola bar
LUNCH	**LUNCH**
Hamburger sandwich French fries, 1 cup Cola, 1½ cups	Hamburger sandwich Medium salad with Thousand Island dressing Fruited low-fat yogurt, 1 cup
SNACK	**SNACK**
	Fig bars, 4 Apple, 1
DINNER	**DINNER**
Pepperoni pizza, 2 slices Lemonade, 1½ cups	Broiled halibut, 4 oz Rotini pasta, 1 cup Soft margarine, 2 tsp Parmesan cheese, 1 tbsp Carrots, ½ cup 1% milk, 1 cup
SNACK	**SNACK**
Potato chips, 1 oz	Cinnamon toast made with whole-wheat bread, 2 slices Hot tea with lemon
2100 kcal 39% energy as fat 13 grams dietary fiber Below adult needs for most vitamins, as well as calcium and iron needs for women	2090 kcal 28% energy as fat 22 grams dietary fiber Meets current established adult nutrient needs for all vitamins, as well as calcium, iron, and other minerals.

Note that focusing on a pattern of low-fat choices based on the Food Guide Pyramid generally increases nutrient adequacy in a diet and also increases the amount of food one can eat.

Large ongoing trials are testing the safety and effectiveness of megadose vitamin E therapy in adult men and women. Some experts recommend that we wait until these trials are finished before recommending widespread megadose vitamin E use. They do not think it is wise to recommend such a practice which has not been proven to be safe and effective using long-term studies. Other experts feel that it is reasonable to recommend this practice, even though we are not absolutely sure it is safe. Some of the public has taken this advice; megadose vitamin E supplement use by adults is common today.

Vitamin and mineral supplements should generally be taken with or just after meals to maximize absorption.

People Most Likely to Need Supplements

Various medical and health-related organizations suggest that the following vitamin and mineral supplementation can be important for certain groups of healthy people:

- Women with excessive bleeding during menstruation may need extra iron.
- Women who are pregnant or breastfeeding may need extra iron, folate, and calcium.
- People with very low energy intakes (less than about 1200 kcal per day) need a range of vitamins and minerals. This is true of some women and older people.
- Some vegetarians may need extra calcium, iron, zinc, and vitamin B-12.
- Newborns, under the direction of a physician, need a single dose of vitamin K.
- People with limited milk intake and sunlight exposure may need extra vitamin D.
- Individuals with lactose intolerance or allergies to dairy products may need extra calcium.

Individuals with certain medical conditions (e.g., vitamin-resistance diseases or long-standing fat malabsorption) and those who use certain medications also may require supplementation with specific vitamins and minerals. Finally, smokers and alcohol abusers may benefit from supplementation, but cessation of these two activities is far more beneficial than any supplementation. Still, a physician should guide all of this therapy.

WHEATLAND CEREAL

Nutrition Facts

Serving Size 1 cup (30g)
Servings Per Container About 11

Amount Per Serving	Wheaties	with ½ cup skim milk
Calories	110	150
Calories from Fat	10	10
	% Daily Value**	
Total Fat 1g*	**1**%	**2**%
Saturated Fat 0g	**0**%	**0**%
Cholesterol 0mg	**0**%	**1**%
Sodium 210mg	**9**%	**11**%
Potassium 120mg	**3**%	**9**%
Total Carbohydrate 23g	**8**%	**10**%
Dietary Fiber 3g	**13**%	**13**%
Sugars 4g		
Other Carbohydrate 16g		
Protein 3g		
Vitamin A	25%	30%
Vitamin C	25%	25%
Calcium	6%	20%
Iron	25%	25%
Vitamin D	10%	25%
Thiamin	25%	30%
Riboflavin	25%	35%
Niacin	25%	25%
Vitamin B_6	25%	25%
Folic Acid	25%	25%
Phosphorus	10%	20%
Magnesium	8%	10%
Zinc	25%	30%
Copper	8%	8%

*Amount in Cereal. A serving of cereal plus milk provides 1g fat, <5mg cholesterol, 270mg sodium, 320mg potassium, 30g carbohydrate (10g sugars), and 7g protein.

**Percent Daily Values are based on a 2,000 calorie diet. Your daily values may be higher or lower depending on your calorie needs:

	Calories:	2,000	2,500
Total Fat	Less than	65g	80g
Sat Fat	Less than	20g	25g
Cholesterol	Less than	300mg	300mg
Sodium	Less than	2,400mg	2,400mg
Potassium		3,500mg	3,500mg
Total Carbohydrate		300g	375g
Dietary Fiber		25g	30g

Figure 7-5
The amount of vitamin and mineral fortification in a typical breakfast cereal. Note that two of the four fat-soluble vitamins are included. Note throughout the chapter that breakfast cereals are a typical source of B vitamins for many of us.

Which Supplement Should You Choose?

Because recent research on a variety of nutrient supplements has revealed a lack of product quality, the USP (United States Pharmacopeia) designation is being extended to an increasing number of nutrient supplements. The USP standards designate strength, quality, purity, packaging, labeling, speed of dissolution, and acceptable length of storage of ingredients for drugs. The purpose of applying them to vitamin and mineral supplements is to establish professionally accepted standards for these products. Consumers who buy nutrient supplements should look for the USP label to ensure quality.

If you decide to take a vitamin and/or mineral supplement, which one should you choose? As a start, choose a supplement that generally contains no more than about 100% of the Daily Values for each vitamin and mineral. Especially avoid products with excess calcium and selenium. Men should use a product that is low in iron or iron free to avoid possible iron overload (see Chapter 8 for details), and older people may want to seek a product that is fortified with extra vitamin B-12 (see Table 7–3). One should read the label carefully to be sure of what is being taken.

Overall, any supplementation should make nutrition sense in terms of nutrient gaps in a diet. A balanced formulation (based on approximately equal % Daily Value quantities) in a supplement is important. Balance will minimize the chance of vitamin and mineral competition as well as possible accompanying toxicity problems, such as the following:

- Excessive intake of vitamin C can cause overabsorption of iron and can contribute to iron toxicity in susceptible people, as well as decrease the ability of certain diagnostic tests to assess the development of diseases.
- Excessive zinc intake can inhibit iron and copper absorption.
- Large amounts of folate can mask signs and symptoms of a vitamin B-12 deficiency (see the other Nutrition Insight in this chapter).

Another consideration in choosing a supplement is avoiding superfluous ingredients, such as para-amino benzoic acid (PABA), hesperidin complex, inositol, bee pollen, and lecithins. These are not needed in our diets. They are especially common in expensive supplements sold in health-food stores and by mail.

TABLE 7-3

Summary of recent recommendations for Daily Vitamin Supplement Use by Adults appearing in reputable publications*

Vitamin D (AI 200 to 600 IU)	Adults with limited sun exposure Adults over age 70 with limited sun exposure Do not exceed 2000 IU total intake†	400 IU (100% DV) 600 IU (150% DV)
Vitamin E (RDA 8 to 10 milligrams)	Healthy adults Adults with diagnosed heart disease Do not exceed 1200 IU	50–400 IU (160%–1300% DV) 400–800 IU (1300%–2600% DV)
Vitamin B-6 (RDA 1.3 to 1.7 milligrams)	Do not exceed 100 milligrams total intake.	2–3 milligrams (100%–150% DV)
Folate (RDA 400 micrograms)	Do not exceed 1 milligram total intake†	400–600 micrograms (100%–150% DV)
Vitamin B-12 (RDA 2.4 micrograms)	Adults over age 50	2–25 micrograms (33%–400% DV)
Vitamin C (RDA 60 milligrams)	Do not exceed 1 gram total intake	250 milligrams (400% DV)

*No specific concern for general supplementation exists for other vitamins. It also should be kept in mind that some respected experts think these recommendations are without merit, as long-term clinical trials have not established safety and effectiveness. They instead emphasize that a varied, balanced diet suffices to maintain health.
†Unless specifically recommended by a physician and then followed for possible toxic effects.
Abbreviations: IU = International Units, DV = Daily Values.
IU values are used because the Daily Values for the specific nutrients are expressed in these units.

Supplements are Regulated Loosely by FDA

Note that unless FDA has evidence that a supplement is inherently dangerous or marked with illegal claims, it will not regulate it closely (see the section on folate for a major exception). Currently, FDA has limited resources and has to act against supplement manufacturers one at a time. So Americans cannot rely on the federal government to protect them from vitamin and mineral supplement overuse. It is best to rely on professional advice.

Like foods, supplements can't carry disease-specific claims unless these assertions are backed by solid scientific evidence and approved by FDA. However, supplements can make general claims about maintaining a healthy body, such as "vitamin A is important to maintain good vision." If so, supplement packages then must alert consumers that these claims have not been evaluated by FDA and that the supplements are not intended to diagnose, treat, cure, or prevent any disease. For consumers this statement should be a red flag that perhaps this supplement is not actually necessary. Note also that some ingredients in herbal products contain chemicals that are naturally harmful, such as certain alkaloids. In other words, "natural" doesn't necessarily mean "safe."

Would the overall health of the nation be improved if our citizens routinely took supplements? Or would this additional intake lead to an unbalanced nutrient state and, in turn, untoward effects? There is no consensus on this question. Consuming a healthy, balanced diet is still the overriding theme, whether supplements are advocated in addition or not at all.

Four web sites to help you evaluate ongoing claims and evaluate safety are:

http://www.acsh.org
http://www.quackwatch.com
http://www.ncahf.org
http://www.nal.usda.gov

The sites are maintained by groups or individuals committed to providing reasoned and authoritative nutrition and health advice to consumers.

THE WATER-SOLUBLE VITAMINS—THE B VITAMINS AND VITAMIN C

Vitamin status can be tested by measuring enzyme activities in red blood cells that require vitamins to function. Such biochemical tests for enzyme activity can be used to determine thiamin, riboflavin, and vitamin B-6 status.

Water-soluble vitamins are more readily excreted than fat-soluble vitamins. Any excess generally ends up in the urine or stool, so consuming the water-soluble vitamins regularly is important. Because they dissolve in water, large amounts of these vitamins can be lost during food processing and preparation. Light cooking such as stir-frying, steaming, and microwaving best preserve vitamin content. A summary of much of what we know about water-soluble vitamins is presented in Table 7–4.

The B Vitamins

The B vitamins are thiamin, riboflavin, niacin, pantothenic acid, biotin, vitamin B-6, folate, and vitamin B-12. Because they often occur in the same foods, a lack of one B vitamin may mean other B vitamins are also low. The B vitamins are all changed into coenzymes, small molecules that interact with enzymes to enable enzymes to function. In essence, the coenzymes contribute to enzyme activity (see Figure 7–1).

As coenzymes, the B vitamins play many key roles in metabolism. The metabolic pathways used by carbohydrates, fats, and amino acids together require input from B vitamins. This makes many B vitamins interdependent because they participate in the same processes (Figure 7–6).

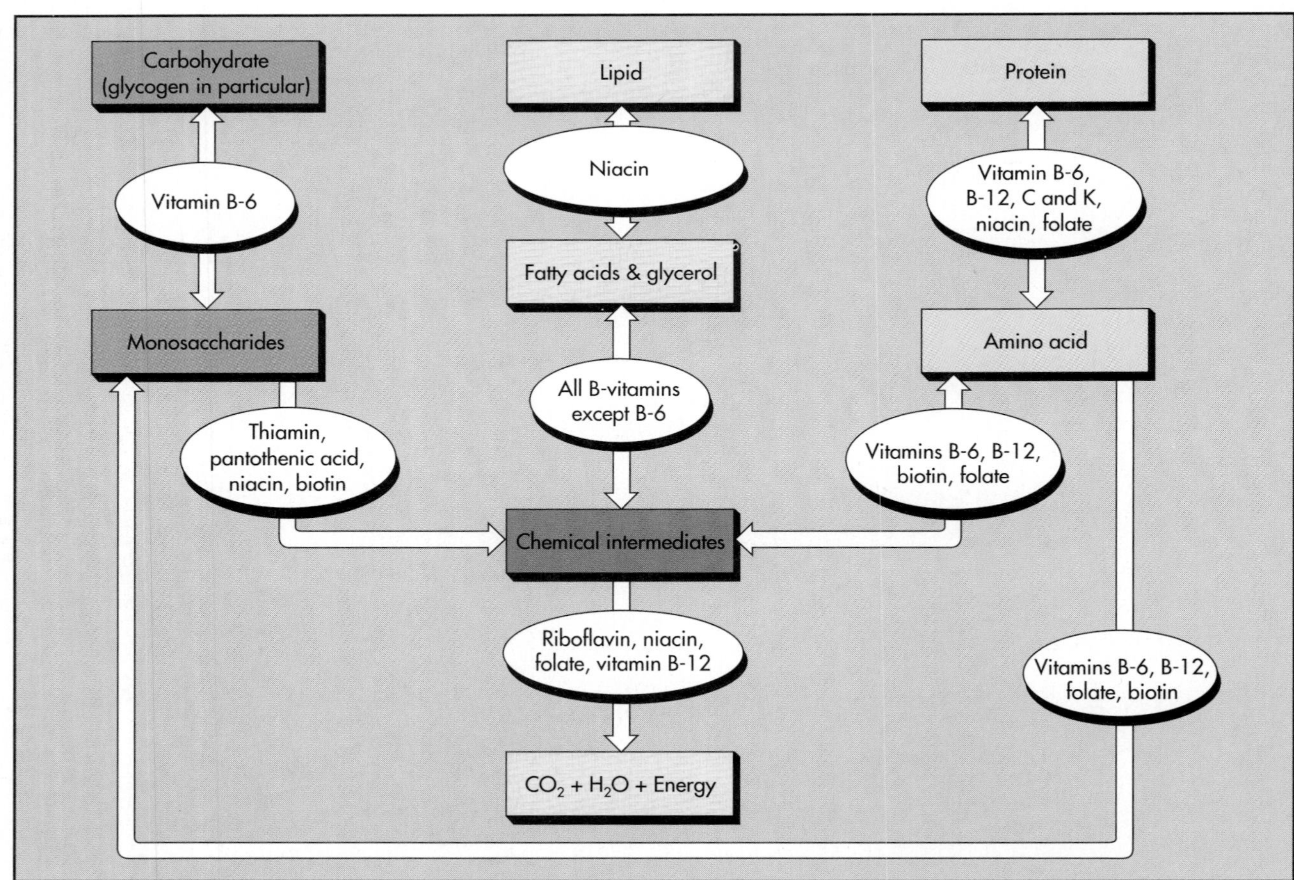

Figure 7–6 *Examples of metabolic pathways for which vitamins are essential. The metabolism of energy-yielding nutrients requires vitamin input.*

TABLE 7-4

A Summary of the Water-Soluble Vitamins, Their Functions, Deficiency Conditions, and Food Sources

Name	Major functions	Deficiency symptoms	People most at risk	Dietary sources*	RDA or AI	Toxicity
Thiamin	Coenzyme involved in carbohydrate metabolism; nerve function	Beriberi: nervous tingling, poor coordination edema, heart changes, weakness	People with alcoholism or in poverty	Sunflower seeds, pork, whole and enriched grains, dried beans, peas, brewer's yeast	1.1–1.2 milligrams	None possible from food
Riboflavin	Coenzyme involved in energy metabolism	Inflammation of mouth and tongue, cracks at corners of the mouth, eye disorders	Possibly people on certain medications if no dairy products consumed	Milk, mushrooms, spinach, liver, enriched grains	1.1–1.3 milligrams	None reported
Niacin	Coenzyme involved in energy metabolism, fat synthesis, fat breakdown	Pellagra: diarrhea, dermatitis, dementia	Severe poverty where corn is the dominant food; alcoholism	Mushrooms, bran, tuna, salmon, chicken, beef, liver, peanuts, enriched grains	14–16 milligrams	Toxicity can begin at over 35 milligrams (flushing of skin especially seen at over 100 milligrams per day)
Pantothenic acid	Coenzyme involved in energy metabolism, fat synthesis, fat breakdown	Tingling in hands, fatigue, headache, nausea	People with alcoholism	Mushrooms, liver, broccoli, eggs; most foods have some	5 milligrams	None
Biotin	Coenzyme involved in glucose production, fat synthesis	Dermatitis, tongue soreness anemia, depression	People with alcoholism	Cheese, egg yolks, cauliflower, peanut butter, liver	30 micrograms	Unknown
Vitamin B-6,† pyridoxine, and other forms	Coenzyme involved in protein metabolism, neurotransmitter synthesis, hemoglobin synthesis, many other functions	Headache, anemia, convulsions, nausea, vomiting, flaky skin, sore tongue	Adolescent and adult women; people on certain medications; alcoholism	Animal protein foods, spinach, broccoli, bananas, salmon, sunflower seeds	1.3–1.7 milligrams	Nerve destruction at doses over 200 milligrams
Folate† (folic acid)	Coenzyme involved in DNA synthesis, other functions	Megaloblastic anemia, inflammation of tongue, diarrhea, poor growth, depression	People with alcoholism, pregnancy, people on certain medications	Green leafy vegetables, orange juice, organ meats, sprouts, sunflower seeds	400 micrograms	None likely; nonprescription vitamin dosage is controlled by FDA
Vitamin B-12† (cobalamins)	Coenzyme involved in folate metabolism, nerve function, other functions	Macrocytic anemia, poor nerve function	Elderly people because of poor absorption; vegans, people with AIDS	Animal foods, especially organ meats, oysters, clams (not natural in plants)	2.4 micrograms	None
Vitamin C (ascorbic acid)	Connective tissue synthesis, hormone synthesis, neurotransmitter synthesis	Scurvy: poor wound healing, pinpoint hemorrhages, bleeding gums	People with alcoholism, elderly who eat poorly	Citrus fruits, strawberries, broccoli, greens	60 milligrams	Doses over 1 gram cause diarrhea and can alter some diagnostic tests

*Fortified breakfast cereals are good sources for most of these vitamins and a common source of B vitamins for many of us.
†These vitamins also participate in homocysteine metabolism, which in turn limits its ability to promote heart disease.

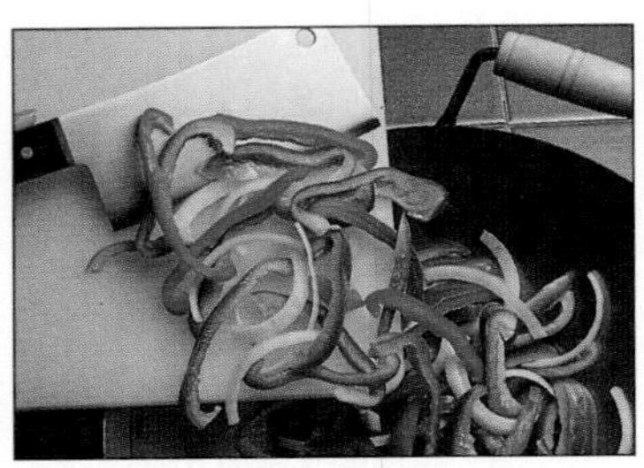

Rapid cooking of vegetables in minimal fluids aids in preserving vitamin content. Stir-frying is one possible method to use.

After being ingested, the B vitamins are first broken down from their coenzyme forms into free vitamins in the stomach and small intestine. The vitamins are then absorbed, primarily in the small intestine. Typically, about 50% to 90% of the B vitamins in the diet are absorbed. Once inside cells the coenzyme forms are resynthesized. Because we make them when needed, there is no need to consume the coenzyme forms themselves.

B Vitamin Intakes of Americans

The nutritional health of most Americans with regard to the B vitamins is generally good. Typical diets in the United States contain plentiful and varied natural sources of these vitamins. In addition, many common foods, such as breakfast cereals, are fortified with one or more of the water-soluble vitamins. In some developing countries, however, deficiencies of the water-soluble vitamins are more common, and the resulting deficiency diseases pose significant public-health problems. (A detailed discussion of nutritional deficiencies worldwide is presented in Chapter 16.)

Despite the generally good B vitamin status of Americans, marginal deficiencies of the water-soluble vitamins may occur in some Americans and others in the western world, especially older people who eat little food. The long-term effects of such marginal deficiencies are as yet unknown, but increased risk of heart disease, cancer, and cataracts of the eye is suspected. However, in the short run, such a marginal deficiency in most people likely leads only to fatigue or other bothersome and unspecific physical effects. With rare exceptions, healthy adults do not develop the more serious B vitamin deficiency diseases from diet alone. The main exceptions are people with alcoholism. The extremely unbalanced diets of some people with alcoholism, in combination with alcohol-induced alteration of vitamin absorption and metabolism, create significant risks for some serious nutrient deficiencies (see the Nutrition Issue in Chapter 14).

In the milling of grains, the seeds are crushed and the germ, bran, and husk layers are removed. This process leaves just the starch-containing endosperm, used to make flour, bread, and cereal products. Since the discarded fractions are rich in many nutrients, the time-honored milling process leads to loss of vitamins and minerals. To counteract this nutrient loss, bread and cereal products made from milled grains are enriched with four B vitamins—thiamin, riboflavin, niacin, and folate—and with the mineral iron. This fortification helps protect Americans from the common deficiency diseases associated with a dietary lack of the added nutrients, but still leaves the products with proportionately less vitamin B-6, magnesium, and zinc than in the whole grains. This is one reason nutrition experts advocate regular consumption of whole-grain products, such as whole-wheat bread, rather than consuming mostly enriched grain products.

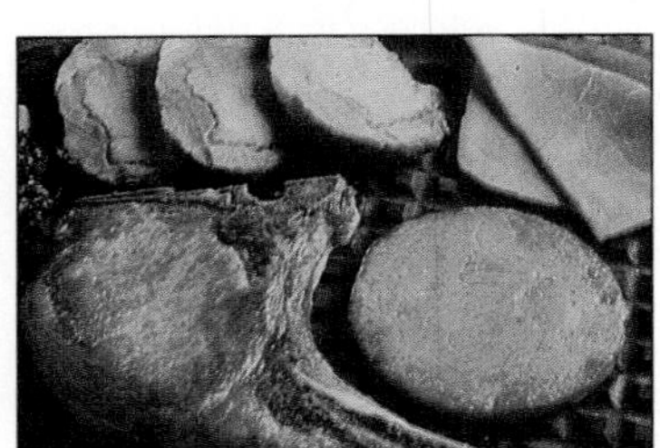

Pork is a good source of thiamin.

Thiamin

Thiamin (formerly called *vitamin B-1*) is used, among other purposes, to release energy from carbohydrate. Its coenzyme participates in reactions in which a carbon dioxide (CO_2) is lost from a larger molecule. This reaction is particularly important in metabolizing glucose, the primary nutrient yielded from carbohydrate digestion (see Figure 7-6).

The thiamin deficiency disease is called ***beriberi,*** a word that means "I can't, I can't" in the Sri Lankan language of Sinhalese. The symptoms include weakness, loss of appetite, irritability, nervous tingling throughout the body, poor arm and leg coordination, and deep muscle pain in the calves. A person with beriberi often develops an enlarged heart and sometimes severe edema.

Beriberi
The thiamin deficiency disorder characterized by muscle weakness, loss of appetite, nerve degeneration, and sometimes edema.

Beriberi is seen where rice is a staple and the polished (white) form is consumed rather than the brown (whole-grain) form. In most parts of the world, brown rice has had its bran and germ layer removed to make white rice, a poor source of thiamin, unless later enriched.

Beriberi results when glucose, the primary fuel for brain and nerve cells, is poorly metabolized. Because the thiamin coenzyme participates in glucose metabolism, body functions associated with brain and nerve action quickly show signs of a thiamin deficiency. Symptoms of depression and weakness can be seen after only 10 days on a thiamin-free diet. Thiamin probably also contributes in other ways to nerve function.

Dietary sources of thiamin

Food item and amount	*Thiamin (milligrams)*
Pork chop, 4 oz	**0.9**
Soy milk, 8 oz	**0.7**
Brewer's yeast, 2 tbsp	**0.6**
Wheat germ, ¼ cup	**0.5**
Ham slices, 2 oz	**0.5**
Canadian bacon, 2 oz	**0.5**
Baked acorn squash, 1 cup	**0.4**
Peanuts, ¼ cup	**0.3**
Orange juice, 8 oz	**0.2**
Vegetarian baked beans, ½ cup	**0.2**

Thiamin in Foods and Needs

Major sources of thiamin include pork products, whole grains (wheat germ), fortified breakfast cereals, enriched grains, green beans, milk, organ meats, peanuts, dried beans, and seeds (Figure 7–7).

The adult RDA for thiamin is 1.1 to 1.2 milligrams per day. Average daily intakes for men exceed this by 50%, and women generally meet the RDA. Some groups, such as poor people and older people, may barely meet their needs for thiamin. A diet dominated by highly processed and unenriched foods, sugar, fat, and alcohol also creates a potential for thiamin deficiency. Oral thiamin supplements are essentially nontoxic since excess thiamin is rapidly lost in the urine.

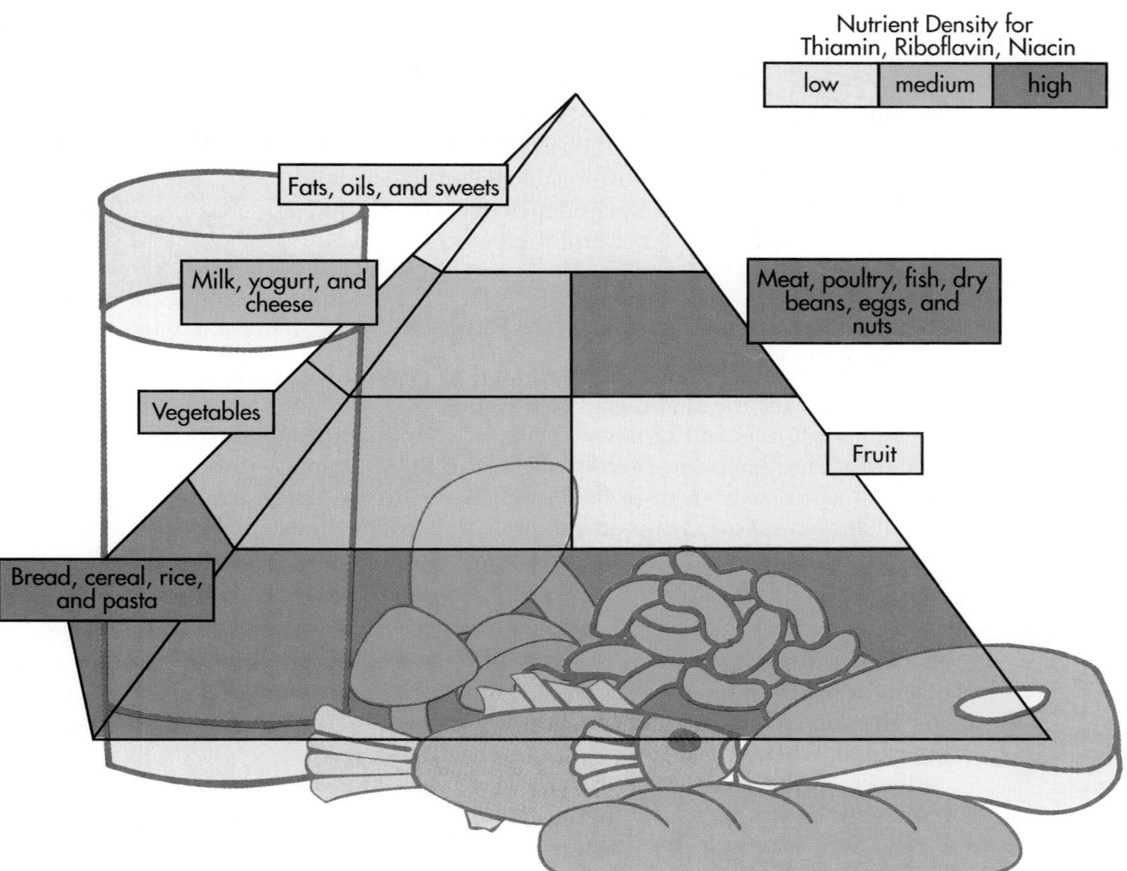

Figure 7–7 *Food sources of thiamin, riboflavin, and niacin from the Food Guide Pyramid. The meat, poultry, fish, dry beans, eggs, and nuts group and the bread, cereal, rice, and pasta group are especially rich sources of these nutrients. The background color of each food group indicates the average nutrient density (milligram per kcal) for the nutrients in that group.*

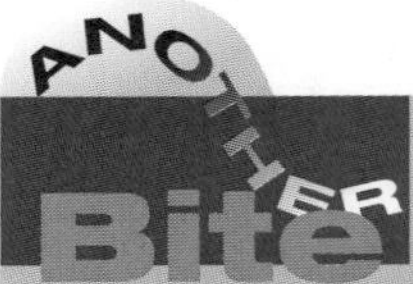

People with alcoholism are at the greatest risk for thiamin deficiency because absorption and use of thiamin are profoundly diminished and excretion is increased by alcohol consumption. Furthermore, the low-quality diet that often accompanies severe alcoholism makes matters worse. Since there is limited thiamin storage in the body, an alcoholic binge lasting 1 to 2 weeks may quickly deplete already diminished amounts of the vitamin and result in deficiency symptoms.

Riboflavin

The name *riboflavin* comes from its yellow color (*flavus* means yellow in Latin). Riboflavin was formerly referred to as *vitamin B-2*.

The coenzymes of riboflavin participate in many energy-yielding metabolic pathways. When cells form cellular energy using oxygen-requiring pathways, such as when fats are broken down and burned for energy, the coenzymes of riboflavin are used (see Figure 7–6). Some vitamin and mineral metabolism also requires riboflavin. In addition, because of its link to activity of certain enzymes, riboflavin has an antioxidant role in the body.

Dermatitis
Inflammation of the skin.

The symptoms associated with riboflavin deficiency include inflammation of the mouth and tongue, **dermatitis,** cracking of tissue around the corners of the mouth (called *cheilosis*), various eye disorders, sensitivity to the sun, and confusion. The first symptoms of a deficiency are inflammation of the mouth and tongue. All symptoms associated with deficiency develop after approximately 2 months on a riboflavin-poor diet. In addition, riboflavin deficiencies probably do not exist by themselves. Instead, a riboflavin deficiency would occur with deficiencies of niacin, thiamin, and vitamin B-6 because these nutrients often occur in the same foods.

Riboflavin in Foods and Needs

Dietary sources of riboflavin

Food item and amount	*Riboflavin (milligrams)*
Fried beef liver, 1 oz	**1.2**
Steamed oysters, 10	**1.1**
Brewer's yeast, 2 tbsp	**0.7**
Low-fat yogurt, 1 cup	**0.5**
Braunschweiger sausage, 1	**0.4**
Milk, 8 oz	**0.4**
Buttermilk, 8 oz	**0.4**
Cooked spinach, 1 cup	**0.3**
Raw mushrooms, 1 cup	**0.3**
Boiled egg, 1	**0.3**

Major sources of riboflavin are milk and milk products, enriched grains, fortified breakfast cereals, meat, and eggs (see Figure 7–7).

The adult RDA of riboflavin is 1.1 to 1.3 milligrams per day. On average, daily intakes of riboflavin are slightly above the RDA. People with alcoholism are the ones who primarily risk riboflavin deficiency because they generally eat nutrient-poor diets. No specific symptoms indicate that riboflavin taken in megadoses is toxic.

Niacin

Niacin is actually composed of a pair of related compounds. Both can function as niacin in the body. Niacin was formerly referred to as *vitamin B-3*.

The coenzyme forms of niacin function in many cellular metabolic pathways. In general, when cell energy is being utilized, a niacin coenzyme is used. Synthetic pathways in the cell—those that make new compounds—also often use a niacin coenzyme. This is especially true for fat synthesis (see Figure 7–6).

Because almost every cellular metabolic pathway uses a niacin coenzyme, a deficiency causes widespread changes in the body. The entire group of symptoms is known as ***pellagra,*** which means rough or painful skin. The symptoms of the disease are **dementia,** diarrhea, and dermatitis (especially on areas of skin exposed to the sun). Later, death often results. Early symptoms include poor appetite, weight loss, and weakness.

Dementia
A general loss or decrease in mental function.

Pellagra became epidemic in southern Europe in the early 1700s when corn, a poor source, became a staple food. It became a major problem in the southeastern United States in the late 1800s and persisted until the late 1930s when standards of living and diets improved. In fact, pellagra is the only dietary deficiency disease ever to reach epidemic proportions in the United States. Today, pellagra is rare in Western societies.

Dietary sources of niacin

Food item and amount	*Niacin (milligrams)*
Steak, 4 oz	**5.6**
Roast turkey, 3 oz	**4.9**
Roast chicken, 3 oz	**4.8**
Ground beef patty, 3 oz	**4.5**
Broiled halibut, 3 oz	**4.2**
Canned tuna, 3 oz	**4.1**
Salmon, 3 oz	**4.0**
Peanuts, ½ cup	**3.1**
Fried beef liver, 1 oz	**1.8**
Raw mushrooms, ½ cup	**1.4**

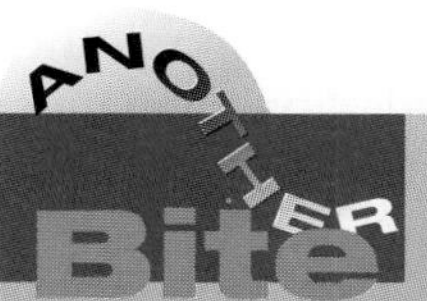

Niacin in corn is bound by a protein that hampers its absorption. Soaking corn in an alkaline solution, such as lime water (water with calcium hydroxide), releases bound niacin and renders it more usable. Hispanic people traditionally soak corn in lime water before making tortillas. This treatment is one reason Hispanic populations never suffered much pellagra.

Niacin in Foods and Needs

Major sources of niacin are poultry, fortified breakfast cereals, beef, wheat bran, tuna and other fish, asparagus, and peanuts (see Figure 7–7). Coffee and tea also contribute some niacin to the diet. Niacin is very heat stable; little is lost in cooking.

Besides the preformed niacin found in protein foods, every 60 milligrams of the amino acid tryptophan is metabolized into about 1 milligram of niacin.

The adult RDA of niacin is 14 to 16 milligrams per day. The RDA is expressed as niacin equivalents to account for niacin received intact from the diet, as well as that made from tryptophan. Intakes of niacin by adults are slightly greater than the RDA, without considering the contribution from tryptophan. Note that tables of food values also ignore this contribution. People with alcoholism and those with rare disorders of tryptophan metabolism are generally the only groups to show a niacin deficiency.

Niacin begins to become toxic at intakes of 35 milligrams of the nicotinic acid form. Effects include headache, itching, and increased blood flow to the skin, causing a general blood vessel dilation or flushing in various parts of the body, especially when intakes are above 100 milligrams per day.

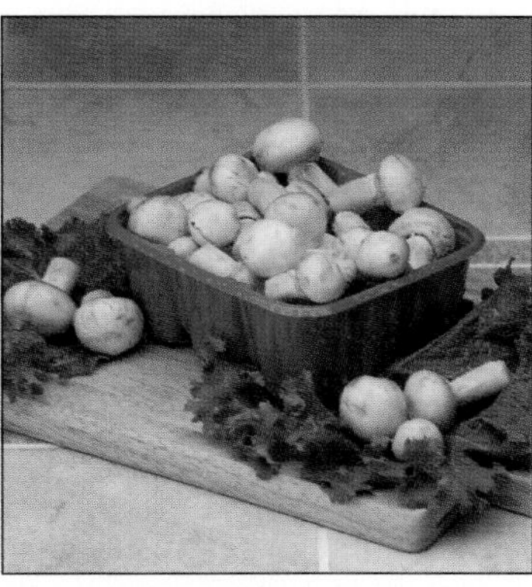

Mushrooms are a good source of niacin.

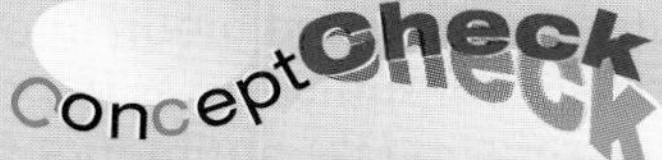

The B vitamins thiamin, niacin, and riboflavin are all important in the metabolism of carbohydrates, proteins, and fats. Energy metabolism in particular requires adequate amounts of coenzymes of these three vitamins. Enriched grains are adequate sources of all three vitamins. Otherwise, pork is an excellent source of thiamin, milk is an excellent source of riboflavin, and protein foods in general—such as chicken—are excellent sources of niacin. Deficiencies of all three vitamins can occur with alcoholism; a thiamin deficiency is the most likely.

Pantothenic Acid

Like the other B vitamins, pantothenic acid helps release energy from carbohydrates, fats, and protein. By forming its coenzyme, called coenzyme A, pantothenic acid

Dietary sources of pantothenic acid

Food item and amount	Pantothenic acid (milligrams)
Sunflower seeds, ¼ cup	**2.3**
Fried beef liver, 1 oz	**1.7**
Raw mushrooms, 1 cup	**1.5**
Brewer's yeast, 2 tbsp	**1.4**
Peanuts, ½ cup	**1.3**
Yogurt, 1 cup	**1.2**
Baked acorn squash, 1 cup	**1.2**
Roast chicken, 3 oz	**0.8**
Cooked broccoli, 1 cup	**0.8**
Milk, 8 oz	**0.8**

allows many energy-yielding metabolic reactions to occur. Coenzyme A makes other molecules much more reactive. For example, coenzyme A must activate fatty acids before they can break down to yield energy. It is also used in the beginning steps of fatty acid synthesis.

Pantothenic acid is so widespread in foods that a nutritional deficiency among healthy people who eat varied diets is unlikely. A full-blown deficiency is so rare that it has possibly been observed only during World War II. Prisoners in the Philippines and Japan displayed a "burning foot" syndrome described as numbness and tingling in the toes and burning and shooting pains in the feet, in addition to other mental and nervous system problems. Other symptoms may include tingling hands, fatigue, headache, sleep disturbances, nausea, and abdominal distress.

Pantothenic Acid in Foods and Needs

Pantothenic acid is present in all foods. *Pantothen* actually means "from every side" in Greek. Good sources of pantothenic acid are sunflower seeds, mushrooms, peanuts, and eggs. Other sources are meat, milk, and many vegetables.

The AI set for pantothenic acid is 5 milligrams per day for adults. The average intake for people in the United States is about 6 milligrams of pantothenic acid per day. A deficiency of pantothenic acid might occur in alcoholism along with a very nutrient-deficient diet. However, the symptoms would probably be hidden among deficiencies of thiamin, riboflavin, vitamin B-6, and folate, so the pantothenic acid deficiency might be unrecognizable. No toxicity is known for pantothenic acid.

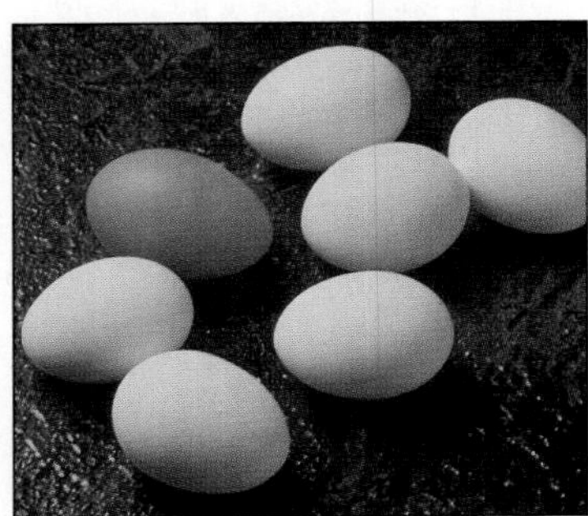

Egg yolks are a source of biotin for many of us.

Biotin

Biotin exists in two active forms in foods. In the ultimate coenzyme form, biotin acts in fat and carbohydrate metabolism.

Biotin assists the addition of carbon dioxide to other compounds. By doing so, it promotes the synthesis of glucose, fatty acids, and DNA, while helping to break down certain amino acids. Symptoms of biotin deficiency include a scaly inflammation of the skin, changes in the tongue and lips, decreased appetite, nausea, vomiting, a form of anemia, depression, muscle pain and weakness, and poor growth.

Biotin in Foods and Needs

Cauliflower, egg yolks, peanuts, and cheese are good sources of biotin. Intestinal bacteria synthesize and supply some biotin, making a biotin deficiency unlikely. However, scientists are not sure how much of the bacteria-synthesized biotin in our intestines is actually absorbed. If the intestinal bacteria are not sufficient, as in people who are missing a large part of the small intestine or who take antibiotics for many months, special attention should be paid to meeting biotin needs. A protein called ***avidin*** in raw egg whites binds biotin and inhibits its absorption. Consuming many raw egg whites eventually leads to the deficiency disease.

The AI for biotin is 30 milligrams per day for adults. Our food supply is thought to provide 100 to 300 milligrams per person per day. Biotin is relatively nontoxic. Large doses have been given over an extended period without harmful side effects to children who exhibit defects in biotin metabolism.

Dietary sources of biotin

Food item and amount	Biotin (micrograms)
Peanut butter, 2 tbsp	**30.1**
Peanuts, ¼ cup	**26.3**
Chili, 1 cup	**9.0**
Boiled egg, 1	**8.0**
Toasted wheat germ, ¼ cup	**7.0**
Rye-Krisp, .5 oz	**6.8**
Wheat bran, ¼ cup	**6.4**
Egg noodles, 1 cup	**4.0**
Swiss cheese, 2 oz	**2.2**
Cauliflower, 1 cup	**1.6**

Vitamin B-6

Vitamin B-6 is actually a family of three compounds. All can be changed to the active vitamin B-6 coenzyme. The general vitamin name is *pyridoxine.*

Functions of Vitamin B-6

The coenzymes of vitamin B-6 are needed for the activity of numerous enzymes involved in carbohydrate, protein, and fat metabolism. Because vitamin B-6 is needed in so many areas of metabolism, a deficiency results in widespread symptoms, such as depression, vomiting, skin disorders, irritation of the nerves, and impaired immune response.

A key function of vitamin B-6 concerns protein because metabolizing any amino acid requires the vitamin B-6 coenzyme. By helping to split the nitrogen group ($-NH_2$) from an amino acid, the coenzyme participates in reactions that allow a cell to synthesize nonessential (dispensable) amino acids.

Another important role of vitamin B-6 is the synthesis of many neurotransmitters. **Neurotransmitters** allow nerve cells to communicate with each other and with other body cells. In the 1950s, infants fed oversterilized commercial formulas developed vitamin B-6 deficiency symptoms, particularly convulsions. Heat destroyed vitamin B-6 in the formulas. Today, manufacturers are more careful to maintain adequate vitamin B-6 content in formulas.

The vitamin B-6 coenzyme is important for the synthesis of hemoglobin, the oxygen-carrying part of the red blood cell. Vitamin B-6 is also necessary for the synthesis of white blood cells, which perform a major role in the immune system.

Finally, vitamin B-6 plays a role in the recycling of homocysteine to the amino acid cysteine. This is important since elevated homocysteine in the blood likely increases the risk for heart disease.

Neurotransmitter
A compound made by a nerve cell that allows for communication between it and other cells.

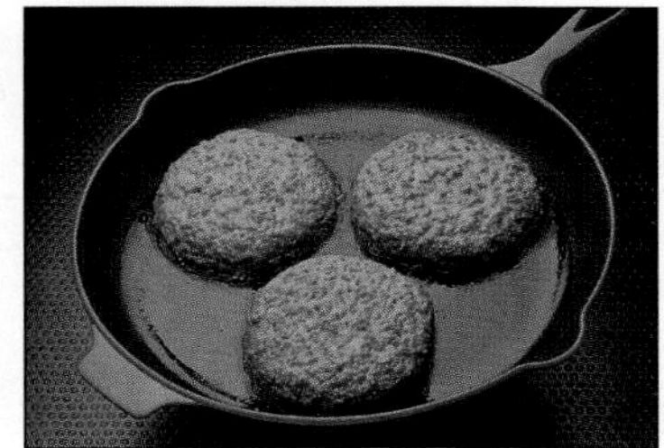

Meats, along with other animal products, are a good source of vitamin B-6.

Vitamin B-6 in Foods and Needs

Major sources of vitamin B-6 are animal products, fortified breakfast cereals, potatoes, and milk. Other sources are such fruits and vegetables as bananas, cantaloupe, broccoli, and spinach (Figure 7–8). Overall, animal sources are the most reliable because the vitamin B-6 they contain is more absorbable than that in plant foods. Food tables listing vitamin B-6 are often incomplete because measuring this vitamin in foods is difficult.

The adult RDA of vitamin B-6 is 1.3 to 1.7 milligrams per day. The RDA is set high in response to high protein intakes (which leads to more protein metabolism) of people in the United States. Average daily consumption of vitamin B-6 for men and women is about equal to the RDA. Reliably separating adequate vitamin B-6 status from an abnormal or deficient state is not yet possible. Still, scientists are concerned that the vitamin B-6 status of some women and older people in general warrants more attention.

Athletes may need slightly more vitamin B-6 because of their increased use of glycogen as a fuel (glycogen metabolism requires vitamin B-6), their increased use of amino acids for fuel, and their high protein intakes. Still, the protein foods in their diets should supply any extra vitamin B-6 needed.

People with alcoholism are susceptible to a vitamin B-6 deficiency because a metabolite formed in ethanol metabolism can displace the coenzyme form from enzymes, increasing its tendency to be destroyed. In addition, alcohol decreases the absorption of vitamin B-6 and decreases the synthesis of its coenzyme form. Cirrhosis and hepatitis (both of which may accompany alcoholism) also disable liver tissue from actively metabolizing vitamin B-6, which in turn decreases synthesis of its coenzyme form.

Dietary sources of vitamin B-6

Food item and amount	*Vitamin B-6 (milligrams)*
Brewer's yeast, 2 tbsp	**0.81**
Salmon, 3 oz	**0.80**
Banana, 1	**0.68**
Avocado, 1	**0.56**
Roast turkey, 3 oz	**0.48**
Roast chicken, 3 oz	**0.48**
Baked potato, 1	**0.47**
Fried beef liver, 1 oz	**0.41**
Watermelon, 1½ cup	**0.33**
Sunflower seeds, ¼ cup	**0.26**

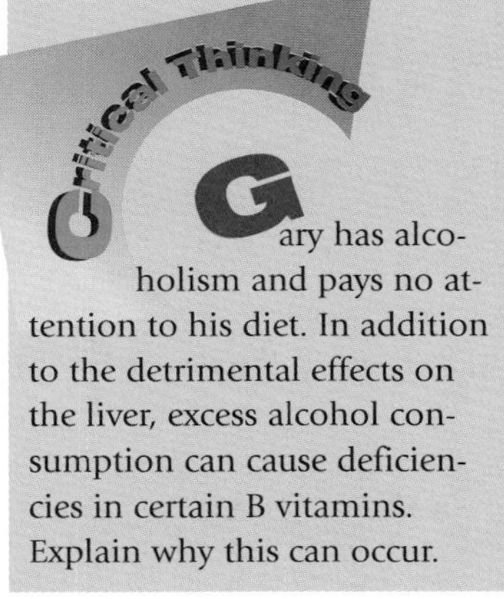

Gary has alcoholism and pays no attention to his diet. In addition to the detrimental effects on the liver, excess alcohol consumption can cause deficiencies in certain B vitamins. Explain why this can occur.

Toxicity of Vitamin B-6

With regard to toxicity, intakes of 2 to 6 grams of vitamin B-6 per day for 2 or more months can lead to irreversible nerve damage, as can long-term intakes of

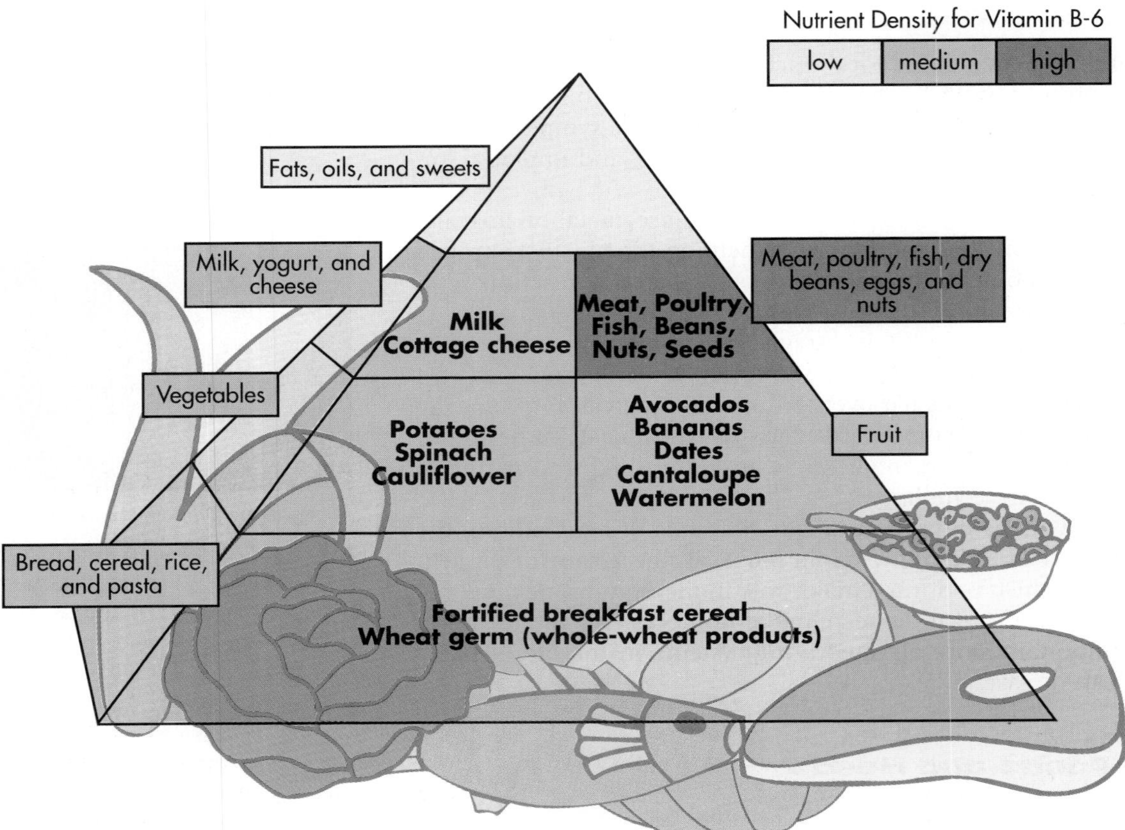

Figure 7–8 *Food sources of vitamin B-6 from the Food Guide Pyramid. The meat, poultry, fish, dry beans, eggs, and nuts group is an especially rich source of this nutrient. The background color of each food group indicates the average nutrient density (milligram per kcal) for vitamin B-6 in that group.*

200 milligrams per day. Use, or more appropriately, misuse, of such megadoses of vitamin B-6 has occurred among body builders and in women attempting to treat themselves for **premenstrual syndrome.** Both uses of vitamin B-6 are ineffective. Symptoms include walking difficulties and hand and foot numbness. Some nerve damage in individual sensory neurons is probably reversible, but damage to the ganglia (where many nerve fibers converge) is probably permanent. With 500 milligram tablets of vitamin B-6 available in health-food stores, taking a toxic dose is quite easy. The Upper Limit for vitamin B-6 intake is set at 100 milligrams per day by the recent DRI revisions.

ConceptCheck

Pantothenic acid and biotin both participate in the metabolism of carbohydrate and fat. A deficiency of either vitamin is unlikely; pantothenic acid is found widely in foods, and our need for biotin is partially met by intestinal synthesis from bacteria. Vitamin B-6 is important for protein metabolism, neurotransmitter synthesis, homocysteine metabolism and other key metabolic functions. Headache, a form of anemia, nausea, and vomiting can result from a vitamin B-6 deficiency. Increased risk of heart disease is also likely. Animal protein foods, fortified breakfast cereals, broccoli, spinach, and bananas are some food sources.

Folate

In the past, folate was referred to as *folic acid* and *folacin*. Today the term *folate* is preferred because it encompasses the variety of food forms of the vitamin.

Functions of Folate

A key role of the folate coenzymes is helping to form DNA. The active coenzymes help in this synthesis by supplying or accepting single carbon compounds. The coenzymes also help metabolize various amino acids and their derivatives, such as homocysteine.

One major result of a folate deficiency is that in the early phases of red blood cell synthesis the immature cells cannot divide because they cannot form new DNA. The cells grow progressively larger because they can still synthesize enough protein and other cell parts to make new cells. When the time comes for the cells to divide, however, the amount of DNA is insufficient to form two nuclei. The cells then remain in a large immature form, known as a **megaloblast.**

Because the bone marrow of a folate-deficient person produces mostly immature megaloblast cells, few mature red blood cells (called ***erythrocytes***) arrive in the bloodstream. When fewer mature red blood cells are present, the blood's capacity to carry oxygen decreases, causing a form of anemia. In short, a folate deficiency causes megaloblastic anemia (also called **macrocytic anemia**).

The changes in red blood cell formation occur after 7 to 16 weeks on a folate-free diet, depending on the person's folate stores. White blood cell formation is also affected but to a lesser degree. In addition, cell division throughout the entire body is disrupted. Clinicians focus primarily on red blood cells because they are easy to examine. Other symptoms of folate deficiency are inflammation of the tongue, diarrhea, poor growth, mental confusion, depression, and problems in nerve function.

Some forms of cancer therapy provide a vivid example of the effects of a folate deficiency on DNA metabolism. A cancer drug, methotrexate, closely resembles a form of folate but cannot act in its place. Because of this resemblance, when methotrexate is taken in high doses, it hampers folate metabolism. In essence, methotrexate crowds out folate in the metabolic pathways. DNA synthesis, and consequently cell division, then decreases. Because cancer cells are among the most rapidly dividing cells in the body, they are among those first affected. However, other rapidly dividing cells, such as intestinal cells and skin cells, are also affected. Not surprisingly, typical side effects of methotrexate therapy are diarrhea, vomiting, and hair loss. These are also typical symptoms of folate deficiency. For other effects of folate on the body see the next Nutrition Insight in this chapter.

Megaloblast
A large, immature red blood cell that results from the particular cell's inability to divide when it normally should.

Erythrocytes
Mature red blood cells. These have no nucleus and a life span of about 120 days; they contain hemoglobin, which transports oxygen and carbon dioxide.

Macrocytic anemia
Anemia characterized by the presence of abnormally large red blood cells.

Folate in Foods and Needs

Green, leafy vegetables (*folate* is derived from the Latin word *folium*, which means *foliage*), organ meats, sprouts, other vegetables, dried beans, and orange juice are the most rich sources of folate (Figure 7–9). The vitamin C in orange juice also reduces folate destruction. Fortified breakfast cereals, milk, and bread also are important sources of folate for many adults.

Food processing and preparation destroy 50% to 90% of the folate in food. Folate is very susceptible to destruction by heat. This underscores the importance of regularly eating fresh fruits and raw or lightly cooked vegetables. As mentioned before, vegetables retain their nutrients best when cooked quickly in minimal water—steaming, stir-frying, or microwaving.

The RDA of folate for adults is 400 micrograms per day. This RDA is based on dietary folate equivalents (DFE). Research has shown that folate present naturally in foods is absorbed only about half as well as synthetic folate added to foods or supplements. Thus to compare folate intake to the RDA, one has to determine how

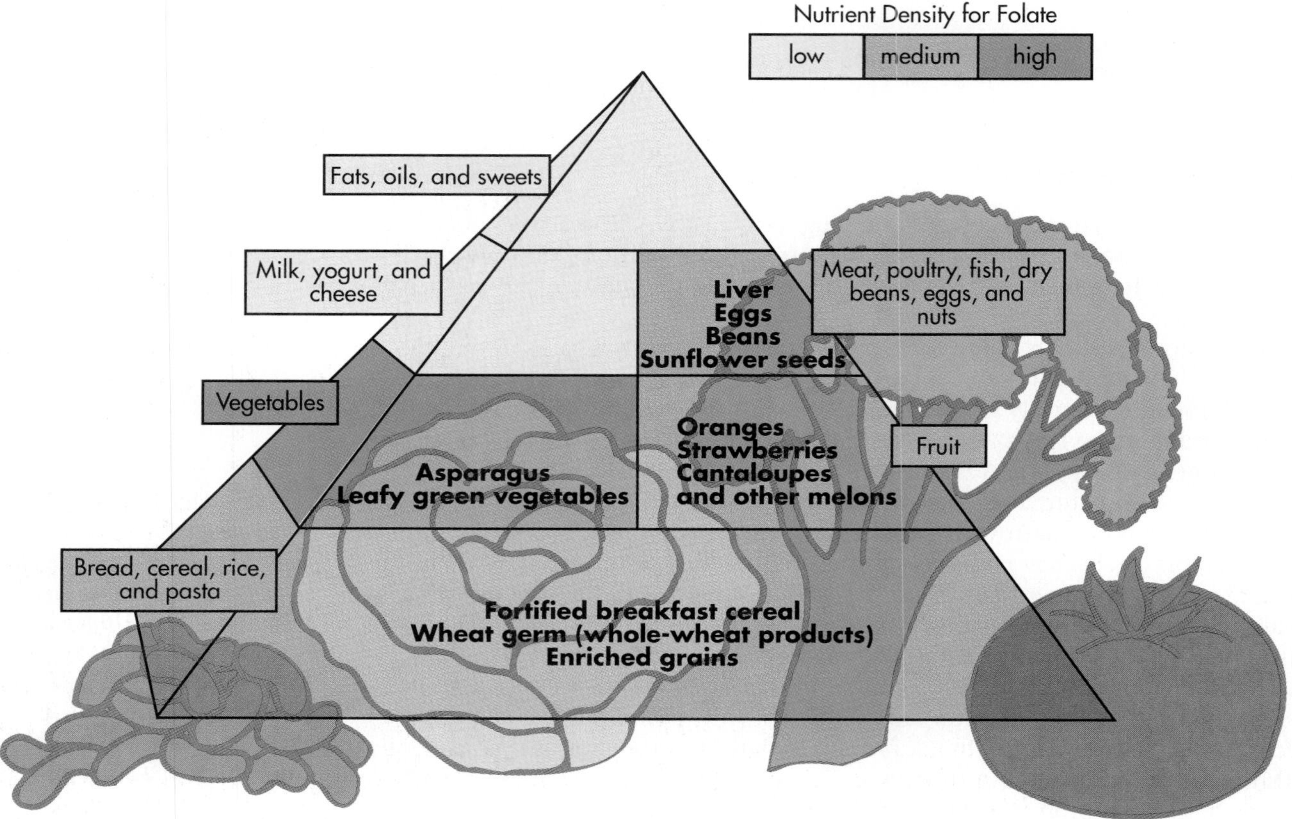

Figure 7–9 *Food sources of folate from the Food Guide Pyramid. The vegetable group is an especially rich source of this nutrient. The background color of each food group indicates the average nutrient density (microgram per kcal) for folate in that group.*

much of a day's food intake comes from food folate and how much comes from synthetic folate added to foods. When in doubt, assume all folate in a diet is in the food form, except that coming from breakfast cereals and refined grain products. Also include in this second category any folate consumed as part of supplements. To calculate the DFE, multiply total synthetic folate intake by 1.7, and add that value to the food folate consumed. For example, if a person consumed 300 micrograms as food folate and 200 micrograms from a breakfast cereal, total folate DFE would be 640 micrograms ([200 × 1.7] + 300). Compared to the RDA of 400 micrograms, one's intake would be sufficient.

Average daily folate intake in the United States is approximately 320 micrograms for men and 220 micrograms for women. With the recent mandate for fortification of grain products with folate, these average intakes should increase by about 85 micrograms per day. Still, intakes for many women will likely remain too low if specific attention is not paid to folate intake.

Folate deficiencies sometimes appear in pregnant women. They need extra folate (600 micrograms per day) to meet an increased rate of cell division and thus of DNA synthesis in their own bodies and that of the developing fetus. Today, prenatal care often includes vitamin and mineral supplements enriched with folate to help compensate for the extra needs associated with pregnancy. Older people are also at risk for folate deficiency, probably because of inadequate folate intake and absorption. Perhaps these people failed to consume sufficient amounts of fruits and vegetables because of poverty or physical problems, such as poor dental health. In addition, folate deficiencies also often occur with alcoholism, due mostly to poor intake and absorption. Symptoms of a folate-related anemia can alert a physician to the possibility of alcoholism.

Dietary sources of folate

Food item and amount	*Folate (micrograms)*
Brewer's yeast, 1 tbsp	**313**
Cooked asparagus, 1 cup	**263**
Cooked lentils, ½ cup	**179**
Romaine lettuce, 1½ cup	**114**
Orange juice, 8 oz	**109**
Cooked spinach, ½ cup	**103**
Cooked broccoli, 1 cup	**78**
Sunflower seeds, ¼ cup	**76**
Cooked beets, ½ cup	**68**
Fried beef liver, 1 oz	**62**

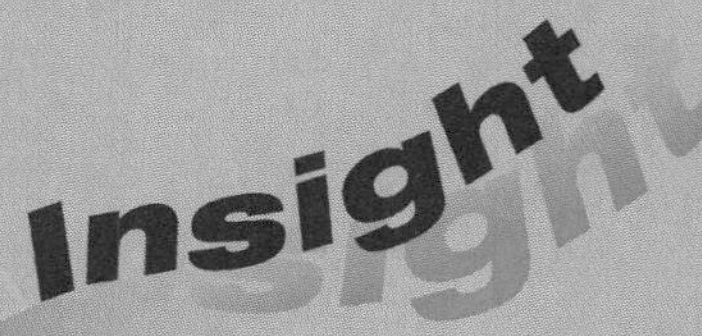

Folate Intake Deserves More Attention

In recent years, effects of folate, other than discussed in detail in the chapter, have lead researchers to believe that folate intake deserves more attention.

Pregnancy and Neural Tube Defects

A maternal deficiency of folate and a genetic predisposition have been linked to development of **neural tube defects** in the fetus (Figure 7–10). These defects include spina bifida (spinal cord or spinal fluid bulge through the back) and anencephaly (absence of a brain). Between 2500 and 3000 infants are so effected annually in the United States. Victims of spina bifida exhibit paralysis, incontinence, hydrocephalus, and learning disabilities. Children born without anencephaly die shortly after birth.

Adequate folate nutriture is crucial for all women of childbearing years since the neural tube closes within the first 28 days of pregnancy, a time when many women are not even aware that they are pregnant. Hence a recommendation is made that ample folate (RDA) be consumed of least 6 weeks before conception. Perhaps as many as 75% of these defects could be avoided by adequate folate status before conception.

Almost all research has been done with folate supplementation, and it appears that even women with varied diets may not consume adequate folate to prevent neural tube defects unless specific attention to folate-rich sources is given. Consuming fortified breakfast cereals is a good practice for meeting folate needs, particularly since they contain a more absorbable form of folate than most food sources. A multivitamin can also supply adequate folate, but women should be careful to monitor the amount of any accompanying vitamin A content.

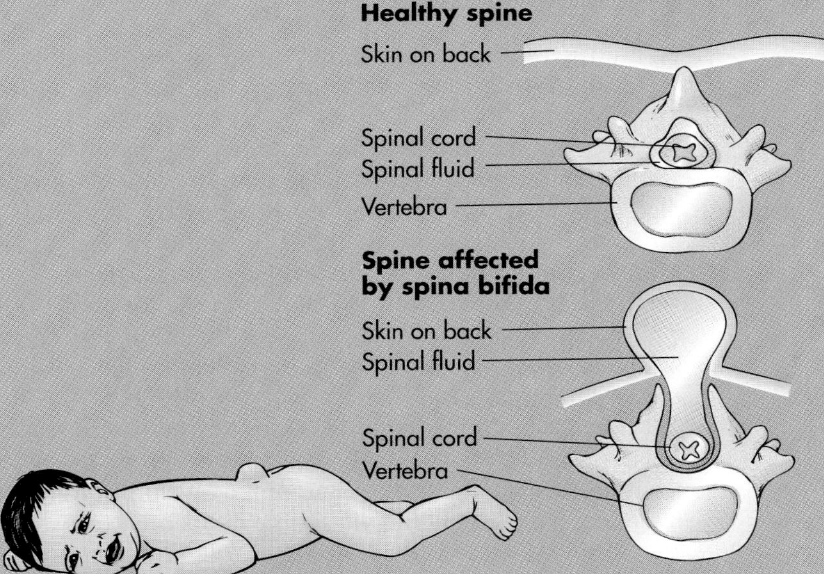

Figure 7–10 *Neural tube defects result from a developmental failure affecting the spinal cord or brain in the embryo. Very early in fetal development a ridge of neural-like tissue forms along the back of the embryo. As the fetus develops, this material develops into both the spinal cord and body nerves at the lower end, and into the brain at the upper end. At the same time, the bones that make up the back gradually surround the spinal cord on all sides. If any part of this sequence goes awry, many defects can appear. The worst is total lack of a brain (anencephaly). Much more common is spina bifida, in which the back bones do not form a complete ring to protect the spinal cord. Deficient folate status in the mother during the beginning of pregnancy greatly increases the risk of neural tube defects.*

Earlier it was noted that most grain products are now fortified with folate. Of course, this is beneficial to most women of childbearing years since it helps prevent birth defects in the case of an unplanned pregnancy. However, because the metabolism and functions of folate and B-12 are linked, regular consumption of large amounts of folate can prevent the appearance of the primary early warning sign of vitamin B-12 deficiency—enlarged red blood cell size. To prevent such masking of vitamin B-12 deficiency, it is the goal of FDA to increase the folate intake of women of childbearing years through grain fortification without producing excessive intake by other groups (over 1 milligram per day). This 1 milligram quantity is the Upper Limit recently set by the DRI revisions. Also, for this reason, FDA limits supplements for nonpregnant adults and food fortification to 400 microgram amounts.

Homocysteine and Heart Disease

Scientists estimate that about 10% of heart disease in the United States may result from excesses of the amino acid derivative homocysteine in the blood. The breakdown of the essential amino acid methionine for the synthesis of various body compounds produces homocysteine. If not recycled, homocysteine can damage the cells that line the blood vessels and in turn trigger the process of atherosclerosis. Folate, vitamin B-12, and vitamin B-6 are all important in the process of recycling homocysteine back to the amino acid forms. Folate receives the most attention in this mechanism of heart disease prevention; some experts suggest that adequate blood folate concentrations could prevent up to 56,000 cardiovascular deaths each year in the United States. In fact, one study found that people in the lowest quarter of blood folate values had a 69% higher risk of heart disease mortality than those in the highest quarter.

Clearly, folate intake demands greater consideration for many of us. In recent years it has become obvious that consuming inadequate amounts of folate is a risky behavior, especially for several population subgroups. These include women of childbearing years, pregnant women, and older persons. Even those who are not a part of any of these groups should examine the amount of folate consumed.

Vitamin B-12

Vitamin B-12 represents a family of compounds that contain the mineral cobalt. All vitamin B-12 compounds are synthesized by bacteria, fungi, and other lower organisms.

The body's complex means of absorbing vitamin B-12 is unique to this vitamin. Vitamin B-12 in food enters the stomach and is released from other materials by digestion, especially by stomach acid. The free vitamin B-12 binds with a substance produced by the salivary glands in the mouth and then later with **intrinsic factor** produced in the stomach. The resulting intrinsic factor/vitamin B-12 complex travels to the last portion of the small intestine for absorption. Utilizing this system, approximately 30% to 70% of dietary vitamin B-12 is absorbed, depending on the body's need for it. Any failure in this system results in only 1% to 2% absorption of dietary vitamin B-12.

Intrinsic factor *A protein-like compound produced by the stomach that enhances vitamin B-12 absorption.*

If a defect in absorption develops, the person usually takes monthly injections of vitamin B-12 to bypass the need for absorption, or megadoses of a supplemental form. In this latter case, the vitamin B-12 absorption defect is overcome by providing enough of the vitamin via simple diffusion across the intestinal tract.

About 95% of all cases of vitamin B-12 deficiencies in healthy people result from defective vitamin B-12 absorption, rather than from inadequate intakes. This is especially true for older people. As we age, our stomachs lose their ability to synthesize the intrinsic factor needed for vitamin B-12 absorption.

Functions of Vitamin B-12

Vitamin B-12 participates in a variety of cellular processes. The most important function is in folate metabolism. Vitamin B-12 is required to convert folate coenzymes to the active forms needed for metabolic reactions, such as DNA synthesis. Without vitamin B-12, reactions that require certain active forms of folate do not take place in the cell. Thus a vitamin B-12 deficiency contributes to a folate deficiency. Another vital function of vitamin B-12 is maintaining the myelin sheaths that insulate nerve fibers from each other. People with vitamin B-12 deficiencies show patchy destruction of the myelin sheaths. This destruction eventually causes paralysis and perhaps death.

In the past the inability to absorb enough vitamin B-12 eventually led to death. Researchers in mid-nineteenth century England noted a form of anemia that caused death within 2 to 5 years of the initial illness, mainly because it destroyed the nerves. They called it **pernicious anemia** (*pernicious* literally means "leading to death"). Clinically the anemia looks much like a folate deficiency anemia as many megaloblasts appear in the bloodstream. The vitamin B-12 anemia is typically called macrocytic anemia.

Pernicious anemia *The anemia that results from a lack of vitamin B-12 absorption; it is pernicious because of associated nerve degeneration that can result in eventual paralysis.*

Besides the anemia, symptoms of pernicious anemia include weakness, sore tongue, back pain, apathy, and tingling in the extremities. Symptoms of nerve destruction generally develop after about 3 years from the onset of the disease. Unfortunately, significant nerve destruction often occurs before the anemia is seen, and this destruction is irreversible. Pernicious anemia and its accompanying nerve destruction generally starts after middle age, affecting up to 10% to 20% of older adults. Both reduced liberation of vitamin B-12 from food due to a fall in stomach acid output and reduced absorption from a fall in intrinsic factor output with aging are to blame.

Infants who are breastfed by vegetarian or vegan mothers are at risk for vitamin B-12 deficiency accompanied by anemia and long-term nervous system problems, such as diminished brain growth, degeneration of the spinal cord, and poor intellectual development. The problems may have their origins during pregnancy, when the mother is deficient in vitamin B-12. Vegan diets supply little vitamin B-12 unless they include vitamin B-12–enriched food or supplements.

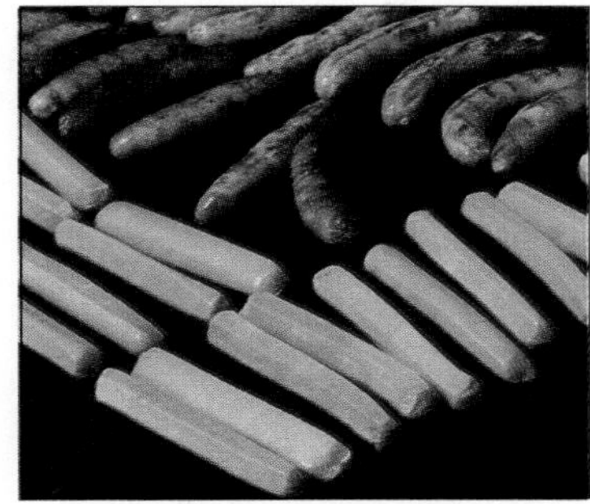

Because they contain organ meat scraps, hot dogs and related products are good sources of vitamin B-12.

Vitamin B-12 in Foods and Needs

Major sources of vitamin B-12 include meat, milk, fortified breakfast cereals, poultry, seafood, and eggs. Especially rich sources of vitamin B-12 are organ meats (especially liver, kidneys, and heart). Adults over age 50 are encouraged to seek a synthetic vitamin B-12 source to aid absorption, which can be limited due to reduced stomach acid output seen in aging. Synthetic vitamin B-12 is not food bound, so it doesn't need stomach acid to aid in liberation from foodstuffs. Thus it will be more readily absorbed than the food form. Breakfast cereals and multivitamin supplements are two possible synthetic sources.

The RDA of vitamin B-12 for adults is 2.4 micrograms per day. On average, men consume 3 times the RDA and women consume two times the RDA. This high intake provides the average meat-eating person with 2 to 3 years' storage of vitamin B-12 in the liver.

It takes approximately 20 years of consuming a diet essentially free of vitamin B-12 for a person to exhibit nerve destruction caused by a diet deficiency. Still, vegans, who eat no animal products, should find a reliable source of vitamin B-12. As noted earlier, older persons are at significant risk for developing pernicious anemia. This develops after a few years of the loss of vitamin B-12 absorption capacity. The quicker appearance is because of the reduced ability to reuse vitamin B-12 that is excreted into the GI tract during digestion, coupled with reduced absorption of dietary sources. Regular physical examinations should test for pernicious anemia. Vitamin B-12 supplements are essentially nontoxic.

Dietary sources of Vitamin B-12

Food item and amount	*Vitamin B-12 (micrograms)*
Fried beef liver, 1 oz	**31.8**
Baked clams, 1 oz	**15.6**
Steamed oysters, 2	**14.4**
Roast beef, 3 oz	**2.0**
Yogurt, 1 cup	**1.4**
Fortified soy milk, 8 oz	**1.0**
Milk, 8 oz	**0.9**
Beef hot dog, 1	**0.9**
Boiled egg, 1	**0.6**
Cooked ham, 3 oz	**0.5**
Ham lunchmeat, 2 oz	**0.4**

People with AIDS also are at risk of vitamin B-12 deficiency, linked to long-standing malabsorption that they often experience. Adequate vitamin B-12 status has been shown in a few studies to lessen the decline in health experienced by those with AIDS.

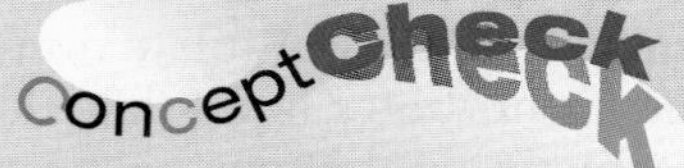

Folate is needed for cell division because it influences DNA synthesis. A folate deficiency results in megaloblastic (macrocytic) anemia, as well as elevated blood homocysteine, inflammation of the tongue, diarrhea, and poor growth. Excess folate intake can mask a vitamin B-12 deficiency since these vitamins work together in metabolism. Folate is found in fruits and vegetables, beans, and organ meats. Emphasizing fresh and lightly cooked vegetables is important because much folate is lost during cooking. Folate needs during pregnancy are especially high; deficiency may lead to neural tube defects in the fetus.

Vitamin B-12 is necessary for folate metabolism. Without dietary vitamin B-12, folate deficiency symptoms, such as macrocytic anemia, develop. In addition, vitamin B-12 is necessary for maintaining the nervous system. Paralysis can develop from a vitamin B-12 deficiency. The absorption of vitamin B-12 requires a number of specific factors. If absorption is inhibited, the resulting deficiency can lead to pernicious anemia and its associated nerve destruction. Concentrated amounts of vitamin B-12 are found only in animal foods; meat eaters generally have a 2- to 3-year supply stored in the liver. Vitamin B-12 absorption may decline as we age. Monthly injections or megadoses can make up for this. Vitamin B-12 also participates with vitamin B-6 and folate in homocysteine metabolism; an adequate intake of all three vitamins minimizes the possibility of development of heart and blood vessel disease related to excess blood homocysteine.

Vitamin C

Scurvy, the vitamin C deficiency disease, was long ago a constant threat to the health of sailors. Its symptoms include weakness, opening of previously healed wounds, slower wound healing, bone pain, fractures, bleeding gums, diarrhea, and pinpoint hemorrhages around hair follicles on the back of the arms and legs. On long sea voyages, captains often lost half or more of their crews to scurvy. In 1740 the Englishman Dr. James Lind first showed that citrus fruits—two oranges and one lemon a day—could cure scurvy. Fifty years after Lind's discovery, rations for British sailors included limes to prevent scurvy.

Vitamin C (ascorbic acid) is a puzzling vitamin. It is found in all living tissues, and most animals synthesize their own from the simple sugar glucose. What is strange is that animals who synthesize vitamin C often make quite a lot of it. For instance, a pig produces 8 grams per day (though we do not benefit from it when we eat pork because it is lost in processing). This amount is over 130 times our human RDA of 60 milligrams. Why some animals make so much vitamin C whereas other animals, including humans, appear to need so little has fueled much controversy.

Vitamin C is absorbed in the small intestine. About 80% to 90% of vitamin C is absorbed when a person eats between 30 and 120 milligrams of it per day. If someone ingests 6 grams (6000 milligrams) per day, absorption efficiency drops to about 20%. A common side effect of megadose vitamin C use is diarrhea. The unabsorbed vitamin C stays in the small intestine and attracts water, finally causing diarrhea.

Functions of Vitamin C

The best understood function of vitamin C is its role in synthesizing the protein collagen. This protein is highly concentrated in connective tissue, bone, teeth, tendons, and blood vessels. It is very important for wound healing. Vitamin C increases the cross-connections between amino acids in collagen, greatly strengthening the tissues it helps form.

A vitamin C deficiency can cause widespread changes in tissue metabolism. Most symptoms of scurvy are linked to a decrease in collagen synthesis. About 20 to 40 days with no vitamin C intake are required for the first symptoms of scurvy to appear.

Vitamin C is one of the cell's water-soluble antioxidants. Recall that vitamin E is a fat-soluble antioxidant for the cell membrane. The antioxidant capabilities of vitamin C can reduce the formation of cancer-causing nitrosamines in the stomach and also keep the folate coenzymes intact, preventing their destruction. Vitamin C and vitamin E work together as free-radical scavengers. Vitamin C also aids in reactivating oxidized vitamin E so that it can be reused. Epidemiological studies suggest that vitamin C is effective in helping prevent certain cancers (such as esophageal, oral, and stomach cancers), heart disease, and cataracts in the eye, probably because of its antioxidant capabilities.

Vitamin C enhances iron absorption by keeping iron in its most absorbable form. The iron in the small intestine's alkaline environment is much more usable than other forms of iron. Thus iron absorption is modestly enhanced. Increasing intake of vitamin C–rich foods is beneficial for those people with poor iron stores. However, one symptom of vitamin C toxicity—with doses of 1 gram or more per day—can be overabsorption of iron, with the potential for iron toxicity.

Vitamin C is vital for the function of the immune system, especially for the activity of certain cells in the immune system. Thus disease states can increase the need for vitamin C, although we don't know what amount above the RDA is needed (if any). Partly on the basis of this observation, Dr. Linus Pauling gained great notoriety by claiming that vitamin C could combat the common cold. He claimed that 1000 milligrams (1 gram) or more of vitamin C daily could reduce the number of colds for most people by nearly half. As a result of the popularity of his books and the respectability of his scientific credentials, millions of Americans supplement their diets with vitamin C.

But does vitamin C reliably and effectively work against colds and other infections? Most medical and nutrition scientists disagree with Pauling's views of vitamin C. Numerous well-designed, double-blind studies have not shown megadoses of vitamin C to reliably prevent colds, though it seems to reduce duration of symptoms by a day or so.

Most vitamin C consumed in large doses ends up in the feces or the urine. Only a small fraction of such large doses can be used. The body is saturated at intakes of about 200 milligrams per day. This means that if more than 200 milligrams of vitamin C is ingested, it is quickly excreted. Finally, vitamin C is also necessary for the synthesis of a number of hormones, neurotransmitters, and other compounds, such as bile acids and DNA.

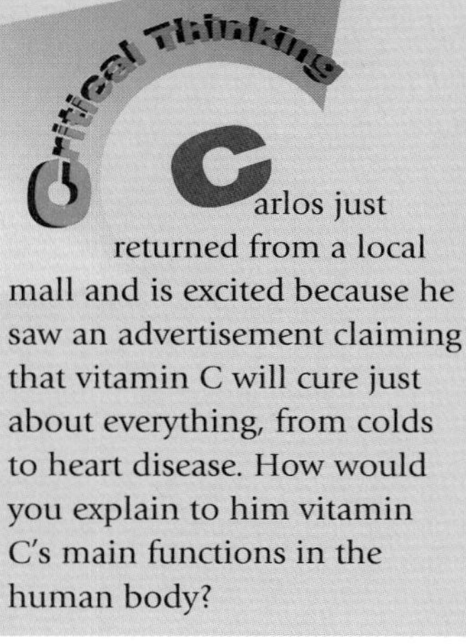

Carlos just returned from a local mall and is excited because he saw an advertisement claiming that vitamin C will cure just about everything, from colds to heart disease. How would you explain to him vitamin C's main functions in the human body?

Vitamin C in Foods and Needs

Major sources of vitamin C are green peppers, cauliflower, broccoli, cabbage, strawberries, papayas, and romaine lettuce. Citrus fruits, potatoes, fortified breakfast cereals, and fortified fruit drinks are also good sources of vitamin C (Figure 7–11). The five to nine servings of fruits and vegetables from the Food Guide Pyramid can easily provide enough vitamin C. Vitamin C is easily lost in processing and cooking as it is very unstable in contact with heat, iron, copper, or oxygen.

The adult RDA of vitamin C is 60 milligrams per day. The 1989 RDA publication (which provides the most recent RDA for vitamin C) recommends that cigarette smokers consume 100 milligrams per day because of the great stress on their lungs from oxygen and toxic by-products of cigarette smoke. Our food supply yields about twice the adult RDA (120 milligrams) of vitamin C per day. Approximately 80 milligrams is derived naturally from foods; the remainder comes from vitamin C added to foods. Nearly all Americans likely meet their daily needs for vitamin C because

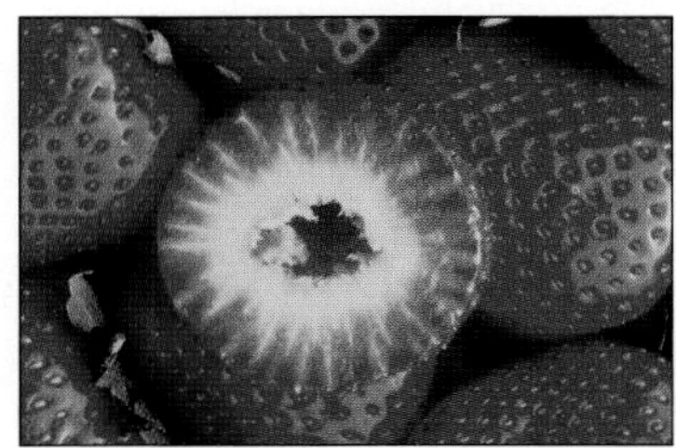

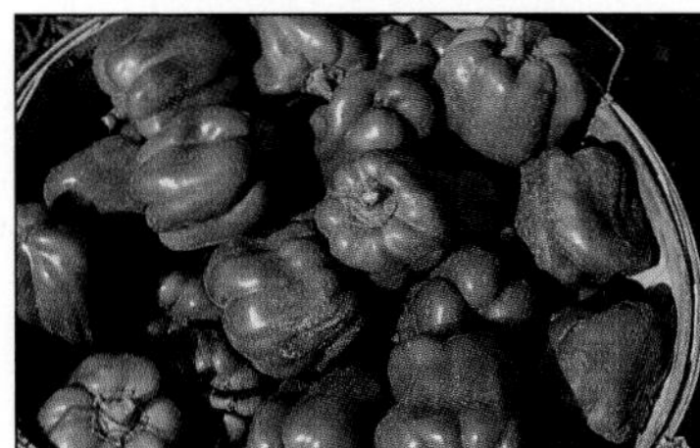

Vegetables such as green peppers are one source of vitamin C, and fruits such as strawberries are another rich source.

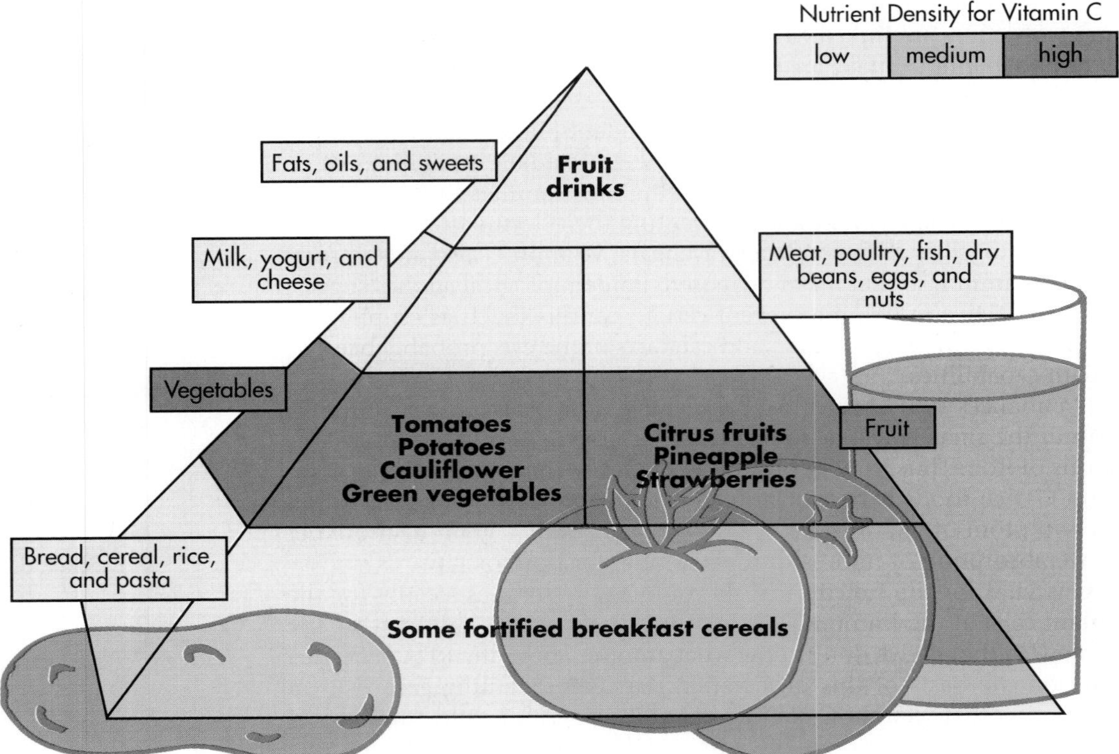

Figure 7–11 *Food sources of vitamin C from the Food Guide Pyramid. The fruit group and the vegetable group are especially rich sources of this nutrient. The background color of each food group indicates the average nutrient density (milligram per kcal) for vitamin C in that group.*

Dietary Sources of Vitamin C

Food item and amount	Vitamin C (mg)
Cooked brussels sprouts, 1 cup	**97**
Strawberries, 1 cup	**82**
Kiwifruit, 1	**74**
Grapefruit juice, 8 oz	**72**
Red peppers, ¼ cup	**71**
Orange, 1	**70**
Green pepper rings, 5	**45**
Tomato juice, 8 oz	**44**
Raw broccoli, ½ cup	**41**
Raw cauliflower, ½ cup	**23**

Hemochromatosis *A disorder of iron metabolism characterized by increased iron absorption and deposition in the liver tissue. This eventually poisons the liver cells.*

men consume an average 120 milligrams per day and women consume 100 milligrams per day. Respected nutrition experts who advocate increased use of vitamin C often recommend intakes of about 200 milligrams per day. Still, this amount can be obtained by sufficient fruit and vegetable intake. Today vitamin C deficiency appears mostly in alcoholic people who eat nutrient-poor diets and in some older persons who also eat poorly.

Toxicity of Vitamin C

Vitamin C is probably not toxic when consumed in amounts less than about 1 gram per day. Regularly consuming more than that may cause stomach inflammation, diarrhea, and iron toxicity (again, caused by overabsorption of iron). This last point is important to note, however, because some people suffer from **hemochromatosis,** a disease characterized by overstorage of iron (see Chapter 8). These people may be harmed if an increased vitamin C intake increases their iron absorption. This is just one of many examples in which recommending a vitamin intake well above the RDA can have conflicting results. Some people may benefit, whereas others may be injured.

If people want to experiment with large doses of vitamin C, they should alert their physician, primarily because high doses of vitamin C can change reactions to medical tests for diabetes or blood in the feces. Physicians may misdiagnose conditions when large doses of vitamin C are consumed without their knowledge.

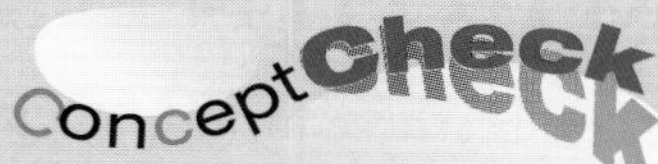

Vitamin C is important in the synthesis of collagen, a major connective tissue protein. A vitamin C deficiency, known as scurvy, causes many changes in the skin and gums, such as small hemorrhages. This is mainly because of poor collagen synthesis. Vitamin C also modestly improves iron absorption, is involved in synthesizing certain hormones and neurotransmitters, and acts as a general body antioxidant. Citrus fruits, green peppers, cauliflower, broccoli, strawberries, and fortified breakfast cereals are good sources of vitamin C. As with folate, eating fresh or lightly cooked foods is important because vitamin C loses a lot of its potency in cooking. High doses of vitamin C can lead to diarrhea and foil various medical tests. These high doses do not prevent the common cold.

Now that you have studied the vitamins, review the Food Guide Pyramid in Chapter 2 and note how each group makes an important vitamin contribution (Figure 7–12).

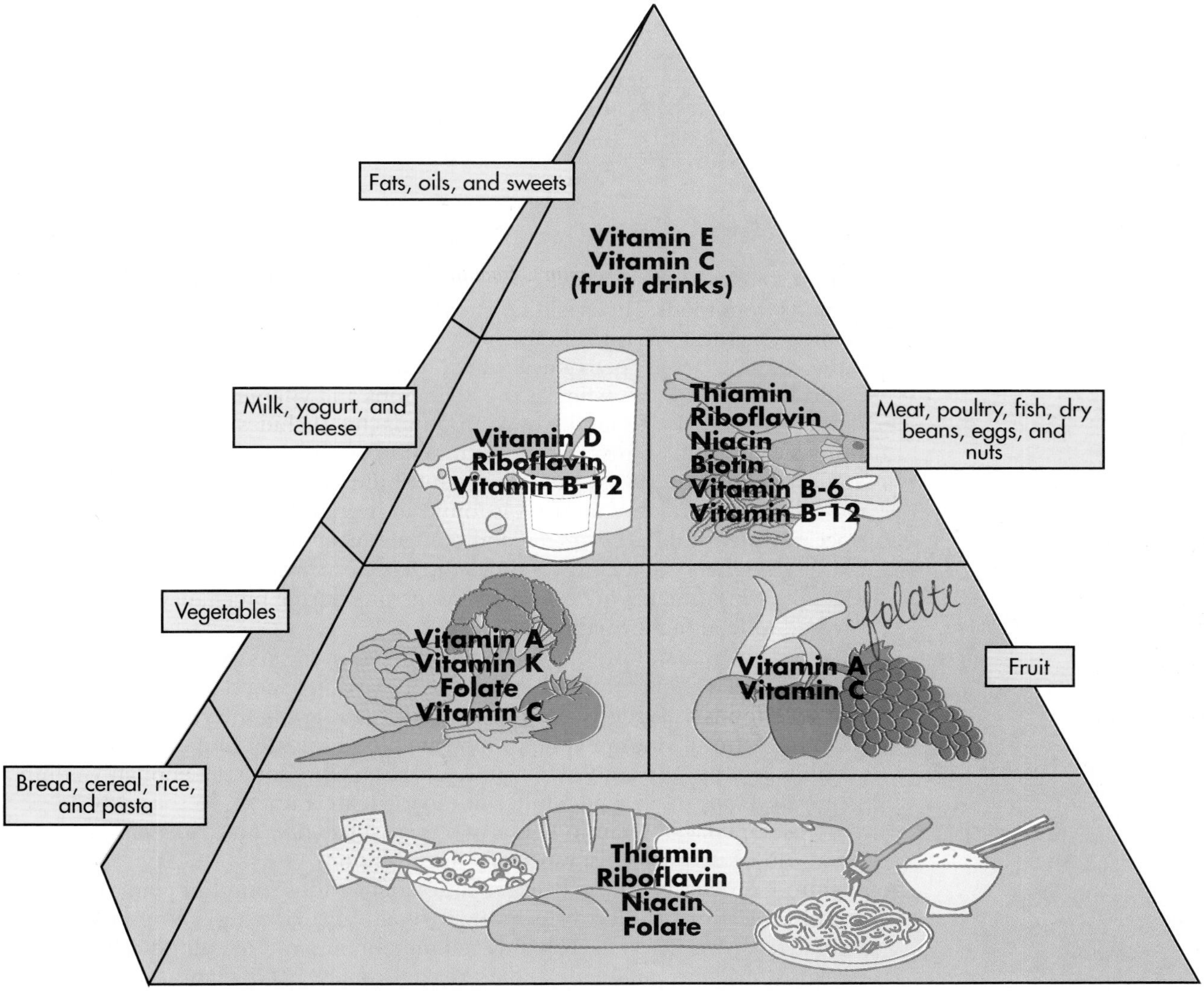

Figure 7–12 *Certain groups of the Food Guide Pyramid are especially rich sources of various vitamins. This is true for the vitamins listed. Each vitamin may be also found in other groups but in lower amounts. Pantothenic acid is also present in moderate amounts in many groups.*

VITAMIN-LIKE COMPOUNDS

A variety of vitamin-like compounds are found in the body. These include the following:

- Choline
- Carnitine
- Inositol
- Taurine
- Lipoic acid

All these vitamin-like compounds are necessary to maintain proper metabolism in the body. They can be synthesized by cells using common building blocks, such as amino acids and glucose. Our diets are also a source. In disease states or periods of active growth, synthesis of vitamin-like compounds may not meet needs, so dietary intake can be crucial. The needs for vitamin-like compounds in certain conditions, such as for premature infants, are being investigated. And even though findings suggest that choline may be an essential nutrient for humans, further research is needed to confirm this. In any case, we consume ample choline, at least 700 to 1000 milligrams per day, to meet our needs. This is in excess of the recently set AI of 550 milligrams per day for men and 425 milligrams per day for women. Although promoted and sold by health food stores, these vitamin-like compounds need not be included in the diet of the average healthy adult.

Summary

- Vitamins are carbon-containing compounds we generally need daily in small amounts from foods. They yield no energy directly, but many contribute to energy-yielding chemical reactions in the body and promote growth and development. Many vitamins act as coenzymes, which help enzymes function. Vitamins A, D, E, and K are fat soluble, whereas the B vitamins and vitamin C are water soluble.
- Vitamin A consists of a family of compounds that includes several forms of preformed vitamin A. Some carotenoids function as antioxidants and can also yield vitamin A when necessary. Vitamin A contributes to vision, immune function, and cell development. Vitamin A is found in liver and fish oils; carotenoids are especially plentiful in dark green and orange vegetables. Vitamin A can be quite toxic, even when taken at just 3 times the RDA, especially preformed vitamin A. High vitamin A intakes are especially dangerous during pregnancy because they can lead to fetal malformation.
- Vitamin D is both a hormone and a vitamin. Human skin synthesizes it using sunshine and a cholesterol-like substance. If we don't spend enough time in the sun, such foods as fish oils and fortified milk can supply the vitamin. The active hormone form of vitamin D helps regulate blood calcium in part by influencing calcium absorption from the intestine. Children who don't get enough vitamin D may develop rickets, and adults with inadequate amounts in the body develop osteomalacia. Vitamin D is a very toxic substance. An intake just 5 times the AI can cause problems, especially in childhood.
- Vitamin E functions primarily as an antioxidant and is found in plant oils. By donating electrons to electron-seeking free-radical (oxidizing) compounds, it neutralizes them. This effect shields cell membranes and red blood cells from breakdown. Claims are made about the curative powers of vitamin E, but more information is needed before megadose vitamin E recommendations for healthy adults can be made with certainty.
- Vitamin K helps blood clot and increases the calcium-binding potential of some organs. Some vitamin K absorbed each day comes from bacterial synthesis in

the intestine, but most comes from foods, primarily green, leafy vegetables. Vitamin K is poorly stored in the body, but our dietary intake alone is usually sufficient. People who can't absorb fat well or who are on antibiotics for long periods may need extra vitamin K.

- Thiamin, riboflavin, and niacin play key roles as coenzymes in energy-yielding reactions. They help metabolize carbohydrates, fats, and proteins. Alcoholism and a poor diet can create deficiencies of these three nutrients. Enriched grain products are common sources of all three of these vitamins.
- Pantothenic acid, which participates in many aspects of cell metabolism, is widely distributed among foods. Biotin, which participates in glucose production, fat synthesis, and DNA synthesis, can be synthesized by bacteria in the intestine. Biotin comes from foods such as eggs, peanuts, and cheese.
- Vitamin B-6 performs a vital role in protein metabolism, especially in synthesizing nonessential amino acids. It also helps synthesize neurotransmitters and performs other metabolic roles, such as metabolism of homocysteine. Headaches, a form of anemia, nausea, and vomiting result from a B-6 deficiency. Increased risk of heart disease is also possible, especially when coupled with inadequate folate or vitamin B-12 intake or both. Generally, women are more likely to have poor vitamin B-6 stores than men. Regular consumption of animal protein foods, and rich plant sources such as broccoli provides needed vitamin B-6. Taking high doses causes malfunction of the nervous system.
- Folate plays an important role in DNA synthesis and homocysteine metabolism. Symptoms of a deficiency include generally poor cell division in various areas of the body, megaloblastic anemia, tongue inflammation, diarrhea, and poor growth. Pregnancy puts high demands for folate on the body; deficiency can result in a neural tube defect in the offspring. A deficiency can also occur in people with alcoholism. Food sources are leafy vegetables, organ meats, and orange juice. Great amounts of folate can be lost in prolonged cooking. Excess folate in the diet can mask a vitamin B-12 deficiency.
- Vitamin B-12 is needed to metabolize folate (and so in addition homocysteine) and maintain the insulation surrounding nerves. A deficiency results in anemia (because of its relationship to folate) and nerve degeneration. Older people often absorb vitamin B-12 inefficiently. If so, they can benefit from monthly injections or megadoses of the vitamin. Generally a dietary deficiency is unlikely because vitamin B-12 is highly concentrated in animal foods, which constitute a major part of the American diet. Vitamin B-12 does not occur naturally in plant foods. Vegans need a supplemental source, and adults over age 50 should consume a synthetic source, such as in fortified breakfast cereals.
- Vitamin C is mainly used to synthesize collagen, a major protein for building connective tissue. A vitamin C deficiency results in scurvy, which is evidenced by poor wound healing, pinpoint hemorrhages in the skin, and bleeding gums. Vitamin C also modestly enhances iron absorption, is a general antioxidant, and is needed for synthesizing some hormones and neurotransmitters. Fresh fruits and vegetables, especially citrus fruits, are generally good sources. Because a great amount of vitamin C is lost in cooking, a good diet should emphasize fresh or lightly cooked vegetables. Deficiencies can occur in people with alcoholism and those whose diets lack sufficient fruits and vegetables. Smoking makes matters worse for people already at risk.

Study Questions

1. Why is the risk of toxicity greater with the fat-soluble vitamins A and D than with water-soluble vitamins?

2 How would you determine which fruits and vegetables displayed in the produce section of your supermarket are likely to provide plenty of carotenoids?
3 What is the primary function of the vitamin D hormone? Which groups of people likely need to supplement with vitamin D, and on what do you base your answer?
4 Describe how vitamin E functions as an antioxidant. Use the term *free radical.*
5 Why is it critical for a surgeon to know the vitamin K status of a patient before operating?
6 The need for certain vitamins increases as energy expenditure increases. Name two such vitamins and explain why this is the case.
7 Take one of the B vitamins that might be low in the American diet and explain why the lack might occur.
8 Which vitamins are lost from cereal grains as a result of the "refining" process? Which vitamins must be replaced by law in the subsequent enrichment process?
9 Although folate itself is not known to have any toxic effects, FDA limits the amount that may be included in supplements and fortified foods. Why?
10 Is it necessary for Americans to consume a great excess of vitamin C to avoid the possibility of a deficiency? Does the intake of vitamin C well above the RDA have any negative consequences?

Further Readings

1 ADA Reports: Position of The American Dietetic Association: vitamin and mineral supplementation, *Journal of The American Dietetic Association* 96:73, 1996.
2 Alaimo K and others: Dietary intake of vitamins, minerals, and fiber of persons ages 2 months and over in the United States: Third National Health and Nutrition Examination Survey, Phase I, 1988–91, *Advance Data* 258:1, 1994.
3 Buring JE, Hennekens CH: Antioxidant vitamins and cardiovascular disease, *Nutrition Reviews* 55:S53, 1997.
4 Can antioxidants save your life? *UC Berkeley Wellness Letter* p. 4, July 1998.
5 Diet and cancer prevention, *American Institute for Cancer Research (AICR) Newsletter* p. 1, Winter 1998.
6 Eskes TKAB: Open or closed? A world of difference: a history of homocysteine research, *Nutrition Reviews* 56:236, 1998.
7 Hall SS: Eat to fight cancer, *Health* p. 106, April 1997.
8 Holick MF: Vitamin D deficiency, the silent epidemic, *Nutrition Action Healthletter* p. 3, October 1997.
9 Holt PR: Modulation of abnormal colonic epithelial cell proliferation and differentiation by low-fat dairy foods, *Journal of the American Medical Association* 280:1074, 1998.
10 Jacques PF and others: Long-term vitamin C supplement use and prevalence of early age-related lens opacities, *American Journal of Clinical Nutrition* 66:911, 1997.
11 Johnston CS, Thompson LL: Vitamin C status of an outpatient population, *Journal of the American College of Nutrition* 17:366, 1998.
12 Levine M and others: Determination of optimal vitamin C requirements in humans, *American Journal of Clinical Nutrition* 62(suppl): 1347S, 1995.
13 Liebman B: 3 Vitamins and a mineral: What to take, *Nutrition Action Healthletter* p. 1, May 1998.
14 Marston W: What's best for breakfast? *Health* p. 34, April 1997.
15 McBean LD: Diet and cancer, *Dairy Council Digest* 68:25, 1997.
16 Meydani M, Meisler JG: A closer look at vitamin E, *Postgraduate Medicine* 102:199, 1997.
17 Oakley GP: Eat right and take a multivitamin, *New England Journal of Medicine* 338:1060, 1998.
18 Rimm EB and others: Folate and vitamin B-6 from diet and supplements in relation to risk of coronary heart disease among women, *Journal of the American Medical Association* 279:359, 1998.
19 Rothman KJ and others: Teratogenicity of high vitamin A intake, *New England Journal of Medicine* 333:1369, 1995.
20 Sharp D: Multivitamins, *Health* p. 106, March 1997.
21 Smith-Warner SA and others: Alcohol and breast cancer in women, *Journal of the American Medical Association* 279:535, 1998.
22 Subar AF and others: Dietary sources of nutrients among U.S. adults, 1989–1991, *Journal of the American Dietetic Association* 98:537, 1998.
23 Utinger RD: The need for more vitamin D, *New England Journal of Medicine* 338:828, 1998.
24 Vitamin and nutritional supplements, *Mayo Clinic Health Letter Supplement* June 1997.

RATE 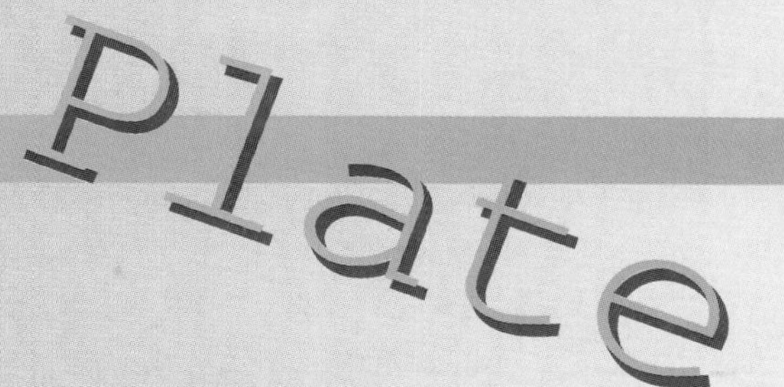

I. Measuring Your Vitamin Intake Against the RDAs

This activity requires you to reexamine the nutritional assessment you did for Chapters 1 and 2. You recorded all the foods and drinks you consumed for 1 day and their quantities. Then you assessed your intake by recording the total amounts of nutrients you consumed. You were then asked to compare your nutrient intake to the RDAs found on the inside front cover of this book. Take your completed assessment and look at your intakes of vitamins A, E, C, B-6, B-12, and thiamin, riboflavin, niacin, and folate. Record these numbers in the table below. Next, record the RDAs for each of these nutrients from your assessment. Then, record the percentage of the RDA you consumed for each vitamin. Lastly, place a +, −, or = in the space provided, reflecting an intake higher than, lower than, or equal to the RDA.

Vitamin	Intake	RDA	% of RDA	+, −, =
A				
E				
C				
Thiamin				
Riboflavin				
Niacin				
B-6				
Folate				
B-12				

ANALYSIS

1. **Which of your vitamin intakes equaled or exceeded the RDA?**

___

2. **Which of your vitamin intakes were below the RDA?**

___

3. **What foods could you eat to improve your dietary intake of vitamins in low amounts in your diet? (Review sources of certain vitamins in this chapter.)**

___

___

II. A Closer Look at Supplement Use

With the current popularity of vitamin and mineral supplements, it is more important than ever that you understand what to look for in a supplement. Use the label below to answer the following questions. Then go to the store and get a general multivitamin and answer these questions again. How do the answers change? Which do you think would be safer to take on a regular basis?

Our protective formula has been extensively researched to bring you the best answer to problems associated with changing seasons.

Suggested use: For best results, begin taking ***Nutramega*** tablets at the very first signs of imbalances in your well-being. During imbalances, take 2 to 3 tablets every three hours. For daily maintenance, take 1 or 2 tablets a day. Or, take as recommended by your health care professional.

WARNING: Not for use by pregnant or nursing women.

KEEP OUT OF THE REACH OF CHILDREN.

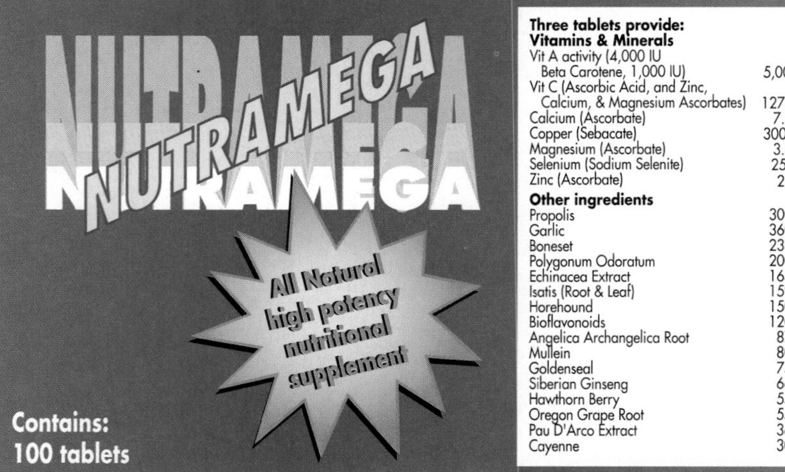

Three tablets provide: Vitamins & Minerals		**% Daily Value**
Vit A activity (4,000 IU Beta Carotene, 1,000 IU)	5,000 IU	100%
Vit C (Ascorbic Acid, and Zinc, Calcium, & Magnesium Ascorbates)	1275 mg	2125%
Calcium (Ascorbate)	7.5 mg	1%
Copper (Sebacate)	300 mcg	15%
Magnesium (Ascorbate)	3.8 mg	1%
Selenium (Sodium Selenite)	25 mcg	30%
Zinc (Ascorbate)	23 mg	153%
Other ingredients		
Propolis	300 mg	
Garlic	360 mg	
Boneset	238 mg	
Polygonum Odoratum	200 mg	
Echinacea Extract	164 mg	
Isatis (Root & Leaf)	159 mg	
Horehound	150 mg	
Bioflavonoids	120 mg	
Angelica Archangelica Root	87 mg	
Mullein	80 mg	
Goldenseal	75 mg	
Siberian Ginseng	66 mg	
Hawthorn Berry	55 mg	
Oregon Grape Root	55 mg	
Pau D'Arco Extract	36 mg	
Cayenne	30 mg	

1. **What is the recommended dosage of this supplement?** ______

2. **Based on the recommended dosage, are there any individual vitamins for which the intake would be greater than 100% of the Daily Value? List these vitamins.** ______

3. **Are there any superfluous ingredients such as herbs or flavors in the supplement? You can often tell this because these ingredients will not have a percent of Daily Value.** ______

4. **Does at least 50% of the vitamin A in the product come from beta-carotene or other carotenoids (to reduce risk of preformed vitamin A toxicity)?** ______

5. **Are there any warnings on the label as to populations who should not consume this product?** ______

6. **Are there any other signs that tip you off that this may not be a safe product?** ______

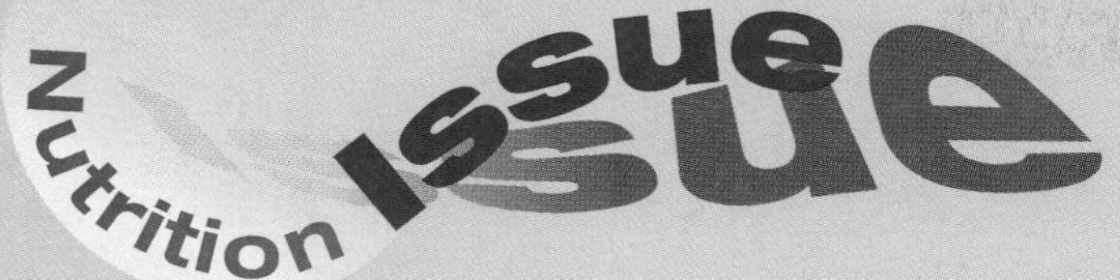

Diet Against Cancer

Cancer is currently the second leading cause of death for American adults and is projected to be the number one cause of early death in the next century, in part because as people live longer the risk of developing cancer increases. It is further estimated that more than 1500 people die each day of cancer in the United States, yielding a cost of about $104 billion from all cancer-related expenses. The top four cancers, causing more than 50% of cancer deaths, are lung, colorectal, breast, and prostate cancers.

Cancer is actually many diseases; these differ in the types of cells affected and, in some cases, in the factors contributing to cancer development (Figure 7-13). For example, the factors leading to skin cancer differ from those leading to breast cancer. Similarly, the treatments for the different types of cancer often differ.

Cancer essentially represents abnormal and uncontrollable division of cells; if untreated or not treatable, it leads to death. Most cancers take the form of tumors, although not all tumors are cancers. A tumor is simply spontaneous new tissue growth that serves no physiological purpose. It can be **benign,** like a wart, or **malignant,** like most lung cancers. The terms *malignant tumor* and *malignant neoplasm* are synonymous with cancer.

Benign
Noncancerous; tumors that do not spread.

Malignant
Essentially to do anything malicious. In reference to a tumor, the property of spreading locally and to distant sites.

Benign tumors are made up of cells similar to the surrounding normal cells and are enclosed in a membrane that prevents them from penetrating other tissues. They are dangerous only if their physical presence interferes with normal functions. A benign brain tumor, for

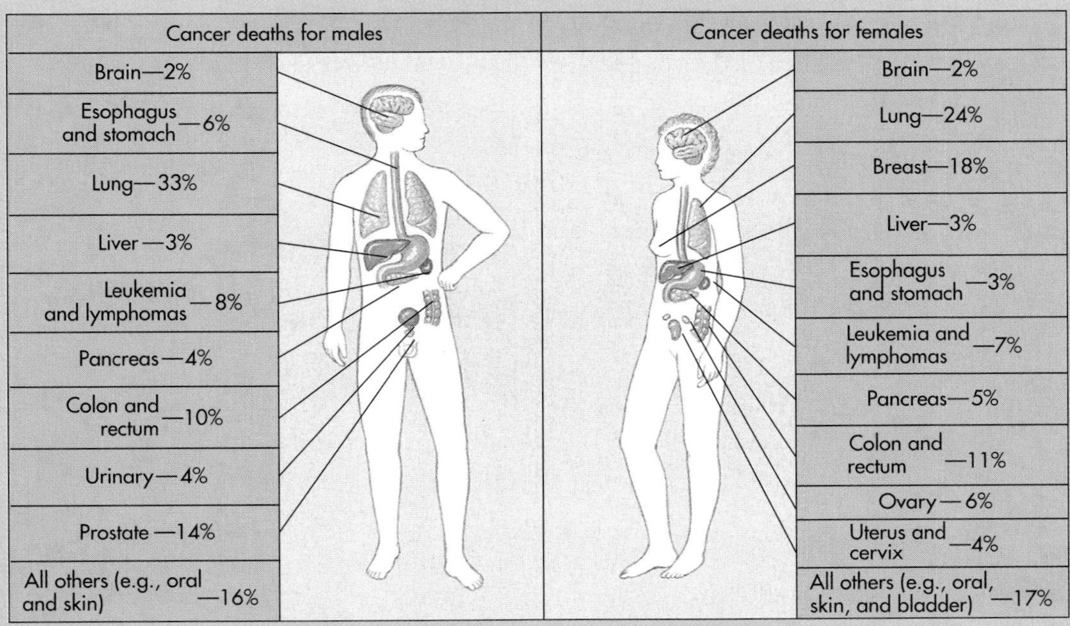

Figure 7-13 *Cancer is actually many diseases. Numerous types of cells and organs are its target. Note that about one-third of all cancers arise from smoking.*
Illustration by William Ober.

example, can cause illness or death if it blocks blood flow in the brain. In contrast, a malignant tumor, or cancer, is capable of invading surrounding structures, including blood vessels, the lymph system, and nervous tissue. It can also spread, or **metastasize,** to distant sites via the blood and lymphatic circulation, thereby producing invasive tumors in almost any part of the body (Figure 7–14). A few cancers, such as leukemia, a form of cancer found in white blood cells, don't produce a mass and so aren't properly classified as tumors. But since leukemic cells exhibit the fundamental property of rapid and inappropriate growth, they are still malignant and therefore represent a form of cancer.

Metastisis
The spreading of disease from one part of the body to another, even to parts of the body that are remote from the site of the original tumor. Cancer cells can spread via blood vessels, the lymphatic system, or direct growth of the tumor.

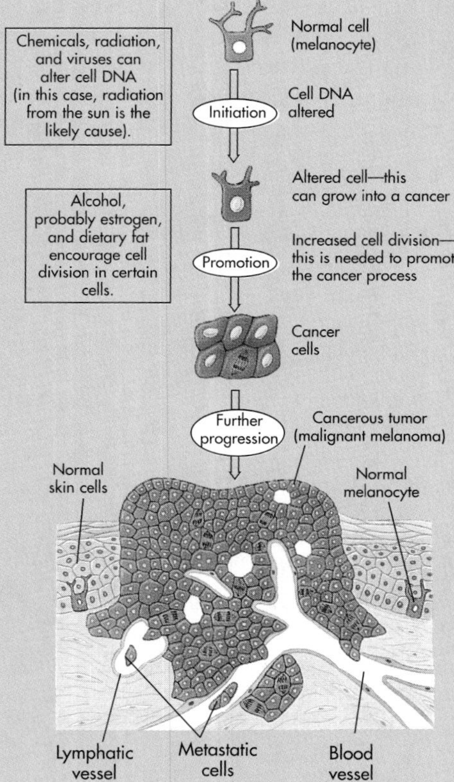

Figure 7–14 *Progression from a normal skin cell to skin cancer through the initiation, promotion, and progression stages. The ball of cells is a developing tumor. As the mass of cells grows, it can invade surrounding tissues, eventually penetrating into both lymph and blood vessels. These vessels carry spreading (metastatic) cancer cells throughout the body, where they can form new cancer sites.*

Both genetics and lifestyle are potent forces that influence the risk for developing cancer. Certain cancers tend to occur in some families more than in others. Thus persons within high-risk families are said to be genetically predisposed, or at risk for developing specific types of cancer. A genetic predisposition is especially important in development of colon cancer and some types of breast cancer. About 30 cancer-susceptibility genes have been isolated. However, experts estimate that only 5% to 10% of all cancers can be explained by inheriting a cancer gene. Thus lifestyle is also a critical factor in most forms of cancer, as evidenced by the variation in cancer rates from country to country. In fact, diet likely accounts for more than 30% to 40% of all cancers.

Although we have little control over our genetic risks for cancer, we do have a great deal of choice in deciding which risks to take with respect to lifestyle, especially with regard to smoking, alcohol abuse, physical activity, and nutrient intake (food choice). It is well established that one-third of all cancers in the United States are due directly to tobacco use. About half of the cancers of the mouth, pharynx, and larynx are associated with heavy use of alcohol. A combination of alcohol use and smoking increases cancer risks even higher. In addition, it has become increasingly apparent that certain dietary factors and degree of physical activity either promote or inhibit cancer. With diet, as with tobacco and alcohol use, imprudent choices today likely cause medical problems tomorrow.

MECHANISMS OF CARCINOGENESIS

To understand how cancer can be prevented, let's first examine how cancer develops in the body. This process involves multiple steps, starting with exposure of a cell to a carcinogen (Table 7–5).

CANCER INITIATION

Cancer begins with a **mutation** of DNA, the genetic material in a cell. As a result, the cell no longer responds to normal physiological controls on cell division. **Cancer initiation** can develop spontaneously, or it can be induced by specific agents. The affected cell now can dictate its own rate of division and is not inhibited from doing so at the expense of

Mutation
A permanent change in a cell's DNA; includes changes in sequence, alteration of gene position, gene loss or duplication, and insertion of foreign gene sequences.

Cancer initiation
The stage in the process of cancer development that begins with alterations in DNA, the genetic material in a cell. This may cause the cell to no longer respond to normal physiological controls.

TABLE 7-5

The Cancer Development Process

CANCER INITIATION

Process: DNA alteration occurs in this relatively short phase (minutes to days).

Causes:

Radiation: e.g., sun overexposure
Cross-links double strands of DNA or breaks them into fragments.
Chemicals: e.g., aflatoxin (mold from peanuts and cereal grains), benzo(a)pyrene (smoke from charbroiled meat fat)
Transformed by body to highly reactive cancer initiators. These compounds are then able to cause mutations in DNA, RNA, and proteins.
Biological agents: e.g., viruses
Promote uncontrolled growth of cells by inserting viral DNA or RNA into normal cells, which alters the cell's genes.

CANCER PROMOTION

Process: DNA alterations are "locked" into the genetic material of cells over a period of months to more than 10 years.

Causes:

Excess estrogen exposure
Excess alcohol
Excess dietary fat
Bacterial infections: e.g., *Helicobacter pylori*

CANCER PROGRESSION

Process: Cells that can grow autonomously appear. These cells spread to surrounding tissue and other sites.

Causes:

Excess energy intake
Lack of early detection
Development of blood supply to the tumor
The tumor uses newly formed capillaries to grow and spread cancer cells to remote sites in the body.

Researchers are attempting to attack cancer from all sides. For example, cancer cells contain an enzyme called telomerase that allows cancer tumors to indefinitely divide by continually lengthening the cap on the ends of DNA strands. This cap shortens as a cell multiplies, eventually preventing further cell division. Studies are ongoing to discover a way to attack telomerase. In addition, angiostatin and endostatin are two natural proteins that are being studied for their ability to inhibit the growth of blood vessels that facilitate cancer metastasis.

surrounding cells. Alteration of DNA can occur within a few minutes to days. Among the factors that can initiate cancer development are radiant energy, certain chemical agents, and biological agents. In addition, some metabolism that occurs in the body can contribute harmful substances. For example, certain products of liver metabolism cause cancer.

Potentially thwarting this process of cancer development are other human genes, called *tumor suppressors.* These may step in to prevent the abnormal growth, slowing cell turnover. However if mutations cause the tumor suppressor to fail, this block against cancer development also fails. Mutations of this and other tumor-suppressor genes are often linked to cancer. Generally speaking, one or more mutations of various genes may be required for a tumor to develop.

CANCER PROMOTION

The initiation stage of carcinogenesis, during which DNA is altered, is relatively short (minutes to days). In contrast, the **cancer promotion** stage may last for months or more than 10 years before the final stage, progression, appears. During the promotion stage the DNA alterations are "locked" into the genetic material of cells.

Cancer promotion *The stage in the cancer process when cell division increases, in turn decreasing the time available for repair enzymes to act on altered DNA and encouraging cells with altered DNA to develop and grow.*

Anything that increases the rate of cell division decreases the chance that the repair enzymes will find the altered part of the DNA in time to do their work. Once a cell multiplies and incorporates its newly altered DNA into its genetic instructions, the repair enzymes can no longer detect the changes in DNA.

Compounds that increase cell division are estrogen, alcohol, and probably high intakes of dietary fat. Bacterial infections in the stomach are also suspected agents, such as with *Helicobacter pylori.*

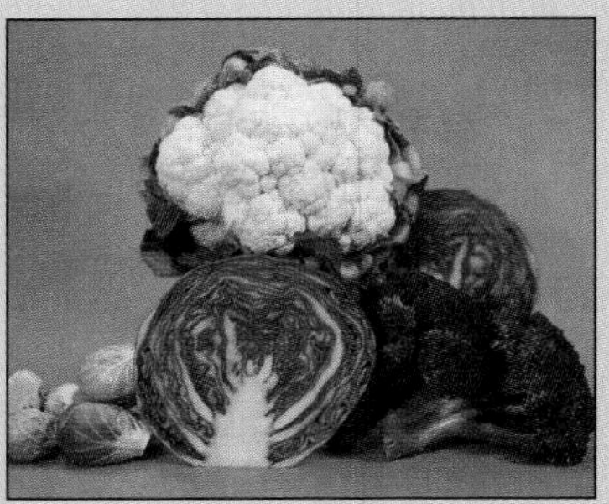

Cruciferous vegetables are rich in cancer-preventing phytochemicals.

Studies with experimental animals have revealed that some substances can inhibit this promotion stage. Compounds present in cruciferous vegetables, onions, garlic, and citrus fruits—as well as vitamin A, vitamin D, and calcium—are thought to do so. Phytochemicals in general were discussed in Chapter 2. Cancer experts agree that a diet rich in fruits and vegetables is a key cancer-preventive measure (Figure 7–15). Relying on supplementation with individual nutrients, such as vitamin A and vitamin C, does not enjoy as much support, partly because this practice doesn't contribute phytochemicals, as food choices supplying these nutrients do.

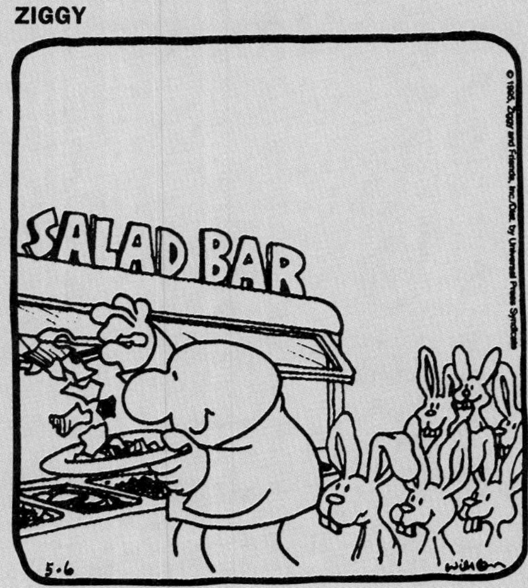

Figure 7–15
Ziggy.

CANCER PROGRESSION

The final stage in carcinogenesis begins with the appearance of cells that can grow autonomously (i.e., without normal controls on growth). During the **cancer progression** stage these malignant, or cancer, cells proliferate, invade the surrounding tissue, and spread (metastasize) to other sites. Early in this stage, the immune system may find the altered cells and destroy them. Or the cancer cells may be so defective that their own DNA limits their ability to grow, and they die. If nothing impedes growth of cancer cells, one or more tumors eventually develop that are large enough to affect body functions, and signs and symptoms of cancer appear (see Table 7–5).

Cancer progression *The final stage in the cancer process, during which the cancer cells proliferate, forming a mass large enough to significantly affect body functions.*

DIET AND CANCER

Cancer quackery aside, a nutritious diet, as well as other factors related to lifestyle, can reduce the risk of cancer initiation and promotion. Some food constituents may contribute to cancer development, whereas others have a protective effect (Table 7–6). First the association between fat/energy intake and cancer is discussed, and then some of the food constituents that may reduce the risk for cancer are covered.

Contribution of Fat and Energy Intakes to Cancer Risk

Excess energy intake, leading eventually to obesity, is related to all major forms of cancer with the exception of lung cancer. This includes cancer of the breast, colon, **endometrium,** and **prostate gland.** The link probably occurs between adipose tissue and the synthesis of estrogen from other hormones in the blood. High concentrations of circulating estrogen in the blood are thought to promote cancer.

A large-scale study called the Women's Health Initiative is testing the hypothesis that a diet with 20% or less energy from fat reduces cancer occurrence in the breast and other sites in adult women (ages 59–70 years). The study is due for completion in 2005. Currently the research community is divided on whether this will be an effective therapy for reducing breast cancer.

A long-standing excess energy intake also may promote cancer. In one study, people with the highest calorie intakes had a 70% higher risk of getting colon cancer than the control group. When animals are fed diets high in fat or total energy, they tend to experience more cancers, especially in the colon and breast. The effect is most apparent when an agent is used to deliberately initiate the cancer process, and the animals then are fed a high-fat or energy-rich diet. Fat and food energy are not considered initiators of cancer, but rather promoters.

The National Cancer Institute (NCI) believes there is a sufficient link between dietary fat and cancer to encourage Americans to reduce fat intake. It recommends initially decreasing dietary fat to about 30% of total energy intake and eventually to 20% or less of total energy if the person is at high risk and can follow such a dietary pattern.

Some nutritionists, however, believe that the NCI has overreacted to the fat and cancer issue. Although epidemiological evidence does link fat and certain forms of cancer, the evidence is not strong. A stronger link actually exists between cancer and total energy in the diet. If rats or mice are treated with a carcinogen to promote either breast or colon cancer and then one group consumes a typical energy intake while a second group consumes a reduced energy intake, the group with the low energy intake will exhibit about a 40% reduction in tumor development. The amount of fat in the diet is not important, as long as energy intake is about 70% of the usual intake of the animals. Energy restriction is currently the most effective technique for preventing cancer in laboratory animals.

The mechanism behind this effect of total energy intake is probably mostly hormonal in nature. Unfortunately, it is very difficult for humans to reduce dietary energy to 70% of usual intake. So while the data obtained from animal studies are interesting, nutritionists do not see any practical way to make recommendations on the basis of these studies. In addition, once cancer is present, energy restriction is no longer helpful.

Cancer-Inhibiting Food Constituents

Many single nutrients may have cancer-inhibiting properties. These anticarcinogens include antioxidants, certain phytochemicals, and dietary fiber (see Table 7–6).

The antioxidant activity of vitamin C and vitamin E helps to prevent formation of **nitrosamines** in the gastrointestinal tract, thus preventing formation of a potent carcinogen. Vitamin E also helps protect unsaturated fatty acids from damage by free radicals. Overall, carotenoids, vitamin E, vitamin C, and selenium function as or contribute to antioxidant systems in the body. These antioxidant systems help prevent the alteration of DNA by electron-seeking compounds.

Nitrosamine
A carcinogen formed from nitrates and breakdown products of amino acids; can lead to stomach cancer.

In addition, phytochemicals from fruits and vegetables, and even tea, block cancer development in some cases. Numerous studies suggest that fruit and vegetable intake reduces the risk of nearly all types of cancer. These foods are normally rich in carotenoids and vitamin C, plus dietary fiber and vitamin E. Adequate vitamin D intake is suspected of reducing breast, colon, and prostate cancer. In sum, a diet that follows the Food Guide Pyramid, so that fruits, vegetables, whole grains, low-fat and nonfat dairy products, and some plant oils are eaten daily, is a rich source of anticarcinogens. It is likely that all of these foods have a "cocktail" effect, in that no one food is likely to prevent cancer alone.

In Chapter 4 the possible role of fiber in preventing colon cancer was introduced. Insoluble fiber decreases transit time so that the stool is in contact with the colon wall for a shorter period of time, thus reducing contact with carcinogens. Soluble fibers may bind bile acids and thus block some recycling of these by the body. Bile acids are thought to contribute to cancer risk by irritating the colon wall, in turn increasing cell division. In addition, dietary fiber (specifically the insoluble fiber content) may increase the binding and excretion of the sex hormones testosterone and estrogen from within the intestines. This is important because of the links between excessive amounts of sex hormones and certain types of cancer, specifically prostate and colon cancer. At the present time, the evidence regarding the importance of fiber in preventing colon cancer is still inconclusive. For now, the recommendation to consume 20 to 35 grams a day is reasonable advice. Liberal use of whole grains, fruits, and vegetables should be sufficient to meet guidelines.

Calcium is also linked to a decrease risk for developing colon cancer. Some studies show that calcium decreases the growth of cells in the colon; therefore it probably decreases the risk of a genetically altered cell developing into a cancer. Calcium may also bind free fatty acids and bile acids in the colon, so they are less apt to interact with cells located there and induce cancer.

THE BOTTOM LINE

A variety of dietary changes will reduce your risk for cancer. Start by making sure that your diet is moderate in energy and fat content and that you consume many fruits and vegetables, whole grains, beans, some fish, and low-fat or nonfat milk products (Table 7–7). In addition, remain physically active, avoid obesity, and moderate alcohol intake if used, and limit intake of animal fat and salt-cured, smoked, and nitrate-cured foods.

TABLE 7-6

Some Food Constituents Suspected of Having a Role in Cancer

Constituent	Dietary sources	Action
POSSIBLY PROTECTIVE*		
Vitamin A	Liver, fortified milk, fruits, vegetables	Encourages normal cell development and differentiation.
Vitamin D	Fortified milk	Increases production of a protein which suppresses cell growth
Vitamin E	Whole grains, vegetable oil, green leafy vegetables	Antioxidant; prevents formation of nitrosamines
Vitamin C	Fruits, vegetables	Antioxidant; can block conversion of nitrites and nitrates to potent carcinogens
Folate	Fruits, vegetables, whole grains	Encourages normal cell development
Selenium	Meats, whole grains	Part of antioxidant system that inhibits tumor growth and kills early cancer cells in the promotion stage
Carotenoids	Fruits, vegetables	Tend to be antioxidants; some of these possibly influence cell metabolism
Indoles, phenols, and other plant substances	Vegetables, especially cabbage, cauliflower, brussels sprouts, garlic, onions, tea (especially green tea)†	May reduce carcinogen activation in the liver and other cells
Dietary fiber	Whole grains, fruits, vegetables, beans	May bind carcinogens in the feces and decrease stool transmit time, thus lowering risk of colon and rectal cancer
Calcium	Milk products, green vegetables	Slows cell division in the colon, binds bile acids and free fatty acids
Omega-3 fatty acids	Cold-water fish, such as salmon and tuna	May inhibit tumor growth
Soy products		Phytic acid present possibly binds carcinogens in the intestinal tract; the genistein component possibly reduces growth and metastasis of malignant cells
Conjugated linoleic acid	Milk products, meats, fish	May inhibit tumor development and act as an antioxidant
POSSIBLY CARCINOGENIC		
Fats	Meats, high-fat milk and milk products, vegetable oils	Linked to increased synthesis of estrogen and other sex hormones, which in excess may themselves increase the risk for cancer. The strongest evidence is for excessive saturated and polyunsaturated fat intake.
Alcohol	Beer, wine, liquor	Contributes to cancers of the throat, liver, bladder and the breast; increased cell turnover and liver metabolism of carcinogens are the main mechanism
Nitrites, nitrates	Cured meats, especially ham, bacon, and sausages	Under very high temperatures will bind to amino acid derivatives to form nitrosamines, potent carcinogens
Multi-ring compounds: Aflatoxin	Formed when mold is present on peanuts and other grains	May alter DNA structure and inhibit its ability to properly respond to physiologic controls; aflatoxin linked to liver cancer.
Benzo(a)pyrene	Charcoal-broiled foods, especially meats	Benzo(a)pyrene linked to stomach and other intestinal cancers

*Many of the actions listed for these possibly protective agents are speculative and have been verified only by experimental animals studies.
†Some are part of the family of cruciferous vegetables, which includes cabbage, brussels sprouts, and broccoli.

TABLE 7-7

One Example of a Diet Intended to Limit Risk for Cancer That Is Low in Fat and Rich in Foods with Anticancer Properties

BREAKFAST

Nonfat milk, 1 cup
Crispy Wheats N' Raisins, 1 cup
Orange, 1
Whole-wheat toast, 1 slice
  with fruit jam, 2 tsp
Hot tea

LUNCH

Sandwich:
  Whole wheat bread, 2 slices
  Monterey Jack cheese, ¾ oz
  Alfalfa sprouts, ½ cup
  Red onion slices
  Mustard
Lowfat yogurt (with fruit), 1 cup
Fig bar cookies, 3
Apple juice, 1 cup

SNACK

Nonfat milk, ½ cup
Graham crackers, 3

DINNER

Salad:
  Romaine lettuce, 1½ cups
    tomato, ½
  Sliced mushrooms, 3
  Oil and vinegar
    dressing, 2 tbsp
Broiled salmon, 3 oz
Brown rice, ¾ cup
Green beans, ¾ cup
Hot tea

SNACK

Banana, 1
Roasted soybeans, ¼ cup

NUTRIENT BREAKDOWN

2200 kcal; 22% kcal as fat

Remember also that if a cancer is left untreated, it can spread quickly throughout the body. When this happens, it is much more likely to lead to death. Thus early detection is critical. Aids to early detection include the following warning signs:

- Unexplained weight loss
- A change in bowel or bladder habits
- A sore that does not heal
- Unusual bleeding or discharge
- A thickening or lump in the breast or elsewhere
- Indigestion or difficulty in swallowing
- An obvious change in a wart or mole
- A nagging cough or hoarseness

There are still other ways to detect cancer early. Colonoscopy examinations for middle-age and older adults, PSA (prostate-specific antigen) tests for men, and Papanicolaou tests (Pap smears) and regular breast examinations (and mammograms starting about age 40) for women are recommended by the American Cancer Society. Finally, to learn still more about cancer, review these sources of credible cancer information on the Internet:

American Cancer Society
http://www.cancer.org
CancerNet
http://www.icic.nci.nih.gov
Oncolink
http://cancer.med.upenn.edu.

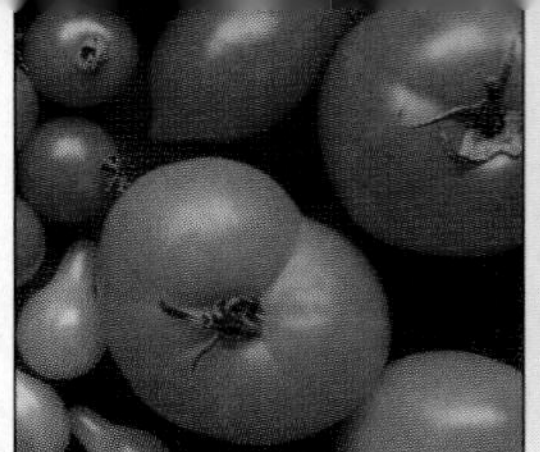

Chapter 8

Water and Minerals

Water—the most versatile medium for all kinds of chemical reactions—constitutes the major portion of our bodies. Without water, our life processes could not exist. If left out of a diet life would cease in a matter of days. We lose about 2 quarts (2 liters) of water daily, and this should be replenished daily because the body does not store water well. We know the resulting constant demand for water as *thirst.*

Many minerals, as is true for water, are vital to health. They contribute to body growth and metabolism, muscle movement, and water balance, among other wide-ranging processes. Researchers are still defining what minerals the body requires and the quantities needed for good health. We are not sure that all the minerals found in our bodies—for example, vanadium and silicon—are necessary to sustain human life. Some minerals, such as lead, may be found in humans only as a contaminant. The mere presence of a mineral in our bodies is not proof that we need it.

Based on the amount we need each day, minerals are categorized as major (requiring over 100 milligrams per day) or trace (requiring 100 milligrams or less per day). These categories do not reflect the importance of those minerals to the body; deficiencies of some trace minerals can cause severe health problems. In this chapter, you will see why the study of water and minerals is critical for understanding human nutrition, and that misuse of supplement forms of minerals easily can lead to toxicity.

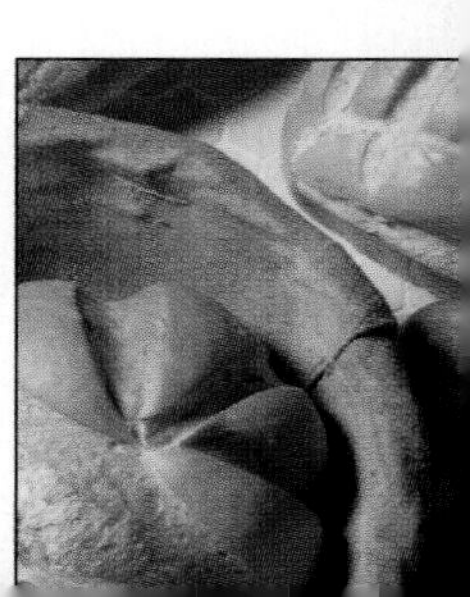

Nutrition Web

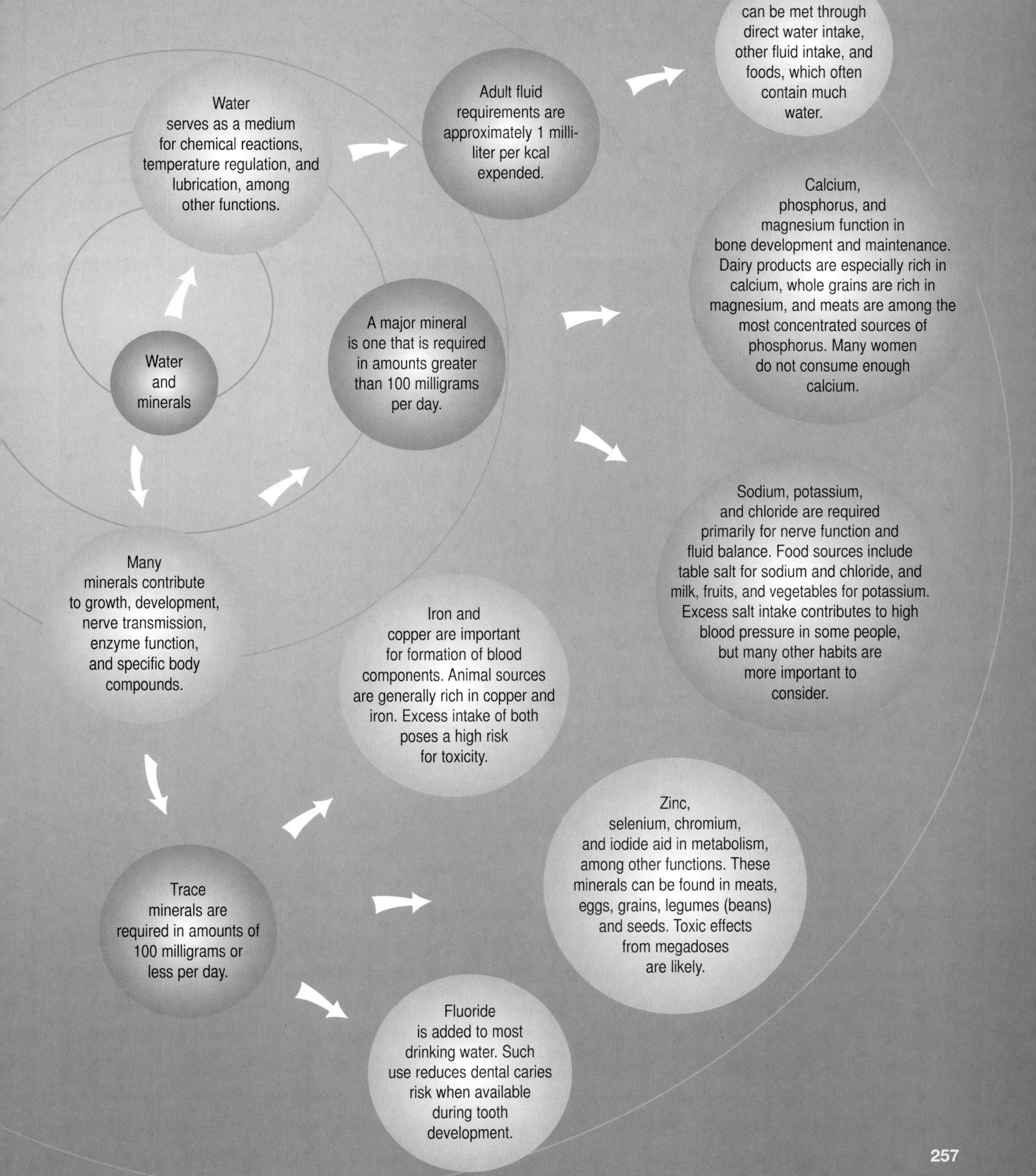

Water and minerals

Water serves as a medium for chemical reactions, temperature regulation, and lubrication, among other functions.

Adult fluid requirements are approximately 1 milliliter per kcal expended.

Fluid needs can be met through direct water intake, other fluid intake, and foods, which often contain much water.

A major mineral is one that is required in amounts greater than 100 milligrams per day.

Calcium, phosphorus, and magnesium function in bone development and maintenance. Dairy products are especially rich in calcium, whole grains are rich in magnesium, and meats are among the most concentrated sources of phosphorus. Many women do not consume enough calcium.

Sodium, potassium, and chloride are required primarily for nerve function and fluid balance. Food sources include table salt for sodium and chloride, and milk, fruits, and vegetables for potassium. Excess salt intake contributes to high blood pressure in some people, but many other habits are more important to consider.

Many minerals contribute to growth, development, nerve transmission, enzyme function, and specific body compounds.

Iron and copper are important for formation of blood components. Animal sources are generally rich in copper and iron. Excess intake of both poses a high risk for toxicity.

Trace minerals are required in amounts of 100 milligrams or less per day.

Zinc, selenium, chromium, and iodide aid in metabolism, among other functions. These minerals can be found in meats, eggs, grains, legumes (beans) and seeds. Toxic effects from megadoses are likely.

Fluoride is added to most drinking water. Such use reduces dental caries risk when available during tooth development.

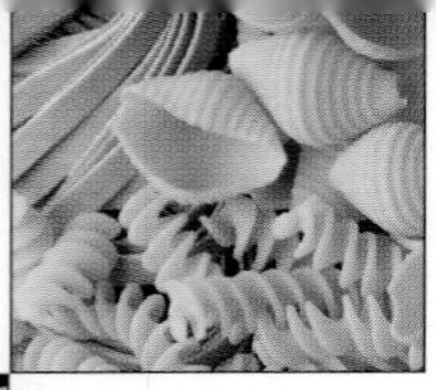
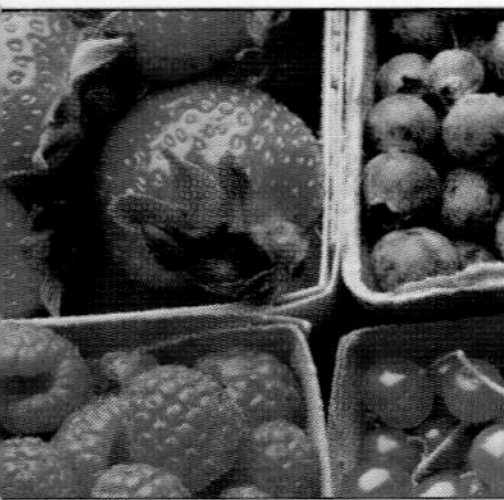

WATER

To appreciate how minerals operate in the body, it helps to understand the nature and general chemical properties of water, as well as specific nutrient-related functions.

Life as we know it could not exist without water. Water is the perfect medium for body processes because it enables chemical reactions to occur. Water even participates directly in many of these reactions. It forms the greatest component of the human body, making up 50% to 70% of the body's weight (about 10 gallons or 40 liters). Lean muscle tissue contains about 73% water. Adipose tissue is about 20% water. Thus, as fat content increases (and the percentage of lean tissue decreases) in the body, total body water content drifts toward 50%.

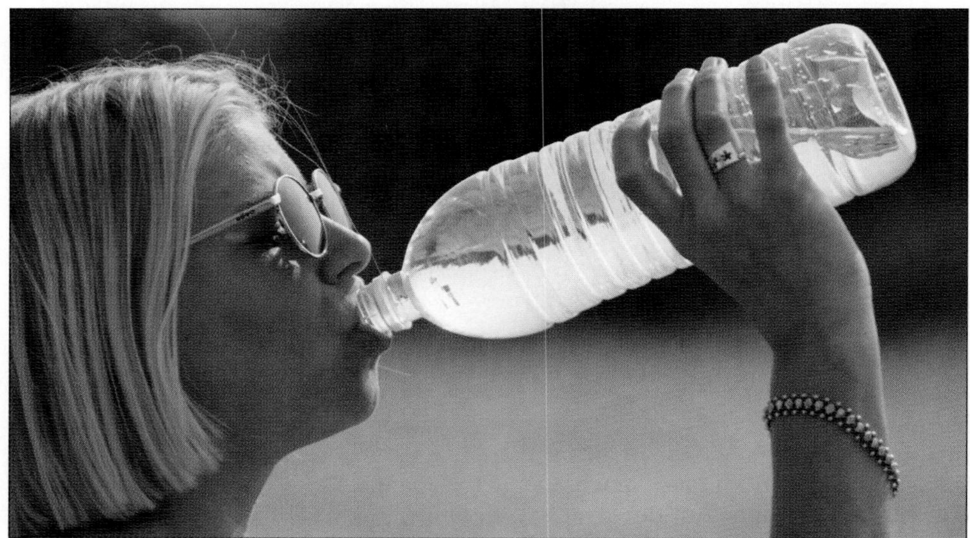

Regular intake of water is essential to replace daily fluid losses. A recent trend in America is to carry this water with us.

Depending on the amount of fat stores present, an adult can survive for about 8 weeks without eating food but only a few days without drinking water. This occurs not because water is more important than carbohydrate, fat, protein, vitamins, or minerals, but rather because we can neither store nor conserve water as well as we can the other components of our diet.

Ion
An atom with an unequal number of electrons and protons. This creates a chemical charge—negative or positive. Negative ions have more electrons than protons; positive ions have more protons than electrons.

Electrolytes
Substances that break down into ions in water and, in turn, are able to conduct an electrical current. These include sodium, chloride, and potassium.

Water in the Body—Intracellular and Extracellular Fluid

Water flows in and out of body cells through cell membranes. Water inside cells forms part of the intracellular fluid—the fluid within the cells. When water is outside cells or in the bloodstream, it is part of the extracellular fluid—that outside cells (Figure 8–1). Because cell membranes are permeable to water, water shifts freely in and out of cells. For example, if blood volume decreases, water can move from the areas inside and around cells to the bloodstream to increase blood volume. On the other hand, if blood volume increases, water can shift out of the bloodstream into cells and the surrounding areas, leading to edema (see Chapter 6).

The body controls the amount of water in the intracellular and extracellular compartments mainly by controlling **ion** concentrations. Ions have electrical charges, and so are called **electrolytes.** Water is attracted to ions, such as sodium, potassium, chloride, phosphate, magnesium, and calcium. By controlling the move-

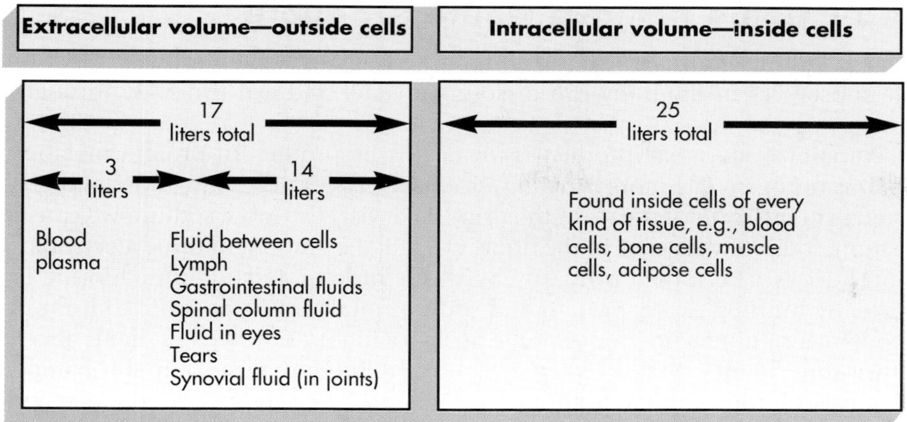

Figure 8–1 *The fluid compartments in the body.*

ments of ions in and out of the cellular compartments, the body maintains the appropriate amount of water in each compartment. Where ions go, water follows.

Positive ions, such as sodium and potassium, end up pairing with negative ions, such as chloride and phosphate. Intracellular water volume depends primarily on intracellular potassium and phosphate concentrations. Extracellular water volume depends primarily on the extracellular sodium and chloride concentrations.

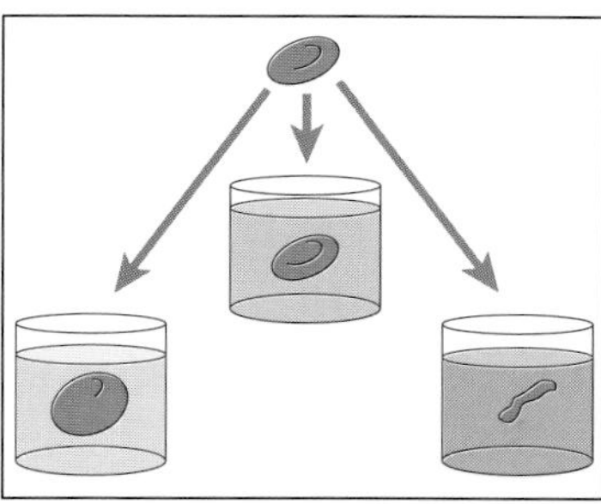

The effects of ion and water balance are easily demonstrated with red blood cells. When water is added to the fluid surrounding the cells, thereby diluting the fluid, water moves into the cells, causing them to expand. Conversely, when particles (e.g., sodium and chloride ions as table salt) are added to the fluid, thereby concentrating it, water moves out of the cells, causing them to shrink. Sugar added to strawberries acts in the same way to draw water out of the fruit.

Water Contributes to Temperature Regulation

Water changes temperature slowly because it has a great ability to hold heat. It takes much more energy to heat water than it does to heat fat. Water molecules are attracted to each, and it takes much energy to separate them. Foods with high water content heat up and cool down slowly. Because water requires so much energy to change states—for example, from a liquid to a gas—it forms an ideal medium for removing heat from the body.

The body secretes fluids in the form of perspiration, which evaporates through skin pores. To evaporate water, heat energy is required. So, as perspiration evaporates, heat energy is taken from the skin, cooling it in the process. Each quart (liter) of perspiration evaporated represents approximately 600 kcal of energy lost from the skin and surrounding tissues. For this reason, fever increases one's need for energy.

About 60% of the chemical energy in food is turned directly into body heat; the other 40% is converted to forms of energy cells can use, and almost all of that energy eventually leaves the body in the form of heat. If this heat could not be dissipated, the body temperature would rise enough to prevent enzyme systems from functioning efficiently. Perspiration is the primary way to prevent this rise in body temperature.

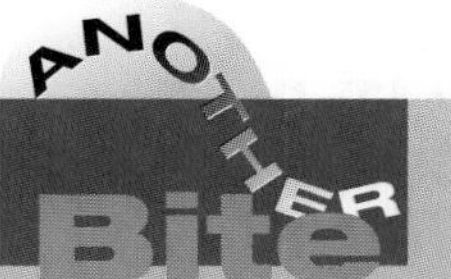

To cool efficiently, perspiration must be allowed to evaporate. If it simply rolls off the skin or soaks into clothing, perspiration doesn't cool us much. Evaporation of perspiration occurs readily when humidity is low. This is why humans often tolerate hot, dry climates far better than they do hot, humid climates.

Water Helps Remove Waste Products

Water is an important vehicle for ridding the body of waste products. Most unusable substances in the body can dissolve in water and exit the body through the urine.

Urea
A by-product of protein metabolism that contains nitrogen.

A major body waste product is ***urea.*** This by-product of protein metabolism contains nitrogen. The more protein we eat in excess of needs, the more nitrogen we excrete—in the form of urea—in the urine. Likewise, the more sodium we consume, the more sodium we excrete in the urine. Overall, the amount of urine a person needs to produce is determined primarily by excess protein and sodium chloride (salt) intake. By limiting excess protein and sodium intakes, it is possible to limit urine output—a useful practice, for example, in space flights. This type of diet is also used to treat some kidney diseases where the ability to produce urine output is hampered.

A typical urine volume is about 1 to 2 liters (1 to 2 quarts) per day, depending mostly on the amount of fluid, protein, and sodium intake. Somewhat more urine output than that is fine, but less—especially less than 600 milliliters (2½ cups)—forces the kidneys to form a very concentrated urine. This is noticeable as a very dark yellow urine. The heavy ion concentration in turn increases the risk of kidney stone formation in susceptible people, generally men. Kidney stones are simply minerals and other substances that have precipitated out of the urine and accumulated in kidney tissues.

Other Functions of Water

Amniotic fluid
Fluid contained in a sac within the uterus. This fluid surrounds and protects the fetus during development.

Water helps form the lubricants found in knees and other joints of the body. It is the basis for saliva, bile, and **amniotic fluid.** Amniotic fluid acts as a shock absorber surrounding the growing fetus in the mother's womb. Ion concentrations vary in each fluid compartment to accommodate specific needs, such as the ability to transfer nerve impulses.

How Much Water Do We Need?

Adults need roughly 1 milliliter of water per kcal expended. We consume about 1 liter (1 quart) of water a day in various liquids, such as fruit juice, coffee, tea, soft drinks, and water itself (Figure 8–2). Foods supply another liter of fluid; many fruits, vegetables, and beverages are more than 80% water (Figure 8–3). Water as a by-product of metabolism provides approximately 350 milliliters (1½ cups) of additional water. This yields a total of about 2.4 liters (10 cups) of water for a 2400 kcal diet, or about 1 milliliter per kcal expended. One way to determine if water intake is adequate is to observe the color of one's urine: it should be pale yellow.

Of the 2.4 liters of water needed, about 1.4 liters is used to produce urine. The rest, about 1 liter, compensates for typical water losses through the lungs (400 milliliters), feces (150 milliliters), and skin (500 milliliters) (see Figure 8–3). Note also

FRANK & ERNEST by Bob Thaves
M.D.
"DRINK A LOT OF LIQUIDS"? WHAT ELSE WOULD I DRINK?
THAVES 11-3
E-mail: FandEBobT@AOL.COM
© 1995 by NEA, Inc.

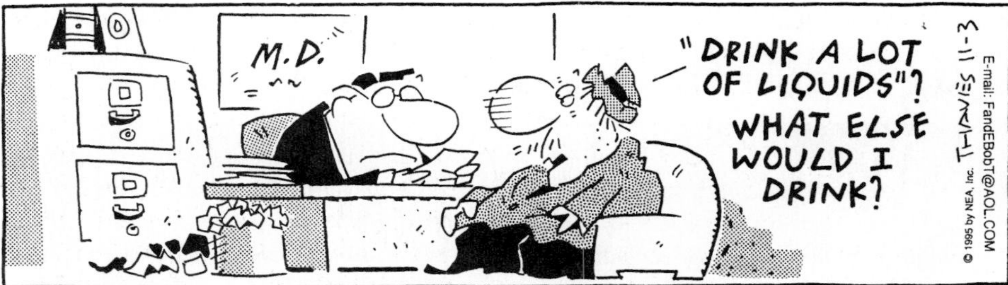

Figure 8–2 *Frank & Ernest.*

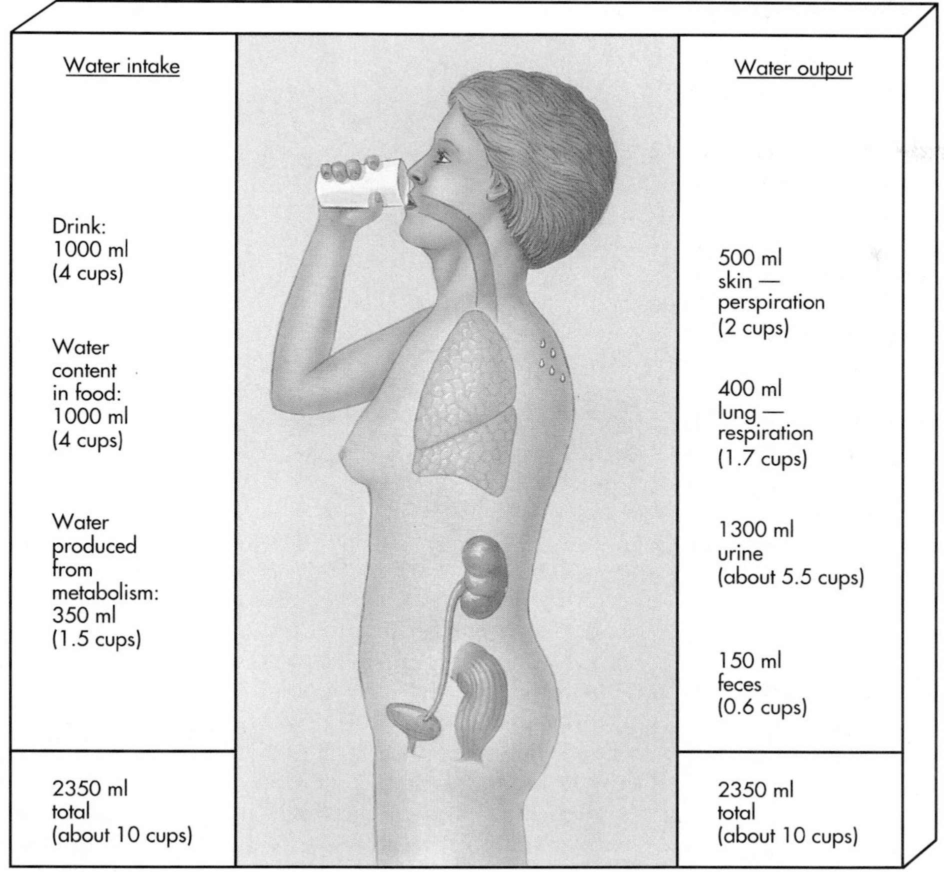

Figure 8-3 *Water balance—intake versus output. We maintain body fluids at an optimum amount by adjusting water intake and output. Most water comes from the liquids we consume. Some comes from the moisture in more solid foods, and the remainder is manufactured during metabolism. Water output includes that lost via lungs, kidneys, skin, and bowels. (Note that ml is the abbreviation for milliliter.)*

Water can be classified by whether it is hard or soft. Hard water generally comes from underground wells and usually contains calcium, magnesium, and iron. The more minerals the water contains the harder it is. Soft water has a low content of these minerals and is often produced by replacing other minerals with sodium.

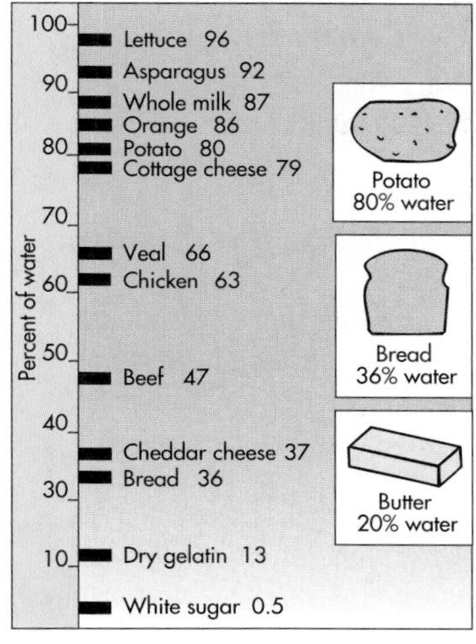

that when we consider the large amount of water used to lubricate the gastrointestinal (GI) tract, the loss of only 150 milliliters of water a day through the feces is remarkable. About 8000 milliliters of water enters the GI tract daily via secretions from the mouth, stomach, intestine, pancreas, and other organs, while the diet supplies an additional 2000 milliliters or more. The kidneys also greatly conserve water. They reabsorb about 97% of the water filtered from waste products.

Thirst

If you don't drink enough water your body often lets you know by signaling thirst. Your brain is communicating the need to drink. This thirst mechanism is not always reliable, however, especially during infancy, illness, in one's older years, and during vigorous exercise. For this reason, athletes should weigh themselves before and after training sessions to determine their rate of water loss and thus their water needs. Replacing at least 75% of this weight loss with fluid is advised, especially as weight loss approaches 2% to 3% or more. Two cups (½ liter) of water weigh about a pound (about half a kilogram) (see Chapter 10 for more details on fluid use in athletics). Ailing youngsters—especially those with fever, vomiting, diarrhea, and increased perspiration—and older persons often need to be reminded to drink plenty of fluids. As Chapter 13 discusses in further detail, infants easily become dehydrated.

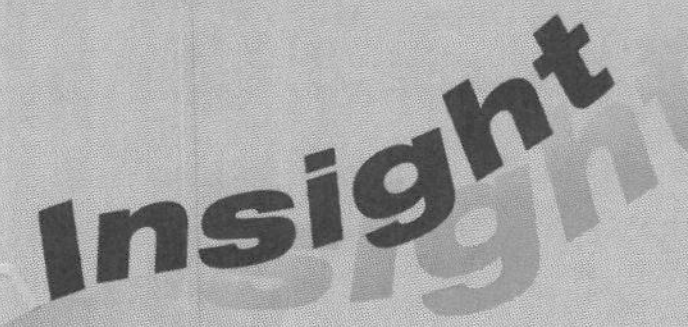

How Safe Is Our Water Supply?

These days, it is common to see 5-gallon bottles of water being delivered to homes. Grocery store shelves are now stocked with many kinds of bottled waters—ranging from simple plastic jugs containing "pure spring water" to fancier, imported varieties of mineral water in glass bottles. In Europe, bottled water is an institution, as popular as soft drinks are in the United States.

Currently, it is quite fashionable to order a bottle of Evian at a restaurant or bar. Not only are people looking for alternatives to alcoholic beverages and soft drinks, but they are also attracted to the perceived health value or taste of bottled water. Is this practice of bottled water use worth the effort and expense?

Because the U.S. water supply is monitored for safety by the Environmental Protection Agency (EPA) and local municipalities, most Americans enjoy a safe water supply from municipal sources. EPA estimates that only about 10 million people may be at risk for contamination due to inadequate filtration of their tap water, primarily those in rural communities. Recent events, however, have shaken the confidence of the public.

In 1993, 400,000 people in Milwaukee became ill and 100 died from water contaminated with *Cryptosporidium*. (A similar outbreak was recently reported in Sidney, Australia.) This protozoan poses little risk to healthy people—other than a case of diarrhea—but this is not true for people who have AIDS or other diseases that compromise function of the immune system (such as some forms of cancer therapy or organ transplant therapy). These high-risk people have, in fact, been advised to boil for at least 1 minute any tap water they use for cooking or drinking to ensure the parasite is destroyed. Alternatively, one can purchase a water filter that screens out *Cryptosporidium* (the National Sanitation Foundation at 800-673-8010 can provide a list of manufacturers) or use bottled water that is certified to be free of this agent (contact the supplier if in doubt). Generally, distilled water or that which has undergone reverse osmosis is parasite free. President Clinton recently signed into law a requirement

Antidiuretic hormone (ADH)
A hormone that is secreted by the pituitary gland and that acts on the kidneys to cause a decrease in water excretion.

Aldosterone
A hormone produced by the adrenal glands that acts on the kidneys to cause sodium, and so water, conservation.

Alcohol inhibits the action of ADH. One reason people feel so weak the day after heavy drinking is that they are very dehydrated. Even though they may have consumed a lot of liquid in their drinks, they have lost even more liquid because alcohol has inhibited ADH. Caffeine also produces a diuretic effect on the body.

What If the Thirst Message Is Ignored?

Once the body registers a shortage of available water, it increases fluid conservation. Two hormones that participate in this process are **antidiuretic hormone (ADH)** and **aldosterone.** The pituitary gland releases antidiuretic hormone (ADH) to force the kidneys to conserve water. The kidneys respond by reducing urine flow. At the same time, as fluid volume decreases in the bloodstream, blood pressure falls. This eventually triggers the release of the hormone aldosterone, which signals the kidneys to retain more sodium and, in turn, more water.

However, despite mechanisms that work to conserve water, fluid is constantly lost via the insensible routes—feces, skin, and lungs. Those losses must be replaced. In addition, there is a limit to how concentrated urine can become. Eventually, if fluid is not consumed, the body becomes dehydrated and suffers ill effects.

By the time a person loses 1% to 2% of body weight in fluids, he or she will be thirsty. And this small water deficit can cause one to feel tired. At a 4% loss of body weight, muscles lose significant strength and endurance. By the time body weight is reduced by 10% to 12%, heat tolerance is decreased and weakness results. At a 20% reduction, coma and death may soon follow.

MINERALS

The metabolic roles of minerals and the amounts of them in the body vary considerably (Figure 8–4). Some minerals, such as copper and selenium, work as cofactors, enabling enzymes to function. Minerals also contribute to many body compounds.

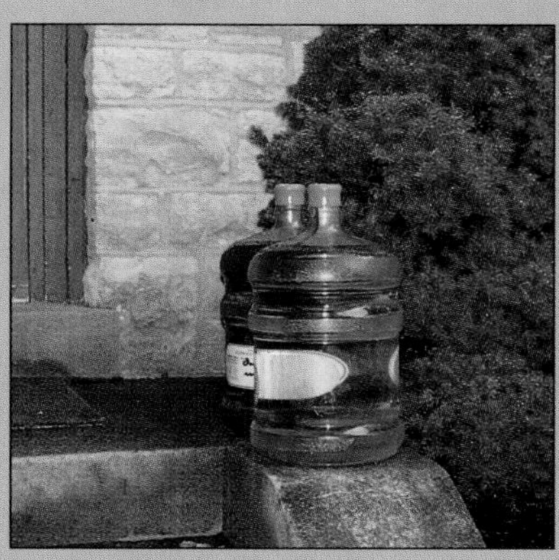

Concern over tap water quality has led some Americans to purchase bottled water. This concern has merit, especially in rural communities.

that water treatment facilities improve filtering procedures in order to reduce the presence of *Cryptosporidium.* As well, these facilities must inform customers of the results of ongoing water quality tests on an annual basis.

As a safeguard against contamination, chlorine and ammonia are added to water to kill bacteria (though such chlorination does not kill *Cryptosporidium*). The addition of such chemicals also has raised concern that drinking water may increase rectal and bladder cancer risk, though there is currently no conclusive proof of such risk. If chlorine in tap water does increase cancer risk, the risk is likely extremely small (perhaps two cases of cancer in 1 million people).

If you find the taste of chlorinated tap water unpleasant or are concerned about the possible cancer risk, you can remove the chlorine from tap water by boiling it or by letting a large container filled with water stand uncovered overnight. In both cases, the chlorine will evaporate, taking its characteristic flavor with it. Alternatively, you can install a filter on the household spigot from which you obtain your water. It should be designed to remove trihalomethanes, common chlorine by-products.

Rural water supplies from wells can also pose a risk for contamination with agricultural runoff—including nitrates and pesticides. Affected people could also consider using a home water filter or bottled water.

Overall, if you are concerned about the safety of your tap water, you can ask the municipal water department for the most current test results just mentioned, or if you have well water (or are just interested), you can have the water tested yourself. Compared with the cost of bottled water or water filters, the testing fee will be insignificant.

As noted in Chapter 15, letting cold water run for a minute or so before taking a drink or before using it in meal preparation is a good way to limit possible lead exposure from household water, especially if the water has been off for more than an hour. For the same reason, avoid using hot tap water for food preparation. Given this practice, most of us can enjoy tap water with peace of mind. For more information on water safety, call the EPA's Safe Drinking Water Hotline at 800-426-4791 or visit the web page http://www.epa.gov/safewater.

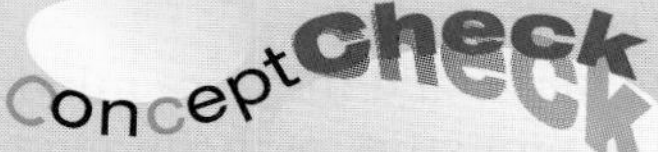

Because the body can neither readily store nor entirely conserve water, we can survive only a few days without it. Water dissolves substances, serves as a medium for chemical reactions and as a lubricant, and aids in temperature regulation. Water accounts for 50% to 70% of body weight and distributes itself all over the body: among lean and other tissues (in both intracellular and extracellular fluids) and in urine and other body fluids. Adults need about 1 milliliter of water or other fluids for each kcal expended. Thirst is the body's first sign of dehydration. If this thirst mechanism is faulty, as it may be during illness or vigorous exercise, hormonal mechanisms also help conserve water by reducing urine output. Excess fluid intake can be hazardous to a person's health. Overall, the U.S. water supply is generally safe; thus, bottled water and home water purification is unnecessary for most of us.

Too much water—whatever amount the kidneys are unable to excrete—can also lead to ill health. However, an excessive amount would have to approach many quarts (liters) each day. When excessive water overwhelms the kidneys' capacity to excrete, blurred vision is one resulting symptom.

For example, iron is a component of hemoglobin in red blood cells. Sodium, potassium, and calcium aid in the transfer of nerve impulses throughout the body. Body growth and development also depend on certain minerals, such as calcium and phosphorus. Water balance requires sodium, potassium, calcium, and phosphorus. At all levels—cellular, tissue, organ, and whole body—minerals clearly play important roles in maintaining body functions.

Minerals are categorized based on the amount we need per day. Generally speaking, if we require greater than 100 milligrams ($\frac{1}{50}$ of a teaspoon) of a mineral, it is considered a **major mineral;** otherwise, it is considered a **trace mineral.** Using

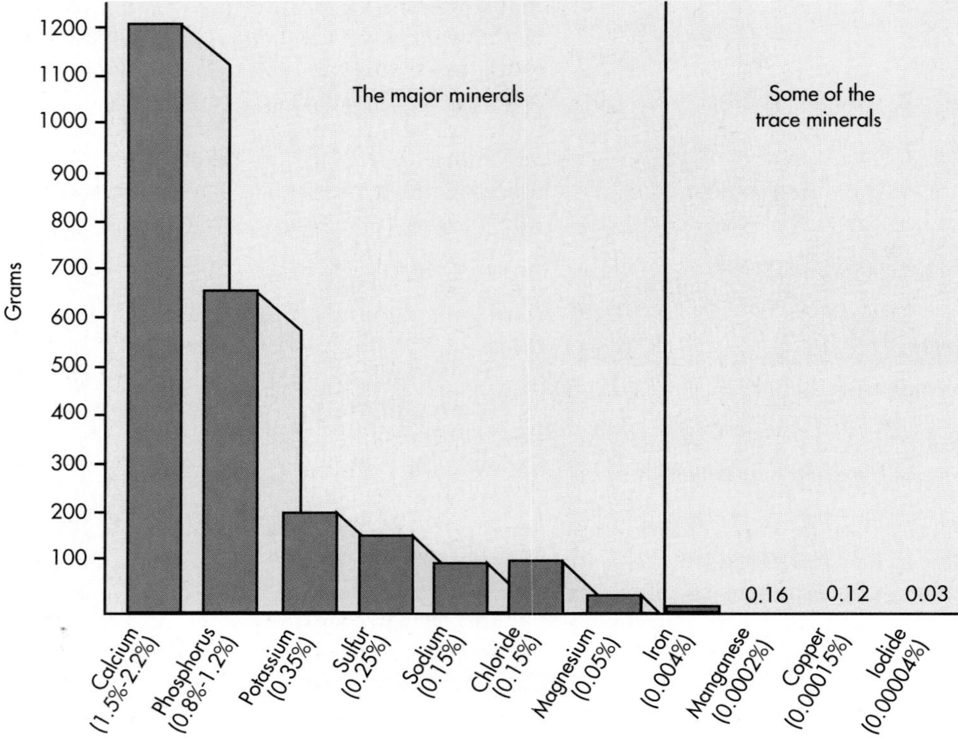

Figure 8-4 *Approximate amounts of various minerals present in the average human body. The percent values in parentheses indicate the amounts as percentages of body weight. Other trace minerals of nutritional importance not listed include chromium, fluoride, molybdenum, selenium, and zinc.*

these criteria, calcium and phosphorus are major minerals and iron and zinc are trace minerals.

The roles and nutritional significance of both the major and the trace minerals are discussed in this chapter. But before examining the properties of the individual minerals, let's consider some topics relevant to all these nutrients.

Mineral Bioavailability

Bioavailability
The degree to which the amount of an ingested nutrient is absorbed and is available to the body.

Foods contain and supply us with many minerals, but our bodies vary in their capabilities to absorb and use available minerals. Although minerals may be present in foods, they are not **bioavailable** unless a body can absorb them. The ability to absorb minerals from a diet depends on many factors. The number listed in a food composition table for the amount of a mineral in a food is just a starting point for estimating the actual contribution the food will make to our mineral needs. Spinach, for example, contains plenty of calcium, but only about 5% of it can be absorbed because of the vegetable's high concentration of *oxalic acid,* a calcium-binder. Usually, about 30% of dietary calcium is absorbed by adults, with the higher percentage coming from dairy products, and in those people consuming moderate amounts of calcium.

Minerals in the average American's diet come from both plant and animal sources. Overall, minerals from animal products are absorbed better, because binders and dietary fiber (as will soon be discussed) are not present to hinder absorption. The mineral content of plants depends on mineral concentration in the soil. Animals, however, may consume foods from multiple soil conditions and may eat a variety of plant products, because the animals are often shipped across country during their growth, so soil conditions have less of an influence. Vegans must be aware of the potentially poor mineral content of some plant foods and choose some concentrated sources of these minerals (see Chapter 6).

Generally the more refined a plant food—as in the case of white flour—the lower its content of minerals. The enrichment process for grains adds only the mineral iron. The selenium, zinc, copper, and other minerals lost when grains are refined are not replaced.

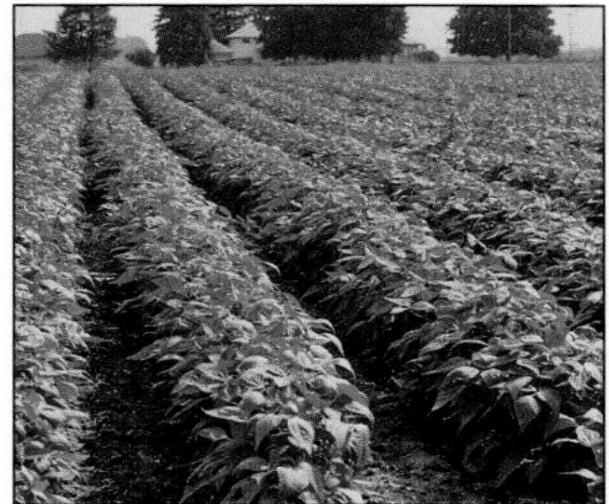

The trace mineral content of plant foods reflects the trace mineral concentration in the soil in which they were grown.

Fiber-Mineral Interactions

Mineral bioavailability can be greatly affected by nonmineral substances in the diet. Components of fiber, especially phytic acid (phytate) in grain fiber, can limit absorption of some minerals by binding to them. Oxalic acid, mentioned before, is another substance in plants that binds minerals and makes them less available to the body. High-fiber diets can decrease the absorption of iron, zinc, magnesium, and probably other minerals. An intake above the recommendation of 20 to 35 grams of dietary fiber per day then can cause problems with mineral status of the body, as noted in Chapter 4.

If grains are leavened with yeast, as they are in bread, enzymes produced by the yeast can break some of the bonds between phytic acid and minerals. This increases mineral absorption. The zinc deficiencies found among some Middle Eastern populations are attributed partly to their consumption of unleavened breads, resulting in low bioavailability of dietary zinc. This is discussed more in a later section.

Mineral-Mineral Interactions

Many minerals are of similar sizes and chemical charges, such as magnesium, calcium, iron, and copper. Having similar sizes and the same chemical charge causes these minerals to compete with each other for absorption, and so they affect each other's bioavailability. Because of this, people should avoid taking individual mineral supplements, unless a medical condition specifically warrants it. This is because an excess of one mineral influences the absorption and metabolism of other minerals. For example, the presence of a large amount of zinc in the diet decreases copper absorption. Food sources pose little risk for mineral interactions.

Vitamin-Mineral Interactions

When consumed in conjunction with vitamin C, absorption of certain forms of iron improves. The vitamin D hormone calcitriol improves calcium absorption. Many vitamins require specific minerals to act as components in their structure and function. For example, the thiamin coenzyme requires magnesium or manganese to function efficiently.

Mineral Toxicities

Excess mineral intake can lead to toxic results, especially with the trace minerals, such as iron and copper. Again, supplement use poses the biggest risk; foods are unlikely causes. This potential for toxicity is yet another reason to carefully consider the use of mineral supplements. Every year, people poison themselves using mineral supplements, even though their intent is to improve health. Many trace minerals are quite toxic at doses not much above typical needs. Mineral supplements exceeding 100% of the Daily Values on the supplement label should be taken only under a physician's supervision, because toxicity and nutrient interactions are possible. In addition, contamination in mineral supplements is a possibility. Use of USP-approved brands lessens this risk.

ConceptCheck

Minerals are vital to the functioning of many body processes. Their bioavailability depends on many factors, including a mineral's interaction with dietary fiber, vitamins, and other minerals. Animal products often yield better mineral absorption than do plants. Still, both animal and plant sources help us meet our mineral needs. Taking megadoses of an individual mineral supplement can greatly diminish the absorption and metabolism of other minerals. In addition, some minerals are potentially toxic in amounts not much in excess of body needs. These are two good reasons to consider carefully any use of mineral supplements.

MAJOR MINERALS

Up to now some general characteristics of minerals and how some of them interact with water in the body have been covered. Now let us review the individual properties of the major minerals in the context of the American diet (Table 8–1).

Sodium (Na)

For your information, the chemical symbols for the minerals discussed are given next to each mineral heading.

We both crave and hear concerns about sodium and its primary dietary source, table salt. Some of this concern is warranted, but it is an essential part of a diet.

The human body absorbs almost all sodium that gets eaten. This sodium then becomes the major positive ion in extracellular fluid and a key factor for retaining body water. Fluid balance throughout the body depends partly on varied sodium and other ion concentrations among the water-containing compartments in the body. Sodium ions also function in nerve impulse conduction and absorption of some nutrients (for example, glucose).

A low-sodium diet—coupled with excessive perspiration, persistent vomiting, or diarrhea—has the ability to deplete the body of sodium. This state can lead to muscle cramps, nausea, vomiting, dizziness, and later to shock and coma. The likelihood of this happening, however, is low because early kidney responses to low sodium status eventually trigger the body to conserve sodium. In addition, people generally eat a lot of sodium. Body conservation of sodium demonstrates how important small amounts are to body functions.

Only when weight loss from perspiration exceeds 2% to 3% of total body weight (or about 5 to 6 pounds) should sodium losses raise concern. Even then, merely salting foods is sufficient to restore body sodium for most people. Endurance athletes, however, may need to consume sports drinks during competition to avoid depletion of sodium (see Chapter 10). Note also that although perspiration tastes salty on the skin, sodium is not highly concentrated in perspiration. Rather, water evaporating from the skin leaves concentrated sodium behind. Perspiration contains about two-thirds the sodium concentration found in blood.

Sodium in Foods and Minimum Requirements

The importance of salt to human health has been recognized since antiquity. Salt was a commodity in the classical world. Indeed, the Latin word *salary* reflects the way a soldier's wages were paid.

About one-third to one-half the sodium we consume is added during cooking or at the table. Most of the rest is added during food manufacturing. Many health authorities are calling for manufacturers to use less sodium so that our total sodium intakes fall. To some extent this is taking place (for example, low sodium soups and crackers). Almost all foods naturally contain a little sodium; the higher amount

TABLE 8-1

A Summary of the Major Minerals

Name	Major functions	Deficiency symptoms	People most at risk	RDA, AI, or minimum requirement	Rich dietary sources	Results of toxicity
Sodium	Functions as a major ion of the extracellular fluid; aids nerve impulse transmission	Muscle cramps	People who severely restrict sodium to lower blood pressure (250–500 milligrams)	500 milligrams	Table salt, processed foods, condiments, sauces, soups, chips	Contributes to high blood pressure in susceptible individuals; leads to increased calcium loss in urine
Potassium	Functions as a major ion of intracellular fluid; aids nerve impulse transmission	Irregular heart beat, loss of appetite, muscle cramps	People who use potassium-wasting diuretics or have poor diets, as seen in poverty and alcoholism	2000 milligrams	Spinach, squash, bananas, orange juice, other vegetables and fruits, milk, meat, legumes, whole grains	Results in slowing of the heartbeat; seen in kidney failure
Chloride	Functions as a major ion of the extracellular fluid; participates in acid production in stomach; aids nerve transmission	Convulsions in infants	No one, probably	700 milligrams	Table salt, some vegetables, processed foods	Linked to high blood pressure in susceptible people when combined with sodium
Calcium	Provides bone and tooth strength; helps blood clotting; aids nerve-impulse transmission; required for muscle contractions	Inadequate intake increases the risk for osteoporosis	Women, especially those who consume few dairy products	1000–1200 milligrams (age over 18 years) 1300 milligrams (age 9–18 years)	Dairy products, canned fish, leafy vegetables, tofu, fortified orange juice (and other fortified foods)	Intakes over 2 grams/day may cause kidney stones and other problems in susceptible people; poor mineral absorption in general
Phosphorus	Required for bone and tooth strength; serves as part of various metabolic compounds; functions as major ion of intracellular fluid	Poor bone maintenance is a possibility	Older people consuming very nutrient-poor diets; people with alcoholism	700 milligrams (age over 18 years) 1250 milligrams (age 9–18 years)	Dairy products, processed foods, fish, soft drinks, bakery products, meats	Impairs bone health in people with kidney failure; results in poor bone mineralization if calcium intakes are low
Magnesium	Provides bone strength; aids enzyme function; aids nerve and heart function	Weakness, muscle pain, poor heart function	Women, and people on certain diuretics	Men: 420 milligrams Women: 320 milligrams	Wheat bran, green vegetables, nuts, chocolate, legumes	Causes weakness in people with kidney failure
Sulfur	Comprises part of vitamins and amino acids; aids drug detoxification	None have been described	No one as long as protein needs are met	None	Protein foods	None likely

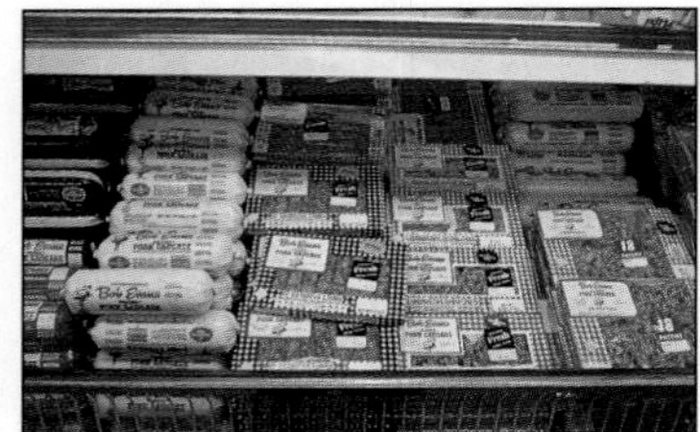

Highly processed foods, particularly processed meats, often have high sodium contents.

Table salt is 40% sodium and 60% chloride. The range of sodium intakes seen in adults of 3 to 6 grams per day translates to 7.5 to 15 grams of salt. A teaspoon of salt contains about 2 grams of sodium (2000 milligrams).

found in milk (about 120 milligrams per cup) is one exception. The more processed food one consumes, generally the higher sodium intake. Conversely, the more home cooking one does, the more sodium control that person has. Major contributors of sodium in the adult diet are white bread and rolls, hot dogs and lunch meats, cheese, soups, and foods with tomato sauce, partly because these foods are eaten so often. Other foods that generally are especially high in sodium include salted snack foods, french fries and potato chips, and sauces and gravies.

If we ate only unprocessed foods and added no salt, we would consume about 500 milligrams of sodium per day. This is also the recommended minimum sodium requirement for adults (see the inside cover for references to mineral needs for other age-groups). Even this is a generous amount, considering that we really need only about 100 milligrams a day.

If we compare 500 milligrams of sodium from unprocessed food with the 3000 to 6000 milligrams or more typically eaten by adults, it is clear that food processing and cooking contribute most of our dietary sodium. As discussed in Chapter 2, nutrition labels list a food's sodium content. When dietary sodium must be severely restricted, these labels become very helpful. Under FDA food-labeling rules, the Daily Value for sodium is 2400 milligrams. FDA established this value because it is consistent with government reports that encourage reduced sodium intakes.

Most humans can adapt to various dietary salt intakes, though very high intakes can be toxic. For most people who eat a typical diet, today's sodium intake is simply tomorrow's urine output. However, approximately 10% to 15% of adults are sodium sensitive. For these people, high sodium intakes contribute to high blood pressure, and lower-sodium diets (about 2 to 3 grams daily) often help correct the problem (see the next Nutrition Insight), but keep in mind that other lifestyle factors also contribute to high blood pressure, and even more so. Scientific groups typically suggest that all adults reduce intake to 2.4 to 3 grams, mostly to limit the risk of later developing high blood pressure. Following this advice also helps maintain healthy calcium status, as sodium intake greater than about 2 grams per day increases urinary calcium loss as the sodium is excreted.

You can evaluate your sodium habits by completing the questionnaire in Table 8–2. The more checks in the "often" or "regularly" columns, the higher your dietary sodium intake. However, not all the habits in the table contribute the same amount of sodium. For example, many natural cheeses are relatively moderate in sodium, whereas processed cheeses and cottage cheese are much higher. You can choose to reduce your sodium intake by cutting back on those items for which you checked "often" or "regularly." You needn't suddenly eliminate foods from your diet. Rather, to moderate sodium intake, choose lower-sodium foods from each food group more often and balance high-sodium food choices with low-sodium ones. It is also important to pay attention to the sodium values listed on food labels, and taste foods before adding salt. In addition, when eating out, avoiding foods commonly prepared with lots of sodium and asking to have sauces served on the side and then using only small amounts are two good ideas.

It is also a good idea to have your blood pressure checked regularly. If you have high blood pressure, you should try to reduce your sodium intake as you follow a comprehensive plan to treat this disease.

It is actually not that hard to eventually adapt to a low-sodium diet. At first, foods will taste quite bland, but eventually you will perceive more flavor as the tongue becomes more sensitive to the salt content of foods. By slowly reducing dietary sodium and substituting oregano, lemon juice, and other herbs and spices, you can eventually become accustomed to a diet that contains only 3 grams of sodium daily but does not result in much of a flavor trade-off. Many new cookbooks offer excellent recipes for flavorful low-sodium foods.

TABLE 8-2

Questionnaire for Evaluating Your Sodium Habits with Respect to Typically Rich Sources

HOW OFTEN DO YOU:	Rarely	Occasionally	Often	Regularly (daily)
1. Eat cured or processed meats, such as ham, bacon, sausage, frankfurters, and other luncheon meats?	☐	☐	☐	☐
2. Choose canned or frozen vegetables with sauce?	☐	☐	☐	☐
3. Use commercially prepared meals, main dishes, or canned or dehydrated soups?	☐	☐	☐	☐
4. Eat cheese, especially processed cheese?	☐	☐	☐	☐
5. Eat salted nuts, popcorn, pretzels, corn chips, or potato chips?	☐	☐	☐	☐
6. Add salt to cooking water for vegetables, rice, or pasta?	☐	☐	☐	☐
7. Add salt, seasoning mixes, salad dressings, or condiments—such as soy sauce, steak sauce, catsup, and mustard—to foods during preparation or at the table?	☐	☐	☐	☐
8. Salt your food before tasting it?	☐	☐	☐	☐
9. Ignore labels for sodium content when buying foods?	☐	☐	☐	☐
10. When dining out, choose foods at restaurants with sauces, or foods that are obviously salty?	☐	☐	☐	☐

The more checks you have in the last two columns, the higher your dietary sodium intake.

Adapted from USDA *Home and Garden Bulletin* No. 232-6, April 1986.

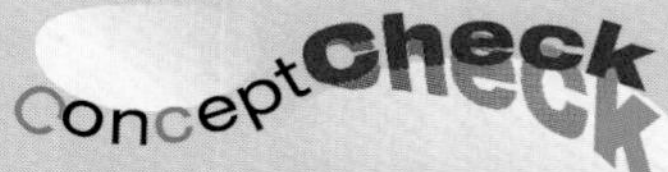

Sodium is the major positive ion of extracellular fluid. It is important for maintaining fluid balance and conducting nerve impulses. Sodium depletion is unlikely, since the typical American's diet has abundant sources of sodium and most of it gets absorbed. The more foods we prepare at home, the more control we have over our sodium intake. The minimum sodium requirement for adults is 500 milligrams per day. The average adult consumes 3000 to 6000 milligrams or more daily. About 10% to 15% of the population is sensitive to sodium. In these people, high blood pressure can develop as a result of high-sodium diets, but many other lifestyle habits are more important. Many scientific groups suggest that for all adults sodium intake should be limited to about 3 grams (3000 milligrams). Sodium in the American diet is provided predominantly through processed foods and salt added in cooking and at the table.

Potassium (K)

Potassium performs many of the same functions as sodium, such as fluid balance and nerve impulse transmission. However, it operates inside, rather than outside, cells. Intracellular fluids—those inside cells—contain 95% of the potassium in the body. Also, unlike sodium, potassium is associated with lower rather than higher blood pressure values. We absorb about 90% of the potassium we eat.

Minerals and High Blood Pressure

One out of four American adults has high blood pressure, as does one out of two in those over age 60. In 1995 alone, consequences of high blood pressure cost almost $24 billion in medical expenses, lost wages, and decreased productivity.

Blood pressure is expressed by two different numbers. The higher number represents **systolic blood pressure,** which is the pressure in the arteries when the heart actively pumps blood. The second value is for **diastolic blood pressure,** which is the artery pressure when the heart is relaxed. Optimal systolic blood pressure is less than 120 millimeters of mercury. Optimal diastolic blood pressure is less than 80 millimeters of mercury. A high diastolic pressure shows a strong relationship to various diseases, as does a high systolic pressure.

High blood pressure (referred to as hypertension in the medical field) is defined as sustained systolic pressure exceeding 140 millimeters of mercury or diastolic blood pressure exceeding 90 millimeters of mercury.

Most cases of high blood pressure (about 95% of cases) have no clear-cut cause. It is described as primary, or essential, in nature (e.g., essential hypertension). Kidney disease, sleep-disordered breathing (sleep apnea), and other causes often lead to the other 5% of cases. African-Americans are more likely than whites to develop high blood pressure and to do so earlier in life. As a result, they also suffer more from high blood pressure–related diseases.

Classification of Blood Pressure for Adults Age 18 Years and Older in Millimeters of Mercury*

Category	Systolic		Diastolic
Optimal	<120	and	<80
Normal	<130	and	<85
High-normal†	130–139	or	85–89
Hypertension			
Stage 1	140–159	or	90–99
Stage 2	160–179	or	100–109
Stage 3	≥180	or	≥110

*Not taking high blood pressure drugs and not acutely ill

†People with diabetes or kidney or heart disease should be treated for high blood pressure at this stage.

Unless blood pressure is measured periodically, development of high blood pressure is easily overlooked. Thus it's described as a "silent" disorder. A physician usually does not treat high blood pressure with medication until the diastolic blood pressure measures at least 90 millimeters of mercury (or the systolic blood pressure reaches 140) on three or more occasions.

Why Control High Blood Pressure?

High blood pressure needs to be controlled mainly to prevent heart disease, kidney disease, strokes and related declines in brain function, poor blood circulation in the legs, and sudden death. All these diseases are much more likely to be found in people with high blood pressure than in people with normal blood pressure. Smoking and elevated blood lipoproteins make these diseases even more likely. People with high blood pressure need to be diagnosed and treated as soon as possible, as the condition generally progresses to a more serious stage over time and also ends up resisting treatment to a greater extent.

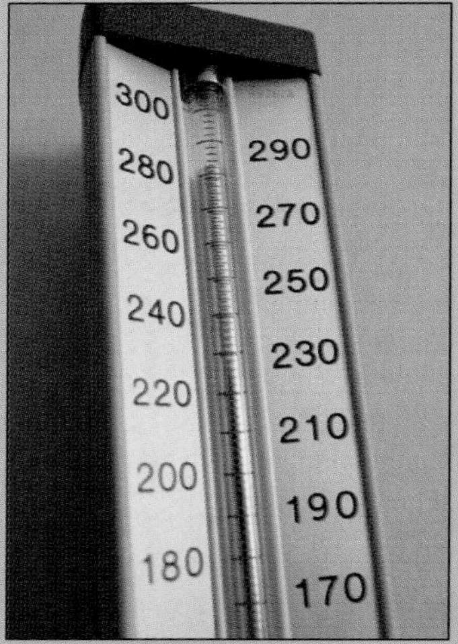

High blood pressure is harmful to many organs in the body. Maintenance of healthy valves is a key to disease prevention throughout life.

Causes of High Blood Pressure

Blood pressure usually increases as a person ages. Some increase is caused by atherosclerosis. As plaque builds up in the arteries, the arteries become less flexible and cannot expand. When vessels remain rigid, blood pressure remains high. Eventually the plaque begins to choke off blood supply to the kidneys, decreasing their ability to control blood volume, and in turn, blood pressure.

Obesity is the main lifestyle cause of high blood pressure, especially in women. High blood insulin associated with insulin-resistant adipose cells is one reason for this. Insulin increases sodium retention in the body and speeds atherosclerosis. Inactivity is the second leading lifestyle cause of high blood pressure. If an obese person can lose weight (often as little as 10 to 15 pounds helps) and engage in regular physical activity, blood pressure often returns to normal.

Alcohol and High Blood Pressure

Excess alcohol intake is the third leading lifestyle cause of high blood pressure, especially in middle-aged males and in African-Americans in general. An intake of two or fewer drinks per day for people with high blood pressure usually does not cause this problem, but the person could experiment with abstinence to see if it improves the overall therapy employed. Some studies suggest, however, that moderate alcohol use reduces the risk of related strokes. This data should not be used to encourage alcohol use in nonconsumers, but moderate drinking does have benefits (see Chapters 5 and 14).

Sodium and Blood Pressure

Sodium intake increases blood pressure in some people, particularly in those who are susceptible to developing the problem. However, only some Americans are very susceptible to sodium-linked increases in blood pressure. Older African-Americans are prime candidates. Sodium is likely the fourth leading lifestyle cause of high blood pressure, but its precise rank is under debate.

The exact mechanism of salt in increasing blood pressure is not clear, but it is thought that excess sodium may cause sodium channels (channels that move sodium into and out of cells) to work too hard. Over time these channels then may begin to fail, so that the kidneys cannot successfully flush all of the excess sodium it receives into the urine.

Other Minerals and Blood Pressure

Minerals such as calcium, potassium, and magnesium also deserve attention when it comes to high blood pressure. In fact, adequate intake of these nutrients may be more important in treating high blood pressure than greatly restricting sodium intake. People often register lower blood pressures—especially the systolic component—when they consume at least the AI for calcium per day, as compared with one-third to one-half that amount. It is reasonable for a person with high blood pressure to experiment, in consultation with a physician, with increasing calcium intake to see if that produces the desired effect.

Potassium intake in the range of about 4 grams also has been shown to moderately decrease blood pressure in people currently consuming far below this amount. Adequate potassium intake yielded by a diet rich in fruits and vegetables also reduces risk of related strokes. Some studies indicate that magnesium also is capable of lowering blood pressure at intakes of about twice the RDA, but overall the results of these studies are inconsistent. Note that increasing the intake of these minerals using supplements is not advised without first consulting a physician.

Other Causes of High Blood Pressure

Other causes of high blood pressure include specific enzymes and hormone-like compounds that are related to kidney function. Medications are available to reduce their effect. Finally, preliminary studies show a link between bone lead concentrations and increased risk of high blood pressure. More information is needed, but it is suspected that even low amounts of lead stored over

TABLE 8-3

A Nutritional Plan to Minimize High Blood Pressure and Stroke Risk*

1. Follow the Food Guide Pyramid. Also consider going beyond this to include more fruit, vegetables, and some nuts (i.e., DASH diet).
2. Make sure to meet nutrient recommendations for calcium, potassium, and magnesium listed in the chapter.
3. Attain and maintain a healthy body weight.
4. Incorporate regular physical activity (at least five times per week).
5. Consume alcoholic beverages in moderation, if at all (two drinks per day maximum).
6. Consume moderate amounts of sodium and see if this helps.
7. Don't smoke.
8. Maintain blood lipoproteins in the normal range (see Chapter 5).

*In addition, make sure to have blood pressure measured on a regular basis (i.e., yearly physician checkups).

decades may damage the kidneys and eventually result in the disease. This is just one of the deleterious effects of lead exposure (see Chapter 15 for more information on lead).

Preventing High Blood Pressure

Many of the risk factors for high blood pressure and stroke are controllable, and appropriate lifestyle changes can reduce a person's risk (Table 8-3). Experts typically recommend trying to lower blood pressure through exercise and lifestyle changes before resulting to blood pressure medications. A trial of up to 12 months of this lifestyle therapy is urged for high-normal and Stage 1 patients. Only after this therapy has failed is the use of medications advocated. And even if medications are needed, lifestyle management is still paramount. Note also that a recent study conducted to see whether dietary factors could influence blood pressure showed that study participants experienced a decrease in blood pressure within days of beginning a specific diet. The response was even similar to that seen with commonly used medications. The diet closely followed the Food Guide Pyramid, with a few additions: one serving of nuts, seeds or legumes per day, two extra servings of fruit per day, and one additional serving of vegetables per day. Sodium intake was kept at 3 grams per day, and alcohol was limited to two servings per week (Table 8-4). For more information, see this web site: http:\\www.nih.gov/news/pr/apr97/Dash.htm.

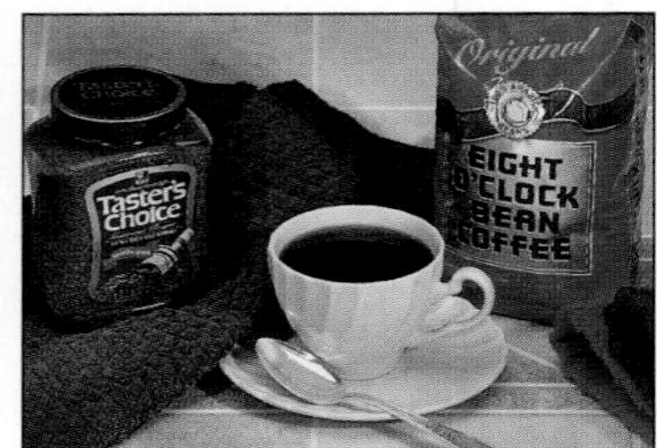

Coffee is a major contributor of potassium to the American diet.

Low blood potassium is a life-threatening problem. Symptoms often include a loss of appetite, muscle cramps, confusion, and constipation. Eventually, the heart beats irregularly, decreasing its capacity to pump blood.

Potassium in Foods and Minimum Requirements

Generally, unprocessed foods are rich sources of potassium. This includes fruits, vegetables, milk, whole grains, dried beans, and meats. Major contributors of potassium to the adult diet include milk, potatoes, beef, coffee, tomatoes and orange juice (Figure 8-5).

TABLE 8-4

The DASH Diet—A Sample Menu (provides approximately 2000 calories)

BREAKFAST	
Shredded Wheat, 1 cup	2 grains
1% low-fat milk, 8 oz	1 milk
Sugar, 1 tsp	
Banana, 1 medium	1 fruit
Grapefruit juice, 4 oz	1 fruit
SNACK	
Pretzels, ¾ oz	1 grain
Diet soft drink, 12 oz	
LUNCH	
Chicken salad, ¾ cup (made with reduced-fat mayonnaise)	1 meat 1 fat
Whole-wheat bread, 2 slices	2 grains
Carrots, 5 baby	1 vegetable
Low-fat yogurt, 1 cup (with artificial sweetener)	1 milk
Applesauce, ½ cup	1 fruit
SNACK	
Mixed nuts, ¾ oz	1 nut
Grape juice, 4 oz	1 fruit
DINNER	
Baked orange roughy, 3 oz	1 meat
Rice, 1 cup	2 grains
Steamed broccoli, 1 cup	2 vegetables
Mixed greens salad, 2 cups (including some other vegetables)	1 vegetable
Light Italian dressing, 1 tbsp	½ fat
Whole-wheat roll, 1 small	1 grain
Margarine, 1 tsp	1 fat
1% low-fat milk, 8 oz	1 milk
SNACK	
Watermelon 1¼ cup	1 fruit

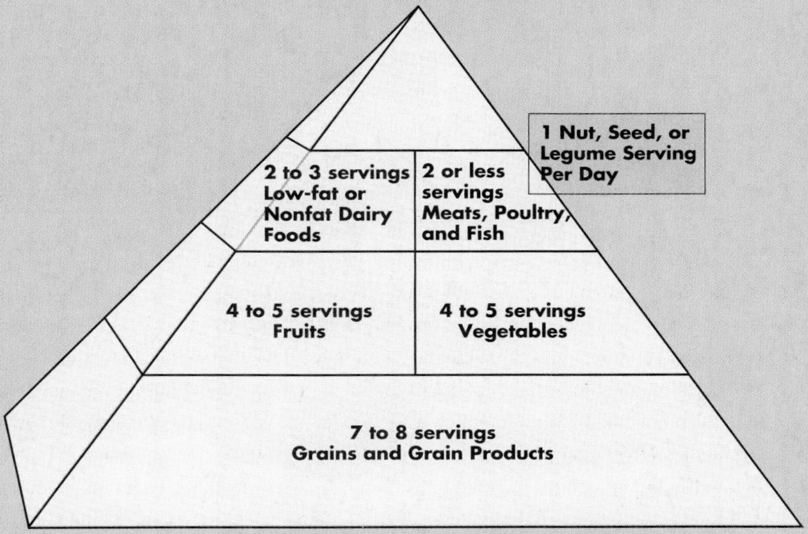

The Dietary Approaches to Stop Hypertension (DASH) diet was found to decrease systolic blood pressure by 5.5 millimeters of mercury (mm Hg) and diastolic blood pressure by 3.0 mm Hg more than the control diet. Overall, this diet provides approximately 18% of energy as protein, 55% as carbohydrate, and 27% as fat, with 6% from saturated fat. The diet contains more fruit and vegetable servings than the Food Guide Pyramid, less fat, and includes a serving of nuts, All DASH participants consumed no more than 3 grams of sodium and up to 2 alcoholic drinks per week. Researchers estimate that if Americans followed the DASH diet, there would be a 15% decrease in heart disease and 27% fewer strokes.

The adult minimum potassium requirement for health is 2000 milligrams (2 grams) per day. Typically an adult gets enough potassium by eating a wide variety of foods. Americans average 2 to 3 grams per day.

Diets are more likely to be low in potassium than sodium because we generally do not add potassium to foods. Some **diuretics** used to treat high blood pressure also deplete the body's potassium. Thus people who take potassium-wasting diuretics need to monitor their potassium intakes carefully. For these people, high-potassium foods—such as fruits, fruit juices, and vegetables—are good additions to the diet, and if recommended by a physician, so are potassium chloride supplements.

Diuretic
A substance that increases the flow of urine.

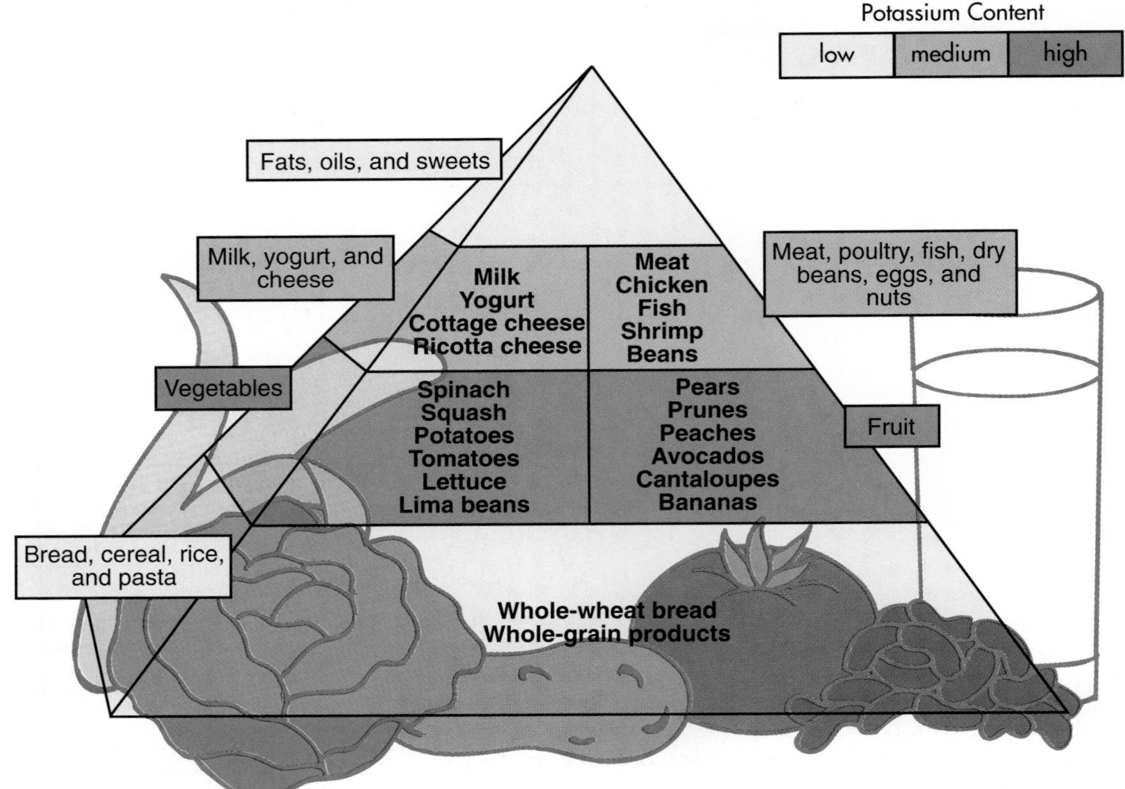

Figure 8-5 *Food sources of potassium from the Food Guide Pyramid. The fruit group and the vegetable group are the best dietary sources of this nutrient, but it is widely distributed in foods. The background color of each food group indicates the amount of potassium in that group.*

A continually deficient food intake, as may be the case in alcoholism, can also result in potassium deficiency. People with anorexia nervosa and bulimia nervosa, whose diets are poor and whose bodies can be depleted of nutrients because of vomiting, are also at risk for potassium deficiency (see Chapter 11). People on very low-calorie diets are also at risk and so are athletes who exercise heavily. As covered in Chapters 9 and 10, all of these people should compensate for potentially low body potassium by consuming potassium-rich foods.

If the kidneys function normally, typical intakes of dietary potassium are not toxic. When the kidneys function poorly, potassium builds up in the blood. This inhibits heart function, causing slowed heartbeats. If untreated, this can be fatal, as the heart eventually stops beating. Consequently, in cases of reduced kidney function, close control of potassium intake becomes critical.

Food Sources of Potassium

Food item and amount	*Potassium (milligrams)*
Baked winter squash, ¾ cup	**780**
Cooked kidney beans, 1 cup	**710**
Baked potato, 1	**610**
Cantaloupe, 1 cup	**490**
Orange juice, 1 cup	**470**
Banana, 1	**470**
Steamed zucchini, 1 cup	**450**
Cooked lima beans, ½ cup	**370**
Raisins, ¼ cup	**300**
Cooked asparagus, 1 cup	**290**

Chloride (Cl)

Chlorine is a very poisonous gas. In our bodies, chloride—an ion form of chlorine—forms an important negative ion for the extracellular fluid. These ions are a component of the acid produced in the stomach and are also used during immune responses as white blood cells attack foreign cells. In addition, nerve function relies on the presence of chloride. As is the case with sodium, most of the body's chloride is excreted by the kidneys; some is lost in perspiration. It is also implicated in the blood pressure–raising ability of sodium chloride.

A chloride deficiency is unlikely, because our dietary sodium chloride (salt) intake is so high. Frequent and lengthy bouts of vomiting—if coupled with a nutrient-poor diet—can contribute to a deficiency, because stomach secretions contain much chloride.

Chloride in Foods and Minimum Requirements

A few fruits and some vegetables are naturally good sources of chloride. Chlorinated water is also a source. However, we consume most chloride as salt added to foods. Knowing a food's salt content allows for a close prediction of its chloride content; recall salt is 60% chloride.

The minimum chloride requirement for health in adults is 700 milligrams per day. Assuming that the average adult consumes at least 7.5 grams of salt daily, that yields 4.5 grams (4500 milligrams) of chloride, an abundance of this ion.

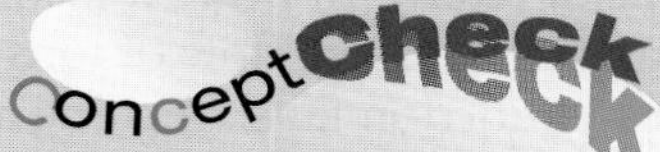

Potassium performs functions similar to those of sodium, except that it is the main positive ion found inside, not outside, cells. Potassium is vital to fluid balance and nerve transmission. A potassium deficiency—caused by an inadequate intake of potassium, persistent vomiting, or use of some diuretics—can lead to loss of appetite, muscle cramps, confusion, and heartbeat irregularities. Fruits and vegetables are generally rich sources of potassium. Potassium intake can be toxic if a person's kidneys do not function properly. Chloride is the major negative ion of extracellular fluid. Chloride also functions in digestion as part of stomach acid and in immune and nervous system responses. Deficiencies of chloride are highly unlikely because we eat so much sodium chloride (salt), the major source.

Calcium (Ca)

All cells need calcium, but more than 99% of the calcium in the body is used to strengthen bones and teeth. This calcium represents 40% of all the minerals present in the body and equals about 2.5 pounds (1200 grams). As calcium circulates in the bloodstream, it supplies the calcium needs of body cells. Growth and bone development require an adequate calcium intake.

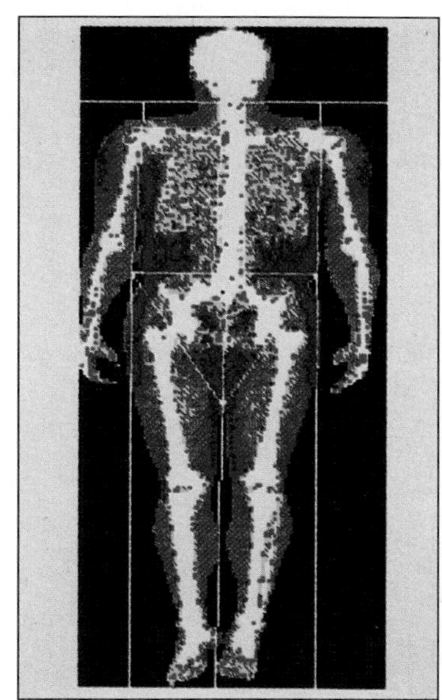

Ninety-nine percent of calcium in the body is in bones.

Unlike sodium, potassium, and chloride, the amount of calcium in the body hinges greatly on its absorption from the diet. Calcium requires an acid environment to be absorbed efficiently. Absorption occurs primarily in the upper part of the small intestine. This area tends to remain acidic because it receives the acidic stomach contents. Much calcium absorption in the upper small intestine depends on the active vitamin D hormone.

Adults absorb about 30% of calcium in the foods eaten, but during times when the body needs extra calcium—such as in infancy and pregnancy—absorption might reach as high as 60%. Young people tend to absorb calcium better than do older people, especially those older than 70. Postmenopausal women generally absorb the least calcium, unless they receive supplements of the hormone estrogen. Estrogen therapy is associated with an increased synthesis of the active vitamin D hormone, which aids calcium absorption. Estrogen also has a direct effect on bones to promote bone health (see the Nutrition Issue).

Many other factors end up enhancing calcium absorption: parathyroid hormone, dietary glucose, and lactose; and normal intestinal motility (flow). Factors limiting calcium absorption include large amounts of phytic acid in dietary fiber from grains; great excess of phosphorus in the diet; polyphenols (tannins) in tea; a vitamin D deficiency; menopause; diarrhea; and old age.

Because we have excellent hormonal systems to control blood calcium, a normal value can be maintained despite an inadequate calcium intake. The bones, however, pay the price. Bone loss caused by insufficient calcium intake proceeds slowly. Only after many years are clinical symptoms apparent. By not meeting calcium needs, some people—especially women—are most likely setting the stage for future bone fractures. However, because we don't know how efficiently each individual absorbs calcium, we often cannot predict who is at the highest risk.

Functions of Calcium

Forming and maintaining bones are calcium's major roles in the body. This is discussed in detail in the Nutrition Issue on osteoporosis. However, calcium is important in many other processes as well. Calcium is essential for blood clotting and for muscle contraction. If blood calcium falls below a critical point, muscles cannot relax after contraction; the body stiffens and shows signs of **tetany.** In nerve transmission, calcium works to release chemical messengers and permits the flow of ions in and out of nerve cells. Without sufficient calcium, nerve function fails, opening another path to tetany. Finally, calcium helps regulate cellular metabolism by influencing the activities of various enzymes and hormonal responses. It is the hormonal regulation of blood calcium that keeps all these processes going, even if you fail to eat enough calcium on a daily basis.

Tetany
A body condition marked by sharp contraction of muscles and failure to relax afterward; usually caused by abnormal calcium metabolism.

Other Possible Health Benefits of Dietary Calcium.

Adequate dietary calcium can reduce the risk of colon cancer, especially in people consuming a high-fat diet (see Chapter 4). Calcium intakes of 800 to 1200 milligrams per day can decrease blood pressure, compared with intakes of 400 milligrams per day or less (see the previous Nutrition Insight). In addition, as covered in Chapter 5, when people with elevated LDL consume a low-fat, low-cholesterol diet, supplementation with calcium at 1200 milligrams per day further reduces LDL. Practical dietary recommendations stemming from all this research indicate that meeting the Adequate Intake (AI) for calcium or exceeding it somewhat may be beneficial for a variety of conditions, not just bone health.

Diets that are low in natural sources of calcium tend also to be low in other essential nutrients found in dairy products such as riboflavin, vitamin A, and potassium. Thus a low calcium intake generally reflects poor dietary patterns. Individuals who increase their calcium intake through foods, rather than supplements, increase their intake of many other nutrients as well.

Calcium in Foods and the AI

Dairy products, such as milk and cheese, provide about 75% of the calcium in American diets. The exception is cottage cheese because most calcium is lost during production. Bread, rolls, crackers, and other foods made with milk products are secondary contributors. Other calcium sources are leafy greens (such as spinach), broccoli, sardines, and canned salmon. However, much of the calcium in some leafy green vegetables, notably spinach, is not absorbed because of the presence of oxalic acid. This effect is not as strong, however, in kale, collard, turnip, and mustard greens. Overall, nonfat milk is the most nutrient-dense (milligrams per kcal) source of calcium because of its high bioavailability and low energy value, with some of the vegetables just noted following close behind (Figure 8–6). The new calcium-fortified versions of orange juice and other beverages, as well as calcium-fortified cottage cheese, breakfast cereals, breakfast bars, and snacks, also follow as close competitors. Another source of calcium is soybean curd (tofu) if it is made with calcium carbonate (check the label). Note that it is the bones in canned fish, such as salmon and sardines, that supply the calcium.

One reason the Food Guide Pyramid contains a milk, yogurt, and cheese group is to supply calcium to the diet. People who do not like milk can use products made with milk, such as chocolate milk, yogurt, cheese, and ice cream. All forms of milk, yogurt, and cheese allow about the same degree of calcium absorption. Moderation

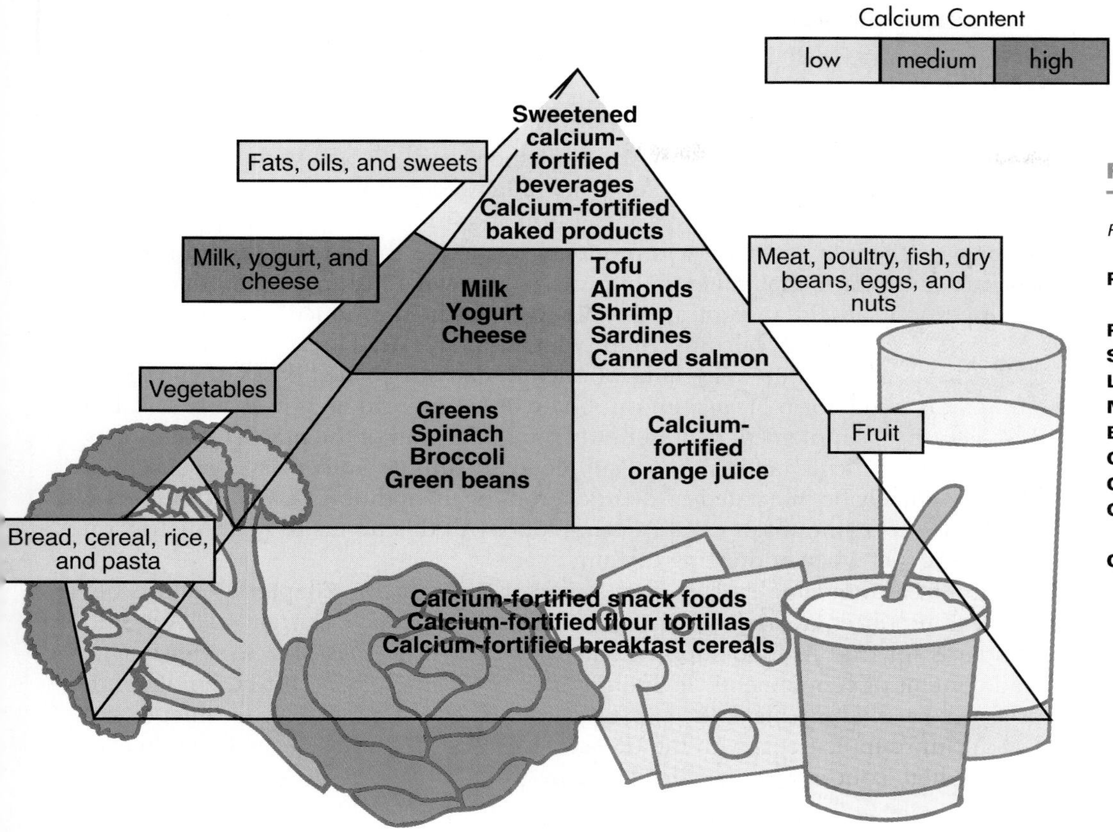

Calcium Content
low
medium
high
Sweetened calcium-fortified beverages
Calcium-fortified baked products
Fats, oils, and sweets
Milk, yogurt, and cheese
Milk
Yogurt
Cheese
Tofu
Almonds
Shrimp
Sardines
Canned salmon
Meat, poultry, fish, dry beans, eggs, and nuts
Vegetables
Greens
Spinach
Broccoli
Green beans
Calcium-fortified orange juice
Fruit
Bread, cereal, rice, and pasta
Calcium-fortified snack foods
Calcium-fortified flour tortillas
Calcium-fortified breakfast cereals

Figure 8–6 *Food sources of calcium from the Food Guide Pyramid. The milk, yogurt, and cheese group includes the richest dietary sources of this nutrient. The background color of each food group indicates the average amount of calcium in that group. Additional calcium-fortified foods appear in stores each year and thus will add to the food sources currently listed for various groups.*

Food Sources of Calcium

Food item and amount	*Calcium (milligrams)*
Parmesan cheese, 2 oz	**670**
Romano cheese, 2 oz	**600**
Swiss cheese, 2 oz	**550**
Low-fat yogurt, 1 cup	**450**
Milk, 1 cup	**300**
Buttermilk, 1 cup	**280**
Cooked spinach, 1 cup	**280**
Canned sardines, 2 oz	**220**
Cooked turnip greens, 1 cup	**200**
Canned salmon (with bones), 3 oz	**180**

in use of either cheese or ice cream as a calcium source is advised, because they are usually high in total and saturated fat. However, some low-fat cheeses and frozen desserts are good calcium sources and have a low fat content.

Information about calcium is mandatory on food labels. The Daily Value for calcium used for food labels is 1000 milligrams.

The AI for calcium for adults ranges from 1000 to 1200 milligrams per day. In the United States, average calcium intakes range from only approximately 600 to 800 for women and 80 to 1000 for men. Thus dietary intakes of calcium by many women, especially young women, are well below the AI, whereas intakes by most men are roughly equivalent to the AI. The greater food consumption by men, to support their higher energy outputs, accounts for part of the difference. An easy way for women to increase calcium intake is to increase their physical activity and in turn their food consumption. It is especially important for vegetarians to focus on eating good plant sources of calcium as well as on the total amount of calcium ingested.

To estimate your calcium intake, use the rule of 300s. Give yourself 300 milligrams to account for calcium in the small amounts provided by a moderate energy intake from foods scattered throughout the diet. Add to that another 300 milligrams for every cup of milk or yogurt or 1.5 ounces of cheese. If you eat a lot of tofu, almonds, or sardines, or drink calcium-fortified beverages, use Appendix A, or your NutraQuest software to get a more accurate account of your calcium intake.

Critical Thinking

Manuela is a vegan. She stopped eating meat and dairy products when she was 12 years old and is now in her mid twenties. She wants to start a family but is concerned about whether she can obtain enough calcium from her diet to ensure her baby's health. She is also concerned that she may be at risk for osteoporosis. How can she consume enough calcium to meet her own and her baby's needs?

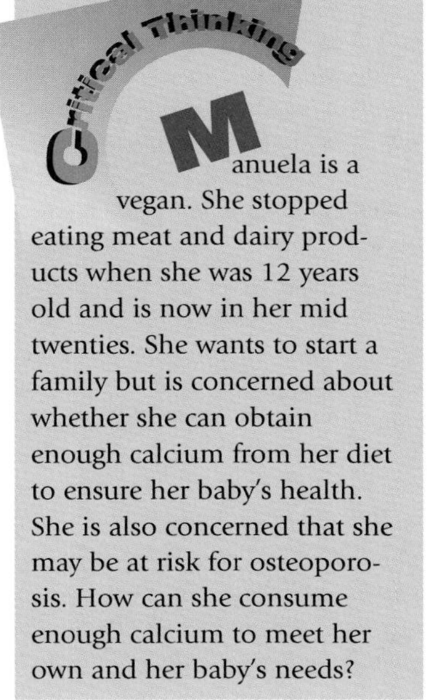

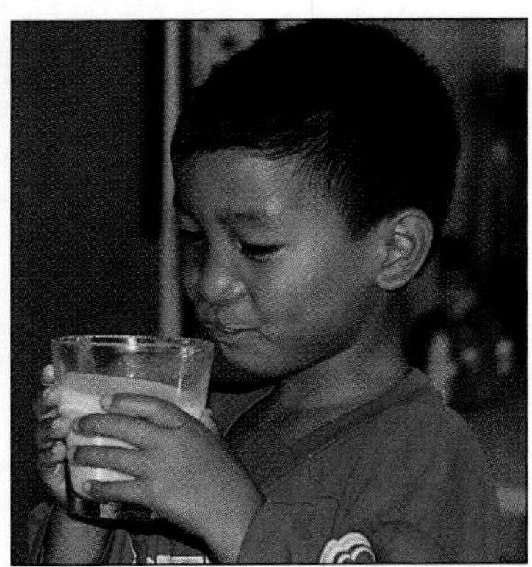

Milk products, and milk itself, are common sources of calcium in the American diet.

Calcium Supplements

Calcium supplements can be used by people who don't like milk or who can't incorporate enough milk products, foods made with milk, or calcium-fortified foods into their diet. Calcium carbonate, the form commonly found in calcium-based antacid tablets, is the most common supplement used. People with ample output of stomach acid should take this supplement between meals in doses of about 500 milligrams. This practice enhances absorption and limits its negative impact on iron absorption. People with low acid production, such as the elderly, should take the calcium carbonate supplement with meals, so that what little acid is produced during digestion can aid absorption. People with low acid production also can use a supplement containing calcium citrate, which is acidic itself, between meals.

Overall, taking 1000 milligrams of calcium daily in divided doses of about 500 milligrams in the form of calcium carbonate or calcium citrate is probably safe, but people using a supplement should notify their physician of the practice. Still, many people have difficulty adhering to a supplement regimen. In contrast, regular food habits can likely be integrated easily into a routine. In addition, it is difficult to consume an excess amount of calcium using foods. All this points to focusing first on improving diet when addressing calcium needs.

Some calcium supplements are poorly digested, because they do not readily dissolve. To test for this, put a supplement in 6 ounces of cider vinegar. Stir every 5 minutes. It should dissolve within 30 minutes.

Some calcium supplements pose a risk for lead toxicity. Chapter 15 points out that lead produces an array of deleterious effects on the body. Currently FDA has no standards for lead in food supplements. However, FDA does plan to regulate the lead content of supplements, including calcium, in the future. Until then, it is important to avoid bonemeal, the worst offender when it comes to lead. Tablet or liquid calcium supplements with the USP seal of approval are less likely than others to contain high concentrations of lead or other contaminants.

An intake of more than 2000 milligrams per day of calcium in some people can cause high blood and urinary calcium concentrations, irritability, headache, kidney failure, soft tissue calcification, kidney stones, decreased absorption of other minerals, and possibly prostate cancer. Note that the Upper Level for calcium intake (set by the recent Dietary Reference Intakes report) is 2500 milligrams per day.

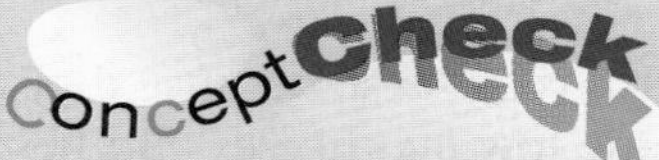

About 99% of calcium in the body is found in the bones. Aside from its critical role in bone, calcium also functions in blood clotting, muscle contraction, nerve-impulse transmission, and cell metabolism. Calcium requires a slightly acid pH and the vitamin D hormone for efficient absorption. Factors that reduce calcium absorption include a vitamin D deficiency, large amounts of dietary fiber (especially excess wheat bran), decreased estrogen in the bloodstream, and old age in general. Blood calcium is regulated primarily by hormones and does not closely reflect daily intake.

Dairy products are rich food sources of calcium. Other foods, such as calcium-fortified beverages, are rich sources as well. Supplemental forms, such as calcium carbonate, are well-absorbed by most people. However, overzealous supplementation can also result in the development of kidney stones and other health problems.

Phosphorus (P)

Although no disease is currently associated with an inadequate phosphorus intake, a deficiency may contribute to bone loss in elderly women. The body absorbs phosphorus quite efficiently, about 70% of dietary intake. This high absorption, plus the wide availability of phosphorus in foods, makes this mineral less important than is calcium in diet planning. The active vitamin D hormone enhances phosphorus absorption, as it does for calcium. Kidney excretion primarily regulates blood phosphorus. This regulating mechanism differs from that of calcium, where changes in the rates of absorption are a more significant factor.

Phosphorus is a component of enzymes, other key metabolic compounds (many of which are involved in energy metabolism), DNA (genetic material), cell membranes, and bone. About 85% of the body's phosphorus is inside bone. The remaining phosphorus circulates freely in the bloodstream and functions inside cells.

Milk products provide much of the phosphorus we consume, as do meat and grain products.

Phosphorus in Foods and the RDA

Milk, cheese, meat, and bread provide most of the phosphorus in the adult diet. Breakfast cereals, bran, eggs, nuts, and fish are also sources. About 20% to 30% of dietary phosphorus comes from food additives, especially in baked goods, cheeses, processed meats, and many soft drinks (about 75 milligrams per 12-ounce—⅓-liter—serving of soft drinks). Next time you have a soft drink, look for a listing of phosphoric acid on the label.

The RDA for phosphorus for adults over age 18 is 700 milligrams daily. Adults eat from about 900 to 1700 milligrams of phosphorus per day. Thus deficiencies of phosphorus are unlikely in healthy adults, especially because it is so efficiently absorbed.

Marginal phosphorus status can be found in premature infants, vegans, people with alcoholism, elderly people on nutrient-poor diets, and people with long-term bouts of diarrhea.

Typical phosphorus intakes in and of themselves do not appear to be toxic for healthy adults, but high amounts can lead to problems in people with certain kidney diseases. In addition, chronic imbalance in the calcium to phosphorus ratio in the diet, resulting from a high phosphorus intake coupled with a low calcium intake, also can contribute to bone loss. This situation most likely arises when the AI for calcium is not met, as can occur in adolescents and adults who regularly substitute soft drinks for milk, or otherwise underconsume calcium. The Upper Level for phosphorus intake is 3 to 4 grams per day.

Food Sources of Phosphorus

Food item and amount	*Phosphorus (milligrams)*
Sardines, 3 oz	**420**
Swiss cheese, 2 oz	**340**
Dried almonds, ½ cup	**340**
Milk, 8 oz	**240**
Broiled salmon fillet, 3 oz	**220**
Roast beef, 3 oz	**210**
Roasted turkey, 3 oz	**180**
Roasted chicken, 3 oz	**170**
American cheese, 1 slice	**160**
Fried beef liver, 1 oz	**130**

Magnesium (Mg)

Magnesium is important for nerve and heart function and aids many enzyme reactions. It is found mostly in the plant pigment chlorophyll, where it functions in respiration. We normally absorb about 30% to 40% of the magnesium in our diets, but absorption efficiency can increase up to about 80% if intakes are low.

Bone contains 60% of the body's magnesium. The rest circulates in the blood and operates inside cells. Over 200 enzymes use magnesium, and many energy-yielding compounds in cells require magnesium to function properly, as does the hormone insulin.

Animals deficient in magnesium become very irritable and, with severe deficiency, eventually suffer convulsions and often die. In humans a magnesium deficiency causes an irregular heartbeat, sometimes accompanied by weakness, muscle pain, disorientation, and seizures. Other possible benefits of magnesium in relation to heart disease include decreasing blood pressure by dilating arteries, preventing heart rhythm abnormalities, and inhibiting blood clotting. People with heart disease should closely monitor intake, especially because they are often on medications such as some diuretics that reduce magnesium status. Keep in mind that a magnesium deficiency develops very slowly, because our bodies store it readily.

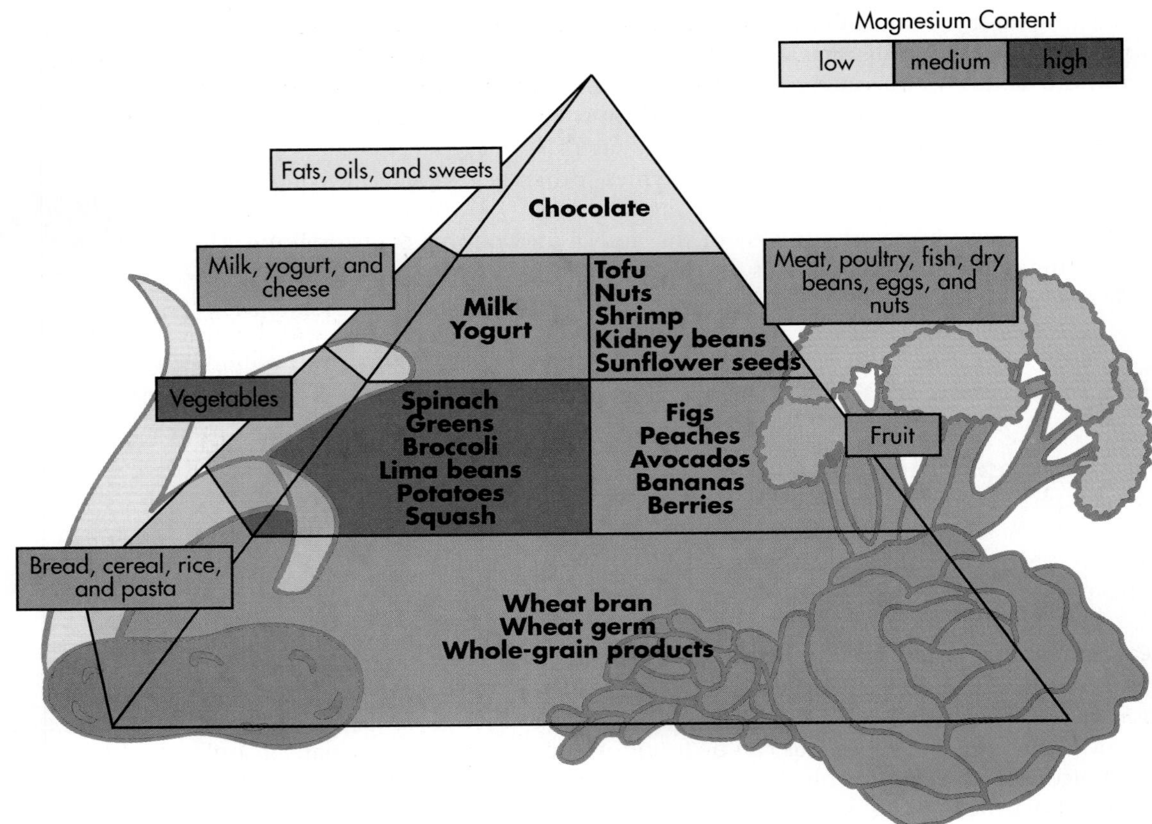

Figure 8–7 *Food sources of magnesium from the Food Guide Pyramid. The vegetable group and whole-grain choices in the bread, cereal, rice, and pasta group are the best dietary sources of this nutrient. The background color of each food group indicates the average amount of magnesium in that group.*

Magnesium in Foods and the RDA

Rich sources for magnesium are plant products, such as whole grains (like wheat bran), broccoli, potatoes, squash, beans, nuts, and seeds. Animal products, such as milk and meats, and even chocolate supply some magnesium although less than the foods in the previous list (Figure 8–7). Two other sources of magnesium are hard tap water, which contains a high mineral content, and coffee.

The adult RDA for magnesium is 420 milligrams per day for men and 320 milligrams per day for women. The Daily Value used for food labeling is 400 milligrams. Adult men consume an average of 350 milligrams daily, whereas women consume closer to 250 milligrams daily. Women especially should find some good sources of magnesium that they like and eat them regularly. A balanced vitamin and mineral supplement generally yields 100 milligrams.

Poor magnesium status is found among users of certain diuretics, as noted above. In addition, heavy perspiration for weeks in hot climates and bouts of long-standing diarrhea or vomiting all cause significant magnesium loss. Alcoholism also increases the risk of a deficiency because dietary intake may be poor and because alcohol increases magnesium excretion in the urine. The disorientation and weakness associated with alcoholism closely resemble the behavior of people with low blood magnesium.

Magnesium toxicity typically occurs only in people who have kidney failure or who overuse over-the-counter medications that contain magnesium, such as certain

Food Sources of Magnesium

Food item and amount	*Magnesium (milligrams)*
Cooked spinach, 1 cup	**130**
Baked acorn squash, 1 cup	**105**
Toasted wheat germ, ¼ cup	**90**
Tofu (soybean curd), 3 oz	**88**
Cashews, ¼ cup	**85**
Cooked blackeyed peas, ½ cup	**45**
Sunflower seeds, ¼ cup	**40**
Cooked kidney beans, ½ cup	**40**
Cooked broccoli, 1 cup	**37**
Whole-wheat bread, 1 slice	**25**

antacids and laxatives. Elderly people are at particular risk, as kidney function may be compromised. The Upper Level for magnesium intake is 350 milligrams per day. Note, however, that this guideline refers only to nonfood sources; it would be difficult to consume a toxic amount of magnesium from foods alone.

Sulfur (S)

Sulfur is found in many important compounds in the body, such as some amino acids (like methionine) and the vitamins biotin and thiamin. Sulfur helps in the balance of acids and bases in the body and is an important part of the liver's drug-detoxifying pathways. Because proteins supply the sulfur we need, sulfur is naturally a part of a healthy diet. Sulfur compounds are also used to preserve foods (see Chapter 15).

ConceptCheck

Phosphorus absorption is quite efficient and is enhanced by the active vitamin D hormone. Urinary excretion mainly controls body content. Phosphorus aids enzyme function and is part of key metabolic compounds and cell membranes. No distinct deficiency symptoms caused by an inadequate phosphorus intake have been reported. Food sources for phosphorus include dairy products, baked goods, and meat. The RDA is met by most Americans. An excess intake of phosphorus can compromise bone health if sufficient calcium is not otherwise consumed. Magnesium is required for nerve and heart function; it also aids activity for many enzymes. Food sources of magnesium are whole grains (wheat bran), broccoli, squash, beef, coffee, beans, nuts, and seeds. People using certain diuretics and people with alcoholism are at greatest risk of developing a deficiency. Many women do not meet the RDA for magnesium. Magnesium toxicity is most likely in people with kidney failure. Sulfur is a component of certain vitamins and amino acids. The protein we consume supplies sufficient sulfur for the body's needs.

TRACE MINERALS

Information about trace minerals is perhaps the most rapidly expanding area of knowledge in nutrition. With the exceptions of iron and iodine, the importance of trace minerals to humans has been recognized only within the last 30 years. Although we need only about 20 milligrams—or less—of each trace mineral daily, they are just as essential to good health as are major minerals.

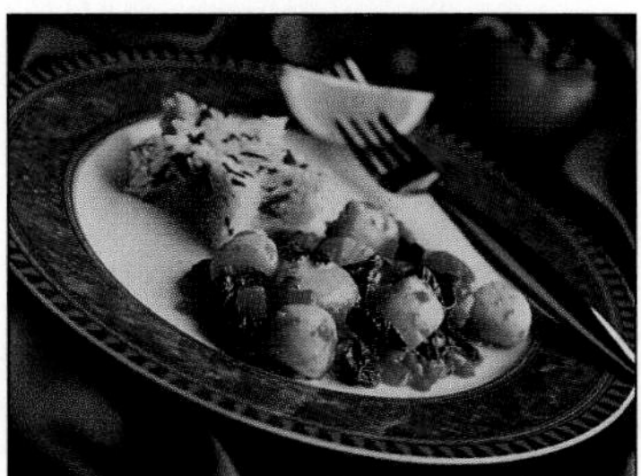

Seafood, like scallops, is a rich source of many trace minerals.

In some cases, discovering the importance of a trace mineral reads like a detective story, and the evidence is still unfolding. As recently as 1961, researchers linked dwarfism in Middle Eastern villagers to a zinc deficiency. Other scientists recognized that a rare form of heart disease in an isolated area of China was linked to a selenium deficiency. In America, some trace mineral deficiencies were first observed in the late 1960s and early 1970s when the minerals were not added to synthetic formulas used for intravenous feeding.

It is difficult to define precisely our trace mineral needs because we need only minute amounts. Highly sophisticated technology is required to measure such small amounts in both food and body tissues.

See Table 8–5 to see what we know about the trace minerals.

Iron (Fe)

The importance of dietary iron has been recognized for centuries. The Persian physician Melampus in 4000 BC gave iron supplements to sailors to make up for iron lost

TABLE 8-5

A Summary of Key Trace Minerals

Mineral	Major functions	Deficiency symptoms	People most at risk	RDA, AI, or ESADDI	Rich dietary sources	Results of toxicity
Iron	Used for hemoglobin and other key compounds used in respiration; used for immune function	Low blood iron; small, pale red blood cells; low blood hemoglobin values	Infants, preschool children, adolescents, women in childbearing years	Men: 10 milligrams Women: 15 milligrams	Meats, spinach, seafood, broccoli, peas, bran enriched breads	Toxicity seen when children consume 60 milligrams or more in iron pills; also in people with hemochromatosis
Zinc	Required for enzymes, involved in growth, immunity, alcohol metabolism, sexual development, and reproduction	Skin rash, diarrhea, decreased appetite and sense of taste, hair loss, poor growth and development, poor wound healing	Vegetarians, elderly people, people with alcoholism	Men: 15 milligrams Women: 12 milligrams	Seafoods, meats, greens, whole grains	Reduces copper absorption; can cause diarrhea, cramps, and depressed immune function (above 45 milligrams per day)
Selenium	Aids antioxidant system	Muscle pain, muscle weakness, form of heart disease	Unknown in healthy Americans	55–70 micrograms	Meats, eggs, fish, seafoods, whole grains	Nausea, vomiting, hair loss, weakness, liver disease (above 200 micrograms per day)
Iodide	Aids thyroid hormone	Goiter; poor growth in infancy when mother is iodide deficient during pregnancy	None in America, because salt is usually fortified	150 micrograms	Iodized salt, white bread, saltwater fish, dairy products	Inhibition of function of the thyroid gland
Copper	Aids in iron metabolism; works with many enzymes, such as those involved in protein metabolism and hormone synthesis	Anemia, low white blood cell count, poor growth	Infants recovering from semi-starvation, people who use overzealous supplementation of zinc	1.5–3 milligrams	Liver, cocoa, beans, nuts, whole grains, dried fruits	Vomiting; nervous system disorders (above 10 milligrams per day)
Fluoride	Increases resistance of tooth enamel to dental caries	Increased risk of dental caries	Areas where water is not fluoridated and dental treatments do not make up for a lack of fluoride	Men: 3.8 milligrams Women: 3.1 milligrams	Fluoridated water, toothpaste, dental treatments, tea, seaweed	Stomach upset; mottling (staining) of teeth during development; bone pain (above 6 milligrams per day)
Chromium	Enhances blood glucose control	High blood glucose after eating	People on intravenous, nutrition, and perhaps elderly people with Type 2 diabetes	50–200 micrograms	Egg yolks, whole grains, pork, nuts, mushrooms, beer	Liver damage and lung cancer (caused by industrial contamination, not dietary excess); best not to exceed 200 micrograms per day
Manganese	Aids action of some enzymes, such as those involved in carbohydrate metabolism	None in humans	Unknown	2–5 milligrams	Nuts, oats, beans, tea	Not defined in humans
Molybdenum	Aids action of some enzymes	None in healthy humans	Unsupplemented intravenous nutrition	75–250 micrograms	Beans, grains, nuts	Unknown in humans

from bleeding wounds during battles. Today, iron deficiency is one of the most common nutrient deficiencies worldwide. Iron is the only nutrient for which adult women have a greater RDA than do adult men. Iron is found in every living cell, adding up to about 5 grams (1 teaspoon) for the entire body.

Absorption and Distribution of Iron

The body uses several mechanisms to regulate iron absorption. Controlling absorption is important, because our bodies cannot easily eliminate excess iron once it is absorbed. Iron absorption from foods varies from about 5% to 10% in healthy people, and 10% to 20% in people with iron deficiency. Overall, iron absorption depends on its form in the food, the body's need for it, and a variety of other factors.

The form of iron in foods especially influences how much is absorbed. About 40% of the total iron in animal flesh is in the form of **hemoglobin** (the same form as in red blood cells) and **myoglobin** (pigment found in muscle cells). This **heme iron** is absorbed more than twice as efficiently as the simple elemental iron, called **nonheme iron.** Nonheme iron is also present in animal flesh, as well as in eggs, milk, vegetables, grains, and other plant foods.

About 10% to 15% of iron in the typical adult diet is heme iron, and usually about 20% is absorbed. Nonheme iron makes up the rest, and usually 2% to 20% is absorbed. Therefore animal flesh, especially red meat, is the best source of iron in the adult diet, because of both its iron content and the amount in the heme form. Consuming heme iron and nonheme iron together increases nonheme iron absorption. A protein factor in meats may also aid nonheme absorption. Overall, eating meat with vegetables and grain products enhances the absorption of all nonheme iron present.

Vitamin C can modestly increase nonheme iron absorption. So when taking an iron supplement, one should consider drinking a glass of orange juice with it. Consuming more foods rich in vitamin C is particularly desirable if dietary iron is inadequate or if blood iron is low. Iron use in the body is also aided by copper, as explained in a later section.

Several dietary factors interfere with our ability to absorb iron. Phytic acid and other factors in grain fibers and oxalic acid in vegetables can all bind iron and reduce its absorption. Polyphenols (tannins) found in tea also reduce iron absorption. It is a good idea to moderate intake of tannins if one has iron deficiency, and keep dietary-fiber intake within 35 grams a day. Zinc also interferes with iron by competing with it for absorption. Finally, high-dose calcium supplements can also bind with iron when both are in the same meal—an important consideration when taking more than 500 milligrams in supplement form per occasion. In fact, experts suggest that adolescents, and menstruating and pregnant women take any calcium supplements at bedtime to avoid this interference.

Overall, the most important factor influencing iron absorption is the body's need for it. In a deficiency state, iron absorption can increase. When iron stores are inadequate, the main blood protein that carries iron readily binds more iron, shifting it from intestinal cells into the bloodstream. If iron stores are adequate and the iron-binding protein in the blood is fully saturated with iron, little will be absorbed from the intestinal cells. It stays bound in the intestinal cells.

By this mechanism, in normal circumstances, iron is absorbed for the most part as needed. If not needed, when intestinal cells are shed at the end of their 2- to 5-day cycle, the iron returns to the lumen of the intestinal tract. This whole process is referred to as a "mucosal block" against excess iron absorption. High doses of iron can still be toxic, but absorption is carefully regulated under typical dietary conditions in most people.

Most iron in the body is contained in the hemoglobin molecules of the red blood cells. Some iron is stored in the bone marrow, and a small portion goes to other body cells, such as the liver, for storage. As iron is needed, it can be mobilized

Hemoglobin
The iron-containing part of the red blood cell that carries oxygen to the cells and some carbon dioxide away from the cells. It is also responsible for the red color of blood.

Myoglobin
Iron-containing compound that binds oxygen in muscle tissue.

Heme iron
Iron provided from animal tissues in the form of hemoglobin and myoglobin. Approximately 40% of the iron in meat is heme iron; it is readily absorbed.

Nonheme iron
Iron provided from plant sources and animal tissues other than in the forms of hemoglobin and myoglobin. Nonheme iron is less efficiently absorbed than heme iron.

from body stores. If dietary intake is inadequate, these iron stores become depleted. Only then do signs of an iron deficiency appear.

Functions of Iron

Iron forms part of the hemoglobin in red blood cells and myoglobin in muscle cells. Hemoglobin molecules in red blood cells transport oxygen (O_2) from the lungs to cells and assist in the return of some carbon dioxide (CO_2) from cells to the lungs for excretion. In addition, iron is used as part of many enzymes, some proteins, and compounds that cells use in energy production. Iron is also needed for brain and immune function, and contributes to drug detoxification in the liver.

Hematocrit
The percentage of blood that is made up of red blood cells.

If neither the diet nor body stores can supply the iron needed for hemoglobin synthesis, the number of red blood cells decreases in the bloodstream. The blood hemoglobin concentration also falls. When both the percentage of red blood cells (called the ***hematocrit***) and the hemoglobin concentration fall, a physician suspects iron deficiency. Physicians also use these two measures to assess iron status, along with the amount of iron and iron-containing proteins in the bloodstream. In severe deficiency, hemoglobin and hematocrit fall so low that the amount of oxygen carried in the bloodstream is decreased. Such a person has anemia, defined as a decreased oxygen-carrying capacity of the blood.

While there are many types of anemia, iron-deficiency anemia is the major type worldwide. About 30% of the world's population is anemic, and about half of those cases are caused by an iron deficiency. Probably about 10% of Americans in high risk categories have iron-deficiency anemia. This appears most often in infancy, the preschool years, and at puberty for both males and females. Growth, with accompanying expansion of blood volume and muscle mass, increases iron needs, making it difficult to consume enough iron. Women are also very vulnerable during childbearing years when menstruation occurs. In addition, anemia is often found in pregnant women, as discussed in Chapter 12. Iron-deficiency anemia in adult men is usually caused by blood loss from ulcers, colon cancer, or hemorrhoids. Finally, athletes can develop anemia, as discussed in Chapter 10.

Clinical symptoms of iron-deficiency anemia primarily include pale skin, fatigue, poor temperature regulation, loss of appetite, and apathy. Insufficient iron for the synthesis of red blood cells and key cell compounds may cause the fatigue. Poor iron stores may also decrease learning ability, attention span, work performance, and immune status even before a person is actually anemic.

More Americans have an iron deficiency than iron-deficiency anemia. Their blood hemoglobin values are still normal, but they have no stores to draw from in times of pregnancy or illness, and basic functioning may not be up to par. That could mean anything from too little energy to perform everyday tasks in an efficient manner to difficulties staying alert in school or on the job.

To speed the cure of iron-deficiency anemia, a person needs to take iron supplements. A physician should also find the cause—an inadequate diet or a bleeding ulcer, for example—so that the anemia does not recur. Changes in diet may prevent iron-deficiency anemia, but supplemental iron is the only reliable cure.

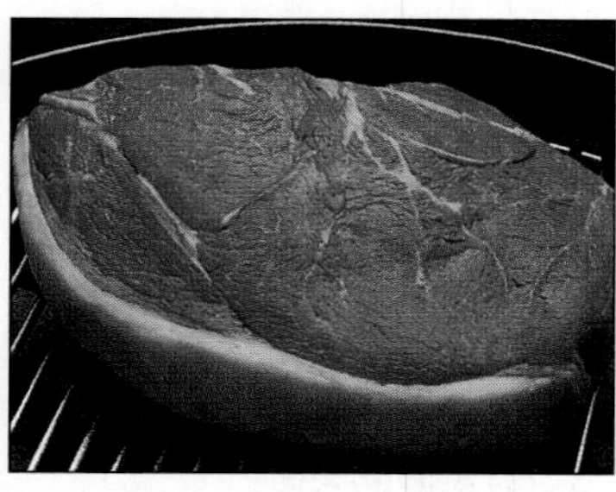

Red meat is a major source of iron in the American diet.

Iron in Foods and the RDA

Animal sources contain some heme iron, the most bioavailable form. These then end up our best iron sources. Iron present in iron supplements is also absorbed well. The major iron sources in the adult diet are fortified breakfast cereals, animal products, and bakery items, such as bread. (Figure 8–8). Most of the iron in these bakery items has been added to refined flour in the enrichment process. Other iron sources are spinach, peas, and legumes, but the iron is less available in these foods than in animal products.

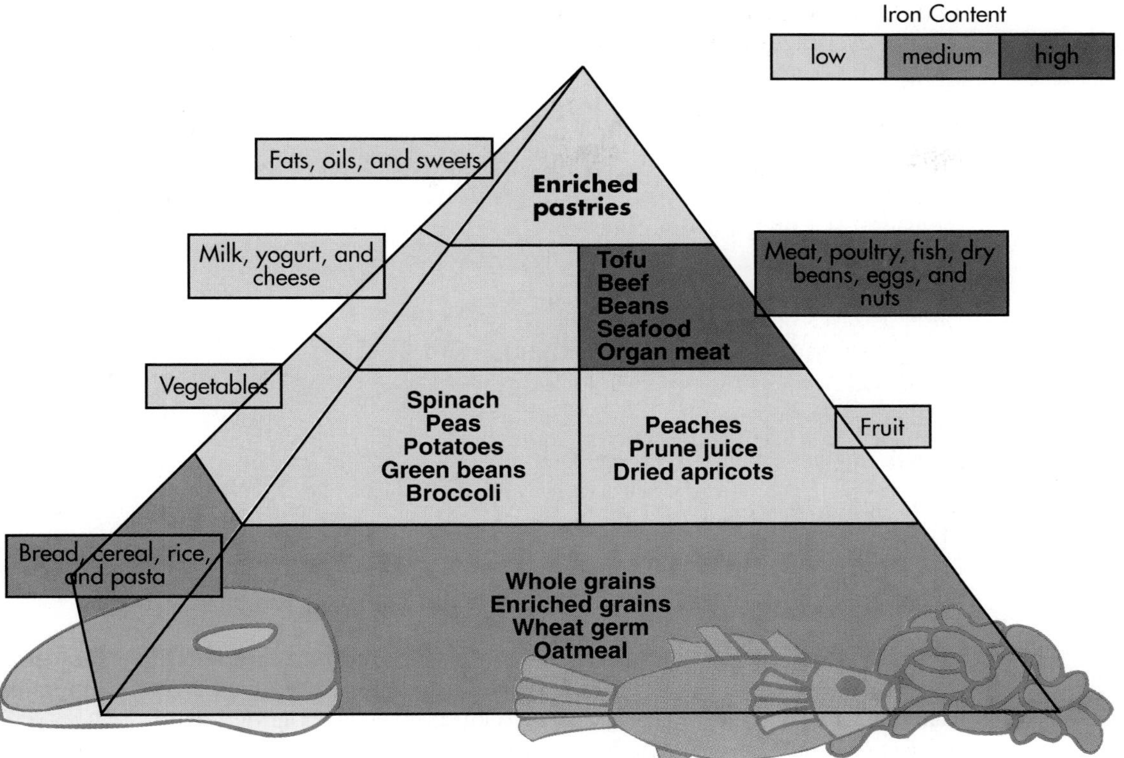

Figure 8–8 *Food sources of iron from the Food Guide Pyramid. The meat, poultry, fish, dry beans, eggs, and nuts group and the bread, cereal, rice, and pasta group are the best dietary sources of this nutrient. The heme iron in the meat, poultry, fish, dry beans, eggs, and nuts group is especially well absorbed. The iron content of a food containing mostly nonheme iron is only an approximate measure of the amount delivered to body cells, as body need greatly influences the absorption of nonheme iron. The background color of each food group indicates the average amount of iron in that group.*

The use of iron-fortified formulas and cereals in the Special Supplemental Food Program for Women, Infant, and Children (WIC) in the United States has been a major contributor to decreasing rates of iron-deficiency anemia in preschool children (see Chapter 12).

Milk is a very poor source of iron. A common cause of iron-deficiency anemia in children is an overreliance on milk, coupled with an insufficient meat intake. Total vegetarians (vegans) are particularly susceptible to iron-deficiency anemia, because of their lack of dietary heme iron.

The daily adult RDA for iron is 10 milligrams for men, as well as for women over 50 years, and 15 milligrams for women ages 19 to 50 years. The RDA value assumes that about 10% of dietary iron is absorbed. If iron absorption exceeds that, less dietary iron is needed.

The higher RDA for young and middle-aged women is primarily because of menstrual blood loss. Women who menstruate more heavily and longer than average may need even more dietary iron, and those who have lighter and shorter flows may need less iron. The variation in menstrual blood loss, and hence, loss of iron, makes it difficult to set an RDA for iron for women.

By recording dietary intakes from a variety of young and middle-aged women, researchers find that most women do not consume 15 milligrams of iron daily. The average daily value is closer to 12 milligrams, while in men it is about 17 milligrams per day. Of course, not all of these women need 15 milligrams or iron daily, because

Food Sources of Iron

Food item and amount	*Iron (milligrams)*
Steamed oysters, 3	**6.9**
Cooked spinach, 1 cup	**6.4**
Cooked kidney beans, 1 cup	**5.2**
Sirloin steak, 4 oz	**3.9**
Pot roast, 4 oz	**3.9**
Fried beef liver, 2 oz	**3.6**
Prune juice, 8 oz	**3.0**
Braunschweiger sausage, 1	**2.7**
Sauerkraut, ½ cup	**1.7**
Cooked green peas, ½ cup	**1.3**

the RDA is set high enough to allow for variations in menstrual flow and absorption rates. Whether male or female, if you are not consuming the RDA for iron, you should be concerned, but not alarmed. Try to consume a diet that meets the RDA for iron, and make sure your physician checks your iron status during regular physical examinations. It is difficult to tell whether a lower iron intake is actually harmful. Although there are very sensitive measures of iron stores in the body, we lack the knowledge to reliably predict the resulting effects on health status when people register low values.

ANOTHER Bite

The adult human body contains about 21 cups (5 liters) of blood. Blood donations are generally 2 cups (500 milliliters). Thus a blood donor gives about a tenth of his or her total supply. Healthy people generally can donate blood two to four times a year without harmful consequences. As a precaution, blood banks first screen potential donors' blood for the presence of anemia.

Toxicity of iron

Although not as common as iron deficiency, iron overload can be serious because it can easily lead to toxic symptoms. Even a large single dose of iron of 60 milligrams can be life-threatening to a 1-year-old. Children are frequently victims of iron poisoning because iron pills and nutrient supplements containing iron are tempting targets on kitchen tables and in cabinets. FDA has recently ruled that all iron supplements must carry a warning about toxicity, and those with 30 milligrams of iron or more per tablet must be individually wrapped.

Smaller does of iron (but still greater than what is needed) over a long period can also cause problems. A form of iron toxicity, for example, has been observed in an African tribe that brews beer in iron pots. Some people of Mediterranean descent have a type of anemia caused by increased destruction of red blood cells; low-dose iron therapy used to treat this disease can lead to toxicity symptoms. Repeated blood transfusions can also lead to iron toxicity.

Hemochromatosis
A disorder of iron metabolism characterized by increased iron absorption and deposition in the liver and heart tissue. This eventually poisons the cells in those organs.

In addition, iron toxicity accompanies the genetic disease called hereditary ***hemochromatosis.*** The disease is associated with a substantial increase in iron absorption. For people with this disease, iron in the body eventually builds up to dangerous amounts, especially in the blood and liver. Some iron is deposited in the muscles, pancreas, and heart. If not treated, the excess iron deposits contribute to severe organ damage, especially in the liver and heart.

Hereditary hemochromatosis requires that a person carry two defective copies of a particular gene to develop the disease. People with one defective gene and one normal gene, called carriers, may also absorb too much dietary iron but not to the same extent as those with two defective genes. About 5% to 10% of Americans of Northern European extraction are carriers of hemochromatosis. Approximately 1 in 250 Americans has both hemochromatosis genes. These numbers are high considering the fact that many physicians regard hemochromatosis as a rare disease and thus do not routinely test for it.

Carriers of one hemochromatosis gene may be prime candidates for heart disease, especially men. As noted in Chapter 5, excess iron in the blood may accelerate atherosclerosis in people with elevated LDL by contributing to oxidation of lipids in the LDL particles. This in turn allows LDL to be taken up more readily by scavenger cells in the blood vessels. However, the importance of iron in stimulating atherosclerosis is still hotly debated. Because of its relatively efficient absorption, dietary heme iron, such as that found in red meats, poses the greatest risk in this regard. To put this relatively new research area into perspective, a reasonable approach is for you to ask to be screened for iron overload at your next visit to a physician (ask for a transferrin saturation test). Because hemochromatosis can go undetected until a person is in their fifties or sixties, some experts recommend screening for anyone over the age of 20. If the disease goes untreated many organs will have literally rusted away by one's fifties or sixties. If you show evidence of hemochromatosis, it would be wise to undergo therapy. This includes regular blood donations and avoidance of both iron-rich foods and iron supplements.

Ideally, consent of a physician should precede any use of iron supplements, especially by men. When iron supplements are advised, there should be adequate follow-up so that supplementation does not exceed what is necessary. Probably the only factor keeping many people with hemochromatosis and carriers of one gene from experiencing serious effects of the disease is that they consume only a moderate amount of iron.

ConceptCheck

Iron is absorbed depending mostly on its form and the body's need for it. Absorption is affected by a "mucosal block," but excess iron intake can override the system, leading to toxicity. Iron absorption increases somewhat in the presence of vitamin C and meat protein and decreases in the presence of large amounts of calcium and some components of grain fiber, such as phytic acid. Iron is used in synthesizing hemoglobin and myoglobin, in supporting immune function, and in energy metabolism. An iron deficiency can cause decreased red blood cell synthesis, which can lead to anemia. It is particularly important for women of childbearing age to consume adequate iron, primarily to replace that lost in menstrual blood. Sources include red meat, pork, liver, enriched grains and cereals, and oysters. Iron toxicity usually results from a genetic disorder called hemochromatosis. This disease causes overabsorption and accumulation of iron, which can result in severe liver and heart damage. Because of the risk of toxicity, any use of iron supplements should be supervised by a physician.

Zinc (Zn)

Although zinc has been recognized as an essential nutrient in farm animals since the early 1900s, zinc deficiency was first recognized in humans in the early 1960s in Egypt and Iran. Zinc deficiencies were determined to cause growth retardation and poor sexual development in some groups of people, even though the zinc content of their diets was fairly high. However, the customary diet contained unleavened bread almost exclusively and little animal protein. Unleavened bread is very high in phytic acid and other factors that decrease zinc bioavailability. Parasite infestation and the practice of eating clay and other parts of soil also probably contributed to the severe zinc deficiency.

In America, zinc deficiencies were first observed in the early 1970s in hospitalized patients who were fed only intravenously. Zinc was not added to solutions at that time, but the protein source in the solutions was based on milk protein or a blood protein, which are both naturally rich in zinc. When the solutions were changed in the early 1970s to include mostly individual amino acids as the protein source, deficiency symptoms quickly developed because amino acid formulas are low in zinc.

Symptoms of adult zinc deficiency include an acnelike rash, diarrhea, lack of appetite, reduced sense of taste and smell, and hair loss. In children and adolescents with zinc deficiency, growth, sexual development, and learning ability may also be hampered. When children show poor growth, they should be checked for inadequate zinc status.

Like iron, zinc absorption is influenced by the foods a person ingests. About 10% to 35% of dietary zinc is absorbed; the higher figure is more likely when animal protein sources are used and when the body needs more zinc. Most people worldwide rely on cereal grains (low in zinc) for their source of protein, energy, and zinc. This makes consuming adequate zinc a problem. In addition, high-dose calcium supplementation with meals causes up to a 50% decrease in zinc absorption. For this reason, groups of people with high calcium needs may need to increase zinc intake as well. Finally, zinc competes with copper and iron absorption.

Functions of Zinc

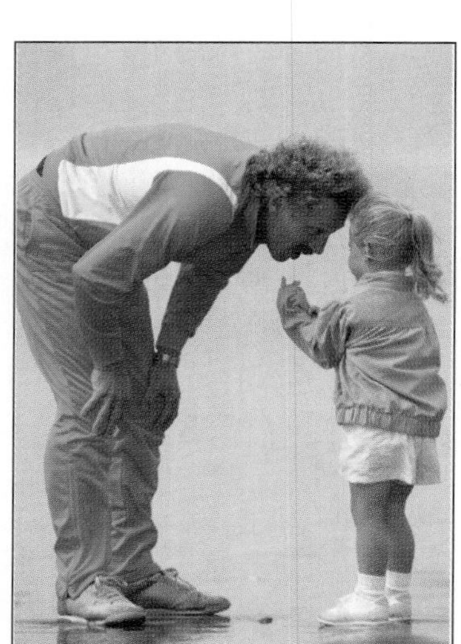

Growth from childhood to adulthood depends in part on our intake of nutrients—zinc is one such nutrient.

More than 300 enzymes require zinc as a cofactor for optimal activity. Adequate zinc intake is necessary to support many bodily functions, such as:

- DNA synthesis and function (some factors that control gene function contain zinc-rich regions that bind DNA)
- Protein metabolism, wound healing, and growth
- Immune function (intakes in excess of the RDA do not provide any extra benefit to immune function)
- Development of sexual organs and bone
- Storage, release, and function of insulin
- Cell membrane structure and function
- Component of superoxide dismutase, an enzyme that aids in the prevention of oxidative damage to cells

Zinc in Foods and the RDA

In general, protein-rich diets are also rich in zinc. Animal foods supply almost half our zinc intake. Major sources of zinc are beef, fortified breakfast cereals, milk, poultry, and bread. As with iron, bioavailability is also important to consider for zinc. Animal foods are again our prime sources because zinc from animal sources is not bound by phytic acid. However, good plant sources of zinc—such as whole grains, peanuts, and beans—should not be discounted. They can deliver substantial amounts of zinc to body cells (Figure 8–9).

The adult RDA for zinc is 15 milligrams for men and 12 milligrams for women. The average American takes in 9 to 15 milligrams of zinc a day, with men showing

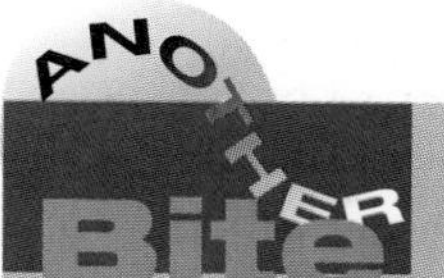

Many companies are singing the praises of zinc as a cold remedy. Products such as Cold Eeze are lozenges that contain zinc, and their claims are based largely on one study done with 100 participants. The 50 individuals in the experimental group took 13.3 milligrams of zinc via the lozenges every 2 hours for the duration of their symptoms. Cold symptoms subsided after 4 days in the experimental group and 7 days in the control group. Nausea was a common side effect of the zinc lozenges. Of nine other followup studies, however, only four have shown beneficial results from zinc. This may be due to bioavailability of various forms of zinc, or simply due to the more bitter flavor of the lozenges used in some studies (placebo effect). Adults can determine if the benefits outweigh the taste. Use in children is not helpful. Any use of such amounts beyond a week or so also is potentially dangerous.

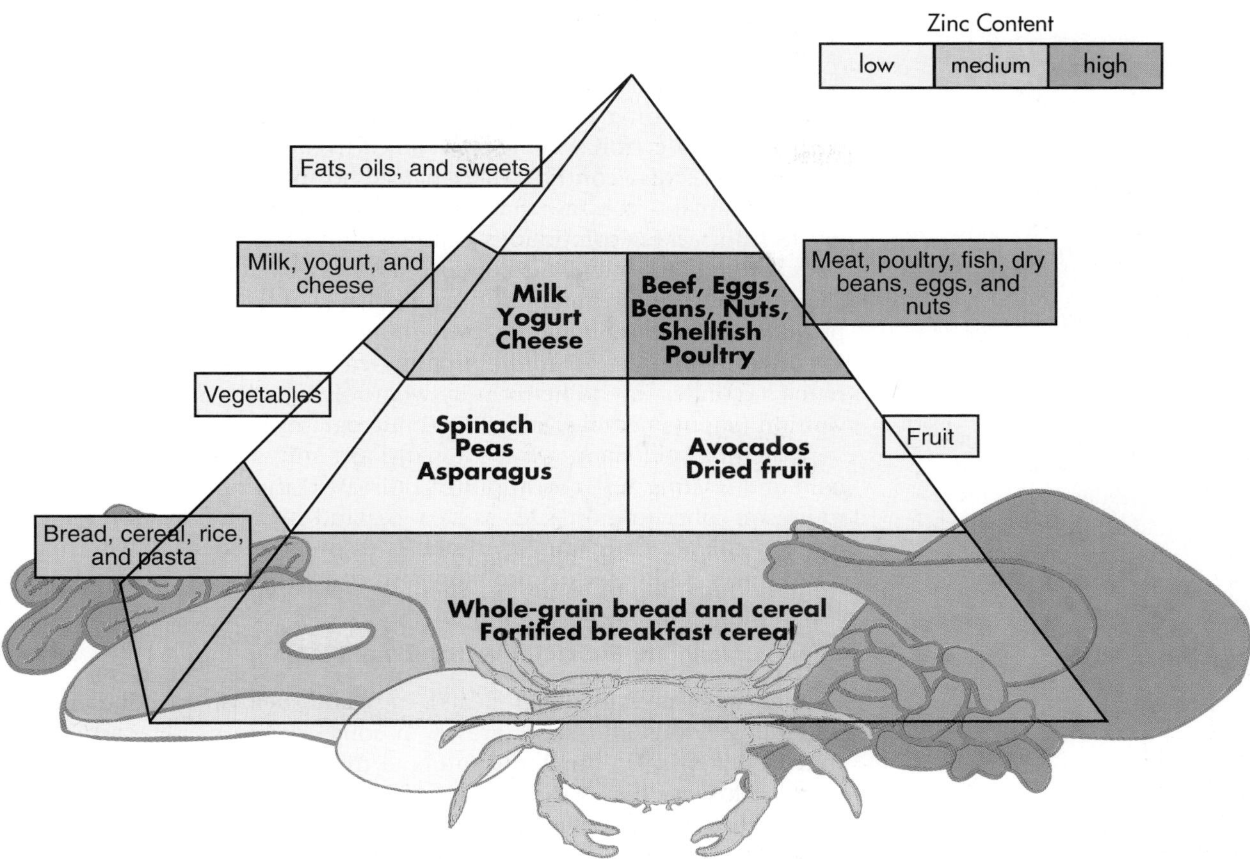

Figure 8-9 *Food sources of zinc from the Food Guide Pyramid. The meat, poultry, fish, dry beans, eggs, and nuts group includes the best dietary sources of this nutrient. Some zinc is supplied by whole grains and fortified breakfast cereals from the bread, cereal, rice, and pasta group. The background color of each food group indicates the average amount of zinc in that group.*

the higher values. This raises concern that many women do not consume enough zinc. Still, there are no indications of moderate or severe zinc deficiencies in an otherwise healthy adult population. It is likely that many Americans—especially women, poor children, vegans, older people, and people with alcoholism—have a marginal zinc status. However, because we lack a sensitive marker for zinc status, a body must be very zinc-depleted for clinical tests to register a deficiency. Furthermore, absorption and excretion can maintain an adequate zinc status even when intakes are somewhat lower than those furnished by typical diets of Americans. However, the long-term effects of marginal zinc intakes are not known. People who show deterioration in taste sensation, recurring infections, poor growth, or depressed wound healing should have zinc status checked.

Excessive zinc intakes, greater than about three to four times the RDA, over time can also lead to problems, as just mentioned. One study has shown that zinc supplements at approximately three to five times the RDA can reduce HDL by about 15%, perhaps by interfering with copper metabolism. That is disturbing for two reasons. First, low HDL is associated with an increased risk of developing heart disease. Second, many people who take zinc supplements do in fact consume an excessive amount. Overall, ideally you should not use megadose zinc supplements unless under close medical supervision. Zinc intakes over 50 to 100 milligrams per day also result in diarrhea, cramps, nausea, vomiting, and depressed immune system function.

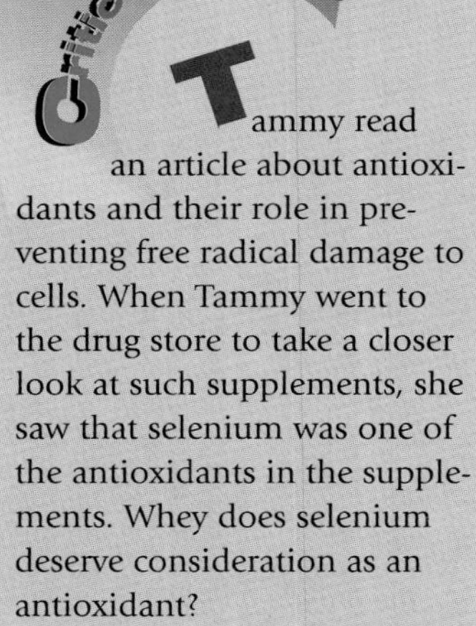

Tammy read an article about antioxidants and their role in preventing free radical damage to cells. When Tammy went to the drug store to take a closer look at such supplements, she saw that selenium was one of the antioxidants in the supplements. Whey does selenium deserve consideration as an antioxidant?

Selenium (Se)

Selenium exists in many forms that are readily absorbed. Selenium's best understood role is aiding the activity of an enzyme that participates in reducing the damage that electron-seeking free radical (oxidizing) compounds can do to cell membranes. It also contributes to thyroid hormone metabolism.

In Chapter 7 you saw that vitamin E helps prevent attacks on cell membranes by electron-seeking compounds. Thus vitamin E and selenium work together toward the same goal. Chapter 7 also discussed how free radical compounds can cause cancer. Although selenium could prove to have a role in cancer prevention, such as prostate cancer, it is premature to recommend megadose selenium supplementation for this purpose. Animal studies in this area are conflicting; current studies with humans are under way to help clarify what role, if any, selenium plays in cancer prevention (supplemental intake of 200 micrograms per day).

Selenium deficiency symptoms in farm animals and humans include muscle pain and wasting and a form of heart disease. Farm animals in areas with low selenium soil concentration, such as New Zealand, and humans in some areas of China develop characteristic muscle and heart disorders associated with inadequate selenium intake. Other factors probably also contribute.

Selenium in Foods and the RDA

Fish, meats (especially organ meats), eggs, and shellfish are good animal sources of selenium. Grains and seeds grown in soils containing selenium are good plant sources. Major selenium contributors to the adult diet are animal and grain products. Because we eat a varied diet of foods supplied from many geographic areas, it is unlikely that low soil selenium in a few locations will mean inadequate selenium in our diets.

The RDA for selenium is 55 to 70 micrograms per day for adults. In general, adults meet the RDA, consuming on average 110 micrograms of selenium each day.

Selenium at daily intakes as low as 900 micrograms per day (15 times the RDA) can cause toxicity symptoms if taken for many months. These symptoms include garlicky breath odor, changes in fingernails, hair loss, nausea and vomiting, and general weakness. Rashes and cirrhosis of the liver may also develop. Because of this potential for toxicity, supplement use of over 200 micrograms per day is not advised.

Food Sources of Selenium

Food item and amount	*Selenium (micrograms)*
Canned tuna, 3 oz	**68**
Sirloin steak, 5 oz	**48**
Shrimp, 4 oz	**45**
Cooked egg noodles, 1 cup	**35**
Roasted ham, 3 oz	**30**
Roasted chicken, 3 oz	**24**
Boiled egg, 1	**11**
Whole-wheat bread, 1 slice	**10**
Oatmeal, ½ cup	**10**
White bread, 1 slice	**8**

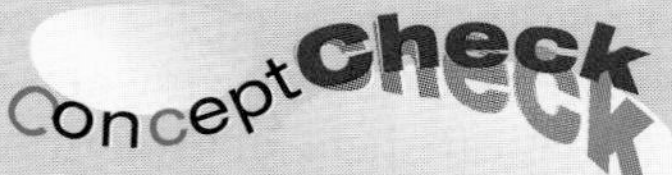

Zinc functions as a cofactor for many enzymes and is important for growth, immune function, and sense of taste. Beef, seafood, and whole grains are good food sources. As in the case of iron, zinc absorption is regulated according to the body's needs for the mineral. If taken in excess amounts, copper competes with zinc for absorption. Selenium activates an enzyme that helps change electron-seeking free radical (oxidizing) compounds into less toxic compounds so these do not attack and break down cell membranes. By helping to dismantle the free radical compounds, selenium works toward the same goal as vitamin E. A selenium deficiency results in muscle and heart disorders. Animal products and grains are good selenium sources; however, the selenium content in plants depends on the selenium concentration in the soil. The misuse of both selenium and zinc supplements can readily lead to toxic results.

Iodine (I)

Iodine in foods is actually found in an ion form, called iodide. During World War I, a link was discovered between a deficiency of iodide and the production of a **goiter,** an enlarged thyroid gland (Figure 8–10). Men drafted from the Pacific Northwest and the Great Lakes Region of the United States had a much higher rate of goiter than did men from other areas of the country. The soils in these areas have very low iodide contents. In the 1920s, researchers in Ohio found that low doses of iodide given to children over a 4-year period could prevent goiter. That finding led to the addition of iodide to salt beginning in the 1920s.

Today, many nations require iodide fortification of salt. In the United States, salt can be purchased either iodized or plain. Check for this on the label of a package of salt next time you are in a grocery store. Some areas of Europe, such as northern Italy, have very low soil levels of iodide, but have yet to adopt the practice of fortifying salt with iodide. People in these areas, especially women, still suffer from goiter, as do people in areas of Central America, South America, and Africa. The World Health Organization estimates that 20 million people in the world have varying degrees of illness caused by iodide deficiency. Eradication of iodide deficiency is a goal of many health-related organizations worldwide.

Goiter
An enlargement of the thyroid gland; this is often caused by insufficient iodide in the diet.

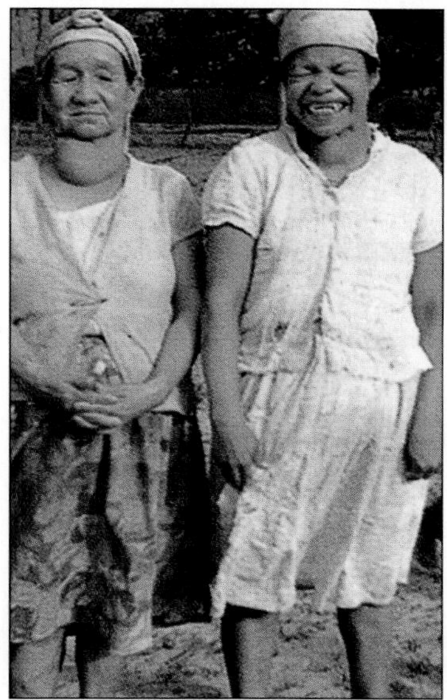

Figure 8–10
Goiter and cretinism in Bolivia. The mother on the left is goitrous, but otherwise normal. The daughter is goitrous, mentally retarded, deaf, and mute.

Function of Iodide

The thyroid gland actively accumulates and traps iodide from the bloodstream to support its hormone synthesis. Thyroid hormones are synthesized using iodide. These hormones help regulate metabolic rate and promote growth and development throughout the body, including the brain.

If a person's iodide intake is insufficient, the thyroid gland enlarges as it attempts to take up more iodide from the bloodstream. This eventually leads to goiter. Simple goiter is a painless condition, but if uncorrected can lead to pressure on the trachea (windpipe), which may cause difficulty in breathing. Although iodide can prevent goiter formation, it does not significantly shrink a goiter once it has formed. Surgical removal may be required in severe cases.

If a woman has an iodide-deficient diet during the early months of her pregnancy, the fetus suffers iodide deficiency because the mother's body uses up the available iodide. The infant then may be born with short stature and develop mental retardation. This stunted growth that results is part of what is known as ***cretinism.*** Cretinism appeared in America before iodide fortification of table salt began. Today, cretinism still appears in Europe, Africa, Latin America, and Asia.

Food Sources of Iodide and the RDA

Saltwater fish, seafood, iodized salt, dairy products, and grain products contain various forms of iodide. Sea salt found in health food stores, however, is not a good source because the iodide is lost during processing.

The RDA for iodide for adults is 150 micrograms. A half teaspoon of iodide-fortified salt (about 2 grams) supplies that amount. Most adults consume more iodide than the RDA—an estimated 170 to 250 micrograms daily, not including that from use of iodized salt at the table. This extra amount adds up because dairies and quick-service restaurants use it as a sterilizing agent, bakeries use it as a dough conditioner, food producers use it as part of food colorants, and it is added to salt.

Amounts of up to 1 to 2 milligrams per day of iodide appear to be safe. However, when very high amounts of iodide are consumed, thyroid gland function is hampered. This can occur in people who eat a lot of seaweed, because some seaweeds contain much iodide.

Dietary Sources of Iodide

Food item and amount	*Iodide (micrograms)*
Iodized salt, ½ tsp	**200**
Baked haddock, 3 oz	**125**
Buttermilk, 1 cup	**98**
Baked cod, 3 oz	**87**
Cottage cheese, ½ cup	**49**
Mozzarella cheese, 1 oz	**34**
Shrimp, 3 oz	**29**
Boiled egg, 1	**22**
Baked perch, 3 oz	**18**
Cheddar cheese, 1 oz	**14**

Copper (Cu)

Copper contributes to the metabolism of iron; it operates in processes that form hemoglobin and transport iron. A copper-containing enzyme aids in the release of iron from storage. Copper is needed by enzymes that create cross-connections in connective tissue proteins. Copper is also needed by other enzymes, such as those that defend the body against free radical (oxidizing) compounds and those that act in the brain and nervous system. Finally, copper performs in immune system function, blood clotting, and blood lipoprotein metabolism. About 55% to 75% of dietary copper is absorbed, with higher intakes associated with lower absorption. This absorption takes place primarily in the stomach and upper small intestine, with copper excretion via the gallbladder. Phytates, certain amino acids, vitamin C, fiber, zinc, and iron may all interfere with copper absorption. Symptoms of copper deficiency include a form of anemia, low white blood cell count, bone loss, poor growth, and some forms of heart disease.

Dietary Sources of Copper

Food item and amount	*Copper (milligrams)*
Steamed oysters, 3	**2.0**
Steamed lobster, 3 oz	**1.7**
Brazil nuts, ½ cup	**1.2**
Brewer's yeast, 3 tbsp	**0.8**
Walnuts, ½ cup	**0.7**
Sunflower seeds, ¼ cup	**0.6**
Cooked kidney beans, 1 cup	**0.4**
Molasses, 3 tbsp	**0.3**
Wheat germ, ¼ cup	**0.2**
Boiled shrimp, 3 oz	**0.2**

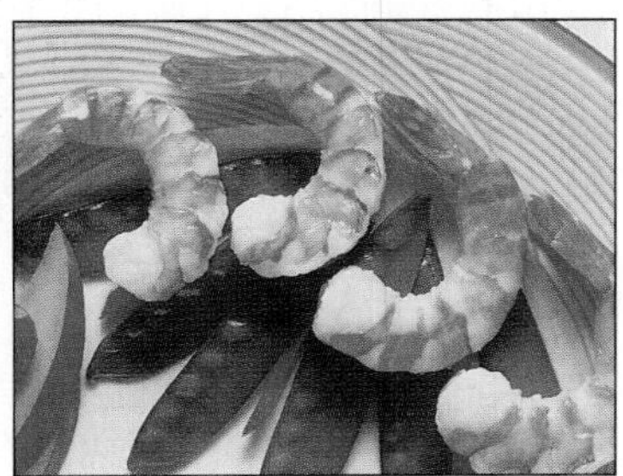

Seafood is one source of copper for a diet.

Copper in Foods and Needs

Copper is found primarily in liver, seafood, cocoa, legumes, nuts, seeds, and whole-grain breads and cereals.

The estimated safe and adequate daily dietary intake (ESADDI) for copper is 1.5 to 3 milligrams daily for adults. The average adult intake is about 1 to 1.5 milligrams per day. Women generally consume the smaller amount. Even so, the copper status of adults appears to be good, though we lack sensitive measures for copper status. It is wise, however, to regularly eat good sources of copper.

The groups most likely to develop copper deficiencies are premature infants, infants recovering from semistarvation on a milk-dominated diet (which is a poor source of copper), and people recovering from intestinal surgery (during which time copper absorption decreases). Recall that a copper deficiency can also result from overzealous supplementation of zinc, because zinc and copper compete with each other for absorption.) Copper can cause toxicity, including vomiting, at single doses of greater than 10 to 30 milligrams. Other forms of toxicity are also possible with megadose uses.

Fluoride (F)

Like chlorine, fluorine (F_2) is a poisonous gas. The fluoride ion (F^-) is the form of this trace mineral essential for human health. This link was found as dentists in the early 1900s noticed a lower rate of dental caries (cavities) in the southwestern United States. These areas contained high amounts of fluoride in the water. The amounts were sometimes so high that small spots on the teeth, called *mottling*, appeared. Even though mottled teeth were quite discolored, they contained very few dental caries. After experiments showed that fluoride in the water did indeed decrease the rate of dental caries, controlled fluoridation of water in parts of the United States began in 1945.

Those of us who grew up drinking fluoridated water generally have 40% to 60% fewer dental caries than people who did not drink fluoridated water as children. Dentists can provide fluoride treatments, and schools can provide fluoride tablets, but it is much less expensive and more reliable to simply add fluoride to a community's drinking water. State and private water sources do not always contain enough fluoride, however. When in doubt, contact your local water plant or have the water in your home analyzed for fluoride content. If it is less than 1 part fluoride per million parts of water (1 ppm), talk to your dentist about the best means for your children to obtain the fluoride they need.

Functions of Fluoride

Dietary fluoride consumed during childhood, when bones and teeth are developing, aids the synthesis of tooth crystals that strongly resist acid. Therefore teeth become very resistant to dental caries. Fluoride also inhibits metabolism and growth of the bacterium that causes dental caries, and fluoride present in saliva directly inhibits tooth demineralization and enhances tooth remineralization.

Fluoride applied to the surface of the teeth by dentists or from toothpaste adds additional protection against dental caries. Thus people of all ages benefit from the topical effects of fluoride, whether or not they consumed fluoridated water or fluoride supplements as children.

High doses of fluoride (20 or more milligrams per day) are being used experimentally in adults to treat severe osteoporosis, especially that seen in the spine. Such high fluoride dosages can cause significant side effects, such as stomach upset and bone pain. Ongoing research is attempting to establish a dose, form, and duration of treatment that aid in increasing bone mass and contribute to reduced fracture risk.

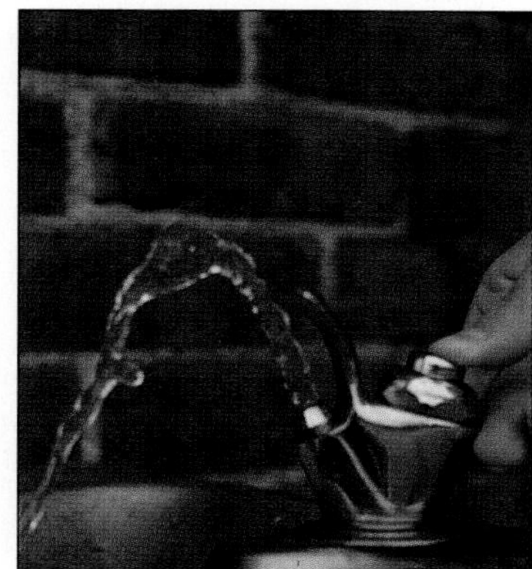

Fluoridated water is responsible for much of the decrease in dental caries throughout the United States in recent years.

Fluoride in Foods and Needs

Tea, seafood, seaweed, and some natural water sources are the only good food sources of fluoride. Most of our fluoride intake comes from fluoride added to drinking water and toothpaste and from fluoride treatments performed by dentists.

The AI for fluoride for adults is 3.1 to 3.8 milligrams per day. This range of intake provides the benefits of resistance to dental caries without causing ill effects. Typical fluoridated water contains about 0.2 milligrams per cup.

A fluoride intake greater than 6 milligrams per day can mottle teeth during their developmental stage, as mentioned above. Children who consume large amounts of fluoridated toothpaste as part of daily tooth care are at greatest risk. Not swallowing toothpaste and limiting the amount used to "pea" size are the best ways to prevent this problem. In addition, children under 6 years should have toothbrushing supervised by an adult. When fluoride intakes reach 20 milligrams per day during tooth development, the tooth structure is weakened and can crumble, however. High fluoride intake in adults does not cause mottling.

ConceptCheck

Iodide is vital for the synthesis of thyroid hormones. A prolonged insufficient intake causes the thyroid gland to enlarge, resulting in a goiter. The use of iodized salt in America has virtually eliminated this condition. Copper functions mainly in iron metabolism and in the cross-bonding of connective tissue. A deficiency can result in a type of anemia. Good food sources of copper are seafoods, legumes, nuts, dried fruits, and whole grains. Fluoride aids in tooth development. When incorporated into the teeth during development, fluoride makes them resistant to acid and bacterial growth, in turn reducing development of dental caries. Fluoride also aids in remineralization of teeth once decay begins. Most of us receive adequate amounts of fluoride from that added to drinking water and toothpaste. A high fluoride intake during tooth development can lead to spotted, or mottled, teeth.

Chromium (Cr)

The importance of chromium in human diets has been recognized only in the past 30 years. There is much we do not understand about this mineral, but chromium deficiency may be related to diabetes in some individuals.

The most-studied function of chromium is the maintenance of glucose uptake into cells. Our current understanding is that chromium enters the cell and acts to enhance the transport of glucose across the cell membrane by interacting with insulin function.

A chromium deficiency is characterized by impaired blood glucose control and elevated blood cholesterol and triglycerides. The mechanism by which chromium influences cholesterol metabolism is not known but may involve enzymes that control cholesterol synthesis. Chromium deficiency appears in people maintained on intravenous nutrition solutions not supplemented with chromium and in children with malnutrition. Because sensitive measures of chromium status are not available, marginal chromium deficiencies may go undetected.

Food Sources of Chromium and Needs

Specific data regarding the chromium content of various foods are scant, and most food composition tables do not include values for this trace mineral. Egg yolks, whole grains (bran), organ meats, other meats, mushrooms, nuts, and beer are good sources. Yeast is also a source. The amount of chromium in foods is closely tied to the local soil content of chromium. To provide yourself with a good chromium intake, regularly choose whole grains in preference to mostly refined grains.

The ESADDI for chromium is 50 to 200 micrograms per day. Average adult intakes in the United States are estimated at about 30 micrograms per day, but could be somewhat higher. Marginal to low chromium intakes (about 20 micrograms per day) may contribute to an increased risk for developing diabetes.

Some research also shows that an intake at the high end of the ESADDI, 200 micrograms per day, may improve blood glucose regulation in Type 2 diabetes, and may raise HDL. More studies are needed on these effects. Chromium toxicity has been reported in people exposed to industrial waste and in painters who use art supplies with a very high chromium content. Liver damage and lung cancer can result. Because of the risk of toxicity, any supplement use should normally not exceed 200 micrograms per day and be supervised by a physician.

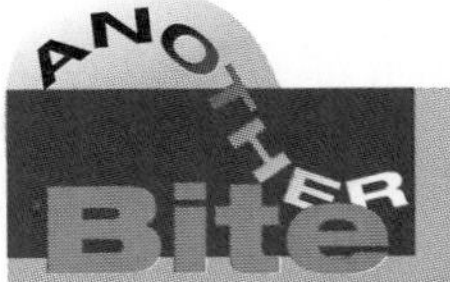

The current promotion of chromium picolinate as an agent to increase lean body mass or act as a weight-loss inducer provides a typical example of misleading use of research results by the health-food industry. The scant positive findings have come from the laboratory of the originator of chromium picolinate. Several well-designed controlled studies, however, have failed to duplicate their findings or have found only a select few individuals (possibly with initially low chromium status whose body composition responded significantly to chromium supplementation. As noted in Chapter 10, any claims for chromium picolinate for weight loss are speculative at best. Still, chromium supplement sales have recently soared to $150 million per year.

Manganese (Mn)

The mineral manganese is easily confused with magnesium. Not only are their names similar, but they also often substitute for each other in metabolic processes. Manganese is needed by some enzymes, such as those used in carbohydrate metabolism. Manganese is also important in bone formation.

No human deficiency symptom is associated with a low manganese intake. Animals on manganese-deficient diets suffer alterations in brain function, bone formation, and reproduction. If human diets were low in manganese, these symptoms would probably appear as well. As it happens, our need for manganese is very low, and our diets tend to be adequate in manganese.

Good food sources of manganese are nuts, rice, oats and other whole grains, beans, and leafy vegetables. The ESADDI for manganese is 2 to 5 milligrams. Average intakes generally fall within this range. Manganese is toxic at high doses, so be cautious with supplement use that exceeds estimated body needs.

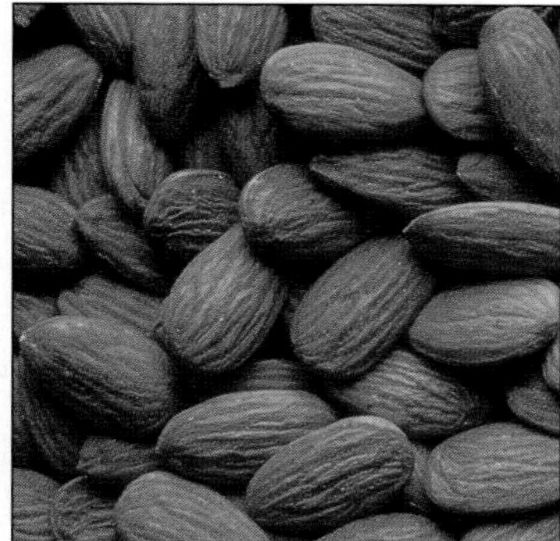

Nuts are a good source of manganese.

Molybdenum (Mo)

Several human enzymes use molybdenum. No molybdenum deficiency has been noted in people who consume normal diets, though deficiency symptoms have appeared in people maintained on intravenous nutrition feedings. These symptoms include increased heart and respiration rates, night blindness, mental confusion, edema, and weakness.

Good food sources of molybdenum include milk and milk products, beans, whole grains, and nuts. The EDADDI for molybdenum is 75 to 250 micrograms, about the same as typical intakes. When consumed in high doses, molybdenum causes toxicity in laboratory animals, with weight loss and decreased growth.

Other Trace Minerals

Although a variety of other trace minerals is found in humans, many of them have not yet been shown to be required. The list of minerals in this category includes boron, nickel, vanadium, arsenic, and silicon (Table 8-6). Widespread deficiency symptoms in humans have never been noted, probably because typical diets provide adequate amounts and they are needed by very few enzymes and metabolic systems. Their potential for toxicity should make one question any supplementation not supervised by a physician. These trace minerals may achieve more importance as more research is reported.

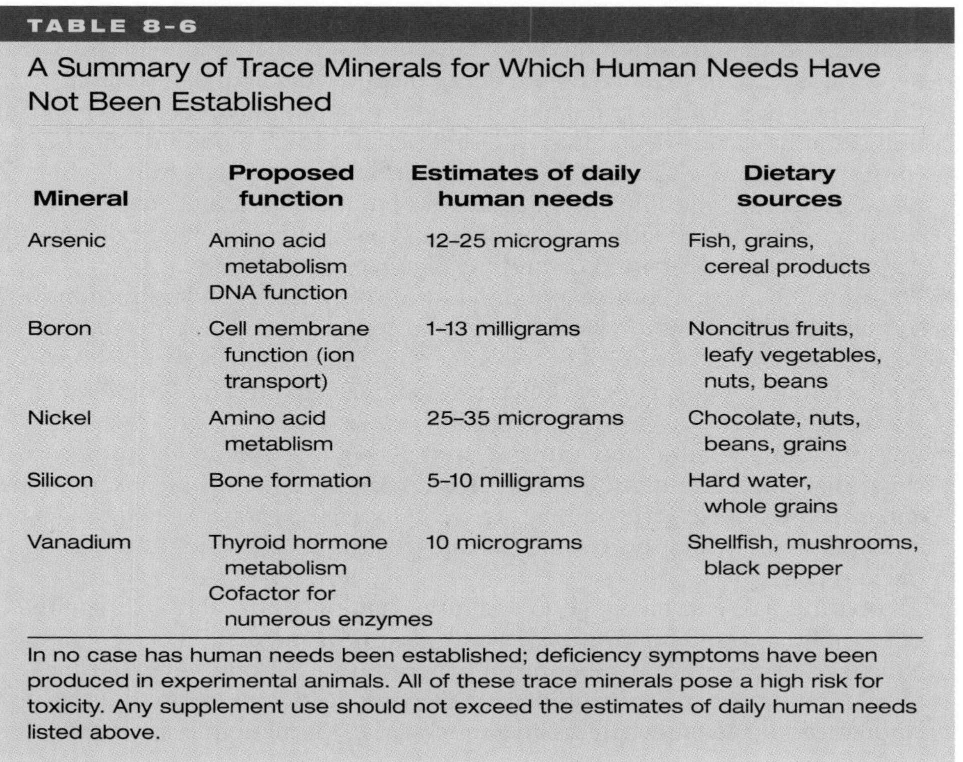

TABLE 8-6

A Summary of Trace Minerals for Which Human Needs Have Not Been Established

Mineral	Proposed function	Estimates of daily human needs	Dietary sources
Arsenic	Amino acid metabolism DNA function	12–25 micrograms	Fish, grains, cereal products
Boron	Cell membrane function (ion transport)	1–13 milligrams	Noncitrus fruits, leafy vegetables, nuts, beans
Nickel	Amino acid metablism	25–35 micrograms	Chocolate, nuts, beans, grains
Silicon	Bone formation	5–10 milligrams	Hard water, whole grains
Vanadium	Thyroid hormone metabolism Cofactor for numerous enzymes	10 micrograms	Shellfish, mushrooms, black pepper

In no case has human needs been established; deficiency symptoms have been produced in experimental animals. All of these trace minerals pose a high risk for toxicity. Any supplement use should not exceed the estimates of daily human needs listed above.

ConceptCheck

Chromium acts to increase the action of the hormone insulin. The amount of chromium found in food depends on soil content. Meats, whole grains, and egg yolks are some good sources. Manganese is a component of bone and used by many enzymes, including those involved in glucose production. Because our need for manganese is low, deficiencies are rare. Nuts, rice, oats, and beans are good food sources. Molybdenum is another trace mineral required by a few enzymes. Good sources include milk, beans, whole grains, and nuts. Deficiencies appear only with intravenous diets. The needs for some other trace minerals—such as boron, nickel, arsenic, and vanadium—have not been fully established in humans. If required, these minerals are needed in such small amounts that our current diets are probably adequate sources of them.

Summary

- Water constitutes 50% to 70% of the human body. Its unique chemical properties enable it to dissolve substances as well as serve as a medium for chemical reactions, temperature regulation, and lubrication. Water also helps regulate the acid-base balance in the body. For adults, daily water needs are estimated at 1 milliliter per kcal expended.
- Overall, the United States enjoys a very safe water supply. However, those with poor immune status should boil water used for drinking and cooking in order to avoid water-borne illness. Bottled water can also be used if desired.
- Many minerals are vital for sustaining life. For humans, animal products are the most bioavailable sources of most minerals. Supplements of minerals exceeding 100% of the Daily Values listed on the label should be taken only under a physician's supervision, because toxicity and nutrient interactions are a likely possibility.
- Sodium, the major positive ion found outside cells, is vital in fluid balance and nerve impulse transmission. The American diet provides abundant sodium through processed foods and table salt. About 10% to 15% of the adult population is sodium-sensitive and is at risk for developing high blood pressure from consuming excessive sodium. One out of four Americans suffers from high blood pressure. Controlling weight and alcohol intake, exercising, decreasing sodium intake, and ensuring adequate potassium, magnesium, and calcium in the diet all can play a part in controlling high blood pressure.
- Potassium, the major positive ion found inside cells, has a similar function to sodium. Milk, fruits, and vegetables are good sources. Chloride is the major negative ion found outside cells. It is important in digestion as part of stomach acid and in immune and nerve functions. Table salt supplies most of the chloride in our diets.
- Calcium forms a part of bone structure and plays a role in blood clotting, muscle contraction, nerve transmission, and cell metabolism. Calcium absorption is enhanced by stomach acid and the active vitamin D hormone. Dairy products are important calcium sources. Women are particularly at risk for not meeting calcium needs.
- Phosphorus aids enzyme function and forms part of key metabolic compounds, cell membranes, and bone. It is efficiently absorbed, and deficiencies are rare, although there is concern about possibly poor intake by some elderly women. Good food sources are dairy products, bakery products, and meats. Sulfur is incorporated into certain vitamins and amino acids. Magnesium is a mineral

found mostly in plant food sources. It is important for nerve and heart function and as an activator for many enzymes. Whole grains (bran portion), vegetables, nuts, seeds, milk, and meats are good food sources.

- Iron absorption depends mainly on the form of iron present and the body's need for it. Heme iron from animal sources is better absorbed than the nonheme iron obtained primarily from plant sources. Consuming vitamin C or meat simultaneously with iron increases nonheme absorption. Iron operates mainly in synthesizing hemoglobin and myoglobin and in the action of the immune system. Women are at great risk for developing iron deficiency, which decreases blood hemoglobin and red blood cell number. When this condition is severe enough to decrease the amount of oxygen carried in the blood, iron-deficiency anemia develops. Iron toxicity usually results from a genetic disorder called hemochromatosis. This disease causes overabsorption and accumulation of iron, which can result in severe liver and heart damage.
- Zinc aids in the action of more than 300 enzymes that are important for growth, development, immune function, wound healing, and taste. A zinc deficiency results in poor growth, loss of appetite, reduced sense of taste and smell, hair loss, and a persistent rash. Zinc is best absorbed from animal sources. The richest sources of zinc are oysters, shrimp, crab, and beef. Good plant sources are whole grains, peanuts, and beans.
- An important role of selenium is decreasing the action of free radical (oxidizing) compounds. In this way, selenium acts along with vitamin E. Muscle pain, muscle wasting, and a form of heart disease may result from a selenium deficiency. Meats, eggs, fish, and shellfish are good animal sources of selenium. Good plant-sources include grains and seeds.
- Iodide forms part of the thyroid hormones. A lack of dietary iodide results in the development of an enlarged thyroid gland or goiter. Iodized salt is a major food source.
- Copper is important for iron metabolism, cross-linking of connective tissue, and other functions. A copper deficiency can result in a form of anemia. Copper is found mainly in liver, seafood, cocoa, legumes, and whole grains.
- Fluoride incorporated into dietary intake during development makes teeth resistant to dental caries. Most Americans receive the bulk of their fluoride from fluoridated water and toothpaste.
- Chromium aids in the action of the hormone insulin. Egg yolks, meats, and whole grains are good sources of chromium. Manganese and molybdenum are used by various enzymes. Clear deficiencies in otherwise healthy people are rarely seen for any of these three nutrients. Human needs for other trace minerals are so low that deficiencies are uncommon.

Study Questions

1. Approximately how much water do you need each day to stay healthy? Identify at least two situations that increase the need for water. Then list three sources of water in the average person's diet.
2. Why are most minerals generally present in higher concentrations in animal foods than in plant foods?
3. What is the relationship between sodium and water balance, and how is that relationship monitored as well as maintained in the body?
4. Identify four factors that influence the bioavailability of minerals from food.
5. What are two similarities and differences between sodium and potassium? Sodium and chloride?
6. In terms of total amounts in the body, calcium and phosphorus are the first and second most abundant minerals, respectively. What function do these minerals have in common?

7 What are the best food sources for zinc and copper?
8 Describe the symptoms of iron-deficiency anemia and explain possible reasons why they occur.
9 Which trace minerals are lost from cereal grains when they are refined? Are any of these nutrients replaced by enrichment?
10 Describe the chief function of fluoride, copper, and chromium in the body.

Further Readings

1 Anderson RA: Effects of chromium on body composition and weight loss, *Nutrition Reviews* 56:266, 1998. See also Anderson RA: chromium, glucose intolerance and diabetes, *Journal of the American College of Nutrition* 17(6):548, 1998.
2 Andrews WC: What's new in preventing and treating osteoporosis? *Postgraduate Medicine* 104(4):89, 1998 (see also pages 215–216).
3 Cadogran J and others: Milk intake and bone mineral acquisition in adolescent girls: randomised, controlled intervention trial, *British Medical Journal* 315:1255, 1997.
4 Colditz GA: Selenium and cancer prevention promising results indicate further trials required, *Journal of the American Medical Association* 276:1984, 1996.
5 Cooper RS and others: The puzzle of hypertension in African-Americans, *Scientific American* p. 56, February 1999.
6 Estell RE: Treatment of postmenopausal osteoporosis, *New England Journal of Medicine* 338:736, 1998.
7 Farley D: Bone builders: support your bones with healthy habits, *FDA Consumer* p. 27, September–October 1997.
8 Filtering the data on water safety, *Health News* p. 4, September 16, 1997.
9 Greeley A: A pinch of controversy shakes up dietary salt, *FDA Consumer* p. 24 November–December 1997.
10 Hetzel BS: Iodine deficiency and fetal brain damage, *New England Journal of Medicine* 331:1770, 1994.
11 Hormone-replacement therapy weighing the benefits and risks, *Harvard Health Letter* 22 (October):1, 1997. (See also February 1999, p. 6.)
12 Kaplan NM: Treatment of hypertension, *American Family Physician* 58:1323, 1998.
13 Kleiner SM: Water: an essential but overlooked nutrient, *Journal of the American Dietetic Association* 99:200, 1999.
14 Kumanyika SK, Cutler JA: Dietary sodium reduction: Is there cause for concern? *Journal of the American College of Nutrition* 16:192, 1997.
15 Liebman B: DASH: a diet for all diseases, *Nutrition Action Healthletter* p. 10 October 1997.
16 Liebman B: Avoiding the fracture zone: calcium, *Nutrition Action Healthletter* p. 1, April 1998.
17 McBean LD: Dairy foods: traditional and emerging health benefits, *Dairy Council Digest* 69(5):25, 1998.
18 Mitchell P: The million-man malady, *American Health* p. 104, March 1998.
19 Nielsen FH: Ultratrace minerals in Shils ME and others (eds) *Modern Nutrition in Health and Disease* 9th edition Baltimore MD, Williams & Wilkins, 1999.
20 Reichman J: The new estrogen option, *American Health* p. 41, April 1998 (see also December 1997, p. 23).
21 Schardt D: Magnesium, *Nutrition Action Healthletter* p. 9, December 1998.
22 Whelton PK and others: Sodium restriction and weight loss in the treatment of hypertension in older people, *Journal of the American Medical Association* 279:839, 1998.

RATE

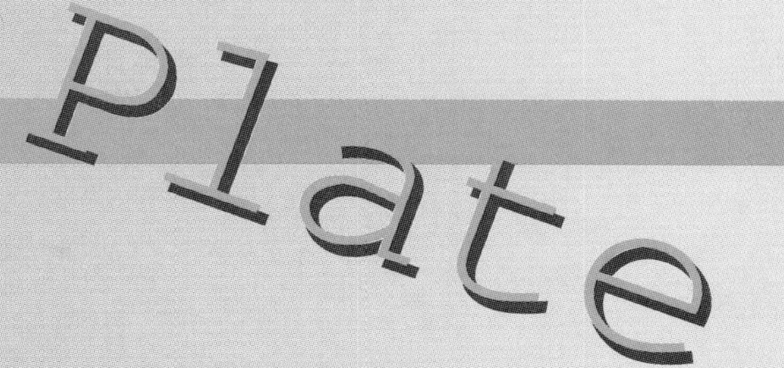

I. How Does Your Mineral Intake Measure Up?

To complete this activity, reexamine your nutritional assessment from Chapter 2. Compare your intake of selective minerals with the RDA, AI, or other established standard. Use your completed nutritional assessment to complete the table below. For each mineral, record your intake, the intake recommended, the percentage of that intake you consumed, and a +, −, or = to indicate an intake higher, lower, or equal to that intake. Note that for sodium and potassium, minimum requirements for health are designated and already recorded in the table (these can also be found on the inside front cover of the book).

Mineral	Intake	RDA/AI	% of Needs	+/−/=
Calcium				
Phosphorus				
Sodium		500 milligrams		
Potassium		2000 milligrams		
Iron				
Zinc				

ANALYSIS

1. Which of your mineral intakes equaled or exceeded the RDA (or other standard set)? Do the nutrients for which you exceeded the desired amounts pose a likely risk for toxicity, based on the total amount consumed?

   ____

2. Which of your intakes were below the RDA (or other standard)?

   ____

3. What foods and cooking practices could be emphasized or de-emphasized to modify your weaknesses? Indicate for each food the specific amount of the missing nutrient(s) supplied.

   ____
   ____
   ____
   ____
   ____

II. Working for Denser Bones

In the Nutrition Issue, you will learn important information about the disease osteoporosis, characterized by thinning and brittle bones.

Osteoporosis affects more than 25 million people in the United States. One-third of all women experience fractures because of this disease, amounting to about 1.5 million bone fractures per year. Given the rise in the number of elderly people in the United States, osteoporosis-related illness and death are anticipated to increase dramatically in coming years.

This is a disease you can do something about. Some risk factors can't be changed, but others can. To what degree are you doing the things that can help prevent this debilitating disease? Answer yes or no to the following questions by placing an X in the appropriate blank.

	Yes	No
1. Do you average at least 20 minutes of sun exposure per day to at least your hands and face to get vitamin D, or do you drink vitamin D–fortified milk regularly?	____	____
2. Do you engage in weight-bearing physical activity (jogging, brisk walking, etc.) for at least 30 minutes on most or all days of the week?	____	____
3. If you are a woman, do you experience regular menstruation?		
4. Do you avoid smoking cigarettes?	____	____
5. Do you avoid regular consumption of large amounts (greater than one to two drinks per day) of alcohol?	____	____
6. Do you consume milk and other dairy products regularly, or substitute other sources to meet at least the AI for calcium?	____	____
7. Do you moderate intake of phosphorus, sodium, protein, and caffeine?	____	____

The more *yes* answers you have, the more you are actively preserving your bone density for the future. Also, remember that this is not just a consideration for women, because if men plan to live well into their eighties and nineties, they are at risk for osteoporosis. In fact, about 14% of all spine fractures and 25% of all hip fractures linked to osteoporosis occur in men.

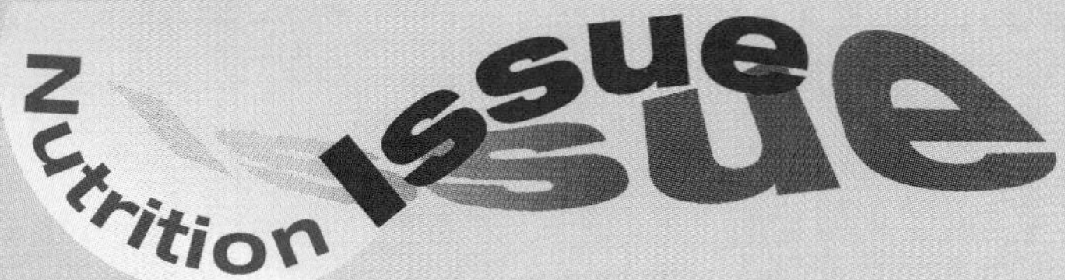

Osteoporosis

Widespread advertising has made it almost impossible for women to ignore **osteoporosis.** The crippling effect this disease has on older persons is now recognized as a major medical problem. The disease affects more than 25 million people in the United States and 200 million worldwide, most of them women. Osteoporosis leads to approximately 1.5 million bone fractures per year, usually in the hip, spine, or wrist. It costs the nation about $13 billion per year in health-care costs. About one-half of Caucasian women (and one-third of all women) experience osteoporosis-related fractures in their lifetimes.

Osteoporosis
Decreased bone mass where no outward cause can be found. Bone composition is essentially normal, just less bone is present. Related to effects of aging, poor diet, and hormonal effects of menopause in women.

The slender, inactive woman who smokes is most susceptible to osteoporosis, but any person who lives long enough can suffer from the disease, including men. About 25% of women older than 50 develop osteoporosis. Among people older than 80, osteoporosis becomes the rule—not the exception. The spine fractures commonly found in women with osteoporosis cause considerable pain and deformity and decrease physical ability (Figure 8–11); hip fractures are seen in both men and women with osteoporosis. Not only is this disease debilitating, it also can be fatal. Up to one-fifth of all older persons who suffer hip fractures eventually die from fracture-related complications.

A QUICK LOOK AT BONE STRUCTURE AND STRENGTH

To better understand the role calcium plays in bone health and osteoporosis, it is important to understand how bone is constructed. Visual observation of the cross-sections of a bone reveals two primary bone structural types: **cortical bone** and **trabecular bone.** These interact within each bone to form quite an engineering marvel of strength (Figure 8–12).

The entire outer surface of all bones is composed of cortical (compact) bone, which is very dense. The shafts of long bones, such as those of the arm, are almost entirely cortical bone. Trabecular (spongy) bone is found in the ends of the long bones, inside the spinal vertebrae, and inside the flat bones of the pelvis. Trabecular bone forms an internal scaffolding network for a bone. It supports the outer cortical shell of the bone, especially in heavily stressed areas, such as joints.

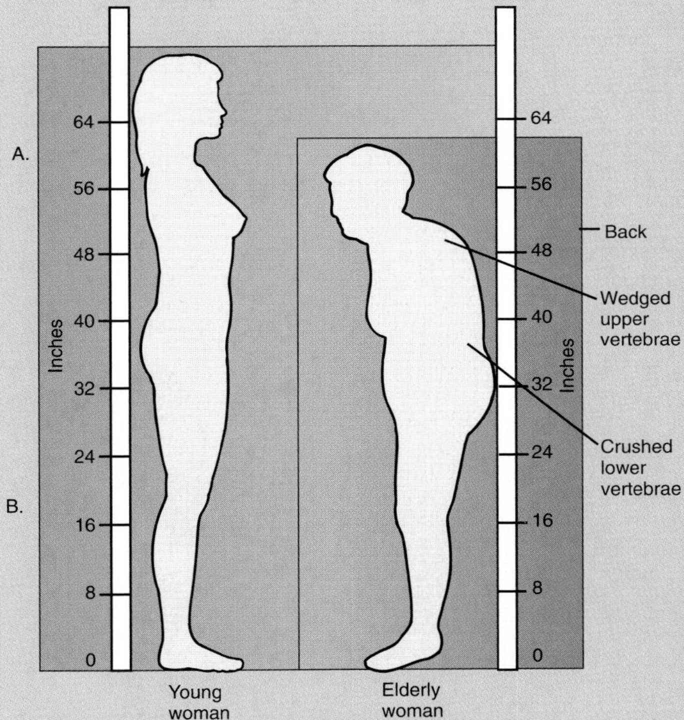

Figure 8–11 *A loss of height and a distorted body shape are commonly seen in osteoporosis. Monitoring changes in adult height is one way to detect early evidence of osteoporosis.*

Bone mass
Total mineral substance (such as calcium or phosphorus) in a cross section of bone, generally expressed as grams per centimeter of length.

Bone mineral density
Total mineral content of bone at a specific bone site divided by the width of the bone at that site, generally expressed as grams per cubic centimeter.

Bone strength depends on a person's **bone mass** and **bone mineral density.** The more bone there is, and especially the more densely packed bone crystals are in the bone, the stronger the bone structure. Another important element of bone strength is the trabecular bone support network inside a bone. It is especially critical for the horizontal trabeculae to extend continuously—without breaks—between the areas of vertical trabeculae. Any break in either the horizontal or more vertical trabecular beams weakens the support system of a bone and increases the risk for bone fracture. And once these beams are broken, there is no way to rebuild them. This is why it is so important to limit bone loss as people age.

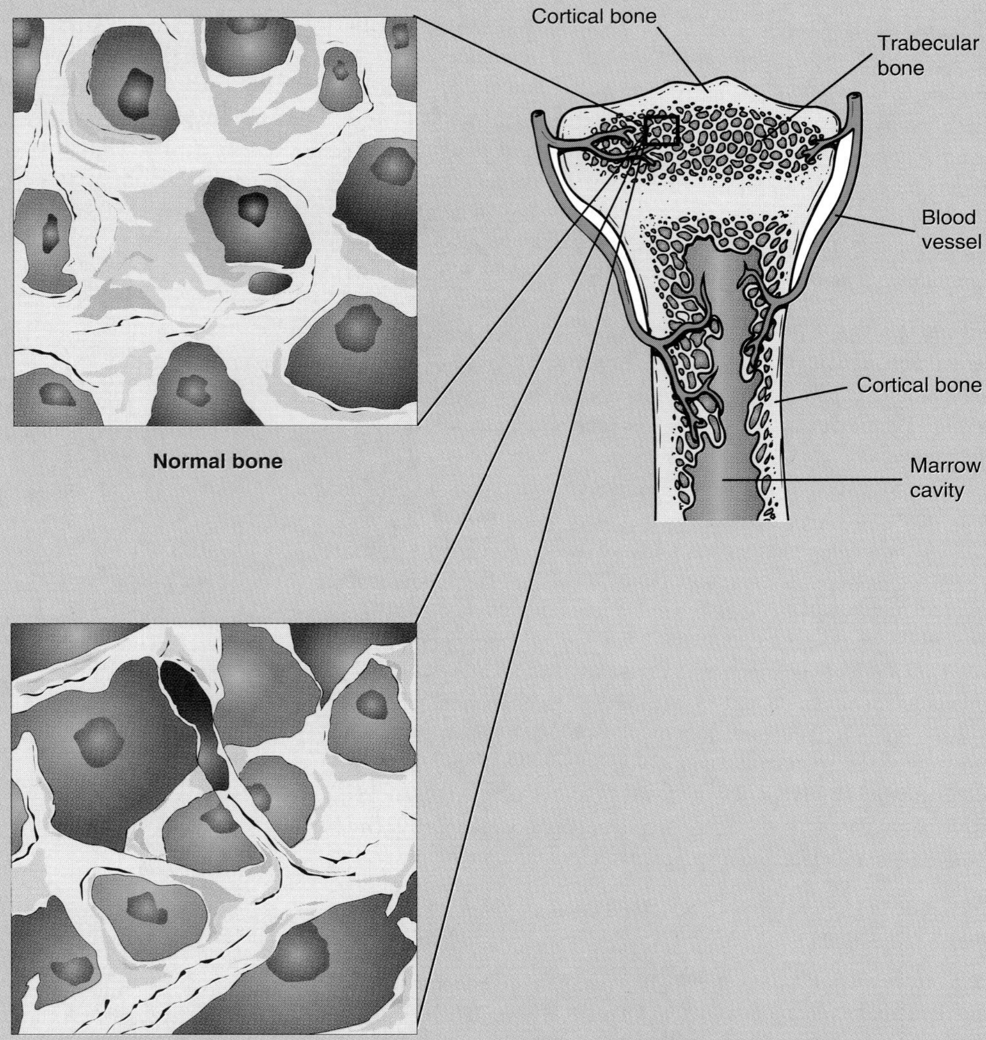

Figure 8–12 *Cortical and trabecular bone. Cortical bone forms the shafts of bones and the outer mineral covering. Trabecular bone supports the outer shell of cortical bone in various bones of the body, as in the upper bone pictured. Note how in the lower picture there is much less trabecular bone. This leads to a more fragile bone, is not reversible to any major extent with current therapies.*

would probably appear as well. As it happens, our need for manganese is very low, and our diets tend to be adequate in manganese.

Good food sources of manganese are nuts, rice, oats and other whole grains, beans, and leafy vegetables. The ESADDI for manganese is 2 to 5 milligrams. Average intakes generally fall within this range. Manganese is toxic at high doses, so be cautious with supplement use that exceeds estimated body needs.

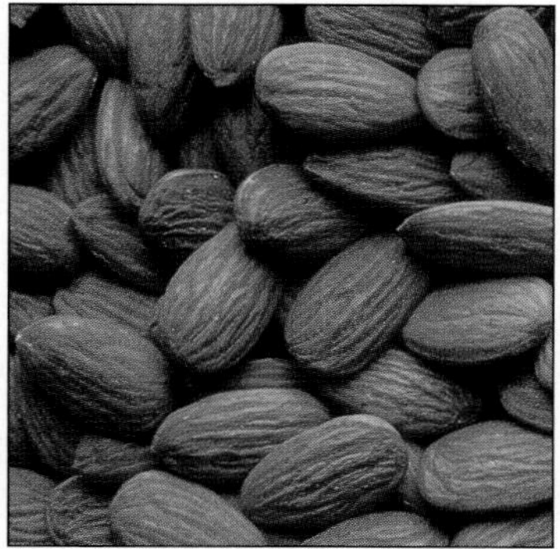

Nuts are a good source of manganese.

Molybdenum (Mo)

Several human enzymes use molybdenum. No molybdenum deficiency has been noted in people who consume normal diets, though deficiency symptoms have appeared in people maintained on intravenous nutrition feedings. These symptoms include increased heart and respiration rates, night blindness, mental confusion, edema, and weakness.

Good food sources of molybdenum include milk and milk products, beans, whole grains, and nuts. The EDADDI for molybdenum is 75 to 250 micrograms, about the same as typical intakes. When consumed in high doses, molybdenum causes toxicity in laboratory animals, with weight loss and decreased growth.

Other Trace Minerals

Although a variety of other trace minerals is found in humans, many of them have not yet been shown to be required. The list of minerals in this category includes boron, nickel, vanadium, arsenic, and silicon (Table 8–6). Widespread deficiency symptoms in humans have never been noted, probably because typical diets provide adequate amounts and they are needed by very few enzymes and metabolic systems. Their potential for toxicity should make one question any supplementation not supervised by a physician. These trace minerals may achieve more importance as more research is reported.

TABLE 8-6

A Summary of Trace Minerals for Which Human Needs Have Not Been Established

Mineral	Proposed function	Estimates of daily human needs	Dietary sources
Arsenic	Amino acid metabolism DNA function	12–25 micrograms	Fish, grains, cereal products
Boron	Cell membrane function (ion transport)	1–13 milligrams	Noncitrus fruits, leafy vegetables, nuts, beans
Nickel	Amino acid metablism	25–35 micrograms	Chocolate, nuts, beans, grains
Silicon	Bone formation	5–10 milligrams	Hard water, whole grains
Vanadium	Thyroid hormone metabolism Cofactor for numerous enzymes	10 micrograms	Shellfish, mushrooms, black pepper

In no case has human needs been established; deficiency symptoms have been produced in experimental animals. All of these trace minerals pose a high risk for toxicity. Any supplement use should not exceed the estimates of daily human needs listed above.

ConceptCheck

Chromium acts to increase the action of the hormone insulin. The amount of chromium found in food depends on soil content. Meats, whole grains, and egg yolks are some good sources. Manganese is a component of bone and used by many enzymes, including those involved in glucose production. Because our need for manganese is low, deficiencies are rare. Nuts, rice, oats, and beans are good food sources. Molybdenum is another trace mineral required by a few enzymes. Good sources include milk, beans, whole grains, and nuts. Deficiencies appear only with intravenous diets. The needs for some other trace minerals—such as boron, nickel, arsenic, and vanadium—have not been fully established in humans. If required, these minerals are needed in such small amounts that our current diets are probably adequate sources of them.

Summary

- Water constitutes 50% to 70% of the human body. Its unique chemical properties enable it to dissolve substances as well as serve as a medium for chemical reactions, temperature regulation, and lubrication. Water also helps regulate the acid-base balance in the body. For adults, daily water needs are estimated at 1 milliliter per kcal expended.
- Overall, the United States enjoys a very safe water supply. However, those with poor immune status should boil water used for drinking and cooking in order to avoid water-borne illness. Bottled water can also be used if desired.
- Many minerals are vital for sustaining life. For humans, animal products are the most bioavailable sources of most minerals. Supplements of minerals exceeding 100% of the Daily Values listed on the label should be taken only under a physician's supervision, because toxicity and nutrient interactions are a likely possibility.
- Sodium, the major positive ion found outside cells, is vital in fluid balance and nerve impulse transmission. The American diet provides abundant sodium through processed foods and table salt. About 10% to 15% of the adult population is sodium-sensitive and is at risk for developing high blood pressure from consuming excessive sodium. One out of four Americans suffers from high blood pressure. Controlling weight and alcohol intake, exercising, decreasing sodium intake, and ensuring adequate potassium, magnesium, and calcium in the diet all can play a part in controlling high blood pressure.
- Potassium, the major positive ion found inside cells, has a similar function to sodium. Milk, fruits, and vegetables are good sources. Chloride is the major negative ion found outside cells. It is important in digestion as part of stomach acid and in immune and nerve functions. Table salt supplies most of the chloride in our diets.
- Calcium forms a part of bone structure and plays a role in blood clotting, muscle contraction, nerve transmission, and cell metabolism. Calcium absorption is enhanced by stomach acid and the active vitamin D hormone. Dairy products are important calcium sources. Women are particularly at risk for not meeting calcium needs.
- Phosphorus aids enzyme function and forms part of key metabolic compounds, cell membranes, and bone. It is efficiently absorbed, and deficiencies are rare, although there is concern about possibly poor intake by some elderly women. Good food sources are dairy products, bakery products, and meats. Sulfur is incorporated into certain vitamins and amino acids. Magnesium is a mineral

Researchers in New Zealand have uncovered what they think is one reason hip fractures are more common in Western countries than in the developing world. Because children in Western countries have higher average nutrient intakes than those in developing countries, they grow faster and to a greater extent. As a result, the part of the thigh bone that fits into the pelvis becomes quite long, and in turn the higher the risk for hip fracture, especially as bone mass decreases with advanced age. This suggests that people in Western countries especially must pursue strategies to avert hip fracture, notably in later years.

BONE MASS IS RELATED TO AGE AND GENDER

Rapid and continual bone growth and calcification occur throughout the adolescent years, ultimately resulting in what is called *peak bone mass.* In the adolescent growth spurt, bone mass is increasing at the rate of about 8.5% per year, Small increases in bone mass then continue between 20 and 30 years of age.

The ultimate amount of bone built by a person is clearly dependent on gender, race, familial patterns seen in the mother and father, and probably other genetically determined factors. In addition, men have higher bone mass value than women, and African-Americans have heavier skeletons than Caucasians. As a direct consequence, men and African-Americans in general have a somewhat lower risk of fractures than other populations. Slender, small-framed Caucasians and Asian women show the lowest bone mass values. Peak bone mass is also related to dietary intake of calcium and other nutrients, such as phosphorus, vitamin A, vitamin D, vitamin K, magnesium, zinc, and copper.

Bone mass varies among young adults, some have much denser bone than others, perhaps because they built more bone when they were young. Some people also may more easily adapt to lower-calcium diets, as has been recently shown in Chinese women in one study. People who have developed more bone by early adulthood can sustain greater age-related bone loss with less fracture risk compared with those who have less bone.

For women, bone loss begins about age 30 and proceeds slowly and continuously to menopause (approximately age 50). It often speeds up at menopause and continues at a high rate for the next 10 years. By age 65 to 70, the rate of bone loss falls to about the same rate as before menopause. In men, bone loss is slow and steady from around age 30. Overall, this bone loss in both males and females progresses without noticeable symptoms.

OSTEOPOROSIS

Failure to maintain enough bone mass in the body can be caused by the vitamin D deficiency disease osteomalacia, the use of certain medications (such as cortisol, antiseizure drugs, and thyroid hormones), and cancer. If these or similar causes are not present, the diagnosis is osteoporosis. Osteoporosis can be roughly classified as type 1 (postmenopausal), which appears in women in the years right after menopause, and type II (senile), which is found in both men and women of advanced age.

All women 65 years and older should be screened for this disease. Medicare covers the cost of the needed **DEXA bone scan.** Younger women are advised to do the same at menopause if they have associated risk factors, or if the results of the screening would help them decide what treatment plan is appropriate.

DEXA bone scan
Method to measure bone density that uses small amounts of x-ray radiation. The ability of a bone to block the path of the radiation is used as a measure of bone density at that bone site. DEXA stands for dual energy, x-ray absorptiometry.

Bone composition in osteoporosis is essentially normal; basically there is just less bone throughout the body. Because these bones have less substance, osteoporosis generally leads to fractures in old age, loss of height, distorted body shape, and loss of teeth.

ESTROGEN REPLACEMENT PLUS CALCIUM IS AN EFFECTIVE APPROACH FOR REDUCING POSTMENOPAUSAL BONE LOSS

Hormone replacement therapy with estrogen (and often with added progestins) is widely recommended for women at menopause to prevent osteoporosis, especially if (1) they have no contraindications to use (such as a history of breast cancer) and (2) they fall in the lower third of bone mass values for their age. Women with intermediate values who do not opt for estrogen treatment should have their bone mass values remeasured at their physician's discretion, typically in 2 to 5 or so years. However, women postponing therapy should realize that alteration of the internal trabecular support system of the bone as a result of bone loss is currently a permanent phenomenon. No available therapy can reverse this problem. Estrogen is also used to reduce the symptoms of menopause. Investigation of such hormone replacement is worthwhile for all women, as many will be postmenopausal for up to a third of their lives. Currently, about 10 million women take estrogen.

Estrogen replacement at menopause greatly slows further bone loss in women. Thus it is reasonable to assume that estrogen replacement therapy will significantly reduce the risk of osteoporosis and related fractures in women who begin treatment right after menopause and continue it thereafter. Estrogen also helps reduce bone loss in older women, even when begun around age 60 years. Unfortunately, the benefits of estrogen all but disappear if later discontinued for more than 5 years.

Estrogen aids bone maintenance in a number of ways. Estrogen is associated with greater synthesis of the active vitamin D hormone. Estrogen also may increase the sensitivity of the intestine to this hormone, in turn improving the action of this hormone and therefore increasing calcium absorption. Finally, the binding of estrogen to sites on bone cells alters synthesis of various local factors produced by white blood cells that influence bone maintenance.

Estrogen therapy is relatively safe for most women but still must be closely supervised by a physician. Resumption of menstruation with some forms of therapy is common, but it subsides after a few years or so. A slight increased risk for certain forms of cancer, notably in the breast and endometrium (the latter if the woman has not had a **hysterectomy**), blood clotting disorders and gallbladder problems have been observed in women on estrogen therapy. Thus close monitoring is needed. Adding progestins to the regimen greatly reduces the risk of endometrial cancer. Current studies are also trying to determine if therapy with lower doses of estrogen than typically used by itself or when coupled with other osteoporosis medications is still as beneficial. This is likely to be the case and should pose less health risk.

Hysterectomy *Surgical removal of the uterus.*

Estrogen replacement therapy is also associated with decreased risk of developing Alzheimer's disease.

An additional benefit of estrogen replacement therapy is a reduction in the risk of heart disease. Heart disease risk climbs sharply after menopause. Estrogen likely blunts this change in part by lowering LDL and raising HDL, as noted in Chapter 5. A direct benefit of estrogen on cells lining the blood vessels is also suspected. In addition, it is possible that estrogen decreases heart disease risk by keeping body fat distribution in the hip area instead of in the upper body (a known risk factor for heart disease).

When the decreased risks for osteoporosis and heart disease are added together, estrogen replacement therapy ends up greatly improving the overall health risk profile for many women, especially those with many risk factors for osteoporosis and heart disease. A woman and her physician should work together to see if that is true for her. Women should also realize that the risk of developing heart disease in one's older years is six times greater than that for developing breast cancer. The Women's Health Initiative trial, currently under way, is designed to help pinpoint the actual net benefit from estrogen replacement experienced by a wide variety of women, and should in turn contribute to this decision making. Results are due by 2006.

Some women cannot take estrogen because they have estrogen-sensitive breasts or uterine tumors. Other therapies, such as taking certain **bisphosphonate compounds** or estrogenlike analogs, are available and quite effective. However, these treatments are still relatively new, more expensive, and often more cumbersome than estrogen therapy.

Bisphosphonates *Compounds primarily composed of carbon and phosphorus that bind to bone mineral and in turn reduce bone breakdown.*

The question that often arises is whether an increased calcium intake can substitute for the use of estrogen or other medications in reducing bone loss in postmenopausal women. Overall, studies have found that taking as much as 2000 milligrams of extra calcium daily (equal to about 7 cups of milk) after menopause does not prevent bone loss in the spine, hip, or wrist as successfully as estrogen replacement does. Although such high intakes of dietary calcium do reduce bone loss in some areas, they are no more effective than calcium intakes closer to the AI in reducing the often significant loss of spinal bone that occurs in the 5 to 10 years immediately after menopause. After that age interval, meeting calcium (and vitamin D) needs is helpful in reducing further bone loss. Thus it is not a question of estrogen versus calcium. Rather, estrogen plus adequate calcium and vitamin D constitutes the most effective treatment currently available, as they work together to preserve bone health.

Research is also ongoing in the area of phytoestrogens, plant compounds that have hormone-like effects in the body. These phytoestrogens can come in the form of isoflavones from soy products, or lignan from grains (flax seed), fruits, and vegetables. It is hoped that these phytoestrogens will act like synthetic estrogen therapy, such as in bone and heart protection. More information is needed to discover the full potential of these foodborne substances.

WILL A NUTRITIOUS DIET IN YOUTH HELP PREVENT OSTEOPOROSIS LATER?

Meeting at least the AI for calcium as part of an overall balanced diet from childhood through adolescence builds a stronger bone structure than does a lower calcium intake. The extent and importance of this difference in bone strength are currently under study, but the information published to date looks promising.

TABLE 8-6

Some Factors Associated with Bone Accretion/Maintenance Versus Increased Age-Related Bone Loss

Accretion/maintenance	Loss	
Male gender	Female gender	
Normal menses	Caucasian or Asian race	Cigarette smoking
Estrogen replacement (or other approved osteoporosis medication)	Lack of menses (generally from postmenopausal status)	Slender figure
African ethnic origin	Early menopause	Bed rest (months)
Thiazide diuretics	Family history of osteoporosis	Anorexia nervosa or bulimia nervosa
Physical activity	Thinner skin	Excessive wheat bran intake
Dietary calcium	Glucocorticoid use	Excessive sodium intake
Vitamin D nutriture	Hyperparathyroidism	Excessive protein, caffeine, and phosphorus consumption if calcium AI is not met
Body weight	Hyperthyroidism	
Overall adequate diet	Thyroid hormone replacement	
Parents with large bone mass	Factors made by white blood cells	
	Alcoholism	

ARE ALL WOMEN AT RISK FOR OSTEOPOROSIS?

Only about one-third of all women experience osteoporosis-related fractures in their lifetimes. Some women just do not live long enough to suffer from osteoporosis. They may experience some bone loss, but their bones still remain reasonably strong throughout their lives. This is especially true of women who die before the age 75.

In addition, some women have much denser bone than others. They probably built more bone when they were young, so they are able to endure greater bone loss without experiencing more fractures. Actually, the reason for such variations in bone mass and fracture risk in women of any age still needs more research. However, researchers have identified numerous factors—including physical activity, excess body weight, and calcium intake throughout life—associated with higher bone mass values in some studies (Table 8-6). Even more factors are associated with low bone mass. One clearly can't focus only on calcium when discussing this disease—many factors are involved.

PROPER PLANNING HELPS PREVENT FRACTURES IN LATER LIFE

As women mature, different strategies for preventing osteoporosis are needed, based on the risk factors present. Young women should see a physician upon any sign of irregular menstruation and should pursue a balanced diet and an active lifestyle with some weight-bearing physical activity (to build/maintain muscle mass).Greater muscle mass linked to physical activity is associated with greater bone mass, as this keeps tension on bone.

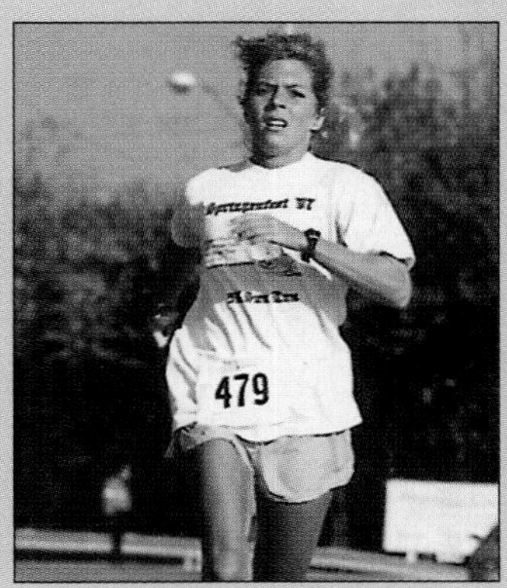

Regular weight-bearing physical activity contributes to bone health.

In young women, regular menstruation is a key factor in bone maintenance, as evidenced by low bone mass in some nonmenstruating female athletes and other women with irregular menstruation, such as those with anorexia nervosa. Physical activity cannot prevent the bone loss associated with irregular menstruation.

Other common risk factors to minimize are smoking and excessive alcohol intake; these work against bone strength. Smoking lowers estrogen in the blood in women, increasing bone loss. Alcohol is toxic to bone cells; alcoholism is probably a major undiagnosed and unrecognized cause of osteoporosis today. Moderation in phosphorus, caffeine, sodium, and protein intake is also advised. These are especially problematic when insufficient calcium is consumed.

At menopause, women should discuss estrogen replacement therapy with a physician. A bone scan at this age is a wise investment in health. They also need to accurately track their height. A decrease of more than 1 inch from premenopausal values is a sign that significant bone loss is taking place.

The NIH has a toll free number for information on osteoporosis (800) 624-BONE. The National Osteoporosis Foundation also will answer your questions about the disease (800-464-6700). Their web site is (http://www.nof.org). Another helpful web site is that of the National Dairy Council (http://www.nationaldairycouncil.org).

Older men and women need to stay physically active (if possible)—including some weight-bearing and resistance activities—and they should meet their AI for calcium (1200 milligrams per day). Older people also need to minimize the risk for falls, especially by limiting their use of medications and alcohol, which might disturb coordination, and should take corrective measures if visual function is impaired. Getting regular sun exposure and consuming food sources of vitamin D also are very important. Supplements containing about 10 to 20 micrograms (400 to 800 IU) are also appropriate if a combination of sun exposure and dietary intake is not sufficient (see Chapter 7).

As you have seen throughout this book, no chronic disease is simple: multiple causes and treatment options are possible. Gaining knowledge as you have allows one to be an active participant in preventive and treatment decisions.

Energy Balance and Imbalance

part 3

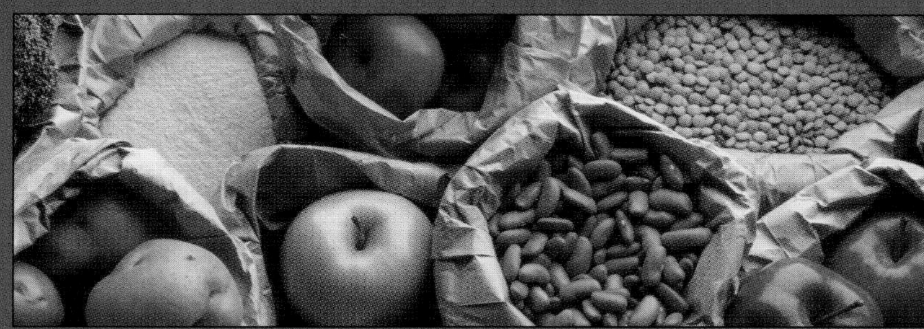

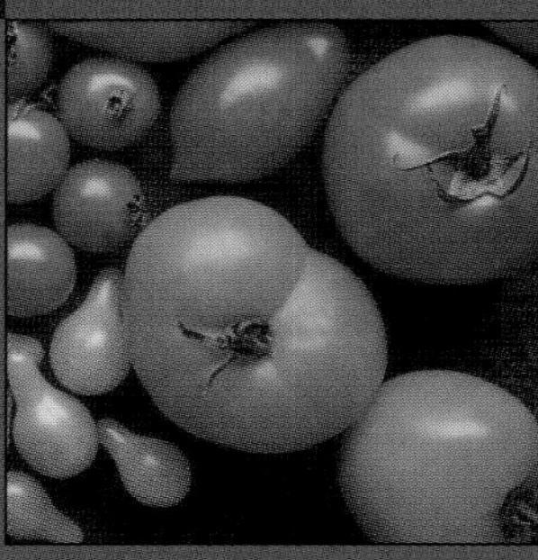

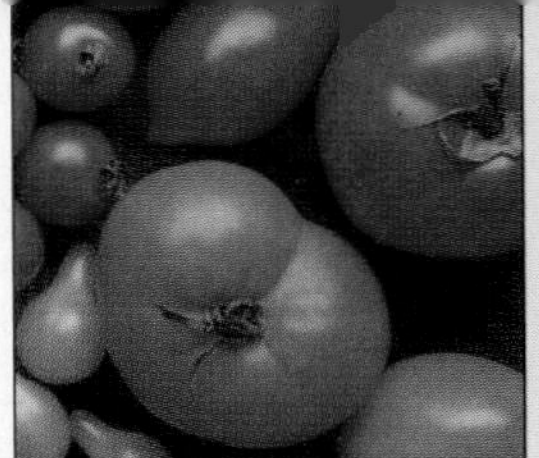

chapter

9 Weight Control

Prevention of obesity has become a major goal of health professionals. There is great concern regarding the increasing number of obese people in America and worldwide. Currently, about 55% of adult Americans and 22% of children weigh too much. This excess weight increases the likelihood of many health problems, such as heart disease, cancer, high blood pressure, certain bone and joint disorders, and Type 2 diabetes.

In the United States, consumers presently pour $40 billion into weight-control products. Most efforts fizzle before bodies become slim. Monotonous, ineffective, and confusing, typical fad diets even endanger some populations, such as children, teenagers, pregnant women, and people with various health disorders.

Yet a more logical approach to weight loss is actually very straightforward: (1) eat less, especially focusing on portion size, (2) perform regular physical activity, and (3) change problematic eating behaviors. This chapter discusses these recommendations to help you understand obesity's effects, causes, and potential treatments. Attention is also given to the treatment of underweight, a comparatively less serious problem in Western society.

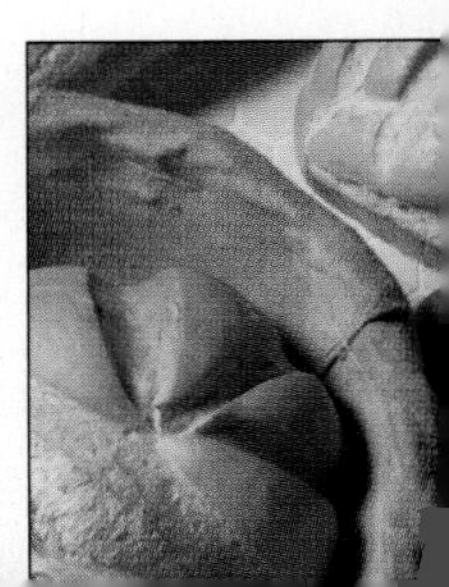

Nutrition Web

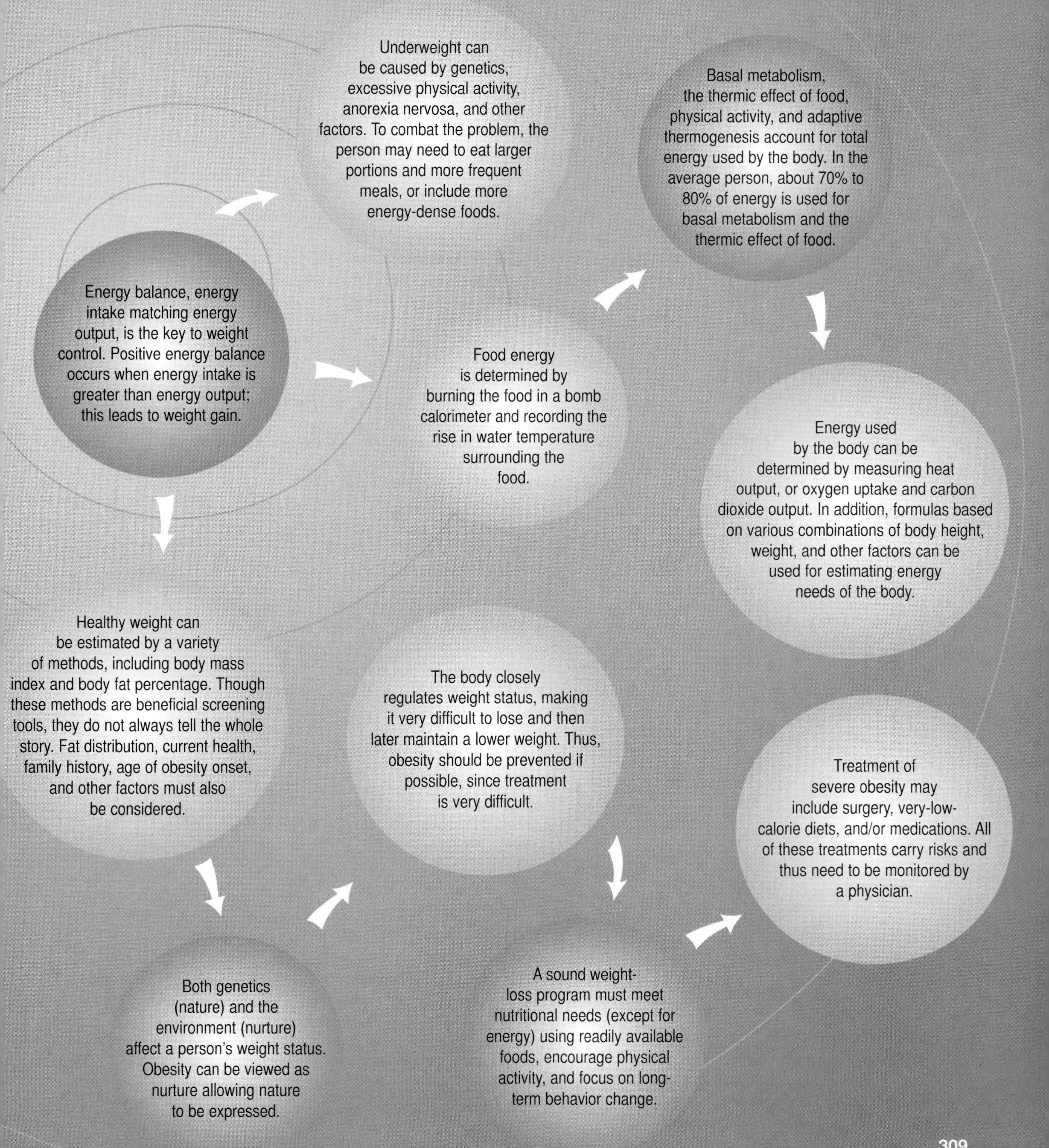

Underweight can be caused by genetics, excessive physical activity, anorexia nervosa, and other factors. To combat the problem, the person may need to eat larger portions and more frequent meals, or include more energy-dense foods.

Basal metabolism, the thermic effect of food, physical activity, and adaptive thermogenesis account for total energy used by the body. In the average person, about 70% to 80% of energy is used for basal metabolism and the thermic effect of food.

Energy balance, energy intake matching energy output, is the key to weight control. Positive energy balance occurs when energy intake is greater than energy output; this leads to weight gain.

Food energy is determined by burning the food in a bomb calorimeter and recording the rise in water temperature surrounding the food.

Energy used by the body can be determined by measuring heat output, or oxygen uptake and carbon dioxide output. In addition, formulas based on various combinations of body height, weight, and other factors can be used for estimating energy needs of the body.

Healthy weight can be estimated by a variety of methods, including body mass index and body fat percentage. Though these methods are beneficial screening tools, they do not always tell the whole story. Fat distribution, current health, family history, age of obesity onset, and other factors must also be considered.

The body closely regulates weight status, making it very difficult to lose and then later maintain a lower weight. Thus, obesity should be prevented if possible, since treatment is very difficult.

Treatment of severe obesity may include surgery, very-low-calorie diets, and/or medications. All of these treatments carry risks and thus need to be monitored by a physician.

Both genetics (nature) and the environment (nurture) affect a person's weight status. Obesity can be viewed as nurture allowing nature to be expressed.

A sound weight-loss program must meet nutritional needs (except for energy) using readily available foods, encourage physical activity, and focus on long-term behavior change.

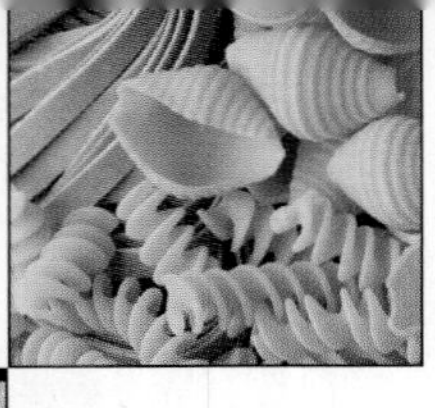

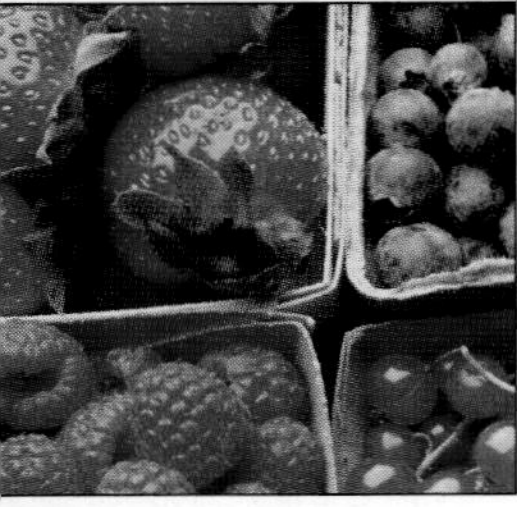

ENERGY BALANCE

Does your weight yo-yo up and down while you aim for your ideal? If the scales keep you emotionally off balance, consider another scale—that of **energy balance.** This balance depends on energy input and energy output, which in turn influence energy stores, primarily the amount of triglyceride in adipose tissue (Figure 9–1). Energy balance can be thought of as an equation: energy consumed minus energy expended. You are in **positive energy balance** when energy consumed is greater than energy expended. The result of positive energy balance is storage of the excess energy in adipose (fat) tissue.

Positive energy balance is necessary during pregnancy because the surplus of energy supports the developing fetus. Infants and children also need to be in positive energy balance to grow. In adults, however, positive energy balance causes creeping weight gain.

Negative energy balance results from an energy deficit. Energy consumed is less than energy expended. Weight loss occurs when a person is in a state of negative energy balance. In adulthood, the weight that is lost consists of a combination of lean and adipose tissue.

As noted in the overview, maintenance of energy balance—energy intake matches energy output—substantially contributes to health and well-being in adults by minimizing the risk for developing many common health problems. Adulthood is often a time of creeping weight gain that can eventually turn into obesity if not checked. However, increasing age is not the primary reason for this weight gain; it is caused primarily by lifestyle, particularly the pattern of excess food intake and too little physical activity. Let's look in detail at the factors that affect the relationship between positive and negative energy balance.

Energy balance
State in which energy intake, in the form of food and/or alcohol, matches the energy expended, primarily through basal metabolism and physical activity.

Positive energy balance
State in which energy intake is greater than energy expended, generally resulting in weight gain.

Negative energy balance
State in which energy intake is less than energy expended, resulting in weight loss.

Energy Intake: The First Half of Energy Balance

Energy needs are met by food intake, represented by the number of calories eaten each day. Early people hunted food to obtain these calories. Today, it is more likely that *food hunts us,* given its wide availability in vending machines, drive-up windows, social gatherings, work setting, and convenient quick-serve restaurants. In recent years, unreasonably large "super-sized" portions in sit-down and quick-service restaurants have especially contributed to this abundance of food energy. Some experts feel these changes have created a "food toxic environment," in that the constant pressure to eat is contributing to weight gain and associated ill health in many of us. More on this later in the chapter.

Determining the Energy Content of Foods

How much food energy is actually contained in a meal? A bomb calorimeter is used to determine the amount of energy in a food (Figure 9–2). The process involves burning a portion of food inside a chamber of the calorimeter that is surrounded by water. As the food burns, it gives off heat, which raises the temperature of the water surrounding the chamber.

The increase in water temperature measured after the food has burned indicates the amount of energy in the food. One kcal is the amount of energy required to increase the temperature of 1 kilogram (about 2.2 pounds) of water by 1° Celsius.

The bomb calorimeter provides values for the amount of energy that can be derived from carbohydrate, fat, protein, and alcohol. Recall that on average carbohydrates yield 4 kcal per gram, proteins 4 kcal per gram, fats 9 kcal per gram, and alcohol 7 kcal per gram.

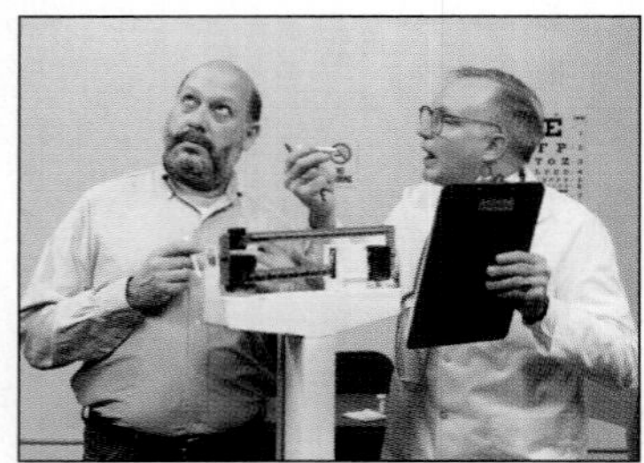

Unfortunately, middle age and weight gain often go together.

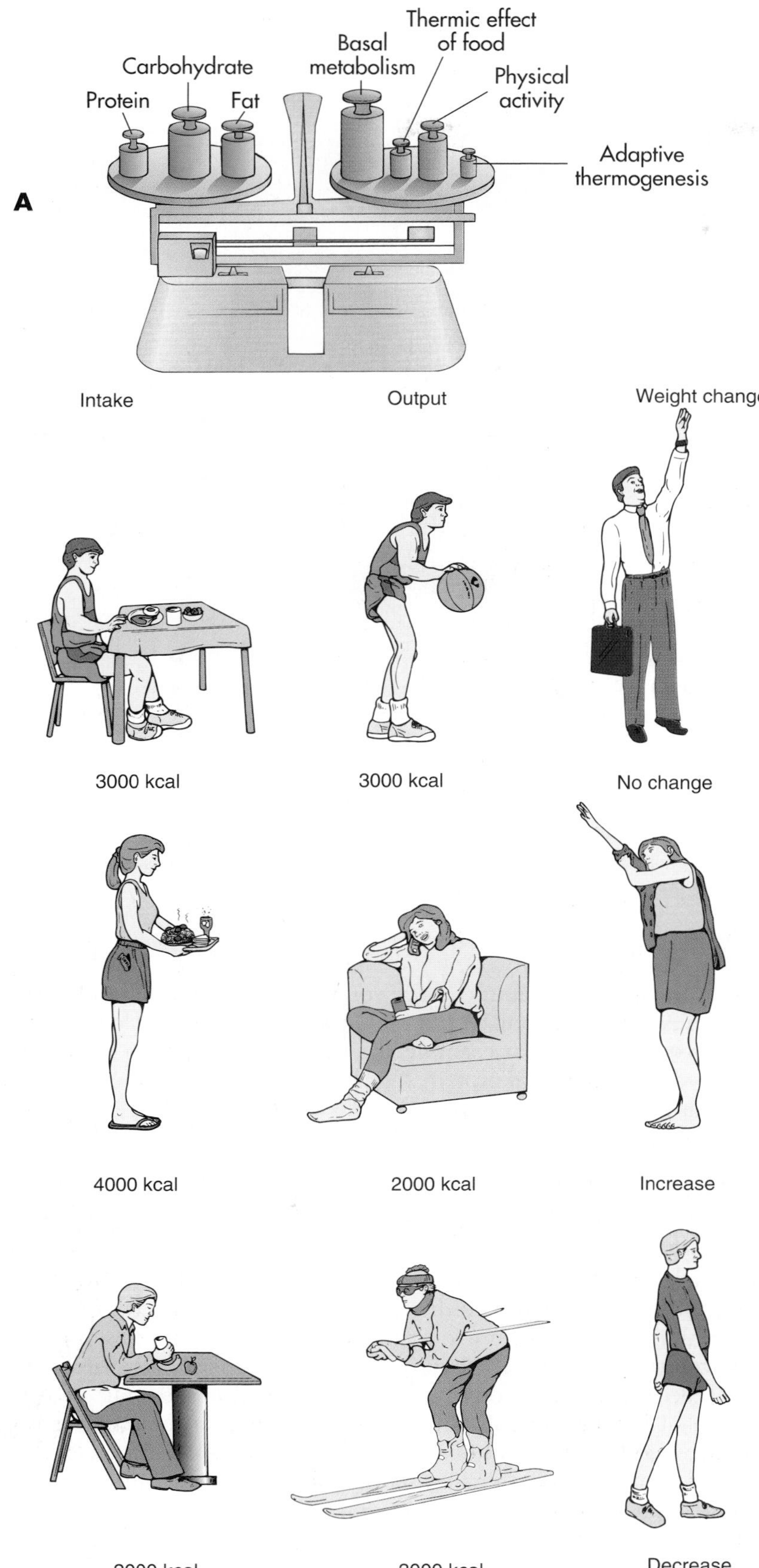

Former Surgeon General Dr. C. Everett Koop is currently spearheading a campaign, called "Shape Up America," to convince overweight people to lose weight and increase physical activity. According to Dr. Koop, obesity is the number two killer in the United States. What many Americans don't understand, he explains, is how serious the problem of excess pounds is: although many Americans are aware that smoking is responsible for more than 400,000 deaths per year, they are not aware that obesity is responsible for nearly as many—300,000—deaths annually in the United States. For more information on the "Shape Up America" campaign see the web site http://www.shapeup.org/sua.

Figure 9-1 *A model for energy balance. The model of a laboratory scale in* **(A)** *incorporates the major variables that influence energy balance. Note that alcohol is an additional source of energy for some of us. The different states of energy balance are shown in* **(B)**.

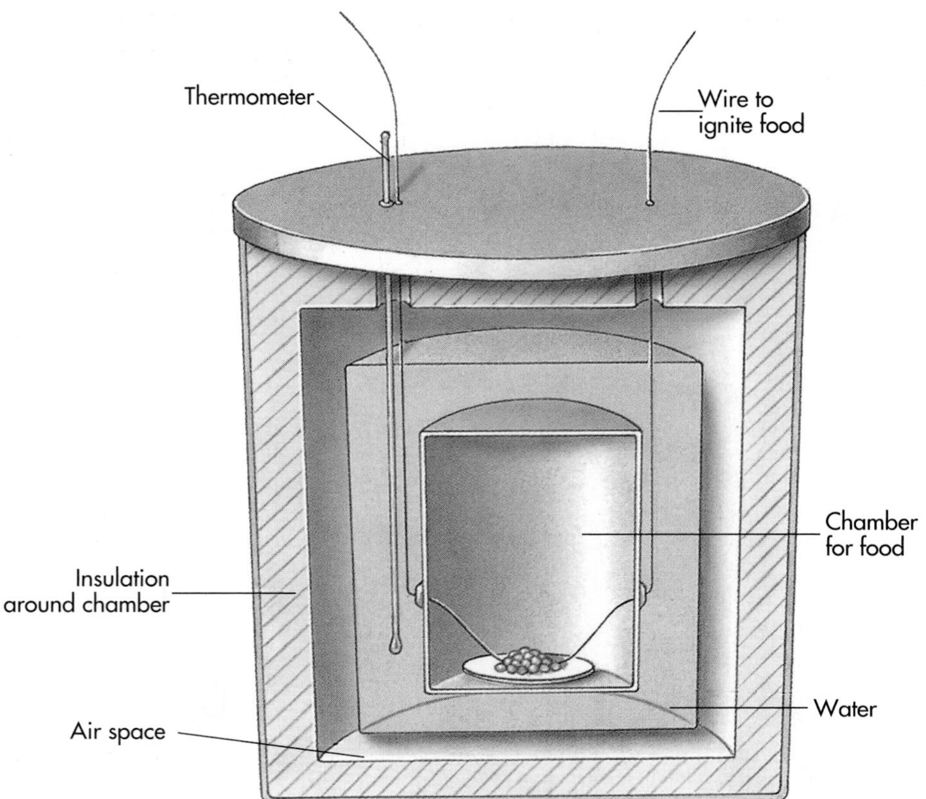

Figure 9-2 *Cross-section of a bomb calorimeter. A dried portion of food is burned inside a chamber charged with oxygen and surrounded by water to determine energy content. As the food is burned, it gives off heat, which raises the temperature of the water surrounding the chamber. The amount of increase in water temperature indicates the number of kcal contained in the food, because 1 kcal equals the amount of heat needed to raise the temperature of 1 kilogram of water 1 degree Celsius.*

As pointed out in Chapter 1, once you know the gram quantities of the energy-yielding substances in a food, you can estimate the total energy content in that food using the energy values. For example, if a banana-flavored rum drink has 20 grams of carbohydrate, 2 grams of protein, 2 grams of fat, and 30 grams of alcohol, it contains about 316 kcal ($[20 \times 4] + [2 \times 4] + [2 \times 9] + [30 \times 7] = 316$).

Bomb Calorimeter Values Tell only Part of the Story

In bomb calorimeter studies, fats produce close to 9 kcal per gram. However, absorbed fats are not immediately utilized to a great extent in the body for energy needs. Instead, much fat goes directly into storage in adipose tissue. We have an essentially unlimited ability to do this.

In contrast, we have a limited ability to store carbohydrate as glycogen. As well, most carbohydrate is used at the time of consumption for energy needs or glycogen synthesis; generally little is converted to fat for storage in the body. This is not to say, however, that infinite amounts of carbohydrate can be consumed: excessive amounts can lead to increased fat synthesis.

With regard to protein, this is used for tissue synthesis, but adults generally eat more than enough protein for this. Beyond body needs and storage capabilities, excess amounts of amino acids are generally metabolized for energy; only some are metabolized to fat.

Based on these observations, experts suggest that ideally fat intake should not exceed the amount of fat burned by the body. Otherwise, fat storage is encouraged, especially when total energy intake exceeds one's needs. Active people can achieve this balance more easily than those who are sedentary can, since physical activity encourages burning of fat and increases energy output. For a person who is sedentary and consumes a large amount of fat, and calories, it is thought that any obesity that results actually represents an adaptation to this high-fat diet. This is because it is thought that only by reaching a certain point of obesity will this sedentary person be able to balance the amount of fat eaten with the amount of fat burned. The greater fat mass present now allows for more release of body fat into circulation, so more fat is available for use. In other words, one needs enough fat mass to be able to burn the equivalent of the great amount of fat consumed. This concept also underscores the importance of maintaining physical activity to encourage the body to burn the fat consumed.

As noted in Chapter 5, it is also easier to overeat high-fat foods because they are energy dense and highly palatable. We can more easily eat a few extra cookies than a few extra apples, even though both may contain about the same amount of food energy. All these findings suggest that to reduce or control body fatness, focus on controlling fat intake, substituting instead moderate amounts of foods naturally rich in starch and dietary fiber.

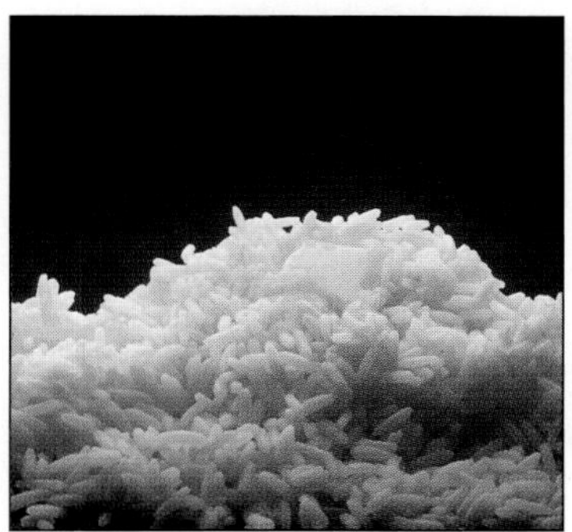

When controlling energy intake, it is important to watch the amount of added fats.

While a person is resting, the percentage of total energy use by various organs is about as follows:

Liver	27%
Muscle	18%
Brain	19%
Heart	7%
Kidney	10%
Other	19%

Energy Use: the Other Side of Energy Balance

So far, some factors related to energy intake have been discussed. Now let's look at the other side of the relationship—energy output.

The body uses energy for three general purposes: basal metabolism, physical activity, and the thermic effect of food. Shivering, the body's reflex to cold, demonstrates another minor form of energy turned into heat production, often called *adaptive thermogenesis* (see Figure 9–1).

Basal Metabolism

Basal metabolism represents the minimal energy expended to keep a resting, awake body alive. This requires about 60% to 70% of total energy use by the body. The processes involved include maintaining a heartbeat, respiration, temperature, and other functions. It does not include energy used for physical activity or digesting foods. Basal metabolism varies about +/− 25% to 30% between individuals.

Basal metabolism
The minimal energy the body requires to support itself, when resting and awake. It amounts to roughly 1 kcal per minute, or about 1400 kcal per day.

Lean body mass
Body weight minus fat storage weight equals lean body mass. This includes organs such as the brain, muscles, and liver, as well as blood and other body fluids.

The amount of energy used for basal metabolism depends primarily on **lean body mass.** That is, basal metabolism is generally higher in people with greater amounts of lean body mass than in those with large proportions of fat mass. The participating tissues—such as muscle, liver, brain, and kidney—show high metabolic activity at rest and have high energy needs. Other influences that determine basal metabolism include the following:

- The amount of body surface (the greater the area, the greater the heat loss)
- Gender (males average higher energy use, because of greater lean body mass)
- Body temperature (fever increases metabolic rate)
- Thyroid hormone (higher amounts increase metabolic rate)
- Aspects of nervous system activity (affects hunger)
- Age (metabolic rate falls as we age through adulthood)
- Nutritional state (eating less slows metabolic rate in the short term)
- Pregnancy (increases metabolic rate)
- Caffeine and tobacco use (increase metabolic rate)

A low energy intake decreases the basal metabolism by about 10% to 20%, or about 150 to 300 kcal per day. This decrease contributes to making losing weight

Smoking cessation increases the risk of adult weight gain and obesity. Smoking cessation is still advised, but a plan to limit weight gain should also be designed. Implementation of some form of regular physical activity can be extremely beneficial in the attempt to keep weight in check. Various health problems associated with smoking, however, make it essential that this population obtain approval from a physician before beginning an intensive exercise regimen.

difficult. In addition, the effects of aging make weight maintenance hard. Basal metabolism declines about 2% each decade past age 30 as actively metabolizing cells slowly and steadily decrease. However, because physical activity helps maintain lean body mass, remaining active as one ages lessens this progression, and in turn helps maintain a high basal metabolism and aids in weight control.

Energy for Physical Activity

Physical activity increases energy expenditure above basal energy needs by as much as 25% to 40%. Unlike basal metabolism, energy expenditure from physical activity varies widely among people.

Climbing stairs rather than riding the elevator, walking rather than driving to the store, and standing in a bus rather than sitting increase physical activity and, hence, energy use. People who fidget use more energy than do those who readily relax.

The alarming rate of obesity in America is caused in part by our general inactivity. We eat little more than people did at the turn of this century, but we are less active. Jobs demand less physical activity, and leisure time is usually spent slouched before a television or computer. What are the alternatives to obesity and inactivity? One answer is *movement!*

Thermic effect of food (TEF)
The increase in metabolism occurring during the digestion, absorption, and metabolism of energy-yielding nutrients; also called diet-induced thermogenesis. This represents 5% to 10% of energy consumed.

Brown adipose tissue
A specialized form of adipose tissue that produces large amounts of heat by metabolizing energy-yielding nutrients without synthesizing much usable energy. The energy is released as heat.

Thermic Effect of Food

In addition to basal metabolism and physical activity, the body uses energy to digest, absorb, and further process food nutrients. Energy used for these tasks contributes to the **thermic effect of food (TEF).** The energy cost of this thermic effect is analogous to a sales tax. It is like being taxed about 5% to 10% for the total energy you eat. To supply the body with 100 kcal for basal metabolism and physical activity needs you must eat more than this, between 105 and 110 kcal. Given a daily energy intake of 3000 kcal, the thermic effect of food would use 180 to 300 kcal. However, the total amount can vary somewhat among individuals.

Adaptive Thermogenesis

The body expends some energy to produce heat in response to a cold environment and as a result of overfeeding. This process is known as *adaptive thermogenesis.* This subject has produced much controversy and interest. In some cases, people who were overfed did not gain the amount of weight that might be expected. Adaptive thermogenesis probably represents a small portion of energy use; about 7% of the total.

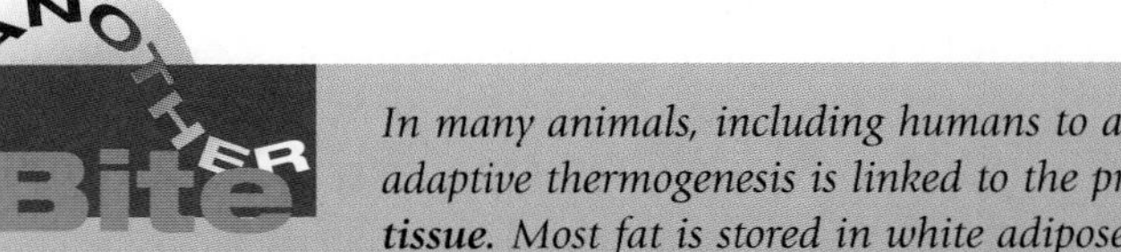

*In many animals, including humans to an undetermined extent, adaptive thermogenesis is linked to the presence of **brown adipose tissue.** Most fat is stored in white adipose tissue. Brown adipose tissue is so named because of its appearance. This tissue yields heat by failing to form much energy (ATP to be specific; see Chapter 10) during the metabolism of energy-yielding nutrients. Most brown adipose cell energy is lost in the form of heat; little is used to perform useful work beyond simply warming the body. Therefore these cells "waste" a lot of potentially useful energy. If you touch an infant's back, you can feel the heat produced by brown adipose tissue. The extent to which brown adipose tissue is both present and operative in adults has not been clearly determined. A lack of increase in brown adipose tissue activity during overfeeding and cold adaptation is associated with obesity in rats. Some evidence suggests that impaired adaptive thermogenesis resulting from abnormalities in the functioning of brown adipose tissue may also contribute to human obesity.*

Overall, a sedentary person uses about 70% to 80% of energy for a combination of basal metabolism and the thermic effect of food. The remainder is used for physical activity and adaptive thermogenesis.

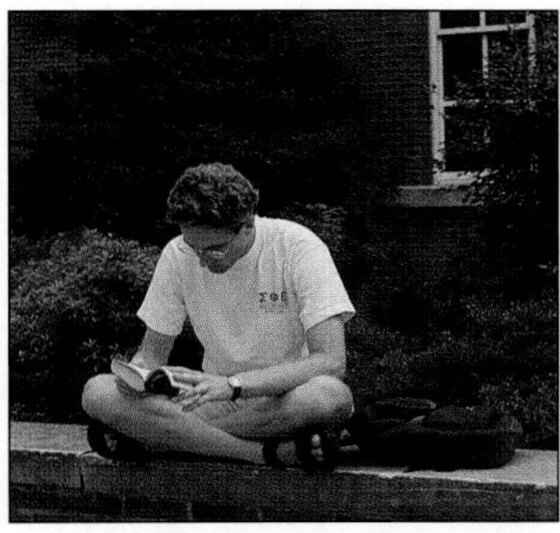

Studying leads to mental stress but puts little physical stress on the body. Hence, energy needs are only about 1.5 kcal per minute.

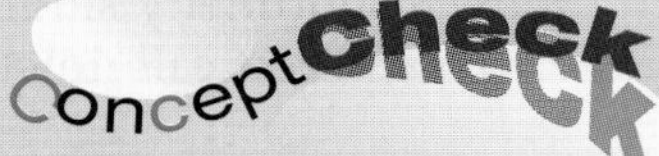

Energy balance compares energy intake with energy output. Energy content of food is expressed in kcal and determined using a bomb calorimeter. This analysis yields the 4-9-4-7 relationship for carbohydrate, fat, protein, and alcohol.

The body uses this energy for four main purposes.

- Basal metabolism represents the minimal amount of energy needed to maintain a body in a resting state. The rate of a person's basal metabolism depends greatly on the amount of lean body mass, the amount of body surface, and other factors.
- Physical activity expenditure represents energy use for total body cell metabolism above what is needed during rest (that is, basal metabolism).
- The thermic effect of food represents the energy needed to digest, absorb, and process absorbed nutrients. This corresponds to about 5% to 10% of energy used for basal metabolism and physical activity.
- Adaptive thermogenesis is heat production in response to cold or overfeeding. A relative lack of brown adipose tissue activity in these circumstances may be associated with human obesity.

In a sedentary person, about 70% to 80% of energy is used for basal metabolism and the thermic effect of food; the remainder is used for physical activity and adaptive thermogenesis.

Determining Energy Use by the Body

The amount of energy a body uses can be measured by both direct and indirect calorimetry, or simply estimated based on weight, degree of physical activity, and age.

Direct and Indirect Calorimetry

Direct calorimetry measures the body heat released by a person. The subject is put into an insulated chamber, often the size of a small bedroom, and body heat released raises the temperature of a layer of water surrounding the chamber. A kcal, as you recall, is related to the amount of heat available to raise the temperature of the water. By measuring the water temperature in the direct calorimeter before and after the body releases heat, scientists can determine the energy expended. This method resembles the bomb calorimeter method for measuring the energy content in food.

Direct calorimetry *A method of determining a body's energy use by measuring heat that emanates from the body, usually using an insulated chamber.*

Indirect calorimetry *A method to measure the energy use by the body by measuring oxygen uptake. Formulas are then used to convert this gas exchange value into energy use.*

Direct calorimetry works because almost all the energy used by the body eventually leaves as heat. However, few studies use direct calorimetry, mostly because of its expense and complexity.

For **indirect calorimetry,** instead of measuring heat output, a technician measures the amount of oxygen a person uses and how much carbon dioxide is produced (Figure 9–3). A predictable relationship exists between the body's use of

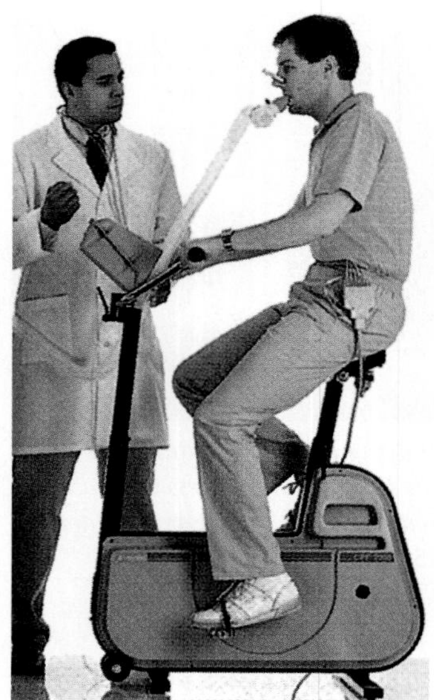

Figure 9-3
Indirect calorimetry. The method of measuring oxygen use and carbon dioxide output can determine energy output during daily activities.

energy and oxygen use. For example, when metabolizing a mixed diet of carbohydrate, fat, and protein—a typical blend of nutrients we use—the human body needs 1 liter of oxygen to burn about 4.85 kcal.

Instruments used to measure oxygen consumption for indirect calorimetry have great versatility. They can be mounted on carts and rolled up to a hospital bed or carried in backpacks while a person plays tennis or jogs. Tables showing energy demands of exercises rely on information gained from indirect calorimetry studies. There are also other methods of determining energy use with indirect calorimetry, but these will not be covered.

Estimating Energy Needs

A rough estimate for energy needs uses a person's weight and degree of physical activity. Total energy needs for a sedentary person are set at 30 kcal per kilogram. The value may then decrease by 100 kcal for every 10 years of age over age 30. People performing moderate activity, such as routine walking, start with 35 kcal per kilogram; those regularly performing heavy activity, as required in some sports play, start at 40 kcal per kilogram. These values can then be adjusted for age, as mentioned previously. For example, a 68-kilogram (150 pound), 40-year-old woman performing moderate activity needs to eat about 2300 kcal ([68 kilogram × 35 kcal/kilogram] − 100) to meet total energy needs.

Rough guidelines for energy needs found in the Food Guide Pyramid publication are as follows:

- Sedentary women and some older adults — 1600 kcal
- Children, teenage girls, active women, most men — 2200 kcal
- Teenage boys, active men, very active women — 2800 kcal
- Young children, pregnant and breast-feeding women — Check with a registered dietitian

These values then need to be fine-tuned based on personal characteristics and experiences, such as amount of physical activity performed.

A simple method of tracking your energy expenditure, and thus your energy needs, is to use the forms in Appendix E. Table 9-6, found later in the chapter, lists the energy costs of various activities. The values account for energy use for basal metabolism, the thermic effect of food, and physical activity.

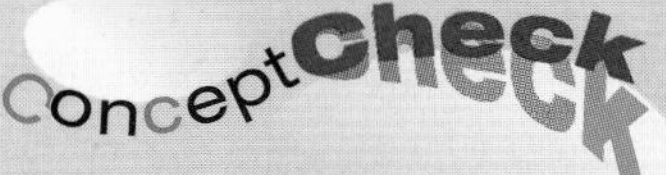

Energy use by the body can be measured by direct calorimetry as heat given off and by indirect calorimetry as oxygen used. Total energy needs can be estimated based on a person's characteristics: weight, age, and amount of physical activity practiced. In addition, the Food Guide Pyramid publication provides rough guidelines for energy intake.

Estimating a Healthy Weight

Numerous methods have been used to set what body weight should be, often called *healthy body weight.* Several types of tables exist, based on weight and one or more factors, including height and body frame size. These tables arise from studies of large population groups. When applied to a population, they provide good estimates of weight associated with health and longevity. These tables, however, do not necessarily refer directly to an individual's weight and health status.

Ideally, family history of obesity-related disease and current health parameters should be considered when establishing a healthy weight for an individual, in addition to weight-for-height. Evidence of the following obesity-related conditions is important:

- High blood pressure
- Elevated LDL
- Family history of obesity, heart disease, or cancer
- Pattern of fat distribution in the body
- Elevated blood glucose

On a more practical note, other questions can be pertinent: What is the least one weighed as an adult, for at least a year? What is the largest size clothing one would be happy with? What weight has one been able to maintain during previous periods of dieting without feeling constantly hungry?

Thus height/weight tables don't tell the whole story. Overall, the individual, under a physician's guidance, should establish a "personal" healthy weight (or need for weight reduction). This assessment can point out how well the person is tolerating from a health standpoint any existing excess weight. Thus current height/weight standards are only a rough guide. Furthermore, a healthy lifestyle may make a more important contribution to a person's health status than the number on the scale. This topic is discussed at greater length later in the chapter with regard to appropriateness of weight loss. In sum, height/weight tables provide a guide for healthy weight, but some fine-tuning is often necessary.

Using Body Mass Index (BMI) to Set Healthy Weight

For the last 50 years weight-for-height tables issued by the Metropolitan Life Insurance Company have been the typical way healthy weight was established. These tables considered gender and frame size, predicting the weight range at a specific height that was associated with the greatest longevity. The latest table (issued in 1983) and methods for determining frame size are in Appendix H.

Currently in the medical and nutrition literature there is less use of the Metropolitan Life Insurance tables and greater use of **body mass index (BMI)** as a weight-for-height standard. In fact, an October 1998 review of obesity assessment and management in a leading nutrition publication (reading no. 8) only referred to body mass index; there was no mention of the Metropolitan Life Insurance Company tables. Still, you may see either in current medical practice. This chapter will focus on body mass index. Research has shown it is the weight-for-height standard that is most closely related to body fat content.

Body mass index *Weight (in kilograms) divided by height squared (in meters). A value of 25 or greater indicates a higher risk for obesity-related health disorders.*

Body mass index is calculated as:

$$\frac{\text{body weight (in kilograms)}}{\text{height}^2 \text{ (in meters)}}$$

An alternate method for calculating BMI is:

$$\frac{\text{weight (pounds)} \times 703.1}{\text{height}^2 \text{ (inches)}}$$

Table 9–1 lists BMI for various heights and weights. Health risks from excess weight begin when the body mass index exceeds 25. A healthy weight-for-height is a BMI 19 to 25. What is your BMI? How much would your weight need to change to yield a BMI of 25? 30? These are general cut-off values for the presence of overweight and obesity, respectively (see later section).

The concept of body mass index is convenient to use because the values apply to both men and women. However, any body weight-for-height standard is actually a crude measure because we are concerned about overfat, not simply overweight, individuals when setting guidelines for healthy weight. The husky athlete is a notable exception; he or she may be overweight but not overfat. For this reason, any weight-for-height measurement should be used only as a screening tool for obesity. Still, overfat and overweight conditions almost always appear together. The focus is on body weight-for-height standards in clinical settings mainly because these are easier to measure than total body fat.

Putting Healthy Weight into Perspective

One current school of thought is to let nature takes its course with regard to body weight. According to this proposal, by trying to lose weight in order to fall within a specific (often unrealistic) height/weight range, people often regain their original weight plus more. In contrast, listening to the body for hunger cues, eating a healthy diet, and remaining physically active eventually helps one maintain an appropriate height/weight value. This concept will be further addressed in the upcoming discussion on treatment for obesity. The clearest idea regarding a healthy weight is that it is personal. Weight has to be considered in terms of health, not simply fashion.

TABLE 9-1

Body Weights in Pounds According to Height and Body Mass Index (BMI)

	BMI (kilograms per square meter)													
	19	20	21	22	23	24	25	26	27	28	29	30	35	40
Height (inches)	Body weight (pounds)													
58	91	96	100	105	110	115	119	124	129	134	138	143	167	191
59	94	99	104	109	114	119	124	128	133	138	143	148	173	198
60	97	102	107	112	118	123	128	133	138	143	148	153	179	204
61	100	106	111	116	122	127	132	137	143	148	153	158	185	211
62	104	109	115	120	126	131	136	142	147	153	158	164	191	218
63	107	113	118	124	130	135	141	146	152	158	163	169	197	225
64	110	116	122	128	134	140	145	151	157	163	169	174	204	232
65	114	120	126	132	138	144	150	156	162	168	174	180	210	240
66	118	124	130	136	142	148	155	161	167	173	179	186	216	247
67	121	127	134	140	146	153	159	166	172	178	185	191	223	255
68	125	131	138	144	151	158	164	171	177	184	190	197	230	262
69	128	135	142	149	155	162	169	176	182	189	196	203	236	270
70	132	139	146	153	160	167	174	181	188	195	202	207	243	278
71	136	143	150	157	165	172	179	186	193	200	208	215	230	286
72	140	147	154	162	169	177	184	191	199	206	213	221	258	294
73	144	151	159	166	174	182	189	197	204	212	219	227	265	302
74	148	155	163	171	179	186	194	202	210	218	225	233	272	311
75	152	160	168	176	184	192	200	208	216	224	232	240	279	319
76	156	164	172	180	189	197	205	213	221	230	238	246	287	328

Each entry gives the body weight in pounds for a person of a given height and BMI. Pounds have been rounded off. To use the table, find the appropriate height in the far left column. Move across the row to a given weight. The number at the top of the column is the BMI for the height and weight. A healthy value is between 19 and 25. Above and below these values health problems generally increase in number and severity.

From Bray GA, Gray DS: *Western Journal of Medicine* 148:429, 1988.

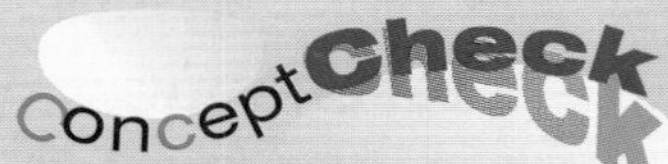

Healthy body weight is generally determined in a clinical setting using a body mass index (or some other weight-for-height standard). The presence of existing weight-related disease and other factors should be considered in determining healthy body weight. Total health and a healthy lifestyle, not simply fashion, should be the major considerations when determining healthy weight.

For more information on weight control, obesity, and nutrition, visit the Weight-control Information Network (WIN) at http://www.niddk.nih.gov/NutritionDocs.html or call 800-WIN-8098. Other web sites include http://www.caloriecontrol.org and http://www.weight.com.

Energy Imbalance

If energy intake exceeds expenditure over time, obesity is likely to result. Often, health problems eventually follow (Table 9–2).

TABLE 9-2

Health Problems Associated with Excess Body Fat

Health problem	Partially attributable to
Surgical risk	Increased anesthesia needs and greater risk of wound infections
Pulmonary disease and sleep disorders	Excess weight over lungs and pharynx
Type 2 diabetes	Enlarged fat cells, which poorly bind insulin and also poorly respond to the message insulin sends to the cell
High blood pressure and stroke	Increased miles of blood vessels found in adipose tissue; increased blood volume; increased resistance to blood flow
Heart disease	Increases in LDL and triglyceride values, low HDL, decreased physical activity
Bone and joint disorders	Excess pressure put on knee, ankle, and hip joints
Gallstones	Increased cholesterol content of bile
Skin disorders	Trapping of moisture and microbes in tissue folds
Various cancers	Estrogen production by adipose cells; animal studies suggest excess energy intake encourages tumor development
Shorter stature (in some forms of obesity)	Earlier onset of puberty
Pregnancy risks	More difficult delivery, increased number of birth defects, and increased needs for anesthesia (if needed)
Reduced physical agility and increased risk of accidents and falls	Excess weight impairs movement
Premature death	A variety of risk factors for disease, listed above

The greater the degree of obesity, the more likely and the more serious these health problems generally become. They are much more likely to appear in people who show an upper-body fat distribution pattern and/or greater than twice healthy body weight (see later chapter discussions).

Underwater weighing
A method of estimating total body fat by weighing the individual on a standard scale and then weighing him or her again submerged in water. The difference between the two weights is used to estimate total body fat.

Bioelectrical impedance
A method to estimate total body fat that uses a low-energy electrical current. The more fat storage a person has, the more impedance (resistance) to electrical flow will be exhibited.

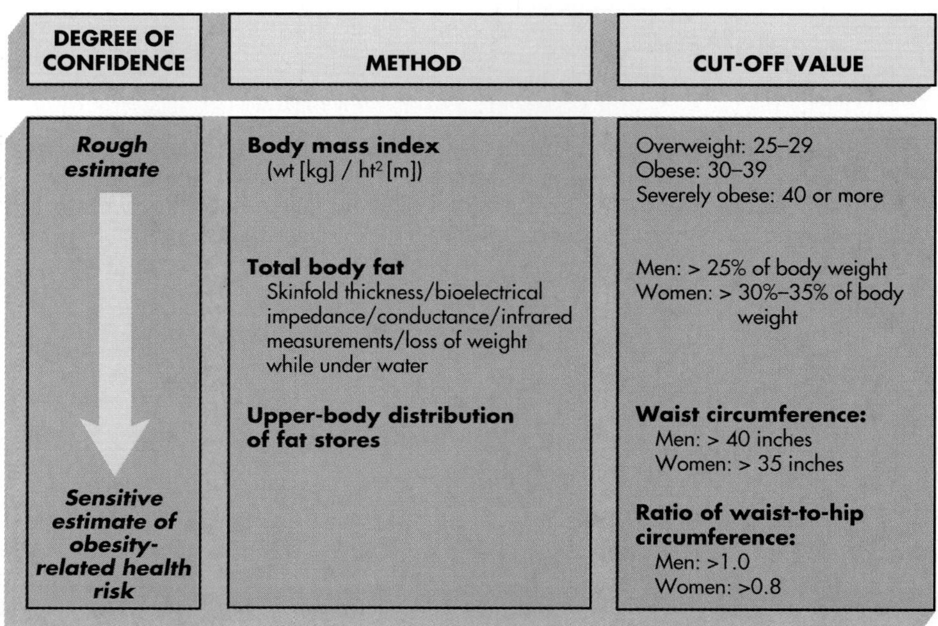

DEGREE OF CONFIDENCE	METHOD	CUT-OFF VALUE
Rough estimate	**Body mass index** (wt [kg] / ht² [m])	Overweight: 25–29 Obese: 30–39 Severely obese: 40 or more
↓	**Total body fat** Skinfold thickness/bioelectrical impedance/conductance/infrared measurements/loss of weight while under water	Men: > 25% of body weight Women: > 30%–35% of body weight
Sensitive estimate of obesity-related health risk	**Upper-body distribution of fat stores**	**Waist circumference:** Men: > 40 inches Women: > 35 inches **Ratio of waist-to-hip circumference:** Men: >1.0 Women: >0.8

Figure 9-4 *Diagnosing the extent of obesity to predict health risk. If a person is obese by any of these measures and has upper-body distribution of fat stores, the risk of complications is greater than if the fat distribution were more in lower body (see late section for detail).*

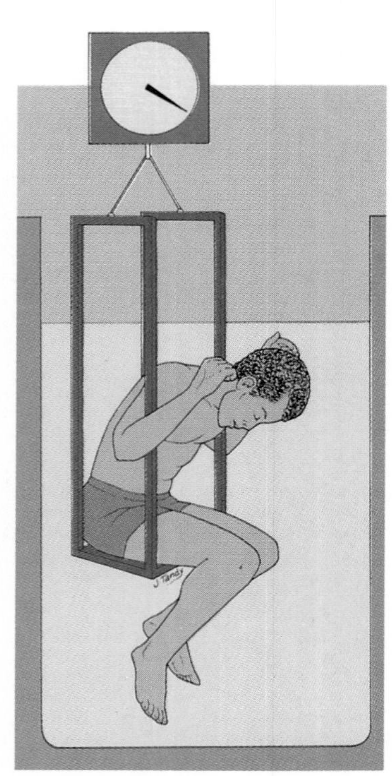

Figure 9-5
Underwater weighing. To get an accurate estimate of body fat, the subject exhales as much air as possible and then holds his breath and bends over at the waist. Once he is totally submerged, the underwater weight is recorded. This weight is then compared to that when not in the water.

Obesity Signifies an Overfat State

Body fat can range from 2% to 70% of body weight. In this regard, men with over 25% body fat and women with over 30% to 35% body fat are considered obese. Desirable amounts are 12% to 20% body fat for men and 20% to 30% fat for women (Figure 9–4). Women need more body fat because some "sex-specific" fat is associated with reproductive functions. This fat is normal and factored into calculations.

Various methods are used to estimate body fat content. **Underwater weighing** (most accurate) works because fat tissue is less dense than lean tissue; because fat floats, the more fat tissue present, the less a person weighs when submerged (Figure 9–5).

Skinfold thickness is the method most widely used to estimate total body fat. Clinicians use special calipers to measure the fat layer directly under the skin at multiple sites (Figure 9–6). After much practice, this method can provide a reasonable estimate of body fat content.

Clinicians have recently begun measuring total body fat using **bioelectrical impedance.** This technique sends a painless, low-energy electrical current to and from the body via wires and electrode patches. Researchers surmise that fat resists electrical flow, so more fat proportionately means greater electrical resistance. Within a few minutes, bioelectrical impedance analyzers convert body electrical resistance into a reasonable estimate of total body fat.

Another new method for estimating total body fat exposes the biceps to infrared light, assessing the interactions with the fat and protein in arm muscle. After only 2 seconds, this flashlight-size device can give an estimate.

Using Body Mass Index to Establish Obesity

When BMI exceeds 25, weight-related health risks often begin, and the person is said to be overweight. A BMI above 30 poses even greater health risks and is

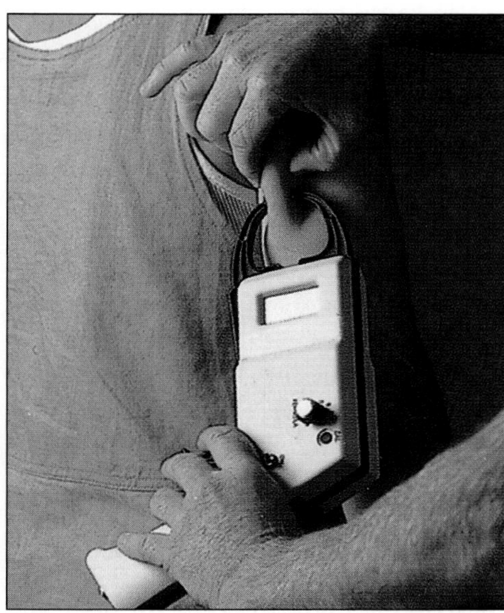

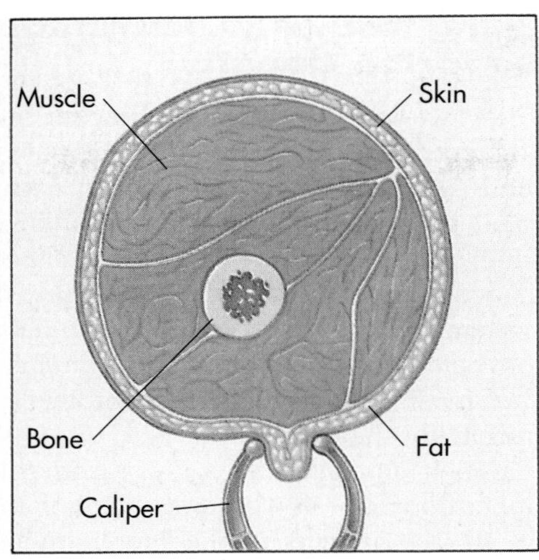

Figure 9-6 *Skinfold measurements. Use of proper technique, calibrated equipment, and some practice skinfold measurements can predict body fat content.*

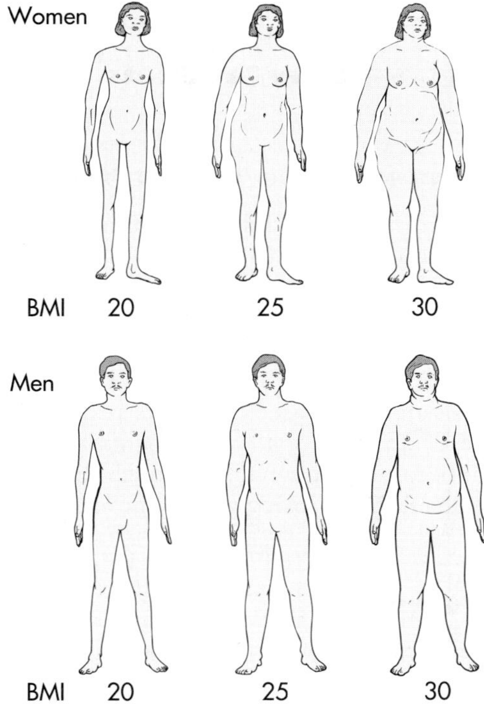

For your reference, estimates of body shapes at different BMI values.

defined as obesity. A value this high suggests that a treatment program should be considered, especially if obesity-related health problems are present. A BMI above 40 represents severe obesity.

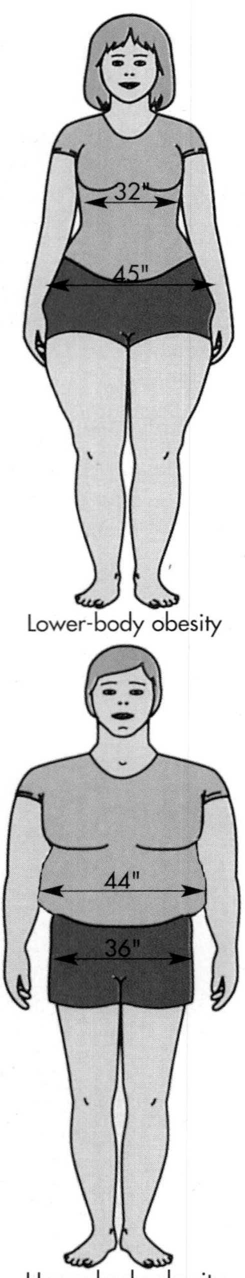

Figure 9–7 *Body fat distribution, showing upper-body and lower-body obesity. The upper-body form brings higher risks for ill health associated with obesity. The woman has a waist circumference of 32 inches and an approximate waist-to-hip ratio of 32 inches by 45 inches, or 0.7. The man has a waist circumference of 44 inches and an approximate waist-to-hip ratio of 44 inches by 36 inches, or 1.2. Thus the man has upper-body obesity based on both measures, but the woman does not.*

Using Body Fat Distribution to Further Describe Obesity

Where we store fat, as well as how much, greatly affects weight-related health risks. Some people store fat in upper-body areas. Others hold fat low. Excess fat in either place generally spells trouble, but each storage space also has its unique risks. Fat deposited in the lower body often resists being shed. However, **upper-body (android) obesity** is related to more heart disease, high blood pressure, and Type 2 diabetes. Whereas other fat cells empty fat directly into general circulation, the fat contents of abdominal fat cells go straight to the liver, by way of the portal vein, before being circulated to the muscles. This process interferes with the liver's ability to clear insulin and also alters lipoprotein metabolism by the liver. Both changes spell trouble for the body.

High blood testosterone (a primarily male hormone) apparently encourages upper-body obesity, as does alcohol intake. This characteristic male pattern of fat storage appears in the "apple-on-a-stick" shape (large abdomen [pot belly] and small buttocks and thighs). A waist circumference (at the umbilicus) more than 40 inches in men and more than 35 inches in women often indicates such a shape. A ratio of waist circumference to hip circumference more than 1.0 in men and 0.8 in women also can indicate upper-body fat storage (Figure 9–7).

Estrogen and progesterone (primarily female hormones) encourage lower-body fat storage and **lower-body (gynecoid or gynoid) obesity**—the typical female pattern. The familiar small abdomen and much larger buttocks and thighs give a pearlike appearance. After menopause, blood estrogen falls, encouraging upper-body fat distribution.

Overall, researchers suggest that women with lower-body fat distribution must be about 20 pounds more obese than men with a "pot belly" shape before they show the same health risks from an overfat state.

Using Age of Onset in the Evaluation of Obesity

When obesity develops in infancy or childhood, numerous adipose cells develop, each with the ability to grow larger. (This is discussed further in Chapter 13, particularly in reference to weight control in childhood.) In adult obesity, fewer adipose cells are usually present, but these contain an excess amount of fat. Still, as obesity progresses in adulthood, adipose cells can increase in number again.

Obesity that develops in childhood is a special concern because the greater number of adipose cells may increase the body's resistance to cutting down fat stores. Adipose cells have a long life span and apparently need to store some fat, so reducing total body fat becomes a tough task. Though the reasons are still puzzling, long-term obesity appears to make losing weight more difficult.

Obesity in Perspective

Obesity may be measured in many ways, but statistics aside, each person has unique characteristics. Treatment needs to account for current energy expenditure, weight-range in adulthood, evidence of Type 2 diabetes, family history of obesity, number of years the person has been obese, and the extent of erroneous nutrition practices. Each person faces possible complications requiring individual treatment plans.

On a positive note, however, only about a 10% weight loss is often needed for many people to experience improvement in health and self esteem. Researchers are calling this a "healthier" weight. Although a person might not achieve a BMI below 25, he or she might still be healthier after a small, lasting degree of weight loss.

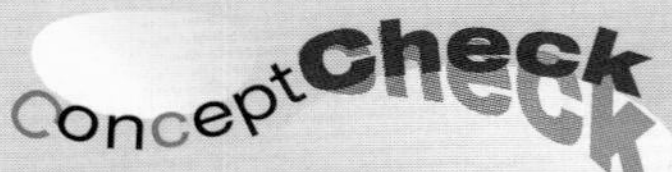

Obesity refers to a state of excessive fat storage. The risk of health problems related to obesity increases under the following conditions:

- A man's percent of body fat exceeds 25%; a woman's exceeds 30% to 35%.
- Body mass index (BMI) is over 25 (calculated as weight in kilograms divided by height squared in meters).

However, if a healthy lifestyle is being followed and no current health problems exist, these guidelines need to be reevaluated.

Body fat storage can be estimated clinically using skinfold thickness or bioelectrical impedance. Fat storage distribution further specifies an obese state as either upper body or lower body. Obesity leads to an increased risk for heart disease, some types of cancer, high blood pressure, Type 2 diabetes, certain bone and joint disorders, and some digestive disorders. The risks for some of these diseases are greater with upper-body fat storage.

Upper-body obesity
The type of obesity, also called android, in which fat is stored primarily in the abdominal area; defined as a waist circumference of greater than 40 inches in men or 35 inches in women, and as well as a waist-to-hip circumference ratio of greater than 1.0 in men and 0.8 in women.

Lower-body obesity
The type of obesity, also called gynoid, in which fat storage is primarily located in the buttocks and thigh area.

Identical twins
Two offspring that develop from a single ovum and sperm and consequently have the same genetic makeup.

Why Some People Are Obese—Nature Versus Nurture

Both genetic traits and psychological factors can increase the risk for obesity. These diverse influences spark controversies concerning which factor yields the greater influence.

How Might Nature Contribute to Obesity?

Identical twins raised apart tend to show similar weight gain patterns, whether lean or obese (Figure 9–8). It appears that nurture—what we learn about eating habits and nutrition, which varies with twins who are raised apart—has less to do with obesity than genes. Twins even tend to accumulate fat in the same body sites. Our genes help determine rates of metabolism and differences in brain chemistry. Both affect weight.

We also inherit specific body types, such as pencil-thin or muscular. The specific body types—known as **endomorphs, mesomorphs,** and **ectomorphs**—greatly determine human size and shape. Endomorphs, with their stocky builds, have short, stubby bones, short trunks, round heads, wide chest and hips, and very short fingers. Ectomorphs, like Abraham Lincoln, are tall and slender with long, thin bones and narrow chests, hips, heads, and fingers. Mesomorphs exhibit a medium, muscular build.

Ectomorphs appear to have an inherently easier time maintaining healthy body weight. Basal metabolism increases as body surface increases. Therefore, taller people use more energy than do shorter ones, even when resting. Some rats and mice inherit a **thrifty metabolism,** one that uses energy frugally. This enables them to store fat more readily than the typical animal. Some people probably inherit a thrifty metabolism as well.

A thrifty human metabolism would require less energy to get through the day. In earlier times, when food supplies were scarce, a thrifty metabolism helped protect against starvation. With today's general abundance of food, operating in this low gear requires a high energy output and wise food choices to prevent obesity.

Genetic influence can be seen by observing a child's parents. A child with no obese parent has only a 10% chance of becoming obese. A child with one obese

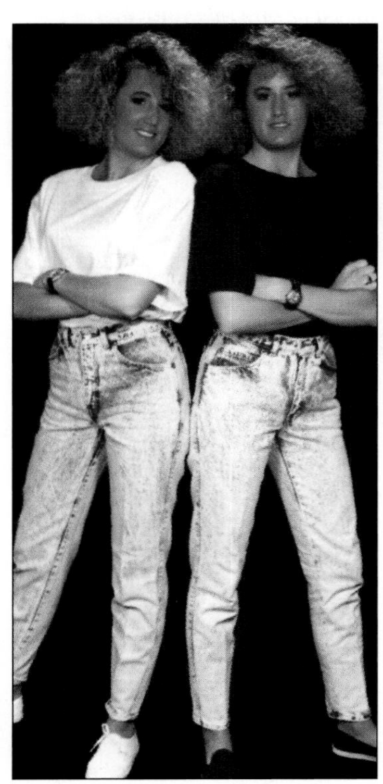

Figure 9–8
Nature or nurture, what causes these twins to have similar body weights?

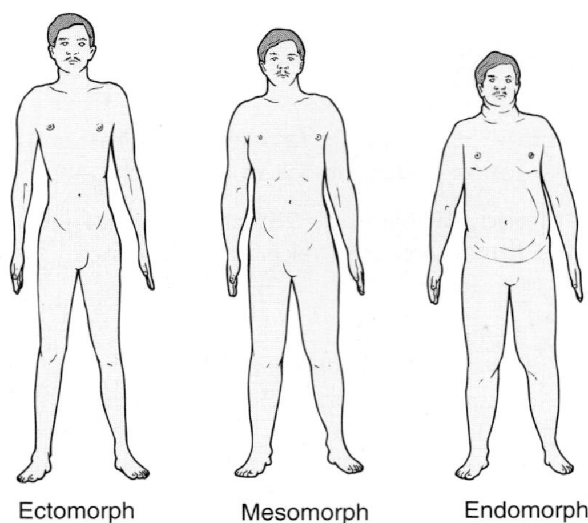

Thrifty metabolism *A metabolism that characteristically conserves more energy than normal so that it increases the risk of weight gain and obesity.*

Fraternal twins *Offspring that develop from two separate ova and sperm and therefore have separate genetic identities, although they develop simultaneously in the mother.*

Little relationship exists between how an infant was fed or how much weight was gained in the first year of life and the presence or absence of obesity in later childhood. Most overweight or obese infants become normal-weight schoolchildren. However, if a child has become obese by 5 years of age, immediate attention is necessary. Obesity in childhood is strongly related to obesity in adulthood.

parent has a 40% risk, and one with two obese parents an 80% risk. It can be argued that these probabilities are related, in part, to the eating behaviors a child learns. **Fraternal twins** vary less in weight than do two unrelated people. This pattern supports the theory that environment, or nurture, affects obesity. Still the close association of body weights between identical twins strongly supports genetic linkage. This varied evidence shows how complicated it is to separate nature from nurture when searching for the causes of obesity (Figure 9–9).

Does Nurture Have a Role?

Environmental factors, such as large portion sizes, ready availability of food, high-calorie diets, and inactivity, shape us as well. Consider that our gene pool hasn't changed much in the last 50 years, but the ranks of obese people have grown. In fact, the number of obese Americans has increased twofold since 1962. In addition, even husbands and wives—who have no genetic link—may behave similarly toward food and eventually assume similar degrees of leanness or chunkiness. Therefore, the family that bonds at the quick-service restaurant counter or when snacking in front of the TV can influence each other's eating habits and, ultimately, fatness.

Is poverty associated with obesity? Ironically, the answer is often yes. Americans of lower socioeconomic status, especially females, are more likely to be obese than those in upper socioeconomic groups. Are cultural expectations or socioeconomic stress the cause of this?

Adult obesity in women is often rooted in childhood obesity. In addition, periods of stress and boredom and excess weight gain in pregnancy contribute to female obesity. Relative inactivity further adds to the problem. These patterns suggest both social and genetic links. Male obesity, however, is not strongly linked to childhood obesity and instead tends to appear after age 30. This common pattern suggests an important role of nurture in obesity.

Nature and Nurture Together

Consider the possibility that obesity is nurture allowing nature to express itself, like an accident waiting to happen (Table 9–3). Some people begin life with a slower

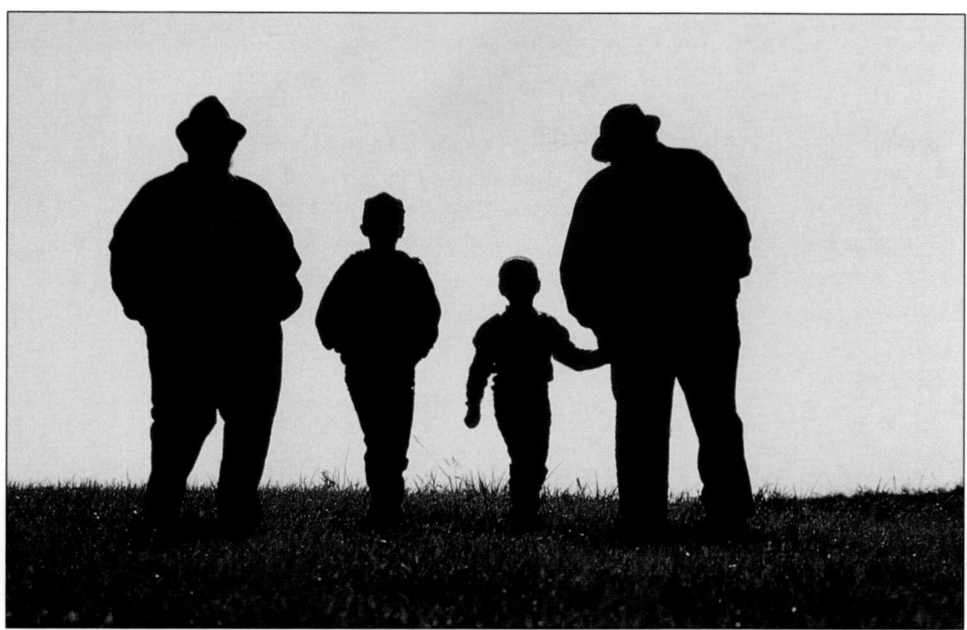

Figure 9-9 *Nature versus nurture. Does the difference in body fat between the grandfathers and the sons arise from nature, nurture, or both?*

metabolism. Put these people in an inactive environment, feed them super-sized portions of high-calorie foods, and praise them for eating. Like any of us, they can be nurtured into gaining weight, which allows their natural tendency for obesity to blossom. The eventual location of the resulting fat storage is strongly influenced by genetics.

If your parents are obese, you're likely to be at risk for obesity all your life. To avoid it will require eternal vigilance. Eat the right foods in the right amounts at the right times for the right reasons. And whatever the answer to the nature versus nurture question is, it is likely that all obese people or those at risk for obesity will face this lifelong struggle as well. Still genes do not control this destiny. With increased physical activity and moderation in food consumption, even those with a genetic tendency toward obesity can maintain a healthy or "healthier" body weight.

The importance of environment in the development of obesity is exhibited in the treatment of Prader-Willi Syndrome. Children with this inherited disorder have an extreme appetite and become extremely obese if food availability is not carefully controlled. If such a child has become obese, however, further careful control of food availability (eg. locking all kitchen cabinets and not allowing the child access to money) can lead to significant weight loss, often 100 pounds or more. This environmental therapy is effective despite the fact that the children maintain their extreme appetite.

ConceptCheck

Genetic background plays a role in obesity, influencing body shape, sites of fat deposition, and rate of basal metabolism. The role of nurture is evident in families, who tend to have similar eating habits, activity patterns, and degrees of fatness. Men tend to develop obesity after age 30, and women tend to have both childhood and adult roots for obesity; this suggests an especially important influence of nurture in men. Because both factors have an impact, it makes sense to assume that nurture serves as a catalyst for expressing or denying a genetic tendency toward obesity.

TABLE 9-3

What Encourages Excess Body Fat Stores and Obesity?

Factor	How fat storage is affected
Age	Excess body fat is more common in adults and middle-aged individuals.
Menopause	Increase in abdominal fat deposition is favored.
Gender	Females have more fat.
Positive energy balance	This is especially important if over a relatively long period.
Composition of diet	High fat intake, excess alcohol intake, and preference for sugary, fat-rich foods are likely to contribute to obesity.
Physical activity	Low or decreasing amount of physical activity ("couch potato") affects energy balance.
Resting metabolic rate	A low value with respect to lean body mass is linked to weight gain.
Thermic effect of food	This is low for some obesity cases.
Use of fat for energy	There is limited fat release into the bloodstream.
Total fat mass	Leptin, produced by adipose tissue, decreases food intake. Greater fat mass leads to greater leptin production.
Ratio of fat to lean tissue	A high ratio of fat mass to lean body mass is associated with weight gain.
Fat uptake by adipose tissue	This is high in some obese individuals and remains high (perhaps even increases) with weight loss.
Variety of social and behavioral factors	Obesity is associated with socioeconomic status, familial conditions, network of friends, busy lifestyles that discourage balanced meals, binge eating, easy availability of inexpensive, "super-sized" high-fat food, dangerous neighborhoods where it is not safe to be outside, pattern of leisure activities, television time, smoking cessation, excessive alcohol intake, and number of meals eaten away from home. These meals are often served in large portions and are high in fat.
Undetermined genetic characteristics	These affect energy balance, particularly via the energy expenditure components, the deposition of the energy surplus as fat or as lean tissue, and the relative proportion of fat and carbohydrate use by the body.
Race	In some ethnic groups, higher body weight may be more socially acceptable.
Certain medications	Food intake increases.
Childbearing	Women may not lose all weight gained in pregnancy, leading to creeping weight gain.
National region	Regional differences, such as high-fat diets and sedentary lifestyles cause more obesity in different places.

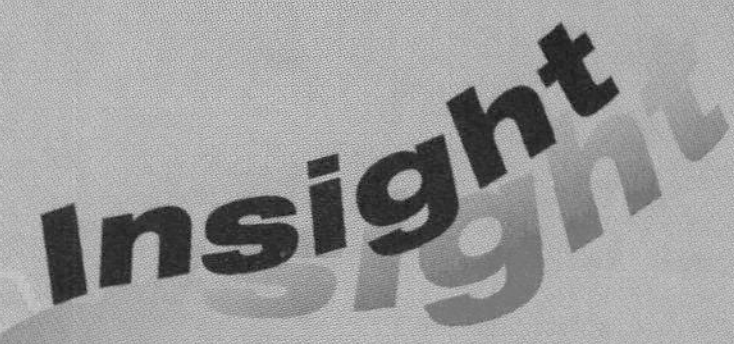

Do You Have a Set Point for Body Weight?

The **set-point** theory espouses the notion that weight is closely regulated by the body. It proposes that humans have a genetically predetermined body weight or body fat content that the body attempts to defend. Some research suggests that the hypothalamus monitors the amount of body fat in humans and tries to keep that amount constant over time. This regulation of body fat content is referred to as a "set point."

Analogies to the tight regulation of blood pressure and body temperature are used to support this concept of set point. You could view the set point as a coiled spring: the further you stray from your usual weight, the harder the force acts to pull you back to that weight.

In the major studies of humans cited to support the set-point theory, volunteers who lost weight through starvation later ate in a way to regain their original weight or a little more. In addition, studies in the 1960s using prisoners with no history of obesity found it was hard for the men to gain weight, and after gaining weight, they quickly returned to their previous weight when returning to their previous habits. Also, after an illness is resolved, a person generally gains lost weight.

Sound physiological evidence also suggests that body weight tends to be regulated. If energy intake is reduced, the blood concentration of thyroid hormone falls, and the metabolic rate slows. In addition, lower body weight decreases the energy cost of each future weight-bearing activity, and the total energy used by lean tissue falls because some of these tissues are also lost. Furthermore, the enzyme used by adipose and muscle cells to take up fat from the bloodstream (lipoprotein lipase) often increases its activity.Through these changes the body resists further weight loss.

If a person overeats, in the short run the metabolic rate tends to increase because total body mass increases. This causes some resistance to further weight gain. People often recognize the body's resistance to weight loss when dieting but do not think much about the resistance to weight gain after eating a big holiday meal. However, in the long run, resistance to weight gain is much less than resistance to weight loss. When a person gains weight and stays at that weight for a while, the body tends to defend the new weight.

Let's explore set-point regulation of weight in concrete terms. The amount we eat varies from day to day. Daily energy intake varies from about 20% (about 400 kcal) below to 20% above a person's 28-day average energy intake. In comparison, even as little as a 2% (40 kcal) overconsumption of energy per day, if continued for 20 years, could result in an over 100-pound gain in fat stores. However, the average weight gain between the ages of 18 and 54 is only about 20 pounds. It appears that some powerful forces encourage a balance of overeating with undereating. Considering also that over a 35-year period an adult eats about 35 tons of food (yielding 30 million kcal), the ability to regulate weight, though imperfect, is still quite impressive.

Arguments against the set-point theory cite the fact that during pregnancy women slowly increase body weight and fat. Also, an average person's weight does not remain constant throughout adulthood; it usually increases slowly, at least until old age. This means that a person must be able to shift his or her set point. It is also argued that if an individual is placed in a different social, emotional, or physical environment, weight can become markedly higher or lower and then is maintained. These arguments suggest that humans, rather than having a set point determined by genetics or number of adipose cells, actually settle into a particular stable weight based on an interaction between nature and nurture influences.

In the final analysis, we must bear much of the responsibility for weight maintenance ourselves. The odds are against the likelihood that, even with a set point helping us, we can avoid creeping weight gain in adulthood without paying attention to this tendency.

TREATMENT OF OBESITY

Obesity should be considered similar to any chronic disease. Treatment requires long-term lifestyle changes, rather than simply taking medicine for 2 weeks, as for a sore throat, or following some quick fix promoted by a fad diet book. People often, however, view a "diet" as something one goes on temporarily, only to resume prior (typically poor) habits once satisfactory results have been achieved. It is for this reason that so many people regain lost weight. In place of this, healthy, active living with appropriate dietary modifications should be the emphasis for both obese and thin people. Let's explore why obesity must be regarded and treated in this way.

Some Basic Premises

As you begin to consider current treatment options for obesity, you should first focus on five important general principles concerning weight loss for adults. (Chapter 13 provides weight-loss strategies for children.)

Much of the Current Mania Surrounding Dieting Is Misdirected

People on diets often fall within a BMI of 19 to 25. Instead of worrying about weight loss, these individuals should be focusing on a healthy lifestyle that allows for weight maintenance. Incorporating needed lifestyle changes and learning to live with one's particular body characteristics—such as an endomorphic shape—should be the overriding goal.

Actually, this dieting mania can be viewed as mostly a social problem, stemming from unrealistic weight expectations (especially for women) and lack of appreciation for the natural variety in body shape and weight. Not every woman can be a size 10, nor can every man look like a Greek god, but all of us can strive for good health and, if physically possible, an active lifestyle.

The Body Defends Itself Against Weight Loss

As noted in the Nutrition Insight, thyroid hormone concentrations and, consequently, basal metabolism drop during weight loss. This fall in metabolic rate is also a consequence of weight loss, caused by a loss of metabolizing tissue. Declines in basal metabolism average 8% to 22% in some studies. This drop contributes to the difficulties of weight loss.

In addition, the activity of the enzyme lipoprotein lipase increases, causing the body to more efficiently take up fat from the bloodstream for storage in adipose cells. Often, fat use for energy needs also remains depressed in people who have recently lost weight. This is a good reason to continue to watch fat intake and remain physically active for weight maintenance. Insulin action on adipose cells also improves with weight loss, which reduces fat release by these cells. Finally, energy use in physical activity falls as weight declines.

Here are some practices that can stimulate metabolism while one is dieting:

- **Perform physical activity regularly throughout the day. Find opportunities for increasing activity, such as quick walks, stair climbing, or calisthenics (sit-ups, push-ups, etc.).**
- **Fidget when sitting and standing.**
- **Eat breakfast, so food intake is spread throughout the day. Each time food is consumed, metabolism increases.**
- **Follow a carbohydrate-rich diet; much of this is further processed by the liver, which uses energy.**
- **Avoid "crash" dieting. Slow weight loss is a better idea because it leads to a smaller decline in metabolism during a diet.**

Weight Cycling Is a Common Phenomenon

Only about 5% of people who follow commercial diet programs actually lose weight and then remain close to that weight. Typically, one-third of the weight lost during dieting is regained within 1 year of the end of dietary restriction, and almost all weight lost is regained within 3 to 5 years. Some programs have slightly higher success rates than 5%, as do some people who simply lose weight on their own. Overall, however, the statistics are grim. Essentially only the surgical approaches to obesity treatment (discussed later) show routine success in maintaining the weight loss. Moreover, the weight gained after dieting includes not only the weight that was lost but often additional weight as well, causing the dieter to be worse off than before. Furthermore, the weight gained may consist primarily of adipose tissue, whereas the weight that was lost consisted more of a mix of adipose and lean tissue. Therefore the long-term effect is not only an increase in total weight but also an increase in percentage of body fat.

Additional negative health consequences are associated with weight cycling (also called yo-yo dieting), such as an increased risk for upper-body fat deposition and profound discouragement and erosion of self-esteem. Nevertheless, experts still encourage obese people to attempt weight loss, if motivated to do so with a strong focus on maintaining that lower weight. Still, dieters need to be aware of the trap of today's crash diet, which too often leads to the next month's weight gain. A weight-loss program should be considered successful only when the subjects involved in the process remain at or close to their lower weights.

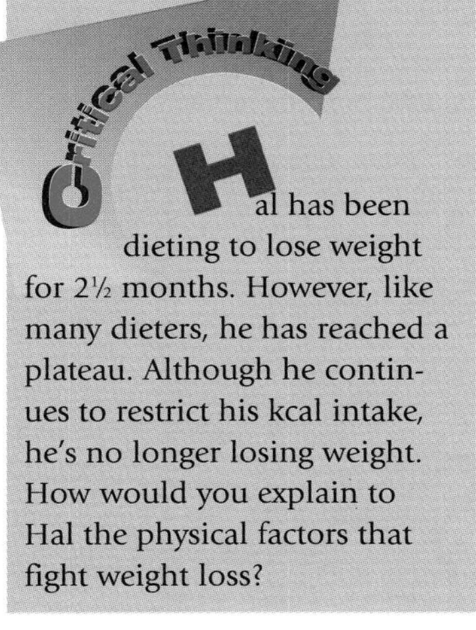

Hal has been dieting to lose weight for 2½ months. However, like many dieters, he has reached a plateau. Although he continues to restrict his kcal intake, he's no longer losing weight. How would you explain to Hal the physical factors that fight weight loss?

Weight Gain In Adulthood Is All Too Common

In adulthood, weight gain is common. Particular prudence should be practiced in these decades, although childhood and adolescent years also deserve attention. Adults should generally set a goal of not gaining greater than about 10 to 16 pounds more than their weight was upon reaching age 21. People who gain weight rapidly should closely monitor food intake and activity patterns to discover the causes and then moderate the increases or reverse the trend in appropriate ways. Later in this chapter, you'll learn how to do this.

Changes in Body Composition Deserve a Primary Focus in Weight Loss

Weight should be lost mostly from adipose stores, not from muscle and other lean tissues. Rapid weight loss at the start of a diet program often represents fluid lost as a result of decreased salt intake and loss of glycogen from the liver and muscles. Much muscle tissue may be lost as well, and this is mostly (about 73%) water. People are fooled when they weigh themselves after starting a fad diet. They lose weight, but very little of it represents fat loss. Any loss of lean tissue means a decrease in basal metabolism and thus a decrease in overall energy expenditure.

All this shows the importance of preventing obesity, because curing the disorder is very difficult. Nutrition experts believe that many people would be healthier if they simply focused on improving food habits, minimizing symptoms of any weight-related chronic disease present (such as high blood pressure), increasing physical activity and not gaining any more weight, rather than remaining focused on a particular body weight and shape. This conclusion is partly made because obtaining and maintaining a substantially lower body weight is so difficult.

Wishful Shrinking—Why Quick Weight Loss Can't Be Mostly Fat

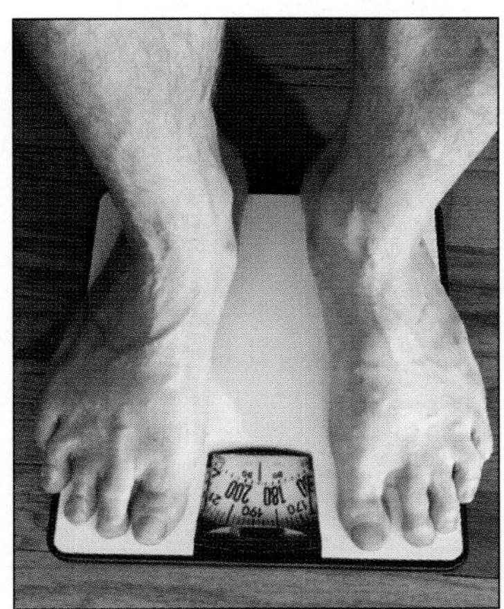

Slow, steady weight loss is one of the characteristics of a sound weight-loss plan.

We know that rapid weight loss cannot consist mostly of fat loss because of the high energy deficit needed to lose a large amount of adipose tissue. The body fat present in adipose tissue contains about 3500 kcal per pound. Fat storage, which includes body fat tissue plus supporting lean tissues, contains approximately 2700 kcal per pound. To lose 1 pound of fat stores (including lean tissue support) per week, energy intake must be decreased by approximately 400 to 500 kcal per day to account for the loss of both body fat and associated lean support tissues that will take place.

Diets that promise 10 to 15 pounds of weight loss per week can't ensure that the weight loss is from fat stores alone. Producing an energy deficit sufficient to lose that amount of fat storage simply isn't practical. Lean tissue, rather than fat, accounts for the major part of the weight lost.

What to Look for in a Sound Weight-Loss Diet

A dieter can try to devise a plan of action by seeking advice from professionals or consulting many current books. Either way, a sound weight-loss program should include three components: control of energy intake, regular physical activity, and acknowledgment that lifelong change in habits is required, rather than simply a short-term weight-loss period (Table 9–4).

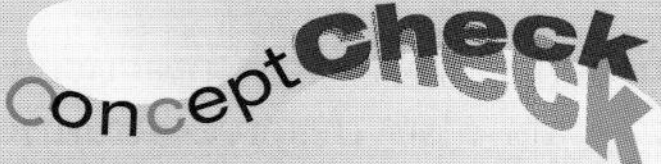

Obesity is a chronic disease that necessitates lifelong treatment. Key points to consider when attempting to treat obesity include the following: (1) The primary focus should be on a healthy lifestyle that can be maintained; (2) the body resists weight loss; (3) typical weight-loss attempts often are followed by weight regain; (4) emphasis should be placed on preventing obesity, since curing this disorder is very difficult; (5) weight should be lost from fat stores, not mostly from lean tissues. Appropriate weight-loss programs have the following characteristics in common: (1) they meet nutritional needs; (2) they can adjust to accommodate habits and tastes; (3) they emphasize readily obtainable foods; (4) they promote changing habits that lead to overeating; (5) they encourage regular physical activity; and (6) they help change obesity-promoting beliefs.

Controlling Energy Intake—The First Key to Weight Loss

Reaching for fruit in a fruit bowl may prevent snacking on fat-laden foods. While having the willpower to resist high-fat foods is desirable, a better alternative may be to avoid the temptation.

A goal of losing 1 to 2 pounds of stored fat per week often requires limiting energy intake to 1000 to 1600 kcal per day for women and 1600 to 2000 kcal for men, with less than 30% of energy intake coming from fat. Recall that adults currently consume about 33% of energy as fat. The range for each gender is due to the varying amounts of physical activity that may be performed. It could also be higher for very active people. Keep in mind that in a very sedentary society, decreasing fat (and calories) is important, because it is difficult to burn much of either without ample physical activity.

Traditionally dieters have counted calories. Many experts recommend counting mostly fat grams, given that control of energy intake also takes place. Chapter 5 contains a table to convert energy intake into an appropriate fat gram allowance. The new food labels simplify the task of counting fat grams. Note that not all food choices need to be low fat. Total fat intake for the day is the focus, as one makes healthy choices based on the Food Guide Pyramid. However, this method will only work if high-calorie fat-free foods—such as fat-free cakes and cookies—are not overeaten, since monitoring total calorie intake is still important.

As discussed in Chapter 5, many of the fat-reduced products flooding the market substitute sugar for fat in order to maintain flavor and consequently end up not much lower in energy content. This makes it easy to gain weight, even on a low-fat diet, without careful portion control of fat-reduced foods.

TABLE 9-4

Characteristics of a Sound Weight-Loss Diet

RATE OF LOSS

1. Slow and steady weight loss, rather than rapid weight loss, is encouraged.
2. Goal is 1 to 2 pounds of loss of fat storage per week.
3. A period of weight maintenance for a few months following a loss of 10% of body weight.
4. Evaluation of need for further dieting before more weight loss begins.

FLEXIBILITY

1. Ability to participate in normal activities (e.g., parties, restaurants).
2. Adaptations to individual habits and tastes.

INTAKE

1. Nutritional needs are met (except for energy).
2. Hunger and fatigue are minimized by providing at least 1200 to 1500 kcal per day (1000 kcal per day may be enough for a very sedentary person).
3. Common foods are included, with no certain foods being promoted as magical.

BEHAVIOR MODIFICATION

1. Maintenance of healthy lifestyle (and weight) is a key concern; there is a lifetime focus.
2. Changes are reasonable and can be maintained.

OVERALL HEALTH

1. Screening by a physician is required for persons with existing health problems, those over 35 years of age who plan to substantially increase physical activity, and those who plan to lose weight rapidly.
2. Regular physical activity, proper rest, stress reduction, and other healthy changes in lifestyle are encouraged.
3. Underlying psychological weight issues are addressed.

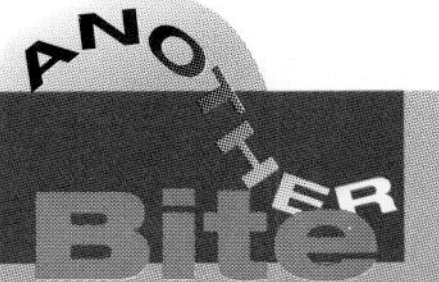

Some experts think that certain fat-reduced foods, such as nonfat sour cream, serve merely to remind dieters what they are missing, driving them back to the high-fat food choice (Figure 9–10). In addition, some studies have shown that people eat more when told a food is fat-reduced, even if it is not. This suggests it may be better to avoid high-fat foods and their fat-reduced counterparts, instead replacing them with a food choice naturally low in fat, such as nonfat yogurt for sour cream or a plain warm bagel for a doughnut.

In any case, dieters should consume at least 1000 kcal daily; fewer than that causes so much hunger that they will probably not be able to stick to the plan. In addition, these low energy intakes will likely result in nutrient deficiencies if a balanced supplement is not taken. A better idea is to first increase physical activity, allowing at least 1200 kcal (ideally, closer to 1500 kcal) to be eaten each day.

An excellent way for a dieter to monitor energy intake at the start of a weight-loss program is by reading labels. Label reading is important, because many foods are more energy-dense than people suppose (Figure 9–11). Another method is to write down food intake throughout the day and then calculate energy intake from the food table in Appendix A in the evening, adjusting future food choices as needed. Because people often underestimate portion size when recording food intake, measuring cups and kitchen scales can help.

THE MIDDLETONS
DIET MILK BONES, DIET DOG FOOD, DIET TREATS!
WHAT NEXT?
!
6-29

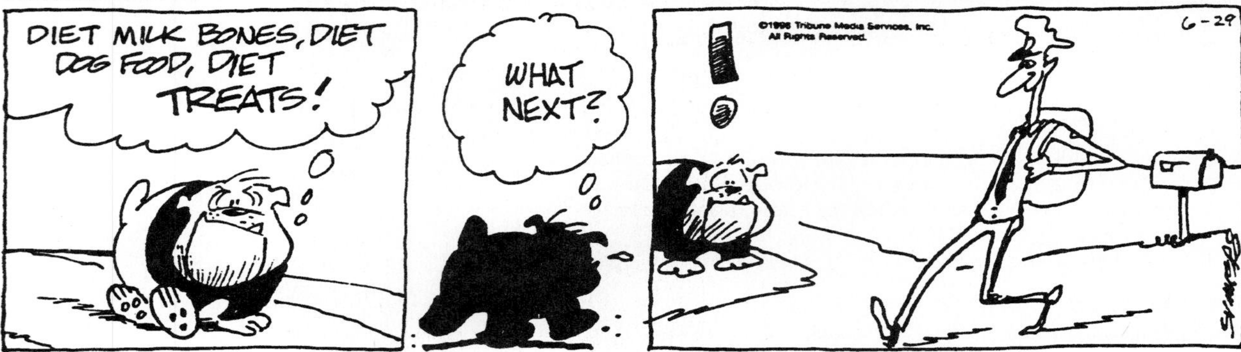

Figure 9–10 *The Middletons.*

PREMIUM LOW-FAT FROZEN YOGURT
CHERRY VANILLA
Nutrition Facts
Serving Size: ½ cup (65g)
Servings Per Container: 16
Amount Per Serving
Calories 100 Calories from Fat 20
% Daily Value*
Total Fat 2g 4%
Saturated Fat 1g 7%
Polyunsaturated Fat 0g
Monounsaturated Fat 1g
Cholesterol 10mg 3%
Sodium 30mg 1%
Total Carbohydrates 17g 6%
Dietary Fiber 0g 0%
Sugars 13g
Protein 3g
Vitamin A 2% • Vitamin C 0%
Calcium 6% • Iron 0%
PREMIUM ICE CREAM
COFFEE
Nutrition Facts
Serving Size: ½ cup (106g)
Servings Per Container: 4
Amount Per Serving
Calories 270 Calories from Fat 150
% Daily Value*
Total Fat 17g 25%
Saturated Fat 11g 54%
Cholesterol 120mg 40%
Sodium 85mg 4%
Total Carbohydrates 20g 7%
Dietary Fiber 0g 0%
Sugars 20g
Protein 5g
Vitamin A 10% • Vitamin C 0%
Calcium 15% • Iron 0%

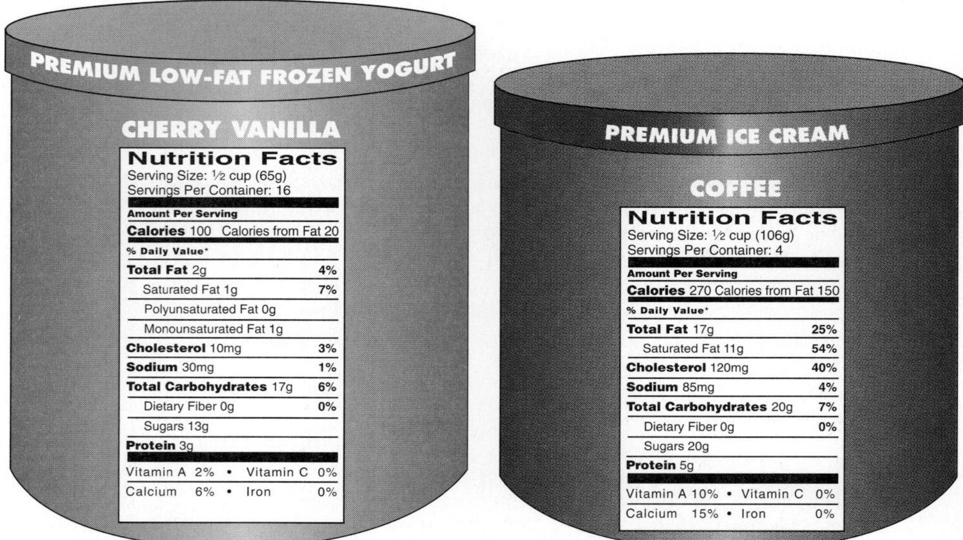

Figure 9–11 *Reading labels helps you choose foods with less fat and calories. Which frozen dessert is the best choice for a person on a weight-loss diet? The % Daily Values are based on a 2000-kcal diet.*

Whatever the method chosen, it is unreasonable to think that measuring food and keeping records will continue for a lifetime. These methods are suggested as a temporary practice for people who need to get accustomed to appropriate portion sizes. Once the eyes and stomach are trained to know what constitutes a specific portion size, it will be possible to then "eyeball" appropriate meals.

Decreasing fat in the diet from 40% to 30% of calories does not result in much compensation. That is, people do not often feel the need to eat large volumes of food to make up for the missing fat. On the other hand, reducing dietary fat to 20% of calories frequently leaves people feeling hungry and leads to the overeating of fat-free foods that are often high in calories. It is only when the dietary fat is replaced by starch-rich carbohydrates and dietary fiber that this compensation can be minimized.

TABLE 9-5

Saving kcal: Ideas to Help Get Started

Check out the following calorie-saving ideas. Then think of other changes to help cut calories.

Instead of	Try	kcal saved
Well-marbled meat (prime rib), 3 oz	Lean meat (eye of round), 3 oz	140
Chicken, ½ breast, batter-fried	Chicken, ½ breast, broiled with lemon	175
Beef stroganoff, ½ cup	Lean roast beef, 3 oz	210
Home-fried potatoes, 1 cup	Baked potato, 1 medium	65
Green bean–mushroom casserole, ½ cup	Cooked green beans, ½ cup	50
Potato salad, ½ cup	Raw vegetable salad, 1 cup	140
Pineapple chunks in heavy syrup, ½ cup	Pineapple chunks canned in juice, ½ cup	25
Bottled French dressing, 2 tbsp	Low-calorie French dressing, 2 tbsp	150
Apple pie, ⅛ of 9″ pie	Baked apple, 1	185
Oatmeal-raisin cookies, 3	Oatmeal-raisin cookie, 1	125
Ice cream, ½ cup	Ice milk, ½ cup	45
Danish pastry, 1	English muffin, ½	150
Sugar-coated corn flakes, 1 cup	Plain corn flakes, 1 cup	60
Whole milk, 1 cup	1% Reduced-fat milk, 1 cup	45
Gin and tonic, 7 oz	Wine cooler made with sparkling water, 6 oz	150
Potato chips, 1-oz bag	Plain popcorn, 1 cup	120
White layer cake with chocolate frosting, 1/12 of 8″ cake	Angel food cake, 1/12 of 10″ tube	185
Regular beer, 12 fl oz	Light beer	40

What Should Be Eaten?

The easiest and healthiest way to eat is to begin with the Food Guide Pyramid, spreading out the food choices into a regular meal pattern (3 or more meals). In addition, when choosing to indulge in sweet or high-fat foods, keep in mind that most of the pleasure comes from the first few bites. Practice savoring these first bites; note the time when the maximum enjoyment has been reached and do not feel the need to eat food beyond that point. Table 9-5 shows how to start reducing energy intake. As you should realize by now, it is best to consider healthy eating a lifestyle change rather than simply a weight-loss plan. One should make reasonable choices, consume appropriate portions, and not expect a miracle overnight.

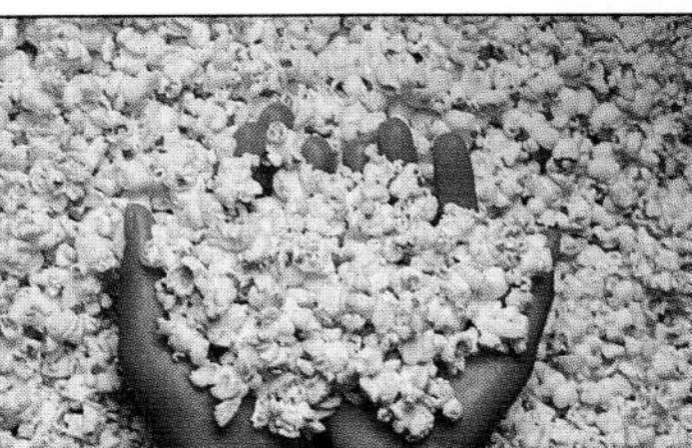

Popcorn is a wise snack choice when eaten in a reasonable quantity.

Regular Physical Activity—A Second Key to Weight Loss and Later Weight Maintenance

Regular physical activity is very important for everyone, especially those who are trying to lose weight or maintain a lower body weight. Fat burning is enhanced. Therefore, it greatly complements a reduction in energy intake for weight loss, but does not substitute for it. Many of us rarely do more than sit, stand, and sleep. Obviously, much more energy is used during physical activity than at rest. In addition, expending only 200 to 300 extra kcal per day above and beyond normal activity, while controlling energy intake, can lead to about a half pound of fat loss per week,

TABLE 9-6

Approximate Energy Costs of Various Activities, and Those Projected for a 150-Pound (68-Kilogram) Person

Activity	kcal per kg per hour	kcal per hour
Aerobics—heavy	8.0	544
Aerobics—light	3.0	204
Aerobics—medium	5.0	340
Backpacking	9.0	612
Basketball—vigorous	10.0	680
Bicycling (5.5 MPH)	3.0	204
Bowling	3.9	265
Calisthenics—heavy	8.0	544
Calisthenics—light	4.0	272
Canoeing (2.5 MPH)	3.3	224
Cleaning (female)	3.7	253
Cleaning (male)	3.5	236
Cooking	2.8	190
Cycling (13 MPH)	9.7	659
Dressing/showering	1.6	106
Driving	1.7	117
Eating (sitting)	1.4	93
Food shopping	3.6	245
Football—touch	7.0	476
Golf	3.6	244
Horseback trotting	5.1	346
Ice skating (10 MPH)	5.8	394
Jogging—medium	9.0	612
Jogging—slow	7.0	476
Lying—at ease	1.3	89
Racquetball—social	8.0	544
Roller-skating	5.1	346
Running or jogging (10 MPH)	13.2	897
Skiing (10 MPH)	8.8	598
Sleeping	1.2	80
Swimming (.25 MPH)	4.4	299
Tennis	6.1	414
Volleyball	5.1	346
Walking (2.5 MPH)	3.0	204
Walking (3.75 MPH)	4.4	299
Waterskiing	7.0	476
Weight lifting—heavy	9.0	612
Weight lifting—light	4.0	272
Window cleaning	3.5	240
Writing (sitting)	1.7	118

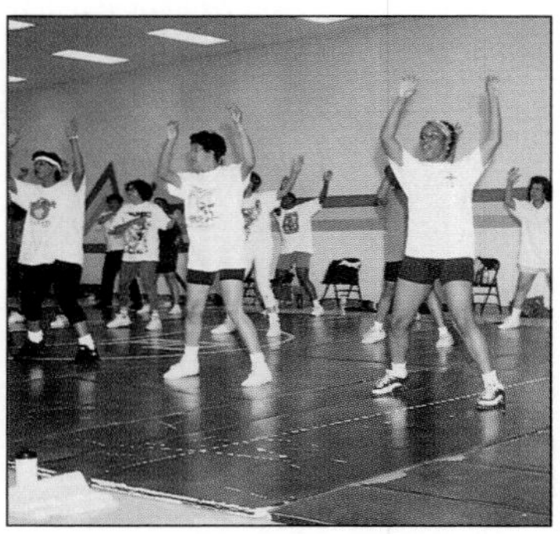

Even a moderate weight loss of 10 to 20 pounds can help improve blood glucose regulation and blood pressure.

or about 25 pounds of fat loss per year. Furthermore, physical activity often boosts overall self-esteem.

Adding any of the activities in Table 9–6 to one's lifestyle leads to more energy expenditure; note that sitting is not a recommended "activity." Duration and regular performance, rather than intensity, are the keys to success with this approach to weight loss. One should search for activities that can be continued over time, and include enough each day to yield about 200 kcal or more. In this regard, walking vigorously 2 miles per day can be as helpful as aerobic dancing or jogging if it is maintained. Moreover, walking is less likely to lead to injuries. Some strength training can also be added to increase lean body mass and, in turn, fat use (see Chapter 10).

The easiest way to increase physical activity is to make it part of a daily routine. To start, one could consider walking every day and then incorporating some regular stair climbing. A simple trick is to park the car farther from school, work, and the shopping mall so one must walk farther.

Behavior Modification—What Makes Us Tick?

Controlling energy intake, so important to weight loss, also means modifying *problem* behaviors. Only the dieter can decide what behaviors keep the person from reaching for the wrong foods at the wrong times for the wrong reasons.

Psychologists often use terms like ***chain-breaking, stimulus control, cognitive restructuring, contingency management***, and ***self-monitoring*** when discussing such behavior modification (Table 9–7). This terminology helps place the problem in perspective and organize the intervention strategy into manageable steps.

Chain-breaking separates behaviors that tend to occur together—for example, snacking on chips while watching television. Dieters may need to break this chain reaction.

Stimulus control puts us in charge of temptations. Options include pushing tempting food to the back of the refrigerator, removing fat-laden snacks from the kitchen counter, avoiding the path by the vending machines, and providing a positive stimulus by keeping low-fat snacks ready to satisfy hunger/ appetite.

Cognitive restructuring changes our frame of mind. For example, after a hard day, one could respond with a walk or satisfying talk with a friend instead of a binge.

Setting some food off limits sets up an internal struggle to resist the urge to eat that food. This hopeless battle can keep us feeling deprived. We lose the fight. Managing food choices with the principle of moderation is best.

Contingency management prepares us for potential pitfalls and high-risk situations. We might rehearse in advance appropriate responses to pressure—like food being passed at a party.

The Rate Your Plate at the end of this chapter allows you to work through a personal behavior change. The activity uses many of the tools described above.

Social Support Aids Behavior Change

Healthy social support is helpful in weight control. Helping others understand how they can be supportive can make weight control easier. Family and friends can provide praise and encouragement. A weight-control professional can keep dieters accountable and help them learn from difficult situations. Long-term contact with a professional can be quite helpful for later weight maintenance. Groups of individuals attempting to lose weight or maintain losses can provide empathetic support.

A Recap

When weight-loss experts pool their collective experience, they identify certain factors that characterize success and failure in weight loss and later weight maintenance. As you've learned from this chapter, success is encouraged by the following measures:

1. Moderation in energy/fat intake. A first step should be use of this intervention to establish weight maintenance behavior before attempting to lose weight.
2. Time and inclination to perform regular physical activity.
3. A sense of control of personal destiny and likelihood of success.
4. Taking charge of the plan with a strong motivation to succeed.
5. Focusing on improved health status to spur success.
6. Positive self-talk (the conversation [internal dialogue] we carry out with ourselves).
7. Social support via family/friends, in turn balancing life with friendships, work, hobbies, and other interests.

Chain-breaking
Breaking the link between two or more behaviors that encourage overeating, such as snacking while watching television.

Stimulus control
Altering the environment to minimize the stimuli for eating—for example, removing foods from sight and storing them in kitchen cabinets.

Cognitive restructuring
Changing one's frame of mind regarding eating—for example, instead of using a difficult day as an excuse to overeat, substituting other pleasures for rewards, such as a relaxing walk with a friend.

Contingency management
Forming a plan of action to respond to a situation in which overeating is likely, such as when snacks are within arm's reach at a party.

Self-monitoring
A process of tracking foods eaten and conditions affecting eating; actions are usually recorded in a diary, along with location, time, and state of mind. This is a tool to help people understand more about their eating habits.

TABLE 9-7

Behavior Modification Principles for Weight Loss

STIMULUS CONTROL

Shopping

1. Shop for food after eating—buy nutritious foods.
2. Shop from a list; limit purchases of irresistible "problem" foods.
3. Avoid ready-to-eat foods.
4. Put off shopping until absolutely necessary.

Plans

1. Plan to limit food intake as needed.
2. Substitute periods of physical activity for snacking.
3. Eat meals and snacks at scheduled times; don't skip meals.

Activities

1. Store food out of sight, preferably in the freezer, to discourage impulsive eating.
2. Eat all food in the same place.
3. Keep serving dishes off the table, especially dishes of sauces and gravies.
4. Use smaller dishes and utensils.

Holidays and parties

1. Drink fewer alcoholic beverages.
2. Plan eating behavior before parties.
3. Eat a low-calorie snack before parties.
4. Practice polite ways to decline food.
5. Don't get discouraged by an occasional setback.

EATING BEHAVIOR

1. Put fork down between mouthfuls.
2. Chew thoroughly before taking the next bite.
3. Leave some food on the plate.
4. Pause in the middle of the meal.
5. Do nothing else while eating (for example, reading, watching television).

REWARD

1. Solicit help from family and friends and suggest how they can help you.
2. Help family and friends provide this help in the form of praise and material rewards.
3. Use self-monitoring records as basis for rewards.
4. Plan specific rewards for specific behavior (behavioral contracts).

SELF-MONITORING

Diet diary

1. Note time and place of eating.
2. List type and amount of food eaten.
3. Record who is present and how you feel.
4. Use diet diary to identify problem areas.

COGNITIVE RESTRUCTURING

1. Avoid setting unreasonable goals.
2. Think about progress, not shortcomings.
3. Avoid imperatives like "always" and "never."
4. Counter negative thoughts with positive restatements.

8. Sustained vigilance in pursuit of goals—realizing it is a lifetime pursuit that must be suited to one's specific needs. It's not a diet but a permanent lifestyle change.
9. Realistic goals that promote gradual change.
10. Keeping track of body weight and body measurements and quickly making changes in a plan if relapse is noticed.
11. Modifying ones environment to facilitate weight loss/maintenance and physical activity.

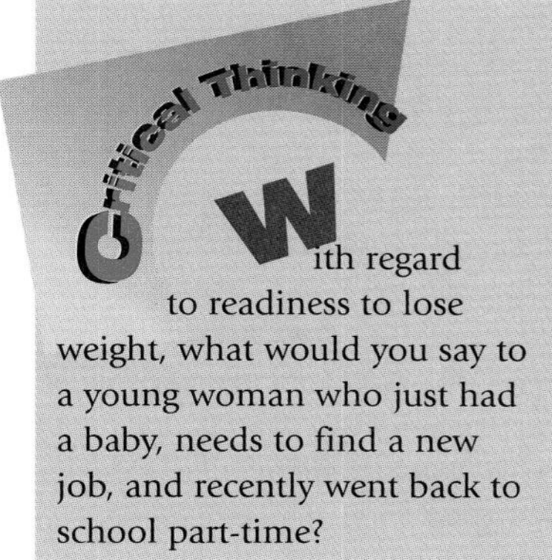

With regard to readiness to lose weight, what would you say to a young woman who just had a baby, needs to find a new job, and recently went back to school part-time?

Failure is encouraged by the following factors:

1. Negative feelings.
2. Out-of-control situations, such as family life or lifestyle that constantly challenges the will to succeed; prior or current practices of bingeing, laxative abuse, or induced vomiting. In these cases professional help should be sought.
3. Reverting to old habits, such as eating primarily foods rich in fat and abusing alcohol.

In the past, dieting emphasized the need for immediate results through unreasonable restrictions, willpower, and perfection. The emphasis today is on a well-balanced diet; regular physical activity; and behavior modification (Figure 9–12). These components should be a part of an overall lifestyle change that is permanent. No foods should be forbidden, and an occasional indulgence should be expected.

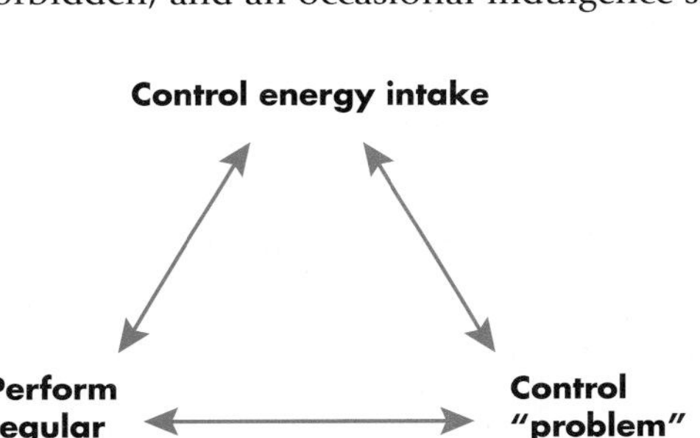

Figure 9–12 *The weight-loss triad. The key to weight loss and maintenance can be thought of as a triangle in which the three corners consist of (1) controlling energy intake, (2) performing regular physical activity, and (3) making needed lifestyle changes. The three corners of the triangle support each other in that without one corner the triangle becomes incomplete. In the same way, without one of the three keys to weight loss, weight loss and later maintenance become unlikely.*

When you read brochures or research reports about specific diet plans, ask not only whether the people lost weight but also whether they maintained much of that weight loss. If this did not happen, then the entire dieting program was in vain.

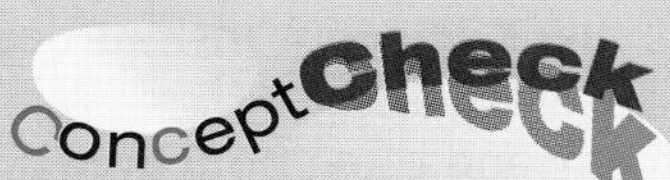

Increasing physical activity as part of daily life should be part of any weight-loss plan. Daily activity such as walking and stair climbing is recommended. Behavior modification can improve conditions for losing weight. One behavior area that requires change is habit chains that encourage overeating, such as snacking while watching television. Another tactic is to modify the environment to reduce temptation; for example, put foods into cupboards to keep them out of sight. In addition, rethinking attitudes about eating—for example, substituting pleasures other than food as a reward for coping with a stressful day—can be important for altering undesirable behavior. Advanced planning to prevent and deal with lapses is vital, as is rallying healthy social support. Finally, careful observation and recording of eating habits can reveal subtle cues that lead to overeating. Overall, weight loss and maintenance is fostered by controlling energy intake, performing regular physical activity, and modifying "problem" behaviors.

Spot-reducing using diet and physical activity is not possible. "Problem" local fat deposits can be reduced in size, however, using suction lipectomy. Lipectomy means surgical removal of fat. A pencil-thin tube is inserted into an incision in the skin, and the fat tissue, such as that in the buttocks and thigh area, is suctioned. This procedure carries some risks such as infection, lasting depressions in the skin, and blood clots that can lead to kidney failure.The procedure is designed to help a person lose about 4 pounds per treatment. Cost is about $1600 per site; total costs range from $2600 to $9000.

Professional Help for Weight Loss

The first professional to see for advice about a weight-loss program is one's primary care physician. Doctors are best equipped to assess overall health and the appropriateness of weight loss. The physician may recommend a registered dietitian for a specific weight-loss plan and answers to diet-related questions. Registered dietitians are uniquely qualified to help design a weight-loss plan because they understand both food composition and the psychological importance of food. Exercise physiologists can provide advice about programs to increase physical activity.

Many communities have a variety of weight-loss organizations. These may include self-help groups, such as Take Off Pounds Sensibly and Weight Watchers. Other programs, such as Jenny Craig, are less desirable for the average dieter. Often the employees are not dietitians or other appropriately trained health professionals. These programs also tend to be expensive because of their requirements for intense counseling or mandatory diet foods and supplements. In addition, the Federal Trade Commission has charged commercial diet-program companies with misleading consumers through unsubstantiated weight-loss claims and deceptive testimonials.

If one decides to use one of these programs it is important to ask about any risks involved, credentials of the staff, and costs of the program (including membership, diagnostic tests, weekly visits, meal replacements, supplements). Also, it is important to find out about the success of previous clients, especially with regard to long-term weight maintenance.

Treating Severe Obesity

Severe (morbid) obesity—having a BMI over 40—requires professional treatment. Because of the serious health problems related to severe obesity, drastic measures may be necessary. Such treatments are recommended only when traditional diets fail. These drastic weight-loss procedures are not without side effects, both physical and psychological, making careful physician monitoring a necessity.

Gastroplasty

Stomach stapling, or **gastroplasty,** is the most common surgical procedure for treating severe obesity. The procedure works by reducing the stomach to the size of a shot glass, about 50 milliliters (2 ounces). Overeating of solid foods is consequently less likely, because rapid vomiting would result. The smaller stomach also promotes more rapid satiety. With the enforced food reduction, about 75% of people with severe obesity eventually lose 50% or more of excess body weight. The surgery's success at long-term loss maintenance often leads to dramatic health improvements, such as reduced blood pressure and correction of Type 2 diabetes. Risk of death from the surgery itself is about 1%.

Gastroplasty has disadvantages. The surgery is costly and often not covered by medical insurance. In addition, follow-up surgery is often needed after weight loss to correct stretched skin that used to be filled with fat. Furthermore, months of difficult adjustments face the dieter who has chosen this drastic approach to weight loss. The elimination of simple carbohydrates (sugar) from the diet is necessary to avoid severe diarrhea. Nutrient deficiencies are also possible if an appropriate diet and nutrient supplement plan is not followed.

This surgery is not reversed, even after the desired weight loss is attained. Thus, however successful for weight loss, gastroplasty still requires major, lifelong lifestyle changes.

Gastroplasty
Surgery performed on the stomach to limit its volume to approximately 50 milliliters, the size of a shot glass.

Very-low-calorie diet (VLCD)
Known also as protein-sparing modified fast *(PSMF), this diet allows a person 400 to 800 kcal per day, often in liquid form. Of this, 120 to 480 kcal is carbohydrate, while the rest is mostly high-biological-value protein.*

Very-Low-Calorie Diets

If more traditional diet changes have failed, treating severe obesity with a very-low-calorie diet (VLCD) is possible. Optifast is one such commercial program.

Nutrition Insight

Medications to Aid Weight Loss

Over-the-counter medications that claim to facilitate weight loss are very profitable. Some can be effective, but so far none can substitute for the basic approach outlined in this chapter to promote weight loss. Diet aids include fiber pills and **phenylpropanolamine.** Phenylpropanolamine is an epinephrine-like drug that can cause a slight decrease in food intake. At a typical dose the degree of appetite suppression varies among people. FDA recommends that phenylpropanolamine be used with caution in people with hyperthyroidism, cardiovascular disorders (including high blood pressure), and diabetes. Adverse reactions may also occur in people taking various other medications or consuming caffeine at the same time.

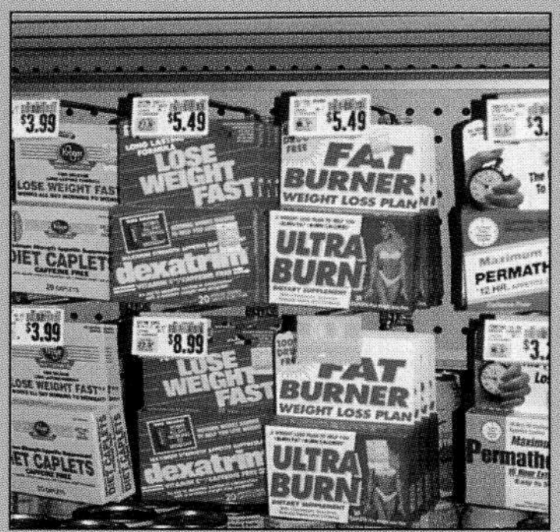

Monitoring energy intake and performing regular physical activity are two keys to weight control. Diet aids sold in grocery stores or pharmacies do not substitute for those behaviors.

Fiber pills can increase bulk in the stomach and ideally lead to satiety. Only soluble fiber, the type found in beans, oats, and guar gum, is effective in decreasing food intake. Bran fiber, such as that found in some fiber pills, is not effective. However, when people consume enough soluble fiber (23 grams) incorporated into crackers to decrease food intake, they also experience significant intestinal gas.

FDA states that people with a BMI of 30 or greater, or those with a BMI of 27 with health problems related to obesity, such as high blood pressure or Type 2 diabetes, are candidates for prescription drug therapy. However, success with this therapy has been shown only for those who also modify behavior and energy intake and increase physical activity. Drug therapy used alone has not been found to be successful.

With regard to the agents employed, phentermine (Adipex-P, Fastin) is available for use. It prolongs the activity of neurotransmitters in the brain. This therapy is effective for some people in the short run but has not yet been proved effective in the long run. Some state medical boards limit use to 12 weeks unless the person is participating in a medical study using the product. The drug should not be used in pregnant or nursing women or those under 18 years of age.

Sibutramine (Meridia) was approved by FDA for weight loss in 1998. It acts to enhance neurotransmitter activity in the brain. The most common side effects are constipation, dry mouth, insomnia, and increase in blood pressure. Preliminary studies have shown that it is effective in helping appropriately screened people lose weight as part of a comprehensive weight control program with careful monitoring for possible problems. The medication orlistat (Xenical) was recently approved by FDA for use in the treatment of obesity in 1999. This medication reduces fat digestion by inhibiting the enzymes responsible for this process. In turn, fat absorption is reduced; more fat than is typical ends up in the feces. The medication must be administered along with a low calorie diet to be useful. To date there is limited information about its long-term safety and effectiveness.

In the mid-1990s there were other medications available that altered neurotransmitters in the brain. These were called fenfluramine (Pondimin) and dexfenfluramine (Redux). FDA pulled these from the market in 1996 because of evidence they caused lung and heart problems and related deaths, especially with use greater than a few weeks. Currently, people who took either of these medications are advised to have a careful medical evaluation to look for potential problems.

After the ban of these medications, some people turned to health-food stores for a substitute—the stimulant ephedra (ma huang) with the mild antidepressant St. John's wort. Ma huang has been linked to over 800 reports of illness and 38 deaths in the United States.

FDA has proposed a maximum daily dosage for ephedrine—the active substance in ephedra—of 24 milligrams per day for no more than 7 days. Beside deaths, ma huang also has been associated with nervous and cardiovascular system effects including high blood pressure, stroke, psychosis, heart attack, seizure, and abnormal heart rhythm. St. John's wort should not be taken with any other antidepressant. Many experts advise staying away from these health-food store combinations until careful testing is done.

Overall, use of medicinal aides as part of a weight-loss program should be carefully thought out, and a physician should regularly monitor the person for potential problems.

Some researchers believe people with body weight greater than 30% above their healthy weight are also appropriate candidates. The diet allows a person to eat 400 to 800 kcal per day, often in liquid form. (These diets were known earlier as protein-sparing modified fasts.) Of this amount, about 30 to 120 grams (120 to 480 kcal) is carbohydrate. The rest is high-quality protein, which supplies about 70 to 100 grams per day (280 to 400 kcal). This low carbohydrate intake often causes ketosis, which may decrease hunger. However, the main reasons for weight loss are the minimal energy allowed and the absence of food choice. About 3 to 4 pounds can be lost per week; men tend to lose at a higher rate than women. When physical activity and weight training augment this diet, a greater loss of adipose tissue occurs. Careful physician monitoring is crucial throughout this very restrictive form of diet therapy. Major health risks include heart problems and gallstones.

Weight regain remains a nagging problem with this type of therapy. If behavioral therapy and physical activity supplement a long-term support program, maintenance of the weight loss is more likely but still difficult. Any program under consideration should include a maintenance plan. Today antiobesity medications also may be included in maintenance phase of the program (see the Nutrition Insight).

TREATING UNDERWEIGHT

Underweight
Body weight for height about 15% to 20% below healthy weight, or a body mass index below about 19. These cutoffs are less precise than for obesity because this condition has been less studied.

Underweight can be caused by a variety of factors, such as anorexia nervosa, cancer, infectious disease, digestive tract disorders, and excessive physical activity. Genetic background may also lead to a higher resting metabolic rate, a small body frame, or both. Significant underweight is also associated with increased death rates, especially when combined with cigarette smoking. Health problems associated with underweight include the loss of menstrual function, complications with pregnancy and surgery, and slow recovery after illness. We frequently hear about the risks of obesity, but seldom of underweight. In our culture, being underweight is much more socially acceptable than being obese.

Sometimes being underweight requires medical intervention. A physician should be consulted first to rule out hormonal imbalances, depression, cancer, infectious disease, digestive tract disorders, excessive physical activity, and other hidden disease, such as anorexia nervosa and bulimia nervosa.

The causes of underweight are not altogether different from the causes of obesity. Internal and external satiety-signal irregularities, rate of metabolism, hereditary tendencies, and psychological traits can all contribute to underweight.

In growing children the demand for energy to support physical activity and growth can cause underweight. During growth spurts in adolescence, active children may not take the time to consume enough energy to support their energy needs. Moreover, gaining weight can be a formidable task for an underweight person. More than 500 extra kcal per day may be required to gain weight, even at a slow pace, in part because of the expenditure of energy in adaptive thermogenesis. In contrast to the weight loser, the weight gainer may need to increase portion sizes and learn to like new energy-dense foods.

When underweight requires a specific intervention, one approach for treating adults is to gradually increase their consumption of energy-dense foods (foods that provide a great deal of energy in a small volume). Italian cheeses, nuts, and granola can be good energy sources with low saturated fat content. Dried fruit and bananas are recommended fruit choices. If eaten at the end of a meal, they don't cause early satiety. Underweight people should replace beverage choices such as diet soft drinks with good energy sources like fruit juices.

Encouraging a regular meal and snack schedule aids in weight gain and maintenance. Sometimes people who are underweight have experienced stress at work or have been too busy to eat. Making regular meals a priority may not only help them attain an appropriate weight, but may also help with digestive disorders, such as constipation, which are sometimes associated with irregular eating times.

Excessively physically active people can reduce activity. If their weight remains low, they may add muscle mass through a resistance (weight-lifting) program, but they must increase their energy intake to support that physical activity. Otherwise, weight gain will be hindered.

If these efforts fail to achieve the desired weight, they should at least prevent health problems associated with being underweight. After achieving that, they may have to accept their very lean frames.

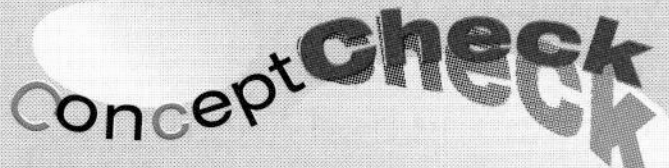

Severely obese people who have failed to lose weight with conservative weight-loss strategies may consider other options. Their doctors may recommend undergoing surgery to reduce the volume of the stomach to approximately 50 millliliters or following a very-low-calorie diet plan containing 400 to 800 kcal per day. Careful physician monitoring is crucial in both cases.

Underweight can be caused by a variety of factors, including genetics, cancer, and anorexia nervosa. Serious health problems should be ruled out by a physician, and treatment may include increasing portion size, eating at regular times, and choosing energy-dense foods.

Summary

- Energy balance is energy intake minus energy output. Negative energy balance occurs when energy output exceeds energy intake, resulting in weight loss. Positive energy balance occurs when energy intake is greater than energy output. The result is weight gain.
- The energy content of food is determined through use of a bomb calorimeter. The food is burned, and in turn raises the temperature of water. The energy sources—carbohydrate, protein, and fat—produce different effects on the body, with fat being most readily stored in adipose tissue.
- Basal metabolism, the thermic effect of food, physical activity, and adaptive thermogenesis account for total energy use by the body. Basal metabolism, which represents the minimum energy expenditure needed to keep the resting, awake body alive, is primarily affected by lean body mass and other factors. Physical activity represents energy use above that expended at rest. The thermic effect of food represents the increase in metabolism to facilitate the digesting, absorbing, and processing of nutrients recently consumed. Adaptive thermogenesis is heat production caused by overfeeding or a cold environment. About 70% to 80% of energy use is accounted for by basal metabolism and the thermic effect of food in a primarily sedentary person.
- Energy use by the body can be measured directly from heat output (direct calorimetry) or indirectly from oxygen uptake (indirect calorimetry). Energy needs of the body can be estimated using formulas based on various combinations of height and weight, with degree of physical activity, and age.
- A person of healthy weight shows good health and performs daily activities without weight-related problems. A body mass index (weight [in kilograms] ÷ height^2 [in meters]) of 19 to 25 is one measure of healthy weight, although weight in excess of this value may not lead to ill health especially when it is not due to an overfat state. This suggests that healthy weight is best determined in conjunction with a thorough health evaluation by a physician.

- ➤ Obesity is usually defined as total body fat percentage over 25% in men and 30% to 35% in women. A body mass index over 30 also represents obesity.
- ➤ Fat distribution partially determines health risks from obesity. Upper-body fat storage is indicated by a waist circumference greater than 40 inches in men and 35 inches in women, or a waist-to-hip circumference ratio greater than 1.0 in men or greater than 0.80 in women. This leads to higher risks of high blood pressure, heart disease, and Type 2 diabetes associated with obesity than does lower-body fat distribution. Other factors, such as age of obesity onset, also need to be considered when evaluating a specific individual.
- ➤ Genetic factors influence the tendency toward obesity. Basal metabolism and body fat distribution both have genetic links. How a person is raised (or nurtured) also influences the tendency toward obesity, Obesity can be viewed as nurture allowing nature to be expressed.
- ➤ The "set-point" theory of weight maintenance states that the body regulates weight very closely, keeping it around a certain "set point." Though it is not impossible to change one's weight for the long term, it is difficult.
- ➤ Those in search of a treatment for obesity should remember these five points: (1) a focus on healthy lifestyle rather than weight loss per se is more appropriate for many potential and current dieters; (2) the body resists weight loss; (3) the emphasis should be on preventing obesity because curing the disorder is very difficult; (4) weight loss should represent mostly a loss of fat storage and not primarily the loss of lean tissues; and (5) rapid weight loss and quick regain can be harmful to physical and emotional health.
- ➤ If energy output exceeds energy intake by about 400 to 500 kcal per day, a pound of fat storage can be lost per week. Decreasing the intake of high-fat foods is one way to obtain this energy deficit, along with increasing physical activity.
- ➤ A sound weight-loss diet meets the dieter's nutritional needs by emphasizing low-fat and nonfat food choices from the Food Guide Pyramid; it adapts to the dieter's habits, consists of readily obtainable foods, strives to change poor eating habits, stresses regular physical activity, and stipulates the participation of a physician if weight is to be lost rapidly or if the person is over 35 years of age and plans to perform substantially greater physical activity than usual.
- ➤ Physical activity as part of a weight-loss program should be focused on duration rather than intensity. Ideally, 200 kcal or more of vigorous activity should be part of each day.
- ➤ Behavior modification, such as stimulus control and self-monitoring, is a vital part of a weight-loss program because the dieter may have had many habits that encourage overeating and thus discourage weight maintenance.
- ➤ Medications to blunt appetite such as phentermine and sibutramine can aid weight-reduction strategies. Use is time limited, generally reserved for those who are obese, and must be administered under strict physician supervision.
- ➤ Underweight can be caused by a variety of factors, such as excessive physical activity and genetic background. When underweight requires medical intervention, a physician should be consulted first to rule out ongoing disease. The underweight person may need to increase portion sizes, learn to like new energy-dense foods, and eat regular meals. A physically active person can reduce excessive activity and substitute some resistance exercise (weight training).

Study Questions

1. Describe how energy content of food is determined. How is this similar to one method of determining total energy content use by the body?
2. Knowing the four contributors to human energy expenditure, propose two hypotheses for the development of obesity, based on the classes of energy expenditure.

3 Define healthy weight in a way that makes the most sense to you.
4 Describe a practical method to define obesity in a clinical setting.
5 What are the two most convincing pieces of evidence that both genetic and environmental factors play significant roles in the development of obesity?
6 Give two arguments for the "set-point" theory of weight maintenance and two against this theory.
7 When searching for a sound weight-loss program, what three key characteristics would you look for?
8 Define the term *behavior modification*. Relate it to the terms *stimulus control, self-monitoring, chain breaking, relapse prevention,* and *cognitive restructuring*. Give examples of each.
9 Why should the treatment of obesity be viewed as a lifelong commitment rather than just a short episode of weight loss?
10 If a friend or relative told you he or she had found a great new vitamin and mineral supplement that claims to allow the loss of 12 pounds in 2 weeks, how would you respond?

Further Readings

1 Albu J and others: Obesity solutions: report of a meeting, *Nutrition Reviews* 55:150, 1997.
2 Astrup A, Flatt JP: Metabolic determinants of body weight regulation. In Bouchard C, Bray GA editors: *Regulation of body weight: biological and behavioral mechanisms,* Philadelphia, 1996, John Wiley & Sons.
3 Bouchard C: Human variation in body mass: evidence for a role of the genes, *Nutrition Reviews* 55 (1):S21, 1997.
4 Campfield LA and others: Strategies and potential molecular targets for obesity treatment, *Science* 280:1383, 1998.
5 Carek PJ and others: Management of obesity: medical treatment options, *American Family Physician* 55:551, 1997.
6 Comuzzie AG, Allison DB: The seareh for human obesity genes, *Science* 280:1374, 1998.
7 Cupp MJ: Herbal remedies: adverse effects and drug interactions, *American Family Physician* 59:1239, 1999.
8 Expert Panel on the Identification, Evaluation, and Treatment of Overweight in Adults, Clinical guidelines on the identification, evaluation, and treatment of overweight and obesity in adults: executive summary. *American Journal of Clinical Nutrition* 68:899, 1998.
9 Foreyt JP, Poston WSC: Diet, genetics, and obesity, *Food Technology* 51 (3): 70, 1997.
10 Gibbs WW: Gaining on fat, *Scientific American* p. 88, August 1996.
11 Grundy SM: Multifactorial causation of obesity: implications for prevention, *American Journal of Clinical Nutrition* 67 (suppl):563S, 1998.
12 Hill JO, Peters JC: Environmental contributors to the obesity epidemic, *Science* 280:1371, 1998.
13 Hirsch J and others: Diet composition and energy balance in humans, *American Journal of Clinical Nutrition* 67 (suppl):551S, 1998.
14 Klem ML and others: A descriptive study of individuals successful at long term maintenance of substantial weight loss, *American Journal of Clinical Nutrition* 66:239, 1997.
15 National Task Force on the Prevention and Treatment of Obesity: Long-term pharmacotherapy in the management of obesity, *Journal of the American Medical Association* 276:1907, 1996.
16 The Pressure to Eat, *Nutrition Action Health Letter.* p. 1, July/August 1998.
17 Rippe JM, et al. Panel discussion: The obesity epidemic—a mandate for a multidisciplinary approach, *Journal of the American Dietetic Association* 98:S56, 1998.
18 Rolls BJ, Miller DL: Is the low fat message giving people a license to eat more? *Journal of the American College of Nutrition* 16:535, 1997.
19 Rosenbaum M and others: Obesity, *New England Journal of Medicine* 337:396, 1997.
20 Shick SM and others: Persons successful at long-term weight loss and maintenance continue to consume a low energy, low fat diet, *Journal of the American Dietetic Association* 98:408, 1998.
21 Stevens J and others: The effect of age on the association between body mass index and mortality, *New England Journal of Medicine* 338:1, 1998.
22 West DB, York B: Dietary fat, genetic predisposition, and obesity: lessons from animal models, *American Journal of Clinical Nutrition* 67 (suppl):505s, 1998.

RATE

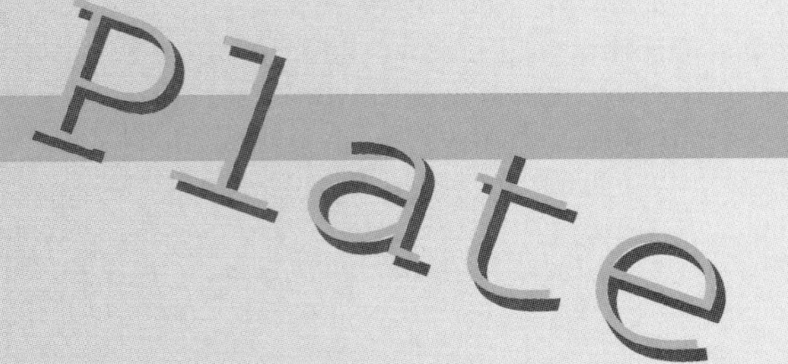

I. A Close Look at Your Weight Status

Determine the following two indices of your body status: body mass index and waist-to-hip ratio.

BODY MASS INDEX (BMI)

Record your weight in pounds: _____ lb.
Divide your weight in pounds by 2.2 to determine your weight in kilograms (kg): _____ kg.
Record your height in inches: _____ in.
Divide your height in inches by 39.3 to determine your height in meters (m): _____ mm.
Calculate your BMI using the following formula:
BMI = Weight (kg)/height(m)^2
BMI = _____ kg/ _____ m^2 = _____

WAIST-TO-HIP RATIO

Use a tape measure to measure the circumference of your waist (at the umbilicus with stomach muscles relaxed) and hips (widest point).
Circumference of waist (umbilicus) = _____ in.
Circumference of hips = _____ in.
Calculate your waist-to-hip ratio using the following formula:
Circumference of waist/circumference of hips
Waist to hip ratio = _____ in/ _____ in = _____

INTERPRETATION

1. **When BMI is greater than 25, health risks from obesity often begin. It is especially advisable to attempt weight loss if your BMI exceeds 30. Does yours exceed 25?**
   Yes _____ No _____
2. **If overweight, a waist-to-hip ratio exceeding 1.0 in men and 0.8 in women indicates upper body fat storage, as does a waist circumference alone of more than 40 inches in men or 35 inches in women. This condition is associated with an increased risk of heart disease, high blood pressure, and Type 2 diabetes.**
   If appropriate, does your ratio or circumference exceed the standard for your gender?
   Yes _____ No _____
3. **Do you feel you need to pursue a program of weight loss?**
   Yes _____ No _____

APPLICATION

From what you've learned in this chapter, what habits could you change in patterns of eating and physical activity to lose some weight and help ensure maintenance of any loss?

____

____

____

II. An Action Plan to Change Weight Status

Now that you have assessed your current weight status, do you feel that you would like to make some changes? Following is a step-by-step guide to behavior change. This process can be useful even for those who are satisfied with their current weight, as it can be applied to changing exercise habits, self-esteem habits, and a variety of other behaviors (Figure 9–13).

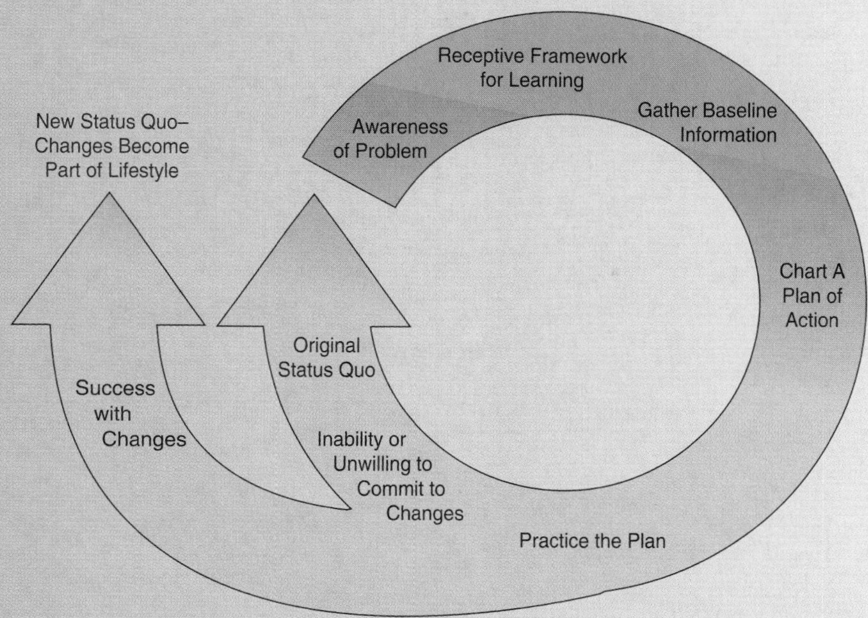

Figure 9–13 *A model for behavior change. It starts with awareness of the problem and ends with the incorporation of new behaviors intended to address the problem.*

BECOMING AWARE OF THE PROBLEM

By calculating your current weight status on the previous page, you have already become aware of the problem, if one exists. From here, it is important to find out more information about the cause of the problem and whether it is worth working toward a change.

1. **Look back at the food diary you completed in Chapter 1. What are some of the factors that most influence your eating habits? Do you eat due to stress, boredom, or feeling depressed? Is volume of food your problem, or do you eat mainly the wrong foods for you? Take some time to assess the root causes of your eating habits.**

2. **Once you have more information about your specific eating practices, you must decide if it is worth changing these practices. A benefits-and-costs analysis can be a useful tool in evaluating whether or not it is worth your effort to make life changes. Use the example below as a guide for listing benefits and costs pertinent to your own situation (Figure 9–14).**

BENEFITS AND COSTS ANALYSIS

1 Benefits of changing eating habits? What do you expect to get, now or later, that you want? What do you get to avoid that would be unpleasant? — *feel better physically and psychologically* — *look better* — — — —	**3 Costs involved in changing eating habits?** What do you have to do that you don't want to do? What do you have to stop doing that you would rather continue doing? — *take time to plan meals and shop* — *must give up some food volume* — —
2 Benefits of not changing eating habits? What do you get to do that you enjoy doing? What do you avoid having to do? — *no need for planning* — *can eat without feeling guilty* — — — —	**4 Costs of not changing eating habits?** What unpleasant or undesirable effects are you likely to experience now or in the future? What are you likely to lose? — *creeping weight gain* — *low self-esteem and poor health* — — —

Figure 9–14 *Benefits and costs analysis applied to increasing physical activity. This process helps put behavior change into the context of total lifestyle.*

SETTING GOALS

What can we accomplish, and how long will it take? Setting a realistic, achievable goal and allowing a reasonable amount of time to pursue it increase the likelihood of success.

1. **Begin by determining the final outcome you would like to achieve. If you are trying to change your eating behaviors to be more healthy, list your reasons for doing so (e.g., overall health, weight loss, self-esteem).**

   Overall goal:

   ____

   ____

   ____

   Reasons to pursue goal:

   ____

   ____

   ____

2. **Now list several steps that will be necessary to achieve your goal. Keep in mind, however, that it is generally best to change only a few specific behaviors at first—walking briskly for 30 minutes 5 times a week, lowering fat intake, using more whole-grain products, and not eating after 7 PM. Attempting small and perhaps easier dietary changes first reduces the scope of the problem and can increase the likelihood of success.**

Steps toward achieving goal:

1. ____
2. ____
3. ____

Note that if you are having trouble deciphering the steps needed to achieve your goal, health professionals are an excellent resource for aid in planning.

MEASURING COMMITMENT

Now that you have collected information and know what is required to reach your goal, you must ask yourself: "Can I do this?" Commitment is an essential component in the success of behavior change. Be honest with yourself. Permanent change is not quick or easy. Once you have decided that you have the commitment required to see this through, continue on to the following sections.

MAKING IT OFFICIAL WITH A CONTRACT

Drawing up a behavior contract often adds incentive to follow through with a plan. The contract could list goal behaviors and objectives, milestones for measuring progress, and regular rewards for meeting the terms of the contract. After finishing a contract, you should sign it in the presence of some friends. This encourages commitment.

Initially plans should reward positive behaviors, and then they should focus on positive results. Positive behaviors, such as regular physical activity, eventually lead to positive outcomes, such as increased stamina.

Below is a sample contract for increasing physical activity (Figure 9–15). Use the blank contract to set up your own incentives. Keep in mind that this sample contract is only a suggestion; you can add your own ideas as well.

Name Alan Young

Goal

I agree to ride my exercise bike
(specify behavior)

under the following circumstances for 30 minutes, 4 times per week
(specify where, when, how much, etc.)
in the evening

Substitute behavior and/or reinforcement schedule I will reinforce myself if I've achieved my goal after a month with a weekend off campus with my roommate.

Environmental planning

In order to help me do this, I am going to (1) arrange my physical and social environment by buying a new jogging suit at the local sporting goods Store

and (2) control my internal environment (thoughts, images) by coordinating riding the bike with the first T.V. watching I do in the evening

Reinforcements

Reinforcements provided by me daily or weekly (if contract is kept):
I will buy myself a new piece of clothing for off campus trip

Reinforcements provided by others daily or weekly (if contract is kept):
at the end of a month if I've completed my goal my parents will buy me a fitness club membership for winter.

Social support

Behavior change is more likely to take place when other people support you. During the quarter/semester please meet with the other person at least three times to discuss your progress.

The name of my "significant helper" is: Mr. and Mrs. Young

This contract should include:

1. Baseline data (one week)
2. Well-defined goal
3. Simple method for charting progress (diary, counter, charts, etc.)
4. Reinforcements (immediate and long-term)
5. Evaluation method (summary of experiences, success, and/or new learnings about self).

Figure 9–15 *Alan's behavior contract. Completing such a contract can help generate commitment to behavior change. What would your contract look like? You'll have a chance to develop one in the Rate Your Plate section later in the chapter.*

PSYCHING YOURSELF UP

Once your contract is in place, you need to "psych yourself up." Discouragement from peers and your own temptations to stray from your plan need to be anticipated. "Psyching yourself up" can enable you to progress toward your goals in spite of others' attitudes and opinions. Almost everyone benefits from some assertiveness training when it comes to changing behaviors. Here are a few suggestions; can you think of any others?

- **No one's feelings should be hurt if you say, "No, thank you," firmly and repeatedly when others try to dissuade you from a plan. Rather, ask them—and yourself—why they want you to eat their way. Your needs are as important as anyone else's.**
- **You don't have to eat a lot to accommodate anyone—your mother, business clients, or the chef. For example, at a party with friends you may feel you have to eat a lot to participate, but you don't. Another trap is ordering a lot just because someone else is paying for the meal.**
- **Learn ways to handle "put-downs"—inadvertent or conscious. An ettective response can be to communicate feelings honestly, without hostility. Tell criticizers that they have annoyed or offended you; that you are working to change your habits and would really like understanding and support from them.**

PRACTICING THE PLAN

Once you've set up a plan, the next step is to implement it. Start with a trial of at least 6 to 8 weeks. Thinking of a lifetime commitment can be overwhelming. Aim for a total duration of 6 months of new activities before giving up. More than once we may have to persuade ourselves of the value of continuing the program. Here are some suggestions to help keep a plan on track:

- ***Focus on reducing, but not necessarily extinguishing, undesirable behaviors.* For example, it's usually unrealistic to say "I'll never eat a certain food again." Better to say "I won't eat that *problem* food as regularly as before."**
- ***Monitor progress.* Note your progress in a diary and reward yourself according to your contract. While conquering some habits and seeing improvement, you may find yourself quite encouraged, even enthusiastic, about your plan of action. That can give you the impetus to move ahead with the program.**
- ***Control environments.* In the early phases of behavior change, try to avoid problem situations, such as parties, coffee breaks, and favorite restaurants. Once new habits are firmly established, you can probably more successfully resist the temptations in these environments.**

REEVALUATION AND PREVENTING RELAPSE

After practicing a program for several weeks to months, it is important to reassess the original plan. In addition, you may now be able to pinpoint other problem areas for which you need to appropriately plan.

1. Begin by taking a close and critical look at your original plan. Does it actually lead to the goals you set? Are there any new steps toward your goal that you feel capable of adding to your contract? Do you need new reinforcements? It may even be necessary to make a new contract. For permanent change, it is worth this time of reassessment.
2. In practicing your plan over the past weeks or months, you have likely experienced relapses. What triggered these relapses? To prevent a total retreat to your old habits, it is important to set up a plan for such relapses. You can do this by identifying high-risk situations, rehearsing a response, and remembering your goals.

You may have noticed a behavior chain in some of your relapses. That is, the relapse may stem from a series of interconnected habitual activities. The way to break the chain is to first identify the activities, pinpoint the weak links, break those links, and substitute other behaviors. Following is a sample behavior chain and a substitute activity list. Consider compiling your own list based on your behavior chains (Figure 9–16).

EPILOGUE

If you have utilized the activities in this section, you are well on your way to permanent behavior change. Recall that this exercise can be used for a variety of desired changes, from quitting smoking, increasing physical activity, or improving study habits. It is by no means an easy process, but the results can be well worth the effort. Overall, the keys to success are motivation (keeping the problem in the forefront of your mind), having a plan of action, securing the resources and skills needed for success, and looking for help from family, friends or a group.

ALTERNATIVE ACTIVITY SHEET

SUBSTITUTE ACTIVITIES

Pleasant activities	1. Singing/washing hair
	2. Reading comics/biking
	3. Sewing/calling a friend
Necessary activities	1. Ironing
	2. Vacuuming
	3. Straightening apartment
Situations when used	1. Wanted ice cream—delayed with bath
	2. Wanted wheat thins—cleaned up apt.
	3. Wanted snack—went for walk
	4. Wanted cookies—did dishes first
	5. Saw leftovers—went for bike ride
	6. Tempted by cookies—set timer
	7. Wanted snack—read comics

BEHAVIOR CHAIN

Identify the links in your eating response chain on the following diagram. Draw a line through the chain where it was interrupted. Add the link you substituted and the new chain of behavior this substitution started.

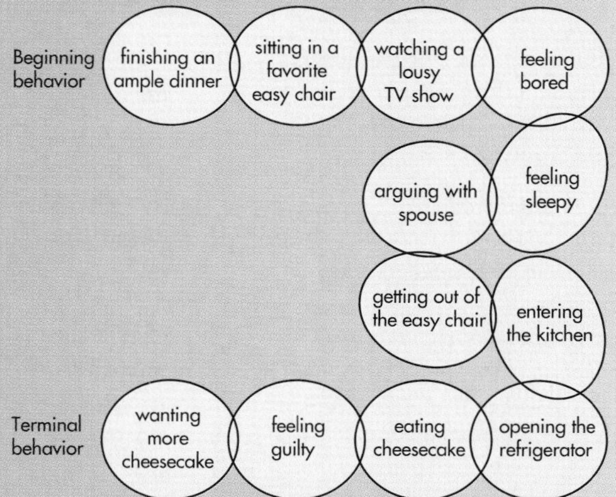

Figure 9–16 *Identifying behavior chains. This is a good tool for understanding more about your habits and pinpointing ways to change unwanted habits. The earlier in the chain you substitute a nonfood link, the easier it is to intervene. Four types of behaviors can be substituted in an ongoing behavior chain.*

1. *Fun activities (taking a walk, reading a book)*
2. *Necessary activities (cleaning a room, balancing your checkbook)*
3. *Incompatible activities (taking a shower)*
4. *Urge-delaying activities (setting a kitchen timer for 20 minutes before allowing yourself to eat)*

Using activities to interrupt behavior patterns that lead to inappropriate eating (or inactivity) can be a powerful means of changing eating habits.

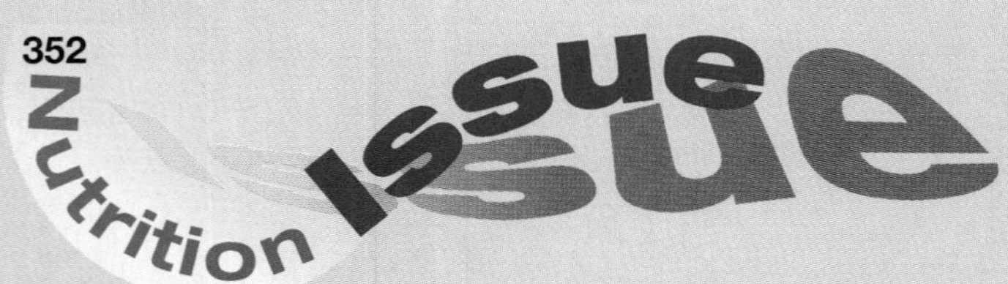

Fad Diets—Why All the Commotion?

Many overweight people try to help themselves by using the latest fad diet book. But as you will see, in the long run most of these diets do not help, and some can actually harm those who follow them (Table 9–8).

You may wonder why fad diet books and dubious weight-loss products marketed through infomercials exist at all. Why doesn't government put a stop to them? Many contain blatant misinformation. However, FDA concerns itself only when products are suspected of doing serious harm, as in the case of earlier forms of liquid protein diets. Overall, ancient advice is still valid: "Let the buyer beware." In addition, FDA does not have enough staff to pursue each new fad diet or investigate each new outrageous product claim. Still, it is illegal in the United States to falsely represent worthless or dangerous cures and medical devices. Thus U.S. citizens can use their rights under federal law to have FDA pursue a seller of a dangerous fad diet book or weight-loss product in an attempt to have it removed from the market.

HOW TO RECOGNIZE A FAD DIET

Earlier in this chapter are listed criteria for evaluating weight-loss programs with regard to their safety and effectiveness. In contrast, fad diets typically share some different common characteristics. Here are a few:

1. They promote quick weight loss. As mentioned before, this loss primarily results from glycogen, sodium, and lean muscle mass depletion. All lead to a loss of body water.
2. They limit food selections and dictate specific rituals, such as eating only fruit for breakfast or cabbage soup every day. The limited selection itself is the reason weight loss occurs. Any diet that causes one to eat less calories than expended will work.
3. They use testimonials from famous people and tie the diet to well-known cities, such as Beverly Hills and New York.
4. They bill themselves as "cure-alls." These diets claim to work for everyone, whatever the type of obesity or whatever the person's specific strengths and weaknesses.
5. They often recommend expensive supplements. Some of these supplements can be harmful because of high doses of vitamin A, vitamin D, or vitamin B-6.
6. No attempts are made at long-term behavior change. Dieters follow the diet until the desired weight is reached and then revert to old eating habits—they are told to eat rice for a month, lose weight, and then return to old habits.
7. They are generally critical of the scientific community, suggesting that physicians and registered dieticians do not really want people to lose weight. They encourage people to look outside the medical establishment for correct advice.

Probably the cruelest characteristic of fad diets is that they essentially guarantee failure for the dieter. These diets are not designed for permanent weight loss. Habits are not changed, and the food selection is so limited that the person cannot follow the diet in the long run. Although dieters assume they have lost fat, they have actually lost mostly muscle and other lean tissue mass. As soon as they begin eating normally again, the lost tissue is replaced. In a matter of weeks, most of the lost weight will come back. The dieter appears to have failed, when actually the diet has failed. This whole scenario can add more blame and guilt, challenging the self-worth of the dieter—and that is very unfortunate. If someone needs help losing weight, professional help is advised. Sound nutrition, regular physical activity, and behavior change are the only interventions that come close to offering hope for weight loss and later weight management, something fad diets rarely offer.

TYPES OF FAD DIETS

Low- or Restricted-Carbohydrate Approaches

This is the most common form of fad diet. The low carbohydrate intake forces the liver to produce needed glucose. The source of carbons for this glucose is mostly protein tissue. Thus a low carbohydrate diet results in protein tissue loss, as well as urinary loss of essential ions, such as potassium. Since protein tissue is mostly water, the dieter loses weight very rapidly. When a normal diet is resumed, the protein tissue is rebuilt and the weight is regained.

Diet plans that use a low-carbohydrate approach are the Dr. Atkins' Diet Revolution, Dr. Stillman's Calories Don't Count Diet, the Scarsdale Diet, the Drinking Man's Diet, Four Day Wonder Diet, and the Air Force Diet. When you see a new fad diet advertisement, look first to see how much carbohydrate it contains. If breads, cereals, fruits, and vegetables are extremely limited, you are probably looking at a low- or restricted-carbohydrate diet.

Low-Fat Approaches

The very-low-fat diet turns out to be a very-high-carbohydrate diet. These diets contain approximately 5% to 10% of energy intake as fat. The most notable is the Pritikin Diet. This approach is not harmful for healthy adults, but it is extremely difficult to follow. People get bored with this type of diet very quickly because they can't eat many of their favorite foods. Dieters primarily eat grains, fruits, and vegetables, which most people cannot do for very long. Eventually the person wants some foods higher in fat or protein. These diets are just too different from the typical American diet for most of us to follow consistently. A popular diet marketed recently, the T-Factor Diet, focuses on restricting fat but is a more moderate approach than the Pritikin diet.

Novelty Diets

A variety of fad diets are built on gimmicks. A rice diet was designed in the 1940s to lower blood pressure; now it has resurfaced as a weight-loss diet. The first phase consists of eating only rice and fruit until you can't stand them any longer. On the Beverly Hills Diet, you eat mostly fruit. Sugar Busters foscuses on the evils of sucrose.

In the last few years a number of diets have become popularized that also focus on reducing carbohydrate intake. The recommended carbohydrate intake is about two-thirds of what most experts recommend (40% versus 60% of calories). The premise is that higher carbohydrate intakes cause excessive insulin output by the body, and this in turn encourages fat storage. Actually eating just about anything causes insulin production. If people have success on these diets, such as *The Zone* or *Protein Power,* it is because the plans are also low in calories. If a person believes enough in a plan such that it provides the motivation to control food intake, any diet will be successful in the short-run. Overall, there is no magic diet prescription that guarantees weight loss: calorie intake in comparison to energy expenditure is an unescapable reality.

The rationale behind these diets is that you can eat only fruit or rice for just so long before becoming bored and, in theory, reducing your energy intake. However, chances are that you will abandon the diet entirely before losing much weight. And even if you continue the diet for a sufficient time period, you will likely regain the weight upon resuming previous eating patterns.

The most bizarre of the novelty diets proposes that "food gets stuck in your body." Fit for Life, the Beverly Hills Diet, and the Eat Great, Lose Weight are examples. The supposition is that food gets stuck in the intestine, putrefies, and creates toxins that invade the blood and cause disease. This is utter nonsense. Nevertheless, the same idea has been promoted in health-food books since the 1800s. Today, Fit for Life suggests that meat eaten with potatoes is not digested and that fresh fruit should be consumed only before noon. These recommendations are absurd. They are gimmicks that appear controversial but are really designed to sell books.

QUACKERY IS CHARACTERISTIC OF FAD DIETS

Fad diets fall under the category of quackery, people taking advantage of others. They usually involve a product or service that costs a considerable amount of money. Often those offering the product or service don't realize that they are promoting quackery, because they were victims themselves. For example, they tried the product and by pure coincidence it worked for them, so they are eager to sell it to all their friends and relatives.

Recent examples of dubious recommendations in the field of weight loss are herbal laxative teas and chromium picolinate. These laxative teas, many of which have oriental-type labels, contain senna, which induces diarrhea. However, this diarrhea does not sufficiently reduce the absorption of calories from the diet. FDA is concerned that these teas may also result in serious injury or death linked to the diarrhea and related intestinal damage that is induced. To date, these teas are linked to the deaths of four young women.

Chromium picolinate, a nutritional supplement, has been touted as an aid for reducing body fat, increasing lean body mass, suppressing hunger, and increasing metabolic rate. However, chromium picolinate has not been approved for weight loss by FDA, nor has the agency seen any convincing data on the claims being made (see Chapter 8).

Numerous other gimmicks for weight loss have come and gone and are likely to resurface. If in the future an important aid for weight loss is discovered, you can feel confident that major journals, such as the *Journal of the American Dietetic Association,* the *Journal of the American Medical Association,* or the *New England Journal of Medicine,* will report it. You don't need to rely on paperback books, newspaper advertisements, or infomercials for new breakthroughs about weight loss (see Figure 9–14).

Usually, quackery harms only the bank account. However, it can lead to life-threatening results. The rule of thumb upon seeing a new diet aid on the market is that if it sounds too good to be true, it is.

TABLE 9-8

Summary of Popular Diet Approaches to Weight Control for the General Public

Approach and examples*	Characteristics and possible negative health consequences
MODERATE CALORIE RESTRICTION	
The Complete Idiot's Guide to Losing Weight	
The Setpoint Diet	Usually 1200–1800 kcal per day, with moderate fat intake
Slim Chance in a Fat World	Reasonable balance of macronutrients
Weight Watcher's Diet	Encourage exercise
The American Heart Association Diet	May employ behavioral approach
Mary Ellen's Help Yourself Diet Plan	
The Beyond Diet	Acceptable if vitamin and mineral supplement is used when energy intake is low and permission of primary physician is granted
The Solution	
Staying Thin	
Nutripoints	
The Good Calorie Diet	
The Callaway Diet	
Living Without Dieting	
Fast Food Diet	
50 Ways to Lose Your Blubber	
Take It Off. Keep It Off	
Make the Connection	
MACRONUTRIENT RESTRICTION	
Low or restricted carbohydrate	
Low:	
Dr. Atkins' Diet Revolution	Generally less than 100 grams of carbohydrate per day
Calories Don't Count	
Wild Weekend Diet	Ketosis; reduced exercise capacity due to poor glycogen stores in the muscles; excessive animal fat intake.
Restricted:	
Miracle Diet for Fast Weight Loss	
Drinking Man's Diet	
Woman Doctor's Diet for Women	
The Doctor's Quick Weight Loss Diet	
The Complete Scarsdale Medical Diet	
Four Day Wonder Diet	
Endocrine Control Diet	
Air Force Diet	
The Zone (and related plans)	
Protein Power	
The Five-Day Miracle Diet	
Healthy for Life	
Low fat	
The Rice Diet Report	Less than 20% of energy from fat
The Macrobiotic Diet (some versions)	Limited (or elimination of) animal protein sources; also all fats, nuts, seeds
The Pritikin Diet	
The Tokyo Diet	
The Palm Beach Lifelong Diet	Little satiety; flatulence; possibly poor mineral absorption from excess dietary fiber; limited food choices sometimes leads to deprivation
The James Coco Diet	Not necessarily to be avoided, but certain aspects of the plan possibly unacceptable
The 35+ Diet	

*Diets may be listed in more than one category if multiple characteristics apply.

TABLE 9-8—cont'd

Summary of Popular Diet Approaches to Weight Control for the General Public

Approach and examples*	Characteristics and possible negative health consequences
7-Week Victory Diet Fat to Muscle Diet T-Factor Diet Fit or Fat Two Day Diet Complete Hip and Thigh Diet The Maximum Metabolism Diet The Pasta Diet The McDougall Plan Ultrafit Diet Stop the Insanity G-Index Diet Eat More, Weigh Less Outsmarting the Female Fat Cell Foods that Cause You to Lose Weight Lean Bodies	
NOVELTY DIETS	
Dr. Abravenel's Body Type and Lifetime Nutrition Plan (or his other books)	Promotes certain nutrients, foods, or combinations of foods as having unique, magical, or previously undiscovered qualities Malnutrition; no change in habits leads to relapse; unrealistic food choices lead to possible bingeing
Sugar Busters Fit for Life The Rotation Diet The Hilton Head Metabolism Diet The Junk Food Diet The Beverly Hills Diet Dr. Debetz Champagne Diet Sun Sign Diet F-Plan Diet Fat Attack Plan Popcorn Plus Diet Jean Simpson's Numbers Diet Autohypnosis Diet The Ultrafit Diet The Princeton Diet The Diet Bible Bloomingdale's Diet The Love Diet Eat to Succeed The Underburner's Diet Eat to Win Two Day Diet Paris Diet Cabbage-Soup Diet Eat Great, Lose Weight Eat Smart, Think Smart *Scent*sational Weight Loss Eat Right for Your Body Type	

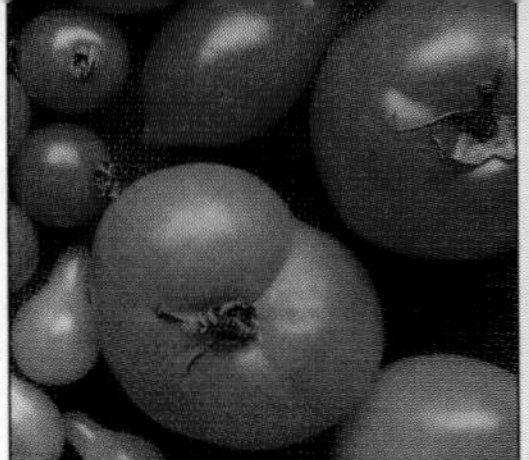

chapter 10

Nutrition
Fitness and Sports

Your muscles and organs use a lot of energy when you dash across the street or smash a backhand across the net. Have you wondered what your body does to transform food into this energy? Understanding where this energy comes from and how it is used is fascinating even if you don't compete in sports.

Then, once your muscles have energy available to them, what determines the type of fuel they use? *You* do, to an extent, depending on how physically fit you are and how hard you perform. Physical fitness, defined as the ability to do moderate to vigorous activity without undue fatigue, affects your fuel use. Diet also has an effect, especially for athletes who expend 2000 or more kcal per day in physical activity.

In this chapter, you will also discover how physical fitness benefits the entire body; it is an essential ingredient in achieving maximal health. Another basic reason to be physically fit is, of course, that it's fun and it feels good. Some people are active simply because they enjoy it, whether they're swimming, playing basketball, or engaging in any of innumerable other activities. Let's now look further at nutrition as it relates to fitness.

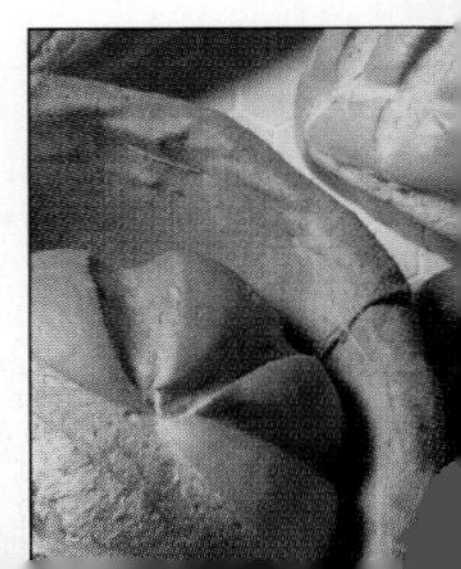

Nutrition Web

Nutrient intake affects one's ability to perform physical activity. Physical activity, in turn, affects nutrient use by the body.

Anyone who exercises regularly should focus one's diet on foods moderate to high in carbohydrates as part of the Food Guide Pyramid.

Athletes should consume enough fluid to minimize loss of body weight and ultimately restore preexercise weight. Sports drinks aid fluid, electrolyte, and carbohydrate replacement. Their use should be considered when continuous activity is expected to last beyond 60 minutes.

Most athletes meet vitamin and mineral needs by the sheer volume of food consumed. Some female athletes are at risk for inadequate iron and calcium intake.

Rather than waiting for a "magic bullet" to enhance performance, athletes should concentrate their efforts on improving training routines and sport technique and consuming well-balanced diets. Adequate fluid and carbohydrate are the primary diet-related ergogenic (work-producing) aids.

A minimum plan for physical activity includes a total of at least 30 minutes per day. A more intense program should begin with warm-up exercises to increase blood flow and warm the muscles and end with cooldown activities. Adding both stretching and resistance exercises complements this more intense program.

At rest and during light activity, muscle cells mainly use fat for fuel, forming carbon dioxide (CO_2) and water (H_2O). For intense exercise of brief duration, muscles use mostly phosphocreatine (PCr) for energy. During more sustained intense activity, carbohydrate use predominates, breaking down to form lactic acid.

For endurance exercise, a mixture of both fat and carbohydrate is used as fuels: carbohydrate is used increasingly as activity intensifies. Little protein is used to fuel muscles.

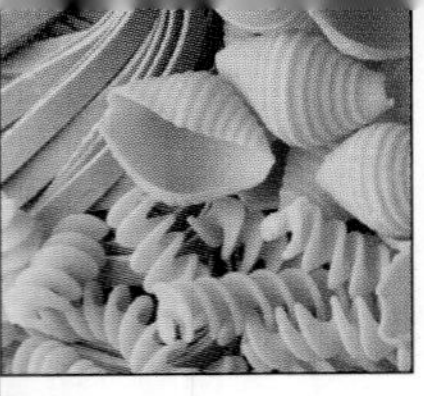

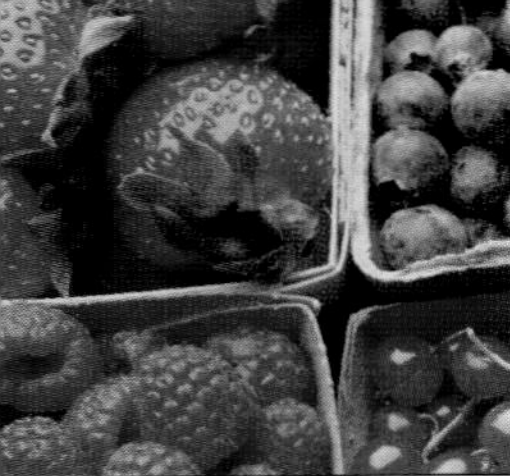

The Close Relationship Between Nutrition and Fitness

The ability to engage routinely in vigorous physical activity requires good health. The ability to perform also depends on a nutritious diet. Adequate fluid and carbohydrate intakes are especially important for enhancing athletic performance.

The benefits of regular physical activity are many: improvement in several aspects of heart function, fewer injuries, better sleep habits and immune function; and improvement in body composition (less body fat, more bone and muscle mass). Physical activity can also reduce stress and positively affect blood pressure and blood glucose regulation. In addition, it aids in weight control and later weight maintenance by increasing overall energy expenditure (Table 10–1).

For the most part, nutrition influences physical activity, and physical activity influences nutrient use and general health. Unfortunately, as noted in Chapter 9, many American adults lead sedentary lives. Did that discussion motivate you to assess your activity patterns and improve them as needed? In other words, will you avoid being simply a spectator throughout your life (Figure 10–1)?

cathy®
by Cathy Guisewite
NO VISIBLE PROGRESS. NO INCREASED STRENGTH.
NO CHEERING CROWD. NO PROUD COACH.
JUST ME, ALONE IN THE LIVING ROOM, WITH ONE SORE MUSCLE SOMEWHERE UNDER THE FAT AND SOME CHEERY PROMISES WRITTEN ON THE SIDE OF A CARDBOARD BOX.
SAY WHAT THEY WILL ABOUT OLYMPIC ATHLETES, THE REAL MEDALS SHOULD GO TO THOSE WHO GET OUT THE AB MACHINE ON DAY TWO.
AB MASTER

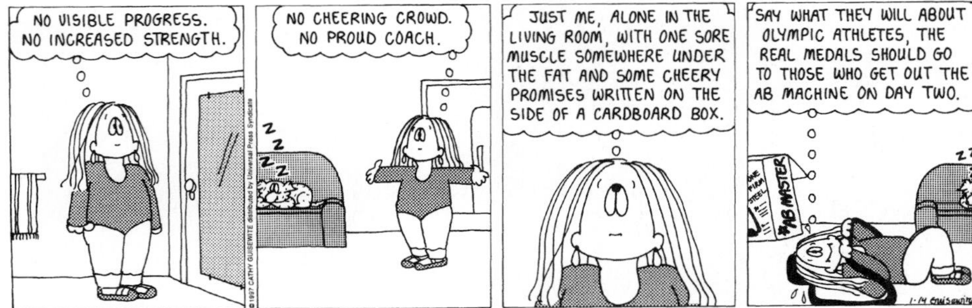

Figure 10–1 *Cathy.*

Applying diet principles to physical activity

Variety: Enjoy many different activities to exercise different muscles.
Balance: Different activities have different benefits, so balance your exercise pattern. For overall fitness, you need exercises that build cardiovascular endurance, muscular strength, and flexibility.
Moderation: Exercise to keep fit without overdoing it. You don't need a heavy workout every day to achieve fitness.

Designing a Fitness Program

For healthy people, a gradual increase to a goal of regular physical activity is recommended. People who are 35 years or older, who have been inactive for many years, or who have an existing health problem should talk to a physician before increasing activity. Health problems that require medical evaluation before beginning an exercise program are obesity, heart disease (or family history of it), high blood pressure, diabetes (or family history), shortness of breath after mild exertion, and arthritis.

Phase 1: Getting Started Means Getting Going

During the first phase of a fitness program, one should begin to incorporate short periods of physical activity into the daily routine. This includes walking, some stair climbing, house cleaning, gardening, and other activities that cause you to "huff and puff" a bit. The goal is a total of 30 minutes of this moderate type of physical activity each day—broken up if need be into increments lasting at least 10 minutes—expending an average of 200 total kcal (see Table 9–6 in the last chapter). Experts suggest starting small, building up to a total of 30 minutes of activity incorporated

TABLE 10-1

Exercise Is Medicine—The Benefits of Regular, Moderate Physical Activity

Cardiovascular health	Increases heart strength and overall cardiovascular function, which decreases chance of developing heart disease. Helps maintain healthy blood pressure. Can increase HDL and lower triglycerides in the blood.
Obesity	Helps maintain lean tissue and promotes loss of fat tissue. Assists in better control of appetite and increases energy expenditure. Helps prevent or reverse development of diseases associated with obesity, including Type 2 diabetes, high blood pressure, and heart disease, even if one can't attain a more healthy weight.
Diabetes	Enhances the action of the hormone insulin, which in turn increases glucose uptake by cells. Contributes to energy balance, which decreases risk of Type 2 diabetes and related complications.
Osteoporosis	Helps strengthen bones and contributes to agility and joint health, which can reduce both the likelihood of falls and injuries caused by falls.
Infections	Reduces susceptibility of respiratory and other infections by enhancing various functions of the immune system.
Cancer	Reduces risk of colon cancer, and possibly breast cancer.
Psychological health	Reduces depression, anxiety, and mental stress, while enhancing a sense of well-being and self image, and improving sleep patterns.

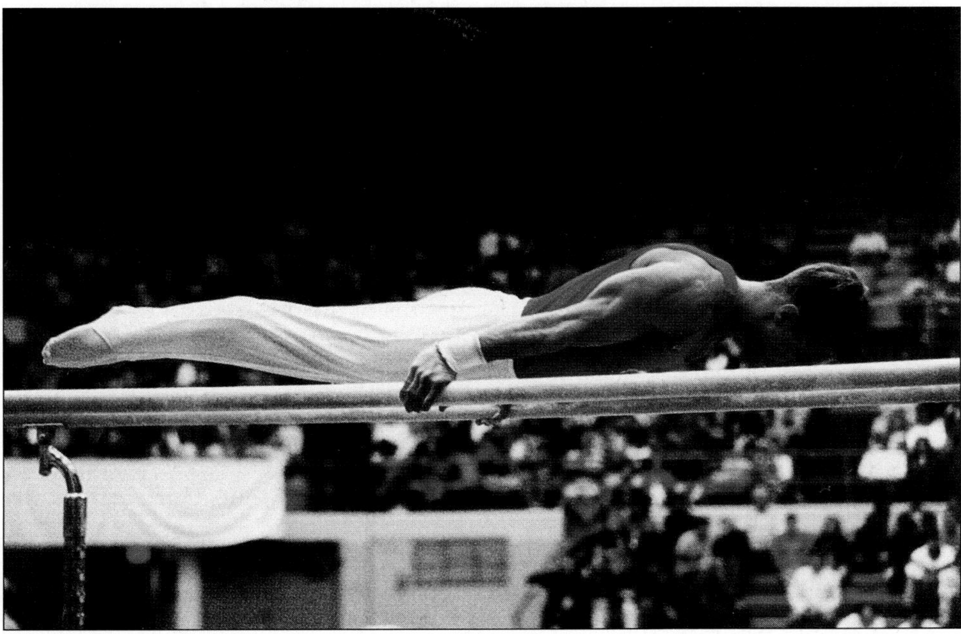

Athletic success hinges on natural ability and training. Meeting nutrient needs supports this effort.

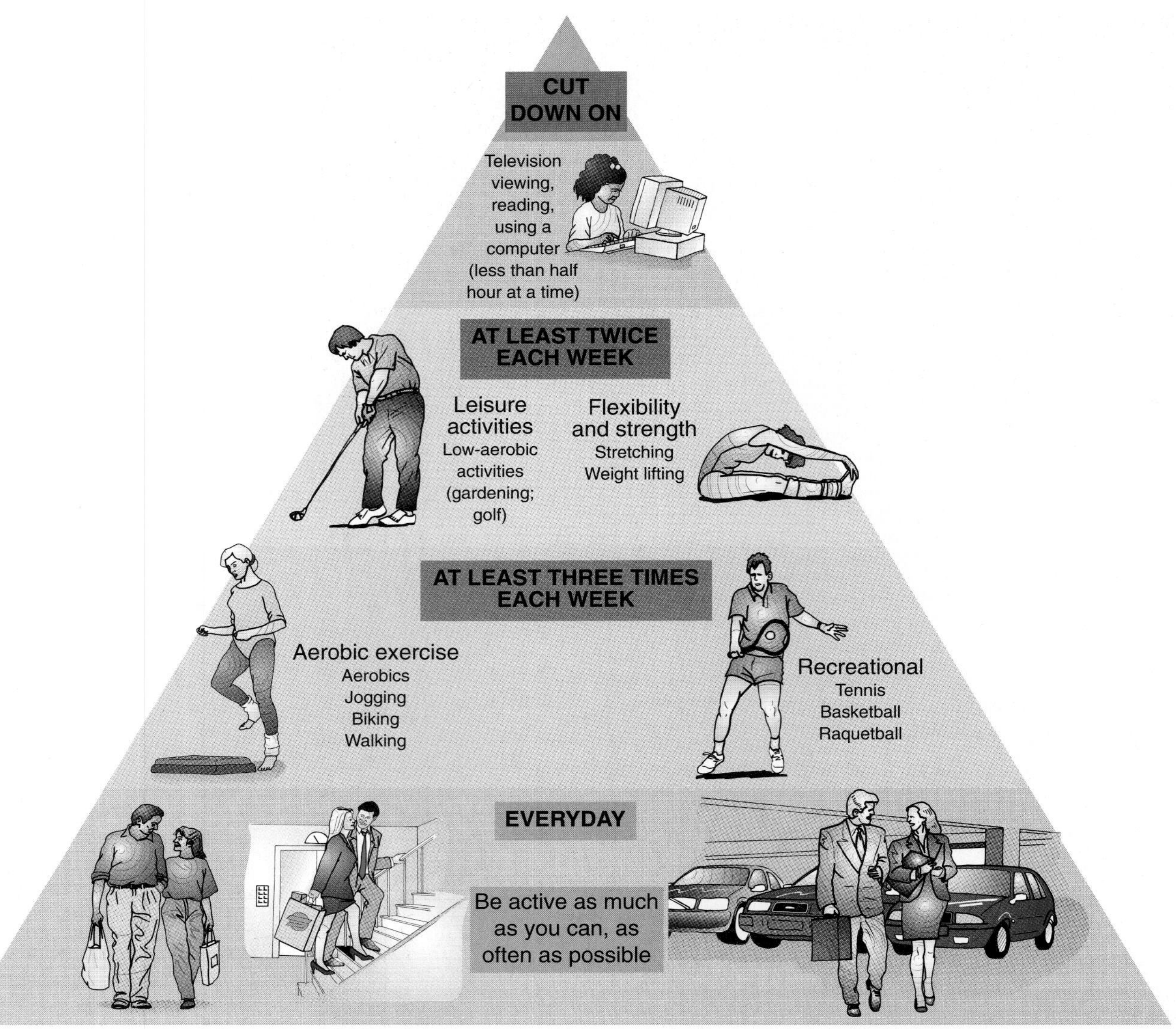

Figure 10–2 *Using the concept of the Food Guide Pyramid, health educators at Park Nicollet Medical Foundation in Minneapolis have created an easy reference—the Physical Activity Pyramid. The recommendations in the pyramid are based on American College of Sports Medicine guidelines.*

into each day's tasks. If there is not much time for activity, one can go for more intensity in the activities that can fit in to get the same benefits (Figure 10–2). Note that only about 1 in 10 adults practices vigorous activities daily, and about half of all adults quit their exercise plan within 3 months of the onset.

The easiest way to increase physical activity is to make it part of a daily routine, similar to other regular activities, such as eating. One does not need to join a gym or attend aerobic classes. Daily activities can meet the Phase 1 goal. Many people find that the best time to exercise is when they need an energy pick-me-up or a break from work. Rather than abandon an exercise program entirely when obstacles impede, one can strive to use any small periods of available time. Once reaping the benefits of exercise, a person will tend to spend more time at it.

Clearly, many of the activities recommended for Phase 1 are not very vigorous. By recommending Phase 1 for those starting an exercise program, fitness experts have not given up on the value of more vigorous physical activity. They're just making concessions to human nature.

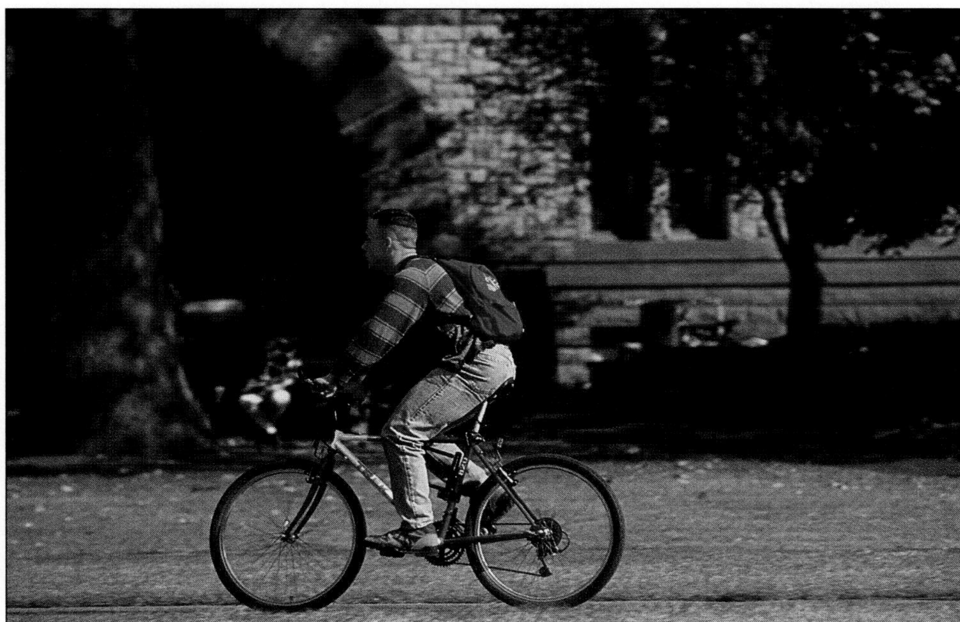

What is the best exercise? One you enjoy.

Phase 2: Seeking Greater Fitness Requires Greater Exertion

Once one can perform regular moderate-intensity activity, attention should turn to more intense activities to reap even more health benefits. Suggested activities include brisk walking, jogging, cycling, and swimming. Based on the latest American College of Sports Medicine guidelines, the goal is 20 to 60 minutes of such vigorous activity 3 to 5 days per week. Some resistance exercise, (for example, push-ups, sit-ups, resistance machines, and weight training) should also be performed 2 to 3 days per week, with a day's rest between each session. Pushing a little past fatigue in these more vigorous exercises of Phase 2 is fine, but when arms or legs start shaking uncontrollably, it's time to ease up. Ignoring pain can almost guarantee an injury. Finally, add some stretching exercises to the routine 2 to 3 days per week.

This basic exercise program should begin with warm-up exercises and stretching, this increases blood flow and warms the muscles. Warming up reduces the risk of injuries. Activities to increase muscular strength, endurance, and flexibility should follow. Cooldown and more stretching exercises finish the program (Table 10–2).

Fitness target heart rates for adults are about 55% to 90% of predicted maximum heart rate (220 minus current age).

Can you pass the U.S. military minimum fitness standards?

25-year-old males: 40 push-ups, 50 sit-ups, and 2 miles in 16:36.

25-year-old females: 17 push-ups, 50 sit-ups, and 2 miles in 19:36.

35-year-old males: 34 push-ups, 38 sit-ups, and 2 miles in 18:18.

35-year-old females: 13 push-ups, 38 sit-ups, and 2 miles in 22:42.

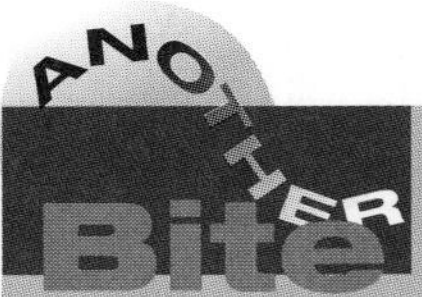

To determine whether you are in the target exercise zone, learn to count your pulse. Placing a hand over your heart is a simple method. However, because clothing may obscure the beat, putting light pressure on either large artery at the side of your neck is best. You can also feel a full pulse at your wrist or inside the bend of the elbow. Count your pulse immediately after stopping exercise because the rate changes very quickly once exercise slows or stops. Find the beat within a second, and count for 10 seconds. Multiply this number by 6 to obtain the count for a full minute. Do not count beyond this because the fall-off rate after exercise is too fast.

TABLE 10-2

Phase 2 Activity Prescription

Warm-up	5–10 minutes of stretching the whole torso. Start with smaller muscle groups (arms) and work toward larger muscle groups (legs and abdomen). 5–10 minutes more of low-intensity exercises, such as walking, slow jogging, or any slow version of anticipated activity. This warms up muscles so that muscle filaments slide more easily over one another and will gradually bring heart rate up to target range.
Workout	20–60 minutes of rhythmic continuous activity at a pace that raises heart rate to within target range. Modify pace or workload as necessary so that the heart rate reaches and does not exceed target range. A good rule of thumb is that one should still be able to converse. Popular aerobic conditioning activities include brisk walking, jogging, swimming, cycling, cross-country skiing, and aerobic dance. Exercises that develop muscular strength and endurance can follow this activity, or alternate with it on different days. These resistance exercises, such as weight training, encourage muscle maintenance and should be done about 2–3 times per week. One set of 8–15 repetitions per exercise is sufficient. Once this is possible, the weight (or resistance) should be increased.
Cooldown	Follow a reverse pattern of warm-up: 5–10 minutes of low-intensity activity and 5–10 minutes of stretching. The same exercises performed during warm-up are appropriate. The cooldown is essential to the prevention of injury and soreness.

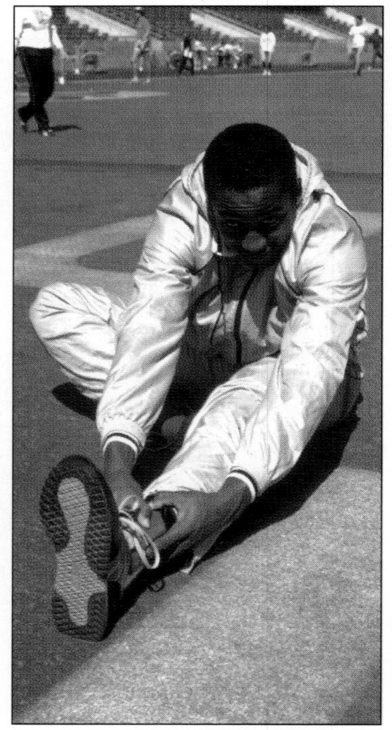

Stretching should be part of warm-up and cooldown activities.

Including several types of enjoyable physical activities in a fitness program is important, as is making sure to start gradually and work up to longer times. Doing too much too soon is a quick way to extinguish enthusiasm and determination. A new trend in exercising is cross-training, in which a variety of exercises are incorporated into a fitness program. For example, 30 minutes of jogging one day might be followed by swimming the next day. Adding variety to a program not only keeps one mentally fresh but also strengthens different muscle groups and reduces risk of injury. This also keeps the program interesting. An exercise partner may offer additional motivation.

Vigorous programs for overweight people should be non-weight-bearing activities, such as swimming, water aerobics, and bicycling. Note also that even if weight loss is not possible, overweight people still benefit from regular physical activity.

Whatever physical activities you choose to include in your fitness program, they should be enjoyable and done regularly and willingly. This way they can become routine. Consider convenience, cost, and options for bad weather so that when motivation wanes, you are not adding further obstacles. Overall, do what you enjoy, but start out small, committing to keep on track and maintaining reasonable expectations. Positive results may take a month or so to be noticeable.

Realize also that harmful side effects may accompany excessive physical activity. The list of complications includes an increased risk of muscular-skeletal injuries, heat illness, sudden death, respiratory infections, gastrointestinal problems, and disturbances in mood and sleeping habits, not to mention impaired performance. These complications are most common in competitive runners, swimmers, and cyclists. Still, although prolonged vigorous exercise poses some health risks, far greater risks exist for those who are and remain primarily sedentary.

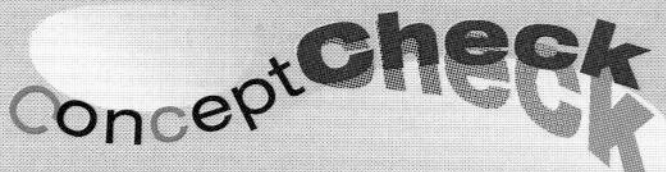

Regular physical activity is a vital part of a healthy lifestyle, ideally constituting a total of at least 30 minutes per day. Including some resistance and stretching activities adds further benefits. People over 35 years should first discuss plans with a physician. Physically active people show lower risks of heart disease, diabetes, obesity, and other common chronic diseases.

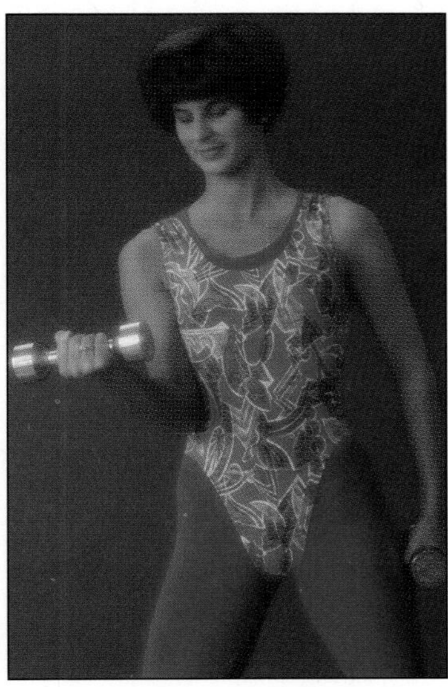

Resistance activities complement more aerobic activities, rounding out a total fitness plan.

Energy Sources for Muscle Use

To allow for the many benefits of locomotion, muscle cells need a specific form of energy for contraction. These and other cells can't directly use the energy released from breaking down glucose or triglycerides. Rather, to utilize the energy in foods, body cells must first convert the energy to a specific form, called **adenosine triphosphate (ATP).**

To store energy, cells make ATP from its breakdown product **adenosine diphosphate (ADP)** and a phosphate group (abbreviated Pi). Again, the cells are using the energy obtained from foodstuffs. Conversely, to release energy from ATP, cells partially break down ATP to ADP and Pi. This releases usable energy for cell functions.

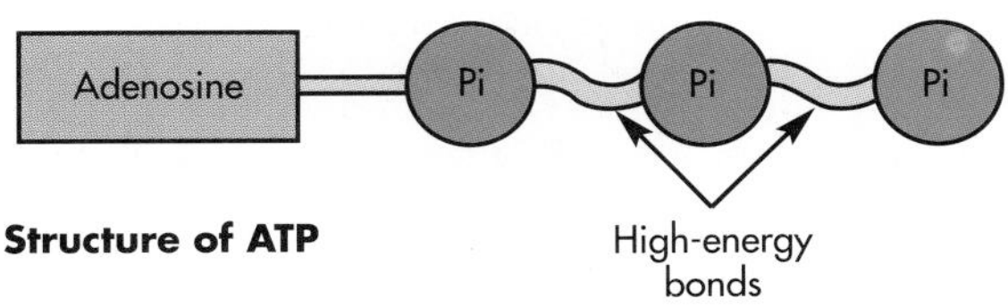

ADP + Energy from Foodstuffs + Pi → ATP
ATP → Energy to do work + ADP + Pi

Essentially, ATP is the immediate source of energy for body functions (Table 10–3). The primary goal in the use of any fuel, whether carbohydrate, fat, or protein, is to make ATP. A resting muscle cell has only a small amount of ATP that can be used. If no resupply of ATP were possible, this stored ATP could keep the muscle working maximally for only about 2 to 4 seconds. Fortunately, another type of high-energy compound—**phosphocreatine (PCr)**—can be broken down to release enough energy to make more ATP. This helps resupply ATP until use of carbohydrate and fat fuels begins in earnest. Overall, cells must constantly and repeatedly use and then re-form ATP, using a variety of energy sources.

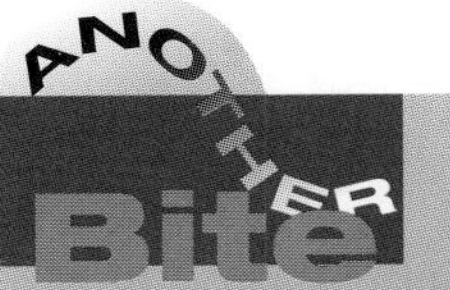

Think about ATP the next time you race after a bus. When you finally sit down, you are exhausted, you breathe hard, and your heart races. Your muscle cells have used up most of their ATP and other high-energy compounds. While you rest, muscle cells begin to resynthesize the ATP used up during your run. Re-forming ATP requires energy. Again, cells get this energy from foodstuffs. If you sit long enough, you can then race off to class using this newly formed ATP.

Adenosine triphosphate (ATP) *The main energy currency for cells. ATP energy is used to promote ion pumping, enzyme activity, and muscular contraction.*

Adenosine diphosphate (ADP) *A breakdown product of ATP. ADP is synthesized into ATP using energy from foodstuffs and a phosphate group (abbreviated Pi).*

Phosphocreatine (PCr) *A high-energy compound that can be used to re-form ATP. It is used primarily during bursts of activity, such as lifting and jumping.*

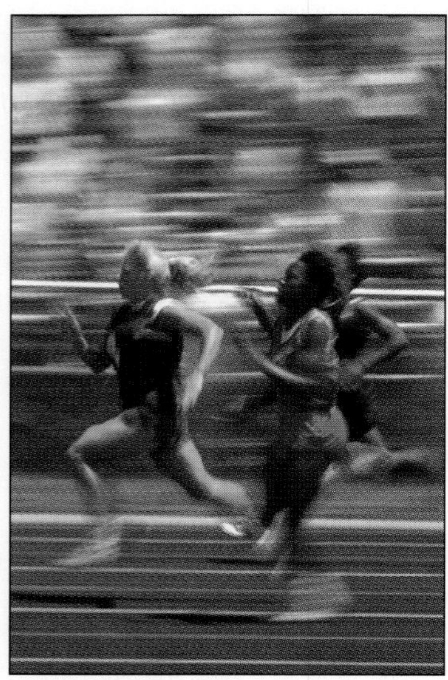

Bursts of muscle activity use a variety of energy sources, including PCr and ATP.

TABLE 10-3

Energy Sources Used by Resting and Working Muscle Cells

Source/system*	When in use	Examples of an exercise
ATP	At all times	All types
Phosphocreatine (PCr)	All exercise initially; extreme exercise thereafter	Shotput, high jump
Carbohydrate (anaerobic)	High-intensity exercise, especially lasting 30 seconds to 2 minutes	200-yard (about 200 meters) sprint
(Carbohydrate (aerobic)	Exercise lasting 2 minutes to 4 to 5 hours; the higher the intensity (for example, running a 6-minute mile), the greater the use	Basketball, swimming, jogging
Fat (aerobic)	Exercise lasting more than a few minutes; greater amounts are used at lower exercise intensities	Long-distance running, long-distance cycling; much of the fuel used in a 30-minute brisk walk is fat
Protein (aerobic)	Low amount during all exercise; moderate amount in endurance exercise, especially once more carbohydrate fuel is not available	Long-distance running

*Note that at any given time more than one system is operating.

Phosphocreatine is the First Line of Defense for Resupplying ATP in Muscles

The instant that breakdown products of ATP begin to accumulate in the contracting muscle, an enzyme is activated to split PCr. This releases energy that can be used to re-form ATP from its breakdown products. If no other source of energy for ATP resupply were available, PCr could probably maintain maximal muscle contractions for about 10 seconds. Because other ATP resupply sources kick in, however, PCr ends up the major source of energy for all events lasting up to about 1 minute.

$$\mathbf{PCr + ADP \rightarrow ATP + Cr}$$

The main advantage of PCr is that it can be activated instantly and can replenish ATP at rates fast enough to meet the energy demands of the fastest and most powerful actions, including jumping, lifting, throwing, and sprinting. The disadvantage of PCr is that not enough of it is made and stored in the muscles for more than a few minutes of use.

Anaerobic
Not requiring oxygen.

Aerobic
Requiring oxygen.

Lactic acid
A three-carbon acid formed during anaerobic cell metabolism; a partial breakdown product of glucose; also called lactate.

Carbohydrate Fuel for Muscles

Carbohydrates are an important fuel for muscles. The most useful form of carbohydrate fuel is the simple sugar glucose, available to all cells from the bloodstream. The breakdown of liver glycogen (a storage form of glucose) helps maintain blood glucose. Breakdown of glycogen stored in a specific muscle also helps meet the carbohydrate demand of that muscle.

When the six-carbon glucose breaks down, the two resulting three-carbon compounds follow one of two main routes. When oxygen supply in the muscle is limited (**anaerobic** conditions) and when the exercise is intense (for example, running 400 meters or swimming 100 meters), the three-carbon compound accumulates in the muscle and is converted to **lactic acid.** About 5% of the energy capable of forming ATP has been extracted at this point.

If plenty of oxygen is available in the muscle (**aerobic** conditions) and the exercise is of moderate to low intensity (for example, jogging or distance swimming), the bulk of the three-carbon compound is shuttled to the **mitochondria** of the cell, where it is further metabolized into carbon dioxide (CO_2) and water (H_2O). This aerobic stage of glucose breakdown yields approximately 95% of the ATP made from complete glucose metabolism to carbon dioxide and water.

Mitochondria
The main sites of energy production in a cell. Structure inside most cells, including muscle cells. Mitochondria also contain the pathway for burning fat for fuel, among other metabolic pathways.

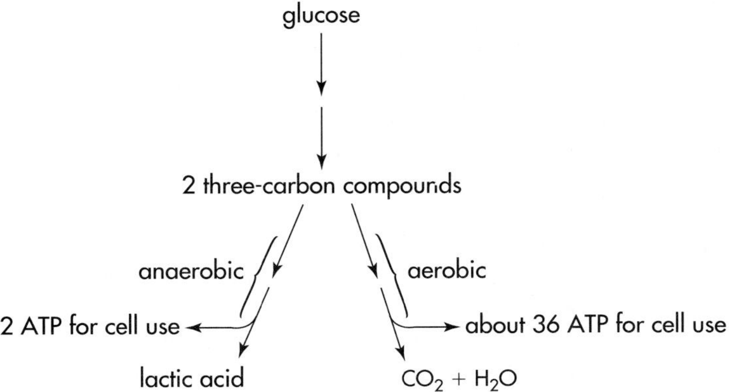

As people start exercising regularly four or five times a week, they experience a "training effect." Initially these people might be able to exercise for 20 minutes before tiring. Months later exercise can be extended to an hour before they feel tired. During the months of training, muscle cells have produced more mitochondria and can burn more fat. As a result, lactic acid production decreases. Because it contributes to muscle fatigue, the less lactic acid produced, the longer the exercise can continue. Part of the training effect derives also from the increased aerobic efficiency of heart and muscle action.

Anaerobic Glucose Breakdown Yields Energy Fast

The advantage of anaerobic glucose breakdown is that it is the fastest way to resupply ATP, other than PCr breakdown. This provides most of the energy for events ranging from about 30 seconds to 2 minutes. The two major disadvantages of the anaerobic process are that (1) the high rate of ATP production cannot be sustained for long events and (2) the rapid accumulation of lactic acid greatly increases the acidity of the muscle. This acid inhibits the activities of key enzymes in the muscle cells, slowing anaerobic ATP production and causing fatigue.

For the most part, lactic acid accumulates in active muscle cells until it is released into the bloodstream. The liver picks up the lactic acid and resynthesizes it into glucose. Glucose can then reenter the bloodstream, where it is available for cell uptake and breakdown. The heart can also use the lactic acid directly for its energy needs, as can less active muscle cells situated near active ones.

Aerobic Glucose Breakdown Yields Energy More Slowly But Does Not Produce Lactic Acid

Aerobic glucose breakdown supplies ATP more slowly than does the anaerobic process, but it releases more energy. Furthermore, the slower rate of aerobic energy supply can be sustained for hours. Moreover, the end products are carbon dioxide and water, not lactic acid. Aerobic glucose breakdown makes a major energy contribution to activities that last anywhere from 2 minutes to 4 or 5 hours (see Table 10–3).

Many researchers have studied various types of carbohydrate feedings to maximize glucose supply to muscles during prolonged exercise. Overall, the techniques have succeeded. Carbohydrate feedings of about 30 to 60 grams per hour during strenuous endurance exercise can aid in maintaining adequate blood glucose, resulting in delay of fatigue by 30 to 60 minutes. This concept is also discussed in a later section.

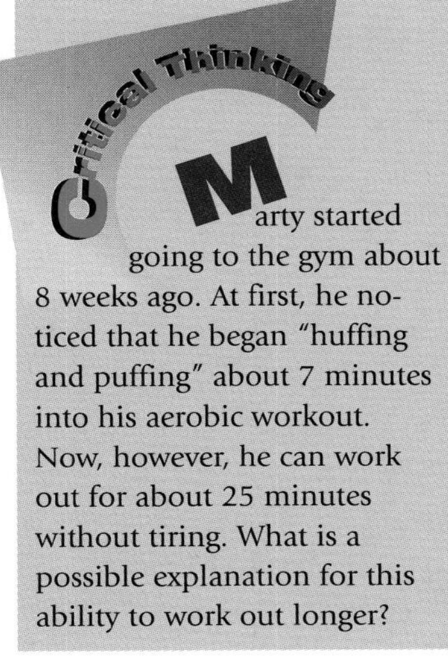

Marty started going to the gym about 8 weeks ago. At first, he noticed that he began "huffing and puffing" about 7 minutes into his aerobic workout. Now, however, he can work out for about 25 minutes without tiring. What is a possible explanation for this ability to work out longer?

Fat: The Main Fuel for Prolonged Low-Intensity Activity

When fat stores in body tissues are broken down for energy, one triglyceride first yields three fatty acids and a glycerol. The majority of the stored energy is found in the fatty acids. During physical activity the fatty acids are released from various fat

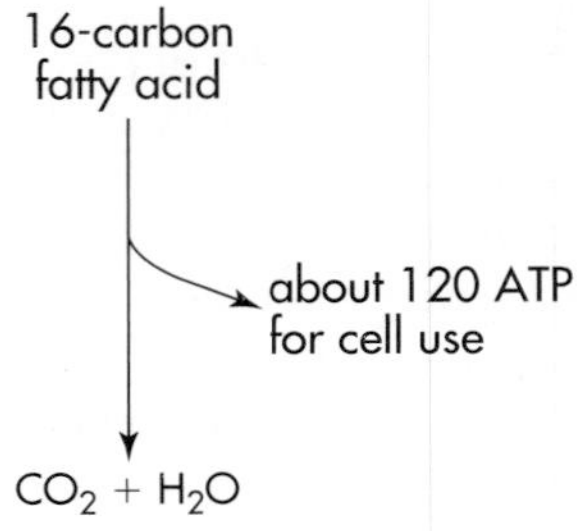

depots into the bloodstream and travel to the muscles, where they are taken into each cell and broken down aerobically to carbon dioxide and water.

The rate at which muscles ultimately use fatty acids partly depends on the concentration of fatty acids in the bloodstream. In other words, the more fatty acids that are released from fat stores into the bloodstream, the more fat will be used by the muscles. Recently, some athletes have attempted to raise their blood concentrations of fatty acids by consuming caffeinated beverages. This practice can actually increase fatty-acid release from the fat depots and is therefore helpful to certain athletes, but it is illegal under International Olympic rules if the amount of caffeine in the body exceeds the equivalent of 6 to 8 cups of coffee (see Table 10–6).

Fat is ultimately not a very useful fuel for intense, brief exercise, but it becomes a progressively more important energy source as duration increases, especially when exercise remains at a low or moderate (aerobic) rate for more than 20 minutes (Figure 10–3). The reason for this is that some of the steps involved in fat breakdown simply cannot occur fast enough to meet the ATP demands of short-duration, high-intensity exercise. If fat were the only available fuel, we would be unable to exercise beyond a fast walk or jog.

The fatty acids can come from all over the body, not necessarily from depots near the active muscles. This is why spot reducing does not work. Exercise can tone the muscles underlying adipose tissue but does not preferentially use those stores. If this was not the case, we would all have lean cheeks and necks, because muscles in that vicinity are regularly used!

The advantage of fat fuel is that it provides tremendous stores of energy in a relatively concentrated form, and we generally have a lot stored. For a given weight of fuel, fat supplies more than twice as much energy as carbohydrate. For very lengthy activities at a moderate pace (for example, hiking) or even sitting at a desk for 8 hours a day, fat supplies about 70% to 90% of the energy required. Carbohydrate use is much less. As intensity increases, such as in a 3-hour marathon run at a competitive pace, muscles use about a 50:50 ratio of fat to carbohydrate. In comparison, for short events, such as a 100-meter sprint or even a 1500-meter race, the contribution of fat used to resupply ATP is minimal. Keep in mind that the only fast-paced (anaerobic) fuel we eat is carbohydrate; slow and steady (aerobic) activity uses carbohydrate, fat, and protein for energy sources.

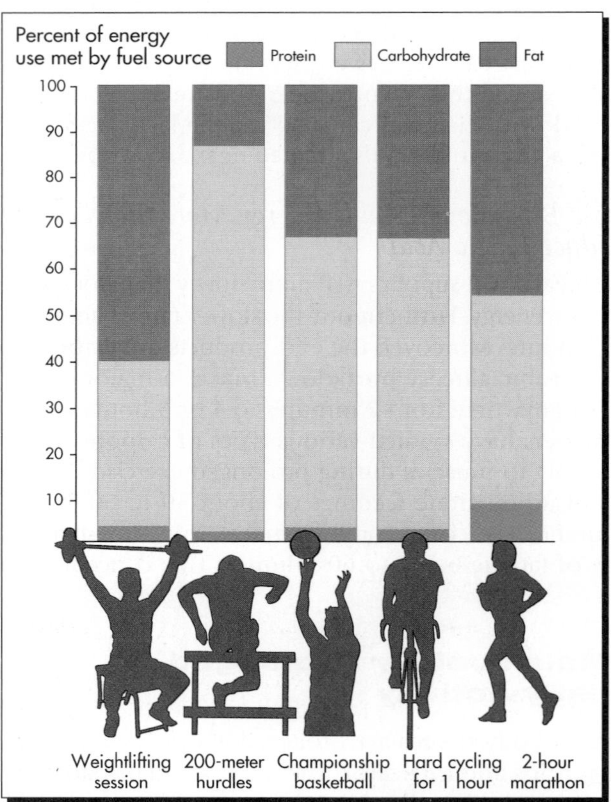

Figure 10–3 *Rough estimates of fuel use during various forms of physical activity.*

Does This Mean We Use Protein to Fuel Activity?

Protein—actually amino acids—can be used for fueling muscles, but as noted in Chapter 6, in most circumstances protein contributes very little to the body's general energy needs. This is also true for the typical energy needs of exercising muscles. However, proteins can contribute somewhat more to energy needs in endurance exercise, perhaps as much as 10% to 15%, especially as carbohydrate stores in the muscles are no longer available. We easily eat enough to supply this amount of fuel. Protein or amino acid supplements are not needed, as discussed in Chapter 6. In fact, it would be difficult for most athletes to eat less than the amount of protein recommended by experts (about 1.2 to 1.6 grams per kilogram body weight). The amount of food eaten supplies much protein (Table 10–4).

Contrary to what many athletes believe, protein is used less for fuel in resistance types of exercise, such as weight lifting, than for endurance exercise, such as running. The primary fuels for the actual act of weight lifting are PCr and carbohydrate. In addition, recent research shows that it is carbohydrate that actually enhances the anabolic effect of weight training, probably by increasing insulin and growth hormone release into the bloodstream.

Athletes who feel they must significantly limit their energy intake, such as gymnasts, or who are vegetarians should specifically determine how much protein they eat, making sure to choose foods that provide a daily protein intake of at least 1.2 grams per kilogram of body weight. Skimping on protein is not a good idea.

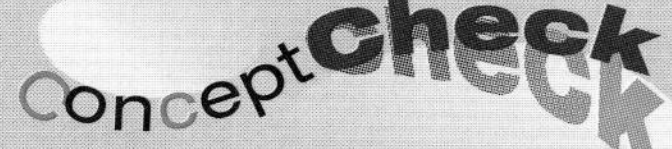

Adenosine triphosphate (ATP) is the main form of energy used by cells. Cells use food energy to form ATP. Phosphocreatine (PCr) can rapidly re-form ATP from its breakdown product adenosine diphosphate (ADP), but PCr supplies are limited. Carbohydrate metabolism to form ATP begins as glucose becomes available from the bloodstream or glycogen breakdown. In a muscle cell, each glucose molecule is broken down through a series of steps to yield either lactic acid or carbon dioxide (CO_2) plus water (H_2O). The process that occurs when glucose is broken down into carbon dioxide and water is called *aerobic* because oxygen is used. The conversion of glucose to lactic acid is called *anaerobic* because no oxygen is used. This latter process allows the cell to quickly re-form ATP and supports the demand for energy during intense exercise. Fat is a key aerobic fuel for muscle cells, especially at low exercise outputs. At rest and light activity, muscles burn primarily fat for energy needs. In comparison, little protein generally is used to fuel muscles. Protein supplies at most 10% to 15% of energy needs during endurance activities.

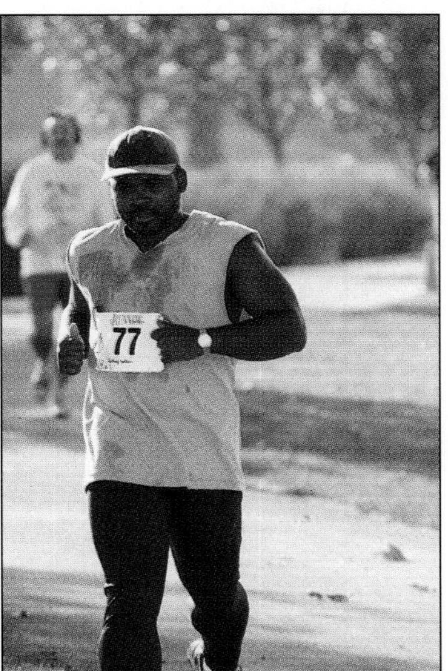

The energy to run comes from carbohydrate, fat, and protein. The relative mix depends on the pace.

Power Food: Dietary Recommendations for Athletes

Athletic training and genetic makeup are two important determinants of athletic performance. A good diet won't substitute for either factor, but as previously mentioned, diet can enhance and maximize an athlete's potential. More important, a poor diet can certainly harm performance.

Determining Needed Food-Energy Intake

Athletes need varying amounts of food energy, depending on each athlete's body size and current body composition and on the type of training or competition being considered. A small person may need only 1700 kcal daily to sustain normal daily activities without losing body weight; a large, muscular man may need 4000 kcal. These rough estimates can be viewed as starting points that each athlete needs to individualize by trial and error.

TABLE 10-4

Sample Daily Menus Based on the Food Guide Pyramid That Provide Various Total Energy Intakes

1500 KCAL DIET
Breakfast

Skim milk, 1 cup
Cheerios, ½ cup
Bagel, ½
Cherry jam, 2 tsp
Margarine, 1 tsp

Lunch

Chicken breast (roasted), 2 oz
Raisins, 2 tbsp
Skim milk, ½ cup
Banana, 1

Snack

Oatmeal-raisin cookie, 1
Low-fat fruit yogurt, 1 cup

Dinner

Spaghetti w/meatballs, 1 cup
Romaine lettuce, 1 cup
Italian dressing, 2 tsp
Green beans, ½ cup
Cranberry juice, 1½ cups

18% protein (68 grams)
64% carbohydrate (240 grams)
19% fat (32 grams)

2000 KCAL DIET
Breakfast

Skim milk, 1 cup
Cheerios, 1 cup
Bagel, ½
Cherry jam, 1 tbsp
Margarine, 1 tsp

Lunch

Chicken breast (roasted), 2 oz
Wheat bread, 2 slices
Mayonnaise, 1 tsp
Raisins, ¼ cup
Cranberry juice, 1½ cups
Banana, 1

Snack

Oatmeal-raisin cookies, 3
Low-fat fruit yogurt, 1 cup

Dinner

Broiled beef sirloin, 3 oz
Romaine lettuce, 1 cup
Italian dressing, 2 tsp
Green beans, 1 cup
Skim milk, ½ cup

17% protein (85 grams)
63% carbohydrate (315 grams)
20% fat (44 grams)

3000 KCAL DIET
Breakfast

Skim milk, 1 cup
Cheerios, 2 cups
Bagel, 1
Cherry jam, 2 tsp
Margarine, 1 tsp
Oat bran muffins, 2

Lunch

Chicken breast (roasted), 2 oz
Wheat bread, 2 slices
Provolone cheese, 1 oz
Mayonnaise, 1 tsp
Raisins, ⅓ cup
Cranberry juice, 1½ cups
Low-fat fruit yogurt, 1 cup

Snack

Banana, 1
Oatmeal-raisin cookies, 3

Dinner

Broiled beef sirloin, 3 oz
Romaine lettuce, 1 cup
Garbanzo beans, 1 cup
Italian dressing, 2 tsp
Spinach pasta noodles, 1½ cups
Margarine, 1 tsp
Green beans, 1 cup
Skim milk, ½ cup

17% protein (128 grams)
62% carbohydrate (465 grams)
21% fat (70 grams)

4000 KCAL DIET
Breakfast

Orange, 1
Cheerios, 2 cups
Skim milk, 1 cup
Bran muffins, 2

Snack

Chopped dates, ¾ cup

Lunch

Romaine lettuce, 1 cup
Garbanzo beans, 1 cup
Alfalfa sprouts, ½ cup
French dressing, 2 tbsp
Macaroni and cheese, 3 cups
Apple juice, 1 cup

Snack

Wheat bread, 2 slices
Margarine, 1 tsp
Jam, 2 tbsp

Dinner

Skinless turkey breast, 2 oz
Mashed potatoes, 2 cups
Pees and onions, 1 cup
Banana, 1
Skim milk, 1 cup

Snack

Pasta, 1 cup
Margarine, 2 tsp
Parmesan cheese, 2 tbsp
Cranberry juice, 1 cup

14% protein (140 grams)
61% carbohydrate (610 grams)
26% fat (116 grams)

5000 KCAL DIET
Breakfast

Cheerios, 2 cups
Bran muffins, 2
Orange, 1
2% milk, 1 cup

Snack

Low-fat yogurt, 1 cup
Chopped dates, 1 cup

Lunch

Apple juice, 1 cup
Chicken enchilada, 1
Romaine lettuce, 1 cup
Garbanzo beans, 1 cup
Alfalfa sprouts, ¾ cup
Grated carrots, ½ cup
Seasoned croutons, 1 oz
French dressing, 2 tbsp
Wheat bread, 2 slices
Margarine, 1 tbsp

Snack

Banana, 1
Bagel, 1
Cream cheese, 1 tbsp

Dinner

2% milk, 1 cup
Beef sirloin, 5 oz
Mashed potatoes, 2 cups
Spinach pasta noodles, 1½ cups
Grated parmesan cheese, 2 tbsp
Green beans, 1 cup
Oatmeal-raisin cookies, 3

Snack

Cranberry juice, 2 cups
Air-popped popcorn, 4 cups
Raisins, ⅓ cup

14% protein (175 grams)
63% carbohydrate (813 grams)
24% fat (136 grams)

The energy required for sports training or competition has to be added to the energy needed to carry on normal activities. This additional energy use averages 5 to 8 kcal per minute for moderate activity; again, this is just an estimate. For example, an hour of bowling requires little energy above that which is required to sustain normal daily living. At the other extreme, a 12-hour endurance bicycle race over mountains can require an additional 4000 kcal per day. Therefore some athletes may need as much as 7000 kcal daily just to maintain body weight while training, whereas others may need 1700 kcal or less.

How Can We Know Whether an Athlete Is Consuming Enough Food Energy?

The first step in assessing energy status is to estimate the athlete's body fat percentage by measuring skinfold thicknesses or using bioelectrical impedance or the underwater weighing technique (see Chapter 9). Body fat should be in the desirable range—that is, about 5% to 15% for most male athletes and 10% to 25% for most female athletes. The next step is daily or weekly monitoring of body weight changes. If body weight starts to fall, food energy should be increased; if weight rises because of increases in body fat, the athlete should be encouraged to eat less.

If the body composition test shows that an athlete has too much body fat, the athlete should lower food intake by about 200 to 500 kcal per day, while maintaining a regular exercise program, until reaching the desirable fat percentage. Reducing fat intake is the best nutrient-related approach. On the other hand, if an athlete needs to gain weight, increasing food intake by 500 to 700 kcal per day will eventually lead to the needed weight gain. A mix of carbohydrate, fat, and protein is advised, coupled with enough training to make sure this gain is mostly from lean tissue, not mostly from added fat stores.

Rapid Weight Loss by Dehydration Is Risky

Wrestlers, boxers, judoists, and oarsmen often try to lose weight so that they can be certified to compete in a lower weight class. This helps them gain a mechanical advantage over an opponent of smaller stature. They usually lose this weight before stepping on the scale for weight certification. Athletes can lose up to 22 pounds (10 kilograms) of body water in 1 day by sitting in a sauna, exercising in a plastic sweat suit, or taking diuretic drugs that speed water loss from the kidneys. Losing as little as 2% to 3% of body weight by dehydration can adversely affect endurance performance. A pattern of repeated weight loss or gain of more that 5% of body weight by dehydration carries some risk of kidney malfunction and heat illness. Death is also a possibility, as was seen in three collegiate wrestlers in late 1997.

To prevent such deaths in the future, the National Collegiate Athletic Association has begun requiring that a minimum safe weight be set by a physician or athletic trainer for each wrestler at the start of the season. Several states also have adopted this practice. If athletes such as wrestlers wish to compete in a lower body weight class and have enough extra fat stores, they should begin a gradual, sustained reduction in food-energy intake long before the competitive season starts. In so doing, the athlete attains a healthier body composition (less fat) while avoiding the potentially harmful and certainly misery-creating effects of severe dehydration. Athletes who have no extra body fat should not attempt to compete at a lower body weight class. Coaches and trainers should be aware of the decreased performance and serious side effects of severe dehydration.

Critical Thinking

Joe is a wrestler who qualified for the lightweight division in his annual high school competition. After a few matches, Joe began to feel dizzy and faint. He was disqualified because he was unable to continue the match. Later, the coach found out that Joe had spent 2 hours in the sauna before weighing in, which had made him dehydrated. What are the consequences of dehydration? What can you suggest as an alternative way to lose weight?

Meeting Carbohydrate Needs in the Training Diet

Anyone who exercises regularly, including the dieter, needs to consume a diet that includes moderate to high amounts of carbohydrates. The diet should include a variety of foods, in accordance with the Food Guide Pyramid. Numerous servings of starches and fruits will provide enough carbohydrate to maintain adequate liver and muscle glycogen stores, especially for replacing glycogen losses from the previous day.

Carbohydrate intake should be at least 5 grams per kilogram of body weight. People engaged in aerobic training and endurance athletes (duration over 60 minutes per day) may need as much as 8 to 10 grams per kilogram. In other words, triathletes and marathon runners should consider eating close to 600 to 700 grams of carbohydrates daily, and even more if necessary, to (1) prevent chronic fatigue and (2) load the muscles and liver with glycogen. This is especially important when performing multiple training bouts in a day, such as swim practice, or heavy training on successive days, as in cross-country running. Table 10–4 showed sample menus, based on the Food Guide Pyramid, for diets providing food energy ranging from 1500 to 5000 kcal per day. Figure 10–4 provides a number of carbohydrate-rich options for meals. In addition, the Exchange System described in Appendix C is a very useful tool for planning all types of diets, including high-carbohydrate diets for athletes.

As you saw in Chapter 9, new fad diets come and go each year. Current plans emphasizing a high protein intake and a low to moderate carbohydrate intake (e.g., *Enter the Zone* or *Protein Power*) would not be appropriate for most athletes. These typically will not supply enough carbohydrate to maintain optimum glycogen stores.

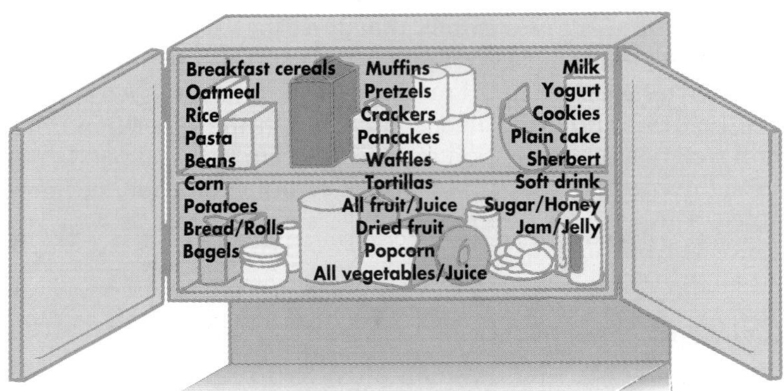

Figure 10–4 *Foods rich in carbohydrate are a key part of a training diet. Many typical foods are carbohydrate-rich. For the specific amount of carbohydrate in each food choice, see Appendix A.*

Note that it is not necessary to give up any specific food when planning a high-carbohydrate diet. Just turn to more of the best (high-carbohydrate foods) and moderate the rest (concentrated fat sources). Sports nutritionists emphasize the difference between a high-carbohydrate meal and a high-carbohydrate–high-fat meal. Before endurance events, such as marathons or triathalons, some athletes seek to increase their carbohydrate reserves by eating potato chips, french fries, banana cream pie, and pastries. Although such foods contain carbohydrate, they also contain a lot of fat. Better high-carbohydrate food choices include pasta, rice, potatoes, bread, and many breakfast cereals (check the label for carbohydrate content). Sports drinks and carbohydrate gels appropriate for carbohydrate loading, such as GatorLode, UltraFuel, and UltraGel, can also help. Consuming only a moderate amount of insoluble dietary fiber (e.g., wheat bran) during the final day of training is a good precaution to reduce the risk of bloating and intestinal gas during the next day's event.

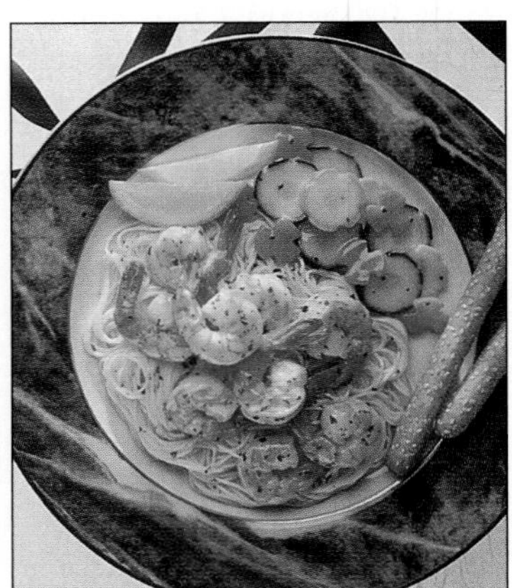

The athlete's plate should be about two-thirds grains and vegetables and one-third protein sources.

As a general rule, athletes should obtain about 60% or more of their total energy needs from carbohydrate, rather than the 50% typical of most American diets, especially when exercise duration exceeds 2 hours. With carbohydrate intakes in this range, intake of fat should fall so that fat provides 20% to 30% of total energy needs. Protein then provides the rest of the total energy—about 12% to 15% of total needs. This approach yields a training diet that is about two-thirds carbohydrate-rich foods and one-third protein-rich foods, with fat mainly from the many other food choices.

A Further Look at Carbohydrate: Carbohydrate Loading

For athletes who compete in continuous intense aerobic events lasting more than 60 minutes or in shorter events repeated over a 24-hour period, undertaking a **carbohydrate-loading** regimen is often advantageous to maximize muscle glycogen fuel. (Note, however, that this duration applies to few athletes.) One possible regimen includes a gradual reduction or "tapering" of exercise intensity and duration, coupled with a gradual increase in dietary carbohydrate as a percentage of energy intake. The procedure can begin 6 days before competition, with the athlete completing a hard workout lasting about 60 minutes. Workouts for the next 4 days then last about 40, 40, 20, and 20 minutes respectively, with exercise intensities being progressively reduced each day. On the final day before competition the athlete rests.

Carbohydrate-loading
A process in which a very high-carbohydrate diet is consumed for about 3 days before an athletic event while tapering exercise duration to try to increase muscle glycogen stores.

The dietary carbohydrate on the first 3 days of this regimen (about 450 grams per day) contributes 45% to 50% of energy intake. The carbohydrate contribution rises to 65% to 75% (about 600 grams per day) for the last 3 days before competition. This carbohydrate-loading technique usually increases muscle glycogen stores by 50% to 85% over typical conditions (that is, when dietary carbohydrate constitutes about 50% of the total energy intake). A typical carbohydrate-loading schedule would look like this:

Days before competition	**6**	**5**	**4**	**3**	**2**	**1**
Exercise time (minutes)	60	40	40	20	20	REST
Carbohydrate (grams)	450	450	450	600	600	600

Total energy intake should decrease as exercise time decreases.

A potential disadvantage of carbohydrate loading is that some water is stored in the muscles with the extra glycogen. In some individuals this additional water weight is sufficient to detract from their sport performance, making carbohydrate loading inappropriate. Athletes considering carbohydrate loading should try it during training (and well before an important competition) to experience its effects on performance. They can then determine whether it is worth the effort.

Carbohydrate loading is safe for adolescents, but the activities for which this technique is useful, such as marathon runs, may not be. Adolescents should obtain the approval of their physician(s) before participating in such a regimen.

When carbohydrate fuel (glycogen) in muscles is eventually used up, maintaining the high initial workload is difficult unless normal blood glucose concentrations are maintained by carbohydrate feedings. Athletes call this point of glycogen depletion "hitting the wall," because further exertion is hampered. Thus when exertion meets or exceeds about 90 minutes, athletes (for example, long-distance runners or cyclists) should consider increasing the amount of carbohydrates stored in muscles.

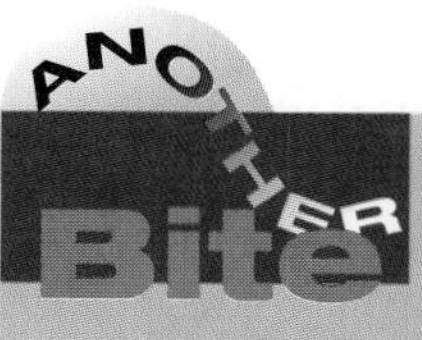

APPROPRIATE ACTIVITIES FOR CARBOHYDRATE LOADING	INAPPROPRIATE ACTIVITIES FOR CARBOHYDRATE LOADING
Marathons	American football games
Long-distance swimming	10-kilometer runs
Cross-country skiing	Walking and hiking
30-kilometer runs	Most swimming events
Triathalons	Single basketball games
Tournament-play basketball	Weight lifting
Soccer	Most track and field events
Cycling time trials	
Long-distance canoe racing	

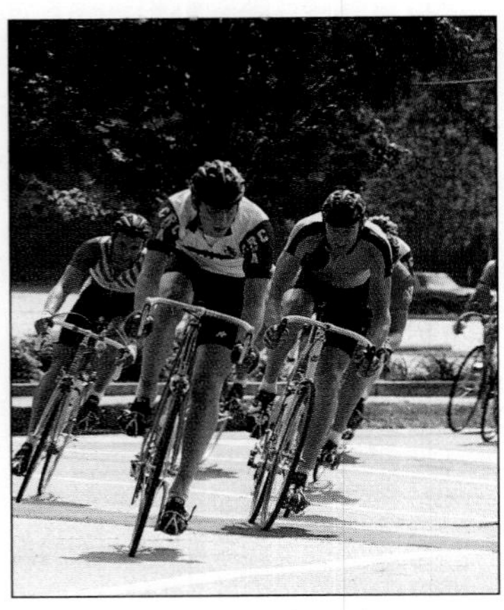

Athletes often expend much energy. Their resulting food intake should easily provide ample protein and other nutrients to support activity.

Vitamin and Mineral Needs for Athletes: Diet Generally Can Meet Extra Needs

Vitamin and mineral needs are the same or slightly higher for athletes compared with sedentary adults. Athletes' needs for vitamin E and vitamin C may be somewhat greater because of the antioxidant protection these nutrients provide in the face of high oxygen use by muscles. Thiamin, riboflavin, vitamin B-6, potassium, magnesium, iron, zinc, copper, and chromium needs may also increase somewhat; these vitamins and minerals play a role in energy metabolism, and some are lost in sweat.

Current research suggests that extra nutrient needs can be met by diet. In addition, because athletes usually have high food-energy intakes, they tend to consume plenty of vitamins and minerals. Athletes who reduce their energy intake to less than 1500 to 1800 kcal to lose weight should however pay close attention to their vitamin and mineral intake. Vegetarian athletes should heed the same warning, as well as athletes undergoing intense training. A good approach for such athletes is to focus on nutrient-dense foods, such as low-fat and nonfat milk, broccoli, tomatoes, oranges, strawberries, whole grains, and kidney beans. Meat-eaters should emphasize lean meat, such as lean beef, turkey, fish, and chicken. Vitamin- and mineral-fortified foods, including many breakfast cereals, are also good choices. Supplemental use of vitamins and minerals is also appropriate, but use should not greatly exceed the Daily Values listed on the labels. Vitamin E use may be an exception. Any use beyond current dietary standards should be discussed first with a physician.

Iron Deficiency Impairs Performance

Athletes, especially female and adolescent athletes, should pay special attention to their iron intake. In all athletes, iron stores can be depleted by both the loss of iron in sweat, urine, and gastrointestinal blood and the increased use of iron required for the elevated production of red blood cells associated with physical fitness. Another less important mechanism of iron loss is foot-strike destruction of red blood cells in the blood passing through the feet; this results from the trauma created at the point of impact when a foot strikes the ground. Young women are at special risk of iron deficiency because of the additional iron loss during menstruation.

If iron stores are not replenished, iron-deficiency anemia and markedly impaired endurance performance can eventually result. Although true anemia (noted as a depressed blood hemoglobin concentration) isn't widespread among athletes, having the blood hemoglobin concentration checked annually and monitoring dietary iron intake is wise, especially for adult women athletes. Vegetarian female athletes should be especially careful to watch iron status. If blood iron is consistently low, athletes are advised to use iron supplements. Iron supplements can improve athletic performance if an athlete is truly anemic, but indiscriminate use of iron supplements is not advised because toxic effects are possible (see Chapter 8).

Calcium Intake Deserves Attention, Especially in Women

Athletes, especially women trying to lose weight by restricting their intake of dairy products, can have marginal or low dietary intakes of calcium. This practice compromises optimal bone health. Of still greater concern are women athletes who have stopped menstruating because their arduous training interferes with the normal secretion of the reproductive hormones. Disturbing reports show that female athletes who do not menstruate regularly have far less dense spinal bones than both nonathletes and female athletes who menstruate regularly. This diminished bone density places them at increased risk for osteoporosis in later life, a subject that is discussed further in the section on the female athlete triad in Chapter 11.

A female runner who does not menstruate regularly may also be more likely to develop a **stress fracture.** Female athletes whose menstrual cycles become irregular should consult a physician to ascertain the cause. Decreasing the amount of training or increasing energy intake and body weight (or doing both) often restores regular menstrual cycles. If irregular menstrual cycles persist, severe bone loss and osteoporosis can result. Extra calcium in the diet does not necessarily compensate for the effects of menstrual loss, but inadequate dietary calcium makes matters worse. Calcium intakes up to 1500 milligrams per day have been suggested, but the most effective measure is to have menstruation resume.

Stress fracture
A fracture that occurs from repeated jarring of a bone. Common sites include bones of the foot.

Meals Before Events Should Emphasize Carbohydrate

To top off muscle and liver glycogen stores, prevent hunger during an event, and provide extra fluid (see next section also), a light meal supplying 300 to 1000 kcal should be eaten about 2 to 4 hours before the event. The longer the period before an event, the larger the meal can be, because more time is available for digestion. A preevent meal should consist primarily of carbohydrate (about 70% of energy: 70 to 175 grams or more), have little insoluble dietary fiber, and include a moderate amount of fat and protein (Table 10–5). Carbohydrate sources such as milk, grapefruit, oatmeal, baked beans, and apples and dates are advocated since these produce a sustained release of glucose during digestion. A preevent meal eaten 1 to 2 hours before an event should be blended to promote rapid stomach emptying.

TABLE 10-5

Convenient Pre-event Meals

Meal	Energy and carbohydrate
BREAKFAST	
Cheerios ¾ cup 2% milk, 1 cup Blueberry muffin, 1 Orange juice, 4 oz	450 kcal 82% carbohydrate (92 grams)
Low-fat fruit yogurt, 1 cup Plain bagel, ½ Apple juice, 4 oz Peanut butter (for bagel), 1 tbsp	482 kcal 68% carbohydrate (84 grams)
Whole-wheat toast, 1 slice Apple, 1 large 2% milk, 1 cup Oatmeal, ½ cup 2% milk, ½ cup	491 kcal 73% carbohydrate (94 grams)
LUNCH OR DINNER	
Chili, 8 oz Baked potato with sour cream and chives Chocolate Frosty	900 kcal 65% carbohydrate (150 grams)
Spaghetti noodles, 2 cups Spaghetti sauce, 1 cup 2% milk, 1½ cups Green beans, 1 cup	761 kcal 66% carbohydrate (129 grams)
Orange, 1 large 2% milk, 1½ cups Chicken noodle soup, 1 cup Saltine crackers, 12 Buttered beans, 1 cup Corn, 1 cup Angel food cake, 1 slice	829 kcal 70% carbohydrate (160 grams)

With regard to the timing of pre-activity meals, the rule of thumb is to allow 4 hours for a big meal (about 1200 kcal), 3 hours for a moderate meal (about 800–900 kcal), 2 hours for a light meal (about 400–600 kcal), and an hour or less for a snack (about 300 kcal).

Because it increases release of insulin, which causes blood glucose to fall, carbohydrate feeding an hour or so before competition was previously thought to adversely affect performance. However, we know now that this practice causes neither premature fatigue nor decreased endurance for most people, especially if they have eaten a few hours before and performed adequate warm-up exercises. In fact, recent studies show positive benefits from preevent carbohydrate feeding. However, some athletes are extremely sensitive to an insulin surge. Athletes should therefore experiment with preevent carbohydrate feedings to determine whether their performance is adversely or positively affected.

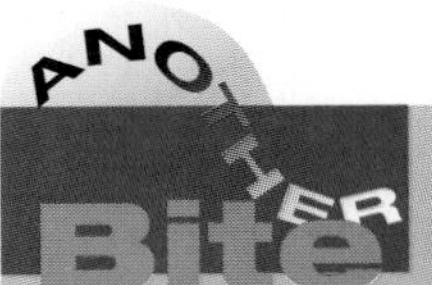

It cannot be emphasized enough that any nutrition strategies should be tested during practice and trial runs before being used in a meet or key event. An athlete should never try a new food or beverage on the day of competition. Some food items and beverages may not be well tolerated, and the day of competition is not the time to find this out.

Maximizing Body Fluids and Energy Stores During Exercise

Water (fluid) needs for an average adult are about 1 milliliter per kcal expended, or about 6 to 8 cups of fluid per day. Athletes need this and generally even more water to maintain the body's ability to regulate its internal temperature and keep itself cool. Much energy released during metabolism appears immediately as heat. Furthermore, heat production in contracting muscles can rise 15 to 20 times above that of resting muscles. Unless body heat is quickly dissipated, **heat exhaustion, heat cramps,** and deadly **heatstroke** may ensue.

Heat exhaustion
Heat illness that occurs when heat stress causes depletion of blood volume from fluid loss by the body. This increases body temperature and can lead to headache, dizziness, muscle weakness, and visual disturbances, among other effects.

Heat cramps
Heat cramps are a frequent complication of heat exhaustion. They usually occur in people who have experienced large sweat losses from exercising for several hours in a hot climate and have consumed a large volume of unsalted water. The cramps occur in skeletal muscles and consist of contractions for 1 to 3 minutes at a time.

Heatstroke
Heatstroke can occur when internal body temperature reaches 105°F. Sweating generally ceases if left untreated, and blood circulation is greatly reduced. Nervous system damage may ensue, and death is likely. Often the skin of individuals who suffer heatstroke is hot and dry.

Virtually all body heat is lost through the evaporation of sweat from the skin. Sweat loss during prolonged exercise ranges from 3 to 8 cups per hour. As the humidity rises, especially when it rises about 75 percent, evaporation slows and sweating become inefficient.

Increased body temperature associated with dehydration is most evident when the amount of water lost exceeds 3% of body weight. This dehydration then leads to a fall in endurance, strength, and overall performance. Wearing football equipment in hot weather can lead to a loss of 2% of body weight in 30 minutes. Marathon runners have been shown to lose 6% to 10% of body weight during a race.

Common symptoms of heat illness include profuse sweating at the outset and then reduced sweating as the illness worsens, headache, dizziness, confusion, nausea, vomiting, muscle weakness, irritability, visual disturbances, elevated body temperature, and flushing of the skin. Anyone experiencing such symptoms should be taken to a cool environment immediately and stripped of excess clothing. Immediate administration of ice packs or cold water is the usual treatment until medical help can be summoned.

To decrease the risk of developing heat-related illness, athletes should replace lost fluids, watch for rapid body-weight changes (2% to 3% or more of body weight), and avoid exercise under extremely hot, humid conditions. Athletes must avoid becoming dehydrated because dehydration during exercise sets the state for heat illness. When possible, fluid intake during exercise should be adequate to minimize body-weight loss and maintain a high volume of pale urine; this practice is a good idea even in the winter, when sweating can go unnoticed. The recommended goal is a loss of no more than 3% of body weight during exercise.

Athletes should first calculate 3% of their body weight and then by trial and error determine how much extra fluid they need to compensate for the amount lost during exercise. This determination will be most accurate if the athlete is weighed before and after a typical workout. For every 1 pound lost, 2 cups of water should be consumed during exercise or immediately afterward. Most athletes find that replacing more than about 75% to 80% of this sweat loss during exercise is uncomfortable.

Thirst is not a reliable indicator of an athlete's need to replace fluid during exercise. An athlete who drinks only when thirsty is likely to take 48 hours to replenish fluid loss. After several days of training, an athlete relying on thirst as an indicator can build up a fluid debt large enough to impair performance.

The following fluid-replacement approach can meet athletes' fluid needs in most cases:

- Freely drink beverages (for example, water, diluted fruit juice, and sports drinks) until 2 hours before an event, even when not particularly thirsty. For events lasting less than 60 minutes, use of water alone is sufficient for fluid replacement.
- About 2 hours before an event, consume about 2 cups of these fluids. This is called *hyperhydration.* The extra fluid in the body will be ready to replace sweat losses as needed.
- During events lasting more than 30 minutes, consume about ½ to ¾ cup of fluid every 15 to 20 minutes as possible. Again, athletes should not wait until they feel thirsty.
- After exercise about 2 cups of fluid should be consumed for every pound lost.

If the weather is hot or humid, even more fluids may be required. Skipping fluids before or during events will almost certainly cause problems!

Two Kansas high school football players and one in North Carolina died in the fall of 1998 from heat illness. Air temperatures were in the 90s to 100s° F during practice. Lack of attention to ongoing hydration caused the deaths.

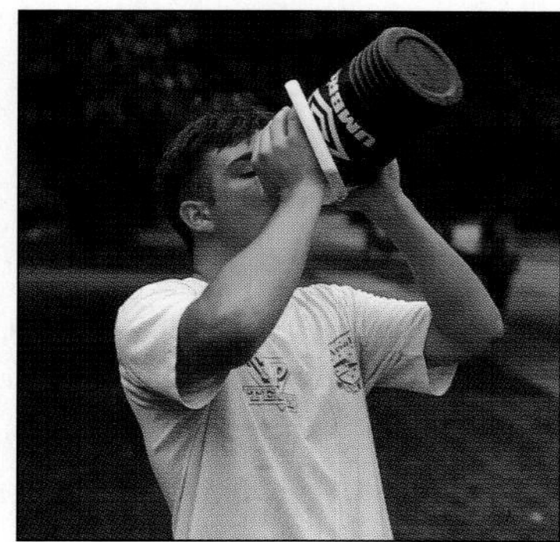

Fluid intake during physical activity is important.

Carbohydrate Intake During Recovery from Exercise

Carbohydrate-rich foods yielding about 70 to 100 grams of carbohydrate should be consumed within 2 hours after extended (endurance) exercise—the sooner the better, because this is when glycogen synthesis is greatest. As well, some protein should be added to this meal, as this aids recovery. This process should then be repeated over the next 2 hours. Athletes who are training intensively can consume a simple sugar candy, sugared soft drink, fruit (for example, raisins) or fruit juice, or a sports-type carbohydrate supplement or gel immediately after training as they attempt to reload their muscles with glycogen. Lunch meat or nuts could provide the protein, or use of a sports bar or sweetened yogurt could provide both protein and carbohydrate. At quick-service restaurants, athletes can order baked potatoes, thicker crust on pizza, and extra rolls and muffins.

Fluid and **electrolyte** (that is, sodium and potassium) intake is also an essential component of an athlete's recovery diet. Fluids and electrolytes help replenish body fluids as quickly as possible, which is especially important if the athlete works out twice a day and the environment is hot and humid. If food and fluid intake are sufficient to restore weight loss, they generally also supply enough electrolytes to meet needs during recovery from endurance activities.

Electrolytes *Compounds that separate into ions in water and, in turn, are able to conduct an electrical current. These include sodium, chloride, and potassium.*

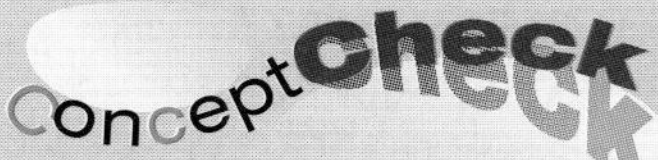

All athletes would do well to plan a diet that follows the Food Guide Pyramid. They should emphasize high-carbohydrate foods, especially in the preevent meal. Protein intake above that available in the usual American diet is generally unnecessary. Nutrient supplements can help correct actual nutrient deficiencies or to compensate for a low nutrient intake. Fluid should be consumed as liberally as possible before, during, and after an event. Endurance athletes may find that a sports-type drink can be helpful for activity lasting more than 60 to 90 minutes.

For more information on sports medicine, visit www.physsportsmed.com on the web. This home page of *The Physician and Sportsmedicine* journal details current issues in sports medicine, including injury prevention, nutrition, and exercise. Also helpful are the web pages of the Gatorade Sports Science Institute: http://www.gssiweb.com, and American College of Sports Medicine http://www.acsm.org.

Nutrition Insight

Sports Drinks: Most Helpful for Endurance Athletes

A question that often arises is whether to drink water or a sports-type drink, such as All Sport, Exceed Energy Drink, Gatorade, PowerAde, and Amino Force, during competition. For sports that require less than 30 minutes of exertion or when total weight loss is less than 5 to 6 pounds, the primary concern is replacing the water lost in sweat, because losses of body carbohydrate stores and electrolytes (sodium, chloride, potassium, and other minerals) are not usually too great. Although electrolytes are lost in sweat, the quantities lost in exercise of brief to moderate duration can easily be replaced later by consuming normal foods, such as orange juice, potatoes, and tomato juice. Keep in mind that sweat is about 99% water and only 1% electrolytes and other substances.

The use of sports drinks is most critical for athletes engaged in sports events lasting longer than 60 to 90 minutes. Prolonged exercise results in large sweat losses and some of the fluid for sweating comes from the bloodstream. If plain water is used to replace the fluid lost from the blood, the concentration of essential electrolytes in the bloodstream may become too diluted. Thus when sports drinks are used to help maintain blood volume, they must contain small amounts of sodium and potassium to avoid electrolyte imbalance. Generally speaking, beverages for the endurance athlete must provide water for hydration, electrolytes to both enhance water and glucose absorption from the intestine and help maintain blood volume, and carbohydrate to provide energy. Beyond 2 to 4 hours of exertion, electrolyte and carbohydrate replacement become increasingly important, especially in hot weather. In fact, sports drinks that contain carbohydrate have been found to delay fatigue during endurance sports with exercise intensities of a 3-hour marathon pace.

The following is but one possible protocol for using sports drinks as part of fluid replacement:

- About 2 hours before endurance exercise, consume 2 cups of water
- Once exercise begins, consume ½ to ¾ cup of a 6% to 8% carbohydrate solution (14 to 19 grams per cup of fluid) about every 15 minutes. The fluid should be cool to enhance palatability. The carbohydrate concentration of many common sports drinks is 6% to 8%, but check the label to be sure (Figure 10–5). If the exercise session is to last more than one hour, the goal for fluid replacement is to yield between 2½ to 5 cups (1600 to 1200 milliliters) of this fluid per hour.

Comparisons of drinks containing **glucose polymers** (glucoses linked together, more properly known as *maltodextrins*), glucose, and sucrose show that all of these carbohydrates have similar positive effects on exercise performance and physiologial function as long as the carbohydrate concentration is in the 6% to 8% range. Drinks in which fructose is the only carbohydrate source are the only exception to this rule. Fructose is absorbed from the intestine more slowly than glucose and often causes bloating and diarrhea.

For the most part, then, the decision to use a sports drink depends primarily on the duration of the activity. As the duration of continuous activity approaches 60 minutes or longer, the advantages from use of a sports drink over plain water begin to emerge.

Quenchmaster
Sports Drink
Nutrition Facts
Serving Size 8 fl oz (240ml)
Servings Per Container 4
Amount Per Serving
Calories 50
% Daily Value*
Total Fat 0g 0%
Sodium 110mg 5%
Potassium 30mg 1%
Total Carbohydrates 14g 5%
Sugars 14g
Protein 0g
Not a significant source of Calories From Fat, Saturated Fat, Cholesterol, Dietary Fiber, Vitamin A, Vitamin C, Calcium, Iron.
* Percent Daily Values are based on a 2,000 calorie diet.

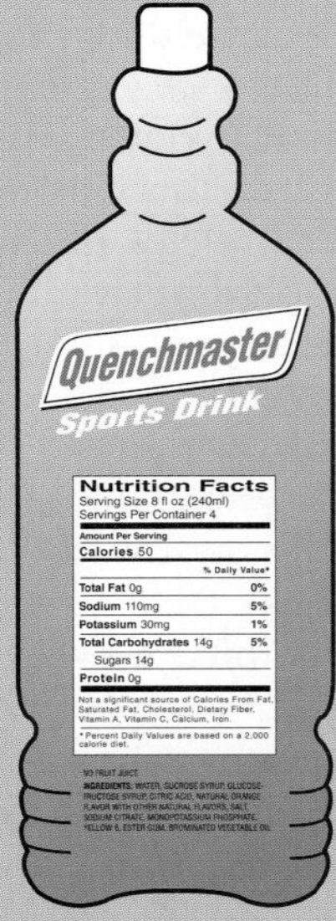

Figure 10–5 *Sports drinks for fluid and electrolyte replacement typically contain a form of simple carbohydrate plus sodium and potassium. The various sugars in this product total 14 grams per 1 cup (240 ml) serving. In percentage terms based on weight, the sugar content is about 6% ([14 grams sugar per serving ÷ 240 grams per serving] × 100 = 5.8%). Sports drinks typically contain about 6% to 8% sugar. This provides ample glucose and other monosaccharides to aid in fueling working muscles, and it is well tolerated. Drinks with a higher sugar content may cause stomach distress.*

Summary

- Regular physical activity is a vital part of a healthy lifestyle, ideally constituting a total of at least 30 minutes per day, including some aerobic and resistance activities. People over 35 years should first discuss plans with a physician. Physically active people show lower risks of heart disease, diabetes, obesity, and other common chronic diseases.
- Adenosine triphosphate (ATP) is the major form of energy used by cells. Human metabolic pathways are able to extract that energy from foodstuffs and store it as ATP energy. Phosphocreatine (PCr) can also provide the energy needed to form ATP in a human cell.
- In carbohydrate fuel use, glucose is broken down into three-carbon compounds, yielding some ATP. The three-carbon compounds can then proceed to an aerobic pathway to form carbon dioxide (CO_2) and water (H_2O) or to an anaerobic pathway to form lactic acid.
- At low workloads, muscle cells use mainly fat for fuel, forming CO_2 and H_2O. For high-output exercise of short duration, muscles use PCr and glucose for energy.
- For endurance exercise, fat and carbohydrate are used as fuels; carbohydrate is used increasingly as activity intensifies. Little protein is used to fuel muscles.
- Anyone who exercises regularly needs to consume a diet that is moderate to high in carbohydrates and consistent with the Food Guide Pyramid. Vitamin and mineral supplements are indicated primarily if a low energy intake makes it difficult to meet nutrient needs or a nutrient deficiency exists.
- Carbohydrate loading can increase usual stores of muscle glycogen. Participants in endurance events that last more than 2 hours benefit most from carbohydrate loading, which basically involves eating a diet very high in carbohydrate for about 3 days before the event.
- Athletes should consume enough fluid both to minimize loss of body weight from fluid loss during exercise and to ultimately restore preexercise weight. A sports-type drink can be helpful for endurance athletes participating in activities lasting more than 60 minutes.

Study Questions

1. How does greater physical fitness contribute to greater overall health? Explain the process.
2. The store of ATP in muscle is rapidly depleted once contraction begins. For physical activity to continue, ATP must be resupplied immediately. Describe how this occurs after initiation of exercise and at various times thereafter.
3. What is the difference between anaerobic and aerobic exercise? Explain why aerobic metabolism is increased by a regular exercise routine.
4. What is glycogen? How does the body obtain it? How is it used during exercise?
5. Are fat stores used as an energy source during exercise? If so, when?
6. What are some typical measures used to assess whether an athlete's energy intake is adequate.
7. List five specific nutrients that athletes need and appropriate food sources from which these nutrients can be obtained.
8. If an athlete wanted to help meet these needs with supplements, what guidelines could you provide to promote safe use.
9. What advice would you give your neighbor, who is planning to run a 50-kilometer (km) race, concerning fluid intake before and during the event?
10. One of your friends, a competitive athlete, asks your opinion about a nutritional supplement sold in a local sporting-goods store. She has read that such supplements, which contain amino acids, can help improve athletic performance. What would you tell her about the general effectiveness of such products?

Further Readings

1 American College of Sports Medicine: Guidelines for Exercise to Maintain Fitness, *Medicine & Science in Sports and Exercise* 30(6):1,1998.
2 Armsey TD, Green GA: Nutrition Supplements: Science vs hype, *The Physician and Sportsmedicine* 25(6):77,1997.
3 Brass EP, Hiatt WR: The role of carnitine and carnitine supplementation during exercise in man and in individuals with special needs, *Journal of the American College of Nutrition* 17:207, 1998.
4 Coleman E: Carbohydrate unloading: a reality check, *The Physician and Sportsmedicine* 25(2):97, 1997.
5 Dunn AL and others: Comparison of lifestyle and structured interventions to increase physical activity and cardiorespiratory fitness, *Journal of the American Medical Association* 281:327, 1999.
6 Eichner ER: Ergogenic aids: what athletes are using—and why, *The Physician and Sportsmedicine* 25(4), 70, 1997.
7 Hawley JA: Fat burning during exercise: can ergogenics change the balance? *The Physician and Sportsmedicine* 26(9):56, 1998.
8 Hyperthermia and dehydration-related deaths associated with intentional rapid weight loss in three collegiate wrestlers—North Carolina, Wisconsin, and Michigan, November–December, 1997, *Journal of the American Medical Association* 279:824, 1998.
9 Jaret P: Getting hooked on an active lifestyle, *Health* p. 59, January–February 1997.
10 Kleiner SM: Eating for peak performance, *The Physician and Sportsmedicine* 25(10):123, 1997.
11 Kujala UM and others: Relationship of leisure-time physical activity and mortality, *Journal of the American Medical Association* 279:440, 1998.
12 Lemon PWR: Is increased dietary protein necessary or beneficial for individuals with a physically active lifestyle? *Nutrition Reviews* 54:S169, 1996.
13 Liebman B: Take a hike, Nutrition Action Health Letter p. 1, January–February 1999.
14 Mason M: Why we don't exercise, *Health* p. 66, July–August, 1998.
15 McBean LD: Physical activity and nutrition: a winning combination, *Dairy Council Digest* 63(3):13, 1998.
16 Schnirring L: ACSM makes advice more flexible, *The Physician and Sportsmedicine* 26(8):16, 1998.
17 Stay stronger longer with weight training, *Harvard Health Letter* p. 1, October 1998.
18 Summary of the Surgeon General's report addressing physical activity and health, *Nutrition Reviews* 54:280, 1996.
19 Thune I and others: Physical activity and the risk of breast cancer, *New England Journal of Medicine* 336:1269, 1997.
20 Williams MH, Branch JD: Creatine supplementation and exercise performance: an update, *Journal of the American College of Nutrition* 17:216, 1998.

RATE 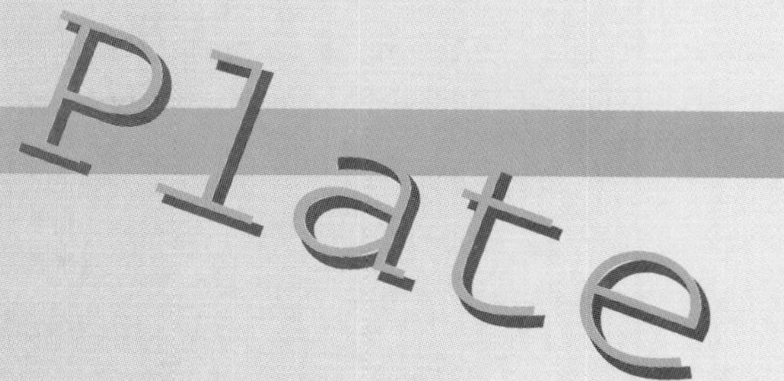

I. How Physically Active Are You?

How physically active are you really? Here are five activity levels based on primarily aerobic activities: (1) sedentary, (2) mostly inactive, (3) moderately active, (4) active, and (5) superactive. Each category is defined below. Your task is to track your activities for the next 3 weeks (even if this class ends before 3 weeks). Assign yourself an activity level each week. Then average the three values and place yourself (X) in the appropriate place on the ladder. Note that you may end up halfway between two classifications.

5. SUPERACTIVE—
One hour of vigorous activity at least 5 days per week. Examples are full-court basketball, mountain climbing, treadmill work, soccer, and other similar activities.

4. ACTIVE—
Thirty minutes of sustained activity at least 5 days per week. Examples are swimming, tennis singles, cycling, jogging, cross-country skiing, and walking briskly.

3. MODERATELY ACTIVE—
Twenty minutes of sustained activity at least 3 days per week or 10 to 15 minutes of sustained activity at least 4 days a week. Examples include tennis doubles, downhill skiing, skating, aerobic dancing, golf, and similar activities.

2. MOSTLY INACTIVE—
Sustained activity fewer than 3 days per week that involves mostly walking. Examples include fishing, bowling, and sporadic jogging.

1. SEDENTARY—
Most activities are limited to sitting or minimal walking.

What kind of program of regular physical activity would allow you to move up the ladder, if appropriate? In addition, some resistance activities a few times a week would add further benefit.

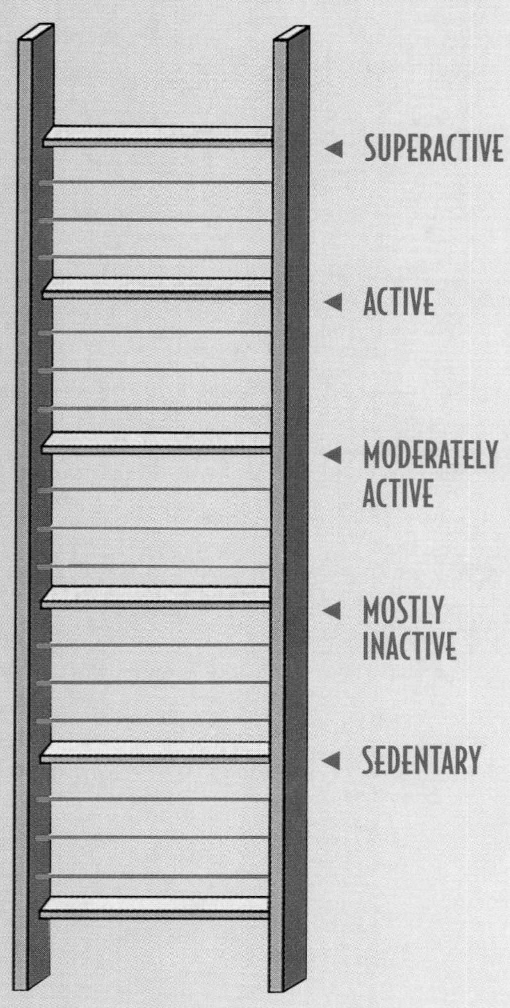

II. Is Your Diet Measuring Up to the Numbers?

In this chapter, several key nutrients were discussed in relation to exercise performance. The following guidelines were mentioned, not only for athletes but for everyone maintaining generally good fitness:

- **Eat a moderate to high amount of carbohydrates (60% or more of total energy intake).**
- **Athletes should eat a minimum of 1.2 grams of protein per kilogram of body weight.**
- **Consume the RDA of vitamins and minerals.**
- **Make sure iron and calcium intake are adequate (especially for women).**
- **Consume enough fluid, especially to maintain weight during prolonged exercise or in hot conditions.**

Review the results of the dietary assessment you completed in Chapter 2. Remember that you assessed 1 day's food intake. Now answer the following questions, whether or not you consider yourself an athlete.

1. **What percentage of your energy intake came from carbohydrate? Was your carbohydrate intake 60% or more of your total energy intake?**

   ____

2. **Did you eat at least 0.8 gram of protein per kilogram of body weight? If you are an athlete, did you consume at least 1.2 grams per kilogram of body weight? Did intake exceed 1.6 grams per kilogram body weight?**

   ____

   ____

3. **Did you consume at least the RDA of all vitamins and minerals assessed, especially iron and calcium? Which ones were below the current nutrient standards?**

   ____

   ____

4. **For nutrients low in your diet, list one rich food source (see Chapters 7 and 8).**

   ____

   ____

5. **Did you consume enough fluid—about 6 to 8 cups for a good starting point?**

   ____

   ____

6. **What can you do to improve your dietary intake to aid general fitness and, if you are an athlete, to promote maximal performance in your chosen event(s)?**

   ____

   ____

   ____

   ____

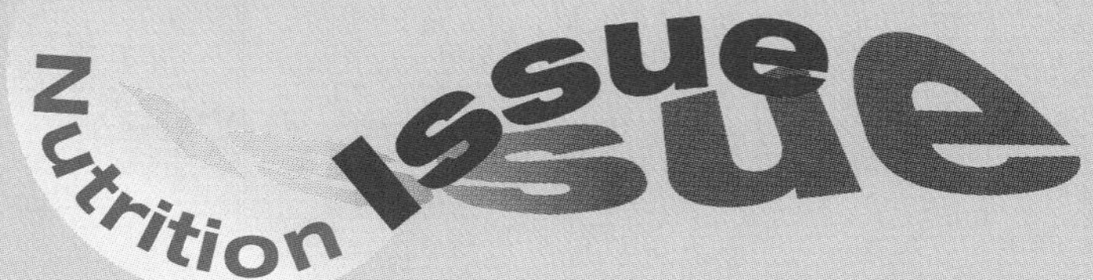

Evaluating Ergogenic Aids to Enhance Athletic Performance

Diet manipulation to improve athletic performance is not a recent innovation. As long as 30 years ago, American football players were encouraged on hot practice days to "toughen up" for competition by liberally consuming salt tablets before and during practice and by not drinking water. Now it is widely recognized that this practice can be fatal. Today's athletes are as likely as their predecessors to experiment; artichoke hearts, bee pollen, dried adrenal glands from cattle, seaweed, freeze-dried liver flakes, gelatin, and ginseng are just some of the ineffective substances now used by athletes in hopes of gaining an **ergogenic** (work-producing) edge.

Still, today's athletes can benefit from recent scientific evidence documenting the ergogenic properties of a few dietary substances. These ergogenic aids include sufficient water, lots of carbohydrates, and a balanced and varied diet consistent with the Food Guide Pyramid. Protein and amino acid supplements are not among those aids, because athletes can easily meet protein needs from foods, as Table 10–4 demonstrated. Clearly, changing average athletes into champions is not possible simply by altering their diets. The use of nutrient supplements should be designed to meet a specific dietary weakness, such as an inadequate iron intake. These and other aids, which often have dubious benefits and may pose health risks, must be given close scrutiny before use. The risk-benefit ratio of these ergogenic aids especially needs to be examined.

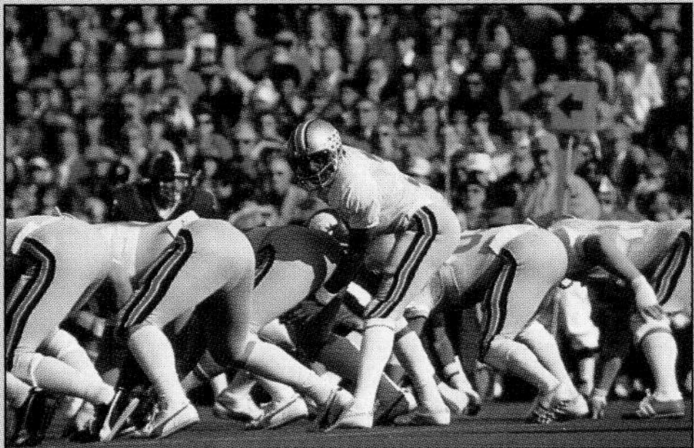

Attention to carbohydrate and fluid needs—along with meeting overall nutrient needs—is the most important ergogenic aid.

As summarized in Table 10–6, no scientific evidence supports the effectiveness of many substances touted as performance-enhancing aids. Many are useless; some are dangerous. Athletes should be skeptical of any substance until it's ergogenic effect is scientifically verified. FDA has a limited ability to regulate these dietary supplements (see the Nutrition Issue in Chapter 1). Even substances whose ergogenic effects have been supported by systematic scientific studies should be used with caution, as the testing conditions may not match those of the intended use. Finally, rather than waiting for a magic bullet to enhance performance, athletes are advised to concentrate their efforts on improving their training routines and sport technique and consuming well-balanced diets as described in this chapter. Adequate fluid and carbohydrate are the primary diet-related ergogenic aids.

Sodium bicarbonate
An alkaline substance basically made of sodium and carbon dioxide ($NaHCO_3$).

Anabolic steroids
A general term for hormones that stimulate development in male sex organs and such male characteristics as facial hair (for example, testosterone).

Growth hormone
A pituitary hormone that produces body growth and release of fat from storage, among other effects.

Carnitine
A compound used to shuttle fatty acids into the cell mitochondria. This allows for the fatty acids to be burned for energy.

TABLE 10-6

An Evaluation of Ergogenic Aids Currently in the Limelight

Substance/ practice	Rationale	Reality
USEFUL IN SOME CIRCUMSTANCES		
Creatine	Increase phospho-creatine (PCr)	Use of 20 grams per day for 5 to 6 days and than a maintenance dose of 2 grams per day may improve performance in those who undertake repeated bouts of bursts of activity, such as in weight lifting. Little is known about the safety of long-term use.
Bicarbonate	Counter lactic acid buildup	Partially effective in some circumstances, such as wrestling, but induces nausea and diarrhea.
Caffeine	Increased use of fatty acids to fuel muscles, promote psychological effects	Drinking 2–3 5-ounce cups of coffee (equivalent to 3–6 milligrams of caffeine per kilogram of body weight) about 1 hour before events lasting about 5 minutes or longer is useful for some athletes; benefits are less apparent in those who have ample stores of glycogen, are highly trained, or habitually consume caffeine; intake of more than about 600 milligrams elicits a urine concentration illegal under Olympic rules (12 micrograms per milliliter).
POSSIBLY USEFUL, STILL UNDER STUDY		
Beta-hydroxy-beta methylbutyric acid (HMB)	Decreased protein carabolism, causing a net growth promoting effect	Research in livestock and humans suggests that supplementation with this may increase muscle mass. Still, safety and effectiveness of HMB use is unknown.
USEFUL IN SOME CIRCUMSTANCES, BUT DANGEROUS OR ILLEGAL		
Anabolic steroids	Increase muscle mass and strength	Although effective, is illegal in the United States; has numerous potential side effects, such as premature closure of growth plates in bones (thus possibly limiting the adult height of a teenage athlete), bloody cysts in the liver, increased risk of heart disease, high blood pressure, and reproductive dysfunction. Possible psychological consequences include increased aggressiveness, drug dependence (addiction), withdrawal symptoms (such as depression), sleep disturbances, mood swings.
Growth hormone	Increase muscle mass	At critical ages may increase height; may also cause uncontrolled growth of the heart and other internal organs and even death; potentially dangerous; requires careful monitoring by a physician.
Blood doping	Either injection of red blood cells harvested earlier from the athlete into the bloodstream or use of medicines to increase red blood cell number in order to try to enhance aerobic capacity	May offer aerobic benefit; very serious health consequences are possible, including thickening of the blood, which puts extra strain on the heart; is an illegal practice under Olympic guidelines.
Gamma hydroxybutyric acid (GHB)	Promoted as a steroid alternative for bodybuilding	FDA has never approved it for sale as a medical product; is illegal to produce or sell GHB in the United states. GHB-related illness includes vomiting, dizziness, tremors, and seizures. Many victims victims have required hospitalization, and some have died. Clandestine laboratories produced virtually all of the chemical accounting for GHB abuse. FDA is working with U.S. Attorney's office to arrest, indict, and convict individuals responsible for the illegal operations.

TABLE 10-6 cont'd

An Evaluation of Ergogenic Aids Currently in the Limelight

Substance/ practice	Rationale	Reality
Androstenedione	Increase muscle mass	Possibly converted to testosterone, which can help build muscle. Its use is banned by the NFL, NCAA, and Olympic Committee. Side effects are acne, fits of rage, baldness, development of breasts in men, stunted growth, and sterility.
Insulin	Promote muscle development and inhibit muscle breakdown	Use can lead to seizures, hypoglycemia, and resulting brain damage. The need for injection can lead to increased risk of hepatitis and other viral diseases. Overall, unsupervised use of this powerful hormone is frought with danger to one's health.
Ephedrine	Increase stamina and exercise performance	Ephedrine (ephedra or ma huang in the herbal form) is currently under scrutiny by FDA due to more than 800 reports of detrimental effects and 38 deaths. FDA is currently reviewing rules that would dictate amount of ephedrine allowed in each pill and taken within a 24-hour period, as well as a warning system on labels. Provisional advice is to consume no more than 24 milligrams per day for a total of 7 days. Ephedrine has caused heart attack, stroke, anxiety, seizure, and death.
NOT EFFECTIVE		
Alcohol	Reduce fatigue, provide energy	Actually impairs performance; can lead to hypoglycemia.
MCT oil (medium chain triglyceride)	Excellent fuel for muscles; transfers directly from GI tract into bloodstream	Can provide a source of energy for muscles, but provides no advantage over carbohydrate intake alone.
Phosphate loading	Improve oxygen delivery to muscles	Not effective.
Inosine	Increase protein and ATP synthesis	Not effective.
Coenzyme Q-10	Increase energy metabolism	Sufficient amount is produced by body.
Carnitine	Shuttle fatty acids into mitochondria of cells	Body cells produce enough; therefore use is ineffective.
Chromium	Enhance insulin function	American College of Sports Medicine states that supplementation is unnecessary. Generally, we eat enough chromium to meet needs.
Other amino acids	Increase bioavailability to promote protein syntheses and lessen muscle loss that occurs during both strength and endurance exercise.	Of no value per se; dietary protein intake is sufficient to meet amino acid needs.
Dehydroepiandrosterone (DHEA)	Increase production of testosterone and provide an anabolic steroid effect	Studies to date are inconclusive. Side effects are masculine traits in women, including hair loss and voice deepening. Men may develop irreversible breast development and prostate gland enlargement. Use is not recommended.
Albuterol	Increase muscle strength and mass	No immediate ergogenic effect for albuterol on either power or endurance.

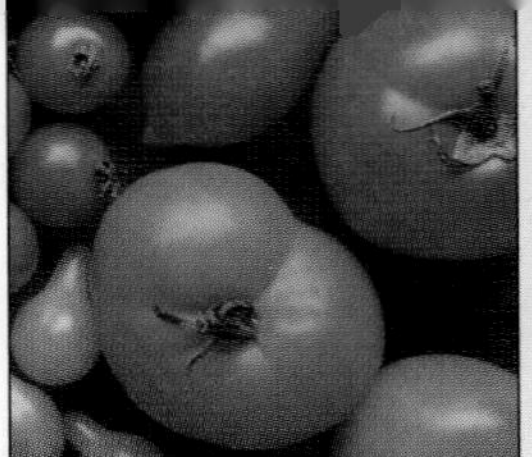

chapter 11

Eating Disorders: Anorexia Nervosa and Bulimia Nervosa

Most of us occasionally eat until we're stuffed and uncomfortable. Faced with savory and tempting foods, we find that we can't easily stop eating. Usually we forgive ourselves, vowing not to overeat the next time. Nevertheless, many of us have problems controlling our weight. Although creeping weight gain can eventually lead to the eating disorder obesity, it is usually associated with simple overeating, coupled with too little physical activity.

In stark contrast, the eating disorders explored in this chapter involve severe distortions of the eating process. Dieting for a week on mostly grapefruit in order to fit into a bikini at spring break does not amount to an eating disorder. Rather, the eating disorders discussed here can develop into life-threatening conditions. What's most alarming about these disorders—anorexia nervosa, bulimia nervosa, female athlete triad, binge-eating disorder, and baryophobia—is the increasing number of cases reported each year.

Some people are more receptive and vulnerable to these disorders than others are, for both psychological and physical reasons. Let's examine the causes and treatments of these conditions in detail, because eating disorders touch many of our lives.

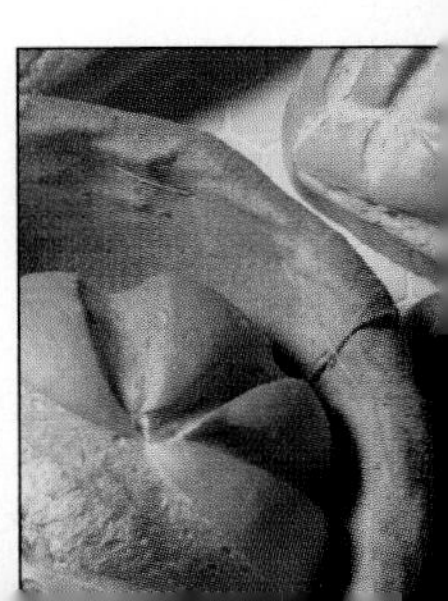

Nutrition Web

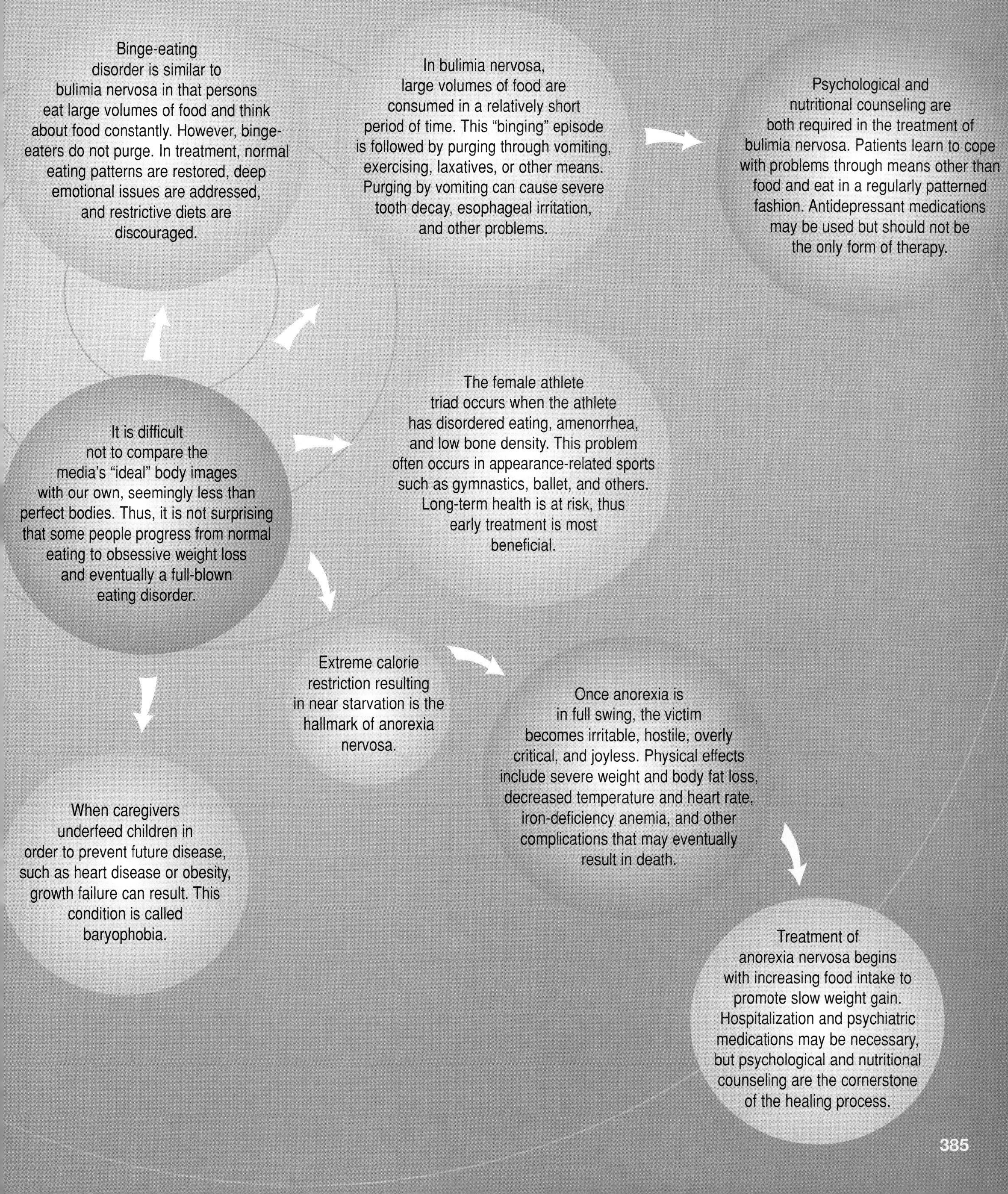

It is difficult not to compare the media's "ideal" body images with our own, seemingly less than perfect bodies. Thus, it is not surprising that some people progress from normal eating to obsessive weight loss and eventually a full-blown eating disorder.

Binge-eating disorder is similar to bulimia nervosa in that persons eat large volumes of food and think about food constantly. However, binge-eaters do not purge. In treatment, normal eating patterns are restored, deep emotional issues are addressed, and restrictive diets are discouraged.

In bulimia nervosa, large volumes of food are consumed in a relatively short period of time. This "binging" episode is followed by purging through vomiting, exercising, laxatives, or other means. Purging by vomiting can cause severe tooth decay, esophageal irritation, and other problems.

Psychological and nutritional counseling are both required in the treatment of bulimia nervosa. Patients learn to cope with problems through means other than food and eat in a regularly patterned fashion. Antidepressant medications may be used but should not be the only form of therapy.

The female athlete triad occurs when the athlete has disordered eating, amenorrhea, and low bone density. This problem often occurs in appearance-related sports such as gymnastics, ballet, and others. Long-term health is at risk, thus early treatment is most beneficial.

Extreme calorie restriction resulting in near starvation is the hallmark of anorexia nervosa.

Once anorexia is in full swing, the victim becomes irritable, hostile, overly critical, and joyless. Physical effects include severe weight and body fat loss, decreased temperature and heart rate, iron-deficiency anemia, and other complications that may eventually result in death.

Treatment of anorexia nervosa begins with increasing food intake to promote slow weight gain. Hospitalization and psychiatric medications may be necessary, but psychological and nutritional counseling are the cornerstone of the healing process.

When caregivers underfeed children in order to prevent future disease, such as heart disease or obesity, growth failure can result. This condition is called baryophobia.

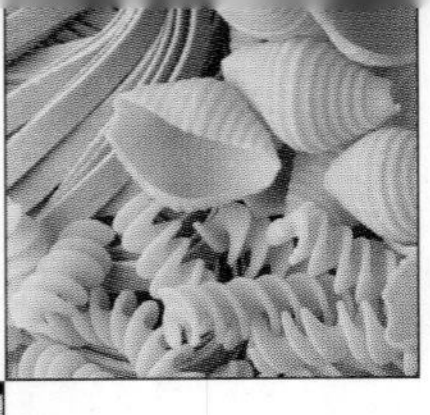

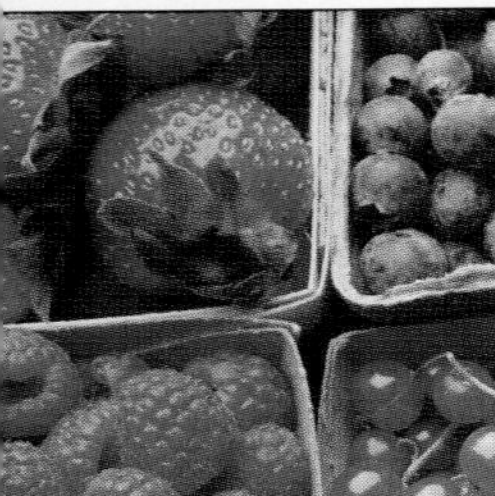

From Ordered to Disordered Eating Habits

In our society we are bombarded daily with images of the "ideal" body. Dieting is promoted to achieve this ideal body—eternally young and acceptable to those around us. Television programs, billboard advertisements, magazine pictures, movies, and newspapers tell us that an ultra-slim body will bring happiness, love, and even success. This is despite the fact that much of society is becoming fatter.

Not comparing the media images with our own is hard. People who are overly susceptible to these messages, for both psychological and physical reasons, may be more likely than others to develop eating disorders.

Given the multiple functions associated with normal eating and the media bombardment about ideal body image, it is not surprising that some people progress from typical responses to hunger and satiety cues, to obsessive weight loss, and then to a full-blown eating disorder, often associated with unusual and strange rituals.

Progression from ordered to disordered eating

Attention to hunger and satiety signals; limitation of energy intake to restore weight to a healthful level

↓

Some "disordered" eating habits begin as weight loss is attempted, such as very restricted eating

↓

Clinically evident eating disorder can be recognized

Food: More Than Just a Source of Nutrients

From birth we link food with personal and emotional experiences. As infants we associate milk with security and warmth, so the bottle or breast becomes a source of comfort as well as food. Even when older, some people continue to derive comfort and great pleasure from food. This is both a biological and a psychological phenomenon. Food can be a symbol of comfort, but eating can also stimulate release of substances called *natural opioids,* which produce a sense of calm and euphoria in the human body. Thus in times of great stress some people will turn to food for a drug-like calming effect.

Food is also used as a reward or a bribe. Haven't you heard or spoken something like the following comments?

You can't play until you clean up your plate.

I'll eat the broccoli if you let me watch TV.

If you love me, you'll eat what I fixed for dinner.

As mentioned in Chapter 1, eating practices may take on religious meanings; signify bonds among cultural, ethnic, and family groups; and be a means to express hostility and affection, prestige, and class values. Similarly, providing, preparing, and distributing food may be a means of expressing love or hatred, or even power, in family relationships.

On the surface, using food as a reward or bribe seems harmless enough. Eventually, however, this practice encourages both caregivers and children to use food to achieve unstated goals. Food may then become much more than a source of nutrients. Regularly using food as a bargaining chip can contribute to abnormal eating patterns. Carried to the extreme, these patterns can lead to disordered eating behavior.

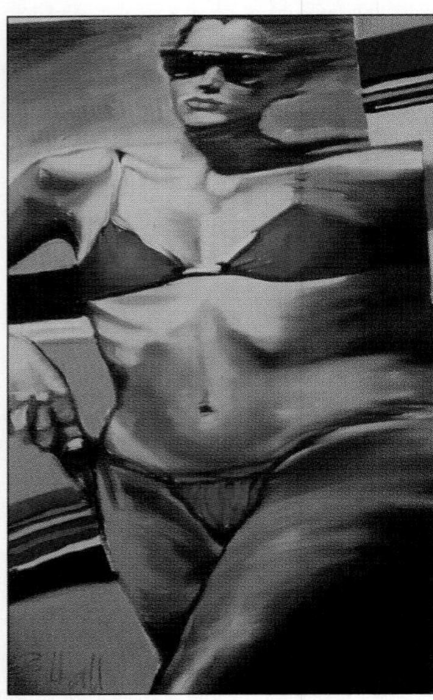

Figure 11-1
Self-image can be ever changing and deceiving. For people with eating disorders, the difference between the real and desired body image may be too difficult to accept.

Overview of Two Common Eating Disorders

The two most common eating disorders—**anorexia nervosa** and **bulimia nervosa**—have been described since the time of the ancient Greeks. Both disorders are psychological problems expressed in part by food practices, and both erode medical, social, and psychological well-being. This section provides a brief description of the characteristics and diagnoses of these disorders. Detailed discussion of these disorders, including their treatment, then follows.

Anorexia nervosa is characterized by extreme weight loss, distorted body image, an irrational, almost morbid fear of weight gain and obesity, and lack of menstrual periods. People with anorexia nervosa typically see themselves as fat even though they are extremely thin (Figure 11-1). The discrepancy between actual and perceived body shape is an important gauge of the severity of the disease.

The term *anorexia* implies a loss of appetite; however, denying one's appetite more accurately describes anorexic behavior. By rough estimate, approximately 1 in 100 Caucasian girls between the ages of 12 and 18 years suffers from anorexia nervosa. The high amount may be due to the tendency for these young females to be diet conscious. It happens less commonly among adult women and African-American women. Men account for only about 5% to 10% of the cases of anorexia nervosa, partly because the ideal image conveyed for men is big and muscular.

Bulimia nervosa (*bulimia* means "great hunger") is characterized by episodes of binge eating followed by attempts to purge the excess energy taken up by the body, usually by vomiting, strict dieting, taking diuretics, **hypergymnasia,** or using laxatives. People with this disorder may be difficult to identify because they keep their binge-purge behaviors secret and their symptoms are not obvious. Between 5% and 17% of adolescent and college-age women suffer from bulimia nervosa. A growing number of male athletes also report these practices, especially those who participate in sports that require achieving weights to fit weight classes, such as boxers, wrestlers, and jockeys. Other activities that may foster eating disorders in men include swimming, dancing, and modeling.

Table 11–1 lists some characteristics of people with anorexia nervosa and bulimia nervosa. People may exhibit some symptoms of an eating disorder but not enough to enable a medical worker to diagnose the disease. Some people show characteristics of both anorexia nervosa and bulimia nervosa, because the diseases overlap considerably (Figure 11–2). About half of the women diagnosed as having anorexia nervosa eventually develop bulimic symptoms, which blurs the distinction. Still, appreciating the differences between the disorders helps in understanding various approaches to prevention and treatment.

Anorexia nervosa
An eating disorder involving a psychological loss or denial of appetite and self-starvation, related in part to a distorted body image and to various social pressures commonly associated with puberty.

Bulimia nervosa
An eating disorder in which large quantities of food are eaten at one time (binge eating) and then purged from the body by vomiting, use of laxatives, or other means.

Hypergymnasia
Exercising more than is required for good physical fitness or maximal performance in a sport; excessive exercise.

TABLE 11-1

Typical Characteristics of Anorexic and Bulimic Persons

Anorexia nervosa	Bulimia nervosa
• Rigid dieting causing dramatic weight loss, generally to less than 85% of what would be expected for one's age • False body perception—thinking "I'm too fat," even when emaciated; relentless pursuit of thinness • Rituals involving food, excessive exercise, and other aspects of life • Maintenance of rigid control in lifestyle; security found in control and order • Feeling of panic after a small weight gain; intense fear of gaining weight • Feelings of purity, power, and superiority through maintenance of strict discipline and self-denial • Preoccupation with food, its preparation, and observing another person eat • Helplessness in the presence of food • Lack of menses after what should be the age of puberty	• Secretive binge eating; never overeating in front of others • Eating when depressed or under stress • Bingeing followed by fasting, laxative abuse, self-induced vomiting, or excessive exercise, generally more often than once a week for a least 3 months • Shame, embarrassment, deceit, and depression; low self-esteem and guilt (especially after a binge) • Fluctuating weight resulting from alternate bingeing and fasting (±10 pounds or 5 kilograms) • Loss of control; fear of not being able to stop eating • Perfectionism, "people pleaser"; food as the only comfort/escape in an otherwise carefully controlled and regulated life • Erosion of teeth, swollen glands • Purchase of syrup of ipecac

This listing can be used in a group discussion to help people assess their risk for developing an eating disorder. Those who exhibit only one or a few of these characteristics may be at risk but probably do not have either disorder. Those who exhibit only one or a few of these characteristics may be at risk but probably do not have either disorder. They should, though, reflect on their eating habits and related concerns and take appropriate action. Note also that many of these characteristics must be present to make the diagnosis of disordered eating. Do not attempt to diagnose these disorders in yourself or others. Instead, use this information to determine whether further professional evaluation is needed.

Based on information in the *Diagnostic and Statistical Manual of Mental Disorders [(DSM-IV)*, Washington, DC, 1994, American Psychiatric Association.

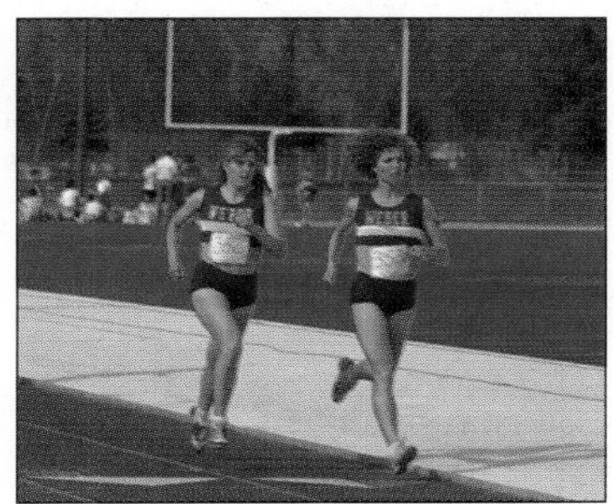

Excessive exercising can be a warning sign of an eating disorder.

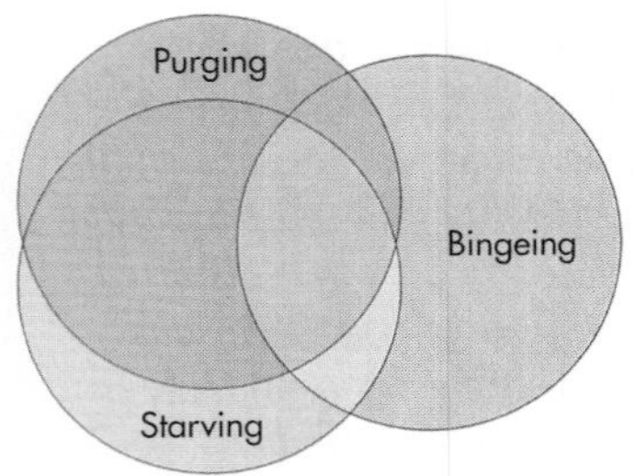

Figure 11–2
The overlap of eating disorders. A combination of binge eating, purging, and/or starving can be found in both anorexia nervosa and bulimia nervosa.

With regard to diagnosis and treatment, only a professional can exclude other possible diseases and correctly evaluate the diagnostic criteria required to make a diagnosis of anorexia nervosa or bulimia nervosa. Once an eating disorder is diagnosed, immediate treatment is advisable. If you know someone with an eating disorder, the best thing you can do is encourage the person to seek professional help. Such help is commonly available at student health centers and student guidance/counseling facilities on college campuses.

There are no simple causes of eating disorders, and there are no simple treatments. The causes are rooted in multiple determinants—biological, psychological, and social. Stress may have an especially strong role in the development of eating disorders. An underlying commonality seems to be the lack of appropriate coping mechanisms as individuals begin to reach adolescence and young adulthood, coupled with dysfunctional family relationships (Figure 11–3).

The Nutrition Issue at the end of this chapter reviews some sociological aspects of these disorders and may help you understand how the disorders develop and why some people are more susceptible than others. As is true for many health problems, both nature and nurture play a role. The increase in the number of cases in recent years supports the importance of nurture.

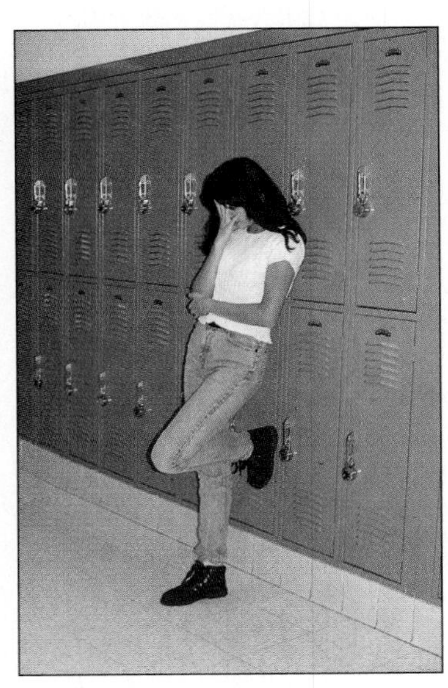

Figure 11–3
The stress of crossing from childhood into adulthood may trigger anorexia nervosa.

Anorexia Nervosa

Anorexia nervosa evolves from a dangerous mental state to an often life-threatening physical condition. As noted earlier, people suffering from this disorder think they are fat and intensely fear obesity and weight gain. They lose much more weight than is healthful. Although food is entwined in this disease, it stems more from psychological conflict.

About 3% to 8% of people with anorexia die prematurely—from suicide, heart ailments, and infections. About half of those with anorexia nervosa recover within 6 years; the rest simply exist with the disease. The longer someone suffers from this eating disorder, the poorer the chances for complete recovery. A young patient with a brief episode and a cooperative family has a better outlook than those without these factors. Prompt and vigorous treatment with close follow-up improves the chances for success.

Anorexia nervosa may begin as a simple attempt to lose weight. A comment from a well-meaning friend, relative, or coach suggesting that the person seems to be gaining weight or is too fat may be all that is needed. The stress of having to maintain a certain weight to look attractive or competent on a job can also lead to disordered eating. Physical changes associated with puberty, the stress of leaving childhood, or loss of a friend may serve as another trigger for extreme dieting. Leaving home for boarding school or college or starting a job can reinforce the desire to appear more "socially acceptable." Still, looking "good" does not necessarily help people deal with anger, depression, low self-esteem, or past experiences with sexual abuse. If these issues are behind the disorder and are not resolved as weight is lost, the individual may intensify efforts to lose weight "to look even better" rather than work through unresolved psychological concerns.

A person with anorexia nervosa may use the disorder to gain attention from the family, sometimes in hopes of holding the family together.

During adolescence, a period of turbulent sexual and social tensions, teenagers seek to establish separate and independent lives. While declaring independence, they seek acceptance and support from peers and parents and react intensely to how they think others perceive them. At the same time, their bodies are changing, and much of the change is beyond their control. Adolescents often lack appropriate coping mechanisms for the stresses of the teen years. In the attempt to take charge of their lives, some teenagers try to maintain extreme control over their bodies, which promotes anorexia nervosa. Genetic factors also appear to increase the risk for anorexia nervosa.

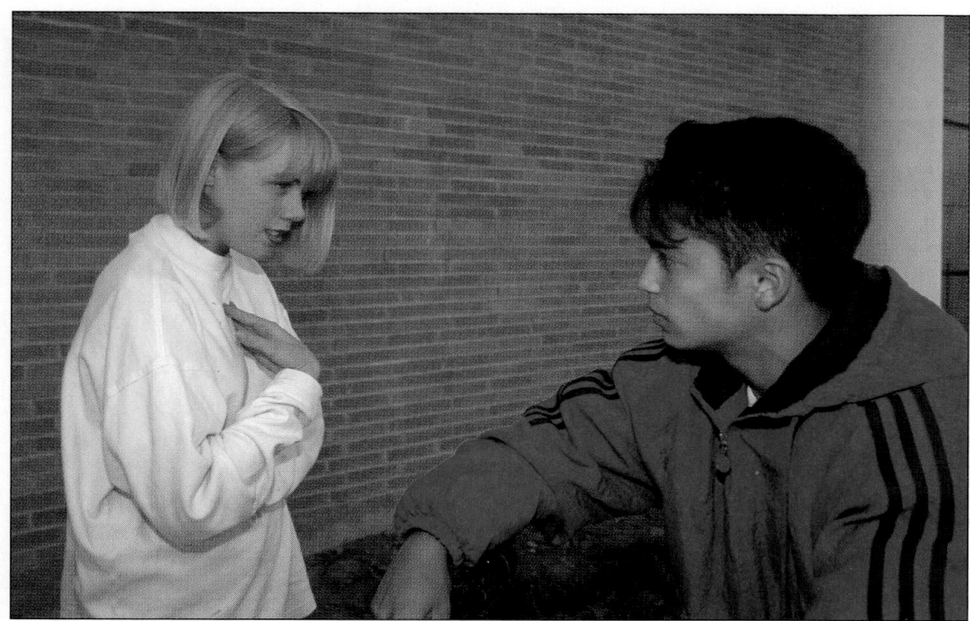

Conflict and physical changes are a common part of adolescence.

Once dieting begins, a person developing anorexia nervosa does not stop. The result is long periods of rigidly self-enforced semistarvation, practiced almost with a vengeance, in a relentless pursuit of thinness. Anorexia nervosa may eventually lead to bingeing on large amounts of food in a short time, then purging. Purging occurs primarily through vomiting, but laxatives, diuretics, and exercise are also used. Thus a person with anorexia nervosa may exist in a state of semistarvation or may alternate periods of starvation with periods of bingeing and purging.

By severely restricting energy intake for long periods, adolescent girls and young adult women greatly compromise their nutritional status, impair their reproductive systems, and retard growth. The harm produced by milder, shorter periods of diet restriction is not clear. Evidence, however, suggests that even moderate diet restriction, if continued, contributes to the risks for various anemias, later pregnancy complications and low-birth-weight infants, and permanently reduced bone density.

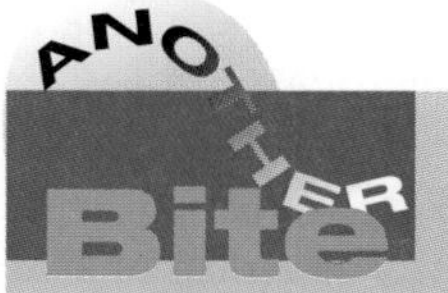

Recently, a 19-year-old patient at the Ohio State University Hospitals was admitted on an emergency basis at a body weight of 60 pounds. She had lost 55 pounds in the last 6 months and was at great risk of impending death. Upon interview, she said she started dieting and could not stop. She was transferred out-of-state to a clinic specializing in eating disorders.

Profile of the Typical Person with Anorexia Nervosa

A person with anorexia nervosa refuses to eat enough. This refusal is the hallmark of the disease, whether or not other practices, such as binge-purge cycles, appear. The most typical anorexic person is a white girl from the middle or upper socioeconomic class. Perhaps her mother also has distorted views of desirable body shape and acceptable food habits. The girl is often described by parents and teachers as "the best little girl in the world."

She is competitive and often obsessive. Her parents set high standards for her. At home, she may not allow clutter in her bedroom. Physicians note that after a physical examination, she may fold her examination gown very carefully, and clean up the examination room before leaving. Even though such behavior may seem obvious, only a skilled professional can tell the difference between anorexia nervosa and other common adolescent complaints, such as delayed puberty, fatigue, and depression.

Nutrition Insight

Anorexia Nervosa: A Case Study

Jill was 17 years old when she was seen at a sports medicine clinic for stress fractures in her feet and lower left leg. At 5 feet 4 inches tall and 89 pounds, she was frail and seemed more like a little girl than a blossoming adolescent. A gymnast with a promising future, this young woman had experienced a number of muscle and skeletal injuries in the previous 6 months. She had stopped having menstrual cycles at age 15, when she weighed about 100 pounds. When asked why she started eating a modest diet consisting of a frozen yogurt banana shake for breakfast, fruit or salad for lunch, and a baked potato with nonfat cottage cheese for dinner, she replied, "Because my coach said that I could fly through the roof on my routines if I lost some weight." That was back when she weighed 113 pounds. Jill's coach called the gymnasts with larger bodies "sows."

Her mother reported that Jill was the type of girl who could never sit still. In addition to her daily routine of an hour run, 30 minutes on the stationary bike, and 2 hours of gymnastics practice, she would do deep knee bends while brushing her teeth and bounce on a minitrampoline while watching TV.

Jill's mother and father had been divorced for 2 years. Although rarely at home because of his sales job, her father criticized her behavior when he was home and would sometimes slap her across the face, frustrated by her imperfection. Jill's mother had multiple sclerosis, and Jill often had to care for her. Despite being popular and well liked by both teachers and students, Jill felt disconnected from people. Jill stated with great pride, "When I strive for perfection and deprive myself of food, I feel strong, secure, and in control." As she sat in the warm clinic with a bulky sweater and baggy slacks, she proclaimed, "The thinner I get, the greater my chances of competing in the Olympics."

The sports medicine staff who saw Jill referred her immediately to the eating-disorder clinic at the local university medical center. Jill's response was to smile, mumble "OK," and quickly leave. Jill's mother doubted that Jill would be willing to go to the clinic.

Parents may not consider a teenager mature enough to make decisions. If the teen disagrees, and the situation is very tense, she may turn to purging or starving as a way to show her power. "You may try to control my life, but I can do anything I want with my body."

In the words of one young woman: "I couldn't get angry, because it would be like destroying someone else, like my mother. It felt like she would hate me forever. I got angry through anorexia nervosa. It was my last hope. It's my own body and this was my last-ditch effort."

A common thread underlying many—but not all—cases of anorexia nervosa is conflict within the family structure, typically manifested by an overbearing mother and an emotionally absent father. When family expectations are always too high—including those regarding body weight—resulting frustration leads to fighting. Overinvolvement, rigidity, overprotection, and denial are typical daily interactions of such families.

Often the eating disorder allows an anorexic person to exercise control over an otherwise powerless existence. Losing weight may be the first independent success the person has had. People with anorexia evaluate their self-worth almost entirely in terms of self-control. Issues of control are central to the development of anorexia nervosa. Some sexually abused children develop anorexia nervosa, believing that if they control their appetite for food, sexual relations, and human contact, they will feel in control and competent and eliminate shameful feelings. Moreover, food restriction, which will arrest development and shut down sexual impulses, may be a strategy to prevent future victimization and guilt feelings in such cases. Often anorexic persons feel hopeless about human relationships and socially isolated because of their dysfunctional families. They substitute the world of food, eating, and weight for the world of human relationships.

Early Warning Signs

A person developing anorexia nervosa exhibits important warning signs. At first, dieting becomes the life focus. The person may think, "The only thing I am good at is dieting. I can't do anything else." This innocent beginning often leads to very abnormal self-perceptions and eating habits, such as cutting a pea in half before eating it. Other habits include hiding and storing food and/or spreading food around a plate to make it look as if much has been eaten. An anorexic person may cook a large meal and watch others eat it while refusing to eat anything.

As the disorder progresses, the range of foods may narrow and be rigidly divided into safe and unsafe ones, with the list of safe foods becoming progressively shorter. For people developing anorexia nervosa, these practices say, "I am in control." These people may be hungry, but they deny it, driven by the belief that good things will happen by just becoming thin enough. It becomes a question of willpower. In addition, many people with anorexia nervosa develop rigid and excessive exercise regimens. They may continue to exercise even when extremely exhausted, suffer injuries, and receive warnings from coaches and physicians to refrain from this type of activity.

Soon people with anorexia become irritable and hostile and begin to withdraw from family and friends. School performance generally crumbles. They refuse to eat out with family and friends, thinking, "I won't be able to have the foods I want to eat," "I won't be able to throw up afterward," or "I won't have time to exercise the calories off."

An anorexic person sees themself as rational and others as irrational. They also tend to be excessively critical of themselves and others. Nothing is good enough. Because it cannot be perfect, life appears meaningless and hopeless. A sense of joylessness colors everything.

As stress increases in the person's life, sleep disturbances and depression are common. Many of the psychological and physical problems associated with anorexia nervosa arise from deficiencies of nutrients, such as thiamin and vitamin B-6, and semistarvation. For this reason a multivitamin and mineral supplement is typically prescribed in therapy. For a female the combination of problems—coupled with lower body weight and fat stores—causes menstrual periods to cease, which is called amenorrhea. This may be the first sign of the disease that a parent notices.

Ultimately an anorexic person eats very little food; 300 to 600 kcal daily is not unusual. In place of food the person may consume up to 20 cans of diet soft drinks and chew many pieces of gum each day.

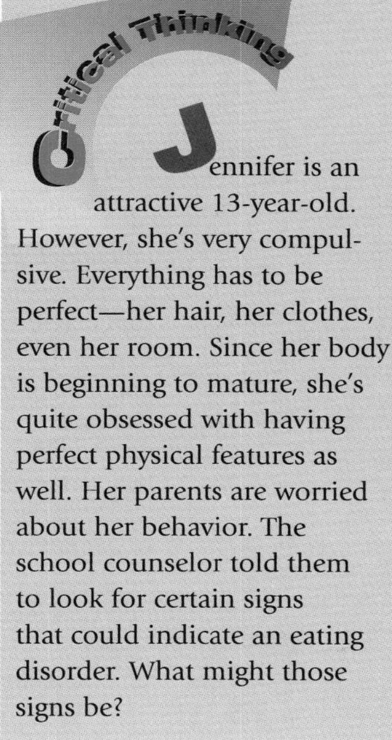

Jennifer is an attractive 13-year-old. However, she's very compulsive. Everything has to be perfect—her hair, her clothes, even her room. Since her body is beginning to mature, she's quite obsessed with having perfect physical features as well. Her parents are worried about her behavior. The school counselor told them to look for certain signs that could indicate an eating disorder. What might those signs be?

Physical Effects of Anorexia Nervosa

Rooted in the emotional state of the victim, anorexia nervosa produces profound physical effects. The anorexic person often appears to be skin and bones. This state of semistarvation disturbs many body systems as it forces the body to conserve as much energy as possible (Figure 11–4). It is this attempt to conserve energy that results in the most physical effects. For this reason, it is possible to put an end to many complications by returning to a state of good nutrition, provided the duration of the insult has not been too long. Following are possible effects caused by hormonal and related responses to semistarvation:

- Lowered body temperature caused by loss of fat insulation.
- Slower metabolic rate caused by decreased synthesis of thyroid hormone.
- Decreased heart rate as metabolism slows, leading to easy fatigue, fainting, and an overwhelming need for sleep. Other changes in heart function may also occur, including loss of heart tissue itself.
- Iron-deficiency anemia from a deficient nutrient intake, which leads to further weakness.
- Rough, dry, scaly, and cold skin from a deficient nutrient intake and related anemia. The skin may also show multiple bruises because of the loss of protection from the fat layer normally present under the skin.
- Low white blood cell count caused by a deficient nutrient intake. This condition increases the risk of infection, one cause of death in people with anorexia nervosa.

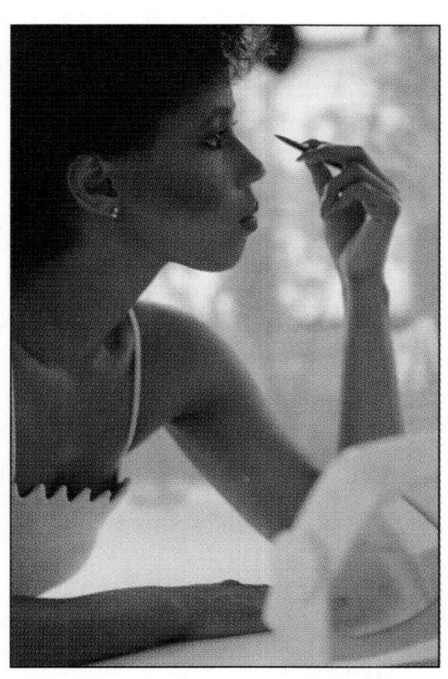

Concern over appearance begins early in life; a focus on healthful outlook with regard to body weight should also begin at this time.

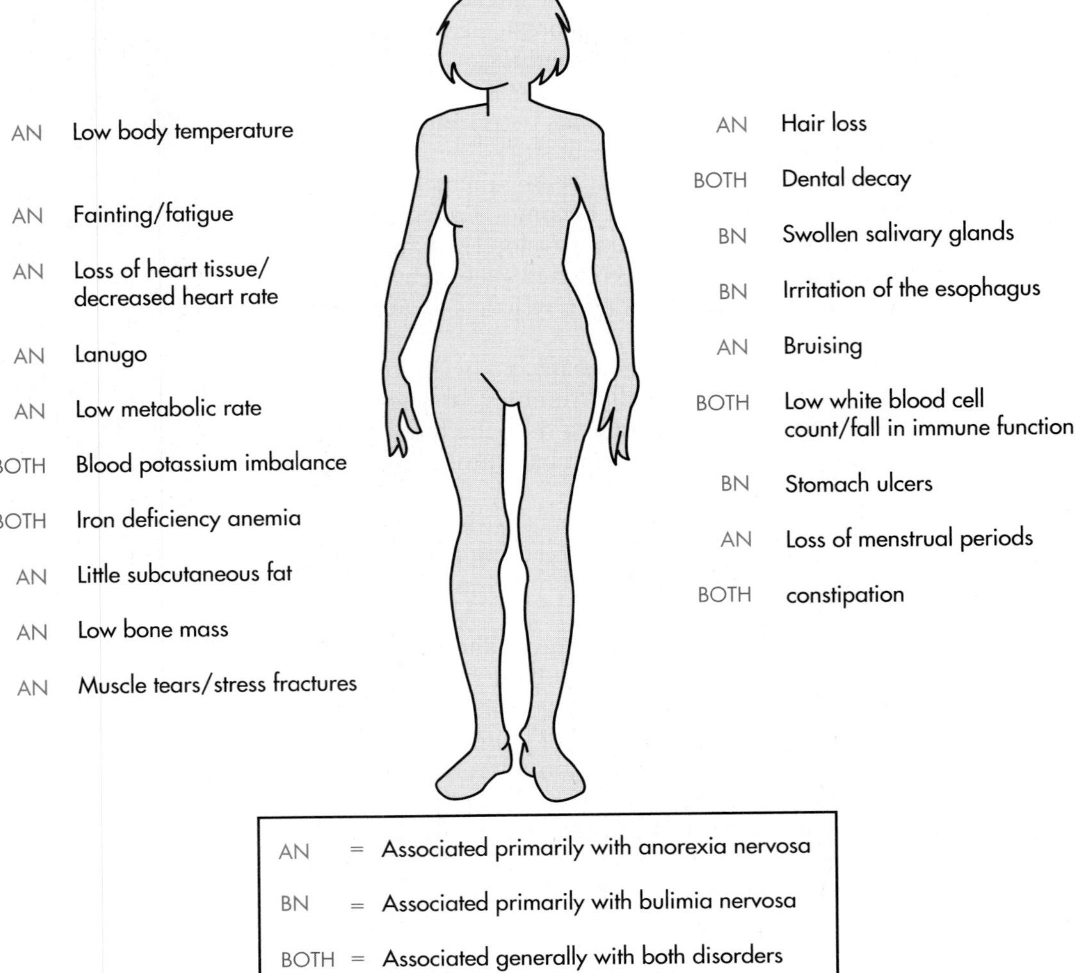

Figure 11–4 *Signs and symptoms of eating disorders. A vast array of physical effects are associated with anorexia nervosa and bulimia nervosa. This figure contains many but is not an exhaustive list of all potential consequences. These physical effects can also serve as warning signs that a problem exists. Professional evaluation is then indicated.*

- Loss of hair caused by a deficient nutrient intake.
- Appearance of **lanugo,** downy hairs on the body that trap air, reducing heat loss and in turn replacing some insulation lost with the fat layer.
- Constipation from semistarvation and laxative abuse.
- Low blood potassium caused by a deficient nutrient intake, loss of potassium from vomiting, and use of some types of diuretics. This increases the risk of heart rhythm disturbances, another leading cause of death in anorexic people.
- Loss of menstrual periods because of low body weight, low body fat content, and the stress of the disease. Accompanying hormonal changes cause a loss of bone mass and increase the risk of osteoporosis later in life.
- Changes in neurotransmitter function in the brain and related depression.
- Eventual loss of teeth caused by frequent vomiting. Until vomiting ceases, one way to reduce this effect on teeth is to rinse the mouth with water right away and brush teeth as soon as possible. Loss of teeth and bone mass can be lasting signs of the disease, even if the other physical and mental problems are resolved.
- Muscle tears and stress fractures in athletes because of decreased bone and muscle mass.

A person with this disorder is psychologically and physically ill and needs help.

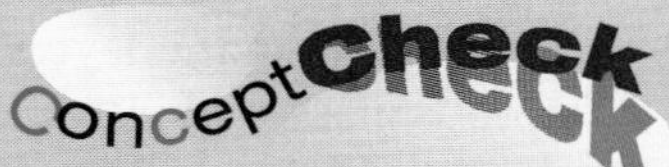

Anorexia nervosa is an eating disorder characterized by semistarvation. It is found primarily—but not exclusively—in adolescent girls, starting at or around puberty. People with anorexia dwindle essentially to "skin and bones" but often believe they are fat. Semistarvation produces hormonal and other changes that lower body temperature, slow the heart rate, decrease immune response, stop menstrual periods, and contribute to hair, muscle, and bone loss. It is a very serious disease that often produces lifelong consequences and may be fatal.

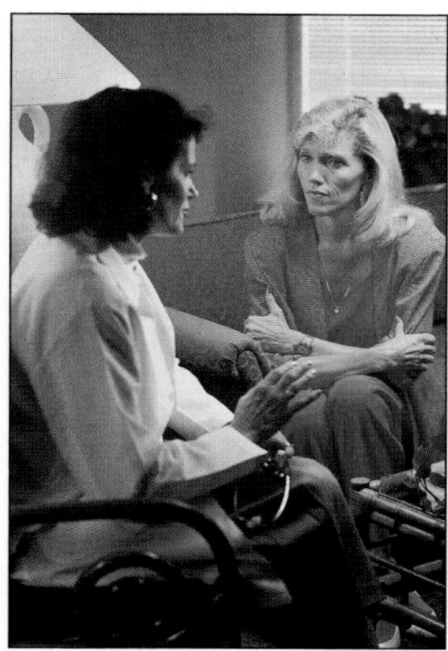

Anorexia nervosa is a potentially fatal disease that requires professional treatment.

Treatment of Anorexia Nervosa

People with anorexia often sink into shells of isolation and fear. They deny that a problem exists. Frequently, their friends and family members meet with them to confront the problem in a loving way. This is called an *intervention*. They present evidence of the problem and encourage immediate treatment. Treatment then requires a team of experienced physicians, registered dietitians, psychologists, and other health professionals working together. The team attempts to work together to restore a sense of balance, purpose, and future possibilities. An ideal setting is an eating disorders clinic in a medical center with inpatient facilities. Hospitalization is generally necessary once a person falls to 70% or below of healthy weight. Still, even in the most skilled hands and using the finest facilities, efforts may fail. As previously stated, anorexia nervosa is usually rooted in psychological conflict. However, a person who has been barely existing in a state of semistarvation cannot focus on much besides food. Dreams and even morbid thoughts about food will interfere with therapy until sufficient weight is regained. This tells us that prevention of anorexia nervosa is of utmost importance.

Nutrition Therapy

The first goal of therapy, then, is to increase food intake, but the therapist must have the patient's cooperation. Otherwise, no long-term benefit will be realized. Nutrition provided through a tube or intravenously is used only if immediate renourishment is required, as these procedures can cause the patient to distrust medical staff. Ideally, weight gain must be gradual and enough to raise the metabolic rate to normal and reverse as many of the physical signs of the disease as possible. Overall, food intake is designed first to minimize or stop any further weight loss. Then the focus shifts to restoring appropriate food habits. After this, the expectation can be switched to ongoing slow weight gain to an individualized goal. A range of 1 to 3 pounds per week is appropriate.

Patients need considerable reassurance during the refeeding process because of uncomfortable effects such as bloating, increase in body heat, and increase in body fat. This is a frightening process, because these changes can lead to feeling out of control.

In addition to helping patients reach and maintain adequate nutritional status, the dietitian on the medical team also provides accurate nutrition information throughout treatment, promotes a healthy attitude toward food, and helps the patient learn to eat based on natural hunger and satiety. The medical team also should assure patients that they will not be abandoned after gaining weight.

Because excessive energy expenditure prevents weight gain, professionals must work with anorexic patients to help them moderate their activity. At many treatment centers, patients are placed on moderate bed rest in the early states of treatment to help promote weight gain.

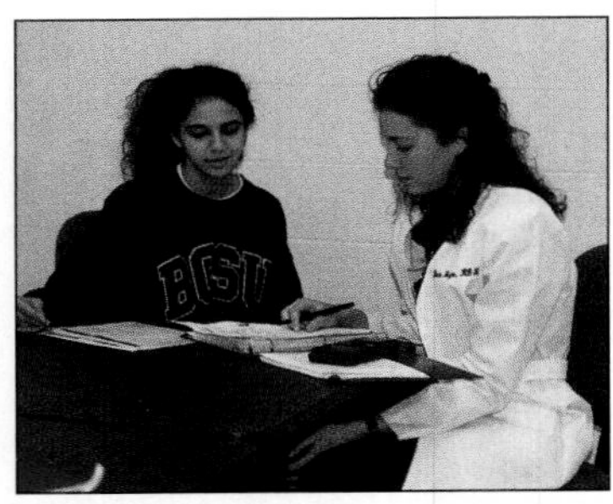

Early treatment for an eating disorder improves chances of success.

Experienced professional help is the key. An anorexic patient may be on the verge of suicide and near starvation. Today, suicide is the most common cause of death in people with anorexia nervosa. In addition, anorexic people are often very clever and resistant. They may try to hide weight loss by wearing many layers of clothes, putting coins in their pockets, and drinking numerous glasses of water.

Psychological and Related Therapy

Once the physical problems of anorexic patients are addressed, the treatment focus shifts to the underlying emotional problems that led to excessive dieting and other symptoms of the disorder. To heal, these patients must reject the sense of accomplishment associated with an emaciated body. If therapists can discover reasons for the disorder, they can develop strategies for restoring normal weight and eating habits by resolving psychological conflicts. Education about the medical consequences of semistarvation is also helpful. A key aspect of psychological treatment is showing affected individuals how to regain control of some facets of their lives and cope with tough situations. As eating evolves into a normal routine, they then can turn to previously neglected activities.

Cognitive behavior therapy *Psychological therapy in which the person's assumptions about dieting, body weight, and related issues are challenged. New ways of thinking are explored and then practiced by the person. In this way the person can learn new ways to control eating disorders behaviors and related life stress.*

Therapists may use **cognitive behavior therapy,** which involves helping the person confront and change irrational beliefs about body image, eating, relationships, and weight. Obviously, issues of sexual abuse need to be addressed as well.

Family therapy is important in treating anorexia nervosa. It focuses on the role of the illness among family members, reactions of individual family members, and ways in which their subconscious behavior might contribute to the abnormal eating patterns. Therapy includes all family members involved with the behavior problem. Frequently a therapist finds family struggles at the heart of the problem. As the disorder resolves, patients must relate to family members in new ways to gain the attention previously tied to the disease. The family needs to help the young person ease into adulthood and accept its responsibilities as well as its advantages.

Self-help groups for anorexic and bulimic people, as well as their families and friends, represent nonthreatening first steps into treatment. People can also attend to get a sense of whether they really do have an eating disorder.

The role of medications in the treatment of anorexia nervosa is very narrow, and they cannot be the sole therapy. Extreme anxiety, relentless depression, or unbearable stomach pain with meals may indicate the need for medication. Overall, though, medications are not known to be highly successful. Instead, food is the drug of choice.

With professional help, many people with anorexia nervosa can lead normal lives. They then do not have to depend on unusual eating habits to cope with daily problems. Although they may not be totally cured, they do recover a sense of normality in their lives. No set answers or approaches exist, because each case is different. Establishing a strong relationship with either a therapist or another supportive person is an especially important key to recovery. Once anorexic patients feel understood and accepted by another person, they can begin to build a sense of self and exercise some autonomy. Then they can progress to substituting healthy relationships with others for a relationship with food, emphasizing alternative coping mechanisms.

A young woman in a self-help group for those with anorexia nervosa explained her feelings to the other group members: "I have lost a specialness that I thought it gave me. I was different from everyone else. Now I know that I'm somebody who's overcome it, which not everybody does."

Concept Check

To relieve the semistarved condition of most anorexic patients, the initial treatment focuses on moderately increased food intake and slow weight gain. Once this is accomplished, psychotherapy can begin to uncover the causes of the disease and help patients develop skills needed to return to a healthy life. Family therapy is an important tool in treatment; while medications have a limited role at best.

Bulimia Nervosa

Bulimia nervosa involves episodes of binge eating followed by attempts to purge the food (energy intake). This eating disorder is most common among young adults of college age, although some high school students are also at risk. Susceptible people often have biological factors and lifestyle patterns that predispose them to becoming overweight, causing them to try frequent weight-reduction diets as teenagers. Like people with anorexia nervosa, those with bulimia nervosa are usually female and successful. Unlike anorexics, however, they are usually at or slightly above a normal weight. Females with bulimia nervosa are also more likely to be sexually active than those with anorexia nervosa.

The person with bulimia nervosa may think of food constantly. In contrast to the anorexic person, who turns away from food when faced with problems, the bulimic person turns toward food in critical situations. Also, unlike those with anorexia nervosa, people with bulimia nervosa recognize their behavior as abnormal. These people often have very low self-esteem and are depressed. Other medical complications that commonly coexist with bulimia nervosa are mood disorders, substance abuse disorders, and anxiety and personality disorders. Lingering effects of child abuse may be one reason for these psychological difficulties. Many bulimic persons report that they have been sexually abused. The world sees their competence, while inside they feel out of control, ashamed, and frustrated.

Bulimic people tend to be impulsive, which may be expressed as stealing, drug and alcohol abuse, self-mutilation, or attempted suicide. Some experts have suggested that part of the problem may actually arise from an inability to control responses to impulse and desire. Some studies have demonstrated that bulimic people tend to come from disengaged families, ones that are loosely organized. Roles for family members are not clearly defined. Too little protection is provided for family members, rules are very loose, and a great deal of conflict exists. Anorexic people tend to have families so actively engaged that roles may be too well defined.

Alicia Machado, 1997's Miss Universe, reported being both anorexic and bulimic at the time she won the crown, stating, "Almost all of us are."

Typical Behavior in Bulimia Nervosa

Many people with bulimic behavior are probably never diagnosed. The strict diagnostic criteria specify that to be diagnosed with bulimia nervosa a person must binge at least twice a week for 3 months. People with bulimia nervosa lead secret lives, hiding their abnormal eating habits. Moreover, it is impossible to recognize people with bulimia nervosa simply from their appearance. Because most diagnoses of bulimia nervosa are based on self-reports, current estimates of the number of cases are probably low. The disorder, especially in its milder forms, may be much more widespread than commonly thought.

Among suffers of bulimia nervosa, bingeing often alternates with attempts to rigidly restrict food intake. Elaborate "food rules" are common, such as avoiding all sweets. Thus eating just one cookie or donut may cause bulimic persons to feel they have broken a rule. Then the objectionable food must be eliminated. Usually this leads to further overeating, partly because it is easier to regurgitate a large amount of food than a small amount. For intake to qualify as a binge, an atypically large amount of food must be consumed in a short period of time and the person must exhibit a lack of control over this behavior.

Binge-purge cycles may be practiced daily, weekly, or at longer intervals. A special time is often set aside. Most binge eating occurs at night, when other people are less likely to interrupt, and usually lasts from ½ to 2 hours. A binge can be triggered by a combination of hunger from recent dieting, stress, boredom, loneliness, and depression. It often follows a period of strict dieting and thus can be linked to intense hunger. The binge is not at all like normal eating; once begun, it seems to propel itself. The person not only loses control but generally doesn't even taste or enjoy the food that is eaten during a binge (Figure 11–5).

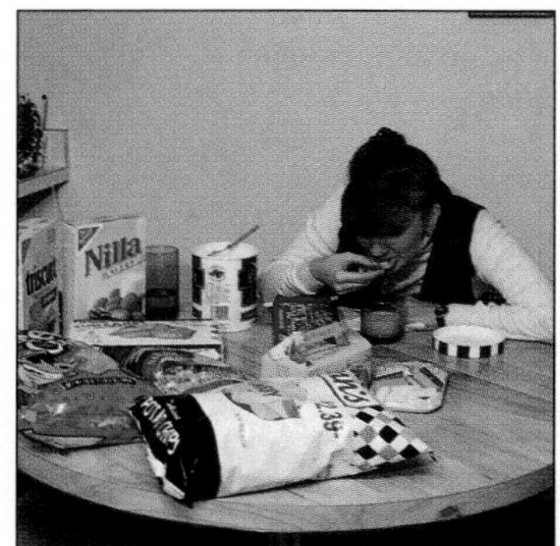

Figure 11–5
The binge-purge cycle can lead to a sense of helplessness.

Frequent binges can lead to enormous food bills for a bulimic person.

Most commonly, bulimic people consume cakes, cookies, ice cream, and similar high-carbohydrate convenience foods during binges, because these foods can be purged relatively easily and comfortably by vomiting. In a single binge, foods supplying 10,000 to 15,000 kcal or more may be eaten. Purging follows in hopes that no weight will be gained. However, even when vomiting follows the binge 33% to 75% of the food energy taken in is still absorbed, which causes some weight gain. When laxatives are used, about 90% of the energy is absorbed. The common belief of bulimic persons that purging soon after bingeing will prevent excessive nutrient uptake and weight gain is clearly a misperception.

Early in the onset of bulimia nervosa, sufferers often induce vomiting by placing their fingers deep into the mouth. They may inadvertently bite down on these fingers. The resulting bite marks around the knuckles are a characteristic sign of this disorder. Once the disease is established, however, a person can often vomit simply by contracting the abdominal muscles. Vomiting may also occur spontaneously.

Another way bulimic people attempt to compensate for a binge is by engaging in hypergymnasia—excessive exercise—to expend a large amount of energy. Some bulimic people try to estimate the amount of energy eaten in a binge and then exercise to counteract this energy intake. This practice, referred to as "debting", represents an effort to control their weight.

People with bulimia nervosa are not proud of their behavior. After a binge they usually feel guilty and depressed. Over time they experience low self-esteem and feel hopeless about their situation (Figure 11–6). Compulsive lying and drug abuse can further intensify these feelings. Bulimic people caught in the act of bingeing by a friend or family member may order the intruder to "get out" and "go away." Sufferers gradually distance themselves from others, spending more and more time preoccupied by and engaging in bingeing and purging.

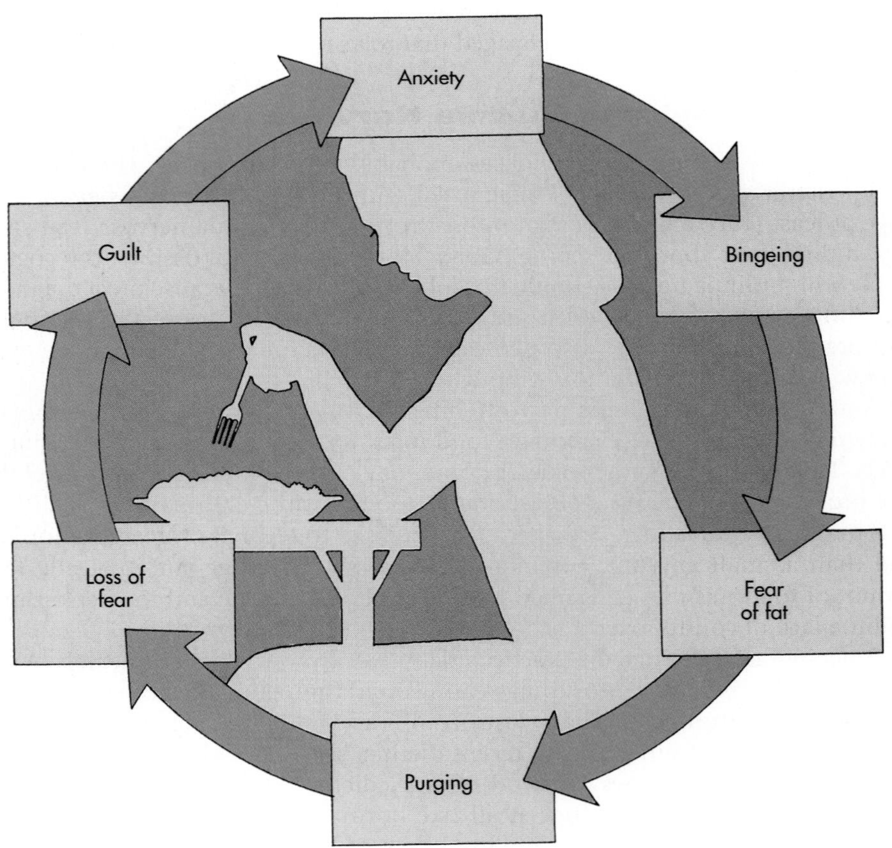

Figure 11–6 *Bulimia nervosa's vicious cycle of obsession.*

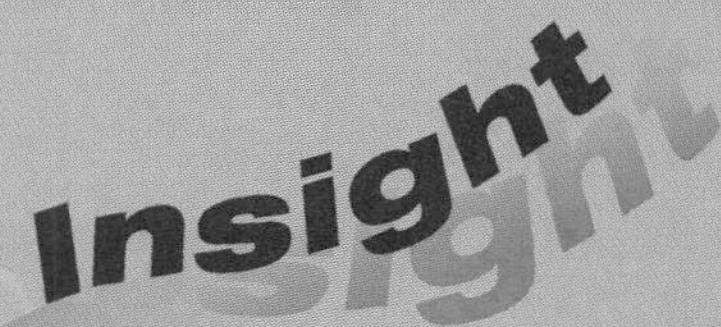

Thoughts of a Bulimic Woman

I am wide awake and immediately out of bed. I think back to the night before, when I made a new list of what I wanted to get done and how I wanted to be. My husband is not far behind me on his way into the bathroom to get ready for work. Maybe I can sneak onto the scale to see what I weigh this morning before he notices me. I am already in my private world. I feel overjoyed when the scale says that I stayed the same weight as I was the night before, and I can feel that slightly hungry feeling. Maybe it will stop today; maybe today everything will change. What were the projects I was going to get done?

We eat the same breakfast, except that I take no butter on my toast, no cream in my coffee, and never take seconds (until Doug gets out the door). Today I am going to be really good, and that means eating certain predetermined portions of food and not taking one more bite than I think I am allowed. I am very careful to see that I don't take more than Doug. I judge myself by his body. I can feel the tension building. I wish Doug would hurry up and leave so I can get going!

As soon as he shuts the door, I try to get involved with one of the myriad responsibilities on my list. I hate them all! I just want to crawl into a hole. I don't want to do anything. I'd rather eat. I am alone; I am nervous; I am no good; I always do everything wrong anyway; I am not in control; I can't make it through the day, I know it. It has been the same for so long. I remember the starchy cereal I ate for breakfast. I am into the bathroom and onto the scale. It measures the same, but I don't want to stay the same! I want to be thinner! I look in the mirror. I think my thighs are ugly and deformed looking. I see a lumpy, clumsy, pear-shaped wimp. There is always something wrong with what I see. I feel frustrated, trapped in this body, and I don't know what to do about it.

I float to the refrigerator knowing exactly what is there. I begin with last night's brownies. I always begin with the sweets. At first I try to make it look like nothing is missing, but my appetite is huge and I resolve to make another batch of brownies. I know there is half of a bag of cookies in the bathroom, thrown out the night before, and I polish them off immediately. I take some milk so my vomiting will be smoother. I like the full feeling I get after downing a big glass. I get out six pieces of bread and toast one side of each in the broiler, turn them over and load them with pats of butter, and put them under the broiler again until they are bubbling. I take all six pieces on a plate to the television and go back for a bowl of cereal and a banana to have along with them. Before the last piece of toast is finished, I am already preparing the next batch of six more pieces. Maybe another brownie or five, and a couple of large bowls full of ice cream, yogurt, or cottage cheese.

My stomach is stretched into a huge ball below my rib cage. I know I'll have to go into the bathroom soon, but I want to postpone it. I am in never-never land. I am waiting, feeling the pressure, pacing the floor in and out of the rooms. Time is passing. Time is passing. It is getting to be time. I wander aimlessly through each of the rooms again, tidying, making the whole house neat and put back together. I finally make the turn into the bathroom. I brace my feet, pull my hair back and stick my finger down my throat, stroking twice, and get up a huge pile of food. Three times, four times, and another pile of food. I can see everything come back. I am so glad to see those brownies because they are so fattening. The rhythm of the emptying is broken and my head is beginning to hurt. I stand up feeling dizzy, empty, and weak. The whole episode has taken about an hour.

From Hall L, Cohn L: *Bulimia—a guide to recovery,* Carlsbad, Calif, 1992, Gurze Books.

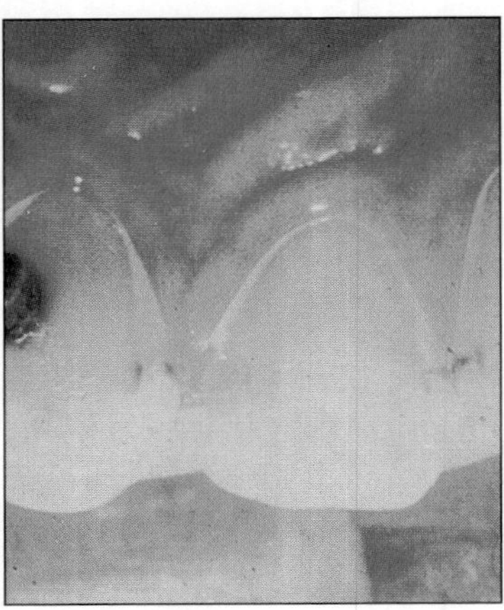

Figure 11–7
Excessive tooth decay is common in bulimic patients.

Health Problems Stemming from Bulimia Nervosa

The vomiting that many bulimic sufferers induce is the most physically destructive method of purging. Indeed the majority of health problems associated with bulimia nervosa arise from vomiting.

- Repeated exposure of teeth to the acid in vomit causes demineralization, making the teeth painful and sensitive to heat, cold, and acids. Eventually the teeth may severely decay, erode away from fillings, and finally fall out. Dental professionals are sometimes the first health professionals to notice signs of bulimia nervosa (Figure 11–7). As noted earlier, until vomiting ceases it is important to rinse the mouth with water after a vomiting episode, especially before brushing the teeth.
- Blood potassium can drop significantly with regular vomiting or use of certain diuretics. This can disturb the heart's rhythm and even produce sudden death.
- Salivary glands may swell as a result of infection and irritation from persistent vomiting.
- Stomach ulcers and bleeding, and tears in the esophagus develop in some cases.
- Constipation may result from frequent laxative use.
- Ipecac syrup, sometimes used to induce vomiting, is poisonous to the heart, liver, and kidneys. It has caused accidental poisoning when taken repeatedly.

Overall, bulimia nervosa is a potentially debilitating disorder that can lead to death, usually from suicide, low blood potassium, or overwhelming infections.

Treatment of Bulimia Nervosa

Though pharmacological agents should not be used as the sole treatment for bulimia nervosa, studies indicate that some medications used to treat depression may be beneficial in conjunction with other therapies.

Therapy for bulimia nervosa, as for anorexia nervosa, requires a team of experienced clinicians. These patients are less likely than those with anorexia to enter treatment in a state of semistarvation. However, if a bulimic patient has lost significant weight, this must be treated before psychological treatment begins. Although clinicians have yet to agree on the best therapy for bulimia nervosa, they generally agree that treatment should last at least 16 weeks. Hospitalization may be indicated in cases of extreme laxative abuse, regular vomiting, and substance abuse.

The first goal of treatment for bulimia nervosa is to decrease the binge amount to in turn decrease the risk of esophageal tears from related purging by vomiting. A decrease in the number of this type of purges will also decrease damage to the teeth.

Nutritional counseling adds two additional goals: correcting misconceptions about food and reestablishing regular eating habits. Patients are given information about bulimia nervosa and its consequences. Avoiding binge foods and not constantly stepping on a scale may be recommended early in treatment. The primary goal, however, is to develop a normal eating pattern. To achieve this goal, some specialists encourage patients to develop daily meal plans and keep a food diary in which they record food intake, internal sensations of hunger, environmental factors that precipitate binges, and thoughts and feelings that accompany binge-purge cycles. Keeping a food diary not only is an accurate way to monitor food intake but also may help identify situations that seem to trigger binge episodes. With the help of a therapist, patients can develop alternative coping strategies.

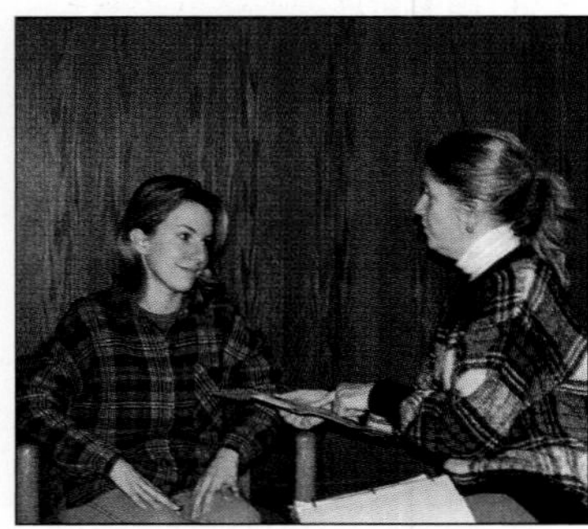

Bulimia nervosa affects many college students. Counselors are aware of this and are available to help.

In general, the focus is not on stopping bingeing and purging per se but on developing regular eating habits. Once this is achieved, the binge-purge cycle should stop by itself. Patients are discouraged from following strict rules about healthy food choices, because this simply mimics the typical obsessive attitudes associated with bulimia nervosa. Rather, encouraging a mature perspective on nutrient intake helps patients overcome this disorder—that is, regular consumption of moderate amounts of a variety of foods balanced among the food groups.

The primary aim of psychotherapy is to improve patients' self-acceptance and help them to be less concerned about body weight. Cognitive behavior therapy is commonly used. For example, to correct the "all-or-none" thinking typical of bulimic persons—if I eat one cookie, I'm a failure and might as well binge—a patient may be asked to test assumptions and beliefs about food and weight. Patient and therapist together examine the validity of such beliefs. The premise of this therapy is that if abnormal attitudes and beliefs can be altered, normal eating will follow. In addition, the therapist guides the person in establishing food habits that will minimize bingeing: avoiding fasting, eating regular meals, and using alternative methods —other than eating—to cope with stressful situations. Group therapy is often useful to foster strong social support. A final goal of therapy is to help bulimic persons accept as normal some depression and self-doubt.

People with bulimia nervosa ultimately must recognize that it is a serious disorder that can have grave medical complications if not treated. Because relapse is likely, therapy should be long term, as mentioned before. Note that those with bulimia nervosa do need professional help because they can be very depressed and are at a high risk for suicide. About 45% of people with bulimia nervosa recover completely from the disorder. Others continue to struggle with it to varying degrees. This fact underscores the need for prevention, because treatment is difficult.

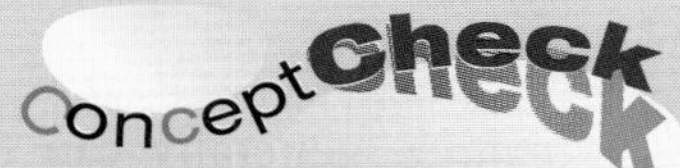

Bulimia nervosa is characterized by episodes of binge eating followed by purging, usually by vomiting. Vomiting is very destructive to the body, often causing severe dental decay, stomach ulcers, irritation of the esophagus, and blood potassium imbalances. Treatment using nutrition counseling and psychotherapy attempts to restore normal eating habits, help the person correct distorted beliefs about diet and lifestyle, and find tools to copy with the stresses of life. Antidepressant medications can aid recovery when added to this regimen.

OTHER DISORDERED EATING PATTERNS

In recent years, three other eating disorders—**female athlete triad, binge-eating disorder** and **baryophobia**—have been recognized as requiring professional treatment. Although these disordered eating patterns share some characteristics with anorexia nervosa and bulimia nervosa, they have some distinctive qualities.

Female athlete triad
A condition characterized by disordered eating, lack of menstrual periods, and low age-adjusted bone density.

Binge-eating disorder
An eating disorder characterized by recurrent binge eating and feelings of loss of control over eating that has lasted at least 6 months. Binge episodes can be triggered by frustration, anger, depression, anxiety, permission to eat forbidden foods, and excessive hunger.

Baryophobia
A disorder of young children and young adults characterized by stunted growth. It results from parental underfeeding in an attempt to prevent development of obesity and heart disease.

Female Athlete Triad

As mentioned previously, women participating in appearance-based and endurance sports are at risk of developing an eating disorder. A recent study of college-age female athletes found that 15% of swimmers, 62% of gymnasts, and 32% of all varsity athletes exhibited disordered eating patterns. Estimates of eating disorders for college women not involved in competitive sports are much lower.

In addition to disordered eating, college women athletes tend to experience irregular menstruation more frequently than other college women. Disordered eating, particularly food restriction and stress, can precipitate this, causing women to have less dense and weaker bones than normal because of lower estrogen and higher cortisol concentrations in the blood. Some of these young women have bones equivalent to those of 50- to 60-year-olds, making them overly susceptible to fractures during both sports and general activities. Much of the bone loss is irreversible.

The combination of disordered eating, lack of menstrual periods, and compromised bone density is called *the female athlete triad.* Those exhibiting the symptoms should get treatment. One treatment plan has the following goals:

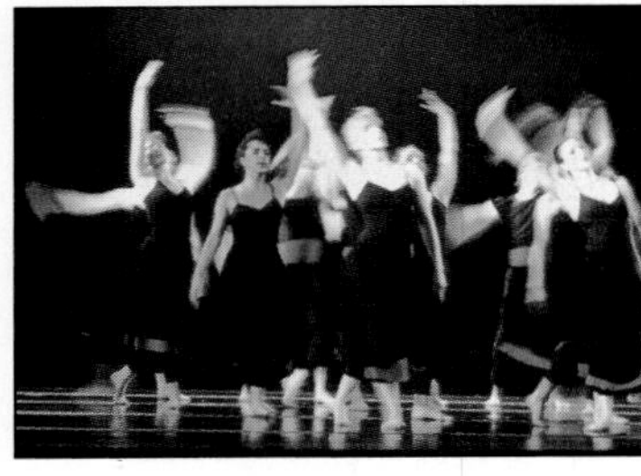

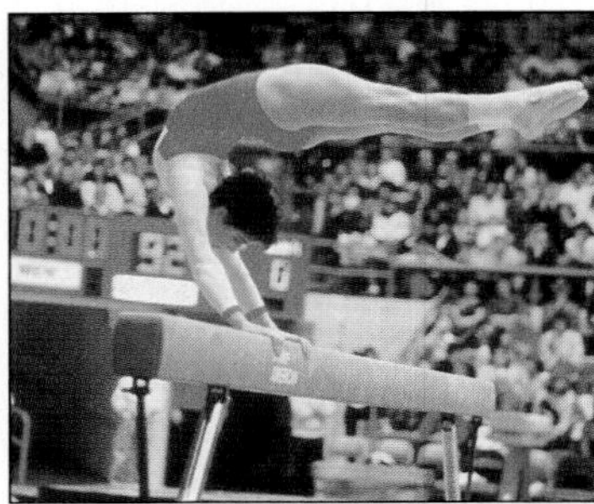

In pursuits where thinness is emphasized, such as ballet and gymnastics, women are at greater risk for developing the characteristics termed the Female Athlete Triad.

- Reduce preoccupation with food, weight, and body fat.
- Gradually increase meals and snacks to an appropriate amount.
- Rebuild the body to a more appropriate weight.
- Establish regular menstrual periods.

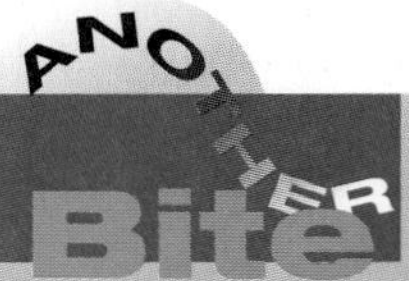

The tragic case of Christy Henrich illustrates why anyone at risk for the female athlete triad should seek professional help. As a young teenager Christy weighed 95 pounds and was 4 feet 11 inches. She showed promise as a gymnast but was told that she was too fat to excel in gymnastics. Christy continued her training but often starved herself, some days consuming just an apple and frequently purging by vomiting. Her success in gymnastics continued, but at age 22 her weight had fallen to 52 pounds, and she died in August 1994 of the effects of long-term semistarvation.

Binge-Eating Disorder

Binge-eating disorder, commonly called *compulsive overeating,* generally can be defined as binge-eating episodes not accompanied by purging (as typifies bulimia nervosa) at least 2 times per week for at least 6 months (Table 11–2).

TABLE 11-2

Some Characteristics of Binge-Eating Disorder

1. Repeated episodes of binge eating, an episode being characterized by both of the following:
   a. Eating in a specific period of time (e.g., within any 2-hour period); the amount of food is definitely larger than most people would eat.
   b. A sense of lack of control during the episodes (e.g., a feeling that one can't stop eating or control what or how much one is eating).
2. During most binge-eating episodes at least three of the following occur:
   a. Eating much more rapidly than usual.
   b. Eating until feeling uncomfortably full.
   c. Eating large amounts of food when not feeling physically hungry.
   d. Eating alone because of being embarrassed by how much one is eating.
   e. Feeling disgusted with oneself, depressed, or very guilty after overeating.
3. The binge eating occurs, on average, at least 2 days a week for 6 months.
4. The behavior is not part of a case of bulimia nervosa or anorexia nervosa.

Based on information in the *Diagnostic and Statistical Manual of Mental Disorders (DSM-IV),* Washington, DC, 1994, American Psychiatric Association.

A female high school athlete recently admitted to a 3-year struggle with anorexia nervosa and bulimia nervosa. Even after her athletic performance declined and she suffered a related sports injury that sidelined her for a year and required surgery, she continued to think that controlling both her weight and eating behaviors would make her the best—academically and physically. This example demonstrates several important points about eating disorders: certain groups of people are at greater risk for developing eating disorders; these people are often high achievers and are very careful about concealing their eating disorder; and eating disorders such as the female athlete triad, bulimia nervosa, and anorexia nervosa frequently overlap.

Approximately 30% of subjects in organized weight-control programs have binge-eating disorder, whereas among the general population only 2% to 5% have this disorder. However, many more people in the general population are likely to have less severe forms of the disorder that do not meet the formal criteria for diagnosis. The number of cases of binge-eating disorder is far greater than that of either anorexia nervosa or bulimia nervosa.

Development and Characteristics of Binge Eating

Individuals with binge-eating disorder often perceive themselves as hungry more often than normal. They usually started dieting at a young age, began bingeing during adolescence or in their early 20s, and did not succeed in commercial weight-control programs. Almost half of those with severe binge-eating disorder exhibit clinical depression.

Typical binge eaters isolate themselves and eat large quantities of a favorite food. Stressful events and feelings of depression, loneliness, or anxiety can trigger this behavior. Giving themselves permission to eat a forbidden food can also precipitate a binge. They sometimes binge on whatever is easy to eat in large amounts—noodles, rice, bread, leftovers. Characteristically, however, binge eaters consume foods that carry the social stigma of "junk" or "bad" foods—ice cream, cookies, sweets, potato chips, and similar snack foods.

In general, people engage in binge eating to induce a sense of well-being and perhaps even numbness, usually in an attempt to avoid feeling and dealing with emotional pain and anxiety. They eat without regard to biological need and often in a recurrent, ritualized fashion. Some people with this disorder eat food continually over an extended period, called *grazing;* others cycle episodes of bingeing with normal eating. For example, someone with a stressful or frustrating job might come home every night and graze until bedtime. Another person might eat normally most of the time but find comfort in consuming large quantities of food when an emotional setback occurs.

Although people with anorexia nervosa and bulimia nervosa exhibit persistent preoccupation with body shape, weight, and thinness, binge eaters do not necessarily share these concerns. Thus neither purging nor prolonged food restriction is characteristic of binge-eating disorder. Some physicians classify binge-eating disorder as an addiction to food, involving psychological dependence. Note that obesity and binge eating are not necessarily linked. Not all obese people are binge eaters, and although obesity may result from trying to numb emotional pain with food, it is not necessarily an outcome.

Binge-eating disorder is most likely to develop in people who never learned to appropriately express and deal with their feelings. Rather than face their problems, they turn to food instead. They continue to do the things that perpetuate the experiences of frustration, anger, and pain. For example, people who regularly become frustrated because they don't assert themselves when necessary may eat to forget their frustration rather than learn to deal with this inhibition and practice assertiveness. The frustration will continue because they never attack the basic problem.

Often, people who practice binge eating have been shaped by families who do not address and express feelings in healthful ways. The parents nurture and comfort their children with food rather than engage in healthy exchanges of self-disclosure of feelings and potential solutions. Members of such families learn to eat in response to emotional needs and pain instead of hunger. Not knowing how to satisfy their personal and emotional needs in more healthful ways, people in these families turn to food.

For some people, frequent dieting beginning in childhood or adolescence is a precursor to binge-eating disorder. During periods when little food is eaten, they get very hungry and obsessive about food. When allowed to eat more food or given permission to go off the diet, they feel driven to eat in a compulsive, uncontrolled way.

Help for the Binge Eater

Those with binge-eating disorder must learn to eat in response to hunger—a biological signal—rather than in response to emotional needs or external factors (such as the time of day or the simple presence of food). Counselors often direct binge eaters to record their perceptions of physical hunger throughout the day and at the beginning and end of every meal. These people must learn to respond to a prescribed amount of fullness at each meal. They should initially avoid weight-loss diets because feelings of food deprivation can lead to more disruptive emotions and a greater sense of unmet needs. Diets are likely to encourage more intense problems with binge eating. Many people with this disorder may experience difficulty in identifying personal emotional needs and expressing emotions. Because this problem is a common predisposing factor in binge eating, communication issues should be addressed during treatment. Binge eaters often must be helped to recognize their own buried emotions in anxiety-producing situations and then encouraged to share them. Learning simple but appropriate phrases to say to oneself can help stop bingeing when the desire is strong.

Self-help groups such as Overeaters Anonymous aim to help recovery from binge-eating disorder. The treatment philosophy parallels that of Alcoholics Anonymous. Overeaters Anonymous attempts to create an environment of encouragement and accountability to overcome this eating disorder. Dietary goals typically range from avoiding restraint in eating to limiting binge foods. Some experts feel that learning to eat all foods—but in moderation—is an effective goal for binge eaters. This practice can prevent the feelings of desperation and deprivation that come from limiting particular foods. There is no set answer, but diet extremism is not needed. Some medications have been found to help reduce binge eating in these individuals by decreasing depression. Overall, people who have this disorder are usually unsuccessful in controlling it on their own. Professional help is advised.

Baryophobia

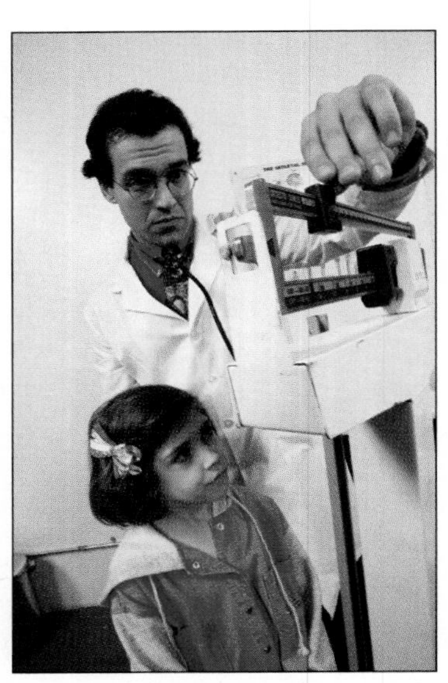

A slowdown in gains in weight and height for one's predicted age can be a sign of baryophobia. If noted, this and other causes deserve further scrutiny.

Some children and young adults who grow more slowly and have a shorter stature than normal may suffer from **baryophobia** (literally, "the fear of becoming heavy"). Decreased growth in children usually results from disease—commonly a hormonal or other metabolic abnormality. In the absence of a recognized disease in such children, the possibility of baryophobia should be investigated. This disorder occurs when children are given the same low-fat, high-carbohydrate diet that adults follow. Adults do this in an attempt to prevent children from developing obesity or heart disease later in life. Today's parents and caregivers, themselves frequently harassed by weight problems, may be determined that the children in their care will avoid such ordeals. Although well-intended, such severely restricted diets are detrimental to children because they don't supply enough energy to sustain an adequate growth rate. In young adults, low-energy diets may be self-imposed to avoid a perceived risk of obesity. Because this disorder results largely from lack of appropriate nutrition information leading to inappropriate food choices, nutritional counseling of caregivers and young adults is the most effective response. Supplying adequate carbohydrate, protein, and other nutrients is the key to promoting growth in both height and weight during childhood and the young-adult years, and it can be done in a healthful manner (see Chapter 13).

PREVENTING EATING DISORDERS

A key to developing and maintaining healthful eating behavior is to realize that some concern about diet, health, and weight is normal. It is also normal to experience variation in what we eat, how we feel, and even how much we weigh. For example, it is not abnormal to experience some minimal weight change (up to 2 to 3 pounds) throughout the day and even more over the course of a week. A large weight fluctuation or ongoing weight gain or weight loss is a more likely indicator that a problem is present. If you notice a large change in your diet, how you feel, or your body weight, it is a good idea to consult with your primary physician. Treating physical and emotional problems early helps lead you to peace of mind and good health.

With a view to society as a whole, many people begin to form opinions about food, nutrition, health, weight, and body image especially during puberty. Parents, friends, and professionals working with young adults should consider the following advise for preventing eating disorders:

- Discourage restrictive dieting, meal skipping, and fasting.
- Provide information about normal changes that occur during puberty.
- Correct misconceptions about nutrition, healthy body weight, and approaches to weight loss.
- Carefully phrase weight-related recommendations and comments, and use with caution.
- Don't overemphasize numbers on a scale. Instead, primarily promote healthful behavior.
- Encourage normal expression of disruptive emotions.
- Encourage children to eat only when they're hungry.
- Teach the basics of proper nutrition and physical activity in school and at home.
- Do not use food as rewards for children.
- Provide adolescents with an appropriate but not unlimited degree of independence, choice, responsibility, and self-accountability for their actions.
- Encourage coaches to be sensitive to weight and body-image issues among athletes.
- Emphasize that thinness is not necessarily associated with better athletic performance.

Our society as a whole can benefit from a fresh focus on healthful food practices and a healthful outlook toward food and weight.

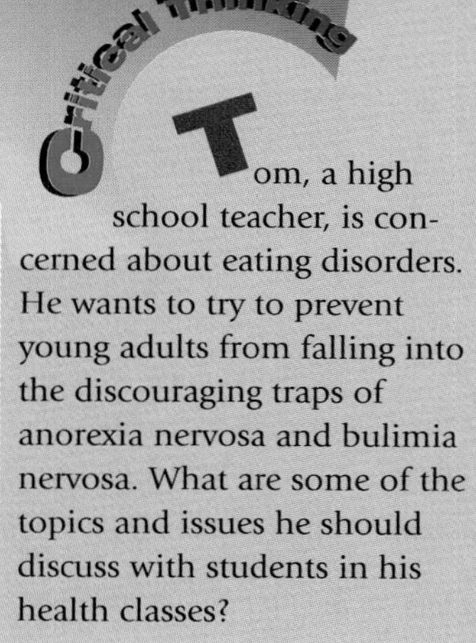

Tom, a high school teacher, is concerned about eating disorders. He wants to try to prevent young adults from falling into the discouraging traps of anorexia nervosa and bulimia nervosa. What are some of the topics and issues he should discuss with students in his health classes?

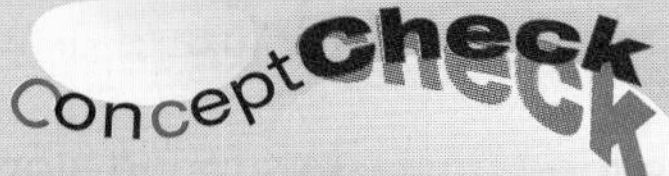

The female athlete triad consists of disordered eating, lack of menstrual periods, and abnormally low bone density associated with female athletes, particularly those in appearance-related and endurance sports. Parents, coaches, teachers, and health professionals need to initiate efforts to prevent and treat this problem. Grazing and food bingeing without purging are two behaviors characteristic of binge-eating disorder. Emotional disturbances are often at the root of this disordered form of eating. Treatment addresses deeper emotional issues, and endorses avoiding food deprivation and restrictive diets, while restoring more normal eating behaviors. Baryophobia describes a condition in which children are underfed by parents in an attempt to limit risk of future disease, such as obesity or heart disease. Growth failure—lack of expected weight and height gains—can result if nutrient intake is not increased to an appropriate amount.

Not only is treatment of eating disorders far more difficult than prevention, these disorders also have devastating effects on the entire family. For this reason, health-care professionals and caregivers should emphasize the importance of an overall healthful diet and moderation as opposed to restriction and perfection.

Along with the more technical articles listed later, you can gain more insight into eating disorders from the following resources designed for the lay public.

Books

Abraham S, Llewellyn-Jones D: *Eating disorders: the facts,* New York, 1997, Oxford University Press.

Cohen MA: *French toast for breakfast: declaring peace with emotional eating,* Carlsbad, Calif., 1995, Gurze Books.

Costin C: *The eating disorders sourcebook,* Chicago, Il, 1996, RGA Publishing Group.

Hirschman JR, Munter CH: *When women stop hating their bodies,* New York, 1995, Ballantine Books.

Hollis J: *Women and food obsession: fat and furious,* New York, 1994, Ballantine Books.

Pipher M: *Hunger pains: the modern woman's tragic quest for thinness,* New York, 1995, Ballantine Books.

Siegel M, Brisman J, Weinshel M: *Surviving an eating disorder: perspectives and strategies for family and friends,* Carlsbad, Calif., 1997, Gurze Books.

Organizations and self-help groups

Academy for Eating Disorders, Montefiore Medical School—Adolescent Medicine, 111 East 210th Street, Bronx, NY 10467; (718) 920-6782

Anorexia Nervosa and Related Eating Disorders, Inc., P.O. Box 5102, Eugene, OR, 97405; (514) 344-1144; http://www.anred.com

The American Anorexia/Bulimia Association, 165 West 46th Street, #1108, New York, NY 10036; (212) 575-6200; http://www.amanbu@aol.com

Eating Disorders Awareness and Prevention, Inc. (EDAP), 603 Stewart Street, Suite 803, Seattle, WA 98101; (206) 382-3587 or (800) 931-EDAP; http://members.aol.com/edapinc

National Association of Anorexia Nervosa and Associated Disorders, Box 7, Highland Park, IL 60035; (847) 831-3438; http://www.medpatients.com/health/20resources/naanad.html

The National Eating Disorders Organization, 6655 South Yale Avenue, Tulsa, OK 74136; (918) 481-4044; http://www.laureate.com

Summary

- Anorexia nervosa is most common among high-achieving perfectionist girls from middle- and upper-class families marked by conflict, high expectations, rigidity, and denial. The disorder usually starts with dieting in early puberty and proceeds to the near-total refusal to eat. Early warning signs include intense concern about weight gain and dieting as well as abnormal food habits, such as cooking food that they won't allow themselves to eat and classifying foods as safe and unsafe. The person likely follows an excessive exercise regimen.
- Anorexic persons become irritable, hostile, overly critical, and joyless; they tend to withdraw from family and friends. Eventually anorexia nervosa can lead to numerous physical effects, including a profound decrease in body weight and body fat, a fall in body temperature and heart rate, iron-deficiency anemia, a low white blood cell count, hair loss, constipation, low blood potassium, and the cessation of menstrual periods. Suicide is the most common cause of death in people with anorexia nervosa.
- Treatment of anorexia nervosa includes increasing food intake to support slow weight gain. Psychological counseling attempts to help patients establish regular food habits and to find means of coping with the life stresses that led to the disorder. Hospitalization and psychiatric medications may be necessary.
- Bulimia nervosa is characterized by bingeing on large amounts of foods at one sitting and then purging by vomiting, laxative use, exercise, or other means. Both men and women are at risk. Vomiting as a means of purging is especially destructive to the body; it can cause severe tooth decay, stomach ulcers, irritation of the esophagus, low blood potassium, and other problems. Bulimia nervosa poses a serious health problem and is associated with significant risk of suicide.
- Treatment of bulimia nervosa includes psychological as well as nutritional counseling. During treatment, bulimic persons learn to accept themselves and to cope with problems in ways that do not involve food. Regular eating patterns are developed as these patients begin to plan meals in an informed, healthful manner. Antidepressant medications can be a helpful addition to the regimen.
- The female athlete triad consists of disordered eating, amenorrhea, and abnormally low bone density and is particularly common in appearance-related and endurance sports. If not corrected, this disorder will eventually lead to decreased athletic performance and general health problems.
- Binge-eating disorder, which is more widespread than either anorexia nervosa or bulimia nervosa, is most common among people with a history of frequent, unsuccessful dieting. Binge eaters typically either practice grazing (i.e., eating continually over extended periods) or bingeing without purging. Emotional disturbances are often at the root of this disordered form of eating. Treatment addresses deeper emotional issues, discourages food deprivation and restrictive diets, and helps to restore normal eating behaviors.

➤ Baryophobia describes a condition in which children are underfed by caregivers in an attempt to limit risk of future disease, such as obesity or heart disease. Growth failure—in weight and height gains—can result if nutrient intake is not increased to appropriate amounts.

Study Questions

1 What are the typical characteristics of a person with anorexia nervosa? What may influence a person to begin rigid, self-imposed dietary patterns?
2 What are the typical components of treatment for anorexia nervosa?
3 List the detrimental physical and psychological side effects of bulimia nervosa. Describe important goals of the psychological and nutrition therapy used to treat bulimic patients.
4 Explain the role of hypergymnasia in eating disorders. What is "debting"? What other methods of purging are used by distorted eater?
5 How might parents significantly contribute to the development of an eating disorder? Suggest an attitude that a parent or adult friend of yours displayed that may not have been conducive to developing a normal relationship to food.
6 Based on your knowledge of good nutrition and sound dietary habits, answer the following questions:
   a How can repeated bingeing and purging lead to significant nutrient deficiencies?
   b How can significant nutrient deficits contribute to major health problems in later life?
7 How, in your opinion, has society contributed to the development of various forms of disordered eating? Provide an example.
8 List the three symptoms that compose the female athlete triad. What is the major health risk associated with amenorrhea in the female athlete?
9 How does binge-eating disorder differ from bulimia nervosa? Describe factors that contribute to the development and treatment of binge-eating disorder.
10 Describe the common characteristics of a parent of a child with baryophobia.

Further Readings

1 ADA Reports: Position of the American Dietetic Association: Nutrition intervention in the treatment of anorexia nervosa, bulimia nervosa, and binge eating, *Journal of the American Dietetic Association* 94:902, 1994.

2 American Psychiatric Association: *Diagnostic and statistical manual of mental disorders (DSM-IV)*, Washington, DC, 1994, American Psychiatric Association.

3 Anderson AE: Recognizing eating disorders, *Nutrition & the M.D.* 24(8):1, 1998.

4 Becker AE and others: Eating disorders, *New England Journal of Medicine* 340:1092, 1999.

5 Bruce B, Wilfley D: Binge eating among the overweight population: a serious and prevalent problem, *Journal of the American Dietetic Association* 96:58, 1996.

6 Eating disorders and exercise: the connection, *Nutrition & the M.D.* 24(7):5, 1998.

7 Eilers GM: Bulimia: my secret no more, *Journal of the American Medical Association* 275:83, 1996.

8 Garner DM, Needleman LD: Sequencing an integration of treatments. In Garner DM, Garfinkel PE, editors: *Handbook of treatment for eating disorders,* 2nd ed., New York, 1997, Guilford Press.

9 Halmi KA; A 24-year old with anorexia nervosa, *Journal of the American Medical Association* 279:1992, 1998.

10 Keel PK: Long-term outcome of bulimia nervosa, *Archives of General Psychiatry* 56:63, 1999.

11 Krowchuk DP and others: Problem dieting behaviors among young adolescents, *Archives of Pediatric & Adolescent Medicine* 152:884, 1998.

12 McDuffe JR, Kirkley BG: Eating disorders. In Krummel DA, Kris-Etherton PM; editors: *Nutrition in women's health,* Gaithersburg, MD, 1996, Aspen Publishers.

13 McGilley BM, Pryor TL: Assessment and treatment of bulimia nervosa, *American Family Physician* 57:2743, 1998.

14 Neumark-Sztainer D: Excessive weight preoccupation, *Nutrition Today* 30:68, 1995.

15 Olivardia R and others: Eating disorders in college men, *American Journal of Psychiatry* 152:1279, 1995.

16 Polivy J: Psychological consequences of food restriction, *Journal of the American Dietetic Association* 96:589, 1996.

17 Steinberg LM: The impact of oral health on diet, *Nutrition & the M.D.* 23(2):1, 1997.

18 Walsh BT, Devlin MJ: Eating disorders: progress and problems, *Science* 280:1387, 1998.

19 Zerbe KJ: Anorexia nervosa and bulimia nervosa, *Postgraduate Medicine* 99:161, 1996.

RATE

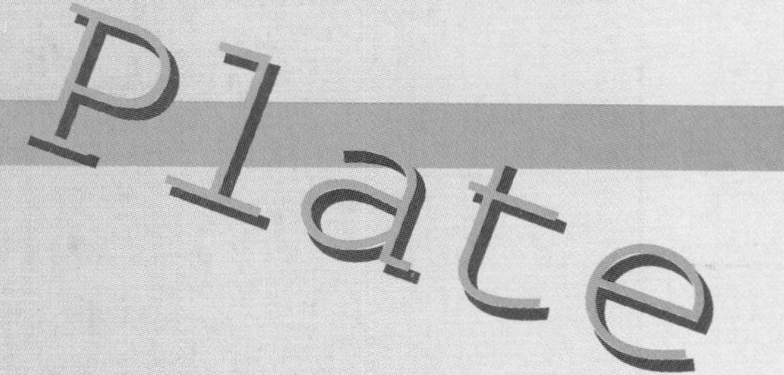

I. Assessing One's Risk of Developing an Eating Disorder

The statements below are based on the primary diagnostic criteria for anorexia nervosa and bulimia. Put an "X" in the space before statements that describe your or a friend's characteristics and lifestyle.

_____ **1. Refuse to keep body weight over a minimal normal weight for age and height.**
_____ **2. Intensely fearful about gaining weight or becoming fat even though you are underweight.**
_____ **3. Feel fat even though quite thin.**
_____ **4. If a female, have missed at least three consecutive menstrual cycles.**
_____ **5. Have recurrent episodes of binge eating.**
_____ **6. Can't control eating behavior during food binges.**
_____ **7. Regularly self-induce vomiting, use laxatives or diuretics, diet strictly or fast, or vigorously exercise for long periods to prevent weight gain.**
_____ **8. Engage in a minimum average of two binge-eating episodes a week.**
_____ **9. Are persistently and excessively concerned with body shape and weight.**

Statements 1 through 4 pertain to anorexia nervosa and 5 through 9 to bulimia nervosa. Complete this activity by answering the following questions:

1. After having completed this checklist, do you feel that you or your friend might have an eating disorder or the potential to develop one?

____

____

2. Do you think many of your friends might have an eating disorder?

____

____

3. What counseling and education resources exist in your area or on your campus to help with a potential eating disorder?

____

____

4. If a friend had an eating disorder, what do you think would be the best way to assist him or her in getting help?

____

____

II. Helping to Prevent Eating Disorders

You have been asked to speak to a junior high school class about eating disorders. What are four major points that you would make to help prevent disordered eating in this population?

1. ______________________________

2. ______________________________

3. ______________________________

4. ______________________________

Here are points you may consider:

1. **Extreme thinness is oversold in the media. Extremely low weight (i.e., BMI of less than 19) is generally not healthy.**
2. **Self-induced vomiting is dangerous. Damage to the teeth, stomach, and esophagus often result.**
3. **Loss of menstrual periods (amenorrhea) is a sign of illness. It is important to see a physician about this. Bone deterioration is a common result.**
4. **Treatment of eating disorders in early phases aids success. These diseases are difficult to treat once firmly established.**

Nutrition Issue

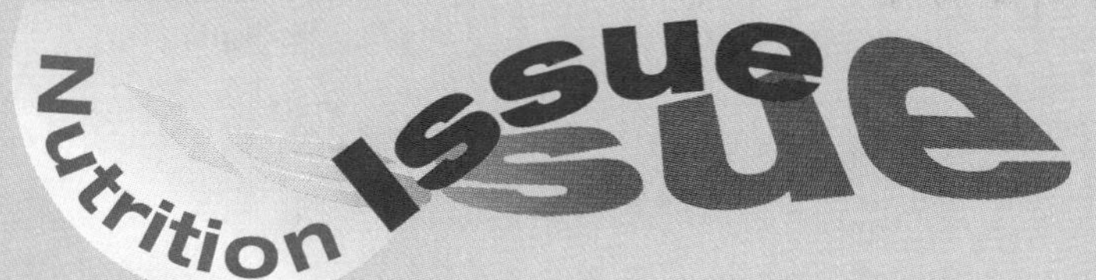

Eating Disorders: A Sociological Perspective

One of the many criteria we use to evaluate ourselves is body image. We identify our body with our self and judge it as we think others see us, knowing that our appearance affects their opinions of us.

Early in life, we develop images of "acceptable" and "unacceptable" body types. Of all the attributes that constitute attractiveness, many people view body weight as the most important, partly because we can control our weight somewhat. Fatness is the most dreaded deviation from our cultural ideals of body image, the one most derided and shunned, even among school children.

Females in particular are likely to diet because they feel strongly about what is acceptable in both size and weight (Figure 11–8). In general, though, most dieting women aren't technically obese. Rather, they diet to correct some perceived flaw or because they simply feel they should weigh less than they do now. Their impulse "to please" fosters this desire to look socially acceptable.

A *Glamour* magazine survey indicated that 80% of the 30,000 respondents were ashamed of their bodies. Those who were dissatisfied primarily wanted to weigh less and have smaller thighs, hips, buttocks, and waists, typical sites of greatest fat deposition in sexually mature women.

CHANGING TIMES

The cultural ideal of the "full-bodied" woman did not survive into the twentieth century in Western society, though it is still in fashion in many nonindustrialized countries, where a large body is a sign of wealth. Over the course of this century the "ideal" female body form in the United States has become progressively thinner. A thin waist with modest hips is the overriding cultural "gold standard," at least as exemplified by models. Our passion for thinness may have its roots in the Victorian era, which specialized in denying "unpleasant" physical realities, such as appetite and sexual desire. Flappers of the 1920s cemented a trend for thinness (Figure 11–9). Even as the ideal gradually moved toward a thinner, more angular body shape, the average weight among the general female population increased.

For Better or For Worse
By Lynn Johnston
WOW! I WONDER WHERE THEY FIND THE GIRLS IN THESE MAGAZINES!
SIGH...
OH, MAN-I WISH I COULD LOOK LIKE THAT!
www.uexpress.com
SHE'S A MODEL, LIZ! IT'S PROBABLY TAKEN 3 HOURS, JUST TO DO HER MAKEUP!
-AN' ANOTHER 3 JUST TO DO HER HAIR!!
SHE'S HAD IMPLANTS, FOR SURE - MAYBE EVEN LIPOSUCTION!!
AN' HER TEETH SURE LOOK CAPPED TO ME!
AN' I BET THE WHOLE PHOTOGRAPH WAS ELECTRONICALLY RETOUCHED BY COMPUTER!
YEAH...
...BUT OTHER THAN THAT— SHE'S PERFECT!

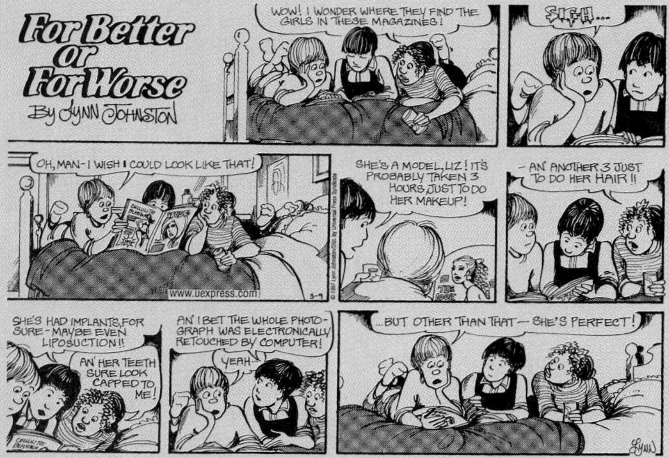

Figure 11–8 *For Better or For Worse.*

FEAR OF THE OBESITY STIGMA

Unfortunately, many Americans today view obesity as a failure of control, willpower, competence, and productivity. At stake are social acceptance and even access to scarce resources, such as good jobs and an attractive spouse. Whether we like it or not, in today's society our appearance says a lot about us, even though the way we were raised and our genetic background are beyond our control. Some people are simply much more likely to become obese than others. Implicit in our societal attitudes is the notion that those who can't control themselves enough to stay slim are unlikely to be good at supervising employees, organizing their work day, and shouldering heavy responsibilities. Clearly, fat is out! A prevailing myth is that thin people are more competent, energetic, and forceful than obese people.

MIXED MESSAGES AND SOCIAL TRENDS

Despite the pressure for thinness, our society is filled with mixed messages. Half the advertisements in women's magazines may describe diets or feature emaciated models, the other half displays tasty foods. Female movie and television stars are almost always utterly thin, often to the degree that it erodes health. Television advertisements encourage us to visit our local quick-service restaurant. There you can buy a hamburger, french fries, and milk shake, totaling approximately 1200 kcal—about the amount of energy our daily basal metabolism uses—without even leaving the car.

In the past several decades, divorce, alcoholism in families, child abuse, school- and work-related stress, socioeconomic changes, and crowded urban conditions have all increased. These changes in our family and social environments encourage children, adolescents, and adults alike to find a release from the pressure. Many find relief in food, which sets the stage for development of an eating disorder.

INTERNALIZING THE THINNESS IDEAL

Eating disorders are usually only a symptom of significant emotional trauma or psychological stress in a person's life. When psychiatrists are able to dig deeper, they find that eating disorders mask serious questions of self-worth, family struggles, and sometimes fears of puberty and the future. The real illnesses are not the eating disorders—though they eventually contribute to poor health—but, rather, the way people feel about themselves. When people internalize the social value favoring thinness and can't meet that goal, their negative self-image is reinforced.

Researchers have linked this preference for a lean body type to the recent surge in eating disorders. As the more full-figured woman was displaced by the ultra-thin woman, the number of eating disorders increased, along with our society's preoccupation with obesity. The cultural pressures toward thinness seem to be stretching the physiological capabilities of many women (and men). For example, researchers surmise that the theoretical body fat content of the "Barbie doll" would not allow for menstruation. Given the natural variability in human basal metabolism and genetic makeup, as well as American's easy access to food and increasingly sedentary lifestyles, it is no surprise that some of us gain weight. In addition, these disorders are rarely seen in developing nations. Therefore it is likely that social changes are causing people predisposed to eating disorders for either biological or emotional reasons to ultimately develop the problems.

GLIMMERS OF HOPE

Because eating disorders stem in part from certain cultural values, changing these values might reduce the pressures predisposing some people to various types of disordered eating behavior. Feminists, for example, assert that true liberation means being free to find one's natural weight. Women who combine careers and motherhood are saying that they have more important things to worry about; some fashion leaders are tolerating more curves; exercise programs are encouraging regular brisk walking, rather than mostly jogging and working out. Some writers, therapists, and registered dietitians are working to help women accept their bodies.

What is the difference between people who can accept themselves—even with a few more pounds than the glamorous people have—and those who chronically diet and feel dissatisfied? Perhaps it is the willingness to recognize that satisfaction comes from within, not from the mirror or the approval of others. The challenge facing many Americans is achieving a healthy body weight without excessive dieting. This means adopting and maintaining sensible eating habits, a physically active lifestyle, and realistic and positive attitudes and emotions while practicing creative ways to handle stress.

A

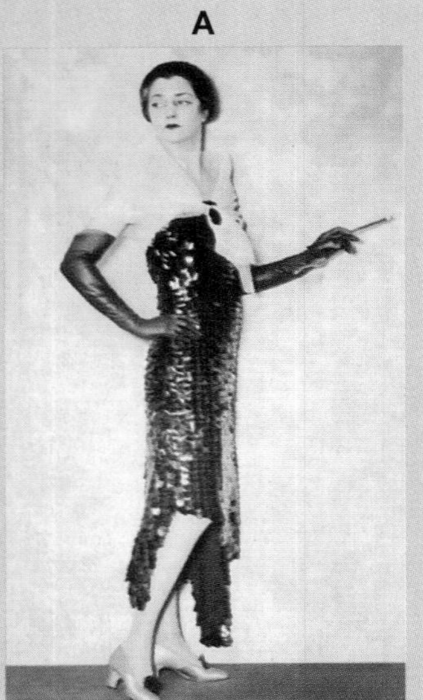

B

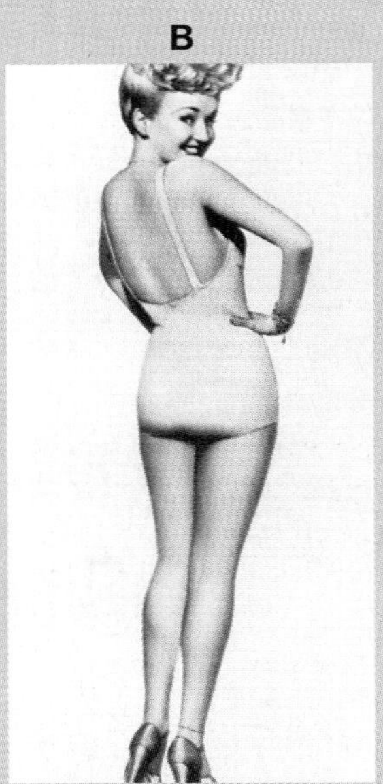

C

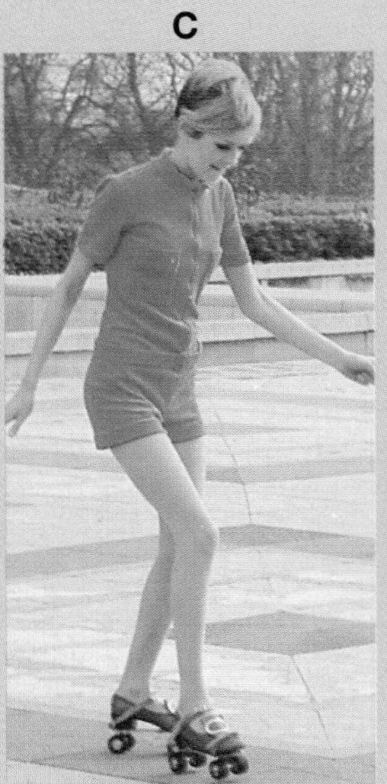

D

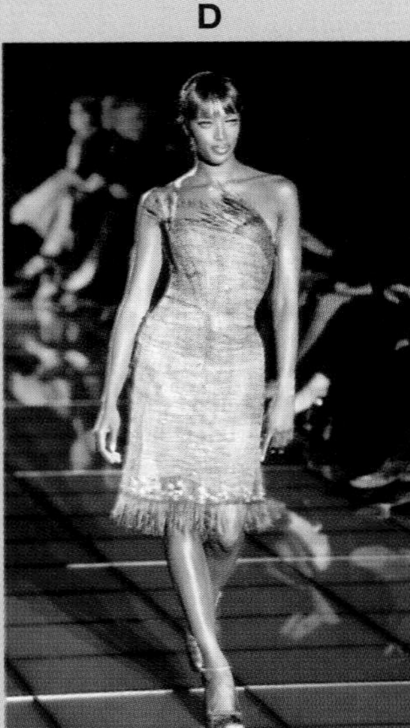

Figure 11-9 *The changing views of body weight. American society has imposed varying stereotypes for body weight, especially for women.* **A,** *The svelte flapper of the 1920s.* **B,** *The "thin but curvaceous" look of the 1940s.* **C,** *Ultra-thin was in during the 1960s.* **D.** *At the turn of this new century, women's fashion is trending toward the image of the muscularly fit with little evidence of body fat.*

part

4

Nutrition: A Focus on Life Stages

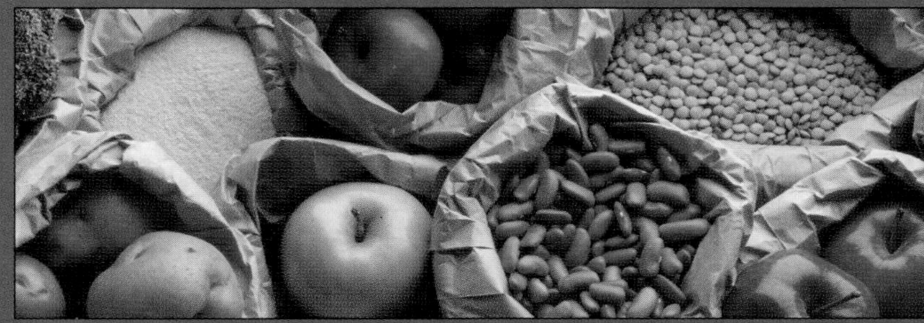

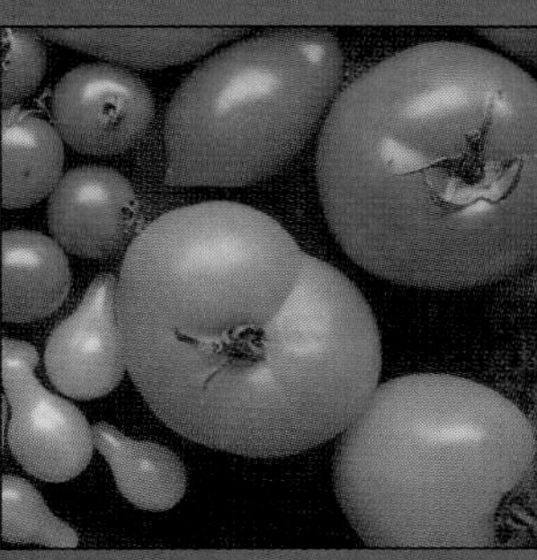

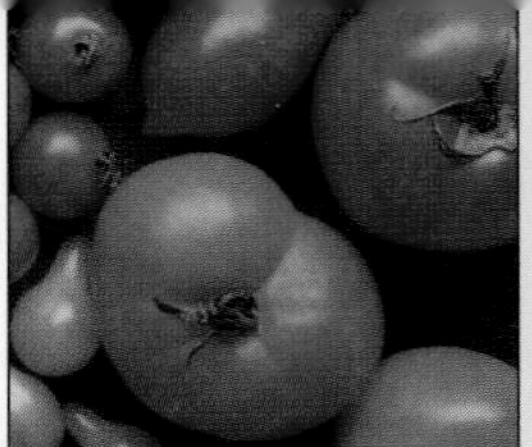

chapter 12

Pregnancy and Breastfeeding

Pregnancy can be a very special time for a couple. Along with the responsibility of shaping a child's health and personality comes the prospective exhilaration of watching the child develop and grow. These parents often feel an overriding desire to produce a healthy baby, which opens them up to new nutrition and health information. The parents-to-be usually want to do everything possible to maximize their chances of having a robust, lively newborn.

Despite these possibilities, the infant mortality rate in the United States is higher than that of 23 other industrialized nations. In the United States about 7 of every 1000 infants per year die before their first birthday, and about 25% to 30% of pregnant women receive inadequate prenatal care in the early months of pregnancy. Teenage mothers are at the highest risk. These are alarming statistics for the country that has the highest per capita expenditure for health care in the world.

Producing a healthy baby is not just a matter of luck. True, some aspects of fetal and newborn health are beyond a parent's control. Still, conscious decisions about social, health, and nutritional factors can significantly affect the baby's health and future. What the parents do relates directly to the likelihood of having a healthy newborn. Then choosing to breastfeed the infant adds further benefit. Let's examine the practices that build toward a healthy baby.

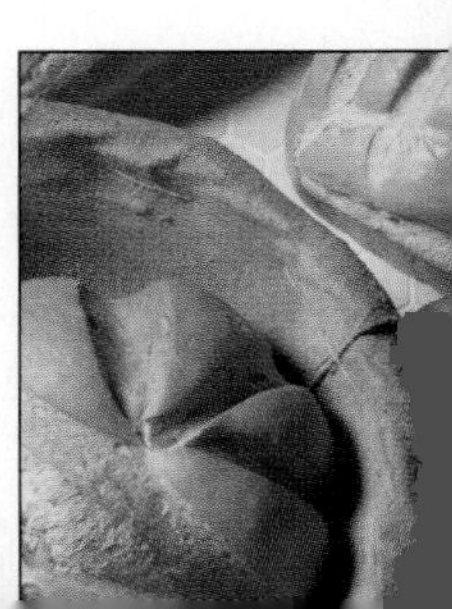

Nutrition Web

Infants born preterm (before 37 weeks of gestation) or with low birth weight (less than 2.5 kilograms, or 5.5 pounds) usually have more medical problems at and following birth than normal infants.

Pregnant teenagers require very careful prenatal and nutritional care. Complications of pregnancy are more common in teenagers than in more mature women because the teenagers have very high physiological demands and often compromised social and economic support.

Poor nutrition and use of some medications, especially in the first trimester, can cause birth defects. If such insults occur later in pregnancy, preterm birth, growth retardation, and altered development may result.

Adequate nutrition is vital during pregnancy and breastfeeding to ensure the well-being of both the infant and the mother.

Extra servings from the milk, yogurt, and cheese group and the meat, poultry, fish, dry beans, eggs, and nuts group of the Food Guide Pyramid are recommended to meet increased nutrient needs in pregnancy. One serving of a fortified breakfast cereal also helps.

Adequate folate intake should be established at least 8 weeks before the time of conception to reduce the risk of neural tube defects. Protein, vitamin, and mineral needs increase during pregnancy. Also, a woman typically needs an additional 300 kcal per day in the second and third trimesters of pregnancy to meet energy needs. Slow weight gain totaling 25 to 35 pounds is a good goal for a woman of healthy weight.

Almost all women are able to nurse their infants.

Iron and folate supplements may be prescribed during pregnancy, as it can be difficult to meet the needs for these nutrients from diet alone. A prenatal supplement generally contributes to both needs.

The nutrient composition of human milk is very different from unaltered cow's milk and much more desirable for human infants. Colostrum, the first fluid produced by the human breast, is very rich in immune factors.

For the infant the advantages of breastfeeding over formula-feeding are numerous, including fewer intestinal, respiratory, and ear infections, and fewer allergies and food intolerances.

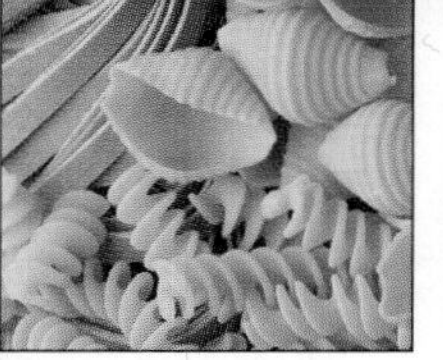
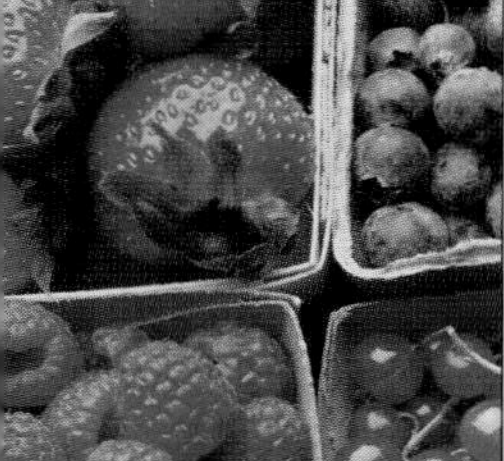

Pregnancy Should Be Planned

Pregnancy deserves planning because many practices or conditions of the mother that can harm the developing infant are modifiable, such as the following:

- Alcohol consumption
- Use of certain medications
- Use of illegal drugs, such as cocaine
- Job-related hazards and stresses
- Smoking
- Inadequate diet, such as too little folate and iron intake
- Excess vitamin A intake and other megadose nutrient supplement use
- Heavy caffeine use
- Lack of medical treatment with HIV-positive status or AIDS
- Ongoing diabetes or high blood pressure

Women need to pay attention to these risks in the months *before* attempts at conception begin. This precaution is necessary because women often do not suspect they are pregnant during the first few weeks after conception and may not seek medical attention until after about the first 2 to 3 months.

Much scientific evidence supports the importance of healthy nutrition and lifestyle habits during pregnancy. Although some aspects of fetal and newborn health are beyond one's control, a woman's conscious decisions about these factors affect her infant's health and future. An adequate vitamin and mineral intake in the months before conception and during pregnancy may help prevent birth defects, such as neural tube defects related to a folate deficiency. Recall that all women capable of becoming pregnant should consume at least 400 micrograms of folate

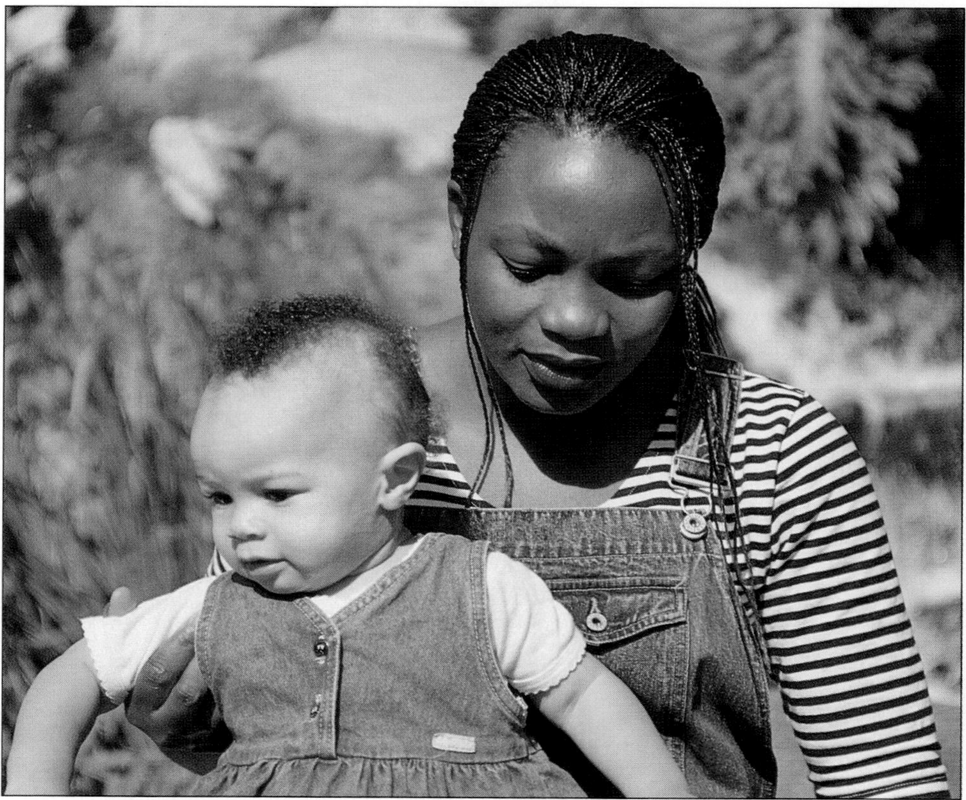

All of us are asked to postpone parenthood until we have the knowledge and the maturity to raise a child.

per day via fortified foods or supplement use (see Chapter 7). Overall, parents should be aware of the role nutrition plays in the development of a healthy infant both before and during pregnancy.

Prenatal Growth and Development

For 8 weeks after its conception, a human **embryo** develops from an **ovum** into a **fetus.** For about another 32 weeks the incomplete fetus continues to develop. When its body finally matures enough, the infant is born. Until birth, the mother nourishes it via a **placenta,** an organ that forms in her uterus to accommodate the growth and development of the fetus (Figure 12–1).

Embryo
In humans, the developing in utero offspring from about the beginning of the third week to the end of the eighth week after conception.

Ovum
The egg cell from which a fetus eventually develops if the egg is fertilized by a sperm cell.

Placenta
An organ that forms in pregnant women. Through this organ oxygen and nutrients from the mother's blood are transferred to the fetus and fetal wastes are removed. The placenta also releases hormones that maintain the pregnant state.

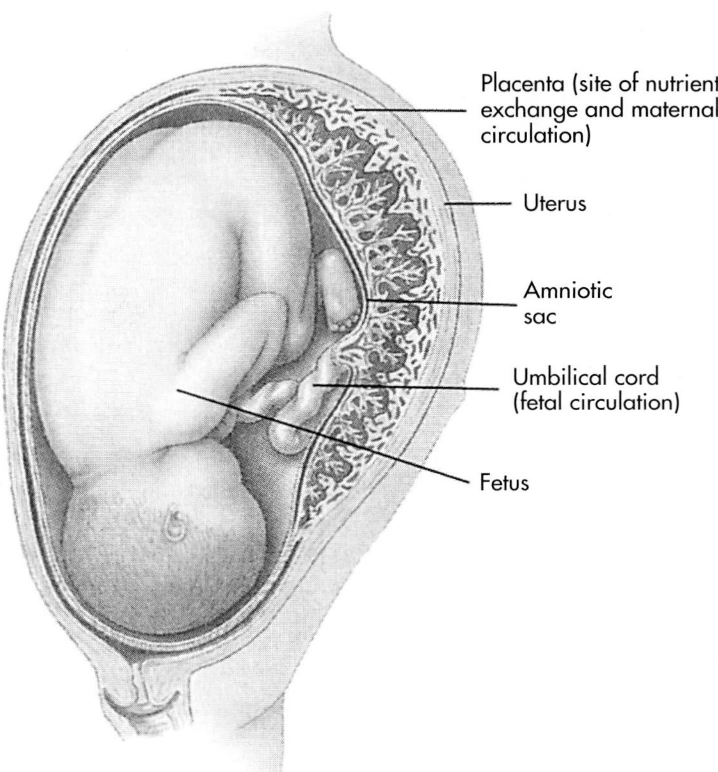

Figure 12–1 *The fetus in relationship to the placenta. The placenta is the organ through which nourishment flows to the fetus.*

Zygote
The fertilized ovum; the cell resulting from union of an egg cell (ovum) and sperm until it divides.

Trimesters
Three 13- to 14-week periods into which the normal pregnancy of 38 to 42 weeks is divided somewhat arbitrarily for purposes of discussion and analysis. Development of the embryo and fetus, however, is continuous throughout pregnancy with no specific physiological markers demarcating the transition from one trimester to the next.

Early Growth—The First Trimester Is a Most Critical Time

In the formation of the human organism, egg and sperm first unite, producing the **zygote** (Figure 12–2). From this point, the reproductive process occurs very rapidly:

- Within 30 hours—zygote divides in half to form 2 cells.
- Within 4 days—cell number climbs to 64 to 128 cells.
- At 14 days—the group of cells is called an embryo.
- Within 35 days—heart is beating, embryo is 1⁄30 of an inch (8 millimeters) long, eyes and limb buds are clearly visible.
- At 8 weeks—the embryo is known as a fetus.
- At 13 weeks (end of first **trimester**)—most organs are formed, and the fetus can move.

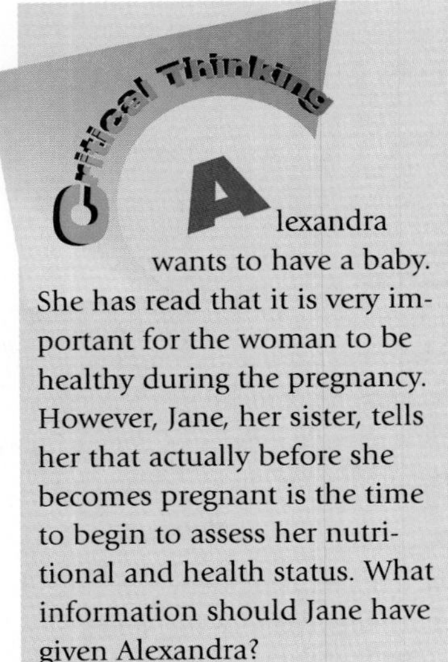

Alexandra wants to have a baby. She has read that it is very important for the woman to be healthy during the pregnancy. However, Jane, her sister, tells her that actually before she becomes pregnant is the time to begin to assess her nutritional and health status. What information should Jane have given Alexandra?

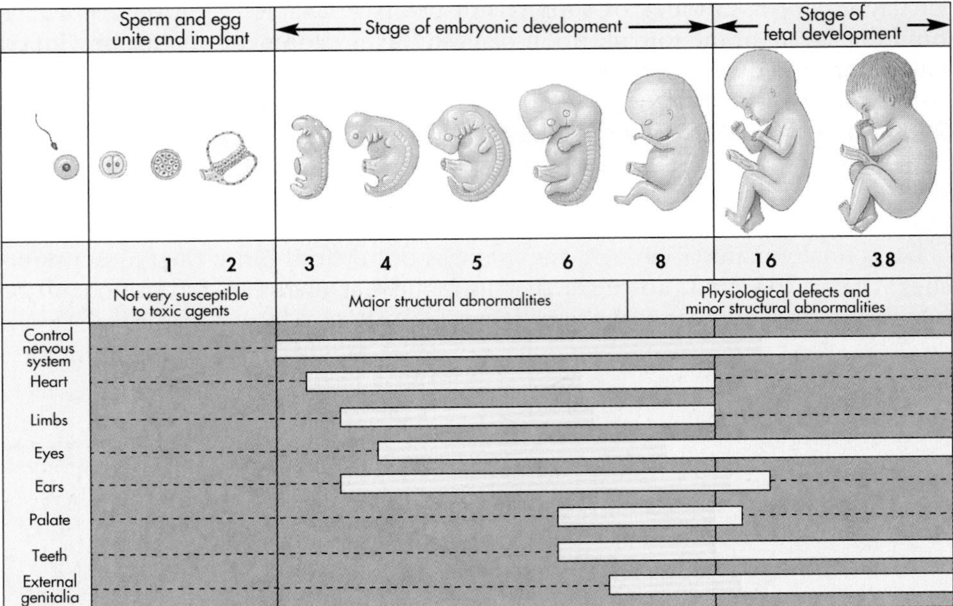

Figure 12–2 *Vulnerable periods of fetal development are indicated with yellow bars. The yellow shading indicates the time of greatest risk to the organ. The most serious damage to the fetus from exposure to toxins is likely to occur during the first 8 weeks after conception. As the chart shows, however, damage to vital parts of the body—including the eyes, brain, and genitals—can also occur during the last months of pregnancy.*

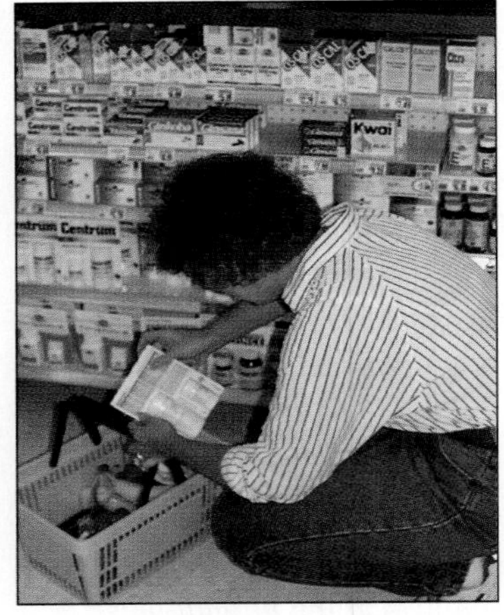

The time to begin thinking about prenatal nutrition is actually before becoming pregnant. This includes making sure that any supplemental use of vitamin A does not exceed 100% of the Daily Value.

For purposes of discussion, the duration of pregnancy—normally 38 to 42 weeks—is divided into three trimesters. Growth begins in the first trimester with a rapid increase in cell number. This type of growth dominates embryo and later fetal development. The newly formed cells then begin to grow larger. Further growth and development then involve mostly increases in cell number.

Nutrition deficiencies and other insults transmitted through the mother to the embryo or fetus—for example, injuries caused by medications and other drugs, smoking and alcohol intake, high intakes of vitamin A, X-ray exposure, or trauma—can alter or arrest the progressing phase of development, particularly in the first trimester (see Figure 12–2). The effects may last a lifetime.

The fetus develops so rapidly during the first trimester that if an essential nutrient is not available, the fetus may be affected even before evidence of the deficiency appears in the mother. For this reason, quality of nutrition is more important than quantity during the first trimester. In other words, women should consume about the same amount of food as usual, but the foods should be more nutrient dense. Though some women lose their appetite and develop nausea during the first trimester, they should try their best to obtain adequate nutrition (see later section).

The Second Trimester

By the beginning of the second trimester a fetus weighs about 1 ounce. Arms, hands, fingers, legs, feet, and toes are fully formed. The fetus has ears and begins to form tooth sockets in its jawbone. With a stethoscope, physicians can detect the fetus' heartbeat. Most bones are distinctly evident through the body, and the fetus may suck its thumb and kick strongly enough to be felt by the mother. As shown in Figure 12–2, the fetus can still be affected by exposure to toxins, but not to the degree seen in the first trimester.

During the second trimester, the mother's breast weight increases by approximately 30% due to deposition of 2 to 4 pounds of fat for breastfeeding. Consequently, undernutrition in the second trimester has a greater effect on the mother than the fetus. For example, if the mother does not meet her nutritional needs during this time, her ability to successfully breastfeed her infant may be affected, as fat stored in the breasts during pregnancy serves as an energy reserve for breastfeeding.

Although a mother's decisions, practices, and precautions during pregnancy contribute to the health of her fetus, she cannot guarantee fetal good health because some genetic and environmental factors are beyond her control. Parents should not hold an unrealistic illusion of control.

The Third Trimester

By the beginning of the third trimester a fetus weighs about 2 to 3 pounds. The third trimester is a crucial time. The fetus will double in length and will increase its weight by about 6 pounds. An infant that is born after about 26 weeks of **gestation** has a good chance of survival if it is cared for in a nursery for high-risk newborns. Sufficient growth and development of the lungs is the key concern of the physician during this time period. In addition, the infant will not contain the mineral (mainly iron and calcium) and fat stores normally accumulated during the last month of gestation. This and other medical problems, such as a poor ability to suck and swallow, complicate nutritional care for **preterm** infants. Note also that infants in this trimester will act as parasites with regard to iron, in that they will deplete the stores of the mother. If the mother is not meeting her iron needs she can end up very depleted after delivery. The fetus also funnels the majority of the mother's blood glucose for its own growth and development during the third trimester, causing the mother to mobilize her fat stores to support energy needs.

At 9 months the fetus weighs about 7 to 9 pounds (3 to 4 kilograms) and is about 20 inches (50 centimeters) long (Figure 12–3). A soft spot in the forehead indicates where the skull bones (fontanelles) are growing together. The bones finally close by the time the baby is about 12 to 18 months of age.

Gestation
The period of intrauterine development of offspring, from conception to birth; in humans, gestation lasts for about 40 weeks after the woman's last menstrual period.

Preterm
An infant born before 37 weeks of gestation; also referred to as premature.

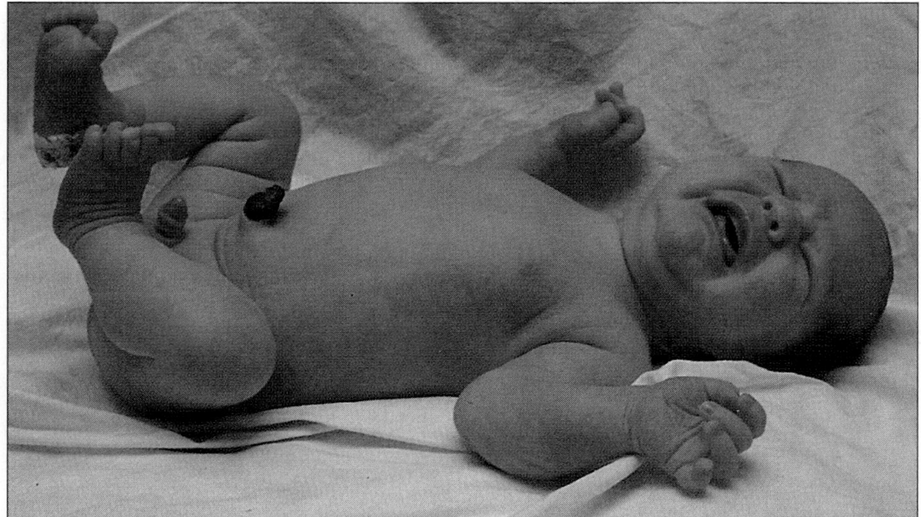

Figure 12–3 *A healthy 1-week-old baby. At birth the baby usually weighs about 7.5 pounds and is 20 inches long.*

Defining a Successful Pregnancy

To define a successful pregnancy, one common goal is protection of the mother's physical and emotional health so that she can return to her prepregnancy health

For Better or For Worse® **by Lynn Johnston**

MICHAEL, YOUR ROOM IS STILL A MESS, YOUR HOME-WORK'S NOT DONE—YOU HAVEN'T DONE A THING!
I KNOW, BUT I WAS THINKING ABOUT IT!

ELIZABETH, TAKE YOUR SHOES OFF THE COUCH! —AND WHY ARE YOU EATING CHIPS WHEN SUPPER WILL BE IN 10 MINUTES?!
I'M HUNGRY NOW!!

WELL, THERE'S SOMETHING TO BE SAID FOR HAVING A KID ON THE WAY, EL'!

IT'S THE ONE TIME YOU HAVE COMPLETE CONTROL OVER THEM!
© 1990 Universal Press Syndicate
10-24
LYNN

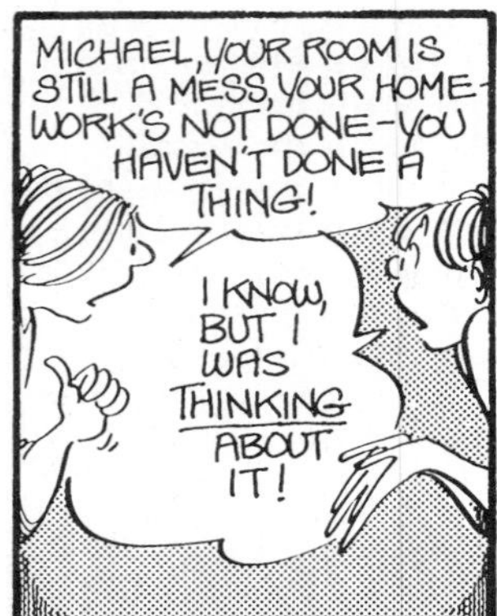

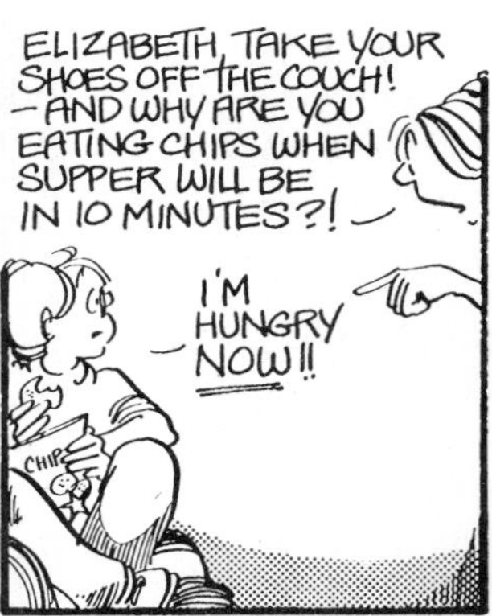

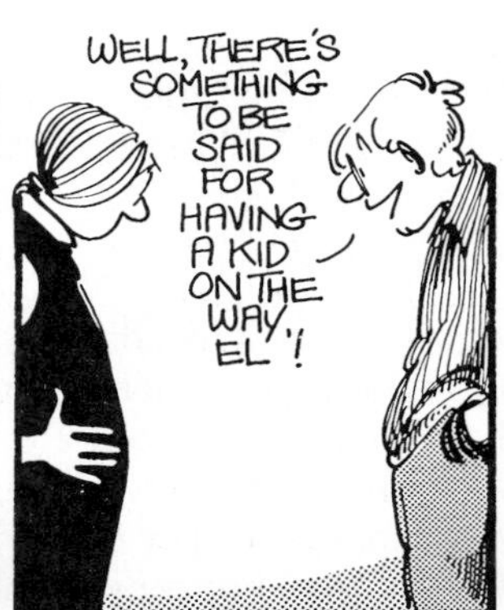

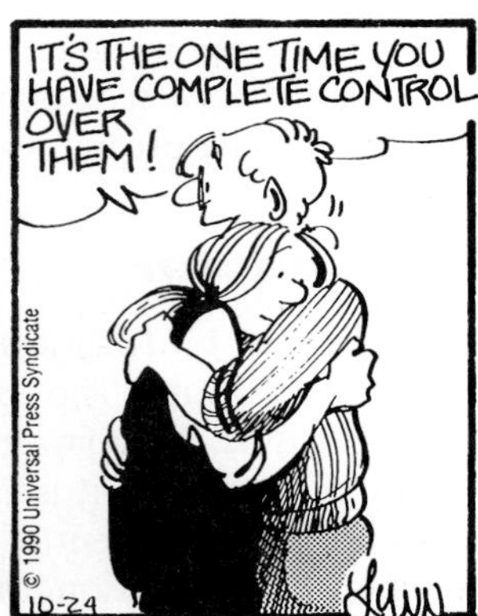

Figure 12–4 *For Better of For Worse*
FOR BETTER OR FOR WORSE © United Feature Syndicate. Reprinted by Permission.

status. As for the infant, two widely accepted goals are (1) a gestation period longer than 37 weeks and (2) a birth weight greater than 5.5 pounds (2.5 kilograms). A gestation period of this length or longer helps insure adequate birth weight and maturation, and hence fewer medical problems are likely to occur.

Low-birth-weight (LBW) infants are those weighing less than 5.5 pounds (2.5 kilograms) at birth. In the United States about 7% of infants are born LBW. Most commonly LBW is associated with preterm birth. About 11% of pregnancies end preterm. Full-term and preterm infants who weigh less than the expected weight for their duration of gestation, the result of insufficient growth, are described as **small for gestational age (SGA).** Infants who are SGA are more likely than normal-weight infants to have medical complications, including problems with blood glucose control, temperature regulation, and growth and development in the early weeks after birth.

The newborn's quality of life must also be considered in rating the success of a pregnancy. Overall, prospective parents should strive toward producing a baby who is born healthy, on time, and with the mental, physical, and physiological capabilities to take advantage of whatever life offers, while also protecting the mother's health (Figure 12–4).

Low birth weight (LBW)
Referring to any infant weighing less than 2.5 kilograms (5.5 pounds) at birth; most commonly results from preterm birth.

Small for gestational age (SGA)
Referring to any infant whose birth weight is less than the expected weight corresponding to the duration of gestation. A full-term newborn weighing less than 2.5 kilograms (5.5 pounds) is SGA. A preterm infant who is also SGA will most likely develop some medical complications.

Hospital-related costs of caring for low-birth-weight newborns total more than $2 billion per year in the United States, ranging from $20,000 to $200,000 per child. Compare this with an average hospital-related cost of $5800 for a normal delivery and an average of $800 for preventive prenatal care.

ConceptCheck

Adequate nutrition is vital both before and during pregnancy to help ensure optimal health of both the mother and her offspring. Organs and body parts in the offspring begin to develop very soon after conception. The first trimester is a critical period when inadequate nutrient intake or alcohol and drug use can result in birth defects.

Infants born after 37 weeks of gestation who weigh more than 5.5 pounds (2.5 kilograms) have the fewest medical problems at birth. To reduce infant and maternal medical problems or death, those involved should take the steps necessary to allow the mother to carry the baby in her uterus for the entire 9 months. Good nutrition and health practices aid in this goal.

The Effect of Nutrition on the Success of Pregnancy

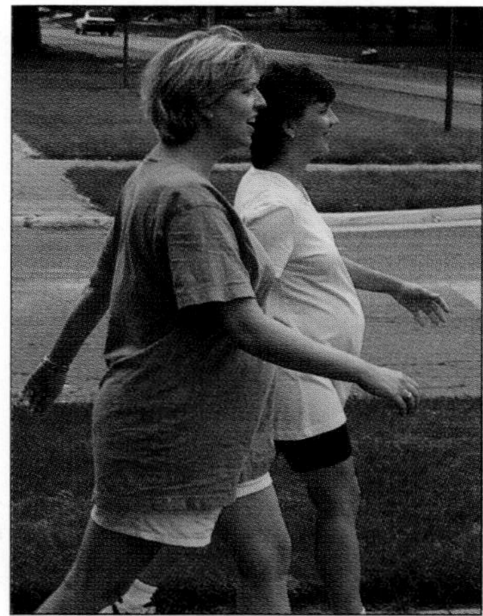

Walking, cycling, swimming, and light aerobics are all suitable exercises during pregnancy.

Is this attention to nutrition worth the effort? Yes, as previously mentioned, evidence shows that the effort is justified. Extra nutrients and energy are for fetal growth, as well as the changes in the mother's body to accommodate the fetus. Her uterus and breasts grow, the placenta develops, her total blood volume increases, the heart and kidneys work harder, and stores of body fat increase.

Though it is difficult to specify what degree of poor nutrition will affect each pregnancy, a daily diet containing only 1000 kcal has been shown to greatly retard fetal growth and development. Increased maternal and infant death rates recently seen in famine-stricken areas of Africa supply further evidence (see Chapter 16).

Genetic background can explain very little of the observed differences in birth weight. Both environmental factors and nutritional factors are more important. The worse the nutritional condition of the mother at the beginning of pregnancy—especially if she is underweight—the more valuable a good prenatal diet and use of prenatal supplements will be in improving the course and outcome of her pregnancy.

Increased Nutrient Needs During Pregnancy

It is important to understand that pregnancy is a time of increased nutrient needs, not restrictions as was once thought. It is equally important to recognize the need for individual assessment and counseling mothers-to-be, as the nutritional and health status of each woman is different. Still, there are some general principles that are true of most women with regard to increased nutrient needs.

Increased Energy Needs

Energy needs during the first trimester are essentially the same as for the nonpregnant woman. In the second and third trimester, on average, a pregnancy requires approximately 300 kcal extra per day. Just 2 cups of fat-reduced milk and a piece of bread can provide those 300 kcal. Though she may "eat for two," the pregnant woman must not double her normal energy intake. She cannot afford a cheeseburger for herself and another for the fetus. Thus, in order to obtain the necessary vitamins and minerals without increasing her energy intake too much, a pregnant woman needs to focus on high-quality nutrient-dense foods. Note that many vitamin and mineral needs are increased by 20% to more than 100% during pregnancy, whereas energy needs during the second and third trimesters represent only about a 15% increase, based on an intake of 2000 kcal per day by nonpregnant women.

If a woman is active during pregnancy, she can add the extra energy she uses to the energy allowance for pregnancy. Her greater body weight requires more energy for activity. Physicians strongly encourage women to continue most activities during pregnancy; except certain calisthenics such as deep knee bends, scuba diving, downhill skiing, weight lifting, and contact sports. Walking, stationary cycling, swimming, and light aerobics are generally advised; though it is not advised that normally inactive women begin an intense exercise program during pregnancy. However, because many women find that they are inactive during the later months of pregnancy, partly because of their increased size, an extra 300 kcal daily is usually enough. Women with high-risk pregnancies may need to restrict their physical activity. To ensure optimal health for both herself and her infant, a pregnant woman should first consult her physician about physical activity and possible limitations.

The American College of Obstetrics and Gynecology suggests the following guidelines for physical activity during pregnancy.

1. **Do not allow heart rate to exceed 140 beats per minute.**
2. **Avoid exercising in hot, humid weather.**
3. **Discontinue exercise that causes discomfort or overheating.**
4. **Drink plenty of liquids to avoid dehydration and overheating.**
5. **After about the fourth month, don't exercise while lying on your back.**
6. **Avoid an abrupt decrease in exertion; In other words, don't just stop and stand around after a hard workout; rather, continue exercising but at a slow pace, gradually reducing pulse rate.**

Pica
The practice of eating nonfood items such as dirt, laundry starch, or clay.

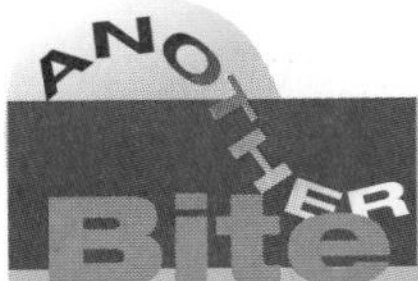

It is a common myth that women instinctively know what to eat during pregnancy. These cravings of the last two trimesters are often related to hormonal changes in the mother, or family traditions. Such "instinct" cannot be trusted, however, based on observations that some women crave nonfood items such as laundry starch and clay, part of what is called ***pica.*** *This practice can be extremely harmful to the mother and the fetus. Overall, though women may have a natural instinct to consume the right foods in pregnancy, humans are so far removed from living by instinct that relying on our cravings to meet nutrient needs is risky. Nutritional advice by experts is more reliable.*

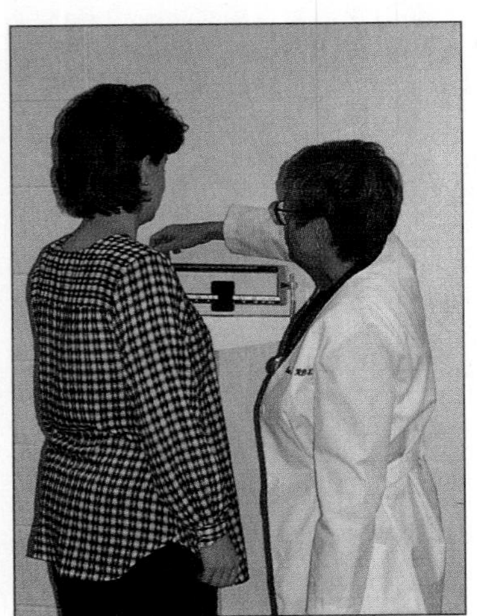
Weight gain is regularly monitored during pregnancy.

Recommended Weight Gain

Adequate weight gain for a mother is one of the best predictors of pregnancy outcome. Her diet should allow for approximately 2 to 4 pounds (0.9 to 1.8 kilograms) of total weight gain during the first trimester and then a subsequent weight gain of 0.75 to 1 pound (0.3 to 0.5 kilogram) weekly during the second and third trimesters.

The recommendations for total weight gain during pregnancy are based on prepregnancy body mass index (BMI). Exceptions to the numbers below include women carrying twins—they should gain 35 to 45 pounds—and adolescents and African-Americans—they should aim for the higher amount in their recommended weight-gain range since they often have smaller babies.

Prepregnancy BMI category	Total weight gain (pounds)	Total weight gain (kilograms)
BMI under 19.8	28–40	12.5–18
BMI 19.8 to 26	25–35	11.5–16
BMI 26 to 29	15–25	7–11.5
BMI over 29	15 or less	7 or less

The weight gain recommended should yield a birth weight of about 7.5 pounds (3.5 kilograms). Although some extra weight gain during pregnancy is usually not harmful, it can set the stage for creeping obesity during the childbearing years if the mother does not return to about her prepregnancy weight. This is especially true if the woman intends to have more than one child. On the other hand, inadequate weight gain generally causes many problems, such as low birth weight and illness. Keeping weekly weight records of weight gain during pregnancy can help assess how much to adjust food intake.

Weight gain during pregnancy, especially in the teenage years, requires regular monitoring so that it approximately follows the pattern in Figure 12–5. If a woman gains too much weight during her pregnancy, she should not be encouraged to lose weight to get back on track. She must still gain more during the final months but should slow the increase in weight to parallel the rise on the prenatal weight-gain chart. This can be done by finding and minimizing sources of unnecessary food energy in the diet. Alternately, if a woman has not gained the desired weight by a given point in pregnancy, she shouldn't gain the needed weight rapidly. Instead, she should slowly gain a little more weight than the typical pattern to meet the goal by the end of the pregnancy.

During pregnancy, women in the United States are more likely to gain excess weight and make poor food choices than to eat too little. Usually the problem is how to limit weight gain, so that they don't have many extra pounds to shed after pregnancy. Excessive weight gain increases risk for complications during pregnancy and encourages excess fetal growth, which makes birth trauma more likely. Loose, accommodating maternity clothes and fluid retention can mask true weight gain during pregnancy.

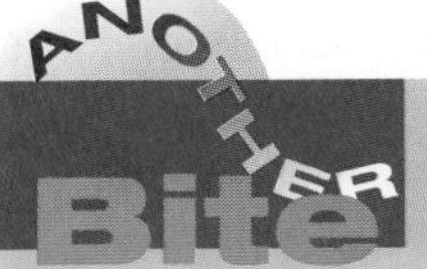

With regard to other weight-related issues, pregnant women who are obese are at an increased risk of high blood pressure and diabetes during pregnancy. The need for surgery and other complications during delivery likewise increase. Thus, these pregnancies require careful monitoring.

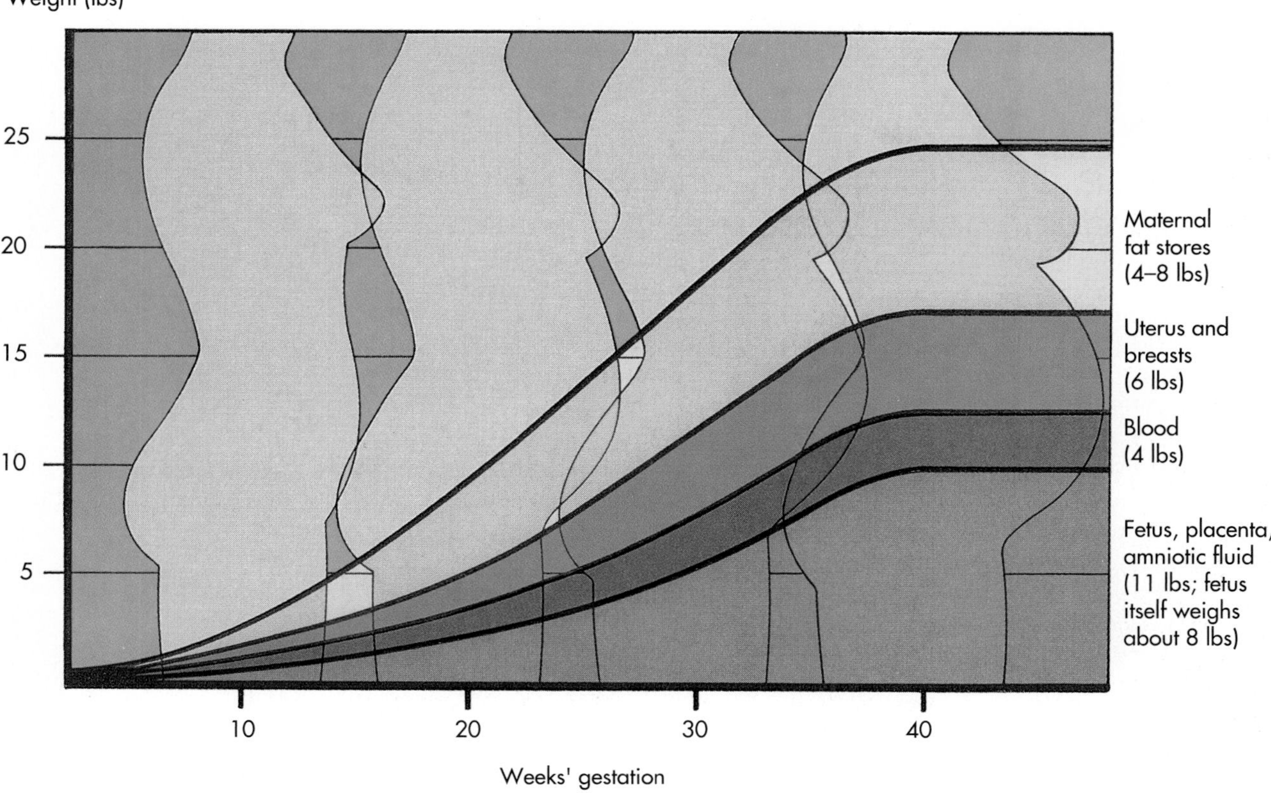

Figure 12–5 *The components of weight gain in pregnancy. A weight gain of 25 to 35 pounds is recommended for most women. Note that the various components total about 25 pounds.*

Increased Protein and Carbohydrate Needs

The RDA for protein increases by 10 to 15 grams daily, depending on age. A glass of milk alone contains 8 grams. Many nonpregnant women already eat at the recommended 60 grams of protein per day and therefore don't need to increase protein intake. However, all women should check to make sure they are actually eating enough protein. Carbohydrate needs are at least 100 grams daily. This amount prevents ketosis, which can harm the fetus (see the next Nutrition Insight). Most women already consume almost twice this amount.

Increased Vitamin Needs

Vitamin needs generally increase; folate deserves the most attention with respect to diet planning. Both fetal and maternal growth in pregnancy depends on an ample supply of folate. Red blood cell formation, which requires folate, increases during pregnancy. Serious folate-related anemia can result if folate intake is inadequate during pregnancy. The RDA for folate increases during pregnancy to 600 micrograms per day. This is a critical goal in the nutritional care of a pregnant woman. As mentioned before, folate deficiency at conception and after has been associated with birth defects, specifically neural tube effects such as spina bifida.

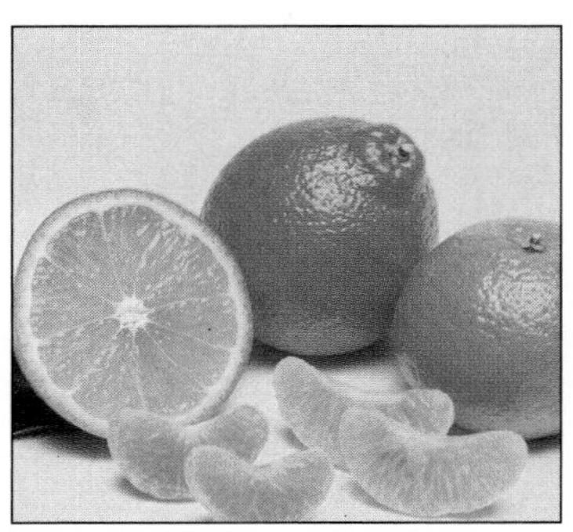

Oranges are a rich source of folate for the prenatal diet.

A woman can meet her folate needs by choosing some folate-fortified foods, along with folate-rich fruits and vegetables as outlined in the Food Guide Pyramid (see later section). Most breakfast cereals and grain products provide folate via the fortification process. A prenatal vitamin and mineral supplement may also be used

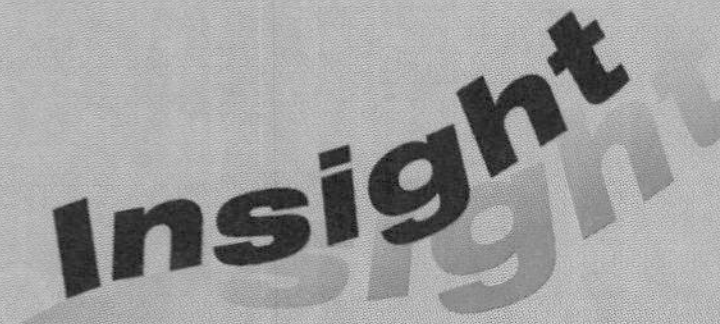

Effects of Factors Other than Nutrition on Pregnancy Outcome

In the United States, about 8 of every 100,000 live births end in the mother's death. It is thought that at least half of all maternal deaths are preventable. For each 100,000 live births, about 720 infants die within the first year. The maternal and infant death rate among African-Americans is more than double the rates among whites in the United States. There are many factors, aside from nutrition, that contribute to poor pregnancy outcomes. Avoiding these factors as possible is important.

Socioeconomic Status. Poverty, inadequate health care and health practices, lack of education, and unmarried status are all associated with problems in pregnancy. Currently, in the United States about 25 % of all births are to unwed mothers.

Closely Spaced Births. Siblings born with less than a year between them are more likely to have low birth weights than are those further apart in age. This danger is especially prevalent among African-American women.

Age Younger than 18. Pregnancies that occur when the mother is younger than 18 are high risk, requiring special monitoring since the mother's body is generally not yet fully developed (see the other Nutrition Insight in this chapter). Overall, mothers who are between 20 and 34 have the best pregnancy outcomes. However, women somewhat older than this still have an excellent chance of producing a healthy infant, if under close medical supervision.

Prenatal Care. Without adequate prenatal care, a woman is three times more likely to give birth to a low-birth-weight baby. Currently, about 10% of women in the United States receive little or no prenatal care.

Lifestyle. Smoking, alcohol consumption (see the Nutrition Issue), use of some medications (ask a physician before taking any medication), and illegal drug use in pregnancy all lead to harmful effects. Smoking, in particular, is linked to preterm birth and low birth weight and appears to increase the risk of birth defects,

to meet the RDA for folate, especially for women with histories of inadequate folate intake, frequent or multiple births, folate-related anemia, or use of medications that increase folate needs.

Women who have previously given birth to an infant with a neural tube defect should consult their physician about the need for folate supplementation; an intake of 4000 micrograms (4 milligrams) per day is advocated in this case but must be taken under a physician's supervision.

Increased Mineral Needs

Mineral needs generally increase during pregnancy, especially for iron. Calcium and zinc also deserve attention.

Iron

Pregnant women need extra iron (30 milligrams per day during the last two trimesters; twice the RDA for nonpregnant women) to synthesize the greater amount of hemoglobin needed during pregnancy and provide iron stores for the fetus. Women often need an iron supplement to meet this need, especially if they don't consume iron-fortified foods, such as breakfast cereals. Because iron supple-

sudden infant death, and childhood cancer. One study has shown that carcinogens in smoke are transmitted to the fetus.

Prenatal Ketosis. Ketosis is not desirable for the growing fetus. Ketones are thought to be poorly used by the fetal brain, possibly slowing fetal brain development. Eating about 100 grams of carbohydrate every day prevents ketosis.

Caffeine Consumption. Caffeine decreases absorption of iron and may reduce blood flow through the placenta. The risk of **spontaneous abortion** has been shown to increase in the first and early in the second trimesters with heavy caffeine consumption (over 300 milligrams or the equivalent of 2 to 3 cups of coffee per day; see Appendix I). Heavy caffeine use during pregnancy may also lead to caffeine withdrawal symptoms in the newborn. It is advisable to limit caffeine intake from such products as coffee, tea, soft drinks (check the label), over-the-counter medicines, and chocolate. Some experts advocate complete avoidance of caffeine during pregnancy.

Aspartame Use. High amounts of phenylalanine (a component of aspartame, for example, Nutrasweet and Equal) in maternal blood disrupt fetal brain development if the mother has a disease known as phenylketonuria (see Chapter 6). If the mother does not have this condition, however, it is unlikely that the baby will be affected by moderate aspartame use. Some experts still recommend caution with regard to aspartame, but total abstinence is not necessary.

Infections. Infection by the bacterium *Listeria monocytogenes* causes mild flulike symptoms, such as fever, headache, and vomiting, about 7 to 30 days after exposure. However, pregnant women, newborn infants, and people with depressed immune function may suffer more severe symptoms, including spontaneous abortion, serious blood infections, and death in up to 25% of cases. Because unpasteurized milk, soft cheeses made from raw milk, undercooked meat, poultry, and seafood, and raw cabbage can be sources of *listeria* organisms, it is especially important that pregnant women avoid these products.

Toxoplasmosis is another infection that causes birth defects. Pregnant women can avoid exposure to the organism that causes toxoplasmosis by having someone else clean the cat's litter box, by avoiding contact with kittens or garden soil, and by not eating raw or undercooked meat.

Many of the risk factors described in this Nutrition Insight are avoidable. The goal of a reduction in maternal and infant deaths requires that more attention be paid to these problems.

ments decrease appetite and can cause nausea and constipation, taking them between meals or just before going to bed is best. Milk, coffee, or tea should not be consumed with an iron supplement because these have substances that interfere with iron absorption. Eating foods rich in vitamin C along with nonheme iron–containing foods helps to increase iron absorption. Pregnant women may also wait until the second trimester, when pregnancy-related nausea generally lessens, to start iron supplementation. Severe iron-deficiency anemia in pregnancy may lead to preterm delivery, low birth weight, and increased risk for fetal death in the first weeks after birth.

Calcium

Calcium is needed during pregnancy to promote adequate mineralization of the fetal skeleton and teeth. Most calcium is required during the third trimester, when skeletal bones are growing most rapidly and teeth are forming. However, attention to calcium intake should start immediately after conception. The current AI for calcium in pregnancy is the same as for women ages 14 to 18 years (1300 milligrams) and that for women age 18–50 years (1000 milligrams). The most practical food sources of calcium are those in the milk, yogurt, and cheese group of the Food Guide Pyramid, calcium-fortified orange juice and other beverages, and various calcium-fortified snacks. Calcium supplements are advised if these options are not chosen. A prenatal supplement generally contains only 200 milligrams of calcium. Thus, use of a prenatal supplement is not a substitute for healthy food choices in meeting calcium needs.

Zinc

Zinc is a mineral important for supporting growth and development. The RDA increases 25% for pregnant women. The protein foods in the diet of a pregnant woman should be able to supply this much zinc. Consuming a fortified breakfast cereal helps out as well. Poor zinc status in pregnancy increases the risk for having a low-birth-weight infant.

A Food Plan for Pregnant Women

One approach to a diet that supports a successful pregnancy is based on the Food Guide Pyramid. It includes at least the following:

- 3 to 4 servings from the milk, yogurt, and cheese group
- 3 servings from the meat, poultry, fish, dry beans, eggs, and nuts group
- 3 servings from the vegetable group
- 2 servings from the fruit group
- 6 servings from the bread, cereal, rice, and pasta group

The servings from the milk, yogurt, and cheese group supply extra protein, calcium, riboflavin, and magnesium. Servings from the meat, poultry, fish, dry beans, eggs, and nuts group supply protein, iron, and zinc, and vegetable protein sources eaten provide much of the extra magnesium needed during pregnancy. The vegetable and fruit group servings provide a variety of vitamins and minerals. One serving from this combination should be a good vitamin C source, and one serving should be a green vegetable or other rich source of folate, such as spinach or orange juice. Selections from the bread, cereal, rice, and pasta group should include some whole-grain varieties. A serving of fortified breakfast cereal is also helpful. See Table 12–1 for a sample menu for pregnancy.

Use of Vitamin and Mineral Supplements by Pregnant Women

Specially formulated supplements for pregnant women are prescribed routinely by most physicians. Use must be supervised by a physician because of their high folate content. In addition to folate, these prenatal supplements typically include the other critical nutrient for pregnancy—iron—and many others as well.

There is no evidence that prenatal supplements cause significant health problems in pregnancy, aside perhaps from the combined amounts of supplementary and dietary vitamin A (mainly during the first trimester). To avoid possible toxicity from vitamin A, no other supplemental source should be used during pregnancy. A maximum total supplemental dose of 5000 IU is recommended.

Prenatal supplements especially contribute to a successful pregnancy for certain women, particularly poor women, teenagers, those with a generally deficient diet, and women carrying multiple fetuses. Still, any use of supplements needs to be directed by a physician. Pregnancy is no time to experiment.

TABLE 12-1

Sample 1800 kcal Daily Menu That Meets Nutritional Needs—Except Calories and Iron—of Pregnant and Breastfeeding Women

	Folate	Calcium	Iron	Zinc
BREAKFAST				
Raisin bran cereal, 1 cup	✓		✓	✓
Orange juice, 1 cup	✓			
1% milk, ½ cup		✓		
SNACK				
Peanut butter, 2 tbsp	✓		✓	✓
Whole-wheat toast, 1 slice	✓		✓	✓
Plain low-fat yogurt, ½ cup		✓		
Strawberries, ½ cup				
LUNCH				
Spinach salad, 1½ cups with 1 tbsp oil and vinegar dressing	✓			
Tomato, ½				
Whole-wheat toast, 1 slice	✓		✓	✓
Provolone cheese, 1½ oz		✓		
SNACK				
Wheat crackers, 4	✓		✓	
1% milk, 1 cup		✓		
DINNER				
Lean hamburger, broiled, 3 oz			✓	✓
Baked beans, ½ cup	✓		✓	✓
Hamburger bun, 1	✓		✓	
Cooked broccoli, ¾ cup	✓			
Soft margarine, 1 tsp				
SNACK				
Bagel, ½	✓		✓	
Jam, 1 tsp				
Hot tea (milk if a teenager)				

*This diet contains 15 milligrams of iron. The vitamin- and mineral-fortified cereal makes an important contribution to meeting nutrient needs. Typically more food energy will be needed and so further food choices will need to be made.

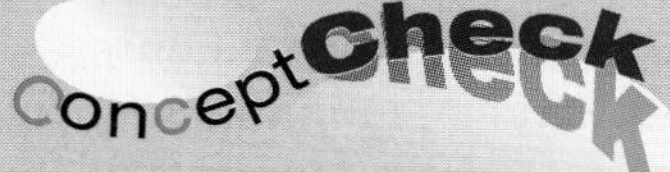

Extra energy and nutrients are used during pregnancy for the growth of the infant and for changes in the mother. Energy needs increase by an average of about 300 kcal per day during the second and third trimesters of pregnancy. Weight gain should be slow and steady up to a total of 25 to 35 pounds for a woman of healthy weight. Protein, vitamin, and mineral needs all increase during pregnancy. Folate, iron, calcium, and zinc are nutrients of particular concern. A balanced diet that follows the Food Guide Pyramid, along with routine prenatal supplement prescriptions for iron, folate, and possibly other nutrients, meets these nutrient needs.

Nutrition Insight

Teenage Pregnancy

About 1 million teenage girls become pregnant at least once before the age of 20, giving the United States the highest teenage pregnancy rate in the Western World—more than twice that of England, France, or Canada. Over 90% of these pregnancies are unintended.

In 1995, surveys showed that 50% of 15- to 19-year-old girls had sexual intercourse at least once, which is up from 29% in 1970. In another survey, 33% of teenage girls did not use any form of contraception during their first act of sexual intercourse.

Minority teenagers with below-average academic skills from families with below-poverty incomes are considerably more likely to become pregnant than other adolescent girls. Often these young mothers are themselves the daughters of teenage mothers and have ended up on the same welfare rolls as their mothers were on. On a positive note, the number of teenage pregnancies has declined about 15% to 20% since 1989.

Teenage pregnancy poses special health problems for both the mother and child. To accommodate their normal growth even when not pregnant, teenagers need an extraordinary nutrient supply. Adolescent girls normally continue to grow taller for 2 years after they begin menstruating and to mature physically for 5 years. Teenage pregnancy adds the needs of the growing fetus to those of the growing mother. They both need considerable amounts of nutrients for their growing bodies.

Diets of teenagers—including those who are pregnant—vary greatly in nutritional adequacy. Many teenagers eat irregularly, skip meals, snack on foods with low nutrient density, and frequently follow restrictive diets.

Pregnant teenagers frequently exhibit a variety of other risk factors that can complicate pregnancy and pose a risk to the fetus. For instance, teenagers are more likely than older women to be underweight at the beginning of pregnancy and to gain fewer than 16 pounds during pregnancy. In addition, their bodies generally lack the maturity needed to safely carry a pregnancy. Teenagers frequently give birth to preterm or LBW infants; about 14% of LBW infants are born to teenagers. This occurs even despite adequate prenatal care. And unfortunately,

Pregnant Vegetarians

Women who practice either lacto-ovo vegetarianism or lacto-vegetarianism generally do not face special difficulties in meeting their nutritional needs during pregnancy. Like nonvegetarian women, they should be concerned primarily with meeting iron, folate, calcium, and zinc needs.

On the other hand, when a total vegetarian (vegan) becomes pregnant, she must carefully plan a diet that includes sufficient protein, vitamin D (or sufficient sun exposure), vitamin B-6, iron, calcium, and zinc and also use a vitamin B-12 supplement. The basic vegan diet listed in Chapter 6 should be modified to include more grains, beans, nuts, and seeds to supply the necessary extra amounts of some of these nutrients. Because iron and calcium are poorly absorbed from most plant foods, iron and calcium supplements are probably necessary, but, to avoid competition for absorption, they should not be taken together. The amounts provided by typical prenatal supplements should suffice to meet iron needs but not calcium needs. The prenatal supplement will also fulfill vitamin D needs if sufficient sun exposure does not take place.

nearly 30% of teens do not even receive prenatal care until the second trimester. Additional complications, such as infant illness or even death, are tied to the teenage mother's day-to-day health practices.

The specific needs of pregnant teenagers vary according to their own growth patterns, body build, and physical activity habits. This makes it difficult to predict their nutrient needs. Clinicians can evaluate the adequacy of their diet by checking for appropriate weight gain during pregnancy and for appropriate food choices. Teenagers should be regularly counseled on nutrition during their prenatal care. They need information about basic nutritional guidelines: the relationship between food and health, the kind and amount of food energy needed to support appropriate weight gain, how to select nutrient-rich foods, appropriate use of prenatal supplements, and preparation for breastfeeding or using commercial infant formulas. They also need to be aware of the risks involved with smoking, drinking alcohol, and using drugs and medications not approved by their physicians.

Programs specifically designed for pregnant teenagers are available in many communities. These typically provide information about community resources; many also offer clothing and supplies for the infant, food resources, transportation for prenatal checkups, and a supportive environment. Nonetheless, even when a teenager successfully delivers a healthy baby, the subsequent impact of parenthood on the mother's education and economic future is often devastating. Few teenage mothers can successfully care for and support themselves and their children. Many young mothers end up forgoing the very education that would qualify them for better jobs, which might permit them to adequately care for and support themselves and their children. Moreover, about 70% of pregnant teenagers are unmarried and don't get married before the birth of their child, further compounding the economic and social difficulties of the young mother and child.

Many efforts are under way to reduce the rate of teenage pregnancy. Prevention is the best medicine. This approach is currently receiving high priority by the federal government. A few broad strategies for public interventions that are designed to reduce the problems associated with teenage pregnancy have been advocated: less acceptance of teenage pregnancy by society in general, an emphasis on sexual abstinence, more sex education and contraceptive services, and better support services for those teenagers who become pregnant. In recent years, teenage sexual activity has been declining and contraceptive use is increasing. It is also important that teens see adult and media support for abstinence and decreased pregnancy rates. In addition, new welfare laws have now been passed requiring teenage mothers on welfare to live at home with a parent or guardian and to stay in school. Ideally these or other solutions will arise as effective measures.

Prenatal Care and Counseling

Education, an adequate diet, and early and consistent prenatal medical care maximize the chances of producing a healthy baby and avoiding the risks covered earlier. If diabetes or high blood pressure are present or developing, these must be carefully controlled to minimize complications in the pregnancy. Women should be concerned about these issues and make appropriate changes before becoming pregnant. Certainly they should be addressed early in pregnancy, and although some women already have good nutritional habits, all should be reminded of diet and lifestyle risks that may harm the growing fetus.

Several U.S. government programs exist to reduce infant mortality by providing high-quality health care and foods. An example of such a program is the Special Supplemental Food Program for Women, Infants, and Children (WIC). This program offers health assessments and foods (or vouchers for foods) that supply high-quality protein, calcium, iron, and vitamins A and C to pregnant and breastfeeding women, infants, and children (to age 5 years) from low-income populations.

On the WIC program, participants' diets have improved markedly, as has the likelihood that women will have a healthy baby. This program is credited with decreasing the cases of iron-deficiency anemia and low-birth-weight infants within the population it serves. Studies have estimated that every dollar spent on the prenatal component of WIC saves about three dollars in public health expenditures for the care of low-birth-weight babies.

Women with acquired immune deficiency syndrome (AIDS) may pass the virus that causes this disease to the fetus during pregnancy or the birth process. About 1 in 3 infected newborns will develop AIDS symptoms and die within just a few years. Mother-infant transmission can be cut significantly if the woman begins taking the drug zidovudine (AZT) by the fourteenth week of pregnancy. Thus screening pregnant women for AIDS and prescribing AZT to those infected are currently advocated.

ConceptCheck

Additional nutrient needs in pregnancy generally can be met by slight modifications of the Food Guide Pyramid. Prenatal supplemental vitamins and minerals are commonly prescribed to further help meet iron folate needs. Taking too many supplements, notably vitamin A, can be hazardous to the fetus. Lacto-ovo or lacto-vegetarians can generally meet the nutrient needs of pregnancy through their diet changes and use of prenatal supplements. Total vegetarians must plan more carefully. Prenatal counseling is most advantageous if begun before pregnancy in order to avoid modifiable risks. Government programs such as WIC are designed to assist poor pregnant women and their children by providing health care and foods.

Critical Thinking

Sandy, who is 4 months pregnant, has been having heartburn after meals, constipation, and difficult bowel movements. As a nutrition student, you understand the digestive system and the role of nutrition in health. What remedies might you suggest to Sandy to relieve her problems?

Physiological Changes Can Cause Discomfort in Pregnancy

During pregnancy, the fetus' needs for oxygen, nutrients, and excretion increase the burden on the mother's lungs, heart, and kidneys. Although a mother's digestive and metabolic systems work very efficiently, some discomfort accompanies the changes her body undergoes to accommodate the fetus.

Heartburn, Constipation, and Hemorrhoids

As muscles relax during pregnancy, women often experience heartburn (see Chapter 3). To decrease symptoms, women should try the following: avoid lying down after eating; eat less fat and avoid irritating, spicy foods; and consume liquid between meals instead of during meals. She should talk to a physician if the problem persists.

Many women also suffer from constipation and hemorrhoids during the pregnancy. The following suggestions may help to reduce this symptom: perform regular physical activity and consume adequate fluid and dietary fiber. She should talk to a physician about the possibility of decreasing iron supplementation if the problem persists.

Edema

Placental hormones and increased blood volume normally cause some swelling (edema) in pregnancy. There is no reason to severely restrict salt to limit mild edema. However, the edema may limit physical activity late in pregnancy and occasionally require a woman to elevate her feet to control the symptoms. Overall, edema generally spells trouble only if high blood pressure and the appearance of much protein in the urine accompany fluid retention (see later section).

Morning Sickness

About 50% of pregnant women experience nausea during the early states of pregnancy. This nausea may be related to the increased sense of smell induced by pregnancy-related hormones circulating in the bloodstream. Although commonly called "morning sickness," pregnancy-related nausea may occur at any time and persist all day.

To help control mild nausea, pregnant women can try the following: avoiding nauseating foods, such as fried or greasy foods; cooking with open windows to dissipate nauseating smells; eating soda crackers or dry cereal before getting out of bed; avoiding large fluid intakes early in the morning; and eating smaller, more frequent meals. Because the iron in prenatal supplements triggers nausea in some women, changing the type of supplement used may provide relief in some cases. If a woman thinks her prenatal supplement is related to morning sickness, she should discuss switching to another supplement with her physician.

Overall, whether it is broccoli or soda crackers, if a food sounds good to a pregnant woman with morning sickness, she should eat it and eat when she can while also striving to follow her prenatal diet. If she has a great deal of difficulty in following her diet, she should alert her physician of this and follow the advice given. Usually nausea stops after the first trimester, but in about 10% to 20% of cases it can continue throughout the entire pregnancy. In cases of serious nausea the preceding practices offer little relief. Vitamin B–6 in amounts about 7.5 times the RDA may be helpful, under a physician's supervision. When appetite is severely reduced or vomiting persists, additional medical guidance is warranted. Hospitalization may be needed if the mother exhibits significant dehydration or weight loss.

Anemia

To supply fetal needs, the mother's blood volume expands up to approximately 50% above normal. The amount of red blood cells expands only about 20% above normal and occurs more gradually. This leaves proportionately fewer red blood cells in a pregnant woman's bloodstream, making it look like she has anemia. This is a normal response to pregnancy, however, rather than the result of inadequate nutrient intake. But, if during pregnancy iron stores and/or dietary iron intake are not sufficient to meet needs, any true iron-deficiency anemia that develops requires medical attention.

Gestational Diabetes

Hormones synthesized by the placenta antagonize the action of the hormone insulin. This antagonism can precipitate **gestational diabetes,** often beginning in weeks 20 to 28, particularly in women who have a family history of diabetes and/or are obese. Gestational diabetes develops in about 4% of pregnancies. Today pregnant women routinely are screened at 24 to 28 weeks for elevated blood glucose concentration 1 hour after consuming 50 grams of glucose. If gestational diabetes is detected, a special diet—especially control of morning carbohydrate intake—and sometimes insulin injections are needed. Regular physical activity is also helpful. Although gestational diabetes often disappears after the infant's birth, it is linked to development of diabetes later in the mother's life, especially if she fails to maintain healthy body weight. Proper control of both gestational diabetes and diabetes present in the mother before pregnancy is extremely important. If not treated, the primary risks are that the fetus can grow quite large and that the pregnancy may result in a cesarean section due to the size of the fetus. Other concerns are potential need for early delivery, increased risk of birth trauma and malformations, as well as low blood glucose in the infant at birth.

Gestational diabetes
A high blood glucose concentration that develops during pregnancy and returns to normal after birth; one cause is placental production of hormones that antagonize regulation of blood glucose by insulin.

Pregnancy-Induced Hypertension

Pregnancy-induced hypertension is a high-risk disorder and occurs in about 7% of pregnancies. In its mild forms it is known as *preeclampsia* and in severe forms as *eclampsia.* Early symptoms include a rise in blood pressure, excess protein in the urine, edema, changes in blood clotting, and nervous system disorders. Very severe effects, including convulsions, can occur in the second and third trimesters. If not controlled, eclampsia eventually damages the liver and kidneys, and mother and fetus may both die. The population most at risk for this disorder includes teenagers, women over the age of 35, and those who have had multiple-birth pregnancies or show poor nutritional status.

Pregnancy-induced hypertension
A serious disorder that can include high blood pressure, kidney failure, convulsions, and even death of the mother and fetus. Mild cases are known as preeclampsia; *more severe cases are called* eclampsia.

Pregnancy-induced hypertension resolves once the pregnancy ends, making delivery the best treatment for the mother. However, since the problem often begins before the fetus is ready to be born, physicians in many cases must employ treatments to prevent the worsening of the disorder. Bed rest and magnesium sulfate are possible treatment methods, though the effectiveness of these and other treatments varies and is often disappointing. Several other treatments are under study, but no definite proof exists for any one approach.

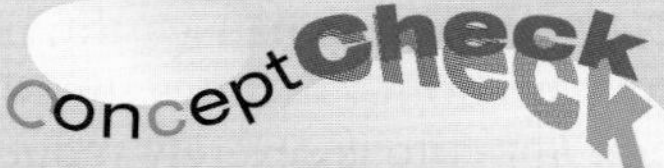

Heartburn, constipation, nausea and vomiting, edema, anemia, and gestational diabetes are possible discomforts and complications of pregnancy. Changes in food habits can often ease these problems. Pregnancy-induced hypertension, with high blood pressure, and kidney and liver damage, can lead to severe complications or even death of both the mother and fetus, if not treated.

Breastfeeding

Breastfeeding one's infant enjoys wide support in the medical community. The American Dietetic Association and the American Academy of Pediatrics recommend breastfeeding exclusively for the first 4 to 6 months with the continued combination of breastfeeding and infant foods through the first year. Recent surveys show, however, that only about 50% of American mothers now nurse their infants in the hospital, and at 6 months only 20% are still breastfeeding their infants. Thus there are many women leaving the hospital breastfeeding, but there is a large dropoff, especially after 2 weeks.

Women who choose to breastfeed usually find it an enjoyable and special time in their lives and in their relationship with their new infant. Bottle feeding with an infant formula is also safe for infants, as discussed in the next chapter, but does not equal the benefits derived from human milk in all aspects. Note that if a woman doesn't nurse her child, breast weight returns to normal very soon after birth.

Ability to Breastfeed

In most cases, problems encountered in breastfeeding are due to a lack of appropriate information, because almost all women are physically capable of nursing their children (see later section for exceptions). Breast size is no indication of success in breastfeeding and generally increases during pregnancy. Most women notice a dramatic increase in the size and weight of their breasts by the third or fourth day of breastfeeding. If these changes don't occur, a woman needs to speak with her physician.

Breastfed infants must be followed closely over the first days of life to ensure that the process is proceeding normally. Monitoring is especially important with a mother's first child, because the mother will be inexperienced with the process of breastfeeding. One result of current practices of rapid hospital discharge is a decreased period of infant monitoring by health-care professionals. Incidents have been reported of infants developing dehydration and blood clots soon after hospital discharge when breastfeeding did not proceed smoothly. New parents especially need guidance about their infant's nutritional and other health-related needs by appropriate professionals in the first days to weeks after hospital discharge.

Interested women should learn the proper technique, what problems to expect, and how to respond to them before the infant is born. Overall, breastfeeding is a learned skill, and mothers need knowledge to nurse safely, especially the first time.

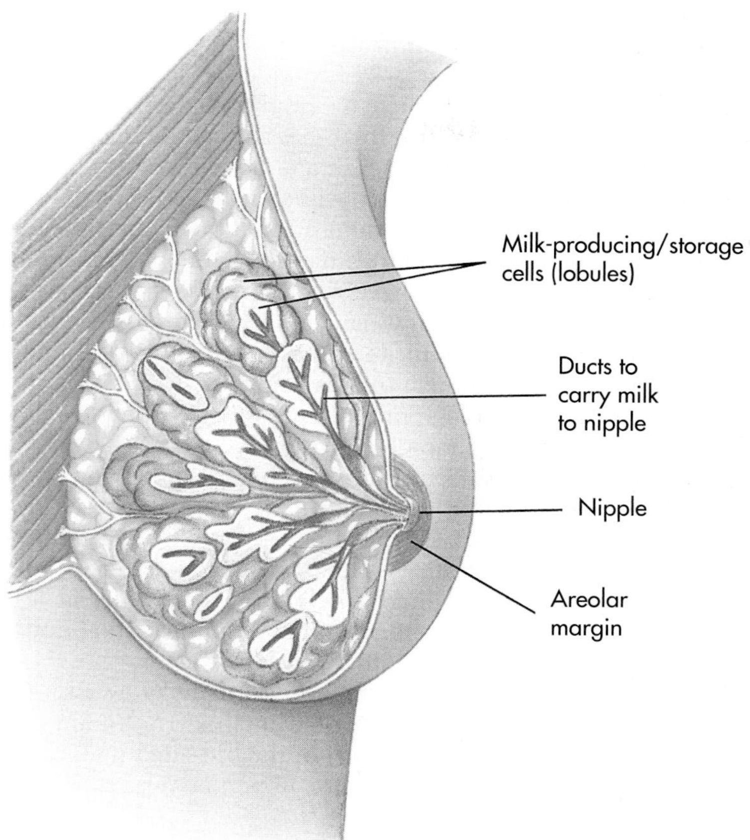

Figure 12–6 *The anatomy of the breast. Many types of cells form a coordinated network to produce and secrete human milk.*

Producing Human Milk

During pregnancy, hormones from the placenta stimulate changes in the breast. For example, breast weight increases by 1 to 2 pounds. After birth the mother produces the hormone **prolactin** to maintain changes in the breast and therefore the ability to produce milk (Figure 12–6).

The hormone prolactin also stimulates the synthesis of milk. Suckling stimulates prolactin release. Milk synthesis then occurs as an infant nurses. The more the infant suckles, the more milk is produced. Milk production closely parallels infant demand. Because of this, even twins can be nursed.

Most protein found in human milk is synthesized by breast tissue. Some proteins also enter the milk directly from the mother's bloodstream. These proteins include immune factors and enzymes. Fats in human milk come from the mother's diet, and some are also synthesized by breast tissue. The sugar galactose is synthesized in the breast, while glucose enters from the mother's bloodstream. Together these sugars form lactose, the main carbohydrate in human milk.

Prolactin
A hormone secreted by the mother that stimulates the synthesis of milk.

Let-down reflex
A reflex stimulated by infant suckling that causes the release (ejection) of milk from milk ducts in the mother's breast.

Oxytocin
A hormone secreted by the posterior part of the pituitary gland. It causes contraction of the musclelike cells surrounding the ducts of the breasts, and the smooth muscle of the uterus.

The Let-Down Reflex

An important brain-breast connection—the **let-down reflex**—is necessary for breastfeeding. The brain releases the hormone **oxytocin** to allow the breast tissues to let down (release) the milk from storage sites. It travels to the nipple area, where a tingling sensation signals the let-down reflex shortly before milk flow begins.

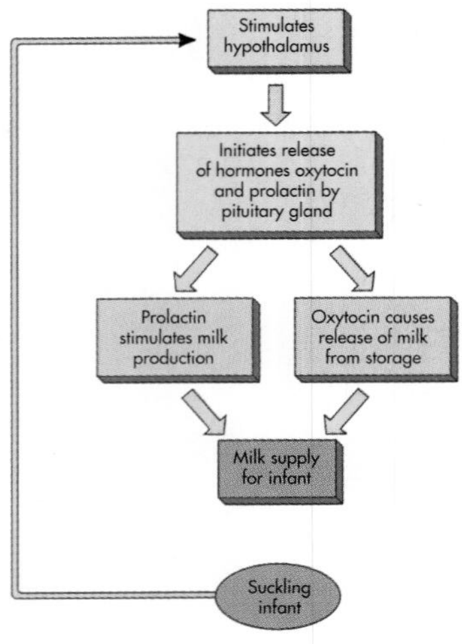

If the let-down reflex doesn't operate, little milk is available to the infant. The infant then gets frustrated and this can frustrate the mother. The let-down reflex is easily inhibited by nervous tension, a lack of confidence, and fatigue. Thus mothers need to find a relaxed environment where they can breastfeed.

After a few weeks, the let-down reflex becomes automatic. The mother's response can be triggered just by thinking about her infant or seeing or hearing another one. At first, however, the process can be a bit bewildering.

Because she cannot measure the amount of milk the infant takes in, a mother may fear that she is not adequately nourishing the infant. As a general rule, a well-nourished breastfed infant should (1) have six or more wet diapers per day after the second day of life, (2) show a normal weigh gain, and (3) pass two to three stools per day that look like lumpy mustard. In addition, softening of the breast during the feeding helps indicate that enough milk is being consumed. Parents who sense their infant is not consuming enough milk should consult a physician immediately because dehydration can develop rapidly.

Disposable diapers can absorb so much urine that it is difficult to judge when they are wet. A strip of paper towel laid inside a disposable diaper makes a good wetness indicator. Or cloth diapers may be used for a day or two to assess whether nursing is supplying sufficient milk.

It generally takes 2 to 3 weeks to fully establish the feeding routine: infant and mother both feel comfortable, the milk supply meets the infant demand, and initial nipple soreness disappears. Establishing the breastfeeding routine requires patience, but the rewards are great. The adjustments are easier if bottle feedings are not introduced until breastfeeding is well established, after at least 3 weeks but preferably not until after 4 to 6 months. Then a supplemental bottle or two of human milk expressed earlier by the mother per day is fine.

Parents need not be concerned that breastfed infants grow a bit more slowly after about 3 months of age than formula-fed infants. The infant's physician is the best judge of whether the rate of growth of the breastfed infant is satisfactory. Essentially the difference is of no consequence, in part because some of it is related to increased fat deposition.

Nutritional Qualities of Human Milk

Unless altered, cow's milk should not be used in infant feeding until the infant is 12 months old. Only human milk (or infant formula) is recommended. Cow's milk is too high in minerals and protein, does not contain enough carbohydrate to meet infant needs, and may trigger development of Type 1 diabetes in infants with a genetic predisposition to the disorder. In addition, the major protein in cow's milk, casein, is harder for an infant to digest than the major protein found in human milk. Finally, certain compounds in human milk presently under study show other possible benefits for the infant. These factors are not present in cow's milk or infant formulas.

Colostrum
The first fluid secreted by the breast during late pregnancy and the first few days after birth. This thick fluid is rich in immune factors and protein.

Meconium
The first thick mucuslike stool passed by the infant after birth.

***Lactobacillus bifidus* factor**
A protective factor secreted in the colostrum that encourages growth of beneficial bacteria in the newborn's intestines.

Colostrum

The first fluid made by a woman's breast is **colostrum.** This thick, yellowish fluid may leak from the breast during late pregnancy and is produced in earnest for a few days to a week after birth. Colostrum contains antibodies and immune-system cells, some of which pass unaltered through the immature GI tract of the infant into the bloodstream. These immune factors and cells protect the infant from some gastrointestinal diseases and other infectious disorders, compensating for its own immature immune system during the first few months of life.

Colostrum facilitates the passage of **menocium,** a stool produced during fetal life. One component of colostrum, the ***Lactobacillus bifidus* factor,** encourages the growth of *Lactobacillus bifidus* bacteria. These bacteria limit the growth of potentially toxic bacteria in the intestine. Overall, breastfeeding promotes the intestinal health of the breastfed infant in this way and in other ways.

Mature Milk

Human milk composition gradually changes until several days after delivery to the composition of mature milk. Human milk looks very different from cow's milk. (Table 13–1 in the next chapter provides a direct comparison.) Human milk is thin and almost watery in appearance and often has a slight bluish tinge. Its nutritional qualities are impressive.

Human milk's main protein forms a soft, light curd in the infant's stomach, easing digestion. Other human milk proteins bind iron, reducing the growth of iron-requiring bacteria. Many of these types of bacteria cause diarrhea. Still other proteins offer the important immune protection already noted.

The lipids in human breast milk are high in linoleic acid and cholesterol, which are needed for brain development. Breast milk also contains long-chain omega-3 fatty acids, such a docosahexaenoic acid (DHA). This unsaturated fatty acid is used for synthesis of tissues in the brain, the rest of the central nervous system, and the eyes. Some evidence indicates that breastfed infants show greater visual acuity and better nervous system development than infants fed commercial formulas, none of which currently contain DHA. This is an active area of research. Breastfeeding for at least 4 months is advocated to obtain this benefit.

Human milk changes in fat composition during each feeding. The consistency of milk released initially (about 60% of the volume) resembles that of skim milk. The next amount (about 35% of the total volume) has a greater fat proportion, similar to whole milk. Finally, the hindmilk (about 5% of the total) is essentially like cream and released after 10 minutes into the feeding. The overall energy content of human milk ends up about the same as that of infant formulas (67 kcal per 100 milliliters). Babies need to nurse long enough (for example a total of about 20 minutes) to get the energy in the rich hindmilk to be satisfied between feedings and grow well.

Human milk also allows for adequate hydration of the infant, provided the baby is exclusively breastfed. A question commonly asked is whether the infant needs additional water, if stressed by hot weather, diarrhea, vomiting, or fever. Providing up to 4 ounces of water a day from a bottle to young breastfed infants is fine in such cases, if the infant's physician agrees. Note that greater amounts of supplemental water can lead to brain disorders, low blood potassium, and other problems, and so can be given only with strict physician's guidance.

A Food Plan for Women Who Breastfeed

Nutrient needs for a breastfeeding mother change slightly if at all from those of the pregnant woman. Exceptions are decreases in folate and iron needs and an increase in the need for energy, vitamins A and C, niacin, and zinc. The diet for breastfeeding women can be the same as that for pregnant women, except teenagers generally should have four servings from the milk, yogurt, and cheese group (see Table 12–1). Iron supplements may be prescribed if anemia developed during pregnancy. Some researchers recommend eating fish twice a week, because the omega-3 fatty acids present in fish are thought to be important for brain development, as just mentioned. Recall from Chapter 5 this is healthy practice for all of us, but for other reasons (primarily heart disease-related).

A reasonable approach for a breastfeeding woman is to eat a balanced diet that supplies at least 1800 kcal per day, has a moderate fat content, and includes a variety of milk products, fruits, vegetables, and whole grains. The woman should drink fluids every time the infant nurses, because adequate hydration encourages ample milk production. If a woman restricts her energy intake too severely, the quantity of milk also decreases. This is not a time to crash diet. More than two alcoholic drinks a day also decreases milk output, as does smoking.

Most substances the mother ingests are secreted into her milk. For this reason she should limit intake of or avoid all alcohol and caffeine and check all medications with a pediatrician. If a woman notices a connection between a food she eats and the infant's later fussiness, she could consider temporarily avoiding that food. Some researchers, on the other hand, feel that the passage of flavors from the mother's diet into her milk affords an opportunity for the infant to learn about the flavor of the foods of its family long before solids are introduced.

Breastfeeding mothers should get their physician's permission before embarking on a vigorous exercise program. Breastfeeding women must also take care to drink plenty of fluids before and after workouts and should avoid exercising when fatigued.

Milk production requires approximately 800 kcal every day. The RDA for energy during lactation is an extra 500 kcal daily above prepregnancy recommendations. The difference between energy needs and intake—about 300 kcal—should contribute to gradual loss of the extra body fat accumulated during pregnancy, especially if breastfeeding is continued for 6 months or more and the woman performs some physical activity. This shows how practical the link is between pregnancy and breastfeeding. Weight loss of 1 to 4 pounds per month in the nursing mother is appropriate, depending on how active the mother is.

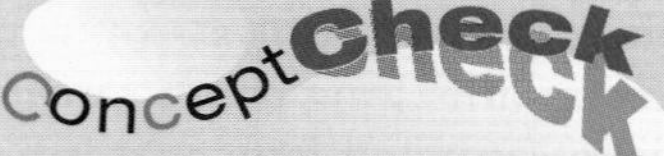

Almost all women have the ability to breastfeed. The hormone prolactin stimulates breast tissue to synthesize milk. Some components of human milk come directly from the mother's bloodstream. Infant suckling triggers a let-down reflex that releases the milk. The more an infant nurses, the more milk is synthesized. The nutrient composition of human milk is very different from that of cow's milk and changes as the infant matures. The first fluid produced, colostrum, is rich in immune factors. The diet for breastfeeding is generally similar to that for pregnancy, except for additional fluids, as well as four servings from the milk, yogurt, and cheese group for teenagers in general.

Pros and Cons of Breastfeeding

As noted already, the vast majority of women are capable of breastfeeding, and infants benefit from it (Table 12–2). Nonetheless, a woman's decision to nurse depends on a variety of factors, some of which may make breastfeeding impractical or undesirable for a woman. Breastfeeding provides distinct advantages, but none so great that a woman who decides to bottle-feed should feel she is significantly penalizing her infant.

TABLE 12-2

Attributes of Breastfeeding

INFANT

- Bacteriologically safe
- Always fresh and ready to go
- Provides immunity while infant's immune system is still immature
- Contributes to maturation of gastrointestinal tract via *Lactobacillus bifidus* factor; decreases chances of diarrhea and respiratory disease.
- Reduces risk of food allergies and intolerances
- Establishes habit of eating in moderation, thus decreasing possibility of obesity later in life
- Contributes to proper development of jaws and teeth for better speech development
- Decreases ear infections
- Facilitates bonding with mother

MOTHER

- Contributes to earlier recovery from pregnancy due to a quicker return of the uterus to the prepregnancy state
- Decreases the risk of ovarian and premenopausal breast cancer
- Lessens the economic strain of purchasing formula
- Facilitates bonding (psychological attachment) with infant

Advantages of Breastfeeding

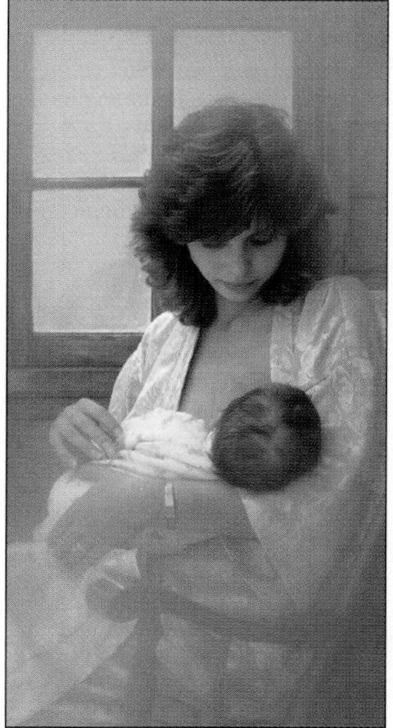

Breastfeeding fosters a closeness and bonding between the mother and the infant.

Human milk is tailored to meet infant nutrient needs for the first 4 to 6 months of life. The possible exceptions are the relative lack of iron and vitamin D. Infant supplements, used under the guidance of a pediatrician, can supply these and are often recommended. Sun exposure also helps compensate for the gap in vitamin D nutriture. If fluoride is not present in adequate amounts in the household water supply or the child is not receiving tap water, a fluoride supplement should be considered after 6 months of age. A dentist should be consulted. Vitamin B–12 supplements are recommended for the breastfed infant whose mother is a complete vegetarian (vegan).

Fewer Infections

Breastfeeding reduces the general risk of infections to the infant. As mentioned, this is partially because of the antibodies in human milk that an infant can use. Breastfed infants also have fewer ear infections because they do not sleep with a bottle in the mouth. Experts strongly discourage allowing infants to sleep with a bottle in their months because when that happens, milk pools there, backs up through the throat, and eventually settles in the ears, creating a growth medium for bacteria. Infant ear infections are a common problem. By avoiding them, parents can decrease discomfort for the infant, avoid trips to the doctor, and prevent possible hearing loss. Tooth decay from nighttime bottles is another likely consequence (see Chapter 13).

Fewer Allergies and Intolerances

Breastfeeding also reduces the chances of allergies, especially in allergy-prone infants (see the Nutrition Issue in Chapter 13). Breastfeeding for even just the first few weeks is beneficial. A longer commitment is better, but the first few months are most critical. Another benefit of breastfeeding is that infants are better able to tolerate human milk than formulas. Formulas must occasionally be switched several times until caregivers find the best one for the infant.

Convenience and Cost

Breastfeeding frees the mother from the time and expense involved in buying and preparing formula and washing bottles. Human milk is ready to go and sterile. This allows the mother to spend more time with her baby. On the other hand, if the mother desires freedom during feeding time to do other things, after the baby is about 1 month old she can express, save, and bottle her own milk for bottle feeding (see below). This is an alternative worth considering.

Barriers to Breastfeeding

A lack of role models, widespread misinformation, fear of appearing immodest, and workplaces outside the home all serve as barriers to breastfeeding.

Misinformation

Probably the major barriers to breastfeeding are misinformation and lack of role models. One positive note has been the widespread increase in the availability of lactation consultants over the past several years. These consultants are a valuable resource for new mothers in the adjustment to breastfeeding. If a woman is interested in breastfeeding, she should also talk to women who have done it successfully. Experienced mothers can be an enormous help to the first-time mother. In almost

Frozen human milk should not be thawed in a microwave. The heat can destroy immune factors in the milk and create hot spots that may scald the infant's tongue.

every community, a group called La Leche League offers classes in breastfeeding and advises women who have problems with it ([800] LALECHE or http://www.lalecheleague.org).

Returning to an Outside Job

Working outside the home can complicate plans to breastfeed. One possibility after a month or two of breastfeeding is for the mother to regularly express and save her own milk. She can express milk by breast pump or manually into a sterile plastic bottle or nursing bag (used in a disposable bottle system). Saving human milk requires careful sanitation and rapid chilling. It can be stored in the refrigerator for about 1 day and be frozen for about 1 month. A schedule of expressing milk and using supplemental formula feedings is most successful if begun after 1 to 2 months of exclusive breastfeeding. After 1 month or so the baby is well adapted to breastfeeding and probably feels enough emotional security and other benefits from nursing to drink both ways.

Some women can juggle both a job and breastfeeding, but others find it too cumbersome and decide to formula-feed. A compromise—balancing some breastfeedings, perhaps early morning and night, with formula-feeding during the day—is possible. However, too many supplemental formula feedings decrease milk production.

Social Concerns

Another barrier for some women is embarrassment about nursing a child in public. Women who feel uncomfortable should be reassured that with appropriate clothing, they can nurse quite discreetly.

Medical Conditions Precluding Breastfeeding

Breastfeeding may be ruled out by certain medical conditions in either the infant or mother. For example, infants with the disease galactosemia or phenylketonuria need special commercial formulas since they are unable to metabolize all of the components in human milk. Both diseases may eventually lead to mental retardation if special formulas are not used.

Mothers who take certain medications that pass into the milk and adversely affect the nursing infant may be advised to avoid breastfeeding. In addition, a woman who has a serious chronic disease (such as tuberculosis, AIDS or HIV-positive status) or who is being treated with chemotherapy medications should not breastfeed.

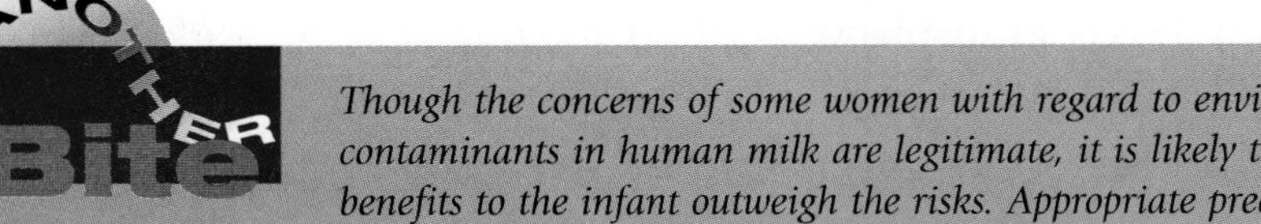

Though the concerns of some women with regard to environmental contaminants in human milk are legitimate, it is likely that the benefits to the infant outweigh the risks. Appropriate precautions for avoiding such contaminants include: (1) avoiding freshwater fish from polluted waters, (2) washing and peeling fruits and vegetables, (3) removing fatty edges of meat, and (4) avoiding rapid weight loss, since contaminants may be released from fatty tissues.

Can a Preterm Infant Be Breastfed?

There is no clear-cut answer to whether a woman can breastfeed a preterm infant. In some cases, human milk is the most desirable form of nourishment, depending on weight and length of gestation. If so, it must usually be expressed from the breast, saved, and then fed through a tube. Fortification of the milk with such nutrients as calcium, phosphorus, sodium, and protein is often necessary to match an infant's rapid growth. In other cases, special feeding problems may prevent the use of human milk or necessitate supplementing it with formula. Sometimes intravenous nutrition is the only option. Working as a team, the pediatrician, neonatal nurses, and registered dietitian must guide the parents in this decision.

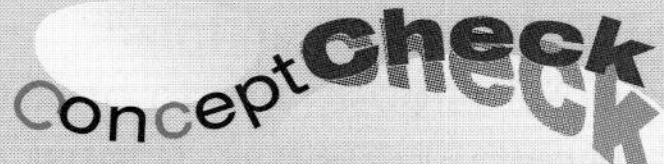

Human milk supplies most of an infant's nutritional needs for the first 6 months, although supplementation with vitamin D and iron may be needed. Breastfeeding is less expensive and often more convenient than formula-feeding. Compared with formula-fed infants, breastfed infants have fewer intestinal, respiratory, and ear infections and are less susceptible to allergies and food intolerances. Despite the advantages of breastfeeding, a lack of role models, misinformation, and social concerns may dissuade a mother from breastfeeding. A combination of breastfeeding and bottle-feeding is possible when a mother is regularly away from the infant. Breastfeeding is not desirable if a mother has certain diseases or must take medication potentially harmful to the infant. The preterm infant, depending on its condition, may benefit from consuming human milk.

Summary

- Adequate nutrition is vital during pregnancy to ensure the well-being of both the infant and mother. Poor maternal nutrition and use of some medications, especially during the first trimester, can cause birth defects. Growth retardation and altered development can also occur if these insults happen later in pregnancy.
- Infants born preterm (before 37 weeks gestation) or those born with low birth weight (less than 2.5 kilograms, or 5.5 pounds) usually have more medical problems at and following birth than normal infants.
- A woman typically needs an additional 300 kcal per day during the second and third trimesters of pregnancy to meet her energy needs. Weight gain should occur slowly, reaching a total of 25 to 35 pounds in a woman of healthy weight. Protein, vitamin, and mineral needs also increase during pregnancy.
- Factors aside from nutrition that influence pregnancy outcome include poverty, close spacing of births, teenage pregnancy, prenatal care, lifestyle, prenatal ketosis, caffeine and aspartame intake, and various infections.
- Extra servings are generally needed from the milk, yogurt, and cheese group, and close attention should be given to the fruit and vegetable groups, and to the meat, poultry, fish, dry beans, eggs, and nuts group of the Food Guide Pyramid. Supplements of iron and folate, in particular, may be required. Adequate intake of folate is important at the time of conception. Any supplement use needs to be guided by a physician, as an excess intake of vitamin A and other nutrients can have harmful effects on the fetus.
- Prenatal care is essential to the health of every fetus. Total vegetarians must plan carefully and consult their physician to meet pregnancy needs.
- Pregnancy-induced hypertension, gestational diabetes, heartburn, constipation, nausea, vomiting, edema, and anemia are all possible discomforts and complications of pregnancy. Often, nutrition therapy can help minimize these problems.
- Pregnant teenagers require very careful prenatal and nutritional care. Complications of pregnancy are more common in teenagers than in more mature women because the teenagers have very high physiological demands and often compromised social and economic support.

- Almost all women are able to nurse their infants. The nutrient composition of human milk is very different from unaltered cow's milk and much more desirable. Colostrum, the first fluid produced by the human breast, is very rich in immune factors.
- For the infant the advantages of breastfeeding over formula-feeding are numerous, including fewer intestinal, respiratory, and ear infections and fewer allergies and food intolerances. Moreover, breastfeeding is also less expensive and possibly more convenient for the mother than formula-feeding. However, an infant can be adequately nourished with formula if the mother chooses not to breastfeed. Breastfeeding is not desirable if the mother has certain diseases or must take medication potentially harmful to the infant. Likewise, breastfeeding is not advised for infants with certain medical conditions, including some preterm infants.

Study Questions

1. Describe how nutritional intake can affect the health of both the mother and the fetus in each trimester of pregnancy.
2. Identify five modifiable behaviors that pose risks to the fetus if continued during pregnancy.
3. Outline current weight-gain recommendations for pregnancy. What is the basis for these recommendations? List two exceptions to these recommendations.
4. List four nutrient needs that increase during pregnancy. How is the Food Guide Pyramid modified to help meet these needs?
5. List three complications of pregnancy and how appropriate nutrition can ease suffering.
6. Why does teenage pregnancy receive so much attention these days? At what age do you think pregnancy would be ideal? Why?
7. Give three reasons why a woman should give serious consideration to breastfeeding her infant.
8. Describe the physiological mechanisms that stimulate milk production and release. How can knowing about these help mothers to nurse successfully?
9. What guidelines can a woman use to determine whether her breastfed infant is receiving sufficient nourishment?
10. How should the basic food plan suitable for pregnancy be modified during breastfeeding?

Further Readings

1 ADA Reports: Position of the American Dietetic Association: promotion of breast-feeding, *Journal of the American Dietetic Association* 97:662, 1997
2 American Academy of Pediatrics: Breastfeeding and the use of human milk, *Pediatrics* 100:1035, 1997.
3 American Academy of Pediatrics: Adolescent pregnancy—current trends and issues: 1998, *Pediatrics* 103:516, 1999.
4 Allen LH: Pregnancy and iron deficiency: unresolved issues, *Nutrition Reviews* 55:91, 1997.
5 Bratton RL: Fetal alcohol syndrome, *Postgraduate Medicine* 98:197, 1995.
6 Erick M: Hyperolfaction and hyperemesis gravidarum: what is the relationship? *Nutrition Reviews* 53:289, 1995.
7 Hinds TS and others: The effect of caffeine on pregnancy outcome variables, *Nutrition Reviews* 54:203, 1996.
8 Jovanovic L: Current management of gestational diabetes, *Nutrition & the M.D.* 24(12):1, 1998.
9 Kalosa KM, Weismiller DG: Nutrition during pregnancy, *American Family Physician* 56(1):205, 1997.
10 Mandelbrot L and others: Perinatal HIV-1 transmission, *Journal of the American Medical Association* 280:55, 1998.
11 Meurer JR and others: Clinical problems and counseling for single-parent families, *American Family Physician* 54:864, 1996.
12 National Academy of Sciences-Institute of Medicine: *Nutrition during lactation,* Washington, DC, 1991, National Academy of Sciences Press.
13 National Academy of Sciences-Institute of Medicine: *Nutrition during pregnancy,* Washington, DC, 1990, National Academy of Sciences Press.
14 Newman J: How breast milk protects newborns, *Scientific American* p. 76, December 1995.
15 Owen AL, Owen GM: Twenty years of WIC: A review of some effects of the program, *Journal of the American Dietetic Association* 97:777, 1997.
16 Seppa N: Exposure to smoke yields fetal mutations, *Science News* 154:213, 1998.
17 Story M, Alton I: Nutrition issues and adolescent pregnancy, *Nutrition Today* 30:142, 1995.
18 Vozenilek GP: What they don't know can hurt them: increasing public awareness of folic acid and neural tube defects, *Journal of the American Dietetic Association* 99:20, 1999.
19 Wang TW, Apgar BS: Exercise during pregnancy, *American Family Physician* 57:1846, 1998.
20 Williams RD: Decreasing the chances of birth defects, *FDA Consumer* p. 12, November 1996.
21 Worthington-Roberts B, Williams SR: *Nutrition in pregnancy and lactation,* Madison, Wis., 1997, Brown & Benchmark.

RATE

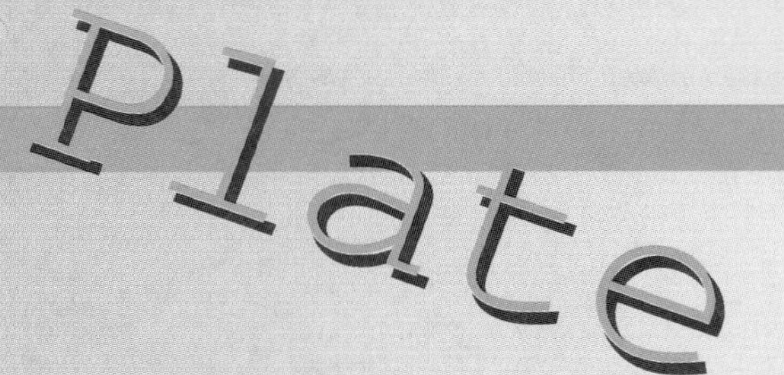

I. Targeting Nutrients Necessary for Pregnant Women

This chapter mentioned that pregnant women may have difficulty meeting their increased needs for iron, folate, calcium, and zinc. List five foods rich in each of these nutrients next to the appropriate heading below. Refer to Chapters 7 and 8 if necessary.

Nutrient	Foods	Nutrient	Foods
Folate	______________	**Calcium**	______________
	______________		______________
	______________		______________
	______________		______________
	______________		______________
	______________		______________
Iron	______________	**Zinc**	______________
	______________		______________
	______________		______________
	______________		______________
	______________		______________
	______________		______________

II. Putting Your Knowledge About Nutrition and Pregnancy To Work

A college friend tells you that she is newly pregnant. You are aware that this friend usually likes to eat the following foods for her meals:

Breakfast
Skips this meal, or eats a granola bar
Coffee

Lunch
Sweetened yogurt
Bagel with cream cheese
Occasional piece of fruit
Regular caffeinated soda

Snack
Chocolate candy bar

Dinner
Pizza, macaroni and cheese, or eggs with toast
Seldom eats a salad or vegetable
Regular caffeinated soda

Snacks
Pretzels or chips
Regular caffeinated soda

1. **Using your software, or Appendix A, evaluate your friend's diet for protein, iron, folate, calcium, and zinc. How does her intake compare to the recommended amounts for pregnancy?**

___

___

___

2. **Now redesign her diet and make sure that her intake meets pregnancy needs for protein, folate, calcium, and zinc. (Hint: fortified foods such as breakfast cereal are generally nutrient-rich foods that can more easily help to meet one's needs.) Increase the iron content as well, but it still may be below the RDA for pregnancy.**

___

___

___

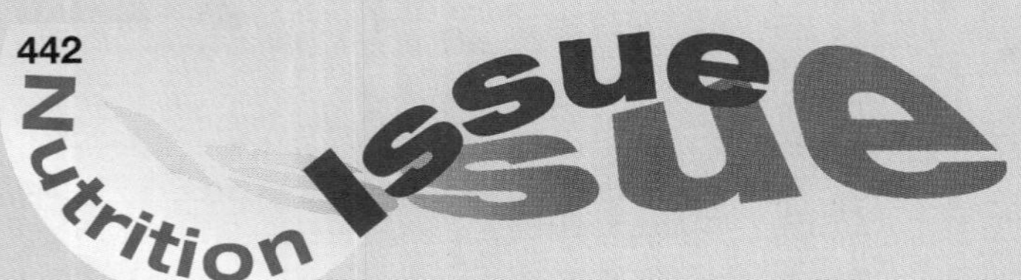

Fetal Alcohol Syndrome

Alcohol is the most common damaging substance to which fetuses are exposed. When a pregnant woman drinks more alcohol than she can metabolize, the excess reaches the embryo (and at later stages the fetus), which has no means of detoxifying it. Women with chronic alcoholism produce children with a recognizable pattern of malformations called **fetal alcohol syndrome (FAS).** A diagnosis of FAS is based mainly on poor fetal and infant growth, physical deformities (especially of facial features), and mental retardation (Figure 12–7). The infant is frequently irritable and may develop hyperactivity and a short attention span. Limited hand-eye coordination is common. Defects in sight, hearing, and mental processing often develop over time.

The range of abnormalities from alcohol exposure varies from the severe effects associated with FAS to reduced birth weight, behavioral effects, growth retardation, and hampered learning ability in infants born to women who report only social drinking. The latter condition, termed fetal alcohol effects (FAE), is not marked by telltale facial abnormalities. For this reasons, parents may not suspect the presence of subtle defects caused by alcohol, even when they exist. FAE can devastate learning potential.

An estimated 3.3 per 10,000 infants born each year exhibit FAS; this has increased since the late 1970s. Many more infants are born annually with FAE. Note that approximately 15% of pregnant women admit to having at least one drink over the past month when asked. Alcohol use is in fact the leading cause of preventable birth defects and mental retardation in the United States and in the Western world as a whole.

Exactly how alcohol causes these defects is not known. One line of research suggests that alcohol, or products produced by metabolism of alcohol, causes faulty migration of cells in the brain during early states of development. In addition, inadequate nutrient intake, reduced nutrient and oxygen transfer across the placenta, cigarette smoking commonly linked to alcohol intake, drug use, and possibly other factors contribute to the overall result. Furthermore, we do not know how much alcohol it takes to produce these adverse effects. Again, for this reason

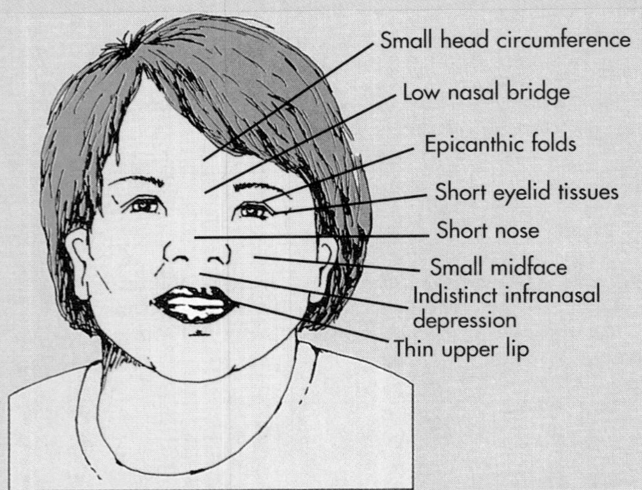

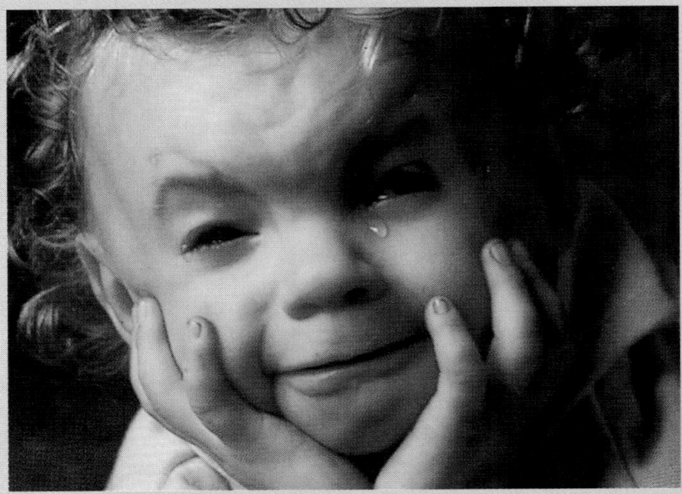

Figure 12–7 *Fetal alcohol syndrome. Milder forms of alcohol-induced changes in the fetus and the infant are known as fetal alcohol effects. The facial features shown are typical of affected children. Additional abnormalities in the brain and other internal organs accompany fetal alcohol syndrome but are not immediately apparent by simply looking at the child.*

many authorities—including the U.S. Surgeon General and the American Medical Association—believe it is best that mothers-to-be avoid alcohol altogether. In other words, there is no safe drinking.

Abstinence is especially important during the first trimester, when key growth and development occur. Alcohol reaches the fetal blood at the same concentration as the mother's blood within 15 minutes of her drinking. However, the effect on the fetus may be up to 10 times greater. For example, just one bout of binge drinking can arrest and alter cell division during critical phases of fetal development. The fetus then may develop an irreversible defect.

Physical damage to the embryo (and later the fetus) results more from first-trimester drinking because the basic structures of tissues and organs develop during this period. Emotional and learning problems stem more from third-trimester drinking because this is when critical further development of the brain occurs. And throughout the pregnancy alcohol interferes with growth. Overall, mothers who drink at least one to two drinks a day throughout pregnancy are much more likely to have growth-retarded infants, and mothers who drink only in late pregnancy are more likely to give birth to preterm infants.

Because alcohol has the capacity to adversely affect each stage of fetal development, the earlier in pregnancy that drinking ceases, the greater the potential for improved outcome. The best course is to consider alcohol an indulgence that must be eliminated from the time of conception until after pregnancy. Currently about half of all women are drinking at the time of conception (that is, before learning they were pregnant). One step in the right direction is the new congressionally mandated warnings about drinking during pregnancy that appear on all alcoholic beverage containers.

Pregnant women should recognize that many cough syrups contain alcohol. Cases have been reported of infants with FAS born to mothers who consumed generous amounts of such cough syrups but no other alcoholic beverages.

Pregnancy lasts only 9 months. In contrast, parents may spend a lifetime caring, often at great expense (estimated at $1.4 million in the United States), for their offspring needlessly handicapped by FAS or FAE. Keep in mind that fetal alcohol syndrome is a completely preventable disease.

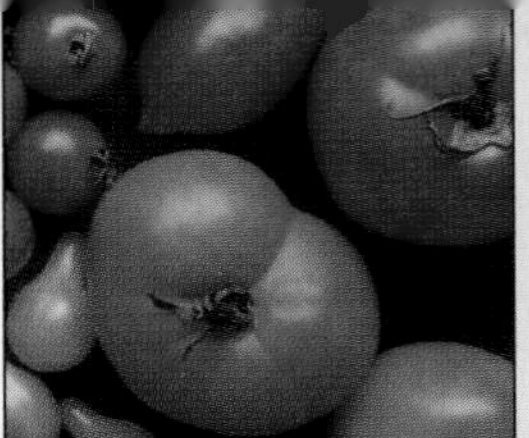

chapter 13

Nutrition from Infancy Through Adolescence

As humans grow through early years into adulthood, our needs for energy and nutrients change. Infants need more energy, protein, vitamins, and minerals per pound of body weight than do adults to support their tremendous growth and development. As growth tapers, children need and eat proportionately less. The erratic eating behaviors of young children pose major challenges for parents and other caregivers. Still, childhood becomes an important time to establish healthful habits, including those related to food choice and physical activity.

The family wields an important influence over the child. Thus education designed to change children's eating behaviors must be directed simultaneously at the main caregivers. They usually determine what foods are purchased and how they are prepared. By stocking a variety of foods at home, introducing different foods regularly, and making mealtimes fun for the whole family, parents and other caregivers can steer children toward lifelong healthful eating patterns.

Maintaining a healthful eating pattern should continue as children grow into teenagers. In exploring all these stages of life, this chapter looks at the key role nutrients play and how food choices should be tailored to meet those needs.

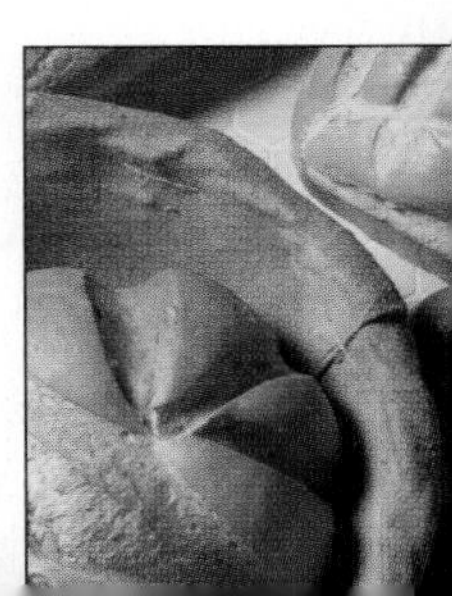

Nutrition Web

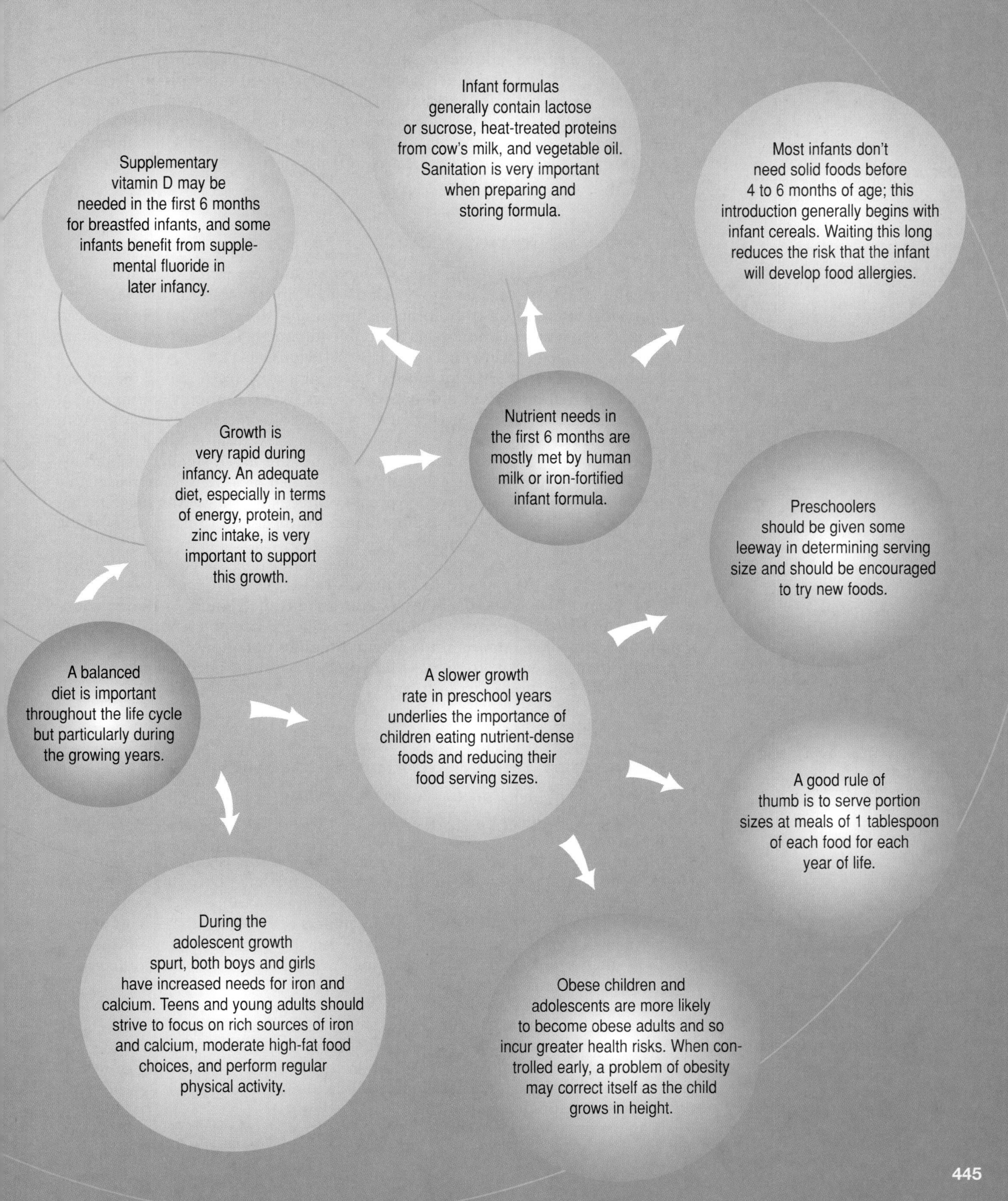

Infant formulas generally contain lactose or sucrose, heat-treated proteins from cow's milk, and vegetable oil. Sanitation is very important when preparing and storing formula.

Supplementary vitamin D may be needed in the first 6 months for breastfed infants, and some infants benefit from supplemental fluoride in later infancy.

Most infants don't need solid foods before 4 to 6 months of age; this introduction generally begins with infant cereals. Waiting this long reduces the risk that the infant will develop food allergies.

Nutrient needs in the first 6 months are mostly met by human milk or iron-fortified infant formula.

Growth is very rapid during infancy. An adequate diet, especially in terms of energy, protein, and zinc intake, is very important to support this growth.

Preschoolers should be given some leeway in determining serving size and should be encouraged to try new foods.

A balanced diet is important throughout the life cycle but particularly during the growing years.

A slower growth rate in preschool years underlies the importance of children eating nutrient-dense foods and reducing their food serving sizes.

A good rule of thumb is to serve portion sizes at meals of 1 tablespoon of each food for each year of life.

During the adolescent growth spurt, both boys and girls have increased needs for iron and calcium. Teens and young adults should strive to focus on rich sources of iron and calcium, moderate high-fat food choices, and perform regular physical activity.

Obese children and adolescents are more likely to become obese adults and so incur greater health risks. When controlled early, a problem of obesity may correct itself as the child grows in height.

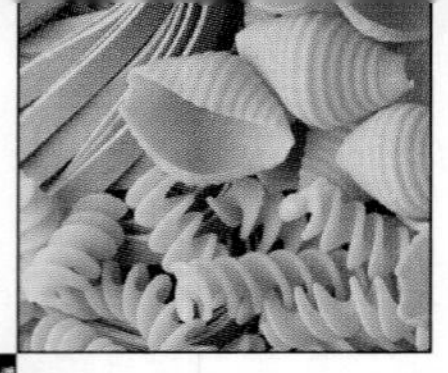

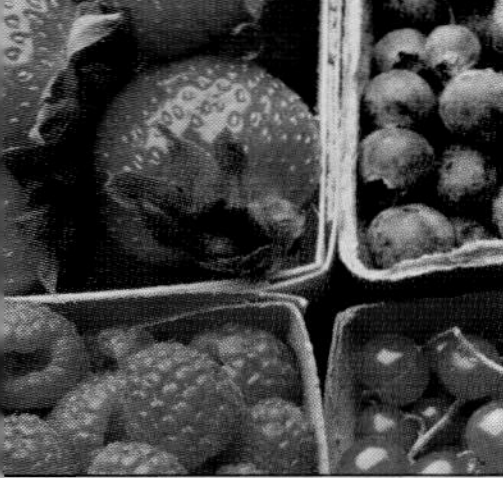

Infant Growth and Physiological Development

During infancy a child's attitudes toward foods and the whole eating process begin to take shape. If parents and other caregivers practice good nutrition and are flexible, they can lead a child into lifelong healthful food habits. Children then need specific attention focused on them; they need to grow in a stimulating environment, and they need a sense of security. Children hospitalized for growth failure gain weight more quickly when loving care accompanies needed nutrients.

The Growing Infant

All babies seem to do is eat and sleep. There's a good reason for this. An infant's birth weight doubles in the first 4 to 6 months and triples within the first year. Such rapid growth requires a lot of both nourishment and sleep. Beyond the first year, growth is slower, it takes 5 more years to double the weight seen at 1 year. An infant also increases in length in the first year by 50% (Figure 13–1).

The human body needs a lot more food to support growth and development than to merely maintain itself once growth ceases. When nutrients are missing at critical phases of growth and development, growth slows and may even stop. From observations of Egyptian mummies, we see that infants were about the same size in 300 BC as they are today. However, adult mummies are much smaller than adults today. Furthermore, the average height of American men in 1700 was approximately 5 feet, 8 inches, while today it is approximately 5 feet, 10 inches. This suggests that people of earlier times generally ate nutrient-poor diets that did not support the growth we typically experience today.

In countries of the developing world today, about half the children are short and underweight for their ages. Poor nutrition—called *undernutrition*—is at the heart of the problem. This occurs to a lesser extent in the United States. In poorer countries, when breastfeeding ceases, children are often fed a high-carbohydrate, low-protein diet. This diet supports some growth but does not allow children to attain their full genetic potential. To grow, children must consume adequate amounts of energy, protein, zinc, and other nutrients.

Children benefit from the love and attention of others.

The Effect of Undernutrition on Growth

As with the fetus in utero, the long-term effects of nutritional problems in infancy and childhood depend on the severity, timing, and duration of the nutritional insult to cell processes.

The single best indicator of a child's nutritional status is gains in height and weight. Mild zinc deficiencies in American children have been linked to poor growth. Improving the diets of these children then leads to improved growth. Overall, eating a poor diet as an infant or child hampers cell division that occurs at that critical stage. Getting an adequate diet later usually won't compensate for lost growth as the hormonal and other conditions needed for growth will not likely be present, and as well bone size is set by about 20 years of age.

Weight primarily reflects current nutrient intake, whereas height is a measure of long-term nutrient intake.

For these reasons a 22-year-old Central American girl who is 4 feet, 8 inches tall cannot attain the adult height of a typical American woman simply by now eating better. Females experience their peak rate of growth before the onset of the menses. Once the time for growth ceases (in women this is about 2 years after they start menstruating), a sufficient nutrient intake will help maintain health and weight but will not make up for all lost growth.

BOYS: BIRTH TO 36 MONTHS
PHYSICAL GROWTH

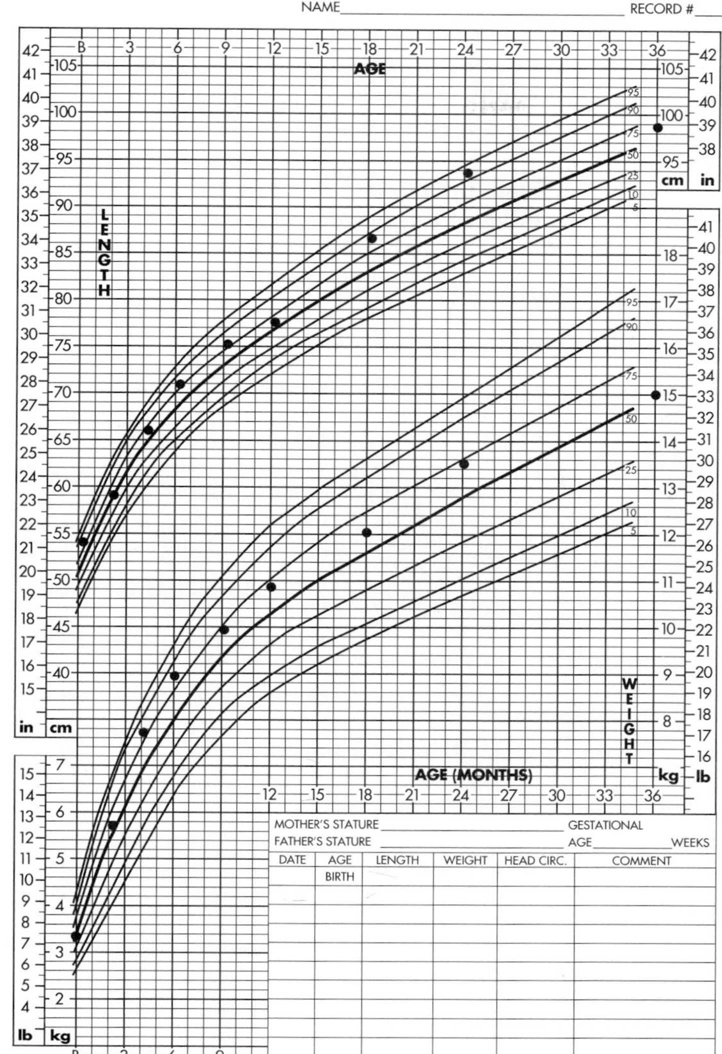

Figure 13–1 *Growth charts used to assess length (height) and weight in young boys. A certain weight and length (height) correspond to a percentile value, which is a ranking of the person among 100 peers. The growth pattern of Dr. Wardlaw's son is plotted to illustrate how this tool is used in medical practice. The federal government is in the process of revising these growth charts. Body mass index will be used as the new weight-height standard.*

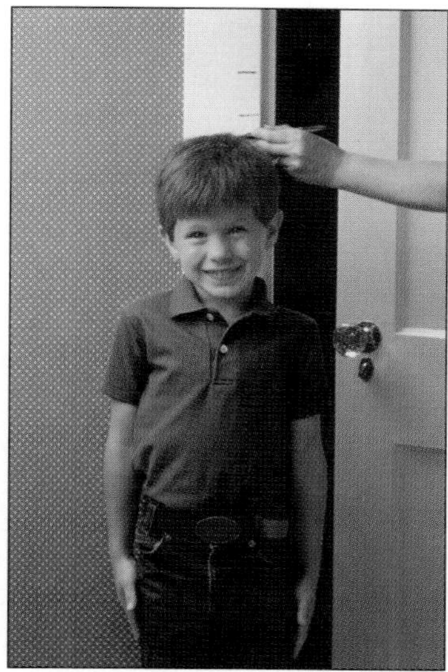

Adequate gains in height are a key marker for nutritional adequacy of a child's diet.

Assessing Infant Growth and Development

Health professionals assess a child's increases in height and weight by comparing them with typical growth patterns recorded on charts. Adequate weight gain in infancy is especially indicative of nutritional health. The current charts contain seven percentile divisions, which represent 90% of children (see Figure 13–1). A percentile represents the rank of the person among 100 peers matched for age and gender. Tony, for example, is at the 90th percentile height for age, meaning that of 100 boys of that age, he is shorter than 10 and taller than 89. A child at the 50th percentile is considered average. Fifty children will be taller than this child; 49 will be shorter. It is important to note that these charts were based primarily on observations of formula-fed infants. Breastfed infants may lag behind these typical patterns but eventually catch up in terms of height.

Children under 2 to 3 years of age are measured with knees unflexed and while lying on their backs, so the term *length* is used rather than *height*.

Height-for-age, weight-for-age, and weight-for-height can be plotted on these charts. Infants and children should have their growth assessed during regular health checkups. Once a pattern is established in infancy and early childhood, such as length (height) for age, the child's measurement should then track along that percentile. If the child's growth doesn't keep up with its various percentile indicators, the physician needs to investigate whether a medical or nutritional problem is impeding the predicted growth.

Infants born preterm may catch up in growth in 2 to 3 years. This requires that the child jump up in the percentiles. If this occurs—especially in length-for-age—it is usually no cause for alarm. On the other hand, jumping percentiles in weight-for-height can be disturbing if the child approaches the 80th to 90th percentiles. Generally a child at the 85th percentile for weight-for-height is considered overweight. Above the 95th percentile, the child is considered obese.

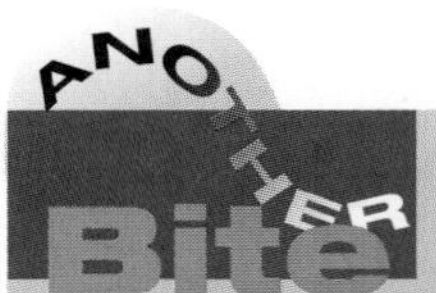

The brain grows faster in infancy than at any other time of life. To accommodate the growth, an infant's head must be very large in proportion to the rest of the body. The rapid growth stops at about 18 months of age. In early physical checkups, a health professional usually measures the head circumference as another means of assessing growth, especially brain growth. How nutritional status affects brain development and intelligence quotient (IQ) is not well understood. We suspect iron deficiency impairs this development. However, studies from Central America suggest that IQ after age 5 years relates more closely to the amount of schooling a child receives than to nutritional intake during childhood.

Adipose (Fat) Tissue Growth

Since 1970 researchers have speculated that overfeeding during infancy may increase adipose (fat) tissue cell numbers. Today we know that adipose cells can also increase as adulthood obesity develops (see Chapter 9). Still, if energy intake is limited during infancy to keep down the number of adipose cells, the growth of other organ systems particularly the brain and related nervous tissue, may also be severely retarded. In addition, most obese infants become normal-weight preschoolers without excessive diet restrictions. For these reasons, it's unwise to restrict diet, and especially fat intake, before 2 years of age. About 40% of energy intake from fat is recommended until that age.

Failure to Thrive

Occasionally an infant doesn't grow much in the first few months. Physical problems that may contribute to retarded growth typically range from poor oral cavity development, infections, and heart irregularities to constant diarrhea associated with intestinal problems. However, more than half the infants who fail to thrive have no apparent disease. Instead the usual cause is poor infant-parent interaction. This stems from misinformation, lack of a parent role model, or apathy about the child's welfare. In general, the problems often arise from the parents' inexperience, rather than intentional negligence.

Infants not only need cuddling; they also respond to voices and eye contact, especially at feeding times. New parents need to appreciate the importance of these practices to their infant's well-being. Some parents also may be over-committed to maintaining a lean child in the hope of preventing future obesity, as discussed in Chapter 11. The result, even though the intention was good, can be failure to thrive.

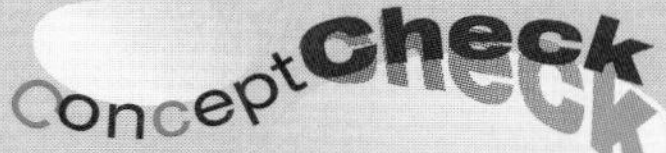

Growth occurs rapidly during infancy: Birth weight doubles in about 4 to 6 months and triples within the first year. Undernutrition in childhood can irreversibly inhibit growth and maturation so that an individual never attains his or her full genetic potential. Infant and child growth is assessed by tracking body weight, length (height), and head circumference over time. It is not desirable for infants to become obese, although no evidence strongly indicates that obese infants become obese adults. However, severe restriction of energy intake is not recommended for infants because it may slow the growth of organ systems. When infants do not grow properly, their failure to thrive may stem from physical disorders or inadequate care, including inappropriate feeding practices.

Infant Nutritional Needs

Infants' nutritional needs vary as they grow, and these differ from adult needs in both amount and proportion. Initially, human milk or commercial iron-fortified infant formula (generally using heat-treated cow's milk as a base) supplies needed nutrients. Solid foods generally are not needed until after 4 to 6 months. Even after solid foods are added, the basis of an infant's diet for the first year is still human milk or commercial infant formula. Because of the critical importance of adequate nutrition in infancy and the difficulties encountered in feeding some infants, more time is spent in this chapter on this development period than on the later periods of childhood.

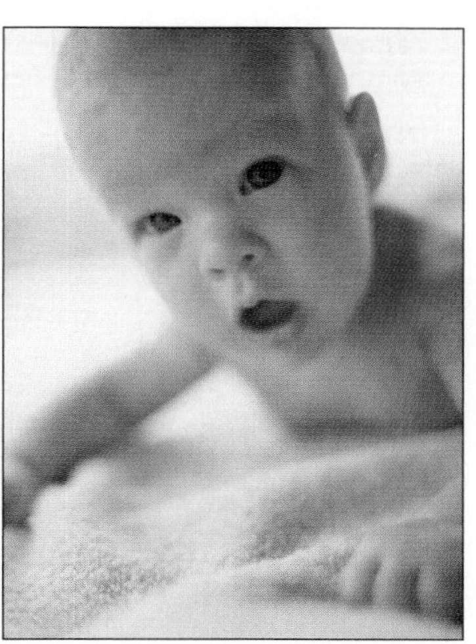

In early infancy nutrient needs are met primarily by human milk or infant formula.

Energy

Infants need about 45 to 50 kcal per pound of body weight daily (98 to 108 kcal per kilogram) to supply them with adequate energy. At 6 months of age this amounts to about 700 kcal daily. Either human milk or commercial infant formula is ideal for the first few months, as both are high in fat and energy content. These supply about 650 kcal per quart of fluid (about 700 kcal per liter; Table 13–1). Later, human milk or infant formula, supplemented by solid foods, can provide even more energy.

The infant's high energy needs are primarily driven by its rapid growth and high metabolic rate. The high metabolic rate is caused in part by the ratio of the infant's body surface to its weight. More body surface allows more heat loss from the skin; the body must use extra energy to replace that heat.

Protein

Daily protein needs vary in infancy from 0.7 to 1 gram of protein for each pound of body weight (1.6 to 2.2 gram per kilogram). The lower amount refers to after 6 months of age. About half of total protein intake should come from essential (indispensable) amino acids. Both goals are satisfied by either human milk or infant formula. Total protein intake should not exceed 20% of energy needs. Excess

Allergy
A hypersensitive immune response that occurs when immune bodies produced by us react with a protein we sense as "foreign" (an antigen).

TABLE 13-1

Composition of Human and Cow's Milk and Infant Formulas (per liter)

Milk or formula	Energy (kcal per liter)	Protein (grams per liter)	Fat (grams per liter)	Carbohydrate (grams per liter)	Minerals* (grams per liter)
MILK					
Human milk	750	11	45	70	2
Cow's milk, whole	670	36	36	49	7
Cow's milk, skim	360	36	1	51	7
CASEIN/WHEY-BASED FORMULAS					
Similac	680	14	36	71	3
Enfamil	670	15	37	69	3
Carnation	670	16	34	73	3
SOYBEAN PROTEIN-BASED FORMULAS					
ProSobee	670	20	35	67	4
Isomil	680	16	36	68	4
PREDIGESTED PROTEIN					
Nutramigen	670	19	26	89	1
Alimentum	680	18	37	68	1
TRANSITION FORMULAS/BEVERAGES†					
Similac Toddler's Best	670	25	33	75	3
Enfamil Next Step	670	17	33	74	3
Carnation Follow-Up	670	17	27	88	3

*Calcium, phosphorus, and other minerals.
†For use after 6 months of age or later (see label).

nitrogen and minerals supplied by high-protein diets would exceed the ability of an infant's kidneys to excrete the resulting metabolic waste products.

In the United States, infant protein deficiency is unlikely, except in cases of mistaken feeding practices, such as when an infant's formula is excessively watered down. Protein deficiency may also be induced by elimination diets used to detect food **allergies** (see the Nutrition Issue at the end of the chapter).

Fat

As already mentioned, infants and children up to 2 years of age should get about 40% of their energy from fat. More than 50% may lead to poor fat digestion. About half the energy supplied by both human milk and infant formula comes from fat. Essential fatty acids should make up at least 3% of total energy. Fats are an important part of the infant's diet because they are energy-dense and vital to the development of the nervous system.

Vitamins of Special Interest

Vitamin K is routinely given by injection to all infants at birth. This dose lasts until the infant's intestinal bacteria are established and begin to synthesize vitamin K. Formula-fed infants receive the rest of the vitamins they need from the formula. Breastfed infants, especially dark-skinned ones, may require a vitamin D supplement if they are not exposed to much sunlight. (Sunlight exposure on human skin activates synthesis of vitamin D; see Chapter 7.) Breastfed infants whose mothers are total vegetarians (vegans) should receive a vitamin B-12 supplement.

Minerals of Special Interest

The iron stores with which children are born are generally depleted by the time birth weight doubles, in 4 to 6 months. The American Academy of Pediatrics recommends that to maintain a desirable iron status, formula-fed infants should be given a commercial iron-fortified formula from birth. Breastfed infants need solid foods to supply extra iron by about 6 months of age. The need for iron is a major consideration in deciding when to introduce solid foods. Some physicians recommend liquid iron supplements from birth or by 1 month of age for breastfed infants. As mentioned, iron deficiency anemia may lead to poor mental development in infants.

Infants need adequate amounts of zinc and iodide to support growth. Human milk and infant formula adequately supply these needs when they supply enough energy to meet needs. In addition, clinicians recommend fluoride supplements to aid tooth development for breastfed infants after 6 months of age. The same holds true for formula-fed infants if the water supply used in home formula preparation—either tap or bottled water—doesn't contain fluoride.

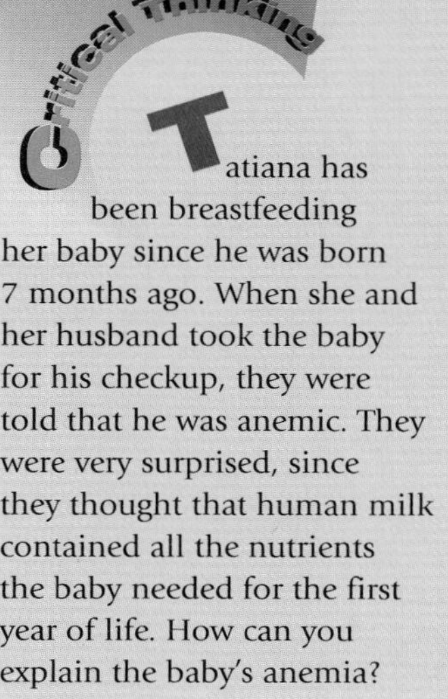

Tatiana has been breastfeeding her baby since he was born 7 months ago. When she and her husband took the baby for his checkup, they were told that he was anemic. They were very surprised, since they thought that human milk contained all the nutrients the baby needed for the first year of life. How can you explain the baby's anemia?

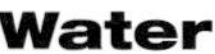

Water

An infant needs about 2 ounces of water and other fluids combined per pound of body weight (about 150 milliliters per kilogram). Infants typically consume enough human milk or formula to supply this amount. However, any conditions that lead to excess water loss—diarrhea, vomiting, fever, hot weather and too much sun—can call for supplemental water.

Infants are easily dehydrated, a condition that has serious effects if not quickly remedied. Dehydration can result in rapidly decreasing kidney function, and the infant may then require hospitalization for rehydration. Special fluid replacement formulas are available to treat dehydration. A physician should guide any use of these products. It is important to remember that excessive fluid can also be harmful, especially to the brain. Overall, it is best to limit supplemental fluids to about 4 ounces (120 milliliters) per day, unless the physician thinks that a greater need exists because of disease or other conditions.

Note that in some grocery stores, bottled water products marketed specifically for infants may be placed alongside infant formulas and electrolyte replacement solutions. This placement may give parents and caregivers the mistaken impression that bottled water products are an appropriate feeding supplement or substitute for infants; they are not and should not be used for such purposes.

ConceptCheck

Most nutrient needs during the first 6 months are met by human milk or infant formula. Breastfed infants may need vitamin D and iron supplements, and formula-fed infants and breastfed infants may need iron if the formula is low in this mineral. Fluoride supplements may be needed by both breastfed and formula-fed infants after 6 months of age. Infants usually receive enough water from the human milk or formula they drink.

Formula Feeding for Infants

Breastfeeding was covered in detail in Chapter 12. Let's now focus on formula feeding. You'll recall that a major advantage of breastfeeding is provision of immune protection to the infant. Another advantage of breastfeeding is the supply of very long-chain fatty acids (those typically found in fish). These fatty acids are found in high concentrations in the eye and brain. Some research suggests that formula-fed infants are at a disadvantage as these fatty acids are not added at this time to commercial formulas. Currently formula manufacturers are studying the safety and importance of doing so. Possible improvements in visual functions and cognitive development are two major effects being studied. Overall, in areas of the world where high standards for water purity and cleanliness are common, formula feeding is a safe alternative for infants, but may not be as beneficial as breastfeeding.

Formula Composition

Casein
Proteins found in milk that form curds when exposed to acid and are difficult for infants to digest.

Whey
Proteins, such as lactalbumin, that are found in great amounts in human milk and are easy to digest.

Standard infant formulas generally contain lactose and/or sucrose for carbohydrate, heat-treated **casein** and **whey** proteins from cow's milk, and vegetable oils for fat (see Table 13–1). Soy protein–based formulas are available for infants who can't tolerate the carbohydrate lactose or the types of proteins found in cow's milk. If the soybean-based formula is not tolerated, the next step is to try a formula that has been treated to partially digest the proteins, such as Nutramigen or Alimentum. A variety of other specialized formulas also are available for specific medical conditions.

Cow's milk as such is not appropriate for infant feeding because of its high protein and mineral content. Cow's milk reflects the greater growth needs of calves. Thus cow's milk must be altered to be safe for infant feeding. Goat's milk, sweetened condensed milk, and evaporated milk as such also are inappropriate for infant feeding.

Some new transition formulas/beverages recently have been introduced for older infants and toddlers (see Table 13–1). Some of these products are intended for use after 6 months of age if the infant is consuming solid foods, whereas others are intended for use only by toddlers. These transition products are lower in fat than human milk or standard infant formulas; their iron content is higher than that of cow's milk, and their overall mineral content is generally more like that of human milk than cow's milk. According to the manufacturers, the advantages of these transition formulas/beverages over standard formulas for older infants and toddlers include reduced cost and better flavor. Parents should consult a physician with regard to use of these products, which to date have seen little use.

Preparation of Formula

Note that not all formula-like products are designed for infant use. A 5-month-old female was admitted to a hospital in Arkansas with symptoms of heart failure, rickets, inflamed blood vessels, and possible nerve damage after being fed Soy Moo (a soy beverage sold in health stores) since 3 days of age. Parents must consult a physician for advice regarding appropriate infant formulas.

Today bottles of formula typically are prepared one at a time using a powdered or concentrated product. Some infant formulas even come in ready-to-feed form. These are poured into a clean bottle and fed immediately.

All utensils used in preparing formula from these preparations should be washed and thoroughly rinsed. Powdered or concentrated formulas are poured into a bottle to which clean, cold water is added (following label directions) and then mixed. The formula is then warmed, if desired, and fed immediately to the infant. Hot water from the faucet should not be used to make formula, since it poses a risk for high lead content (see Chapter 15). Cold water poses much less risk.

Refrigerating diluted formula for 1 day is safe. However, formula left over from a feeding should be discarded because it will be contaminated by bacteria and enzymes in the infant's saliva. If well water is used, it should be boiled before making formula for at least the infant's first 3 months of life, and also be analyzed for excessive concentration of naturally occurring nitrates, which can lead to a severe form of anemia. Boiling and then cooling tap water is also advised by some groups, based on recent evidence that even municipal water may contain microbes that can harm the vulnerable, such as infants (see Chapter 15).

Feeding Technique

Because infants swallow a lot of air along with either formula or human milk, it's important to burp an infant after either 10 minutes of feeding or 1 to 2 ounces (30 to 60 milliliters) from a bottle, and again at the end of feeding. Spitting up a bit of milk is normal at this time. Once fed, infants generally should be placed on their backs. If an infant tends to spit up a lot after feeding, the physician may recommend placement on one side. In this case the caregiver would need to place a rolled-up blanket or foam wedge on each side of the infant in order to support that position. In no case should an infant be placed face down unless a physician recommends otherwise; this is a major risk factor for the development of sudden infant death syndrome (SIDS). Placement on the back is the most protective against SIDS with regard to the two positions recommended.

A study of SIDS in Sweden showed increased risk with low maternal age, multiparity, maternal smoking, and male infants. Smoking appears to be the greatest risk factor. Other risk factors may include soft mattresses and loose blankets, and an irregular heartbeat.

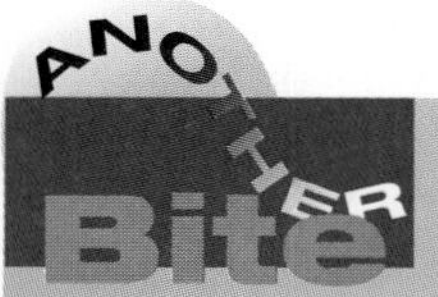

When the infant begins acting full, bottle feeding should be stopped, even if some milk is left in the bottle. Common cues that signal that an infant has had enough formula (or solid as well in later infancy) include turning the head away, inattention, falling asleep, and becoming playful. Generally the infant's appetite is a better guide than standardized recommendations concerning feeding amounts.

Development of Feeding Skills in the Older Infant

By 6 to 7 months the infant has learned to grab and transfer objects from one hand to the other. At about this time teeth begin to appear, and the infant begins to handle finger foods with some dexterity. Dry toast, sliced in strips, offers hours of enjoyment.

By age 7 to 8 months, infants can push food around on a plate and play with a drinking cup, can hold a bottle and self-feed a cracker or piece of toast. In mastering these manipulations, infants develop self-confidence and self-esteem. It's important that parents be patient and support these early feeding attempts, even though they appear inefficient.

At around 10 months of age, infants practice in earnest self-feeding finger foods and drinking from a cup. Feeding time is often very messy. Food is used as a means to explore the environment. By the first birthday, their bodies have developed sufficiently to accommodate crawling, probably walking, and self-feeding. Although attempts at feeding are still erratic, developing children take great pride in doing more things independently. As children drink from a cup more frequently, fewer bottle feedings and/or breastfeedings are necessary. The added mobility of walking should naturally lead to gradual weaning from the bottle or breast.

To ease efforts in feeding solid foods, at this stage of development consider the following tips:

- Use a baby-sized spoon; a small spoon with a long handle is best.
- Hold the infant comfortably on the lap, as for breastfeeding or bottle feeding, but a little more upright to ease swallowing. When in this position, the infant expects food.

Nutrition Insight

Dietary Guidelines for Infant Feeding

In response to various controversies surrounding infant feeding, the American Academy of Pediatrics has issued a number of statements concerning infant diets. The following guidelines are based on these statements:

- **Build to a variety of foods.**
  For the first months of life, human milk is all an infant needs. When the infant is ready, start adding new foods one at a time. During the first year, the goal is to teach an infant to enjoy a variety of nutritious foods. A lifetime of healthy eating habits begins with this important first step.

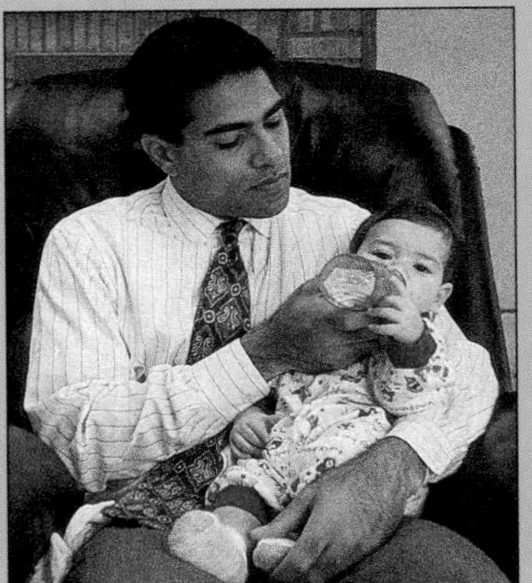

Careful attention during feeding allows the caregiver to pick up on the infant's signal as to when the feeding should cease.

- **Pay attention to your infant's appetite to avoid overfeeding or underfeeding.**
  Feed infants when hungry. Never force an infant to finish an unwanted serving of food. Watch for signs that indicate hunger or fullness.
- **Infants need fat.**
  Although fat is the cause of many adult health problems, it's an essential source of energy for growing infants. Fat also helps the brain and nervous system develop.
- **Choose fruits, vegetables, and grains, but don't overdo high-fiber foods.**
  Although many adults benefit from higher-fiber diets, they are not good for infants. They are bulky, filling, and often low in energy. The natural amounts of fiber and nutrients in fruits, vegetables, and grains are appropriate as part of a healthy infant diet.
- **Infants need sugars in moderation.**
  Sugars are an additional source of energy for active, rapidly growing infants. Foods such as human milk, fruits, and juices are natural sources of sugars and other nutrients as well. Foods that contain artificial sweeteners should be avoided; they don't provide the energy growing infants need.
- **Infants need sodium in moderation.**
  Sodium is a necessary mineral found naturally in almost all foods. As part of a healthy diet, infants need sodium for their bodies to work properly.
- **Choose foods containing iron, zinc, and calcium.**
  Infants need good sources of iron, zinc, and calcium for optimum growth in the first 2 years. These minerals are important for healthy blood, proper growth, and strong bones.

The recommendations in this chapter are consistent with these guidelines. In essence, there is no evidence that very restrictive diets during infancy have positive effects, whereas their hazards are well documented.

- Put a small dab of food on the spoon tip and gently place it on the infant's tongue.
- Convey a calm and casual approach to the infant, who needs time to get used to food.
- Expect the infant to take only two or three bites of the first meals. Anything more than that is real success.

By the end of the first year, finger-feeding becomes more efficient, drinking from a cup improves, and chewing is easier as more teeth erupt. Foods in the diet begin to resemble a Food Guide Pyramid pattern (Table 13–2). Still, experimentation and unpredictability are to be expected.

TABLE 13-2

Sample Daily Menu for a 1-Year-Old Child*

BREAKFAST

Applesauce, 1–2 tbsp
Cheerios, ¼ cup
Whole milk, ½ cup

SNACK

Hard-cooked egg, ½
Wheat toast, ½ slice with ½ tsp margarine
Orange juice, ½ cup

LUNCH

Roasted chicken (minced), 1 oz
Rice, 1–2 tbsp with ½ tsp margarine
Cooked peas, 1–2 tbsp
Whole milk, ½ cup

SNACK

Cheese, ½ oz
Wheat crackers, 4
Whole milk, ½ cup

DINNER

Hamburger (crumbled), 1 oz
Mashed potatoes, 1–2 tbsp with ½ tsp margarine
Cooked carrots, 1–2 tbsp (cut in strips, NOT coins)
Whole milk, ½ cup

SNACK

Banana, ½
Oatmeal cookies, 2 (no raisins)
Whole milk, ½ cup

Nutritional analysis

Total energy (kcal)	1100
% energy from:	
Carbohydrate	40%
Protein	19%
Fat	41%

*This diet plan is just a start. A 1-year-old may need more or less food. In those cases, serving sizes should be adjusted. The milk can be fed by cup; some can be put into a bottle if the child has not been fully weaned from the bottle. The juice should be fed in a cup.

Introducing Solid Foods

The time to introduce solid foods into an infant's diet hinges on a few important factors:

Nutritional need—Calorie needs increase as the infant ages. Solid foods help meet that need especially in the second 6 months of life. As well, iron stores are exhausted by about 6 months of age. Either solid foods or iron supplements are then needed to supply iron if the child is breastfed or fed a formula not supplemented with iron. Iron, however, is not the only nutrient missing from human milk and unfortified infant formulas. Vitamin D and fluoride (the latter after 6 months of age) may also deserve attention. Still, before 4 to 6 months, it's unnecessary to add solid foods.

Physiological capabilities—Infants cannot readily digest starch before 3 months. As they age, their digestive capabilities increase. Kidney function likewise is quite limited until about 4 to 6 weeks of age. Until then, waste products from high amounts of dietary protein or minerals are difficult to excrete.

Physical ability—Three markers indicate that a child is ready for solid foods: (1) the disappearance of the extrusion reflex (thrusting the tongue forward and pushing food out), (2) head and neck control, and (3) the ability to sit up with support. These usually occur around 4 to 6 months of age, but they vary with each infant.

Preventing allergies—An infant's intestinal tract can readily absorb whole proteins from birth until 4 to 5 months of age. Thus early exposure to many types of proteins—particularly proteins in cow's milk and egg whites—may predispose a child to future allergies and other health problems, because some types of these proteins may be absorbed intact. For this reason, it's best to minimize the number of different types of proteins in a child's diet, especially during the first 3 months.

With these considerations in mind, the American Academy of Pediatrics recommends that solid foods not be introduced until 4 to 6 months of age, and that infants receive no cow's milk as such before 1 year.

In general, a child starting solid foods should weigh at least 13 pounds (6 kilograms) and should be drinking more than 32 ounces (1 liter) of formula daily or breastfeeding more than 8 to 10 times within 24 hours. This description generally applies to 6-month-old infants and to some 4-month-old infants.

Parents may believe that the early addition of solid foods will help the infant sleep through the night. This achievement is a developmental milestone; the amount of food consumed by the infant is irrelevant.

Before 4 to 6 months, infants are not physically mature enough to consume much solid food. Attempts to push down solid foods have sometimes led to force-feeding with a feeder (a giant syringe) or mixing infant cereal with milk and putting it in a bottle. Even if these are traditional alternatives in your family, there is no reason to carry on these practices. The inconvenience alone should make one consider whether all the effort is worth it. This practice is unnecessary nutritionally, tedious, and possibly dangerous for the infant because it increases the risk of allergies and choking or inhaling food when crying. Even so, many children are already eating solids before 4 months of age. Only occasionally does a rapidly growing infant—one who consumes more than 32 ounces (1 liter) of formula daily—need solid foods at 4 months to meet high energy needs. And if so, these are to be fed by spoon, not by mixing with formula and feeding with a bottle.

Which Solid Foods Should Be Fed First?

Before 6 months of age the first solid foods should be iron-fortified cereals (single protein source like rice, not mixed protein sources). A good idea is to offer foods after some breastfeeding or formula feeding, when the edge has been taken off the infant's hunger. This practice aids in early spoon-feeding. Rice cereal is the best cereal to begin with because it's least likely to cause allergies. (Figure 13–2). After the age of 6 months the first food is not such an important issue. Some pediatricians may recommend lean ground (strained) meats for more absorbable forms of iron. After a week of feeding and the infant shows no problems, another type of cereal or perhaps a cooked and strained (blended) vegetable, meat, fruit, or egg yolk can then be added. It is best to add vegetables before fruits. If fruits are offered first, the infant will prefer the sweet taste and likely resist vegetables. Each feeding step builds on the last. Although yogurt and cottage cheese are also well tolerated and their consistencies make them good candidates for early foods, they are not good sources of iron.

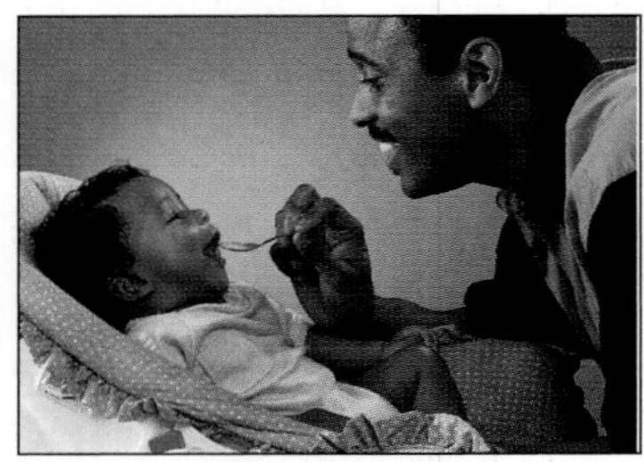

In the early stages of solid food introduction, these foods complement rather than replace human milk or infant formula in the diet.

Waiting about 7 days between new foods is important because it can take that long for evidence of an allergy or intolerance to develop. See the Nutrition Issue for more details about food allergies. It is also important not to introduce mixed foods such as meat with vegetables, until each component of the mixed food has been given separately. Otherwise, if an allergy or intolerance develops, it will be difficult to identify the offending food. Note that many babies outgrow food sensitivities in childhood. A variety of strained foods is available for infant feeding. Single-food items are more desirable than mixed dinners and desserts, which are less nutrient-dense. Most brands have no added salt, but some fruit desserts contain a lot of added sugar.

As an alternative, plain foods from the table—vegetables, fruits, and meats (no seasoning added)—can be ground up in an inexpensive plastic baby food

RICE

CEREAL FOR BABY

Nutrition Facts
Serving Size 1/4 cup (15g)
Servings Per Container About 15

Amount Per Serving	
Calories 60	
Total Fat	0.5mg
Sodium	0mg
Potassium	20mg
Total Carbohydrate	12g
Fiber	0g
Sugars	0g
Protein	1g

% Daily Value	Infants 0–1	Children 1–4
Protein	4%	4%
Vitamin A	0%	0%
Vitamin C	0%	0%
Calcium	15%	10%
Iron	45%	60%
Thiamin	45%	30%
Riboflavin	45%	30%
Niacin	25%	20%
Phosphorus	10%	6%

INGREDIENTS: RICE FLOUR, SOY OIL-LECITHIN, TRI- AND DICALCIUM PHOSPHATE, ELECTROLYTIC IRON, NIACINAMIDE, RIBOFLAVIN (VITAMIN B-2), THIAMIN (VITAMIN B-1).

Serving size

Serving sizes for infant foods are based on the average amount eaten at one time by a child under 2 years.

Total fat

Shows the amount of total fat in a serving of the food. Unlike labels on adult foods, labels on infant foods do not list calories from fat, saturated fat, or cholesterol. Since infants and toddlers under 2 years need fat, the labels do not include details on fat content. Parents should not attempt to limit their infant's fat intake.

Daily Values

Food labels for infants and children under 4 years list the Daily Value percentages for protein, vitamins, and minerals. Unlike labels on adult foods, Daily Values for fat, cholesterol, sodium, potassium, carbohydrate, and fiber are not listed because these values have not been set for children under 4 years.

Figure 13–2 *The labels on infant foods, like those on adult foods, contain a Nutrition Facts panel. However, the information provided on infant food labels differs from that on adult food labels, especially with respect to saturated fat and cholesterol intake (see Figure 2–2 for a comparison).*

Typical solid food progression starting at 4 to 6 months*

Week 1	**Rice cereal**
Week 2	**Add strained carrots**
Week 3	**Add applesauce**
Week 4	**Add oat cereal**
Week 5	**Add cooked egg yolk**
Week 6	**Add strained chicken**
Week 7	**Add strained peas**
Week 8	**Add plums**

***Extending the rice cereal step for a month or so is advised if solid food introduction begins at 4 months of age. Note also that at any point signs of allergy or intolerance develop, substitute another similar food item.**

grinder/mill. Another option is to pureé a larger amount of food in a blender, freeze it in ice-cube portions, store in plastic bags, and defrost and warm as needed. Careful attention to cleanliness is necessary. Infant foods made at home should be ground before seasonings are added to please the rest of the family. The infant doesn't notice the difference if salt, sugar, or spices are omitted. It's best to introduce infants to a variety of foods, so that by the end of the first year the infant is consuming many foods—milk, meats, fruits, vegetables, and grains.

As early as possible, by about 8 months or so, juices and infant formula should be offered in a cup. Drinking from a cup helps prevent nursing bottle syndrome. As an infant plays with a bottle, the carbohydrate-rich fluid bathes the teeth, providing an ideal growth medium for bacteria. Bacteria on the teeth then make acids that dissolve tooth enamel. Infants should never be put to bed with a bottle or placed in an infant seat with a bottle propped up. When children are allowed to do this, fluid

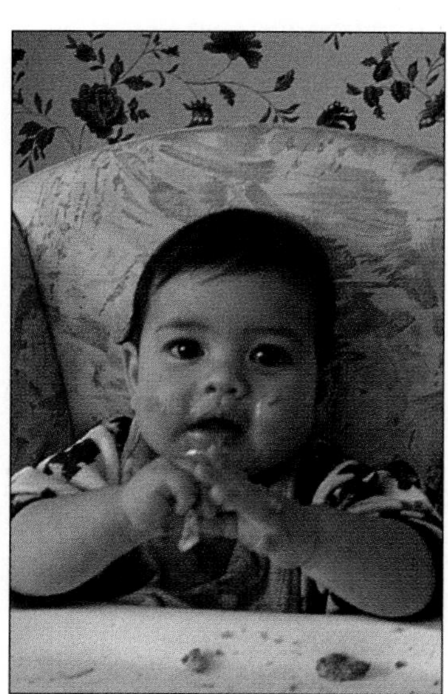

Early feeding attempts should be encouraged, even though they're messy.

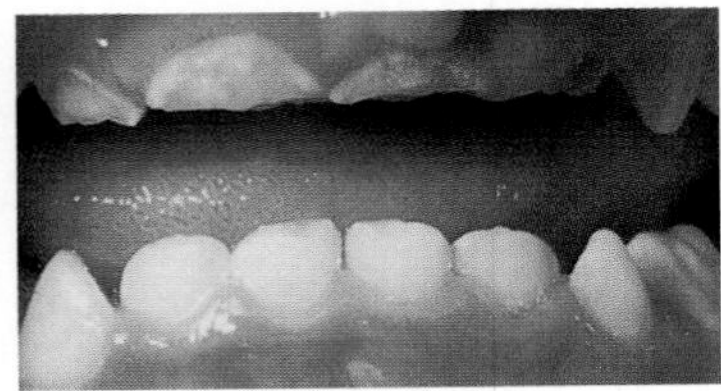

Figure 13–3 *Nursing bottle syndrome. An extreme example of tooth decay caused by nursing-bottle syndrome. This child was probably often put to bed with a bottle. The upper teeth have decayed almost all the way to the gum line.*

(even milk) pools around the teeth, increasing the likelihood of dental caries (Figure 13–3). Again, infants need careful attention when being fed. Propping bottles does not constitute careful attention.

What Not to Feed an Infant

Following are several foods and practices to avoid when feeding an infant:

- *Honey and corn syrup*—These products may contain *Clostridium botulinum*. This can lead to botulism, which can be fatal in children under 1 year old (see Chapter 15).
- *Very salty and very sweet foods*—Infants don't need a lot of sugar or salt added to their foods. They enjoy bland foods much more than do adults.
- *Excessive infant formula or human milk*—After 6 months, solid foods should play a greater role in satisfying an infant's increasing appetite, as they contain considerably more iron than do human milk, cow's milk, and low-iron formulas. About 24 to 32 ounces (¾ to 1 liter) of human milk or formula daily is ideal after 6 months, with food supplying the rest of the infant's energy needs.
- *Foods that tend to cause choking*—These foods include hot dogs (unless finely cut into sticks, not coin shapes), candy, whole nuts, grapes, coarsely cut meats, raw carrots, popcorn, and peanut butter. Caregivers should not allow younger children to gobble snack foods during playtime and should supervise all meals.
- *Cow's milk, especially low-fat or nonfat cow's milk*—Beyond 2 years, children can drink 1% or 2% milk, because by then they are consuming enough solid foods to supply energy and fat needs.
- *Foods that tend to cause allergies*—egg whites, chocolate, nuts, and cow's milk.
- *Feeding excessive amounts of apple or pear juice*—The fructose and sorbitol contained in these juices can lead to diarrhea, because they are slowly absorbed. Also, if fruit juice or related drink products are replacing formula or milk in the diet, the infant may not be receiving adequate amounts of calcium and other minerals that are essential for bone growth. In fact, studies have shown a link between excessive amounts of fruit juice and diminished weight and/or height in some children, and obesity in others. Thus these products should be used sparingly. Infants can usually safely consume 4 to 8 ounces of juice in the course of a day, with no more than 2 to 4 ounces given at a time. Diluting juices with an equal part of water is a good idea, but it should be begun early, before the infant becomes accustomed to full-strength juices.

A summary of infant feeding recommendations:

Breastfed infants

- **Breastfeed for 6 months or longer if possible. Then introduce infant formula if and when breastfeeding declines or ceases.**
- **Add iron-fortified cereal at about 4 to 6 months of age.**
- **Investigate the need for fluoride, iron, and vitamin D supplements.**
- **Provide a variety of basic, soft foods after 6 months of age, advancing to a varied diet.**

Formula-fed infants

- **Use infant formula for the first year of life, preferably an iron-fortified type.**
- **Add iron-fortified cereal at about 4 to 6 months of age.**
- **Investigate the need for a fluoride supplement if the water supply is not fluoridated.**
- **Provide a variety of basic, soft foods after 6 months, advancing to a varied diet.**

ConceptCheck

Infant formulas generally contain lactose or sucrose, heat-treated proteins from cow's milk, and vegetable oil. Formulas may or may not be fortified with iron. Sanitation is very important in preparing and storing formula. Solid foods should not be added to an infant's diet until the child is both ready for and needs solid food, usually not before 4 to 6 months of age. The first solid food can be iron-fortified infant cereals, with very gradual; additions of other foods—one at a time each week. Some foods to avoid giving infants in the first year are honey, corn syrup, cow's milk (particularly low-fat and nonfat milk), egg whites, nuts, chocolate, very salty or sweet foods, foods that may cause the child to choke (eg candy, whole nuts, popcorn), and excessive amounts of fruit juice or related products.

Health Problems Related to Infant Nutrition

Parents, other caregivers, and clinicians should be alert for a variety of potential health problems related to infant nutrition so corrective action can be taken quickly. In some cases such problems stem from inappropriate feeding practices and inadequate nutrient intakes, including the following:

- Diet providing insufficient iron
- Absence from the diet of an entire food group of the Food Guide Pyramid as solid foods are introduced and become the main source of nutrients
- Drinking raw (unpasteurized) milk, which may be contaminated with bacteria or viruses
- Drinking goat's milk in later infancy, which is low in folate, iron, vitamin C, and vitamin D; if used, it must be pasteurized and given in conjunction with a balanced nutrient supplement
- Failure to begin drinking from a cup by 1 year of age
- Continuing to feed from a bottle past 18 months of age
- Intake of supplemental vitamins or minerals above 100% of the appropriate RDA or other standard
- Drinking much fruit juice before 6 months of age as a substitute for commercial infant formula or human milk

Now let's look more closely at four common infant health problems that cause concern for caregivers. Parents and other caregivers usually need to consult with a physician in dealing with these conditions. The web site of the American Academy of Pediatrics (http://www.aap.org) and that of the American Medical Association called KidsHealth (http://www.ama-assn.org/insight/h_focus/nemours/index.htm), are two other resources.

Colic

Repeated crying episodes lasting 3 or more hours that don't respond to typical remedies—such as feeding, holding, or diaper changes—are characteristic of infants who develop **colic.** Colic affects 10% to 30% of all infants, so it is neither uncommon nor abnormal. Colicky infants typically cry during the late afternoon and early evening, and their nighttime sleeping is almost always disturbed by crying spells. In addition, these infants frequently pass gas rectally, clench their fists, draw up their legs, hold the body straight, and want to be held. The only good news is that colic usually goes away after a few months.

Colic
Sharp abdominal pain that generally occurs in otherwise healthy infants and is associated with periodic inconsolable crying spells.

Parents can do several things to help reduce excessive crying. For instance, many infants tend to become quiet and alert when held snugly to the shoulder. Parents should also check to see whether the infant is tired or bored or wants to suckle. Some infants can be calmed by rhythmic sounds or movement, or with pacifiers.

Breastfeeding of colicky infants should continue. A temporary decrease or cessation in consumption of dairy products, caffeine, chocolate, and vegetables such as broccoli and onions by a breastfeeding mother may help reduce colic in her infant. Formula-fed infants with severe colic are sometimes helped by changing from a standard formula to a soy-based or predigested protein formula (see Table 13–1). In addition, physicians may prescribe certain medications to calm colicky infants and reduce gas buildup.

Diarrhea

Diarrhea in infants, characterized by numerous loose stools in a day, results from various causes, including bacterial and viral infections. In the United States, about

500 infants die each year of simple dehydration resulting from diarrhea, and about 210,000 are hospitalized for this reason. For prevention of dehydration, infants with diarrhea should be given plenty of fluids, as advised by a physician. Specialized electrolyte-replacement fluids, such as Pedialyte, may be recommended for very short-term use. These contain glucose, sodium, potassium, chloride, and water.

Once diarrhea subsides, a bottle-fed infant may be switched to a soy-based, lactose-free formula for a few days. This allows time for the intestine to produce sufficient lactase enzyme to digest the large amount of lactose typically found in formulas. A breastfed infant should continue at the breast for the duration of the diarrhea. If solid foods are consumed, the physician may also prescribe a BRAT diet (bananas, rice, applesauce, toast) for short-term use; note this is not a nutritionally adequate diet for long-term use.

Milk Allergy

Cow's milk contains more than 40 proteins that can cause allergic reactions in infants. Although some of these proteins are inactivated by heating (scalding) milk others are very heat stable. A "true" milk allergy develops in about 1% to 3% of formula-fed infants. Such infants may experience vomiting, diarrhea, blood in the stool, constipation, and other symptoms. As mentioned, if milk allergy is suspected, a formula-fed infant can be switched to a soy-based formula. In 20% to 50% of cases, however, use of soy formula provides only temporary relief, because the soy protein eventually triggers an allergic reaction in some infants. In such cases a predigested-protein formula will be necessary (see Table 13–1). If the child is breastfeeding, the mother may experiment with eliminating cow's milk from her diet. Fortunately, such an allergy seldom lasts beyond 3 years of age.

Iron-Deficiency Anemia

Iron-deficiency anemia typically occurs in older infants who consume few solid foods and whose diets are dominated by cow's milk, which contains little iron and causes intestinal bleeding in young infants. Iron stores are then quickly depleted by the daily need to synthesize new red blood cells. The best way to prevent iron-deficiency anemia is to feed an iron-fortified commercial formula beginning at birth if formula is used; to start an infant on iron-fortified cereals and meats at about 4 to 6 months; and to limit formula to 16 to 25 ounces (500 to 750 milliliters) daily at this time. If anemia does develop, medicinal iron is used under a physician's guidance.

Feeding Preterm Infants

Preterm infants are fed either a specially designed formula or human milk. As noted in Chapter 12, nutrients may be added to human milk to increase its protein, mineral, and energy content. Preterm infants must be fed immediately because their bodies store little fat or carbohydrate.

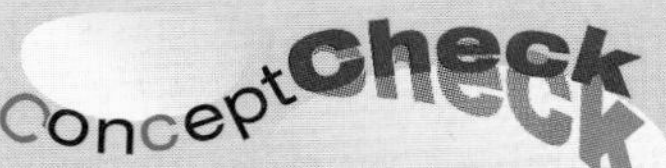

Colic is commonly associated with inconsolable crying. Switching to an infant formula made with soy or predigested proteins may reduce colic. It may also be helpful for breastfeeding mothers to decrease or avoid intake of dairy products, caffeine, chocolate, and certain vegetables, under a physician's guidance. Diarrhea requires additional fluids to prevent dehydration. Infants who can't tolerate the proteins in standard cow's milk formula can be switched to an infant formula containing soy protein or predigested protein. Introducing iron-containing solid foods at an appropriate time and avoiding use of cow's milk as such during the first year can generally prevent iron-deficiency anemia in infants.

Preschool Children

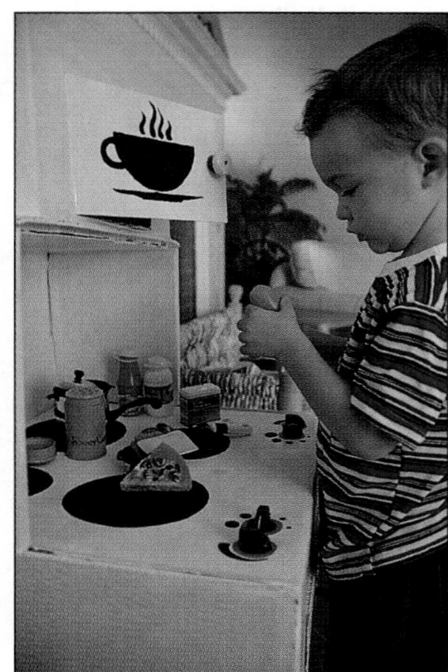

Interest in food starts early in life.

The rapid growth rate that characterized infancy tapers off quickly during the subsequent few years. The average annual weight gain is only 4.5 to 6.6 pounds (2 to 3 kilograms), and the average annual height gain is only 3 to 4 inches (7.5 to 10 centimeters) between the ages of 2 and 5. As a toddler's growth rate tapers off, eating behavior changes. For example, the decreased growth rate leads to a decreased appetite compared with infants.

Because of the reduced appetite of preschool children, choosing nutrient-dense foods is particularly important with children who eat relatively little. This is a good time to emphasize some whole grains, fruits, and vegetables without increasing fat and simple sugar intake. A whole-grain breakfast cereal with limited fat and sugar is an excellent choice. There is no need to decrease fat or simple sugar intake severely, but fatty and sweet food choices should not overwhelm more nutritious ones.

How to Help a Child Choose Nutritious Foods

The preschool years are the best time for a child to start a healthful pattern of living and eating, focusing on regular physical activity and nutritious foods. Parents and other caregivers are role models: if they eat a variety of foods, the children will eat a variety of foods.

One way adults can encourage young children to eat nutritious, well-balanced meals is to serve new foods and repeat exposure to them. If a child observes adults and older children eating and enjoying a food, there's a good chance he or she will eventually accept it. The dinner hour is a good time for children to experience new foods and to develop their own likes and dislikes. Preschool children especially tend to be wary of new foods. One reason is that their taste buds are more sensitive than those of adults. In addition, they have a general distrust of unfamiliar foods.

Children generally like certain foods—especially those with crisp textures and mild flavors—and familiar foods. Young children are especially sensitive to hot-temperature foods and tend to reject them. Preschoolers eventually develop skill with spoons and forks and can even use dull knives (Table 13–3). However, it's still a good idea to serve some finger foods. A goal should be to make mealtime a happy, social time. Share enjoyment of healthful foods. A regular family meal daily—whether breakfast, lunch, or dinner—is an appropriate setting for children to learn about healthful eating and to build good eating habits.

Childhood Feeding Problems

Tensions between parents, or between parents and children, often contribute to eating problems. Getting to the root of family problems and creating a more harmonious family atmosphere are important steps toward resolving many childhood feeding problems. Children like predictable schedules and environments. In addition, parents must often be educated as to what to expect of a preschool child and what food-related goals to set. Let's consider some typical complaints and concerns of parents, the causes of the problems, and suggestions for correcting them.

Two-year-olds commonly prefer particular foods, but parents needn't worry about this. A child may switch from one specific food focus (often called a jag) to another with equal intensity. If the caregiver continues to offer choices, the child will soon begin to eat a wider variety of foods again, and the specific food focus will disappear as suddenly as it appeared.

"My Child Won't Eat as Much or as Regularly as He Did as an Infant."

This behavior is typical of preschoolers, because their growth rate slows after infancy and thus they don't need as much food. Table 13–3 shows a general food plan, based on the Food Guide Pyramid, that is appropriate for preschool and school-age children. Note that until about 5 years of age, serving sizes in the vegetable group, fruit group, and meat, poultry, fish, dry beans, eggs, and nuts group can be

TABLE 13-3

Food Plan for Preschool and School-Age Children Based on the Food Guide Pyramid

Food group	No. of servings	Approximate serving size* Age 1-2	Age 3-4	Age 5-6	Age 7-12
Milk, yogurt, and cheese	3	½–¾ cup or 1 oz	¾ cup or 1½ oz	1 cup or 2 oz	1 cup or 2 oz
Meat, poultry, fish, dry beans, eggs, and nuts	2 or more	1 oz or 1–2 tbsp	1½ oz or 3–4 tbsp	1½ oz or ½ cup	2 oz or ½ cup
Vegetables	3 or more	1–2 tbsp	3–4 tbsp	½ cup	½ cup
Fruit	2 or more	1–2 tbsp or ½ cup juice	3–4tbsp or ½ cup juice	½ cup or ½ cup juice	½ sup or ½ cup juice
Bread, cereal, rice, and pasta	6 or more	½ slice or ½ cup	1 slice or ½ cup	1 slice or ¾ cup	1 slice or ¾ cup

*Use as a starting point. Increase serving size as energy yields dictate, but maintain variety in the diet by making sure all food groups are still appropriately represented.

Adapted from Food and Nutrition Service, US Department of Agriculture: *Meal pattern requirements and offer versus serve manual,* FNS–265, 1990.

estimated as 1 tablespoon per year of life. Normal-weight children have a built-in feeding mechanism that adjusts hunger to regulate food intake at each stage of growth. If a child is developing and growing normally and the caregiver is providing a variety of healthful foods, all can be confident the child isn't starving.

In addition, parents should recognize that this is an important age for children to explore the world around them. Even good eaters are sometimes more interested in exploring than eating. There's room for occasional indulgences, a skipped meal or two, or once-in-a-while "less-than-ideal" choices. It's eating and lifestyle habits over the course of a month and lifetime that matter.

"My Child Is Always Snacking, Yet She Never Finishes Her Meal."

Children have small stomachs. Offering them six or so small meals succeeds better than limiting them to three meals each day. When we eat isn't nearly so important as what we eat. If nutritious snacks are readily available, these would be good to offer at midmorning or midafternoon when the child becomes hungry (Table 13–4).

When a child refuses to eat, it's best not to overreact. Most children don't starve themselves to any point approaching physical harm. When children refuse to eat, have them sit at the table for a while; if they still aren't interested in eating, remove the food and wait until the next scheduled meal or snack.

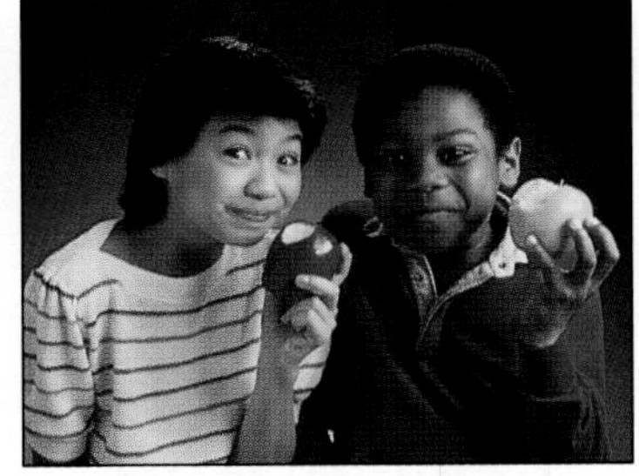

Childhood is an ideal time to begin to enjoy healthy foods.

"My Child Never Eats His Vegetables."

Children generally eat enough fruit but not an adequate amount of vegetables. A one-bite policy can be encouraged, and guidelines can be set to discourage fussing over unfamiliar foods. It takes time for a child to become enthusiastic about a new food, but with continual exposure and a positive role model, chances are good that the child will grow to like it. Having the child help choose and prepare the vegetables might also help.

TABLE 13-4

Ideas for Nutritious Snacks and Beverages

Snack	Serving suggestion	Snack	Serving suggestion	Snack	Serving suggestion
Fresh raw vegetables	Serve with a dip of cottage cheese or yogurt blended with dried buttermilk dressing	Flour tortillas	Spread with refried beans or canned chili, sprinkle with grated cheese and broil; top with chili sauce	Parfait	Make with yogurt, fruit, and granola
Celery	Spread with peanut butter and sprinkle on raisins, shredded carrots, or finely chopped nuts	Ready-to-eat cereals	Use brands low in sugar and containing fiber; serve with raisins	Gelatin	Add fruit or vegetable juice, vegetables, fruits, or cottage cheese
Bananas	Dip in sweetened yogurt or spread with peanut butter and roll in coconut, chopped nuts, or granola	Pita bread	Place sliced meat, cheese, lettuce, and tomato in open pocket	Frozen fruit cubes	Freeze puréed apple-sauce or fruit juice into cubes
Sliced apples or crackers	Serve with a dip of peanut butter, honey, nuts, raisins, and coconut	English muffins or pita bread	Top with spaghetti sauce, grated cheese, and meats; broil or bake and cut in fourths	Fruit fizz	Add club soda to juice instead of serving soft drinks
Bagels	Spread with cream cheese or peanut butter and top with chopped bananas, crushed pineapple, or shredded carrots	Potato skins	Sprinkle with shredded cheese, broil, and top with yogurt and bacon bits	Fruit shake	Blend milk with fresh fruit (bananas, berries, or a peach) and a dash of cinnamon or nutmeg
Quick bread or muffins	Make with carrots, zucchini, pumpkin, bananas, nuts, dates, raisins, lemons, squash, or berries	Canned chili	Heat and top with onions, lettuce, and tomato; use as dip for Italian or French bread, biscuits, or cornbread	Yogurt frost	Combine fruit juice and yogurt; add fresh fruit if desired
		Kabobs	Make with any combination of fruit, vegetables, and sliced or cubed cooked meat (remove toothpicks before serving)	Hot chocolate	Make hot chocolate or cocoa with milk chocolate and a dash of cinnamon
		Popcorn	Serve plain or make 3 quarts and sprinkle with ¼ cup grated cheese and ½ tsp garlic or onion salt	Seeds	Shelled sunflower seeds
				Fish	Tunafish on crackers
				Canned soup	Cup of vegetable or minestrone; nice on a cold winter day

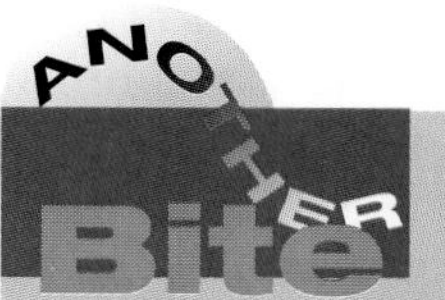

Children cannot and should not be forced to eat. They need to develop independence and identities separate from their parents. In other words, children have to choose for themselves—a practice that should be encouraged. No one food is an essential part of a diet. Hunger is still the best means for getting a child to eat. It may be effective to feed children vegetables at the start of a meal, when they are hungriest, and offer new foods with familiar ones. A platter of raw or lightly cooked carrots, broccoli, green and red peppers, cabbage, and mushrooms eaten as a snack with friends can do a lot to remedy a vegetable problem. A 4- or 5-year-old child can safely eat raw vegetables without fear of choking. Recall that children often are more sensitive than adults to strong flavors and odors. Nutritious dips "sell" vegetables to many children. Vegetables may acquire more appeal when children help prepare them. And, as with any food, it is important to remember that children have likes and dislikes too.

Do Children Need a Vitamin/Mineral Supplement?

Major scientific groups, such as the American Dietetic Association and the American Society for clinical Nutrition, believe that vitamin and mineral supplements are unnecessary for healthy children; it's better to emphasize a wide variety of foods. However, a child who is ill or has a very erratic food preference pattern or appetite may need a balanced nutrient supplement not exceeding 100% of Daily Values on the label, especially if these conditions persist. Diets for children who eat totally vegetarian fare should focus especially on protein, vitamin D, vitamin B-12, calcium, iron, and zinc. Parents generally offer children conservative amounts of nutrient supplements, so toxicity is unlikely. Still, giving supplements is often unnecessary, especially in light of today's typically highly fortified breakfast cereals, which children often eat.

If current childhood feeding practices are to become more healthful, the focus should shift from high-fat food choices to lower-fat choices, and to the bottom half of the Food Guide Pyramid, including whole grains, fruits, and vegetables.

Nutritional Problems in Preschool Children

Chapter 4 noted that it's unlikely that use of sugar is the cause of hyperactivity or antisocial behavior in most children.

Three nutrition-related problems found in preschool children are iron-deficiency anemia, constipation, and dental caries. Proper diet can help correct or relieve these conditions substantially.

Iron-Deficiency Anemia

Childhood iron-deficiency anemia is most likely to appear in children between the ages of 6 and 24 months. It can lead to a decrease in both stamina and learning ability, because the oxygen supply to cells decreases. Another effect is lowered resistance to disease. Fortunately, childhood anemia is fairly uncommon here, probably because of children's use of iron-fortified breakfast cereals. Also deserving of credit is the Special Supplemental Food Program for Women, Infants, and Children (WIC), sponsored by the federal government. This program emphasizes the importance of iron-fortified formulas and cereals and distributes them—along with nutrition education—to low-income parents of infants and preschool children considered to be at nutritional risk.

The best way to prevent iron-deficiency anemia in children is to regularly feed them foods that are adequate sources of iron. Iron-fortified breakfast cereals and a few ounces of lean meat are convenient means of getting more iron into a child's diet. The high proportion of heme iron in many animal foods allows the iron to be more readily absorbed than is iron from plant foods. Consuming a vitamin C source along with the less readily absorbed iron in plants and supplements will aid absorption.

Constipation

Although constipation may be associated with disease, some young children experience constipation that is unrelated to any medical condition. Dietary interventions include eating more dietary fiber and drinking more fluids. Excessive milk intake could be reduced to see if that helps. Foods to emphasize for dietary fiber are fruits, vegetables, whole-grain breads and cereals, and beans. The current daily dietary fiber goal for children between ages 3 and 18 years is the child's age plus 5 grams. After that age typical adult recommendations are appropriate (see Chapter 4). Fluid recommendations are 5 cups per day for toddlers, and up to 9 cups per day for older children.

Dental Caries

A well-planned diet goes a long way in reducing the risk for dental caries in young children. Earlier it was mentioned that infants are prone to nursing bottle syndrome, which can lead to excessive tooth decay. The following tips can help reduce dental problems in children:

- Begin oral hygiene when teeth start to appear.
- Seek early pediatric dental care.
- Drink fluoridated water.
- Use fluoridated toothpaste twice daily.
- Snack in moderation.
- Have a dentist apply tooth sealants if needed.
- If toddlers or preschoolers desire chewing gum, sugarless is the best choice as this has been shown to actually reduce the incidence of dental caries.

Chapters 4 and 8 provide a fuller description of diet and dental health. If needed, those discussions will aid in putting this list of recommendations into perspective.

Modifying Childhood Diets to Reduce Future Disease Risk

Earlier chapter covered the role of diet in development of heart disease and hypertension and the recommendations concerning diet to reduce the risk for these diseases. Parents sometimes wonder whether similar diet modifications are appropriate and beneficial during childhood.

Diets Designed to Limit the Risk of Heart Disease

We know that development of atherosclerosis begins in childhood. Children in the United States currently derive about 33% of their energy from fat with about 13% of energy from saturated fat. Today two schools of thought exist with regard to children and heart disease in preschool and later school years. The National Cholesterol Education Program suggests that children 2 years and older consume no more than 30% of energy as fat, 10% of energy as saturated fat, and 300 milligrams of cholesterol. (Note that this is the same recommendation it gives to adults.) The American Academy of Pediatrics recommends that children eat a similar diet by age 5 years, and cautions against including less than 30% of energy as fat. However, other researchers have recently proposed that fat simply be gradually reduced from about 40% of energy intake in infancy to the 30% figure by the time a child's linear growth ceases (at about age 16 to 18 years). Note that if diets contain about 30% of energy as fat and are carefully planned (i.e., they follow the Food Guide Pyramid), normal childhood growth can be expected. Parents can choose which path to follow in conjunction with their child's physician. In general it's unnecessary to discourage children from consuming nutrient-dense foods such as milk and meat just because they contain some fat. The overriding message is moderation in fat intake.

USDA recently adapted the Food Guide Pyramid for children 2- to 6-years old.
- **2 servings milk, yogurt and cheese**
- **2 servings meat, poultry, fish, dry beans, eggs, and nuts**
- **2 servings fruits**
- **3 servings vegetables**
- **6 servings bread, cereal, rice, and pasta**

Low-Sodium Diets

Scientific data neither confirm nor refute the notion that eating less sodium will reduce the risk of future hypertension. Moderation in sodium consumption does help build good health habits for the future—especially if the person later develops high blood pressure and needs to eat even less sodium. If children become accustomed to less salt, they'll be less inclined to eat very salty foods as adults. This reduction in salt also contributes to better calcium retention in the body, as covered in Chapter 8.

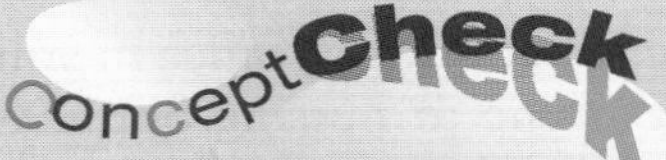

The rapid growth rate of an infant's first year slows during the toddler and preschool years (ages 2 to 5). As a child's appetite decreases, adults need to serve nutrient-dense foods and allow the child to decide how much to eat. Sudden shifts in food preferences are to be expected. Snacking is fine if attention is given to the selection of healthful foods and good dental hygiene. Vitamin and mineral supplements are usually not needed—a plan following the Food Guide Pyramid should meet nutrient needs. Children need plenty of iron-rich foods to prevent iron-deficiency anemia. Adequate dietary fiber and fluid help prevent constipation. Developing heart-healthy habits after the age of 2 years is advocated by some experts, but highly restrictive diets are not appropriate during childhood. Diets for children who eat totally vegetarian fare should focus on protein, vitamin D (or regular sun exposure), vitamin B-12, calcium, iron, and zinc content.

School-Age Children

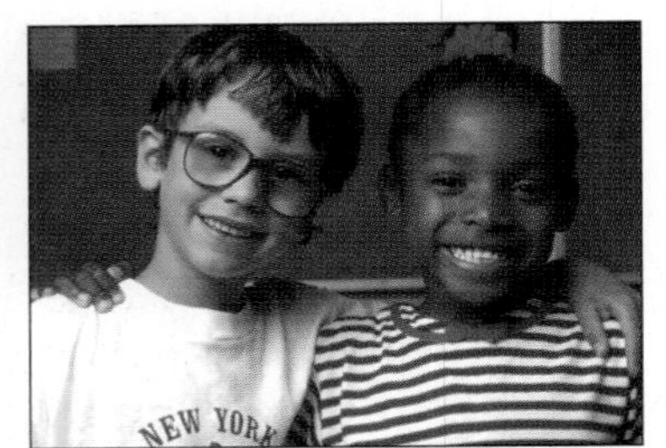

Breakfast benefits the school-age child in many ways, nutritional and behavioral.

In general, the nutritional concerns and goals applicable to school-age children are the same as those discussed in relation to preschoolers. The Food Guide Pyramid continues to be a good basis for diet planning, with an emphasis on moderating fat intake and ensuring adequate iron and calcium intake. The only difference is that serving size increases as energy needs increase (see Table 13–3). Now let's look at several nutritional issues of particular concern during the school-age years.

Breakfast, Fat Intake, and Snacks

Once children enter school, their eating patterns become more scheduled and consumption of regular meals—especially breakfast—becomes an important focus. Though there is controversy over the true benefit of breakfast on cognitive ability, children who eat breakfast will likely more easily meet needs for vitamins and minerals over children not eating breakfast. To influence morning test performance it currently appears that breakfast must be eaten within a half hour of a test; the rise in blood glucose is thought to change performance.

Breakfast menus need not be limited to traditional fare. A little imagination can spark the interest of the most reluctant child. Instead of conventional breakfast foods, parents can offer leftovers from dinner, pizza, spaghetti, soups, yogurt with trail mix on top, chili, or sandwiches for starters.

There is general agreement that diets of school-age children should include a variety of foods from each major group, while not necessarily excluding any specific food because of its fat content. Overemphasis on fat-reduced diets during childhood has been linked to an increase in eating disorders and encourages an inappropriate "good food," "bad food" attitude.

Steering children toward healthful foods, in school and at home, is likely to be more successful if they are exposed to nutrition education. Such education can help children understand why eating a proper diet will make them feel more energetic, look better, and work more efficiently. One recent survey of school children highlights the need for nutrition education. On the day of the survey, 40% of the children ate no vegetables, except for potatoes or tomato sauce; 20% ate no fruits; and 75% snacked at least twice. Some 36% of the students ate at least four different types of snack foods. Another recent study showed that only 1% of about 3,300 children 2 to 19 years met their recommended servings from all five Food Guide Pyramid groups. Clearly, the diets of many school-age students can stand general improvement, particularly with regard to fruit, vegetable, grain, and milk choices. The web site http://ificinfo.health.org/index3.htm provides much information on promoting healthy eating habits in children.

Critical Thinking

Tim refuses to eat breakfast before school. He doesn't like cereal, toast, or any of the other usual breakfast foods. What can Tim's parents do to ensure that he eats nutritious foods before leaving for school?

Nutrition Insight

Childhood Obesity

In the United States about 22% of school-age children place above the 85th percentile in weight-for-height and are considered overweight, and the number of cases is currently increasing. In the short run, ridicule and embarrassment are the main consequences of such obesity. Significant health problems associated with obesity, such as heart disease, Type 2 diabetes, and high blood pressure usually don't appear until adulthood. Still, childhood obesity should not be ignored since about 40% of obese children (and about 80% of obese adolescents) become obese adults. Significant weight gain generally begins either between ages 5 and 7 or during the teenage years.

Current research points to many potential causes of childhood obesity. Recall the nature versus nurture discussion in Chapter 9. Some infants are born with lower metabolic rates; they use energy more efficiently and in turn can more easily save energy intake for fat storage. Thus childhood obesity is linked to heredity. Obesity in children also has a correlation to sibling and maternal obesity.

Researchers believe that although diet is still an important factor, inactivity is the key to the increase in childhood obesity. The TV generation now glues itself to the tube for an average of 24 hours a week, including hours of advertisements for high-fat and sugar-laden foods; many children spend another 10 hours or so playing computer and video games. The Academy of Pediatrics recommends a limit of 14 hours of TV and computer time per week. In addition, excessive snacking, overreliance on quick-service restaurants, parental neglect, lack of safe areas to play, latchkey conditions, and high-fat/high-energy food choices most likely contribute to childhood obesity.

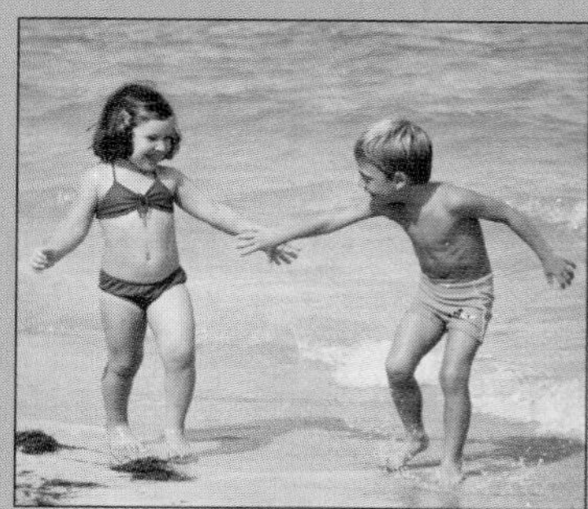

Many children start out life at an appropriate weight-for-height. A goal should be to retain that healthy proportion.

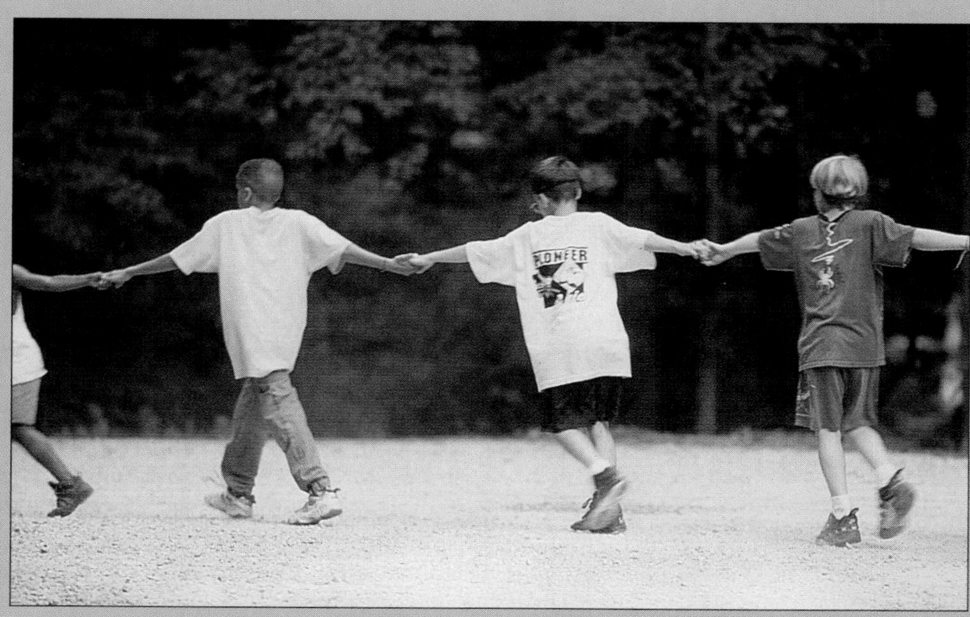

Children benefit from opportunities to be physically active.

Treating the Obese Child

The initial approach in treating an obese child is to assess how much physical activity he or she engages in. If a child spends much free time in sedentary activities (such as watching television or playing video games), more physical activities should be encouraged—30 minutes or more of moderate to intense physical activity per day for children and adolescents. An overall active lifestyle will help children not only to attain a healthy body weight but also maintain a healthy body weight later in life. Two good ideas are getting the family together for a brisk walk after dinner and finding an after-school sport the child enjoys.

Moderation in energy intake is important, especially limitation of high-fat and high-energy foods, such as sugar-laden carbonated beverages and high-fat milk. These are leading calorie contributors to the diets of many children. The focus should be on more nutrient-dense foods and healthy snacks.

Resorting to a weight-loss diet is usually not necessary. In the short run, it's best to emphasize changing habits. Children have an advantage over adults in dealing with obesity; their bodies can use stored energy for growth. Thus if weight gain can be moderated, increases in height and resulting lean body tissue may reduce the percentage of body weight accounted for as stored fat, yielding a more healthful weight-to-height ratio. This is one reason it's desirable to treat obesity in childhood. Further growth can contribute to success.

If a child will still be obese after attaining ultimate adult height, a weight-loss regimen may be necessary. This is especially appropriate after the adolescent growth spurt. Weight loss should be gradual, perhaps ½ pound per week. If weight loss is necessary in younger children, the child should be watched closely to ensure that the rate of growth continues to be normal. The child's energy intake shouldn't be so low that gains in height diminish.

Obese children often need to find a new way to relate to foods, especially snack foods. An important family rule could be that children are allowed to eat only while sitting at the dining table or in the kitchen. This could stop endless hours of snacking in front of the television and make all family members more conscious of when they are eating. It also might be helpful to put portions of snack foods on plates rather than allow snacking to go on indefinitely, as often happens when children eat directly from a full box of crackers or cookies.

A child's self-esteem is extremely fragile. Obesity itself affects the child's psyche. Humiliation doesn't work; it only makes the child feel worse. Support, admiration, and encouragement of the child's efforts at weight control are more effective and should be emphasized.

Finally, it is important to understand that not all female children are designed to look like runway models nor male children to look like professional athletes. In other words, some children will simply weigh more than others. A healthful lifestyle with plenty of physical activity and nutritious foods remains the key concern.

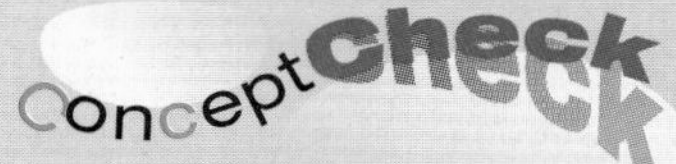

The school-age child is advised to follow the Food Guide Pyramid, moderating choices high in fat and simple sugars. Breakfast is an important meal to refuel the body for a new school day and to help ensure fulfilling nutrient needs for the day. Attention to regular physical activity and healthy diet should help prevent/treat childhood obesity and build a desirable lifestyle pattern for later life.

The Teenage Years

Generally girls begin a rapid growth spurt between the ages of 10 and 13, and boys experience rapid growth between the ages of 12 and 15. Nearly every organ in the body grows during these periods. Most noticeable are increases in height and weight and development of secondary sexual characteristics. Girls usually begin menstruating (reach menarche) during this growth spurt, and they grow very little beyond 2 years after menarche. Early-maturing girls may begin their growth spurt as early as age 7 to 8, whereas early-maturing boys may begin growing by age 9 to 10.

During the growth spurt, girls gain about 10 inches (25 centimeters) in height and boys gain about 12 inches (30 centimeters). Girls also tend to accumulate both lean and fat tissue, whereas boys tend to gain mostly lean tissue. This growth spurt provides about 50% of ultimate adult weight and about 15% of ultimate adult height.

As the growth spurt begins, teenagers begin to eat more. If teens choose nutritious food, they can take advantage of their increased hunger and easily satisfy their nutrient needs. As with older age groups, the Food Guide Pyramid provides the basis for meeting these nutrient needs, with the major difference being three servings of milk and milk products.

Nutritional Problems and Concerns of Teens

Anorexia nervosa and bulimia nervosa were covered in detail in Chapter 11. Other nutritional problems are more common during the teen years. A recent survey of high school students showed that only a little over 25% had eaten five servings of fruits and vegetables on the previous day. At the same time, the dietary fat content of teenagers is three to four percentage points higher than suggested amounts, and they are eating approximately 25% more sodium than recommended. Another concern is that many teenage girls stop drinking milk, so they may not consume enough calcium to allow for maximal mineralization of bones through their early twenties. Young women who don't consume enough calcium, typically from a low intake of milk products, are likely to develop osteoporosis later, as discussed in Chapter 8. In their place are soft drinks, currently the fifth leading contributor to calories in the diets of teenagers.

The AI for calcium for both males and females between ages 9 and 18 years is 1300 milligrams per day, compared with 800 milligrams per day for younger children. Unfortunately, most teenage girls do not consume the AI for calcium. Again, three servings per day from the milk, yogurt, and cheese group are recommended for all teenagers and young adults.

A further concern is iron deficiency. Iron-deficiency anemia sometimes appears in girls after they start menstruating and in boys during their growth spurt. About 10% of teenagers have low iron stores or related anemia. Teens who strive to forge an identity by adopting dietary patterns unfamiliar to their families—vegetarianism, for example—may not know enough about the alternate diet pattern to keep from developing health problems, such as iron-deficiency anemia. It's important that teenagers choose good food sources of iron, such as lean meats, whole grains, and enriched cereals. Teenage girls, particularly those with heavy menstrual flows, need to eat good sources of iron (or regularly consume an iron supplement). Iron-deficiency anemia is a highly undesirable condition for a teen. It can produce increased fatigue and decreased ability to concentrate and learn. School and athletic performance may suffer.

Acne is a common teen concern—about 80% of teens experience it. Although it's popularly believed that eating nuts, chocolate, and pizza can make acne worse, scientific studies have failed to show a strong link between any dietary factor and acne. It is important to note that many acne medications contain analogs of vitamin A. Though these treatments can be quite effective, the close supervision of a physician is crucial as these vitamin A analogs can be toxic. As previously mentioned in chapter 7, vitamin A itself is no help in treating acne, and excess amounts of vitamin A or related analogs can cause birth defects. Thus teens on these vitamin A medications should not become pregnant.

A Closer Look at the Diets of Teenage Girls

Teenagers in general are apt to adopt fad diets, eat away from home or miss meals completely, and snack a lot. Teenage girls especially are very concerned with weight gain, appearance, and social acceptance. Recent government statistics revealed that female students were significantly more likely to report currently trying to lose weight (44%) than were male students (15%). Moreover, 27% of female students who considered themselves the right weight reported they were currently trying to lose weight. It is important for teenage girls to realize that weight gain in the form of increased body fat is to be expected in the adolescent growth spurt.

As previously mentioned, a strictly vegetarian diet must be monitored for adequate energy, protein, iron, B-12, calcium, and vitamin D. This becomes particularly important in teenagers, as their diets are often already compromised.

WHEN YOU'RE YOUNG, EVERYTHING SEEMS POSSIBLE...
EXCEPT FOR MIDDLE AGE.
http://macnelly.com

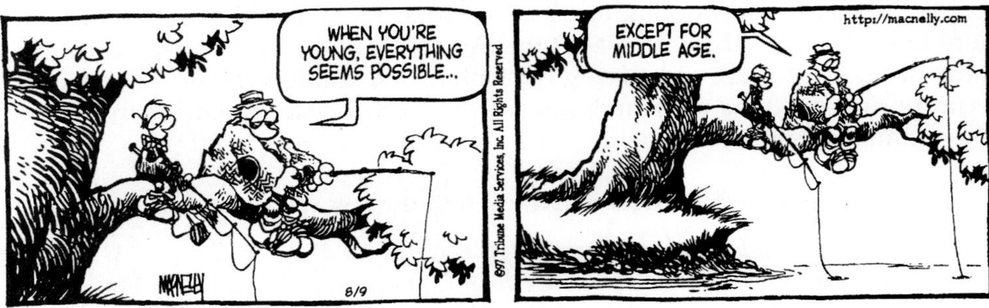

Figure 13–4 *Shoe.*

In an attempt to reach personal goals, teenage girls may eat dangerously little, select just a few items, and frequently skip meals altogether. If their limited food choices then consist of french fries, soft drinks, and pastries, little room is left for foods that are rich nutrient sources. It's not only calcium and iron that teenage girls need to be concerned about—they often don't consume enough folate, zinc, and vitamins A and C. Common use of diet pills and the increasing number of bulimia nervosa cases further add to these nutritional problems.

Helping Teens Eat More Nutritious Foods

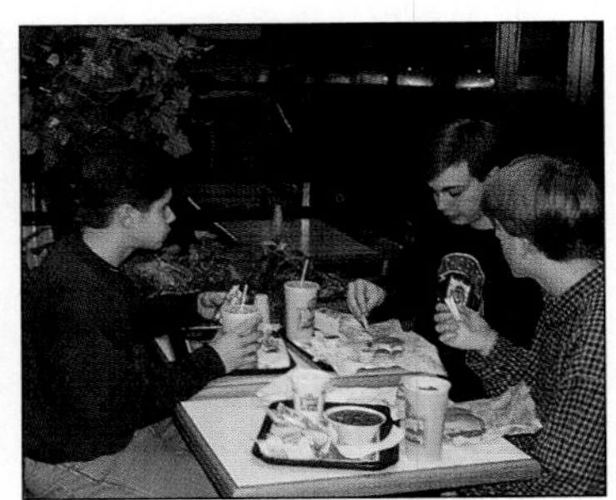

The teenage years are noted for snacking and eating at quick-service restaurants. With reasonable food choices, teenagers can have healthful diets while still enjoying snacks and socializing at their favorite hangouts.

Teenagers face a variety of challenges. They pursue their independence, experience identity crises, seek peer acceptance, and worry about physical appearance. All of these factors affect food choice. Advertisers take advantage of this by pushing a vast array of products—candy, gum, soft drinks, and snacks—targeted toward the teenage market.

Teens often don't think about the long-term benefits of good health. They have a hard time relating today's actions to tomorrow's health outcomes. Many teenagers tend to think they can just change habits later; there's no hurry (Figure 13–4).

Still, healthful teen food habits don't have to include giving up favorite foods. Small portions of these foods can complement larger portions of nonfat and low-fat dairy products, lean meats, vegetable proteins, fruits, vegetables, and whole-grain products.

As reviewed in Chapter 5, choosing healthful foods is becoming easier in many of today's quick-service restaurants. Some restaurants have evolved beyond hamburgers, french fries, and milk shakes to include a variety of vegetables, salad bars, and ethnic foods. In addition, some restaurants are trying to cater to their more health-conscious clientele. Still, many of the meal selections remain high-calorie options when compared with the amounts of other nutrients provided. Teens who eat regularly at quick-service restaurants should choose meals carefully to meet their nutrient needs without exceeding their energy needs.

Overcoming the Teenage Mind-Set

One strategy for working with teenage boys is to stress the importance of nutrition and physical activity for physical development—especially muscular development—and for fitness, vigor, and health. With teenage girls, one approach is to help them understand how to choose nutrient-dense foods and activities that lead to better health while maintaining a healthy weight. For teenagers, it's more effective to focus on the benefits of healthful foods and regular physical activity they can reap right now than to talk about health hazards that may or may not happen at some later time.

Are Teenage Snacking Practices Harmful?

Teens often obtain one-fourth to one-third of all their energy and major nutrients from snacks. Unfortunately, recent studies find just what you might expect—that teens snack mostly on potato and corn chips, cookies, candies, and ice cream. Key reasons for snacking include an opportunity to get out and socialize with friends, accessibility, hunger, and celebrating a special event. Teenagers can obtain many nutrients from snacking. Even quick-service restaurants offer some good choices. By choosing wisely and eating in moderation, teens can eat at quick-service restaurants and still consume a very healthful diet. Snacks and quick-service restaurants themselves are not the problem; poor food choices are.

Poor dietary habits formed during teenage years often continue into adulthood, giving rise to an increased risk of chronic diseases, such as heart disease, osteoporosis, and some types of cancer. Getting this message across to teenagers is an important and challenging task for parents and health professionals.

Alcoholism, a significant health problem that may have its roots in the teen years, is covered in detail in Chapter 14. Smoking—another habit that compromises health—also often begins in teen years, and is currently increasing in this age group.

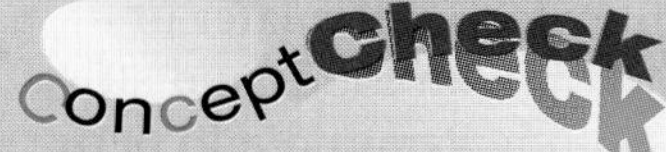

A second period of rapid growth occurs during the teen years. Girls generally start this growth spurt earlier than boys. The Food Guide Pyramid should guide meal planning. Common nutritional problems in these years arise from poor food choices and include inadequate calcium intake in girls, iron-deficiency anemia, and sometimes excessive intake of total fat and saturated fat. Because changes occur so rapidly during these years, and in so many areas—psychological, social, and physical—it may be difficult to stress the importance of nutrition to teenagers. Moderation in fat intake and portion size are two goals to consider when choosing snacks and meals in quick-service restaurants.

Summary

- Growth is very rapid during infancy. An adequate diet, especially in terms of energy, as well as the nutrients protein and zinc, is essential to support normal growth. Undernutrition can cause irreversible changes in growth and development. Growth in infants and children can be assessed by measuring body weight, height (or length), and head circumference over time.
- Nutrient needs in the first 6 months can be met by human milk or iron-fortified infant formula. Supplementary vitamin D and iron may be needed in the first 6 months for breastfed infants, and many infants may need supplemental fluoride after 6 months of age.
- Infant formulas generally contain lactose or sucrose, heat-treated proteins from cow's milk, and vegetable oil. These formulas may or may not be fortified with iron. Sanitation is very important when preparing and storing formula.
- Most infants don't need solid foods before about 4 to 6 months of age. Solid food should not be added to an infant's diet until the nutrients are needed, the GI tract can digest complex foods, the infant has the physical ability to control tongue thrusting, and the risk of developing food allergies has decreased.
- The first solid food given should be iron-fortified infant cereals (or ground meats). Other single foods can be added gradually, at the rate of about one each week. Some foods to avoid giving infants in the first year include honey and corn syrup, cow's milk (especially fat-reduced varieties), egg whites, nuts, chocolate, very salty or sweet foods, or foods that may cause choking.

- Introducing iron-containing solid food at the appropriate time and not offering cow's milk until 1 year of age can generally prevent iron-deficiency anemia in late infancy.
- A slower growth rate in preschool years underlies the importance of children's eating nutrient-dense foods and reducing their food serving sizes. Choosing iron-rich foods, such as lean red meats, is important at this age. Portion sizes at meals of 1 tablespoon of each food for each year of life is a good rule of thumb.
- Preschoolers should be given some leeway in determining serving size and should be encouraged to try new foods. Highly restrictive diets designed to reduce the risk of heart disease or high blood pressure are not recommended for preschoolers or older children, unless prescribed by a physician.
- Obese children and adolescents are more likely to become obese adults and so incur greater health risks. Parents can provide healthful food choices, while children should control portion sizes. When controlled early, a problem of obesity may correct itself as the child continues to grow in height.
- During the adolescent growth spurt, both boys and girls have increased needs for iron and calcium. Inadequate calcium intake by teenage girls is a major concern because it can set the stage for development of osteoporosis later in life. Teenagers generally should moderate their intake of high-fat foods and strive to meet the serving recommendations of the Food Guide Pyramid and perform regular physical activity.

Study Questions

1. Why does nutritional deficiency in the first few months of life have such a profound effect on later years?
2. List four nutrients that are in high demand for an infant. How are each of these demands met (and not exceeded) by human milk or formula?
3. Outline three key factors that help determine when to introduce solid foods into an infant's diet. What is the recommended order in which to begin feeding solid foods?
4. Describe three possible health problems in infancy along with the potential cause(s) and nutrition-related solutions.
5. What kind of eating changes can parents expect when their infant becomes a toddler? How should these changes be handled?
6. Describe the two "schools of thought" with regard to lowering fat intake in the diets of toddlers. What would you do with your own child?
7. What three factors are likely to contribute to obesity in a typical 10-year-old child?
8. Describe three pros and cons of snacking. What is the basic advice for healthful snacking from childhood through the teenage years? How can foods from quick-service restaurants be incorporated into such a plan?
9. Which two nutrients are of particular interest in planning diets for teenagers? Why does each deserve to be singled out?
10. List three nutrients of concern for a teenage vegetarian, and a vegetarian food source for each.

Further Readings

1 ADA Reports: Position of the American Dietetic Association: Dietary guidance for healthy children aged 2 to 11 years, *Journal of the American Dietetic Association* 99:93, 1999.
2 Balon AJ: Management of infantile colic, *American Family Physician* 55:235, 1997.
3 Berenson GS and others: Association between multiple cardiovascular risk factors and atherosclerosis in children and young adults, *New England Journal of Medicine* 338:1650, 1998.
4 Birch LL: Children's food acceptance patterns, *Nutrition Today* 31:234, 1996.
5 Carroll JL, Siska ES: SIDS: Counseling parents to reduce risk, *American Family Physician* 57:1566, 1998.
6 Cowell C: Nutritional concerns for preschool-age children, *Topics in Clinical Nutrition* 11(3):38, 1996.
7 de Andraca I and others: Psychomotor development and behavior in iron-deficient anemic infants, *Nutrition Reviews* 55:125, 1997.
8 Garza C, Frongillo EA: Infant feeding recommendations, *American Journal of Clinical Nutrition* 67:815, 1998.
9 Glinsmann WH and others: Dietary guidelines for infants: a timely reminder, *Nutrition Reviews* 54:50, 1996.
10 Harel Z and others: Adolescents and calcium: what they do and do not know, and how much do they consume, *Journal of Adolescent Health* 22:225, 1998.
11 Johnson DB: Nutrition in infancy: evolving views on recommendations, *Nutrition Today* 32:63, 1997.
12 Leyden: Therapy for acne vulgaris, *New England Journal of Medicine* 336:1156, 1997.
13 McBean LD: How to grow a healthy child, *Dairy Council Digest* 69:31, 1998.
14 Moran R: Evaluation and treatment of childhood obesity, *American Family Physician* 59:861, 1999.
15 Picciano MF and others: How to grow a healthy child, *Nutrition Today* 34(1):6, 1999.
16 Skinner JD and others: Transitions in infant feeding during the first year of life, *Journal of the American College Nutrition* 16:209, 1997.
17 Spencer JP: Practical nutrition for the healthy term infant, *American Family Physician* 54:138, 1996.
18 Stehlin IB: Infant formula second best but good enough, *FDA Consumer*, p. 17, June 1996.
19 Subar AF: Dietary sources of nutrients among U.S. children, 1989–1991, *Pediatrics* 102:913, 1998.
20 Taylor SL and others: Food allergies and avoidance diets, *Nutrition Today* 34(1):15, 1999.
21 Van Itallie TB: Predicting obesity in children, *Nutrition Reviews* 5:155, 1998.
22 Willatts P and others: Effect of long-chain polyunsaturated fatty acids in infant formula on problem solving at 10 months of age, *The Lancet* 352:688, 1998.

RATE

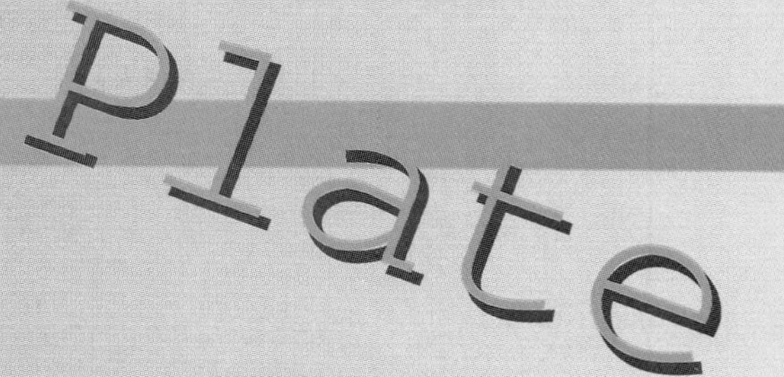

I. Getting Young Bill to Eat

Bill is 3 years old, and his mother is worried about his eating habits. He absolutely refuses to eat vegetables, meat, and dinner in general. Some days he eats very little food. He wants to eat snacks most of the time. His mother wants him to eat a formal lunch and dinner to make sure he gets all the nutrients he needs. Mealtime is a battle because Bill says he isn't hungry, but his mother wants him to eat everything served on his plate. He drinks five or six glasses of whole milk per day because that is the one food he adores.

When his mother prepares dinner, she makes plenty of vegetables, boiling them until they are soft, hoping this will appeal to Bill. Bill's dad waits to eat his vegetables last, regularly telling the family that he eats them only because he has to. He also regularly complains about how dinner has been prepared. Bill saves his vegetables until last and usually gags when his mother orders him to eat them. Bill has been known to sit at the dinner table for an hour until the war of wills ends. Bill's mother serves casseroles and stews regularly because these are her best dishes. Bill likes to eat breakfast cereal, fruit, and cheese and will regularly request these foods for snacks. However, his mother tries to deny his requests so he will have an appetite for dinner. Bill's mother comes to you and asks you what she should do to get Bill to eat.

ANALYSIS

1. **List four mistakes Bill's parents are making that contribute to Bill's poor eating habits.**

____

____

____

____

2 **List four strategies they might try to promote good eating habits in Bill.**

____

____

____

____

II. Evaluating a Teen Lunch

Below are two typical teen lunches and nutritional information for each.

Meal 1	Amount	Item
	2 pieces	Cheese pizza
	1 each	Milk chocolate candy bar
	20 fl oz	Cola

Meal 2	Amount	Item
	1	Hamburger with condiments
	30 each	French fries
	20 fl oz	Cola

	Meal 1	Meal 2	Nutrient needs for teens
kcal	990	1000	3000 males 2200 females
Protein (grams)	32	20	59 males 44 females
Vitamin C (milligrams)	5	18	60
Vitamin A (RE)	300	10	1000 males 800 females
Iron (milligrams)	3	4	12 males 15 females
Calcium (milligrams)	545	100	1300

1. Keeping in mind that meals should meet about one-third of nutrient needs, what are the shortcomings and excesses of these meals? (i.e., given the nutritional information, compare these meals to one-third the RDA for calories, protein, vitamin C, vitamin A, and iron, and the AI for calcium). ______________________________

____

____

2. How would you change these meals to improve balance and to meet the nutrient needs above? (Hint: use your software program or Appendix A). ______________________________

____

____

3. Reflect on your food choices as a teenager. Do you think your meal choices were balanced and varied? Why or why not? What could you have done to improve your nutritional habits at that time? ______________________________

____

____

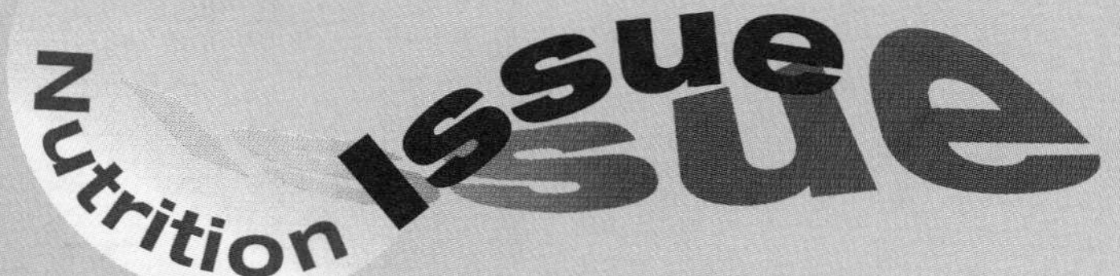

Food Allergies and Intolerances

Adverse reactions to foods—indicated by sneezing, coughing, nausea, vomiting, diarrhea, hives, and other rashes—are broadly classed as food allergies (also called *hypersensitivities*) or **food intolerances.** Allergies involve responses of the immune system designed to eliminate foreign proteins, called **allergens.** The symptoms experienced by susceptible people, such as rapid increase in heart rate and shortness of breath, are the result of this battle. In contrast, the symptoms of food intolerances do not result from a true allergic reaction. Rather, food intolerances are caused by an individual's inability to digest certain food components or by the direct effect of a food component or contaminant on the body. It is important to understand the difference between food allergies and food intolerances. Let's examine each process, first allergies and then intolerances, so you can learn how to reduce the risk of becoming a victim of the food you eat.

Food intolerance
An adverse reaction to food that does not involve an allergic reaction.

Allergen
A foreign protein, or antigen, that induces excess production of certain immune system antibodies; subsequent exposure to the same protein leads to allergic symptoms. While all allergens are antigens, not all antigens are allergens.

FOOD ALLERGIES: SYMPTOMS AND MECHANISM

Allergic reactions to foods occur more frequently in females than males, and especially during infancy and young adulthood. Experts estimate that up to about 1% to 2% of adults and up to about 6% to 8% of children are allergic to certain foods. Three types of reactions may occur after ingestion of problem foods by susceptible people:

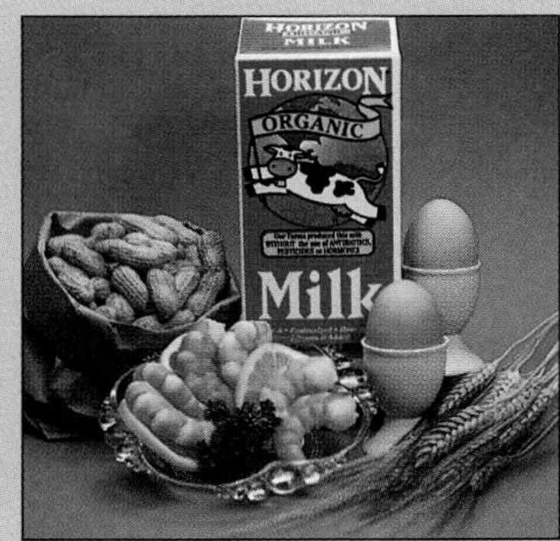

Eggs, wheat, milk, nuts and seafood pose the greatest risk for food allergies in childhood.

- *Classic*—itching, reddening skin, asthma, swelling, choking, and a runny nose
- *GI tract*—nausea, vomiting, diarrhea, intestinal gas, bloating, pain, constipation, and indigestion
- *General*—headache, skin reactions, tension and fatigue, tremors, and psychological problems

Any reaction that is milder than these distinct allergic ones is referred to as a **food sensitivity.**

Allergic reactions vary not only in the body system affected but also in their duration, ranging from seconds to a few days. A generalized, all-systems reaction is called **anaphylactic shock.** This severe allergic response results in lowered blood pressure and respiratory and GI tract distress. It can be fatal. Although any food can trigger anaphylactic shock, the most common culprits are peanuts, tree nuts (walnuts, pecans, etc.), shellfish, milk, eggs, soybeans, wheat, and fish. For a smaller number of people, avoiding foods like peanuts or shellfish is a matter of life and death.

Food sensitivity
A mild reaction to a substance in a food that might be expressed as light itching or redness of the skin.

Anaphylactic shock
A severe allergic response that results in lowered blood pressure and respiratory and GI tract disorders. It can be fatal.

Almost all food allergies are caused by proteins in milk, eggs, corn, nuts (especially peanuts), seafood, soy products, and wheat. Other foods sometimes identified with adverse reactions include meat and meat products and cheese.

Testing for a Food Allergy

Diagnosis of a food allergy can often be a difficult task (Table 13–5). It requires the help of a skilled physician. The first step in determining whether a food allergy is present is to record in detail a history of symptoms, time from ingestion to onset of symptoms, most recent reaction, quantity and nature of food needed to produce a reaction, and the food suspected of causing a reaction. A family history of allergic diseases can also help, as allergic reactions tend to run in families.

The next step is to eliminate from the diet for 1 to 2 weeks all foods that appear to be causing the allergy,

TABLE 13-5

Assessment Strategies for Food Allergies

History	Includes description of symptoms, time between food ingestion and onset of symptoms, duration of symptoms, most recent allergic episode, quantity of food required to produce reaction, suspected foods, and allergic diseases in other family members.
Physical examination	Look for signs of an allergic reaction (rash, itching, intestinal bloating, etc.)
RAST test	Determine presence of immune bodies in blood that bind to allergens tested. Skin tests can also be used; a drop of antigen is placed on the skin where it has been scratched or punctured. If a person is allergic to the test antigen, a red eruption will develop.
Elimination diet	Establish a diet lacking the suspected offending foods and stay on it for 1 to 2 weeks or until symptoms clear.
Food challenge	Add back small amounts of excluded foods one at a time, as long as anaphylactic shock is not a possible consequence.

The American Academy of Allergy and Immunology has a 24-hour toll-free hot line (800-822-2762) to answer questions about food allergies and to help direct people to specialists who treat the problem. Free information on food allergies is available by writing to The Food Allergy Network, 4744 Holly Ave., Fairfax, VA 22030. The telephone number is (800) 929-4040; the web site is http://www.foodallergy.org

plus all other foods suspected of causing an allergy based on the person's food history. Once a diet is found that causes no symptoms, called an **elimination diet,** foods that are known not to trigger anaphylactic shock can be added back one at a time. Any reintroduced food that causes significant symptoms to appear is identified as an allergen for the person.

Elimination diet
A restrictive diet that systematically tests foods that may cause an allergic response by first eliminating them for 1 to 2 weeks and then adding them back one at a time.

Treatment of Food Allergies

Once potential allergens are identified, the best treatment is to avoid them, especially for people with zero tolerance. Careful reading of food labels is essential for many allergic people and advisable for all. A major challenge for the clinician treating a person with a food allergy is to make sure that what remains in the diet can still provide essential nutrients. A registered dietitian can help guide the diet-planning process.

If an allergy-prone woman is pregnant or breastfeeding, she should avoid offending foods—like eggs, milk, and peanuts—because allergens can cross the placenta during pregnancy. Allergens will also be secreted in her milk. She should work with her physician and registered dietitian to make sure she still consumes an adequate diet. In addition, when food allergies run in the family, women are advised to breastfeed their infants exclusively for 6 months. Human milk contains factors that play a role in maturation of the small intestine. Formula-fed infants, especially those on formulas based on cow's milk, have a greater risk for developing allergies. Breastfeeding then should continue for as long as possible, preferably to 1 year.

The **prognosis** for food allergies that first appear before 3 years of age is good. About 80% of young children with food allergies outgrow them before 3 years. Food allergies diagnosed after 3 years of age, however, are often more long-lived, but not always. In these cases about 33% of people outgrow their food allergies within 3 years. For others, the condition may be prolonged; some food allergies can last a lifetime, especially for peanuts and seafood. Periodic reintroduction of offending foods can be tried every 6 to 12 months or so to see whether the allergic reaction has decreased.

Prognosis
A forecast of the course and end of a disease.

FOOD INTOLERANCES

Food intolerances are adverse reactions to food that do not involve allergic mechanisms. Generally, larger amounts of an offending food are required to produce symptoms of an intolerance than to trigger allergic symptoms. Common causes of food intolerances include:

- Constituents of certain foods (e.g., red wine, tomatoes, grapefruit and apple juice, and pineapples) that have physiological effects such as changes in blood pressure or increased drug activity
- Certain synthetic compounds added to foods, such as sulfites, (e.g., in wine) food-coloring agents, and monosodium glutamate (MSG)

- Food contaminants, including antibiotics and other chemicals used in the production of livestock and crops, as well as insect parts not removed during processing
- Toxic contaminants resulting from ingestion of improperly handled and prepared foods containing *Clostridium botulinum*, *Salmonella* bacteria, or other food-borne microbes (see Chapter 15)
- Deficiencies in digestive enzymes, such as lactase.

Almost everyone is sensitive to one or more of these causes of food intolerance, many of which produce GI tract symptoms.

The basic treatment for food intolerances is to avoid specific offending components. However, total elimination often is not required because people generally are not as sensitive to compounds causing food intolerances as they would be to allergens. For instance, a slight amount of sulfites in a glass of wine may be tolerable, whereas a large amount may cause a reaction.

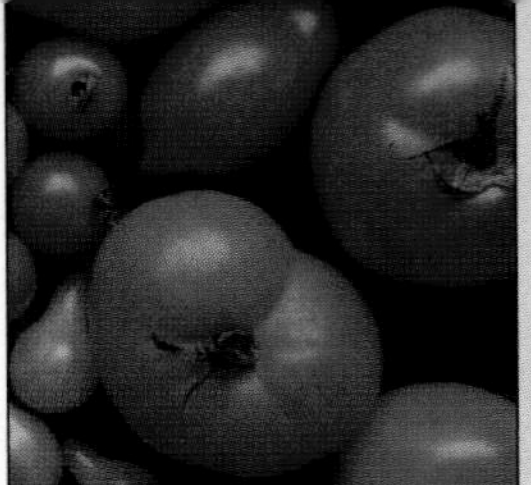

Chapter 14

Nutrition During Adulthood

Eating is one of our great pleasures. Guided by common sense and moderation, eating well is also a means to good health. Most of us want a long, productive life, free of ongoing illness. Yet, many people from early middle age onward suffer heart disease, strokes, Type 2 diabetes, osteoporosis, and other chronic diseases. We can slow the development of, and in some cases even prevent, these diseases by pursuing a diet that works against them. This action is most profitable if we begin early and continue throughout adulthood. We serve ourselves best—as individuals and as a nation—by striving to maintain vitality even in the later decades of life. This concept was first explored in Chapter 1 and is discussed again in this chapter concerning the special nutrition issues surrounding older persons.

Keep in mind that present day-to-day health practices can significantly influence health during later life. Although genetics does play a role, as discussed in Chapter 1, many health problems that occur with age are not inevitable; they result from disease processes that influence physical health. Much can be learned from healthy older people whose attention to health and physical activity—along with a genetic propensity and a little luck—keeps them active and vibrant well beyond typical retirement years. Successful aging is the goal. Age fast or slow—it is partly your choice.

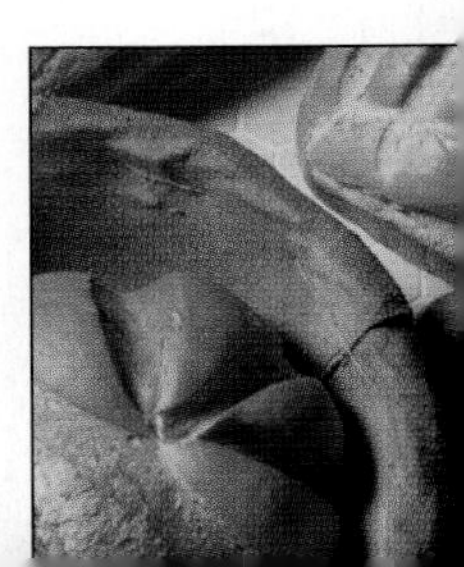

Nutrition Web

Delaying symptoms of and disabilities from chronic disease for as many years of adult life as possible is a laudable life goal. Nutrient intake and regular physical activity play a part in this process.

Aging likely results from automatic cellular changes and environmental influences, such as genetic damage, free-radical reactions, hormonal changes, alterations in immune function, elevated blood glucose, and excess energy intake.

Related problems of older people are loss of teeth, a reduction in the senses of taste, thirst, and smell, changes in gastrointestinal tract function, and deterioration in heart and bone health. Diet and lifestyle changes can help compensate.

Scientists are only now beginning to study specific nutrient requirements for older people. Diet plans should be based on the Food Guide Pyramid and Dietary Guidelines, with consideration for present health problems, decreased physical abilities, presence of drug-nutrient interactions, possible depression, alcoholism, and economic constraints.

If one is of legal age, small amounts of alcohol are permissible in a diet. However, more than one to two drinks per day can contribute to many health problems.

Because of decreased mobility, minimal social contact, and an inability to prepare foods, many older people benefit from congregate meal sites, home-delivered food, and other related services in their area that support nutritional health.

Nutrients such as vitamin D, vitamin E, vitamin B-6, folate, vitamin B-12, zinc, and calcium, along with dietary fiber, deserve special attention in diet planning in later life. Carefully planned supplementation is appropriate if diet changes don't suffice, but this does not substitute for healthy dietary habits.

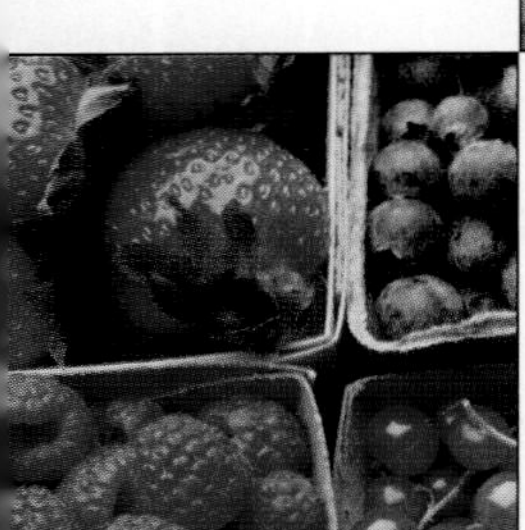

Our Adult Years

Many adults in America today have turned a healthful diet and moderate physical activity into lifetime pursuits. Coupled with avoiding tobacco products, sleeping an adequate amount, drinking enough fluid, and limiting stress, these actions contribute to a healthful, long life. It is important to begin these habits early in adult life so as to avoid or minimize many of the typical health problems seen in older adults and discussed in this chapter.

A Diet for the Adult Years

One diet approach that optimizes long-term nutritional health emphasizes low-fat and nonfat milk products, some lean meats, plant proteins, a rich variety of fruits and vegetables, and generous amounts of whole-grain breads and cereals. The Food Guide Pyramid in Chapter 2 is a blueprint for this diet. Then to further refine these food choices, also apply the latest Dietary Guidelines issued by the USDA/DHHS, and discussed in Chapter 2.

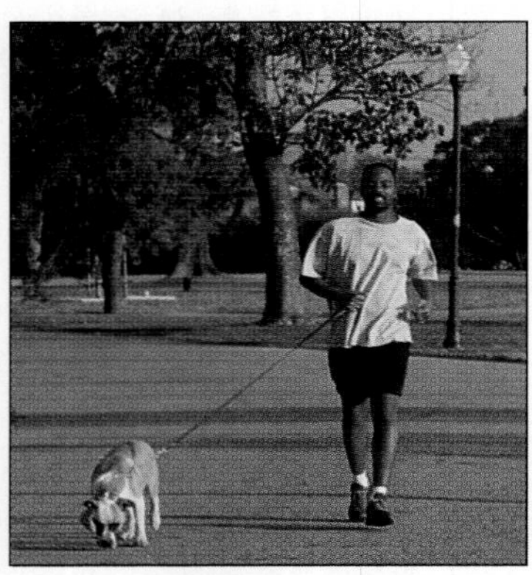

Many adults find that regular physical activity adds an important dimension to their lives.

Figure 14–1 depicts those two tools for diet design. The practices recommended can accommodate many cultural dietary patterns (see the Nutrition Issue in Chapter 1). They are broad enough to allow you to include all the foods you enjoy in an eating plan—you just may have to eat some foods less frequently than others or in smaller portions, depending on your health needs and preferences. Moderation, rather than elimination, should be your overriding consideration.

Are Adults Following These Diet Recommendations?

In general, American adults, both young and old, are trying to follow many of the diet recommendations listed. Since the mid-1950s adults have consumed less saturated fat as more people substitute nonfat and low-fat milk for cream and whole milk. Adults eat more cheese, however, which is usually a concentrated form of saturated fat. Since 1963 adults have eaten less butter, fewer eggs, less animal fat, and more vegetable fats and oils and fish. These changes generally follow the recommendations to reduce the intake of saturated fat and cholesterol and instead emphasize unsaturated fat. Today, animal breeders are raising much leaner cattle and hogs than in 1950, which helps. Our demand for chicken, a relatively lean source of animal protein, has skyrocketed.

Other aspects of the average U.S. diet are more mixed. The latest nutrition survey of eating habits shows that the major contributors of energy to the adult diet are white bread, beef, milk, doughnuts, cakes and cookies, soft drinks, chicken, cheese, salad dressing, mayonnaise, margarine, and sugars/syrups/jams. If the trend in diets were truly toward decreasing sugar and saturated fat, and increasing dietary fiber, many of these foods could hardly appear at the top of the list.

Appendix B reviews diet planning guidelines issued by the Canadian government for Canadians. In addition, Chapter 1 discussed *Healthy People 2000*, a U.S. federal agenda aimed at disease prevention and health promotion for Americans.

A list following suggestions for improvement covered in this book would stress low-fat and nonfat milk, whole-wheat bread and whole-grain cereals, lean meat and tuna, nuts and kidney beans, some fish, and oranges, carrots, romaine lettuce, broccoli, and green beans. What would your list look like?

Your task is to identify and change lifestyle practices most likely to cause illness and chronic disease. You began that process in Chapter 1. You can determine whether needed changes include switching to whole-grain cereal and walking briskly every day for 30 or more minutes. These practices both promote overall health.

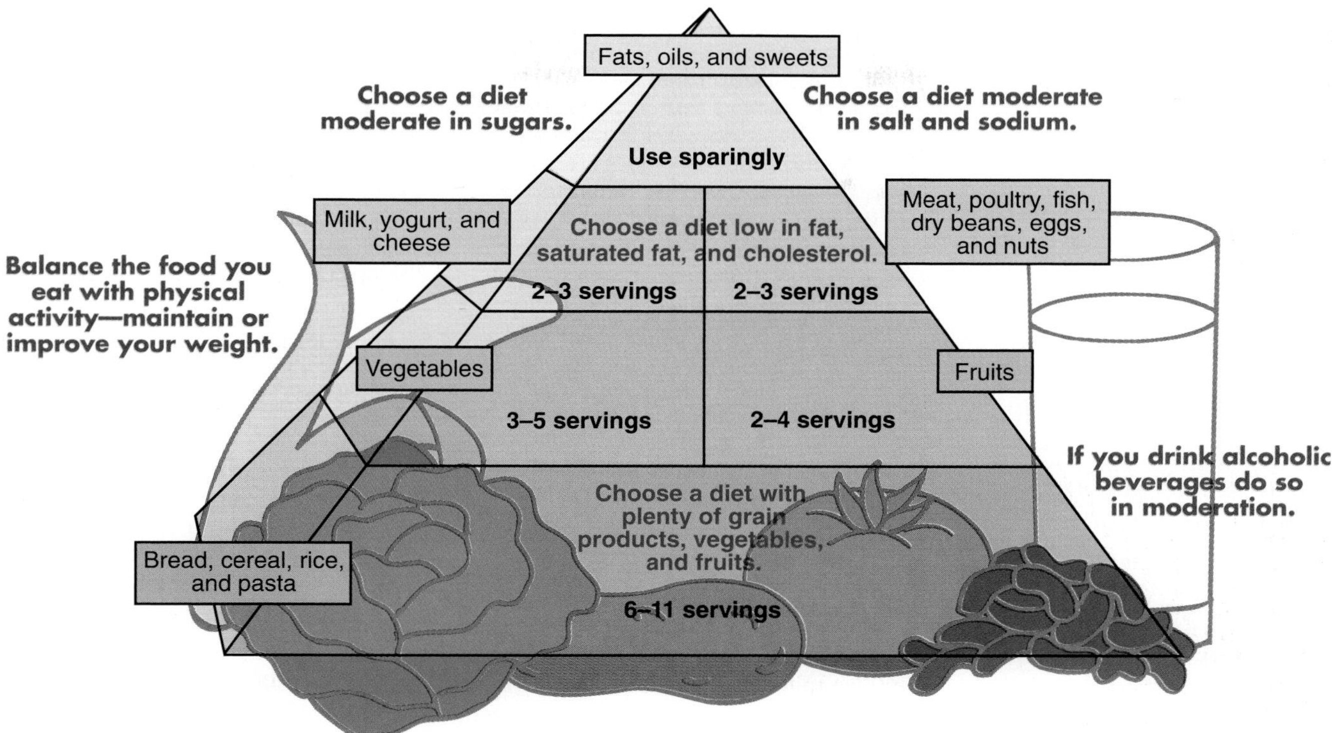

Figure 14–1 *Using the tools provided by the Food Guide Pyramid and Dietary Guidelines is one way for adults to plan a healthy diet.*

The overriding consideration should be quality and length of life and the impact dietary changes might have on them. Now is the time to design and begin to practice this plan. Adulthood, and the sooner the better, is a key time to learn more about one's risk factors for chronic diseases and do something about each one where possible.

A Note of Caution

Not all nutrition and health researchers agree with the blanket guidelines set by major health and science institutions. Some scientists do not think that general recommendations for the public can be justified for sugar, sodium, and cholesterol intake. Rather, they believe these recommendations need to be individualized.

Although it can be argued that individualized dietary recommendations for such nutrients as sodium are best, that approach would be quite costly for the nation. General recommendations are appropriate if they benefit most people while not hampering the health of others. Not all people will benefit equally from following the general recommendations—for example, moderation in sodium intake—but no one is likely to be harmed. The dietary change may cause some inconvenience and necessitate the formation of new eating habits for some people. Nevertheless, we should all consider the general dietary recommendations, personalizing the advice when possible under the guidance of our health-care advisors.

ConceptCheck

A basic plan to promote health and prevent disease includes eating a balanced, varied diet, performing regular physical activity, abstaining from smoking, limiting or abstaining from alcohol intake, obtaining adequate fluid and sleep, and limiting or learning ways to deal with stress more effectively. More specific dietary guidelines direct people to eat a variety of foods; maintain healthy weight; choose a diet low in fat, saturated fat, and cholesterol; choose a diet with plenty of vegetables, fruits, and grain products; use sugars only in moderation; use salt and sodium only in moderation; and, if you drink alcoholic beverages, do so in moderation. Some scientists believe that these guidelines do not necessarily constitute an individual "prescription."

A Focus on the Older Years

How long do your family members generally live? Of those who died early in adulthood, can you pinpoint some causes? Do you plan to live longer than your parents did or will? How long will that be? Some basic statistics can help you predict this.

Life Span

Life span
The potential oldest age a person can reach.

Life span refers to the maximal number of years humans live. As far as we know, this hasn't changed in recorded time. The longest human life documented to date is 122 years. In contrast, the domestic dog has a life span of 20 years, and a rat, 5 years.

Life Expectancy

Life expectancy
The average length of life for a given group of people born in a specific year (such as this year).

Life expectancy is the time an average person born in a specific year, such as 1999, can expect to live. Currently, life expectancy in America is about 73 years for men and about 80 years for women, with a span of "healthy years" of about 64. Furthermore, if you survive to the age of 80, you can tack on another 7 to 9 years of life expectancy. Worldwide the highest average life expectancy is 82 years for women and 76 years for men in Japan.

Life expectancy hasn't always been this long; for primitive humans, it was about 20 to 35 years. It increased to about 49 years in Medieval England and remained so until the turn of this century. During the last 80 years, life expectancy for nearly all peoples of the world has increased, mainly because of changes in the principal causes of death.

At the turn of this century, infectious diseases commonly caused death. Vaccines and antibiotics have tremendously lowered death from disease. The decline in infant and childhood deaths, coupled with better diets and health care, has allowed more people to age first into maturity and then into older years; especially in developed countries. Now the principal causes of death in Western societies are related to heart disease and cancer (Table 1-1).

Historically the trend in America has been toward an ever-older population. During colonial times, half the population was over 16 years of age. By 1990, half were over 33. By 2050, half could be over 43, and approximately 20% of the entire U.S. population will be 65 years and older, twice as many as reach 65 today. This age—65 years—is arbitrarily listed as a dividing line for the beginning of later life because one can qualify for full Social Security benefits. When old age occurs, however, it varies for each of us according to health and independence. Some people are quite healthy and independent at age 65, whereas others are disabled and greatly dependent on assistance for activities of daily living.

Among the older population the group constituting those aged 85+ years is the fastest growing segment. Between 1997 and 2050 the population aged 85+ years is expected to increase from about 3.4 million to more than 19 million. This is the first time in history any society will need to deal with such a large population of older people.

The "Graying" of America

The "graying" of America just described poses some potential problems. Today, while people older than age 65 account for 13% of the U.S. population, they account for more than 25% of all prescription medications used, 40% of acute care hospital stays, and 50% of the federal health budget. Hip fractures alone cost our nation about $10 billion per year. Of older persons, 85% have nutrition-related problems, such as heart problems, Type 2 diabetes, high blood pressure, osteoporosis, and obesity.

Postponing these chronic diseases for as long as possible will help control health-care costs. The more independent, healthy years people live, the better life can be for them and the less they burden the health-care system, which will increasingly have to scramble to accommodate a growing elderly population. Note that the diseases that commonly accompany old age—osteoporosis and atherosclerosis, for example—are not an inevitable part of aging. Many can be prevented or managed, for the most part. Some people do die of old age, not as a direct result of disease.

What Actually Is Aging?

One view of aging describes it as processes of slow cell death beginning soon after fertilization. When we are young, aging is not apparent because the major metabolic activities are directed toward growth and maturation. We produce plenty of active cells to meet physiological needs. During late adolescence and adulthood the body's major task is to maintain cells. Inevitably, though, cells age and die. Eventually, as more cells die, the body can't adjust to meet all physiological demands. Body functioning begins to decrease (Figure 14–2). Still, organs usually retain enough **reserve capacity** so that for a long time the body shows no outward disease. Although no symptoms appear, subclinical disease may develop, and if the disease is allowed to progress unchecked, organ function and then body function eventually deteriorate noticeably.

Reserve capacity
The extent to which an organ can preserve essentially normal function despite decreasing cell number or cell activity.

The aging process is clearly illustrated by changes for many people in the function of the enzyme lactase. For some people, lactase activity in the small intestine slows during childhood. Generally, however, clear symptoms of the deficiency—gas and bloating after generous milk consumption—do not appear until adulthood. Although lactase output decreases in these cases, perhaps from birth, enough enzyme is present to digest the lactose consumed until adulthood.

Cells age probably because of automatic cellular changes and environmental influences. Even in the most supportive of environments, cell structure and function inevitably change. Eventually, cells lose their ability to regenerate the internal parts they need, and they die. As more and more cells in an organ system die, organ function decreases. After age 14 months, human brain cells are continually lost, but we have enough reserve capacity to maintain mental function throughout life. **Kidney nephrons** are also continually lost. In some people this loss leads to eventual kidney failure, but most of us maintain sufficient kidney function. Again, in aging, there is first a reduction in reserve capacity. Only after that is exhausted does actual organ function noticeably decrease.

Kidney nephrons
Unit of kidney cells that filters wastes from the bloodstream and deposits them into the urine.

The causes of this aging are still a mystery. Most likely, aging results from an interaction of genetic background and the changes listed in Table 14–1. Even very

TABLE 14-1

Current Hypotheses About the Causes of Aging

Errors occur in copying the genetic blueprint (DNA)

Once sufficient errors in DNA copying accumulate, a cell can no longer synthesize the major proteins needed to function and it therefore dies.

Connective tissue stiffens

Parallel protein strands, found mostly in connective tissue, chemically bond and cross-link to each other. The bonding decreases flexibility in key body components altering organ function (e.g. joints and arteries stiffen).

Electron-seeking compounds damage cell parts

Electron-seeking free radicals can break down cell membranes and proteins. One way to prevent some damage from these compounds is to consume adequate amounts of vitamins E and C, selenium, and carotenoids. Use of supplements to help meet these needs is discussed later in the chapter.

Hormone function changes

The blood concentration of many hormones, such as testosterone in men and estrogen in women, fall during the aging process. Replacement of these and other hormones is possible; research is ongoing (see the Nutrition Insight).

Glycosylation of proteins

Blood glucose, when chronically elevated, attaches to various blood and body proteins. This decreases protein function and can encourage immune system attack on such altered proteins. Such problems are typical of people with poorly controlled diabetes.

The Immune system loses some efficiency

The immune system is most efficient during childhood and young adulthood, but with advancing age it is less able to recognize and counteract foreign substances, such as viruses, that enter the body. Nutrient deficiencies, particularly of protein, vitamin E, vitamin B-6, and zinc, also hamper immune function (see Chapter 3).

Autoimmunity develops

Autoimmune reactions occur when white blood cells and other immune bodies fail to distinguish between substances normally present in the body and invading foreign proteins. White blood cells and other immune bodies then begin to attack body tissues in addition to foreign proteins. Many diseases, including some forms of arthritis, involve this autoimmune response.

Death is programmed into the cell

Each human cell can divide only about 50 times. Once this number of divisions occurs, the cell automatically succumbs. This degradation occurs by design, probably as a way for the body to regulate cell number. One mechanism for this limitation is that DNA shortens in length with every cell division. Recall from Chapter 7 that cancer cells defeat this shortening, in turn allowing for immortal growth.

Excess energy intake speeds body breakdown

Underfed animals, such as spiders, mice, and rats, live longer. Scientists have yet to pinpoint the exact mechanisms that allow for life extension in calorie-restricted animals (see the Nutrition Insight).

healthy people have a shortened life expectancy if they are exposed to sufficient environmental stress, such as radiation and certain chemical agents like industrial solvents. Because cell aging and diseases such as cancer are aggravated by environmental factors, it makes good sense to avoid such risks as excessive sunlight exposure and hazardous chemicals. Again, as has been stressed, we have some control over how quickly we age.

With regard to vitamins, as noted in Chapter 7 some scientists suggest that each day adults should consume from 250 to 500 milligrams of vitamin C, and 100 to 800 IU of vitamin E, as an additional means to prevent chronic age-related disease. For minerals, 200 micrograms of selenium per day has been promoted (see Chapter 8). This advice is reasonable to consider if one's physician approves of the

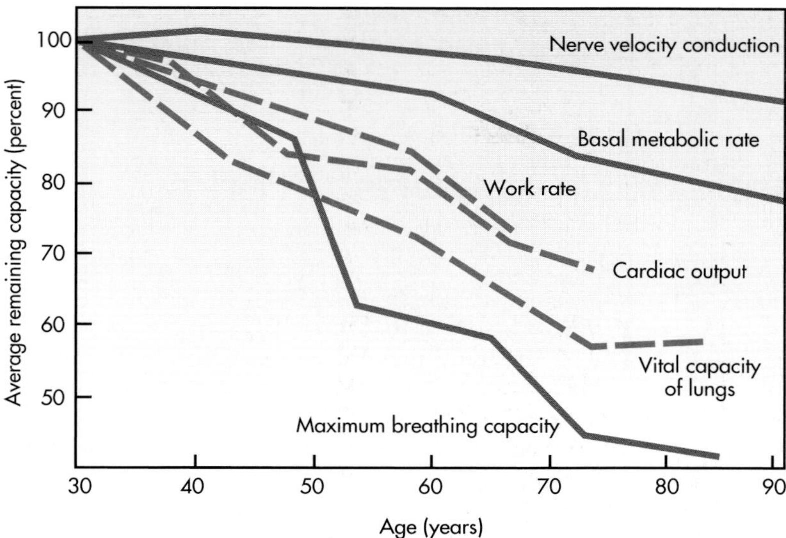

Figure 14-2 *Declines in physiological function seen with aging. The decline in many body functions is especially evident in sedentary people.*

practice, but does not enjoy universal support by nutrition experts at this time. In addition, this emphasis on supplements doesn't substitute for the other practices recommended in the introductory section in this chapter. Recall the discussion of the health-promoting effects of phytochemicals in Chapter 2. Few of these are present in supplements. In addition, the longest lived peoples in the world—for example rural people in China—do not use supplements, as these are not routinely available. This observation reinforces the importance of diet and an active lifestyle for both disease prevention and extending of one's healthy years of life.

Overall, use of any supplement or related product to slow aging should be seen as experimental and necessitates careful supervision by a physician to look out for possible ill effects. You can get a free fact sheet on supplements and aging by going to the web site for the National Institute on Aging at http://www.nih.gov/nia or by calling (800) 222-2225.

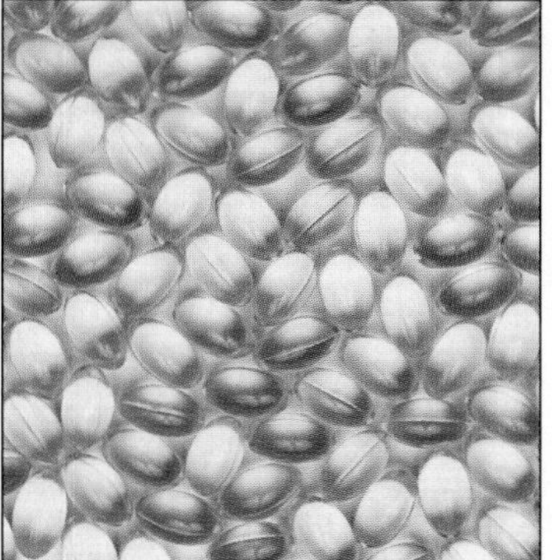

Nutrient supplements can complement, but should not substitute for a more comprehensive plan to maintain health as one ages.

ConceptCheck

Although life span has not changed, life expectancy has increased dramatically over the past century. In many societies this means an increasing proportion of the population is, and will be, over 65 years of age. Avoiding continually rising health-care costs and maximizing satisfaction with life require postponing and minimizing chronic illness. Aging begins early in life and probably results from both automatic cellular changes and environmental influences. Some current hypotheses of aging suggest these possible causes: errors in DNA accumulate, connective tissue stiffens, electron-seeking free-radical compounds break down cell parts, hormonal and immune systems don't function well, and autoimmune responses and high blood glucose damage key body compounds. Diet can play a role in slowing some of these processes. Use of supplements, medical therapies and energy restriction to do so are in experimental phases.

Insight

Reversing the March of Time—What Works to Slow Aging?

Effective Interventions

Healthy Diet

Some of the longest-lived peoples of the world live in Japan and China. Researches suggest that a diet based on rice, fish, vegetable protein sources, fruits, vegetables, and limited meat contributes to this record longevity in Japan. In China a diet based on rice, corn, vegetables, and tea is a likely reason. Use of supplements to correct nutrient deficiencies also has been shown to improve the span of healthy years in older people in the United States (see later section).

Spartan Energy Intake

For many years, scientists have known that underfed animals live longer. All other nutrient needs are met, but calories are restricted. Scientists have not yet pinpointed the exact mechanism that allows for life extension in calorie-restricted animals, but they speculate that modified glucose use, decreased free-radical damage, changes in gene function, less cell metabolism, and a variety of other factors contribute to longer life. Researchers are currently studying rhesus monkeys that are on a 30% lower energy intake than typical rhesus monkeys. Though the calorie-restricted monkeys have lower blood pressure, blood cholesterol, and triglycerides, and higher HDL after 17 years, it is too soon to analyze the full implications of this severe restriction. On the downside, the monkeys have the same appetite as typical monkeys, making them somewhat desperate for food; their bone density is reduced; and their reproductive ability is in question.

Like the rhesus monkeys above, humans housed in Biosphere II had to follow a limited diet because they overestimated their ability to grow their own food. They experienced declines in body weight, blood pressure, blood cholesterol, and blood glucose on the spartan 1800-kcal diets. These parameters remained at the low end of healthy values. It is unknown whether adults in general would voluntarily restrict themselves to this degree in order to obtain the same health benefits (Figure 14–3).

Aerobic and Strength-Training Physical Activity

Older adults who exercise regularly to their capacity add from months to years to their life. From simple brisk walking to water aerobics and light weightlifting—any activity is helpful. Physical activity increases muscle strength and mobility, improves mental outlook, eases daily tasks that require some strength, improves sleep and balance, slows bone loss, and increases joint movement, reducing injuries. However, when older adults stop their weight-training and exercise programs, gains in muscle strength are quickly lost. This illustrates the importance of regular physical activity throughout life.

THE MIDDLETONS
OH NO! BUD JONES, MY OLD ARMY PAL, PASSED AWAY.
HE WAS YOUR AGE, WASN'T HE?
YEAH- IT MAKES YOU THINK! YOU'VE GOT TO GRAB LIFE BY THE HORNS! GO FOR THE BRASS RING!
SIEZE THE DAY!
©1996 Tribune Media Services, Inc. All Rights Reserved
LEAVE THAT GALLON OF ROCKY ROAD, I'VE GOT SOME LIVING TO DO!
5-13

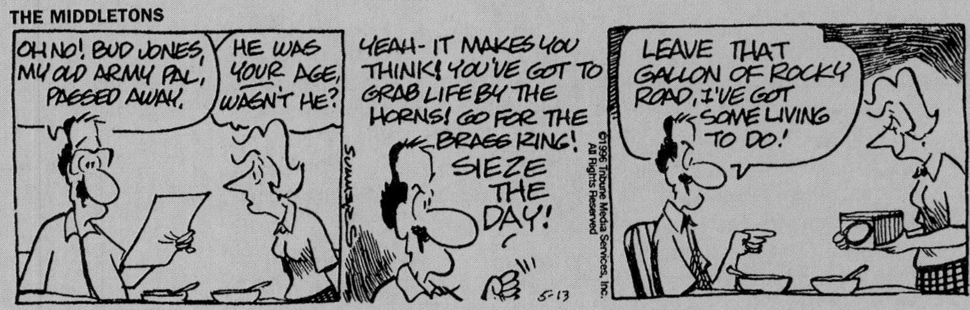

Figure 14–3 *The Middletons.*

After obtaining their physician's approval to get started, older people can seek out programs to begin strength and aerobic training at community recreation centers or the local YMCA or YWCA. Most of these organizations have qualified trainers who can help set up a program. Dumbbells are inexpensive and thus ideal for performing weight training at home. Chapter 10 provides some general advice on this topic, including advice for warm-up, stretching, and cooldown activities. Overall, much of what we associate with aging in terms of physical health results from long-standing sedentary lifestyles.

Estrogen Replacement in Women

Estrogen replacement in women has been shown to extend life up to about 40 months. There are risks to such estrogen use, as reviewed in Chapter 8, but many older women are appropriate candidates for the therapy. It is wise for older women to investigate whether such use is in their best interest.

Experimental Medical Therapies

Growth Hormone

A fall in growth hormone concentration is also being investigated as a potentially treatable hormonal cause of aging. Growth hormone stimulates protein synthesis in cells, such as muscle cells, as well as produces various other effects in the body. However, replacing growth hormone has wide-ranging, unpredictable effects and is very costly. Studies so far support the hypothesis that growth hormone–related loss of lean body mass plays a role in aging. Still, once treatment with growth hormone in adults is stopped, gains in lean body mass are lost.

The risks and benefits of this treatment probably will be known within 2 or 3 years, but it could take another 5 to 10 years to determine the best dosage. Growth hormone therapy has been associated with significant adverse side effects, such as **carpal tunnel syndrome** and breast development in men, and possibly high blood pressure, diabetes-like symptoms, and colon cancer. All these problems may limit its clinical usefulness in older people. Growth hormone is currently available only by prescription.

Testosterone

Testosterone concentration declines with age. This decline in testosterone is linked to a decline in muscle strength. Studies support the concept that a subgroup of older males may benefit from testosterone therapy. Postmenopausal women, especially those who have undergone surgical menopause, may also be candidates for testosterone therapy if estrogen therapy alone does not reduce menopausal symptoms. Note that there are some side effects with use, such as masculinizing effects in women, a decline in HDL in the blood, and prostate gland enlargement. Treatment is still in the experimental phase and currently is not generally recommended due to possible side effects.

Dubious, Unregulated, and Potentially Dangerous Interventions

The 1994 Dietary Supplement Health and Education Act passed in 1994 opened the door for sale of previously banned substances. (Recall that this was discussed in Chapter 1.) As long as the manufacturers claim these products to be "food supplements," they avoid the need for careful premarket testing of safety and efficacy. Thus use of any of the following substances requires careful physician monitoring for potential ill effects. In addition, since these products are not closely regulated by FDA, purity and potency are often different than the label suggests. One cannot have the same confidence in their use as with prescription medications. The latter are carefully regulated for purity and potency and provide full disclosure of potential benefits and risks.

DHEA

The hormone *dehydroepiandrosterone (DHEA)* circulates at extremely high concentration in young adults and falls after the age of 30. This change has led to speculation that DHEA decline plays a role in aging. However, the physiological function of this steroid hormone is unclear, and long-term effects of using products containing this hormone are also unknown. Unfortunately, many Americans do not know that DHEA can cause acne, irritability, fall in HDL in the blood, insomnia, masculinization of women, prostate gland enlargement, and possibly prostate and breast cancer. Until

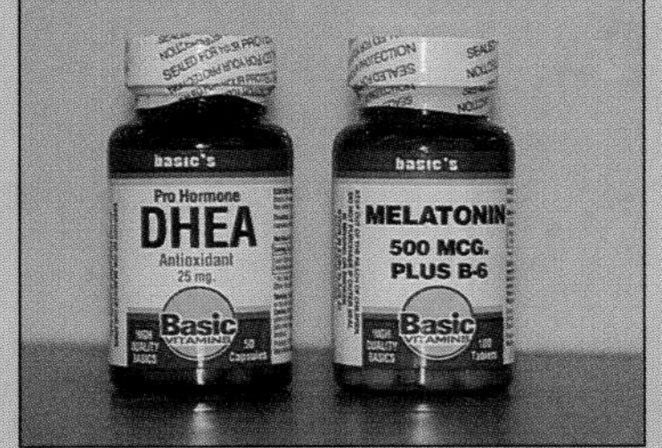

A variety of products are advocated to slow aging. No research to date supports such effectiveness in humans.

long-term studies ensure the safety of DHEA, extreme caution should accompany any use of this still mysterious hormone. Note that many adult men show prostate gland enlargement, making DHEA use for them a very risky proposition.

Melatonin

Production of the hormone melatonin declines after puberty. Melatonin is known for its ability to induce sleep; preliminary laboratory animal studies suggest that it may also slow the aging process. Still, few if any of the studies showing this antiaging property are reliable enough to prove this claim. Leading melatonin researchers note that little is known about the long-term effects of this treatment on humans; there is evidence that it reduces ovulation in women. In fact, French, British, and Canadian governments have banned its sale. Overall, until it is shown to be safe and effective, it is premature to take melatonin preparations in the hope of slowing the aging process.

Coenzyme Q-10

Coenzyme Q-10, an enzyme used in energy metabolism, is very popular in Japan and is also sold in the United States. Early studies were promising in showing that the enzyme worked as an antioxidant, slowed aging, and treated heart failure, but the studies were small and short term. More research is needed to prove any benefits from Coenzyme Q-10. The body produces much Coenzyme Q-10, and it is widely distributed in the food supply.

In summary, there is no pill that substitutes for a healthy diet and physical activity. Some medical interventions look promising for selected persons; physician monitoring is crucial in all cases.

The Effects of Aging on the Nutritional Health of Older People

Older adults vary more in health status among themselves than do persons in any other age-group. This means that chronological age is not so useful in predicting physical health status (physiological age). As noted earlier, among people aged 65 and over, some are totally independent, healthy people, whereas others are frail and require almost total care. To predict the nutritional problems of an older person, it is necessary to know the extent of physiological change caused by aging and whether the person shows early warning signs for long-term poor nutrition. As you examine how aging affects body systems and how these changes contribute to nutritional health, note the suggested ways to lessen health risks in your life and adopt changes in diet to counteract problem conditions (Table 14–2).

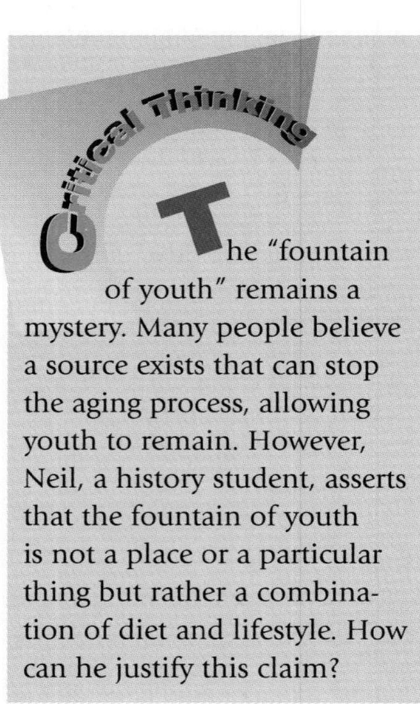

The "fountain of youth" remains a mystery. Many people believe a source exists that can stop the aging process, allowing youth to remain. However, Neil, a history student, asserts that the fountain of youth is not a place or a particular thing but rather a combination of diet and lifestyle. How can he justify this claim?

Decreased Appetite and Food Intake

Decreases in body weight are common in adults age 65 to 90, who may not eat enough to meet energy needs. Many causes of inadequate food intake in older people are possible. Researchers suggest that biological origins, such as changes in blood-borne factors that influence feeding, account for some of this (see Chapter 1 for a review of these factors). Changes in taste and smell may also be important. In addition, social aspects play a role in reduced food intake. Many older people live alone, a circumstance that is associated with less food consumption.

To maintain health, older adults need to address the issue of declining weight. Significant weight loss in older people, sometimes termed the "dwindles," increases risk of illness and death. It may also indicate ongoing illness and reduced tolerance to medication, or simple withdrawal from life itself. Even in apparently healthy older individuals, successful weight maintenance may require an increased conscious control over food intake relative to that of younger individuals. Consuming energy-dense snacks between meals is one strategy, such as nuts, yogurt, oatmeal cookies, and bananas. Later in the chapter other ideas are presented.

TABLE 14-2

Typical Physiological Changes Experienced by Older Adults and Recommended Diet Lifestyle Responses

Change	Response
Decrease in appetite and food intake	Monitor weight and strive to eat enough to maintain healthy weight (see Table 14–4 for ideas)
Decline in sense of taste and smell	Vary the diet and experiment with herbs and spices
Loss of teeth	Work with dentist to maximize chewing ability; modify food consistency as necessary
Decreased sense of thirst	Consume about 6 to 8 cups of fluid each day, and watch for evidence of dehydration (e.g., minimal urine output)
Constipation	Consume 20 to 35 grams of dietary fiber daily, choosing primarily fruits, vegetables, and whole grains; meet fluid needs (as above)
Decline in lactase production	Limit milk serving size; consume yogurt or cheese; seek other calcium sources (see Chapter 8 for ideas)
Iron-deficiency anemia	Include some lean meat in the diet; ask one's physician to monitor blood iron status
Decline in liver function	Consume alcohol in moderation, if at all
Decline in insulin function	Maintain healthy body weight and perform regular physical activity
Decline in kidney function	Modify protein and other nutrients in diet when advised by physician
Decline in immune function	Meet nutrient needs, especially protein, vitamin E, vitamin B-6, and zinc.
Decline in lung function	Don't smoke tobacco products; perform regular physical activity
Decline in vision	Consume fruits and vegetables regularly to gain benefit of carotenoids and vitamin C
Decrease in lean tissue	Meet nutrient needs, and perform regular physical activity, including some resistance activity (see Chapter 10)
Decrease in cardiovascular function	Keep blood lipids and blood pressure within desirable range, using diet and medications when needed (see Chapter 5 and 8); stay physically active.
Decrease in bone mass	Meet nutrient needs, especially calcium and vitamin D, and perform regular physical activity (see Chapter 8)

What we see as the physiological changes associated with aging is the sum of natural processes and lifestyle practices. By adopting practices that minimize a decline in body function in the adult years, we invest in our future health.

The Senses of Taste and Smell

Sensitivity to taste and smell often decreases with age, starting at about age 60. Food may require stronger seasonings. An inadequate diet and possibly zinc deficiency can also contribute to a loss of taste, however. Therefore a poor appetite should never be dismissed as a characteristic of old age. Many causes can be remedied by measures such as making sure to vary the diet and adding extra seasonings and condiments.

Pharmaceutical companies have recently begun to market liquid meal-replacement formulas to older adults. Previously, these products were primarily used in hospitals and nursing homes. These products are protein rich and have a fat content similar to 2% or whole milk, with added vitamins and minerals. It generally takes 4 cups (1 liter) or more of the product to yield the Daily Values for vitamins and minerals, at an energy cost of about 1000 kcal. Many of these products have an unusual taste because of the vitamins that have been added. Older adults can decide if the convenience, cost, and taste make this a wise diet choice.

Dental Health

About 30% or more older people in the United States have lost all their teeth. Attention to dental hygiene and dental care throughout life greatly lessens this risk. Gum disease commonly causes tooth loss. Replacement dentures enable some to chew normally, but many older adults—especially men—have denture problems. Solving individual dietary needs requires identifying foods that need to be modified in consistency. When people have problems chewing, the nutrient-dense snacks just mentioned can help, as well as cutting food into small pieces. Sometimes just allowing extra time for chewing and swallowing encourages more eating.

Thirst

Older adults often partially lose their sense of thirst and in turn don't drink enough fluids. They are then more likely to become dehydrated, a condition that leads to confusion and sometimes hospitalization. It is important for them to consume enough fluids, and if necessary, they should be monitored to ensure they do so. About 6 to 8 cups of fluid daily is a good goal. This amount must be adjusted if diuretics are used or in certain other medical conditions.

Gastrointestinal Tract

The main intestinal problem for older people is constipation (see Chapter 3 for a review of this problem). To keep the intestinal tract performing efficiently, older people generally need to consume more dietary fiber than they characteristically did in their youth. The goal is approximately 10 to 13 grams per 1000 kcal in the diet but generally no more than 35 grams on a daily basis. Regular consumption of nuts, fruits, vegetables, beans, and whole grains provides enough dietary fiber. They should also drink enough fluid to move along masses that could form from high fiber intake. Physical activity likewise helps keep things moving smoothly. Because medications can induce constipation, a physician should be consulted if constipation might be related to a medication.

As noted earlier, lactase production frequently decreases with age. Chapter 4 listed several options for people with lactose intolerance. The stomach has less acid output as people age, usually limiting, in turn, absorption of vitamin B-12, and eventually, to pernicious anemia. People over 50 years of age are now advised to seek a vitamin B-12 fortified food source, such as a breakfast cereal, or take a supplement that contains vitamin B-12. This use of such synthetic sources of vitamin B-12 helps compensate for the fall in absorption seen in older years (see Chapter 7).

Less stomach acid may also hamper iron absorption. Other conditions that affect the body's iron status occur with regular use of aspirin, which frequently causes blood loss in the stomach, and use of antacids, which may bind iron. Ulcers and hemorrhoids can also cause blood loss. Careful attention to iron status is necessary in these cases.

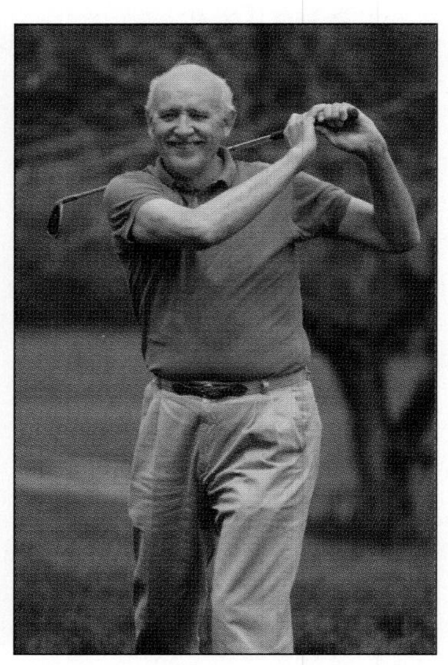

Age is no reason not to continue whatever physical activity is possible. This contributes to many aspects of health, including that of the GI tract.

Liver, Gallbladder, and Pancreas

With age the liver functions less efficiently. When there is a history of significant alcohol consumption, fat buildup in the liver accounts for some decline. Alcohol abuse is a problem among a small but significant group of older individuals who may continue this pattern from earlier in life or develop heavy drinking patterns and alcoholism later. Later development of this problem sometimes arises from the loneliness and social isolation of retirement or loss of a spouse. Alcohol-related sickness is greater in older people, so the health consequences of this excess are considerable. Also, older adults are more likely to take medications that increase alcohol's deleterious effects. If cirrhosis then ultimately develops, the liver functions even less efficiently (see the Nutrition Issue at the end of this chapter).

When its function significantly deteriorates, the liver cannot efficiently detoxify many substances. The possibility for vitamin A toxicity in turn increases. Elderly people should be warned not to take excessive amounts of vitamin A.

The gallbladder also functions less efficiently as we age. Gallstones may dam up the bile to be secreted through the gallbladder, causing it to pool and back up into the liver instead. Gallstones can also interfere with fat digestion by allowing less bile into the small intestine. A low-fat diet or surgery may be necessary.

Although the digestive function of the pancreas may decline with age, the pancreas has a large reserve capacity. A sign of a failing pancreas is high blood glucose, which occurs under several different conditions. Glucose may circulate in the bloodstream, instead of being taken up by cells, because the pancreas secretes less insulin or because cells resist insulin actions—especially adipose (fat) cells in obese people with upper-body fat storage. Another cause can be insufficient chromium intake. Where appropriate, improved nutrient intake, regular physical activity, and weight loss can improve insulin action and blood glucose regulation.

Since 1958 the number of Americans with Type 2 diabetes has tripled, mostly because the population is getting older and more obese. Currently about 16 million Americans have Type 2 diabetes, an increase of 5 million since just 1983.

Kidney Function

Over time the kidneys filter wastes more slowly as they lose nephrons (filters). As noted in Chapter 6, kidneys deteriorate more often in people who have regularly eaten excessive protein. The deterioration significantly decreases the kidneys' ability to excrete the products of protein breakdown, and may eventually require medical therapy.

Lung Function

Lung efficiency declines somewhat with age and is especially pronounced in older people who have smoked and continue to smoke tobacco products. The decrease in lung efficiency contributes to a general downward spiral in body function; breathing difficulties limit physical activity and endurance and frequently discourage eating. Besides not smoking, being physically active helps prevent lung problems. People need not lose their capacity to breathe deeply, as long as sufficient aerobic activity is part of their regular routine.

Hearing and Vision

Hearing and vision both decline in aging. Hearing impairment occurs mainly in members of industrial societies with urban traffic and aircraft noise and loud music. Elderly people may also avoid social contacts because they can't hear.

Degenerating eyesight, frequently caused by retinal degeneration, can affect a person's ability to physically get to a grocery store, locate the foods desired, read labels for nutritional content, and prepare the foods at home. Regular consumption of foods rich in carotenoids, in particular dark green, leafy vegetables, such as kale, collard greens, spinach, Swiss chard, mustard greens, and romaine lettuce, decreases the risk of developing retinal degeneration. Corn, pumpkin, zucchini, and oranges can be added to the list. These vegetables are rich in lutein and/or zeaxanthin, two carotenoids found in the portion of the eye subject to damage from age-related degeneration. Such vision changes may make people afraid to socialize, be active, or take care of important routines of daily life, such as shopping. Recall from Chapter 7 the role vitamin C plays in reducing cataracts in the eye. This benefit serves as another reason adults should have a diet rich in fruits and vegetables.

In addition to physical exercise, some experts recommend that the elderly exercise their minds by doing jigsaw and crossword puzzles, playing bridge, and participating in a variety of other thought-provoking activities. These activities help retain brain function, just as physical exercise helps maintain physical function.

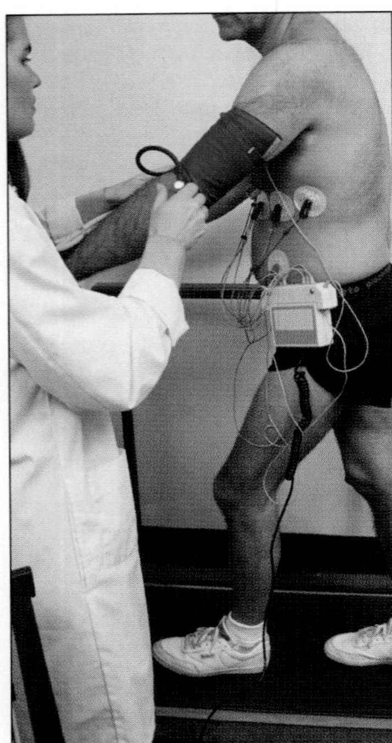

Anyone over 35 years of age is advised to obtain physician approval before beginning a program of vigorous physical activity. The physician may suggest an exercise treadmill test be done to assess exercise tolerance.

Decrease in Lean Tissue

Some muscle cells shrink and others are lost as muscles age; some muscles lose their ability to contract as they accumulate fat and collagen protein. Lifestyle greatly determines the rate of muscle mass deterioration. As you might predict, an active lifestyle tends to maintain muscle mass, whereas a very inactive one encourages its loss. Ideally an active lifestyle should include some resistance activity (weight training) throughout life. The latter reduces muscle loss in older people. In addition, maintaining adequate muscle mass provides a reserve for illness. This then contributes to one's recovery back to health. After obtaining their physician's approval to get started, older people should seek out programs to begin strength and aerobic training.

Older adults also benefit from physical activity because it stimulates food intake by raising energy expenditure. By eating more, they increase their chances of consuming adequate amounts of nutrients. Overall, much of what we associate with aging in terms of physical health results from long-standing sedentary lifestyles.

Increases in Fat Stores

As lean tissue decreases with age, the body often takes on more fat. Much of this results from overeating and minimal physical activity. If obesity results, this is not desirable, especially because it can raise blood pressure and blood glucose. Obesity can also make walking and performing daily tasks more difficult. Although a small fat gain in adulthood may not compromise health, large gains are often problematic.

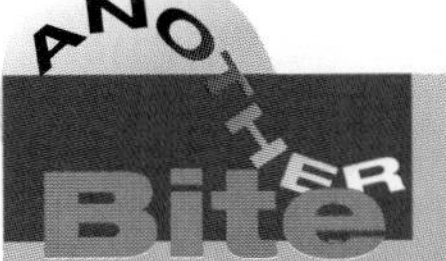

In early adulthood and middle age, significant weight gain is a major problem. Late in life, weight loss—especially if unintentional—is more of a concern. Weight loss in older people often means increased risk of death. It may also indicate increased sickness and poor tolerance of medications. When assessing weight in older people, compare present weight with the previous year's weight.

Cardiovascular Health

The heart often pumps blood less efficiently in older people, usually because of insufficient physical activity. Poor heart conditioning allows fatty and connective tissues to infiltrate the heart's muscular wall. This decline in **cardiac output** is not inevitable with aging; it does not occur as much among older people who remain physically active.

Heart attack and stroke, the major causes of death in all adults, are caused primarily by atherosclerosis and high blood pressure. You already know the main way to limit the buildup of atherosclerotic plaque: keep your LDL and total cholesterol/HDL ratio in the desirable range (see Chapter 5). New evidence shows that a diet very low in fat (vegan diet) can cause some plaques to decrease in size. Other studies use diet and medications to lower blood cholesterol, which in turn reduces the amount of plaque in the arteries supplying the heart. This suggests that a heart-healthy diet is more important during middle to late adulthood than researchers previously thought. Consuming sufficient vitamin B-6, folate, and vitamin B-12 is also important to avoid elevated blood homocysteine, an additional risk factor for heart disease.

Cardiac output
The amount of blood pumped by the heart.

Treating elevated LDL in an older person who has other illnesses, such as chronic lung disease and **dementia,** which are likely to shorten life as well as hamper its quality, is probably inappropriate. But if a healthy 70-year-old who is likely to live another 10 to 15 years has both elevated LDL and evidence of heart disease or suffered a heart attack, an eating and exercise plan is probably in order to reduce the chance of more problems. Note also that the advisability of fat restrictions for the very old (those older than 85 years of age) for the prevention of chronic disease is questionable. Dietary modifications should be made instead to respond to the current disease state, such as the presence of diabetes or failing kidney function.

Dementia
General persistent loss or decrease in mental function.

High blood pressure is heavily implicated in both stroke and heart attack in older adults. The Nutrition Insight in Chapter 8 reviews the roles of diet and lifestyle interventions on blood pressure, such as eating a balanced diet (especially one rich in fruits and vegetables high in potassium), walking briskly and otherwise performing regular physical activity, maintaining healthy weight, and moderating alcohol intake.

Bone Health

Chapter 8 discussed the decline in bone health associated with aging. Recall that bone loss in women occurs primarily after menopause. Bone loss in men is slow and steady from middle age throughout later life. Estrogen replacement at menopause is the most reliable treatment to lessen bone loss in women. Other medication regimens are also possible. Further measures to prevent bone loss can be started earlier and continued throughout life—maintaining adequate calcium and vitamin D nutriture (see later section), not smoking, and drinking alcohol moderately, if used. Underweight women are at especially high risk for developing osteoporosis. Performing weight-bearing activity, such as walking, also helps sustain bone.

Very severe osteoporosis limits the ability of older people to move about, shop, prepare food, and live normally. They eat less and get fewer nutrients. Older people should also work with their physicians to develop a plan for limiting falls. Falls may be caused by the side effects of medication, gait and balance disorders, impaired vision, and environmental hazards (e.g., icy steps, loose throw rugs).

Other Factors That Influence Nutrient Needs in Older Adults

Medications and old age often go together. Medications can improve health and quality of life, but some of them also affect nutrient needs at all ages, including the later years. Sixty-six percent of the elderly population regularly take prescription drugs; many drugs affect appetite or absorption of nutrients. Often, people must take several medications for long periods. They should make sure to work with their physician and pharmacist to coordinate all medications taken. Pharmacists can advise when to take drugs—with or between meals—for greatest effectiveness.

Up to 10% or slightly more of older adults experience significant depression. That—combined with isolation and loneliness as family and friends die, move away, or become less mobile—frequently contributes to apathetic eating and weight loss. People living alone do not necessarily make poor food choices, but they often consume less energy, in part from skipping meals. Older men are especially prone to this habit. About one-third of all older people not in nursing homes live alone. Depression can be a downward spiral in which poor appetite produces weakness that leads to even poorer appetite (Figure 14–4). In older adults the resulting poor nutritional state can produce further mental confusion and increased isolation and loneliness.

Grapefruit juice can affect the potency of some prescription medications, such as certain blood pressure medications, tranquilizers, antihistamines, and others. For this reason a physician or pharmacist should be consulted before grapefruit juice is used by those on prescription medication.

Former President Jimmy Carter recommends that older adults stay connected to life to maximize health. This can include volunteering one's services and helping one's friends through their elder years.

Depression is often treatable, but medication alone will not help those who are experiencing major life changes such as the death of a spouse. Adequate social support also is essential.

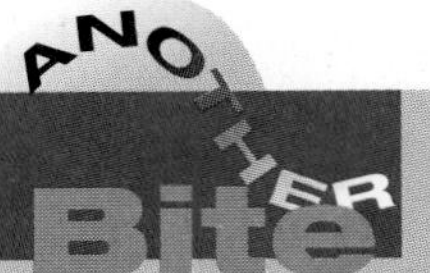

The disease known as Alzheimer's often takes a terrible toll on the mental and eventual physical health of older people. In general terms, Alzheimer's disease is best described as a progressive brain disorder marked by an inability to remember, reason, or understand what is going on. Age is the primary risk factor. Scientists propose causes, including altered cell development and altered brain proteins. Two medications are approved for lessening Alzheimer's symptoms, but they show only limited benefits. Dietary concerns revolve around making sure the person eats enough food to maintain healthy weight and overall nutrient needs and observation of the person's meals to make sure meal habits do not pose a health risk (e.g., holding food in one's mouth or forgetting how to swallow). Warning signs of Alzheimer's disease are recent memory loss that affects job performance, difficulty performing familiar tasks, problems with language, disorientation to time and place, faulty or decreased judgment, problems with abstract thinking, misplacing things, changes in mood or behavior, changes in personality, and loss of initiative. To find out more about Alzheimer's disease you can go to the web site for the Alzheimer's Association at http://www.alz.org, or call (800) 272-3900. You can also call the National Institute on Aging's Alzheimer's Disease Education and Referral Center at (800) 428-4380.

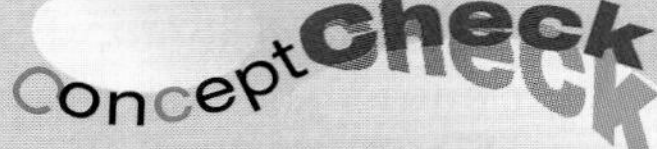

Nutritional problems common to aging adults relate to both the process of chronic diseases and the normal decrease in organ function that occurs with time. All these organ systems and functions can decrease as we age: appetite; sense of taste, smell, thirst, hearing, and sight; digestion and absorption; liver, gallbladder, pancreas, kidneys, lungs, heart; and the immune system. In addition, bone mass and muscle mass gradually decrease, the latter largely because of a deficient diet and inactivity. Appropriate diet changes and regular physical activity can often help reduce the impact of these results of aging.

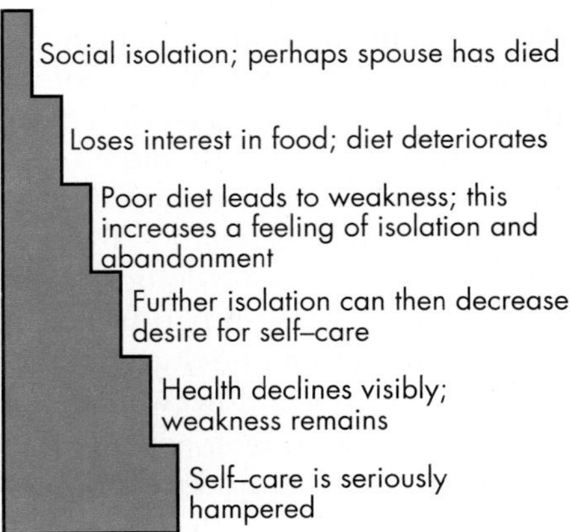

Figure 14–4 *The decline of health often seen in older adults. This decline needs to be prevented whenever possible.*

To What Extent Do Nutrient Needs Change in Later Life?

Only during the last few years has much research focused on this question (Table 14–3). Because the DRIs and remaining 1989 RDAs apply only to healthy people, many older people—for example, those who have ulcers or are heavy aspirin users—are not covered by these standards. Indeed it is particularly tricky to develop nutrient standards that are valid for most older people because so many are ill and/or regularly take medication.

TABLE 14-3

Comparisons of RDAs and AIs of Some Nutrients Between Young and Older Adults

Nutrient	Difference	Advice for consumption
Vitamin B-6	+0.2–0.4 milligrams per day (1.5 to 1.7 milligrams vs 1.3 milligrams)	Consume fortified foods, such as breakfast cereals, or use a balanced supplement.
Vitamin B-12	Obtain synthetic source, up to about 25 micrograms per day.	Consume fortified foods, such as breakfast cereals, or use a balanced supplement.
Vitamin D*	+5–10 micrograms (200 to 400 IU) (400 to 600 IU vs 200 IU)	Use of a supplement would be the most reliable source (up to 600 IU per day). Fortified milk and sun exposure are other options.
Calcium*	+200 milligrams (1200 milligrams vs 1000 milligrams)	Consume more milk products, or find a fortified source, such as orange juice. Supplements in doses less than 500 milligrams per pill are appropriate as well.

*A recent study found that meeting the new recommendations for calcium and vitamin D reduced bone loss and related hip fractures. Older adults need to be aware of the importance of meeting calcium and vitamin D needs.

Researchers have suggested that the current nutrient standards for healthy older people are probably too high for vitamin A; a bit too low in protein (for active people about 1 gram per kilogram of body weight is advised); and likely sufficient for the other vitamins and minerals.

Still, a well-planned diet that follows the Food Guide Pyramid can meet the nutrient needs for older people within about 1600 to 1800 kcal, except for probably folate, vitamin B-12, and calcium. It would take at least three servings from the milk, yogurt, and cheese group for calcium—a recommendation that most older people would find difficult to meet. Calcium-fortified foods can help when necessary (see Chapter 8 for details). Meeting the folate and vitamin B-12 standards also is aided by use of fortified foods, such as breakfast cereals. Use of a balanced nutrient supplement is also appropriate, but it should be low in or free of iron. Women after menopause have iron needs that are the same as men, as they no longer lose iron in menstruation. Recall from Chapter 2 that men should not take a supplement containing iron as they consume enough and it can easily accumulate to toxic amounts in the body. This now applies to women, as they experience minimal iron loss in the postmenopausal state. Finally, if megadose vitamin E use is indicated, this will require a separate supplement.

Planning a Diet for Older People

To supply energy needs for males age 51 and older, the 1989 RDA publication suggests 2300 kcal; for females, the recommendation is 1900 kcal. (These values are based on a 170-pound, 68-inch-tall man and a 143-pound, 63-inch-tall woman.)

Studies show that older men eat closer to 1800 to 2100 kcal, whereas women eat about 1300 to 1600 kcal. Thus diet plans for older adults should focus on nutrient-rich foods. A good practice is to decrease sugar and fat consumption to increase the diet's nutrient density and to make sure dietary fiber intake is adequate. In addition, some protein should come from lean meats to help meet vitamin B-6 and zinc needs, two nutrients of special concern. Fluid needs are about 6 to 8 cups (about 2 liters) per day.

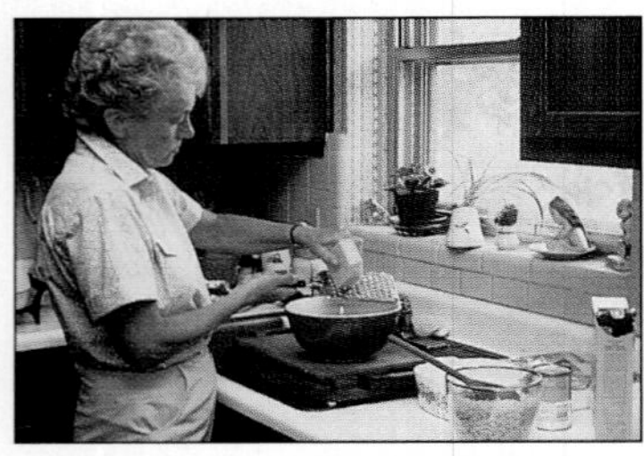

Cooking for just one or two people can be challenging. Consuming half of what is prepared and freezing the other half is one tip.

Singles of all ages face logistical problems with food: purchasing, preparing, storing, and using food with minimal waste are challenging. Economy packages of meats and vegetables are normally too large to be useful for a single person. Many singles live in small dwellings, some without kitchens and freezers. Creating a diet to accommodate a limited budget and facilities and a single appetite requires special considerations. Following are some practical suggestions for diet planning for singles:

- If you own a freezer, cook large amounts, divide into portions, and freeze.
- Buy only what you can use; small containers may be expensive, but letting food spoil is also costly.
- Ask the grocer to break open a family-sized package of wrapped meat or fresh vegetables and separate it into smaller units.
- Buy only several pieces of fruit—perhaps a ripe one, a medium-ripe one, and an unripe one—so that the fruit can be eaten over a period of several days.
- Keep a box of dry milk handy to add a nutritious punch to recipes for baked foods and other foods for which this addition is acceptable.

Nutritional deficiencies and protein-energy undernutrition have been identified among some aging populations, particularly those in nursing homes or long-term care facilities and those who are hospitalized. These nutritional problems increase the risk for many diseases, including bed sores (pressure ulcers), and compromise recovery from illness and surgery. Feeding sick, infirm, and mentally confused people is time-consuming and demanding work that requires special training. Friends, relatives, and health personnel should look for poor nutrient intake in all older people, including those who live in nursing home settings. About 40% of adults now age 65 will spend some time in a nursing home. Family members have a unique opportunity to make sure nutrient needs are met by looking for weight maintenance based on regular, healthful meal patterns. If problems arise in instituting a healthful diet, registered dietitians can offer professional and personalized advice.

Overall, healthy nutrition (and lifestyle habits) benefits older adults in many ways. It delays the onset of some diseases; improves management of some existing diseases; hastens recovery from many illnesses; can increase mental, physical, and social well-being; and often decreases the need for and length of hospitalization. Thus a healthy diet should be a vital part of the health maintenance program for older people. A variety of strategies can promote healthful eating in later life (Table 14–4). These should focus on presenting nutritious, tasty foods in a pleasant environment.

Community Nutrition Services for Older People

Health-care advice and services for older people can come from clinics, private practitioners, hospitals, and health maintenance organizations. Home health-care agencies, adult day-care programs, adult overnight-care programs, and **hospice** centers (for the terminally ill) can supply daily care. Professionals in the above-mentioned organizations can help identify older people whose health needs may require extra attention. Figure 14–5 shows a valuable screening tool, based on the acronym "DETERMINE." When this tools suggests a problem, careful follow-up by a physician is indicated.

DETERMINE

- ***D**isease*
- ***E**ating poorly*
- ***T**ooth loss or mouth pain*
- ***E**conomic hardship*
- ***R**educed social contact and **i**nteraction*
- ***M**ultiple medications*
- ***I**nvoluntary weight loss or gain*
- ***N**eed for assistance with self care*
- ***E**lder at an advanced age*

TABLE 14-4

Guidelines for Healthful Eating in Later Years

- Eat regularly; small, frequent meals may be best. Use nutrient-dense foods as a basis for each menu.
- Find out which convenience foods and labor-saving devices can be of help.
- Try new foods, new seasonings, and new ways of preparing foods. Don't use just convenience foods and canned goods.
- Keep some easy-to-prepare foods and snacks, such as canned fruit and frozen yogurt, on hand for times when you feel tired.
- Have a treat occasionally, perhaps an expensive cut of meat or a favorite fresh fruit.
- Eat in a well-lit or sunny area; serve meals attractively; use foods with different flavors, colors, shapes, textures, and smells.
- Arrange things so food preparation and clean-up are easier.
- Eat with friends, relatives, or at a senior center when possible.
- Share cooking responsibilities with a neighbor.
- Use community resources for help in shopping and other daily care needs.
- Stay physically active.
- If possible, take a walk before eating to stimulate appetite.
- When necessary, chop, grind, or blend hard-to-chew foods. Softer, protein-rich foods can be substituted for meat when poor dental function limits normal food intake. Prepare soups, stews, cooked whole-grain cereals, and casseroles.
- If your eating movements are limited, cut the food ahead of time, use utensils with deep sides or handles, and obtain more specialized utensils if needed.

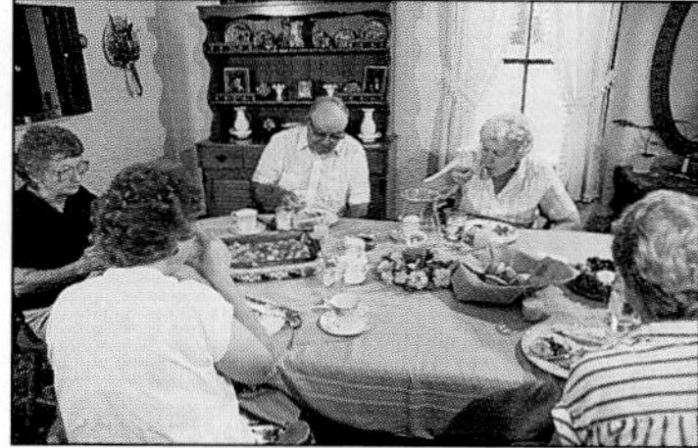

Older people benefit from the friendship of others at meals.

Nutrition programs for those age 60 and over offer congregate meal programs, which provide lunch at a central location, and home-delivered meals (often known as Meals-on-Wheels if sponsored by the local private or public agencies). About 2.3 million Americans are served each year. Currently about 85% of the meals use the home-delivered method. Federal commodity distribution is available in some areas of the United States to low-income older people. Food stamps can benefit older people whose incomes are below the poverty level. Food cooperatives and a variety of clubs and social organizations provide additional aid.

Many eligible older people are missing meals and are poorly nourished simply because they don't know of available programs. Irregular meal patterns and weight loss, often caused by difficulties in preparing food, are warning signs that undernutrition may be developing. An effort should be made to identify and inform poorly nourished people of community services.

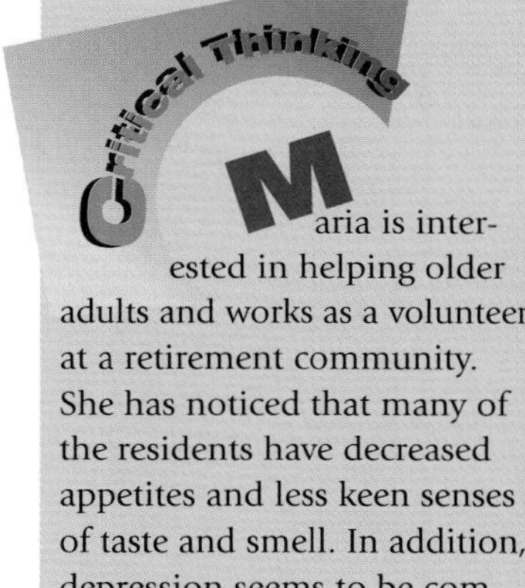

Maria is interested in helping older adults and works as a volunteer at a retirement community. She has noticed that many of the residents have decreased appetites and less keen senses of taste and smell. In addition, depression seems to be common among the residents. How can Maria explain these observations?

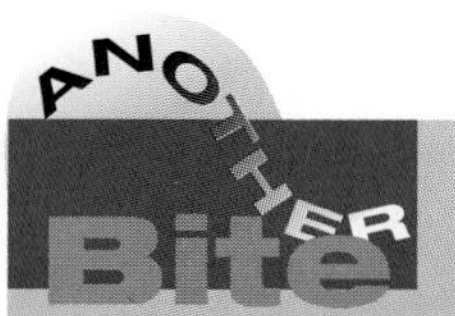

Congregate meal programs can positively influence the nutritional status of otherwise homebound people. Still, congregate meal programs provide at most one meal a day and usually not every day of the week. If people come to depend on them exclusively, they eat too few meals. The problem with home-delivered meals is that the one or two meals delivered may never be eaten, and if not eaten on delivery and left at room temperature, they may become unsafe to eat later. Thus these programs can help older adults but probably don't meet all their nutritional needs.

To learn more about meal programs for senior citizens in your area, call the Administration on Aging's Elder Care Locator, (800) 677-1116 or the web site of the Administration on Aging http://www.aoa.dhhs.gov/.

The ideal is to remain healthy and live independently for as long as possible without becoming socially isolated. Personal living situations can greatly determine whether an older person is well-nourished. For some, just getting to the store or

A Nutrition Test for Older Adults

Here's a nutrition check for anyone over age 65. Circle the number of points for each statement that applies. Then compute the total and check it against the nutritional score.

1. The person has a chronic illness or current condition that has changed the kind or amount of food eaten. (2 points)
2. The person eats fewer than two full meals per day. (3 points)
3. The person eats few fruits, vegetables, or milk products. (2 points)
4. The person drinks 3 or more servings of beer, liquor, or wine almost every day. (2 points)
5. The person has tooth or mouth problems that make eating difficult. (2 points)
6. The person does not have enough money for food. (4 points)
7. The person eats alone most of the time. (1 point)
8. The person takes three or more different prescription or over-the-counter drugs each day. (1 point)
9. The person has unintentionally lost or gained 10 pounds within the last 6 months. (2 points)
10. The person cannot always shop, cook, or feed himself or herself. (2 points)

Nutritional score:

0–2: Good. Recheck in 6 months.

3–5: Marginal. A local agency on aging has information about nutrition programs for the elderly. The National Association of Area Agencies on Aging can assist in finding help; call (800) 677-1116. Recheck in 6 months.

6 or more: High risk. A doctor should review this test and suggest how to improve nutritional health.

Figure 14–5 *A nutrition checklist for elderly people.*

Reprinted with permission by the Nutrition Screening Initiative, a project of the American Academy of Family Physicians, the American Dietetic Association and the National Council on Aging, Inc., and funded in part by a grant from Ross Products Division, Abbott Laboratories.

carrying groceries may be a major problem. Relatives and friends can be a real help. Special transportation arrangements may also be available through a local transit company or taxi service.

Even more insights for helping older persons can be found on the web site of the American Geriatrics Society (http://www.americangeriatrics.org/).

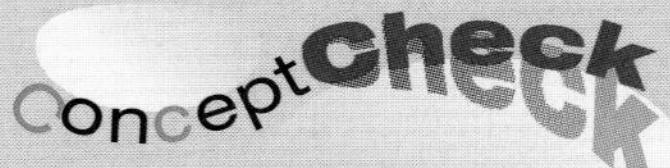

Specific nutrient requirements for older adults are only now being extensively studied. Diet plans should be modified for decreased physical abilities, presence of drug-nutrient interactions, possible depression, and economic constraints. Particular attention should be paid to the opportunity for sun exposure and intake of the vitamins D, B-6, folate, and B-12, as well as the minerals calcium and zinc, and dietary fiber. A nutrient-dense diet along with the use of some fortified foods, such as breakfast cereals, helps to meet these needs. Careful use of supplements is also appropriate. In the United States, many nutrition services—such as congregate and home-delivered meals—are available to help our aging population obtain a healthful diet.

Summary

- A goal for all of us should be to delay symptoms of and disabilities from chronic diseases for as many years as possible. Good nutritional habits, especially those that follow the Food Guide Pyramid and Dietary Guidelines, play a role in this process.
- Although maximum life span hasn't changed, life expectancy has increased dramatically over the past century. For many societies, this means that an increasing proportion of the population is over 65 years of age. As health-care costs rise, the goal of delaying disease becomes even more important for all of us.
- Aging begins before birth. Cell aging probably results from automatic cellular changes and environmental influences, such as DNA damage. Add to this list damage caused by electron-seeking free-radical compounds, high blood glucose, hormonal changes, and alterations in the immune system as possible causes.
- Nutritional problems of older adults are related to the presence of chronic diseases and to the normal decreases in organ function that occur with time. These include loss of teeth, lessened sensitivity in the senses of taste and smell, changes in gastrointestinal tract function, and deterioration in heart and bone health. Although disease affects nutritional state, the reverse is also true. Undernutrition adversely affects immune function, allowing for infection.
- Scientists are only now beginning extensive study of specific nutrient needs for older people. Diet plans should be based on a nutrient-dense approach and individualized for existing health problems, decreased physical abilities, presence of drug-nutrient interactions, possible depression, and economic constraints. Specific nutrients, such as vitamin D, vitamin B-6, folate, vitamin B-12, zinc, and calcium, along with dietary fiber, often deserve special attention in diet planning.
- There are many options available for procurement of food for the elderly, especially for those who are nutritionally compromised. Most communities have congregate or home-delivered meal systems, food stamps, and other provisions for those who qualify.

Study Questions

1. List four of the Dietary Guidelines and give an example of why each one may be difficult for the elderly to implement. What are some solutions to these barriers?
2. What is the difference between life span and life expectancy? As life expectancy increases, what consequence affects the entire population?
3. Name three hormones associated with aging and the attributes of each. What are the risks associated with taking these hormones?

4 Describe two hypotheses proposed to explain the causes of aging and note evidence for each in your daily life experiences.
5 List four organ systems that can decline in function in later years, along with a diet/lifestyle response to help cope with the decline.
6 Defend the recommendation for regular physical activity during late adulthood, including some resistance activity (weight training).
7 How might nutrition needs of older people differ from those of younger people? How are their needs similar? Be specific.
8 What three resources in a community are widely available to aid older adults in maintaining nutritional health?
9 Describe some early warning signs of undernutrition in the elderly and note some of the nutrition implications that arise as this process advances.
10 List four of the screening tools for ill health in the elderly that are part of the acronym DETERMINE. Briefly justify the inclusion of each.

Further Readings

1 Angell M, Kassirer JP: Alternative medicine—the risks of untested and unregulated remedies, *New England Journal of Medicine* 339:839, 1998.
2 Birrer RB: Depression and aging too often do mix, *Postgraduate Medicine* 104(3):143, 1998.
3 Blumberg J: Nutritional needs of seniors, *Journal of the American College of Nutrition* 16:517, 1997.
4 Burge SK: Alcohol-related problems: recognition and intervention, *American Family Physician* 59:361, 1999.
5 Dawson-Hughes B and others: Effect of calcium supplementation on bone density in men and women 65 years of age or older, *New England Journal of Medicine* 337:670, 1997.
6 Hakim AA and others: Effects of walking on mortality among nonsmoking retired men, *New England Journal of Medicine* 338:94, 1998.
7 Harris TB and others: Carrying the burden of cardiovascular risk in old age: associations of weight and weight change with prevalent cardiovascular disease, risk factors, and health status in the Cardiovascular Health Study, *American Journal of Clinical Nutrition* 66:837, 1997.
8 Jensen GL, Rogers J: Obesity in older persons, *Journal of the American Dietetic Association* 98:1308, 1998.
9 Johns-Cupp M: Melatonin, *American Family Physician* 56:1421, 1997.
10 Kleiner SM: Strategies for energetic aging, *The Physician and Sportsmedicine* 26(11):69, 1998.
11 Kerschner H, Pegues JAM: Productive aging: a quality of life agenda, *Journal of the American Dietetic Association* 98:1445, 1998.
12 Living longer, *Mayo Clinic Health Letter* 17(1):1, 1999.
13 McBean LD: Special dietary needs of mature Americans, *Dairy Council Digest* 69:19, 1998.
14 Mlot C: Running on one-third empty: primates on a low-cal diet are in a metabolic slow lane, perhaps to longer life, *Science News* 151:162, 1997.
15 Schaefer DC: Constipation in the elderly, *American Family Physician* 58:907, 1998.
16 Should you start taking over-the-counter hormones? *Tufts University Health & Nutrition Letter*, p.4, July 1997.
17 Tan RS, Bransgrove L: Testosterone replacement therapy, *Postgraduate Medicine* 103(5):247, 1998.
18 Thun MJ and others: Alcohol consumption and mortality among middle-aged and elderly U.S. adults, *New England Journal of Medicine* 337:1705, 1997.
19 Vallee BL: Alcohol in the western world, *Scientific American*, p. 79, June 1998.
20 Vita AJ and others: Aging, health risks, and cumulative disability, *New England Journal of Medicine* 338:1035, 1998.
21 Wellman NS and others: Elder insecurities: poverty, hunger, and malnutrition, *Journal of the American Dietetic Association* 97(suppl 2):S120, 1997.
22 When food just doesn't taste the way it used to, *Tufts University Health & Nutrition Letter*, p. 8, February 1998.

RATE

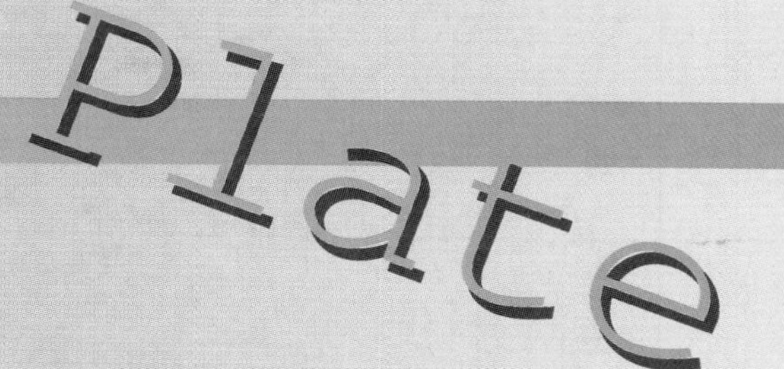

I. Adulthood Issue: Could You or Someone You Know Have a Problem with Alcohol?

The Nutrition Issue in this chapter discusses ethanol, commonly known as *alcohol.* Problem drinking often has its seeds in the teen years. Significant health consequences of this typically arise in adulthood. A prominent contributor to 5 of the 10 leading causes of death in the United States, misuse of alcohol is one of our most preventable health problems. The social consequences of alcohol dependency include divorce, unemployment, and poverty. The following questionnaire was developed by the National Council on Alcoholism. With this assessment you can examine whether you or someone you know might need help. Answer the following questions by placing an "X" in the appropriate blank.

	Yes	No
1. Do you occasionally drink heavily after disappointment, a quarrel, or when someone gives you a hard time?	______	______
2. When you have trouble or feel under pressure, do you drink more heavily than usual?	______	______
3. Have you ever noticed that you're able to handle liquor better than you did when you first started drinking?	______	______
4. Do you ever wake up the morning after you've been drinking and discover that you can't remember part of the evening before, even though your friends tell you that you didn't pass out?	______	______
5. When drinking with other people, do you try to have a few extra drinks when others won't know it?	______	______
6. Are there certain occasions when you feel uncomfortable if alcohol isn't available?	______	______
7. Have you recently noticed that when you begin drinking, you're in more of a hurry to get the first drink than you used to be?	______	______
8. Do you sometimes feel a little guilty about your drinking?		
9. Are you secretly irritated when your family or friends discuss your drinking?	______	______
10. Have you recently noticed an increase in the frequency of memory blackouts?	______	______
11. Do you often find that you wish to continue drinking after your friends say they've had enough?	______	______
12. Do you usually have a reason for the occasions when you drink heavily?	______	______
13. When you're sober, do you often regret things you have done or said while drinking?	______	______
14. Have you tried switching brands or following different plans to control your drinking?	______	______

15. Have you often failed to keep promises you've made to yourself about controlling or stopping your drinking? ________ ________
16. Have you ever tried to control your drinking by changing jobs or moving to a new location? ________ ________
17. Do you try to avoid family or close friends while you're drinking? ________ ________
18. Are you having an increasing number of financial and work problems? ________ ________
19. Do more people seem to be treating you unfairly without good reason? ________ ________
20. Do you eat very little or irregularly when you're drinking? ________ ________
21. Do you sometimes have the "shakes" in the morning and find that it helps to have a little drink? ________ ________
22. Have you recently noticed that you can't drink as much as you once did? ________ ________
23. Do you sometimes stay drunk for several days at a time? ________ ________
24. Do you sometimes feel very depressed and wonder whether life is worth living? ________ ________
25. Sometimes after periods of drinking do you see or hear things that aren't there? ________ ________
26. Do you get terribly frightened after you have been drinking heavily? ________ ________

INTERPRETATION

These are all symptoms that may indicate alcoholism. "Yes" answers to several of the questions indicate the following stages of alcoholism:

Questions 1–8:	Potential drinking problem
Questions 9–21:	Drinking problem likely
Questions 22–26:	Definite drinking problem

It is vital that people assess themselves honestly. If you or someone you know demonstrates some or a number of these symptoms, it is important that help be pursued. If there is even a question in your mind, go talk to a professional about it. Alcohol abuse is one of many problems adults, including older people, face.

II. Older Adult Issue: Helping Older Adults Eat Better

During their lifetimes, most people usually eat meals with families or loved ones. As elderly people reach even older ages, many of them are faced with living and eating alone. In a study of the diets of 4400 older Americans, one man in every five living alone and over age 55 ate poorly. One of four women between the ages of 55 and 64 years followed a low-quality diet. These poor diets can contribute to deteriorating mental and physical health. Consider the following example of the living situation of an older adult:

Neal, a 70-year-old man, lives alone in a house in a local suburban area. He lost his wife 1 year ago. He doesn't have many friends; his wife was his primary confidante. His neighbors across the street and next door are friendly, and Neal used to help them with yard projects in his spare time. Neal's health has been good, but he has had trouble with his teeth recently. His diet has been poor, and in the last 3 months his physical and mental vigor has deteriorated. He has been slowly lapsing into a depression and so keeps the shades drawn and rarely leaves his house. Neal keeps very little food in the house, because his wife did most of the cooking and shopping and he just isn't that interested in food.

If you were one of Neal's relatives and learned of Neal's situation, what six things could you do or suggest to help improve his nutritional status and mental outlook? Look back into the chapter to get some ideas.

1. ______________________________

2. ______________________________

3. ______________________________

4. ______________________________

5. ______________________________

6. ______________________________

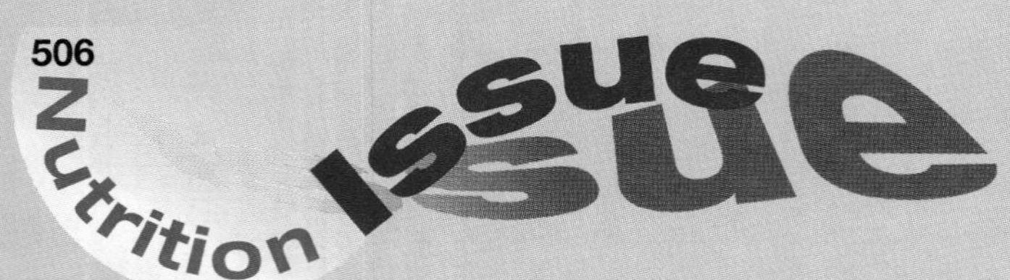

Alcohol—Metabolic, Nutritional, and Social Implications

Alcohol use is an issue requiring careful examination by all of us, including the aged. While moderate drinking decreases the risk for heart disease and stroke, excessive consumption of alcohol is by far the most common drug abuse—wrecking families and friendships; spurring risky behaviors, suicide, and rape and other violence on college campuses; and filling jails. This misuse of alcohol costs American society more than 100,000 lives, with about one-fourth of them from highway deaths, and accounts for as much as $75 billion per year in health-care expenditures. About 15 million Americans currently have alcoholism; about 3 million are over age 60 years. From early adulthood through later years, excess alcohol intake has an enormous detrimental effect on nutritional and overall health. Many of us have witnessed this destruction firsthand.

The reason for this reduction in heart disease and stroke risk with regular alcohol use is still debatable, but probably involves an increase in HDL in the blood and a reduction in blood clotting and overall stress. Certain compounds in red wine may also act as antioxidants and thus may make this source of alcohol more potent in reducing heart disease and stroke risk than others. Singling out red wine is controversial, however, as some experts feel that the upscale lifestyles of typical wine drinkers is also part of the reason for greater longevity.

The American Medical Association defines alcoholism as an illness characterized by significant impairment directly related to persistent, excessive use of alcohol. Impairment can involve physiological, psychological, and social dysfunction. Causes of alcoholism include genetic, psychosocial, and environmental factors.

Some studies suggest that as much as 50% of a person's risk for alcoholism comes from genetic factors. Children of people with alcoholism have a fourfold increased risk of alcoholism, even when adopted by people with no history of alcoholism. This suggests that people with a family history of alcoholism need to be especially alert for evidence of the early signs of alcohol dependence. Ability to "hold one's liquor" is one indicator for genetic risk and is an important screening tool for potential alcohol problems. Still, children of people with alcoholism account for only a fraction of the alcohol abusers in the United States. Any one of us can become addicted if we drink long enough and hard enough.

ALCOHOL IN THE BODY

After a person drinks an alcoholic beverage, his or her blood concentration of alcohol rises rapidly. Alcohol, technically known as *ethanol,* is readily absorbed into the blood from all parts of the gastrointestinal tract. You've probably been warned, with good reason, not to drink on an empty stomach. Alcohol absorption depends partly on the rate of stomach emptying. Food slows the stomach's emptying rate and stimulates secretions, such as gastric acid, which dilute the alcohol and slow its absorption into the bloodstream.

While the liver is metabolizing alcohol, it cannot rapidly metabolize medications, such as sedatives. Consequently, high amounts of alcohol mixed with some sedatives may cause a person to lapse into a coma and die.

A social drinker who weighs 150 pounds and has normal liver function metabolizes about 7 to 14 grams of alcohol per hour. This is about 8 to 12 ounces of beer or

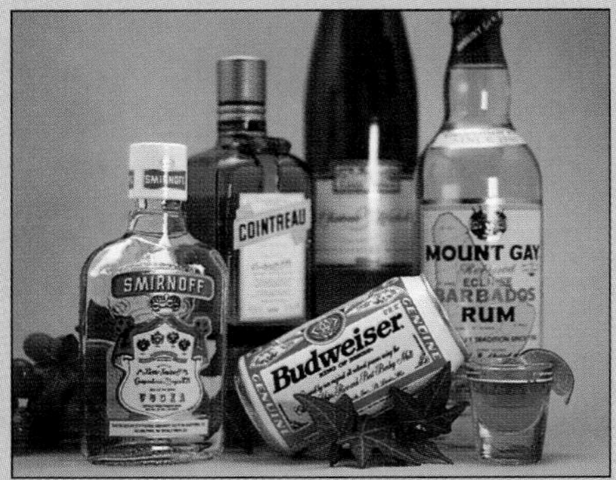

Alcoholic beverages are high in food energy and low in or devoid of essential nutrients. Moderation is important, if used at all.

TABLE 14-5

Energy, Carbohydrate, and Alcohol Content of Alcoholic Beverages*

Beverage	Amount (ounces)	Alcohol (grams)	Carbohydrates (grams)	Energy (kcal)
BEER				
Regular	12	13	13	146
Light	12	11	5	99
DISTILLED				
Gin, rum, vodka, whiskey, tequila	1.5	15	—	105
Brandy, cognac	1.0	9	—	64
WINE				
Red	3	8	2	64
White	3	8	1	60
Dessert, sweet	3	14	11	138
Rosé	3	8	1	63
Manhattan	3	26	3	191
Martini	3	27	—	189
Bourbon & Soda	3	11	—	78
Whiskey Sour	3	15	5	122

*There is little to no fat or protein contribution to energy content.
From USDA.

half an ordinary-sized drink (Table 14–5). When the rate of alcohol consumption exceeds the liver's metabolic capacity, blood alcohol rises and symptoms of intoxication appear (Table 14–6).

When a man and woman of similar size drink the same amount of alcohol, the woman retains more alcohol in her bloodstream; women cannot metabolize as much alcohol in their stomach cells. They also have lower amounts of liver enzymes that metabolize alcohol. In addition, women more quickly develop alcohol-related ailments, such as cirrhosis of the liver, than men with the same drinking history.

Alcohol then goes on to affect the brain more than any other organ. Acting as a sedative, alcohol tends to relieve the drinker's anxiety, cause slurred speech, reduce coordination in walking, impair judgment and sleep, and encourage uninhibited behavior. The mechanism for these effects is thought to be linked to changes in neurotransmitter synthesis and altered cell membrane fluidity in the brain. Because alcohol lowers inhibition, it appears to act as a stimulant, but in fact it is a powerful depressant. As William Shakespeare wrote, "It stirs up desire, but takes away the performance." Because it reduces secretion of the body's antidiuretic hormone, alcohol increases urination. It also causes the blood vessels to dilate, releasing body heat.

ALCOHOL AND OVERALL HEALTH

About 32% of all Americans have three drinks or less each week, and about 22% have two drinks or less a day. Only about 11% have more than two drinks a day. Although the public health impact of alcohol abuse is still being calculated, misuse of alcohol, in and of itself, is one of the most preventable health problems in the United States. Excessive consumption of alcohol contributes significantly to 5 of the 10 leading causes of death in the United States—

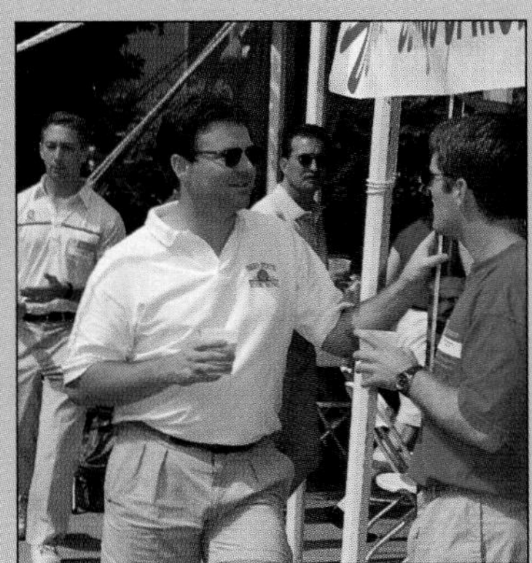

Alcohol intake encourages fat deposition, especially in the abdominal region.

TABLE 14-6

Blood Alcohol Concentration and Symptoms

Concentration*	Sporadic drinker	Chronic drinker	Hours for alcohol to be metabolized
50 (party high)	Congenial euphoria; decreased tension	No observable effect	2–3
75	Gregarious	Often no effect	
100 (0.1%)	Uncoordinated; legally drunk (as in drunk driving) in most states; note that 0.08% is legal drunkenness in a growing number of areas in the United States	Minimal signs	4–6
125–150	Unrestrained behavior; episodic uncontrolled behavior; legally drunk at 0.15% in all states	Pleasurable euphoria or beginning of uncoordination	6–10
200–250	Alertness lost; lethargic	Effort required to maintain emotional and motor control	10–24
300–350	Stupor to coma	Drowsy and slow	
Over 500	Some will die	Coma	Over 24

*Milligrams of alcohol per 100 milliliters of blood.

Modified from Wyngaarder JB, Smith LH: *Cecil textbook of medicine,* fourth edition, Philadelphia, 1988, WB Saunders. Used with permission.

certain forms of cancer, cirrhosis of the liver, motor vehicle and other accidents, suicides, and homicides. Tobacco interacts with alcohol in a way that reinforces its effects in causing esophageal and oral cancer. In addition, excessive alcohol drinking increases the risk of some types of heart disease, high blood pressure (especially in African-Americans), nerve diseases, nutritional deficiencies, damage to a pregnant woman's fetus, abdominal obesity, and many other disorders. (Figure 14-6). A major cause of lasting mental retardation that begins in infancy stems from fetal exposure to alcohol (see Chapter 12).

Social consequences of dependence on alcohol include family violence, divorce, unemployment, and poverty. An estimated 27 million American children are more likely to develop abnormally in psychosocial skills and relationships because their parents abuse alcohol.

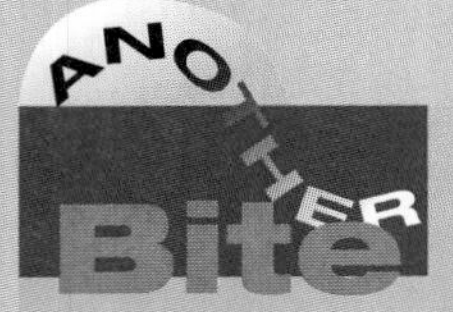

Typical nutrient deficiencies seen in alcoholism are thiamin, riboflavin, niacin, vitamin B-6, folate, vitamin B-12, vitamin C, vitamin A, vitamin D, and vitamin K. Also possible are calcium and zinc deficiencies. These arise from a combination of deficient diets, poor absorption, and alterations in liver function. Eventually, protein-energy malnutrition, as evidenced by weight loss and emaciation, also may develop.

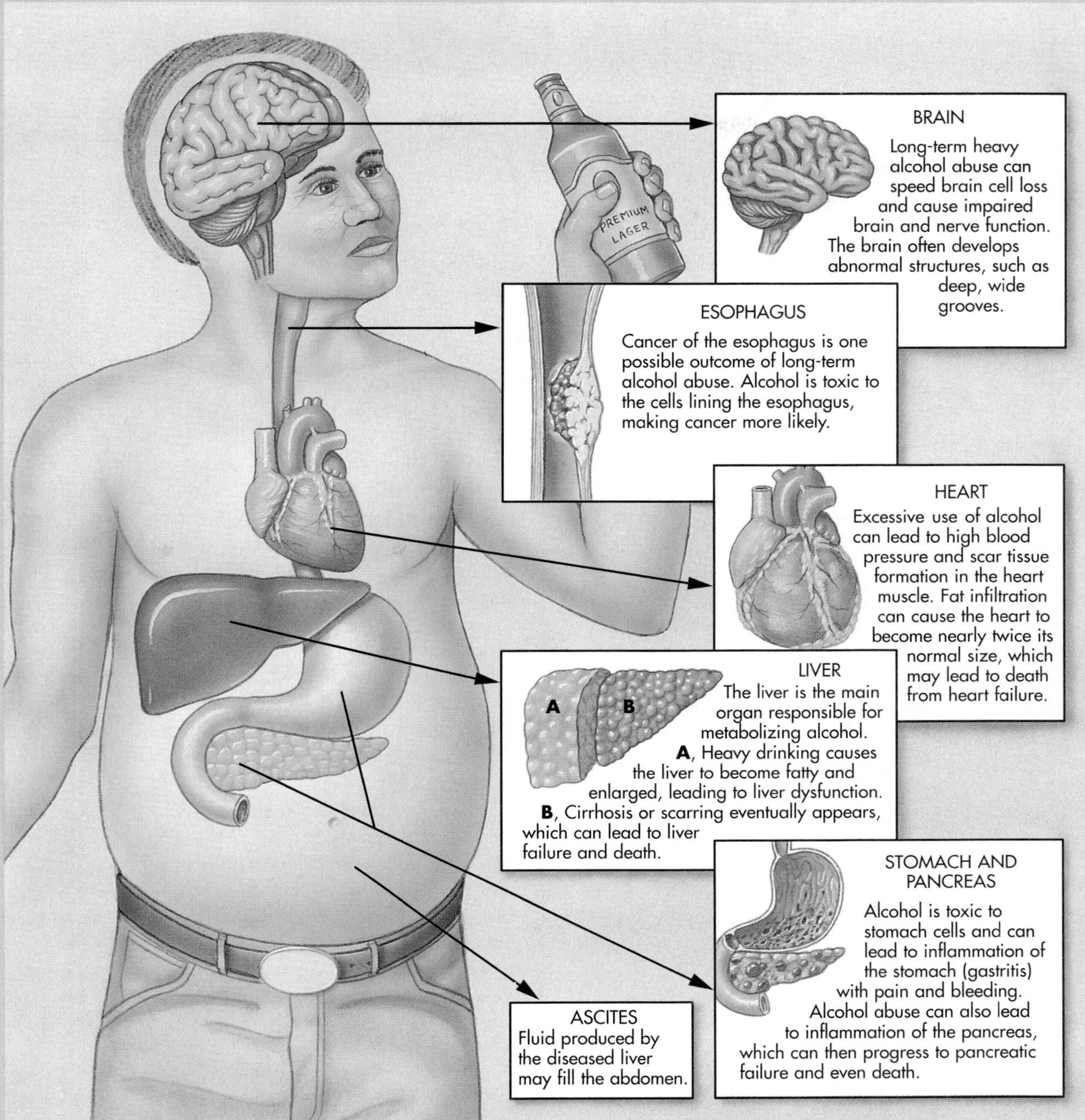

Figure 14-6 *Effects of alcohol abuse on the body. The mind-altering effects of alcohol begin soon after it enters the bloodstream. Within minutes, alcohol numbs nerve cells in the brain. Heart muscle strains to cope with alcohol's depressive action. If drinking continues, rising blood alcohol causes impaired speech, vision, balance, and judgment. With an extremely high blood-alcohol content, respiratory failure is possible. Over time, alcohol abuse increases the risk of liver and pancreas failure and certain forms of heart disease and cancer.*

All this must tell us—use alcohol cautiously and in moderation, if at all. Drinking even small amounts of alcohol can lead to dependence. Sometimes, there is only a fine line between social drinking and alcoholism.

People aged 20 to 40 drink the most alcohol. Excessive drinking often begins earlier; many high school seniors report having consumed alcohol in the past month; about 5% call themselves daily drinkers. The earlier in life that alcohol abuse begins, the more likely alcoholism will result.

CIRRHOSIS

Long-term alcohol use causes liver cirrhosis, a chronic and usually relentlessly progressive disease characterized by fatty infiltration of the liver. Eventually the fat chokes off the blood supply, depriving the liver cells of oxygen and nutrients. Liver cells then die and are replaced by connective (scar) tissue. In America, most cases of cirrhosis are caused by alcohol consumption. Cirrhosis develops in about 12% to 31% of cases of alcoholism. In addition to the amount and duration of alcohol consumption, genetic factors and individual differences determine the body's response to alcohol. Once a person has cirrhosis, there is a 50% chance of death within 4 years, which is a worse prognosis than in many forms of cancer. Most of the deaths from alcoholic cirrhosis occur in people ages 40 to 65.

There are a number of possible mechanisms that underlie the liver damage from alcohol abuse, such as production of free radicals that damage liver cells. A major metabolite of alcohol may also contribute to liver destruction.

No specific amount of alcohol consumption guarantees cirrhosis. One observable pattern is that cirrhosis commonly results from a 15-year consumption of approximately 80 grams of alcohol per day. This is equivalent to 7 beers per day (Table 14–5). Some evidence suggests that damage is caused by a dose as low as 40 grams per day for men and 20 grams per day for women. Early stages of alcoholic liver injury are reversible, but advanced stages usually are not.

A nutritious diet helps prevent some complications associated with alcoholism, but usually alcoholism wreaks serious destruction on the body in spite of an adequate diet. Laboratory animal studies show clearly that even when a nutritious diet is consumed, alcoholism can lead to cirrhosis. Still, deficient nutritional status compounds the problem of cirrhosis as it makes the liver more vulnerable to toxic substances by depleting supplies of antioxidants, such as vitamin C, which can reduce free-radical damage to the liver if present in adequate amounts.

Binge drinking is common among college students (4 or more [for women] to 5 or more [for men] drinks per occasion). This is a major cause of suicide, hazing deaths, and academic failure. About 40% of college students practice binge drinking. Each year this leads to death in otherwise healthy young adults. Such deaths occurred twice in 1997.

GENERAL GUIDELINES FOR ALCOHOL USE

Neither the Surgeon General's office, the National Academy of Science, nor the USDA/DHHS recommends drinking alcohol. All groups caution that if adults do consume alcohol, they should (1) drink alcohol only in moderation with meals (no more than two drinks a day for men and one for women or people over 65 years of age); (2) avoid drinking any alcohol before or while driving, operating machinery, taking medications, or engaging in any other activity requiring sound judgment; and (3) avoid drinking alcohol while pregnant. Although this obviously isn't a plea for teetotalers to start drinking, people who have a drink or so a day and are not prone to abuse should know that there's nothing wrong with moderate drinking as long as they are of legal age and aren't putting themselves or others at risk.

Unfortunately, however, when some of us allow ourselves to drink, we end up drinking too much. A family history of alcoholism especially questions the benefit of even moderate use. Furthermore, people who regularly take certain medications (such as aspirin or anticonvulsants) or who have family history of breast cancer or other alcohol-related cancers, high blood pressure, high blood triglycerides, diabetes, a sleep disorder or ulcers should consult a physician first before they choose to drink.

DO YOU HAVE A PROBLEM WITH ALCOHOL?

Asking a person about the quantity and frequency of alcohol consumption is an important means of detecting abuse and dependence. The following questionnaire (CAGE) is popular for use in routine health care.

Cage Questionnaire to Screen for Alcohol Abuse

C: Have you ever felt you ought to ***Cut*** down on drinking?
A: Have people ***Annoyed*** you by criticizing your drinking?
G: Have you ever felt bad or ***Guilty*** about your drinking?
E: Have you ever had a drink first thing in the morning to steady your nerves or get rid of a hangover ***(Eye-opener)?***

More than one positive response to the CAGE questionnaire suggests an alcohol problem. Another key point to probe is tolerance. Does it take more to make you inebriated than it did in the past? Finally, asking questions about frequency of drinking completes the screening.

TREATMENT

Once a diagnosis of alcohol abuse or dependence is established, a physician should arrange appropriate treatment and counseling for the patient and family. An important goal of counseling is to identify ways to compensate for loss of pleasures from drinking. This helps the drinker confront the immediate problem of how to stop drinking. Total abstinence must be the ultimate objective. For people with alcoholism, there is no such thing as "controlled drinking." A problem drinker cannot return safely to social drinking. The person should enter an Alcoholics Anonymous (AA) program or a reputable therapy program for people with alcoholism. For more information, one can check with a local mental health treatment center for programs available in the community or call (800) 245-4656. In addition, one may visit the Alcoholics Anonymous web page at http://www.alcoholics-anonymous.org and that of the Al-Anon Family Groups, Inc. (http:\\www.al-anon.alateen.org).

The spouse should join the treatment program as well. Success is usually proportionate to participation in AA, other social agencies' programs, and religious counseling. About 2 years of treatment should be expected.

Current research does not support the generally negative public opinion about the prognosis for alcoholism. In most job-related alcoholism treatment programs, where workers are socially stable and—because of the risk to jobs and pensions—well motivated, recovery rates reach 60% or more. This remarkably high cure rate is probably accounted for by early detection. Once a person moves from problem drinking to an advanced stage of alcoholism, success rates seldom exceed 40% to 50%. Early identification and intervention remain the most important steps in the treatment of alcoholism. The federal government is a great resource for such information:

Substance Abuse and Mental Health
Services Administration
The National Clearinghouse for
Alcohol and Drug Information
800/729-6686
or
http:\\www.health.org.

The medication disulfiram (Antabuse) can help the person with alcoholism to make the essential decision to stop drinking. An early step in alcohol metabolism is blocked by the action of this drug. As a result, a highly toxic alcohol by-product accumulates in the blood, when alcohol is consumed. This produces nausea, vomiting, diffuse flushing, and a shocklike reaction. FDA recently approved naltrexone (Revia) as another agent to aid in the treatment of alcohol dependence. This agent reduces the craving for alcohol and blunts the associated inebriation ("high") from alcohol intake.

part

5

Nutrition: Beyond the Nutrients

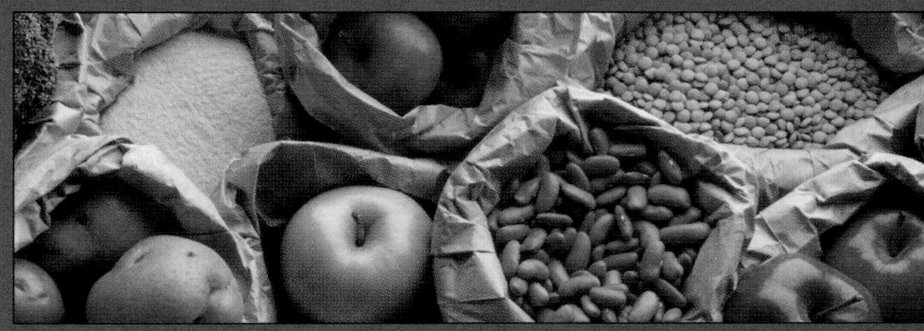

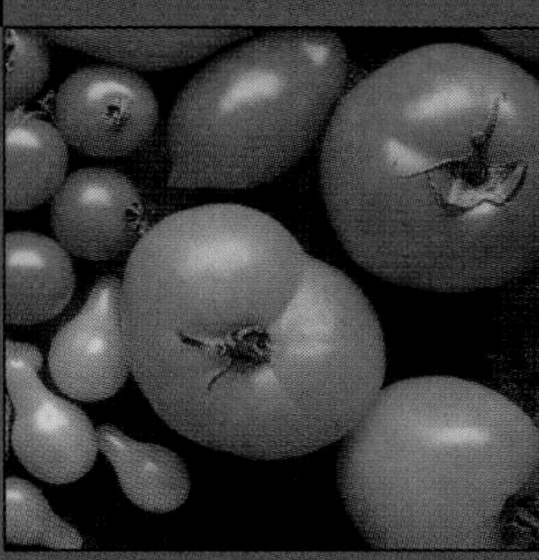

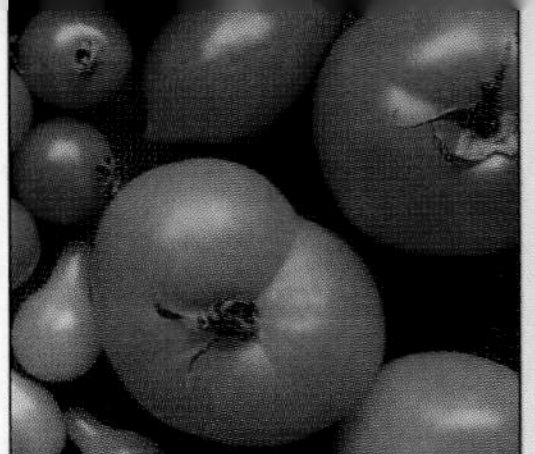

chapter

15

Food Preservation and Safety Issues

At the turn of the century, conditions in Chicago's meat-packing industry were sickening. Moldy, spoiled meat was commonly doused with borax to cover up the smell, and glycerine was added to make it look fresh. By 1906 increasing public pressure forced the passage of the first Food and Drug Act in the United States. Federal inspection then safeguarded the public from worm-infested and diseased meat and generally improved food preparation standards.

Today food safety warnings appear everywhere. Attention has turned to more contemporary food safety concerns, such as microbial and chemical contamination. On the one hand, we are told to eat more fruits, vegetables, fish, and poultry; and on the other hand, we are warned that these foods may contain dangerous substances. Only 20% of 500 people recently surveyed said they felt very confident that the food they bought was safe to eat. So we still must ask, "How safe is our food?"

Scientists and health authorities agree that Americans enjoy a relatively safe food supply. Over the past 90 or so years, tremendous progress has been made in food safety. Nonetheless, microbes and certain chemicals in foods still can pose a health risk. This chapter focuses on these food-related hazards—how real they are and how to minimize their effect on your life. Note that you bear much responsibility for this—government agencies and industry can do only so much.

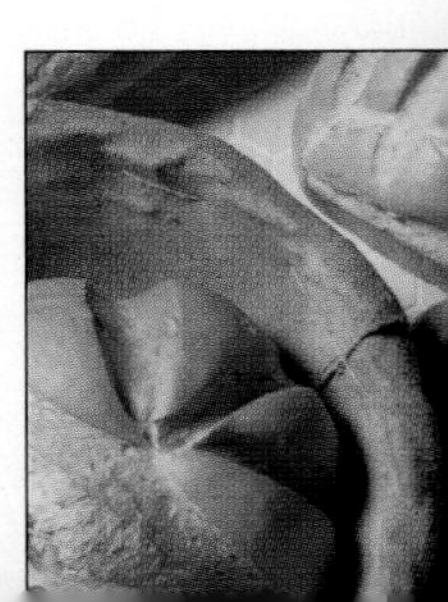

Nutrition Web

Bacteria and other microbes in food pose the greatest risk for foodborne illness. In the past, salt, sugar, smoke, fermentation, and drying were used to protect against foodborne illness. Today thorough cooking, pasteurization, and temperature control (keeping hot foods hot and cold foods cold) provide additional insurance.

Cross-contamination, the transfer of microbes from one food to another, commonly causes foodborne illness, especially when bacteria on raw animal products contact foods that can support their growth. Because of the risk of cross-contamination, no perishable food should be kept at room temperature for more than 1 to 2 hours (depending on the environmental temperature), especially if the food may have come in contact with raw animal products.

Treatment for foodborne illness usually requires drinking lots of fluids, avoiding contact with food while diarrhea is present, washing hands thoroughly, and getting bed rest. Antibiotics also may be prescribed. Botulism and hepatitis A are two types of foodborne illness that require prompt medical attention.

A variety of environmental contaminants can be found in foods. Because most of them dissolve in fat, exposure can be minimized by trimming fat from meats and discarding fat that is rendered during cooking of meats, fish, and poultry. In addition, it's helpful to wash fruits and vegetables thoroughly and discard the outer leaves of leafy vegetables.

Food additives are used primarily to extend shelf life by preventing microbial growth and destruction of food components by oxygen, metals, and other substances. In most cases the Delaney Clause allows FDA to ban manufacturers from adding to foods any substance that causes cancer.

Toxic substances occur naturally in a variety of foods, such as green potatoes, raw fish, and some types of mushrooms. In many cases, cooking foods limits their toxic effects.

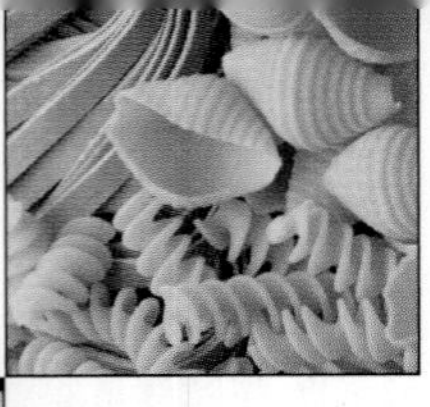

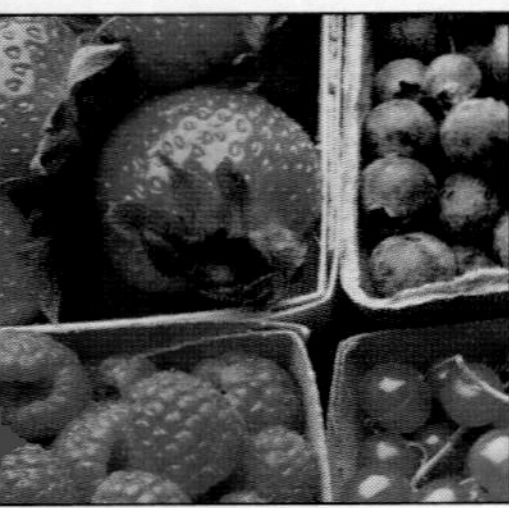

Setting the Stage

During the early stages of urbanization in the United States, contaminated water and food—notably milk—were responsible for many large outbreaks of typhoid fever, septic sore throat, scarlet fever, diphtheria, and other devastating human diseases. These experiences led to the development of processes for purifying water, treating sewage, and **pasteurizing** milk. Since that time, safe water and milk have become universally available, with only occasional problems for either.

The greatest health risk today from food is contamination from **bacteria** and, to a lesser extent, from various forms of **fungi** and viruses. These microbes can all cause **foodborne illness** (Table 15–1). For example, one child died and 50 others became ill from a particularly toxic strain of *Escherichia coli* (*E. coli*) bacteria that was attributed to contaminated apple juice. In another case, 170 children became ill when served strawberries in their school lunch program that were contaminated by hepatitis A virus. In early 1999 75 people were sickened and 17 died—including 5 unborn children—from eating lunch meat and hot dogs contaminated with *Listeria* bacteria.

Since microbial contamination of food is by far the more important issue for our day-to-day health it will be discussed first. This chapter will then cover the use and safety of food additives. Note that food additives cause only about 4% of all cases of foodborne illness in the United States.

Pasteurizing
The process of rapidly heating food products to kill disease-causing microorganisms.

Bacteria
A group of single-cell microorganisms; some produce poisonous substances that cause illness in humans. They contain only one chromosome and lack many organelles found in human cells. Some can live without oxygen and survive by means of spore formation.

Fungi
Simple parasitic life forms including molds, mildews, yeasts, and mushrooms. They live on dead or decaying organic matter. Fungi can grow as single cells, like yeast, or as a multicellular colony as seen with molds.

Foodborne illness
Sickness caused by ingestion of food containing toxic substances produced by microorganisms.

Foodborne Illness

About one-third to one-half of all cases of diarrhea in the United States, upward of 33 million each year, are induced by foodborne organisms. Overall, these agents sicken up to 81 million Americans per year, at a cost of up to $37 billion annually in medical expenses and lost productivity, and lead to about 9000 deaths.

Most people experience a brief but distressing episode of diarrhea from foodborne illness, such as so-called traveler's diarrhea. Foodborne illness generally presents no real long-term health risk for the average person, but for many it can be serious. Some people suffer greatly from foodborne illness, including the following:

- Infants and children
- The elderly
- Those with liver disease, diabetes, or HIV infection (and AIDS)
- Cancer patients
- Pregnant women
- People taking immunosuppresant agents (e.g., posttransplant patients)

Some bouts of foodbourne illness, coupled with the previous conditions, are lengthy and lead to food allergies, seizures, blood poisoning (from **toxins** or microbes in the bloodstream), or other illnesses.

Because foodborne illness often results from unsafe handling of food at home, we each bear much responsibility for preventing foodborne illness. Usually it is not possible to tell by taste, smell, or sight that a particular food contains harmful microbes, so you might not even be aware that food caused your distress. In fact, your last case of diarrhea may have been caused by something you ate.

Why Is Foodborne Illness Such a Concern?

The risk of contracting foodborne illness is worth your attention, because—in addition to problems from consumers' mishandling food—recent trends have added new causes. First, there is greater consumer interest in eating raw or undercooked foods of animal origin. In addition, more people receive medication that suppresses their ability to combat foodborne infectious agents. Another factor is the continuing increase of the elderly population.

TABLE 15-1

Organisms That Cause Foodborne Illness: Their Sources, Symptoms, and Prevention

Organism	Source	Symptoms	Prevention methods
BACTERIA			
Staphylococcus	Found in nasal passages and in cuts on skin. Toxin is produced when food contaminated by bacteria is left for extended time at room temperature. Meats, poultry, egg products, tuna, potato and macaroni salads, and cream-filled pastries pose greatest risk.	Onset: 2–6 hours after eating. Diarrhea, vomiting, nausea, and abdominal cramps. Mimics flu. Lasts 24–36 hours. Treatment includes bed rest and fluids. Rarely fatal.	• Sanitary food-handling practices. • Thorough cooking of foods. • Prompt and proper refrigeration of foods. • Keeping cuts on skin covered.
Salmonella	Found in raw meats, poultry, eggs, fish, unpasteurized milk, and products made with these items. Multiplies rapidly within 8 hours at room temperature. The bacteria themselves are toxic.	Onset: 5–72 hours after eating. Nausea, fever, headache, abdominal cramps,diarrhea, and vomiting. Treatment includes bed rest and fluids. Can be fatal in infants, the elderly, and the sick. Otherwise, deaths rare.	• Sanitary food-handling practices. • Thorough cooking of foods. • Prompt and proper refrigeration of foods. • Avoid cross-contamination of foods, especially when handling foods likely to contain *Salmonella.* • Consumption of fresh juices that are pasteurized.
Clostridium perfringens	Found throughout the environment, sometimes in spore form. Generally found in meat and poultry dishes. Multiplies rapidly when foods are present in large quantities and are left for extended period of time at room temperature, especially stew and gravy. The bacteria themselves are toxic.	Onset: 8–24 hours after eating (usually 12 hours). Abdominal pain and diarrhea. Symptoms last a day or less, usually mild. Can be more serious in older or ill people. Treatment includes bed rest and fluids.	• Sanitary handling of foods, especially meat and meat dishes, gravies, and leftovers. • Thorough cooking and reheating of foods, boil gravy. • Prompt and proper refrigeration.
Clostridium botulinum	Found throughout the environment. However, bacteria produce toxin only in a low-acid, oxygen-free environment, such as in canned food. Green beans, mushrooms, corn, and beef have been sources. Honey and corn syrup may carry spores.	Onset: 12–36 hours after eating. Symptoms include double vision, inability to swallow, speech difficulty and progressive paralysis of the respiratory system. OBTAIN MEDICAL HELP IMMEDIATELY. BOTULISM CAN BE FATAL. AN ANTIDOTE MAY BE HELPFUL IF ADMINISTERED PROMPTLY.	• Using proper methods for canning low-acid foods. • Avoiding commercial cans that have leaky seals or are bent, bulging, or broken. • Destroying toxin after can or jar is opened by boiling contents hard for 20 minutes, but discarding if toxin is suspected (off-odors and milky fluid are signs).
Campylobacter	Found on poultry, beef, and lamb, and can contaminate the meat and milk. Chief food sources are raw poultry and meat and unpasteurized milk.	Onset: 2–5 days after eating, or longer Diarrhea, headache, abdominal cramping, fever, and sometimes bloody stools. Lasts 2–7 days. Treatment includes bed rest and fluids.	• Thorough cooking of foods, especially those that may possibly carry the bacteria. • Sanitary food-handling practices. • Avoid unpasteurized milk.
Listeria	Found in soft cheeses, lunch meats, hot dogs, and unpasteurized milk.	Onset: 7–30 days. Fever, headache, vomiting, and sometimes more severe symptoms possible, especially in infants, pregnant women, and those with depressed immune function function such as in AIDS.	• Thorough cooking of foods. • Sanitary food-handling practices. • Avoiding unpasteurized milk.
Yersinia	Found throughout nature; carried in food and water. They multiply rapidly at both room and refrigerator temperatures. Generally found in raw vegetables, meats, water, and unpasteurized milk.	Onset: 2–3 days. Fever, headache, nausea, diarrhea, and general malaise Mimics flu and appendicitis.	• Thorough cooking. • Sanitizing cutting instruments and cutting boards before preparing foods to be eaten raw. • Avoiding unpasteurized milk and untreated water.

TABLE 11-1—cont'd

Escherichia coli (0157:H7 and other strains)	Undercooked beef, especially ground beef. Fruits, vegetables (e.g., alfalfa sprouts), and yogurt are also sources.	Onset: 2–4 days. Bloody diarrhea, abdominal cramps, kidney failure.	• Thorough cooking, especially of beef. • Avoiding unpasteurized dairy products and juice.
Vibrio vulnificus	Raw seafood, especially raw oysters.	Onset: 6–72 hours. Diarrhea, fever, weakness, blood infection, death.	• Thorough cooking of seafood.
Vibrio cholerae	Human carriers, infected shellfish, contaminated water and food	Onset: 2–3 days. Vomiting, severe watery diarrhea, which can lead to dehydration and cardiovascular collapse; death.	• Handwashing after defecating.
Shigella	Transmitted via fecal-oral route and somewhat to food and water	Onset: 1–3 days. Abdominal cramps, diarrhea, fever, bloody stools.	• Handwashing and sanitary food production.
VIRUSES			
Hepatitis A virus	Found in shellfish harvested from contaminated areas and foods that are handled a lot during preparation and then eaten raw. Recently found in frozen strawberries.	Onset: 30–60 days. Jaundice, fatigue. May cause liver damage and death.	• Sanitary handling of foods. • Use of pure drinking water. • Adequate sewage disposal. • Thorough cooking of foods.
Norwalk, human rota-virus	Found in the human intestinal tract and expelled in feces. Contamination occurs: (1) when sewage is used to enrich garden/farm soil (2) by direct hand-to-food contact during the preparation of meals (3) when shellfish-growing waters are contaminated by sewage	Onset: 1–7 days. Severe diarrhea, nausea, and vomiting. Respiratory symptoms. Usually lasts 4–5 days, but may last for weeks.	• Sanitary handling of foods. • Use of pure drinking water. • Adequate sewage disposal. • Adequate cooking of foods.
PARASITES			
Trichinella spiralis	Found in pork and wild game.	Onset: weeks to months. Muscle weakness, fluid retention in face, fever flulike symptoms.	• Thorough cooking of wild game. Pork may also be contaminated, but rarely.
Anisakis	Found in raw fish.	Onset: 12 hours. Stomach infection, severe stomach pain.	• Thorough cooking of fish.
Tapeworms	Found in raw beef, pork, and fish.	May cause abdominal discomfort, diarrhea.	• Thorough cooking of all animal products. • Avoiding raw fish dishes, such as sushi. • Consuming commercially frozen fish.
Cyclospora	Carried to food via contaminated water; Guatemalan raspberries suspected in recent outbreaks.	Onset: 1 week Prolonged diarrhea, vomiting, muscle aches, fatigue. May be fatal in the very young and elderly.	• Irradiation (not yet in practice). • Boiling contaminated water.
FUNGI			
A group of toxic compounds (mycotoxins) produced by molds, such as aflatoxin B-1 and ergot	Found in foods that are relatively high in moisture. Chief food sources: beans and grains that have been stored in a moist place.	Can cause liver and/or kidney disease.	• Checking foods for visible mold and discarding those that are contaminated. • Cheese is one exception. Simply cutting a wide margin around the mold is a safe practice. • Properly storing susceptible foods.

This list is not inclusive of all potential causes of foodborne illness, but does include the major ones of concern.

Furthermore, the food industry tries where possible to increase the shelf life of products. A longer shelf life at room temperature allows more time for bacteria in foods to multiply. Some bacteria grow even at refrigeration temperatures. Partially cooked—and some fully cooked—products pose a particular risk, because refrigerated storage may only slow, not prevent, bacterial growth.

The risk of illness from foodborne microbes increases as more of our foods are prepared by centralized kitchens outside the home. Supermarkets especially have become major food processors over the past decade and now offer a variety of prepared foods from specialty meat shops, salad bars, and bakeries. With the increasing number of two-income families, more people are looking for convenient, easy-to-prepare nutritious foods. Supermarkets offer entrées that can be served immediately or reheated. The foods are usually prepared in central kitchens or processing plants and shipped to individual stores. If a food product is contaminated in the central kitchen or processing plant, patrons of stores over a wide area can suffer foodborne illness.

The centralization of food production by the food processing industry also adds to the risk of foodborne illness. For example, a malfunction in an ice cream plant in 1994 resulted in 224,000 suspected cases of *Salmonella* bacterial infections, linked to use of contaminated milk. In 1998, 209 people spread across 11 states were sickened—47 of which had to be hospitalized—from consuming a toasted oat cereal contaminated with the same microbe.

A recent survey showed that restaurants are part of the problem: only 13% implemented the voluntary FDA Food Code for cooking temperatures for meat, eggs, fish and poultry. It is no surprise then that in 1993 at least four people died and 700 because ill in Washington and surrounding western states after eating at a chain of quick-service restaurants. The source of the problem was undercooked hamburger contaminated with the bacterium *E. coli* 0157:H7. Overall, the growth of large-scale food production and distribution technologies has introduced new and different foodborne risks.

Still another cause of increased foodborne illness in America is greater consumption of ready-to-eat foods imported from foreign countries. In the past, food imports were mostly raw products processed here under strict sanitation standards. Now, however, we import more processed foods—such as cheese from France and seafood from Asia—some of which are contaminated. Most of these imports are not carefully inspected. Federal authorities are currently examining whether more rigorous inspection procedures are needed for these imports. It is likely that tougher standards will soon be imposed.

Use of antibiotics in animal feeds is increasing the severity of cases of foodborne illness. This use encourages bacteria to develop resistant strains, those that can grow even if exposed to typical antibiotic medicines.

Finally, more cases of foodborne disease are reported now because scientists are more aware of the roles of various players in the process. In addition, physicians are more likely to suspect foodborne contaminants as a cause of illness. Every decade the list of microorganisms suspected of causing foodborne illness lengthens (see Table 15–1). Furthermore, we now know that food, besides serving as a good growth medium for some microorganisms, simply transmits many others as well. Seafood especially is receiving greater scrutiny and surveillance by FDA in this regard. In addition, FDA is launching a $500,000 campaign to educate consumers about the risks of eating raw oysters. For more information about these risks, contact FDA's Seafood Hotline at 1-800-FDA-4010, or one through the American Seafood Institute at 1-800-328-3474 between 9 AM and 5 PM Eastern time on weekdays. The latter provides free information on the purchase, preparation, and nutritional value of seafood products.

Overall, this discussion is not meant to be a scare tactic. Many people avoid foodborne illness each year. However, the more you know about the problem, the

When traveling to developing countries it is recommended that you "boil it, peel it, or don't eat it." Ironically, up to 70% of our fruits and vegetables during certain seasons comes from these countries. In other words, you do not have to travel to acquire traveler's diarrhea or other foodborne risks. In response, we should carefully inspect and wash produce, as we would in a foreign country. In addition, it is important to fully cook all seafood, as much of this is imported.

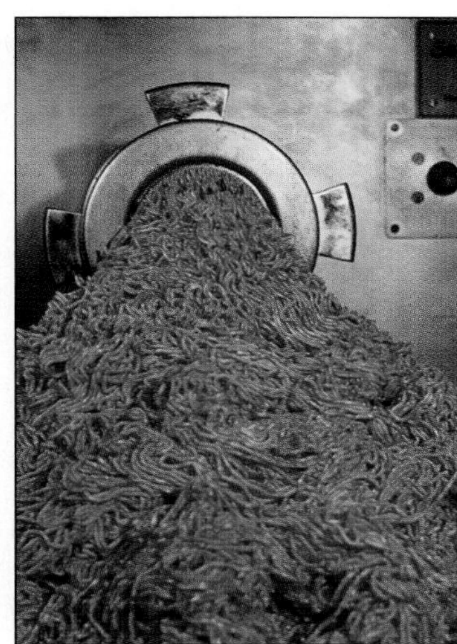

Food contaminated in a central plant can go on to produce illness in people in surrounding states or even across the nation. In the case of hamburger, it is important to cook it thoroughly—160°F (71°C), with brown color throughout and clear juices.

greater ability you have to protect yourself and count yourself among those free of such illness.

Irradiation
A process in which radiation energy is applied to foods, creating compounds (free radicals) within the food that destroy cell membranes, break down genetic material, link proteins together, limit enzyme activity, and alter a variety of other proteins and cell functions that can lead to food spoilage. This process does not make the food radioactive.

Aseptic processing
A method by which food and container are simultaneously sterilized; it allows manufacturers to produce boxes of milk that can be stored at room temperature.

Food Preservation—Past, Present, and Future

For centuries, salt, sugar, smoke, fermentation, and drying have been used to preserve food. Ancient Romans used sulfites to disinfect wine containers and preserve wine. In the age of exploration, European adventurers traveling to the New World preserved their meat by salting it. Most preserving methods worked on the principle of decreasing free water—that is, the amount of water not bound to other components in the food. Bacteria need abundant stores of water to grow; yeasts and molds can grow with less water, but some is still necessary. Adding sugar or salt decreases free water by binding to it. The process of drying drives off free water.

Decreasing the water content of some high-moisture foods, however, causes them to lose essential characteristics. To preserve such foods—cucumbers (pickles), cabbage (sauerkraut), milk (yogurt), and grape juice (wine)—fermentation has been a traditional alternative. Selected bacteria are used to ferment the foods. The fermenting bacteria make acids and alcohol, which minimize the growth of other microbes.

Today we can add pasteurization, sterilization, refrigeration, freezing, **irradiation,** canning, and chemical preservatives to the list of food preservation techniques. A new method of food preservation—**aseptic processing**—simultaneously sterilizes the food and package separately before the food enters the package. Liquid foods, such as fruit juices, are especially easy to process in this manner. With aseptic packaging, boxes of sterile milk and juices can remain on supermarket shelves, free of microbial growth, for many years.

Food irradiation is also a fairly recent development. For more than a decade FDA has permitted limited irradiation of certain food products. The radiation used does not make the food radioactive, as some consumers believe. However, the energy is strong enough to break chemical bonds, destroy cell walls and cell membranes, break down genetic material, and link proteins together. Irradiation thereby controls growth of insects, microorganisms, and parasites in foods. FDA recently approved its use for raw red meat to reduce risk of *E. coli* and other infectious pathogens. USDA also recently endorsed the practice. Prior to this only pork and chickens were so treated. Irradiation also extends the shelf life of spices, dry vegetable seasonings, meats in general, and fresh fruits and vegetables.

Irradiated food, except for dried seasonings, must be so labeled (see margin). Foods treated this way are safe in the opinion of FDA and many other health authorities. Japan, France, Italy, and Mexico all use food irradiation technology. To date, consumer acceptance of food irradiation in the United States is mixed, and the number of irradiated products on the market are few.

International label for noting prior irradiation of the food product.

Foodborne Illness: When Undesirable Microbes Alter Foods

Foodborne illness is caused by specific toxin-producing bacteria and other microbes. Many different types of bacteria cause foodborne illness, such as *Bacillus, Campylobacter, Clostridium, Escherichia, Listeria, Vibrio, Yersinia, Salmonella, Staphylococcus,* and others (Table 15–2). Because each teaspoon of soil contains about 2 billion bacteria, we are constantly at risk for foodborne illness. Luckily, as far as we know, only a small number of all bacteria actually pose a threat. It is important that you be aware of the specific agents.

TABLE 15-2

Some Recent Examples of Cases of Foodborne Illness

BACTERIA	• Five people fell ill from *Salmonella* after eating fish cakes in which the breading, which was mixed with raw egg, was not fully cooked. Eight people became sick after consuming tiramisu, a dessert that contains raw eggs. • A man in Arkansas developed botulism after eating stew that was cooked and then kept at room temperature for 3 days. He spent 49 days in the hospital—42 of them on mechanical ventilation. Refrigeration to reduce growth of the bacteria and thorough cooking are two keys to preventing development of *C. botulinum* in these foods. • Lettuce shredded in a Texas plant and then placed in large plastic bags was the cause of the largest *Shigella* bacterial outbreak ever reported in the United States. At least 347 people became ill. A cruise was cut short when more than 600 people developed shigellosis and one person died. • More than 5000 people were sickened by *E. coli*-contaminated potato salad in Chicago. • A teenage boy and his father experienced abdominal pain, vomiting, and diarrhea within 30 minutes of eating 4-day-old homemade pesto. The pesto had been reheated and left out a number of times during the 4-day period. It was apparently contaminated with *Bacillus cereus.* The boy died of liver failure as a result. • Since 1992, 17 people in Florida have died of *Vibrio vulnificus* infection after eating raw oysters. Half or more cases of such infections result in death, especially in people at high risk for foodborne illness. Eating any raw or lightly (partially) cooked seafood poses a high risk, especially that harvested from the Gulf Coast from April through October. • The first documented foodborne illness caused by *Listeria* organisms in North America occurred in commercially prepared coleslaw. Later, incidents that involved 48 deaths were associated with soft "Mexican-style" cheeses. Because pasteurization destroys *Listeria* organisms, reports of contaminated milk and cheese products suggest that contamination occurred following pasteurization, probably from the addition of unpasteurized milk. Lunch meat and hot dogs also have been shown to cause *Listeria* infections.
VIRUSES	• Norwalk viruses are probably responsible for about 30% to 40% of all cases of viral intestinal infection in adults. The infection is typically found in nursing homes. Recently, outbreaks caused by contaminated ice occurred in Pennsylvania and Delaware. Another outbreak of Norwalk virus was attributed to an infected bakery worker who stirred a vat full of buttercream frosting with his bare hand and arm.
PARASITES	• Illness linked to contaminated water in metropolitan Milwaukee and Sidney, Australia, was traced to *Cryptosporidium.* This parasite is found in many species of birds and animals and in their feces. Consumption of water or food contaminated with the parasite can cause cryptosporidiosis, a rare but potentially serious disease. A group attending a dinner banquet developed diarrhea after 3–9 days. Eight of 10 stool specimens obtained from the group of 54 ill banquet attendees were positive for *Cryptosporidium.* Green onions not washed before use at the restaurant were the likely cause. Food workers at the restaurant reported they did not consistently wash green onions before using them to prepare food or serving them to patrons. • Guatemalan raspberries have been associated with approximately 1000 cases of *Cyclospora* in the United States and Canada. Authorities speculate that contaminated water used with pesticides caused the outbreak (this is not known for certain). Following two outbreaks, the United States banned the fruit until further precautions can be taken. Authorities are currently examining the use of irradiation, which would kill the *Cyclospora,* but this practice is not currently in use.

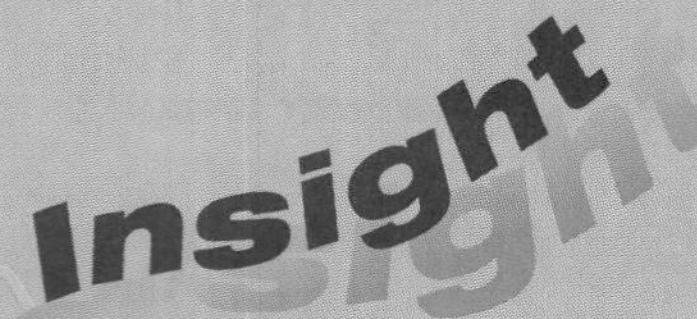

A Closer Look at Agents That Cause Foodborne Illness

Bacteria

Bacteria pose the greatest risk for foodborne illness. These organisms cause health problems either directly by invading the intestinal wall and producing an infection or indirectly by producing a **toxin** in food that later harms us. Most of these toxins are not detectable by human sight or smell and may remain on food even after bacteria have died. Thus, although a food appears safe, bacteria or bacterial toxins still may be present that cause illness.

The optimum temperature for most disease-causing bacteria is about 98°F (body temperature; 37°C). A few bacteria can thrive in almost freezing temperatures, while others thrive in very high temperatures. Some bacteria survive these and other harsh environmental conditions through **spore** formation. Spores are dormant reproductive cells capable of later forming into adult organisms without the help of another cell. In the spore state, bacteria can remain stable for months or years. Sufficient cooking kills bacteria and spores, and the toxins produced as well. Irradiation of foods such as beef also works.

Viruses

A well-known example of foodborne illness caused by a virus is hepatitis A. Viruses in general cannot metabolize, grow, or move by themselves. Instead, they must use a living host cell to reproduce, and cannot grow in food once it is harvested or slaughtered because it is no longer alive. Because viruses cannot multiply in foods, they must enter in sufficient amounts through contamination, such as bits of animal feces that contaminate foods. Similar contamination can occur in seafood, such as oysters, that live in sewage-containing waters. Thorough cooking and handwashing are two methods of preventing viral foodborne illness. Irradiation of foods also works.

General Rules for Preventing Foodborne Illness

You can greatly reduce the risk of foodborne illness by following some very important rules. It's a long list, because many risky habits need to be addressed.

Recent evidence of Mad Cow Disease in Great Britain is of little concern in the United States. USDA has banned the import of cattle from Great Britain since the late 1980s; no case of the disease has been noted in the United States. As a precaution, however, FDA is implementing a ban on the recycling of animal tissue from ruminant animals (e.g., cows, goats, sheep) for animal feed. These are suspected carriers of the disease.

Purchasing Food

- When shopping, select frozen foods and perishable foods last, such as meat, poultry, or fish. Always have these products put in separate plastic bags so that drippings don't contaminate other foods in the shopping cart. Then, don't let groceries sit in a warm car; this allows bacteria to grow. Get the perishable foods home and promptly refrigerate or freeze.
- Don't buy or use food from flawed containers that leak, bulge, or are severely dented or buy or use food from jars that are cracked or have loose or bulging lids. Don't taste or use food that has a foul odor or spurts liquid when the can is opened; the deadly *Clostridium botulinum* toxin may be present.
- Purchase only pasteurized juice, milk, and cheese. This is especially important for pregnant women because highly toxic bacteria—such as *Campylobacter*—and viruses that can harm the fetus thrive in unpasteurized products.
- Purchase only the amount of produce needed for a week's time. The longer you keep fruits and vegetables, the more time available for bacteria to grow.

Fungi

Fungi of concern in food safety do not specifically infect people. Instead, some fungi, such as certain mushrooms, contain poisons. Molds, which make up most of fungi, produce toxins called **mycotoxins** as they grow on foods. The best-known mycotoxins are the aflatoxins, found on moldy grains and peanuts; these cause cancer.

Fungi are hardy organisms. They can live in acid and alkaline conditions and can grow in concentrated salt and sugar solutions. Fungi require minimal moisture to grow; they can obtain water from the medium on which they live or from the atmosphere. When the atmosphere becomes dry, they can go into a resting state or form spores. As spores, fungi can be scattered by the wind or carried by animals. When an airborne spore lands on an appropriate target, such as a ripe orange, the spore germinates and begins to grow, producing the typical mold observed on spoiled fruit.

Cooking does not destroy mycotoxins present. Thus, it is best to throw out moldy foods; for cheese it is fine to just cut a wide margin around the moldy section.

Parasites

Parasites are higher forms of life and include the protozoans, flukes, nematodes, roundworms, and tapeworms. They enter the body through the intestinal tract. In the United States, the parasite most apt to be in the food supply is *Trichinella spiralis.* This tiny organism may be present in raw and undercooked pork and pork products, such as sausage. Trichinosis is rare today, probably because people realize that pork must be cooked thoroughly to kill the nematode worm that causes it, and modern sanitary feeding practices have reduced *Trichinella* in hogs. About a hundred cases of trichinosis per year are reported in the United States. However, other cases may be unreported. In addition to pork, bear meat and other raw meats are potential sources. It is seldom found in commercial meat.

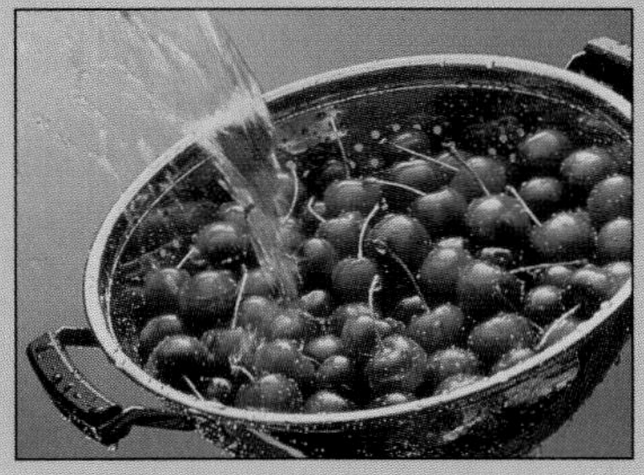

Wash fruit well before use to reduce possible bacteria, parasite, and pesticide exposure.

An early developmental stage in the life history of some parasites is the larval stage. **Larvae** of parasites may be present in some foods, such as meats, and when eaten can lead to illness. Thorough cooking destroys larval and adult parasite stages. Irradiation of foods destroys these organisms as well.

- When purchasing precut produce, avoid those that look slimy, brownish, or dry; these are signs of improper holding conditions.

Preparing Food

- Thoroughly wash hands with hot, soapy water before and after handling food, and after using the bathroom. This practice is especially important when handling raw meat, fish, poultry, or eggs.
- Make sure counters, cutting boards, dishes, and other equipment are thoroughly cleaned and rinsed before use. Then be especially careful to use hot, soapy water to wash surfaces and equipment that have come in contact with raw meat, fish, poultry, and eggs as soon as possible to remove *Salmonella* and *Campylobacter* bacteria that may be present. Current investigations show that the kitchens in many homes need much more attention to overall sanitation.
- If possible, cut foods to be eaten raw on a clean cutting board reserved for that purpose. Then clean this cutting board using hot, soapy water. If the same board must be used for both animal products and other foods, cut any potentially contaminated items, such as chicken, last. After cutting animal products, wash the cutting board thoroughly.

USDA recommends cutting boards with unmarred surfaces that are made of easy-to-clean, nonporous materials, such as plastic, marble, or glass. If you prefer a wooden board, reserve it for a specific purpose; for example, set it aside for

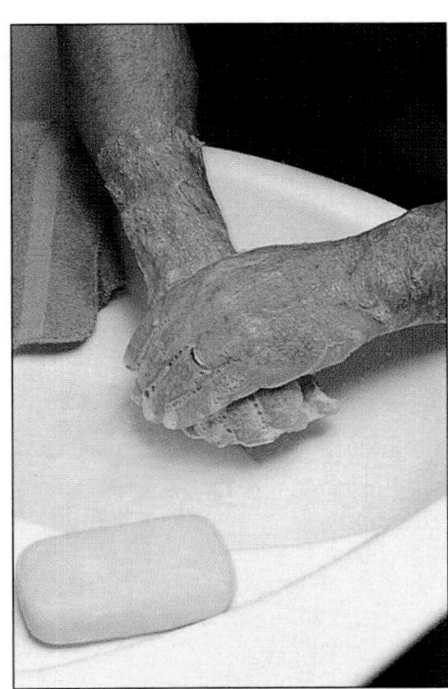

Washing hands thoroughly with hot water and soap should be the first step in food preparation.

Critical Thinking

Jon wants to buy a cutting board for his new kitchen. He's been looking at all of the possibilities: plexiglas, plastic, and wood. How would you advise him so that he can minimize the risk of any foodborne illness from his food preparation?

cutting raw meat and poultry. Then keep a separate board for chopping produce or slicing bread to prevent these products from picking up bacteria from raw meat. Note that many foods are served raw, so any bacteria clinging to them are not destroyed.

Furthermore, USDA recommends that all cutting boards, plastic or wood, be replaced when they become streaked with hard-to-clean grooves or cuts, which may harbor bacteria. In addition, both wood and plastic boards should be sanitized once a week in a solution of 2 teaspoons chlorine bleach per quart of water. Flood the board with the solution, let it sit a few minutes, and then rinse thoroughly.

- When thawing foods, do so under cold running water, in the refrigerator for 1 to 3 days, or in a microwave oven. Also cook foods immediately if the product was thawed under cold water or in the microwave. Never let frozen foods thaw unrefrigerated all day or night. Also, marinate food in the refrigerator.
- Avoid coughing or sneezing over foods, even when you're healthy. Cover cuts on hands with a sterile bandage. This helps stop *Staphylococcus* from entering food.
- Carefully wash fresh fruit and vegetables under running water to remove dirt and bacteria clinging to the surface, using a vegetable brush if the skin is to be eaten. People recently became ill from *Salmonella* that was introduced from melons used in making a fruit salad and from oranges used for fresh-squeezed orange juice. The bacteria were on the outside of the melons and oranges.
- Completely remove moldy portions or soft/rotten portions of food, or preferably don't eat the food. **When in doubt, throw the food out.** Mold growth is prevented by properly storing food at cold temperatures and using the food within a reasonable length of time—within 3 days for leftovers. (Figure 15–1).
- Use refrigerated ground meat and patties in 1 to 2 days and frozen meat and patties within 3 to 4 months.

Garfield ®
by Jim Davis
HOPE YOU DIDN'T EAT THE MEAT LOAF, GARFIELD
IT'S BEEN IN THE FRIDGE FOR SIX MONTHS
ANYBODY WHO EATS THAT HAS ONLY MINUTES LEFT
JUST ENOUGH TIME FOR DESSERT THEN
JIM DAVIS 10-3

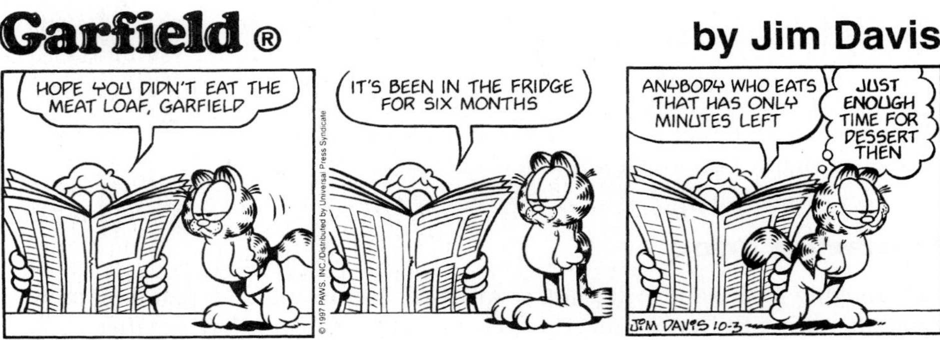

Figure 15–1 *Garfield.*

Cooking Food

- Cook food thoroughly, especially beef, fish, and pork (160°F [71°C]), poultry (180°F [82°C]), and eggs (until the yolk and white are hard). This is the single most important practice. Cooking destroys most foodborne bacteria, such as toxic strains of *E. coli,* whereas freezing only halts growth. A good general precaution is to eat no raw animal products. USDA answers questions about safe use of animal products ([800] 535-4555, 10 AM to 4 PM weekdays, Eastern time).

  Seafood also poses a risk of foodborne illness. Use fresh fish within 1 to 2 days of purchase. Properly cooked fish should flake easily and be opaque or dull and firm. If it's translucent or shiny, it's not done.

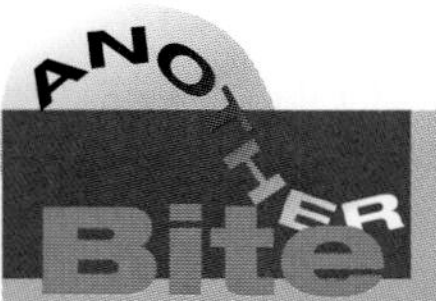

Raw fish dishes, such as sushi, can be safe for most people to eat if they are made with very fresh fish that is commercially frozen and then thawed. The freezing is important to eliminate potential health risks from parasites. FDA recommends that the fish be frozen to an internal temperature of −10°F for 7 days. If you choose to eat uncooked fish, purchase the fish from reputable establishments that have high standards for quality and sanitation. People at high risk for foodborne illness would be wise to avoid raw fish products.

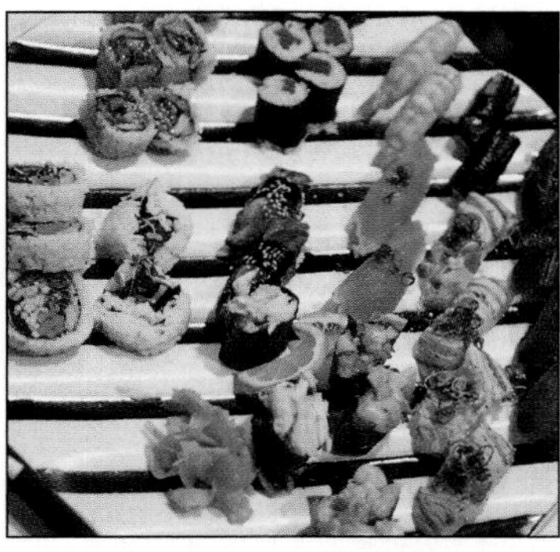

Sushi, like all raw fish or meat dishes, is a high-risk food. For maximum protection from foodborne illness, animal foods should be cooked thoroughly before eating.

- Cook stuffing separately from poultry (or wash poultry thoroughly, stuff immediately before cooking, and then transfer the stuffing to a clean bowl immediately after cooking). Make sure the stuffing reaches 165°F (74°C). Again, *Salmonella* and *Campylobacter* are the major concerns with poultry.
- Once a food is cooked, consume it right away, or cool it to 40°F (4°C) within 2 hours. If it is not to be eaten immediately, in hot weather (85°F and above) make sure this cooling is done within 1 hour. Do this by separating the food into as many shallow pans as needed to provide a large surface area. This reduces the risk of *Clostridium perfringens*–related illness. Be careful not to recontaminate cooked food by contact with raw meat or juices from hands, cutting boards, dirty utensils, or in other ways.
- Serve meat, poultry, and fish on a clean plate—never the same plate that was used to hold the raw product. For example, when grilling hamburgers, don't put cooked items on the same plate that was used to carry the raw product out to the grill.
- Cook food completely at the picnic site, with no partial cooking in advance.
- Follow all canning procedures listed with the appliance. Not doing so with low-acid foods, such as asparagus, beets, mushrooms, corn, green beans, and meats poses a risk for *Clostridium botulinum* growth.
- Reduce the risk of bacteria surviving during microwave cooking by:
  Covering food with glass or ceramic when possible to decrease evaporation and heat the surface;
  Stirring and rotating food at least once or twice for even cooking. Then, allow microwaved food to stand, covered, after cooking is completed to help cook the exterior and equalize the temperature throughout;
  Using the oven temperature probe or a meat thermometer to check that food is done (insert it at several spots to make sure);
  Using the oven's defrost setting if thawing meat in the microwave. Ice crystals in frozen foods are not heated well by the microwave oven and can create cold spots that later cook more slowly.

The World Health Organization's golden rules for safe food preparation

1. Choose foods processed for safety.
2. Cook food thoroughly.
3. Eat cooked foods immediately.
4. Store cooked foods carefully.
5. Reheat cooked foods thoroughly.
6. Avoid contact between raw and cooked foods.
7. Wash hands repeatedly.
8. Keep all kitchen surfaces meticulously clean.
9. Protect foods from insects, rodents, and other animals.
10. Use pure water.

The USDA recently boiled these down to four actions:

1. Clean. Wash hands and surfaces often.
2. Separate. Don't cross-contaminate.
3. Cook. Cook to proper temperatures.
4. Chill. Refrigerate promptly.

Storing and Reheating Cooked Food

- Keep hot foods hot and cold foods cold. Hold food below 40°F (4°C) or above 140°F (60°C) (Figure 15–2). Foodborne illness microbes thrive in more moderate temperatures (60° to 100°F [16° to 43°C]). Some microbes can even grow in the refrigerator. Again, don't leave cooked or refrigerated foods, such as meats and salads, at room temperature for more than 2 hours (or 1 hour in hot weather) because that gives microbes an opportunity to grow. Store dry food at 60°F to 70°F (16°C to 21°C).
- Reheat leftovers to 165°F (74°C); reheat gravy to a rolling boil to kill *Clostridium perfringens* bacteria that may be present. Merely reheating to a good eating temperature isn't enough to kill sufficient bacteria.

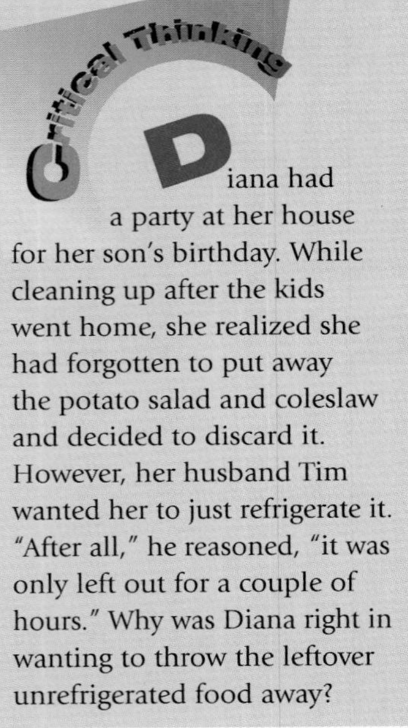

Diana had a party at her house for her son's birthday. While cleaning up after the kids went home, she realized she had forgotten to put away the potato salad and coleslaw and decided to discard it. However, her husband Tim wanted her to just refrigerate it. "After all," he reasoned, "it was only left out for a couple of hours." Why was Diana right in wanting to throw the leftover unrefrigerated food away?

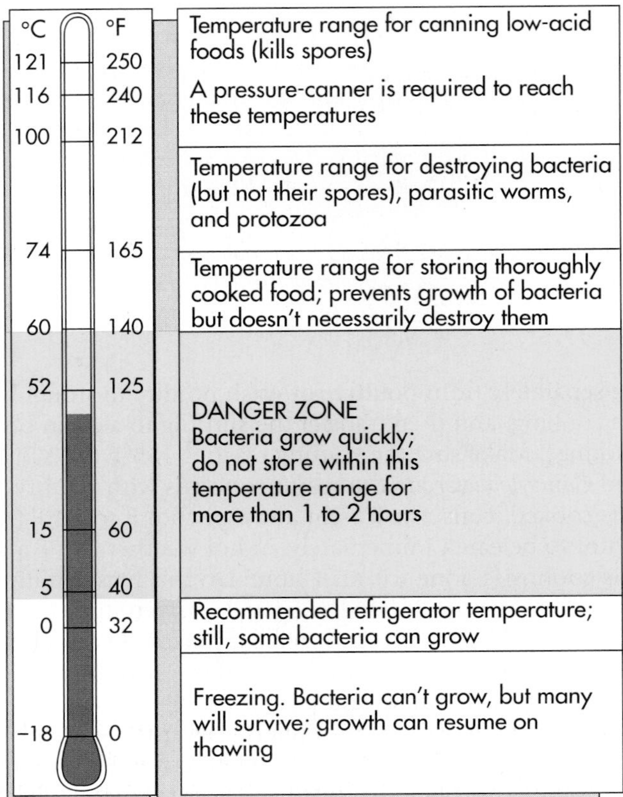

Figure 15–2 *Effects of temperature on microbes that cause foodborne illness.*
(Adapted from *Temperature Guide to Food Safety: Food and Home Notes,* No. 25, Washington, DC, June 20, 1977, USDA.)

- Store peeled or cut-up produce, such as melon balls, in the refrigerator.
- Make sure the refrigerator stays below 40°F (4°C). Either use a refrigerator thermometer or keep it as cold as possible without freezing milk or lettuce.

Microbes that cause foodborne illness commonly enter food through cross-contamination—from one source to another—and grow in temperatures favorable to them. Potential sources of cross-contamination in the kitchen also are dirty kitchen towels and sponges—especially sponges. Clean (and replace) these regularly. Overall, it's essential to practice sanitary food-handling procedures when preparing any food.

To emphasize the importance of preventing cross-contamination, consider that 14 people were recently sickened by *Campylobacter* after eating in a restaurant. Inspection of the restaurant indicated that the countertop surface area was too small to separate raw poultry and other foods adequately during preparation. The cook reported cutting up raw chicken for the dinner meals before preparing salads, lasagna, and sandwiches as luncheon menu items. Lettuce for salads was then shredded with a knife, and the cook wore a towel around her waist that she frequently used to dry her hands. The lettuce or lasagna was probably contaminated from the raw chicken through the unwashed or inadequately washed countertop. Dirty hands and cooking utensils also were suspected causes.

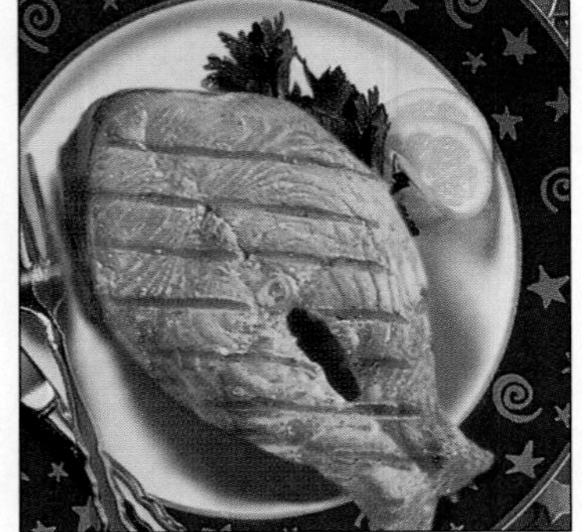

Fresh fish should be carefully refrigerated and used soon after purchase—within 1 to 2 days.

As one final precaution, watch for safe food-handling techniques when you eat out. Check that foods in a salad bar are iced; custard and pudding pies are chilled; hot foods served on a hot food bar are in fact hot; and vending machines are checked regularly, especially those containing sandwiches and milk. Send back any meat, poultry, seafood, or fish that does not appear thoroughly cooked. Food stored and served in dormitory cafeterias should also be properly handled.

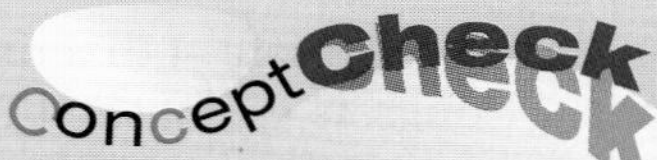

Bacteria and the toxins they produce pose the greatest risk for foodborne illness. In the past the addition to foods of sugar and salt, as well as smoking and drying, were used to prevent the growth of microorganisms. Today we know that ensuring cleanliness, keeping hot foods hot and cold foods cold, and cooking foods thoroughly offer additional protection from foodborne illness. Treat all raw animal products, cooked food, and raw fruits and vegetables as potential sources of foodborne illness.

To prevent foodborne intoxication from *Staphylococcus* organisms, cover cuts on hands and avoid sneezing on foods. To avoid *Salmonella* and *Campylobacter* infection, separate raw meats, especially poultry products to destroy any *Salmonella* or *Campylobacter* bacteria present. To avoid intoxication from *Clostridium perfringens,* rapidly cool leftover foods and thoroughly reheat them. To avoid intoxication from *Clostridium botulinum,* carefully examine canned foods. Overall, don't allow cooked food to stand for more than 1 to 2 hours at room temperature. For other causes of foodborne illness, precautions already mentioned generally apply as well. In addition, carefully handle raw animal products so that their juices do not contaminate other foods; consume only pasturized juice and poultry products; wash all fruits and vegetables; and thoroughly wash your hands with soap and water before and after preparing food, and after using the bathroom.

Food Additives

By the time you see a food on the market shelf, it usually contains substances added to make it more palatable or increase its nutrient content or shelf life. Manufacturers also add some substances to foods to make them easier to process. Other substances may have accidentally found their way into the foods you buy. All these extraneous substances are known as *additives,* and although some may be beneficial, others can be harmful. All purposefully added substances must be evaluated by FDA or other federal agencies.

Why Are Food Additives Used?

Most additives are used to limit food spoilage. Food additives, such as potassium sorbate, are used to maintain the safety and acceptability of foods by retarding the growth of problem microbes implicated in foodborne illness.

Additives are also used to combat some enzymes that lead to undesirable changes in color and flavor in foods but don't cause anything so serious as foodborne illness. This second type of food spoilage occurs when enzymes in a food react to oxygen—for example, when apple and peach slices darken or turn rust color as they are exposed to air. Antioxidants are a type of preservative that retards the action of oxygen-requiring enzymes on food surfaces. These preservatives are not necessarily novel chemicals. They include vitamins E and C and a variety of sulfites. Finally, additives are used to adjust acidity, improve flavor and color, leaven, provide nutritional fortification, thicken, and emulsify food components.

Without the use of some food additives, it would be impossible to safely produce massive quantities of foods and distribute them nationwide or worldwide, as is now done. Despite consumer concerns about the safety of food additives, many have been extensively studied and proved safe when federal guidelines for their use are followed.

Intentional Versus Incidental Food Additives

Food additives are classified into two types: **intentional food additives** (directly added to foods) and **incidental food additives** (indirectly added as contaminants). Both types of agents are regulated. Currently, more than 2800 different substances are intentionally added to foods. As many as 10,000 other substances enter foods as contaminants. This includes substances that may reasonably be expected to enter food through surface contact with processing equipment or packaging materials.

Intentional food additives
Additives knowingly (directly) incorporated into food products by manufacturers.

Incidental food additives
Additives that appear in food products indirectly, from environmental contamination of food ingredients or during the manufacturing process.

Some definitions here might help you:

Toxicology The scientific study of harmful substances
Safety The relative certainty that a substance won't cause injury
Hazard The chance that injury will result from use of a substance
Toxicity The capacity of a substance to produce injury or illness at some dosage

The GRAS List

In 1958 all food additives used in the United States and considered safe at that time were put on a **generally recognized as safe (GRAS)** list. Congress established the GRAS list because it believed manufacturers did not need to prove the safety of substances that were already generally regarded as safe by knowledgeable scientists. Since that time FDA has been responsible for proving that a substance does not belong on the GRAS list.

Some substances on the list have been reviewed. A few, such as cyclamates, failed the review process and were removed from the list. Recently the additive red dye No. 3 was banned because it is linked to cancer. Many chemicals on the GRAS list have not yet been rigorously tested, primarily because of expense. These chemicals have received a low priority for testing, mostly because they have long histories of use without evidence of toxicity or because their chemical forms do not suggest they are potential health hazards.

Generally recognized as safe (GRAS) *A list of food additives that in 1958 were considered safe for consumption. Manufacturers were allowed to continue to use these additives, without special clearance, when needed for food products. FDA bears responsibility for proving they are not safe, but can remove unsafe products from the list.*

Are Synthetic Chemicals Always Harmful?

Nothing about a natural product makes it inherently safer than a synthetic (manmade) product. Many synthetic products are simply laboratory copies of chemicals that also occur in nature (see the discussion in Chapter 16 on biotechnology for some examples). Moreover, although human endeavors contribute some toxins to foods, such as synthetic pesticides and industrial chemicals, nature's poisons are often even more potent and prevalent. Some cancer researchers believe that we ingest more natural toxins produced by plants than we do synthetic pesticide residues. This comparison doesn't make synthetic chemicals any less toxic, but it does lend perspective.

Consider vitamin E, which is often added to food to prevent rancidity of fats. This chemical is safe when used within certain limits. However, high doses have been associated with health problems in certain people (see Chapter 7). Thus even well-known chemicals we are comfortable using can be toxic in some circumstances and at some concentrations.

Testing Food Additives for Safety

Food additives are tested for safety on at least two animal species, usually rats and mice. Scientists determine the highest dose of the additive that produces *no observable effects* in the animals. These doses are proportionately much higher than humans are ever exposed to. The maximum dosage is then divided by at least 100 to establish a margin of safety for human use. The rationale of using a 100-fold margin is that we assume humans are at least 10 times more sensitive to food additives than are laboratory animals and that any one person might be 10 times more sensitive than another. This very broad margin ensures in most cases that the food additive in question will cause no harmful health effects in humans.

One important exception applies to the schema for testing intentional food additives: If an additive is shown to cause cancer, even though only in very high doses, no margin of safety is allowed. The food additive cannot be used, because it would violate the **Delaney Clause** in the 1958 Food Additive Amendments. This clause prohibits intentionally adding to foods a compound that was introduced after 1958 and causes cancer. Very few exceptions to this clause are allowed; the few are discussed in a following section.

Note that this 100-fold margin of safety is over 30 times that for vitamin A, when you compare the RDA to a potentially toxic dose for pregnant women.

Incidental food additives are another matter altogether. FDA cannot simply ban various industrial chemicals, pesticide residues, and mold toxins from foods, even though some of these contaminants can cause cancer. These products are not purposely added to foods—they are present whether we like it or not. FDA sets an acceptable amount for these substances. Basically, an incidental substance found in a food cannot contribute to more than one cancer case during the lifetimes of 1 million people. If a higher risk exists, the amount of the compound in a food must be reduced until the guideline is met.

Obtaining Approval for a New Food Additive

Today, before a new substance can be added to foods, FDA or other federal agencies must approve its use. Besides rigorously testing an additive to establish its safety margins, manufacturers must provide information that (1) identifies the new additive, (2) gives its chemical composition, (3) states how it is manufactured, and (4) specifies laboratory methods used to measure its presence in the food supply at the amount of intended use.

Manufacturers must also offer proof that the additive will accomplish its intended purpose in a food, that it is safe, and that it is to be used in no higher amount than needed. Additives cannot be used to hide defective food ingredients, such as rancid oils; deceive customers; or replace good manufacturing practices. A manufacturer must establish that the ingredient is necessary for producing a specific food product.

Today, sugar, salt, corn syrup, and citric acid constitute 98% of all additives (by weight) used in food processing.

Common Food Additives

A list of food additive categories appears in Table 15-3. Let's look at some of the specific categories of additives to learn more about the substances employed.

TABLE 15-3

Food Additive Categories

Anticaking agents	Formulation aids: carriers, binders, fillers, plasticizers	Processing aids (cont.): catalyst, flocculants, filter aids, crystallization inhibitors
Antimicrobial agents	Fumigants	Propellants
Antioxidants	Humectants	Sequestrants
Color and adjuncts	Leavening	Solvents and vehicles
Conditioners	Lubricants and release agents	Stabilizers and thickeners
Curing and pickling	Nonnutritive sweeteners	Surface active agents
Dough strengtheners	Nutritive sweeteners	Surface-finishing agents
Drying agents	Oxidizing and reducing agents	Synergists
Emulsifiers	pH control	Texturizers
Enzymes	Processing aids: clarifying, clouding	
Firming agents		
Flavor enhancers		
Flavoring agents		
Flour treating		

Alternative Sweeteners

Currently saccharin, acesulfame (Sunette) and sucralose are the only nonnutritive sweeteners used in foods. Because aspartame (Nutrasweet) yields energy, it is considered a nutritive sweetener (see Chapter 4). Saccharin is a relatively weak carcinogen for rats when administered over two generations. The cancers are found primarily in the bladder. However, population studies of humans have not found an increased risk of developing bladder cancer from exposure to saccharin. Still, a cancer-warning label must appear on any product that contains saccharin. This is one of the exceptions to the Delaney Clause; FDA is prevented from banning it by the U.S. Congress, which responded to constituent desires.

When buying food products, especially perishables, check the product date for safety. Four types of dates are commonly used. The pack date is the day the product was manufactured. The pull or sell date indicates the last date the product should be sold. It allows some time for storing food at home before eating. Check the expiration date of foods stored at home, because that is the last date the food can safely be stored on the shelf. Last, baked goods may have a freshness date, indicating that the product may safely be eaten for a short time after the date but may not taste the same.

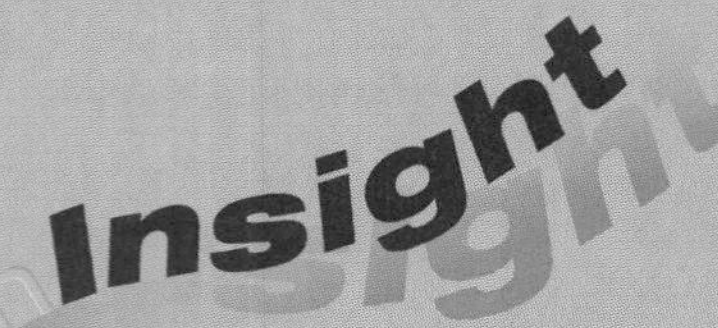

Caffeine—Is There an Ax to Grind?

Why all the controversy over a cup of coffee? Can't we come to one definite conclusion? Researchers have spent a great deal of time on the study of caffeine, the substance of greatest concern in the favorite beverage of many of us. So why do recommendations change from year to year?

Many factors complicate the study of caffeine intake, not the least of which is the memory of study participants. On average we consume 75% of our caffeine intake as coffee, 15% as tea, 10% as soft drinks, and 2% as chocolate. But researchers need a more detailed picture of individuals' specific habits, so they ask people to remember consumption patterns from 10 years ago or more. Do you remember how many cans of soft drinks you drank a day 10 years ago? Do you remember all the sources of caffeine you consumed, or how many cups of regular versus decaf coffee you drank 3 years ago?

Another factor that complicates research is that heavy coffee drinkers often have other deleterious health habits such as heavy alcohol consumption, smoking, and high-fat diets. In addition, smokers are likely to drink more coffee because their blood is cleared of caffeine faster than nonsmokers. Are the health consequences found in heavy coffee drinkers due to caffeine, or is it possible that these other harmful habits are the true cause? In addition, caffeine is not often consumed by itself. With the recent popularity of trendy coffee shops that serve everything from mocha java to flavored lattes, it is difficult to separate caffeine intake from cream, sugar, artificial sweeteners, and flavorings. So what is the conscientious coffee drinker to think? Let's explore the myths and facts of caffeine intake as it is known today.

Caffeine can cause anxiety, increased heart rate, insomnia, increased urination, constipation or diarrhea, and gastrointestinal upset. In addition, those already suffering from ulcers may experience irritation due to increased acid production, those who have panic attacks may find that caffeine worsens the symptoms, and those prone to heartburn may find that caffeine worsens this symptom because it relaxes sphincter muscles in the stomach and esophagus. Some people need very little caffeine to feel such effects, and the dosage for children is likely even lower than for adults.

Withdrawal symptoms are also very real. Former coffee drinkers may experience headache, nausea, and depression for a short time after discontinuing use. These symptoms can be expected to peak at 20 to 48 hours following the last intake of caffeine. Symptoms hold true even for those trying to quit as little as one cup of coffee a day. Slow tapering of use over a few days is recommended to avoid this problem.

Are there more serious consequences of consuming caffeine regularly. It has been hypothesized that caffeine consumption can lead to certain types of cancer, such

Antimicrobial Agents

Sodium benzoate, sorbic acid, and calcium propionate are common preservatives. Sorbic acid is a potent inhibitor of molds and fungal growth. Calcium propionate, a natural part of some cheeses, inhibits mold growth.

Antioxidants

This type of food preservative helps delay food discoloration from oxygen exposure, such as occurs when potatoes are diced. It also helps keep fats from turning rancid. Two widely used antioxidants are BHA (butylated hydroxyanisole) and BHT (butylated hydroxytoluene). Vitamin E and related compounds also serve as antioxidants.

Sulfites, a group of sulfur-based chemicals, are widely used as antioxidants in foods. Some people (1 in 100 according the FDA estimates) are extremely sensitive to sulfites and may have difficulty breathing, wheeze, and vomit, as well as develop hives, diarrhea, abdominal pain, cramps, and dizziness. As a result, FDA now limits the use of sulfites on raw fruits and vegetables—especially with use in salad bars.

as pancreatic and bladder cancers. The association of caffeine with cancer has not been supported in recent literature. At this time it appears that there is no major connection between caffeine and cancer.

The limelight also has been drawn away from caffeine with regard to heart disease and coffee consumption. Heavy use does increase blood pressure for a short period of time. Coffee consumption also has been linked to increased LDL and triglycerides. This association was found to be caused by cafestol and kahweol, two oils in ground coffee, as discussed in Chapter 5. However, since 1975 filtered and instant coffees have become popular, and these products do not contain the harmful oils. When researchers correct for tobacco use in coffee drinkers, no distinct correlation is seen between filtered or instant coffee consumption and increased risk for heart disease. It is prudent, though, to limit the amount of coffee from French coffee presses and from expresso, as these beverages are not filtered.

Women are thought to be at higher risk for a variety of deleterious effects with caffeine consumption, including osteoporosis, and birth defects and miscarriages in their offspring. It is true that heavy caffeine use increases the amount of calcium excreted in urine. For this reason, it is important that heavy coffee drinkers check their diets for adequate calcium sources. FDA currently recommends that the complete elimination or at least limitation of caffeine by pregnant women. Though there is currently no convincing evidence of an association between caffeine consumption and birth defects, some studies do show a higher likelihood for miscarriages in women consuming more than 150 mg of caffeine per day (Appendix I lists the caffeine content of foods). In addition, women who are trying to become pregnant may want to avoid caffeine, as a significant increase in risk of infertility has been seen with consumption of approximately two cups of coffee or four cans of cola per day. For these reasons, the American Medical Association and consumer groups recently called on FDA to ensure that the amount of caffeine be labeled when it is present in a product.

In contrast to these possibly harmful effects of caffeine consumption, many people are convinced of the benefits of a "cup of joe." Though some women testify to the idea that caffeine improves premenstrual symptoms, currently no study proves this theory. Some weight-loss drugs used to contain caffeine, under the assumption that it made the drugs more effective. FDA has since banned this use as it was found to be ineffective. You may have heard that caffeine can improve physical performance. This has been shown in highly trained athletes; recall that use of large amounts of caffeine is banned in international events (see Chapter 10). For those who are below professional status, though, no benefit has been shown.

Though the debate over caffeine will likely continue as long as Americans drink coffee, current research does not support many of the concepts previously thought of as fact. These studies are, in fact, reinforcing the idea of moderation—the equivalent of about two to three cups of coffee per day. Remember that there are no good or bad foods, but anything in excess can have damaging effects, caffeine and coffee included, and more so in some people than others.

FDA also requires manufacturers to declare the presence of sulfites on labels of packaged foods containing appreciable amounts. Labels on wine bottles often list a sulfite warning.

Colors

Color additives don't improve nutritional qualities, but they can make foods more visually appealing. Food colorings cannot be used to deceive consumers—for example, by covering blemishes, concealing any inferiority, or misleading people in any way. Although colorings are arguably unnecessary additives, manufacturers have satisfied FDA that color is "necessary" for the production of certain foods.

Controversy has surrounded the use of some food colors Currently the safety of using tartrazine (FD&C yellow No. 5) is disputed. It has caused allergic symptoms—such as hives, itching, and nasal discharge—in sensitive individuals, especially in people allergic to aspirin. Although few Americans are sensitive to tartrazine, FDA requires manufacturers to list FD& C yellow No. 5 on labels of food products containing it. Some red dyes have also raised alarms, and some have been banned.

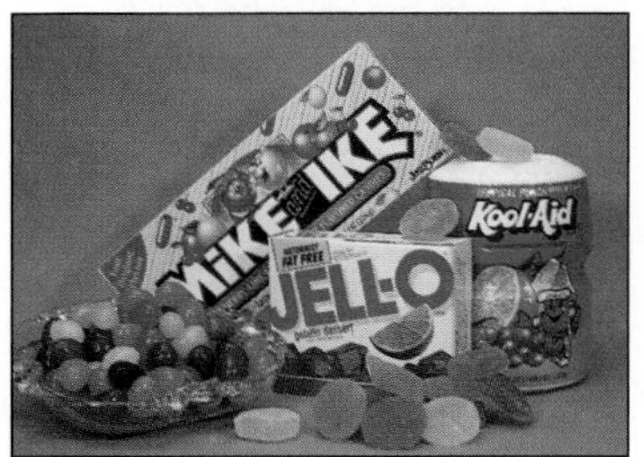

Color additives make some foods more desirable. Their use must be noted on the label so people sensitive to certain varieties can avoid that substance.

Currently FDA requires manufacturers to list all forms of synthetic colors on the labels of foods that contain them. Pigments extracted from plant sources are exempted from specific description on food labels.

Flavors and Flavoring Agents

Both naturally occurring and artificial agents can impart more flavor to foods. These agents include extracts from spices and herbs, as well as synthetic agents. You've probably recognized flavors of some spices and of liquid derivatives of onion, garlic, cloves, and peppermint in foods. To met the demand of industry, manufacturers have developed synthetic flavors that not only taste like natural flavors but also have the advantage of stability. Often artificial flavors, such as butter and banana flavors, have the same chemical composition as the natural flavor.

Flavor Enhancers

Flavor enhancers are substances such as monosodium glutamate (MSG) that help bring out the natural flavors of foods, such as in Chinese food and packaged gravy. Note that the glutamate portion is simply a nonessential amino acid. A small percentage of people are sensitive to the glutamate in MSG and, after exposure, experience flushing, chest pain, facial pressure, dizziness, sweating, rapid heart rate, nausea, vomiting, high blood pressure, and headache. The onset of symptoms occurs about 10 to 20 minutes after ingestion and may last from 2 to 3 hours. Infants are the most sensitive to MSG, in part because infants have not yet developed a complete blood-brain barrier. This means they cannot fully exclude such substances as MSG from the brain.

People who find themselves sensitive to MSG should avoid it. It may be present alone (look for the word *glutamate*), as well as in any isolated protein source (caseinate, texturized vegetable protein, etc.), yeast extract, bouillon, soup stock, and seasonings. Tomatoes, mushrooms, and parmesan cheese are also sources of free glutamate. Fortunately, most of us find that moderate use of MSG or glutamate in foods poses no significant risk to our health. FDA is currently contemplating label requirements for MSG.

Nutrient Supplements

Vitamin and mineral supplements are added to foods to improve their nutritional quality. Sometimes they replace nutrients lost in processing, as occurs when enriching flour.

Vitamin A is added to margarine and some forms of milk. Vitamin D is added to some dairy products. Potassium iodide is added to salt, and calcium and folate to some flours, fruit juices, and other products. Breakfast cereals often contain a variety of added nutrients, as do some fruit juices and related beverages.

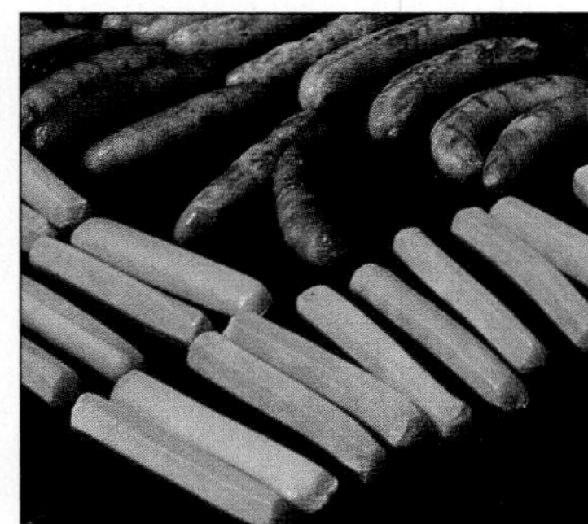

Cured meats derive their pink color from nitrates. The National Cancer Institute advises consuming these foods in moderation, as the nitrates/nitrites present some cancer risk.

Curing and Pickling Agents

The similar compounds, nitrates and nitrites, are used as preservatives, especially to prevent growth of *Clostridium botulinum*. Sodium and potassium nitrates and nitrites are used to preserve meats such as bacon, ham, salami, and hot dogs. Nitrates and nitrites have been used for centuries, in conjunction with salt, to preserve meat. An added effect of nitrates is their reaction with pigments in meat to form a bright pink color. This gives ham, hot dogs, and other cured meats their characteristic appearance.

Nitrate consumption from both cured foods and natural vegetables has been associated with the synthesis of nitrosamines in the stomach. Some nitrosamines are cancer-causing agents, particularly for the upper airway and esophagus. The actual risk appears to be low.

Federal agencies surmise that consumers take for granted a margin of microbial safety gained from nitrite use in cured meats. People often serve these meats cold or at least underheated. Consequently, these agencies have chosen not to ban nitrate or nitrite use in foods but rather to change manufacturing practices to lower amounts of preformed nitrosamines and suggest moderation in the use of these food products. Since 1975 there has been an 80% decrease in the amount of nitrites in cured meats.

The addition of vitamin C (sodium ascorbate) to cured meats, such as bacon, is one way to reduce the amount of nitrosamines formed in foods. This is a common manufacturing practice today. Other antioxidants used, such as sodium erythrobate, also inhibit synthesis of nitrosamines.

You might wonder why, if nitrates and nitrites form chemical substances that can cause cancer, they aren't banned by the Delaney Clause. In the United States, USDA regulates the use of chemicals in meats. The laws that govern USDA regulation of foods are separate from those that govern FDA regulation. Because of this, the Delaney Clause does not apply to USDA actions. Currently USDA sees no clear threat to public safety from the regulated use of nitrates and nitrites in meats, so no action has been taken.

Conclusion

In general, if you consume a variety of foods in moderation, the chances of food additives jeopardizing your health are minimal (Figure 15–3). Pay attention to your body. If you suspect an intolerance or sensitivity, consult your physician for further evaluation. Remember that, in the short run, you are more likely to suffer either from poor food-handling practices that allow bacteria to grow in food or from consuming raw animal foods than from consuming additives. Excess energy, saturated fat, sodium, and other potential "problem" nutrients in our diets pose the greatest long-term risk.

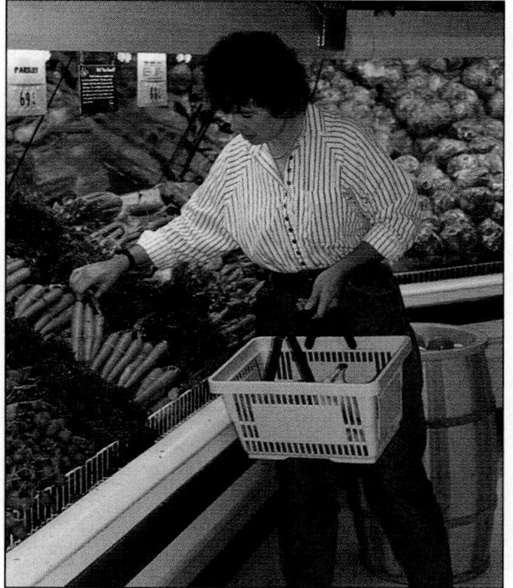

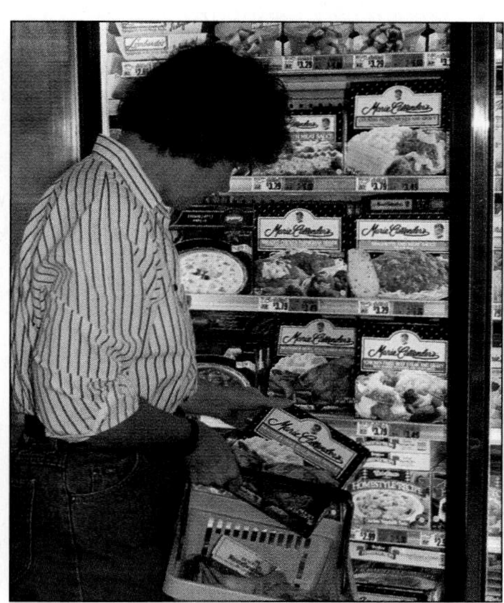

Figure 15–3 *Depending on food choices, a diet can be either (A) essentially free of or (B) contain food additives. For most of us, this specific concern regarding food choice is not worth worrying about.*

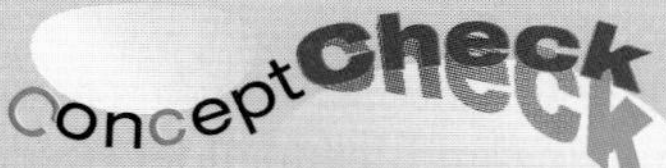

Food additives are used to reduce spoilage from microbial growth, oxygen, and other processes. Additives are also used to adjust acidity, improve flavor and color, leaven, provide nutritional fortification, thicken, and emulsify food components. Additives are classified as intentional (direct), which are purposely added to foods, and incidental (indirect), which turn up in foods from environmental contamination or various manufacturing practices. The amount of an additive allowed in a food is limited to $\frac{1}{100}$ of the highest amount that has no observable effect when fed to animals. The Delaney Clause allows FDA to limit intentional addition of cancer-causing compounds to food under its jurisdiction. Also limited by law are the permissible amounts of carcinogens that incidentally enter foods.

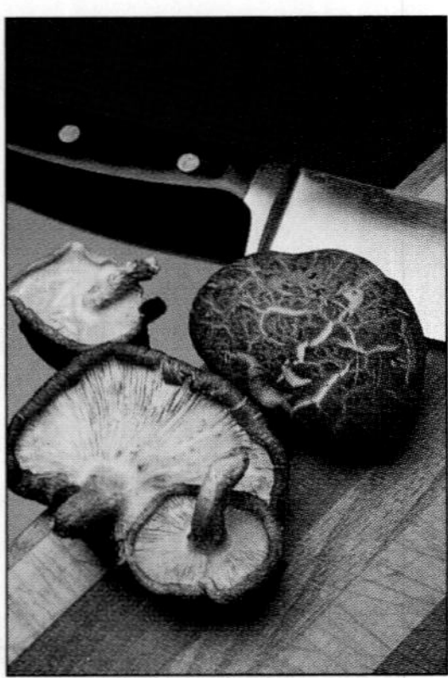

When hunting wild mushrooms, know what you are looking for. Many varieties contain deadly toxins.

Substances That Occur Naturally in Foods and Can Cause Illness

Foods contain a variety of naturally occurring substances that can cause illness. Here are some of the more important examples:

Safrole—found in sassafras, mace, and nutmeg; causes cancer.
Solanine—found in potato shoots and green spots on potato skins; inhibits the action of neurotransmitters.
Mushroom toxins—found in some species of mushrooms; can cause stomach upset, dizziness, hallucinations, and other neurological symptoms. The more lethal varieties can cause liver and kidney failure, coma, and even death. FDA regulates commercially grown and harvested mushrooms. These are cultivated in concrete buildings or caves. However, there are no systematic controls on individual gatherers harvesting wild species, except in Michigan and Illinois.
Avidin—found in raw egg whites; binds the vitamin biotin in a way that prevents its absorption.
Thiaminase—found in raw clams and mussels; destroys the vitamin thiamin.
Glycyrrhizic acid—found in pure licorice extracts; causes high blood pressure.
Tetrodotoxin—found in puffer fish; causes respiratory paralysis.
Protease inhibitor—found in raw soybeans; inhibits digestive enzymes.
Oxalic acid—found in spinach; binds calcium and iron.
Herbal teas—containing senna or comfrey; can cause diarrhea and liver damage.

People have coexisted for centuries with these naturally occurring substances and have learned to avoid some of them and limit intake in other cases. Today they pose little health risk. Farmers know potatoes must be stored in the dark so that solanine won't be synthesized. Furthermore, we've developed cooking and food preparation methods to limit the potency of other substances. Nevertheless, it's important to understand that some potentially harmful chemicals in foods occur naturally.

Environmental Contaminants in Food

A variety of environmental contaminants may be found in foods. Table 15-5 in the Nutrition Issue lists ways to limit pesticide residue in the diet. Aside from pesticide residues and products of fungal growth, though, other important contaminants deserve attention.

Lead

Ingesting lead can cause anemia, kidney disease, and damage to the nervous system and can interfere with nerve impulse conduction. Lead toxicity is a particular problem for children because they absorb it to a greater degree than adults, and it is associated with IQ deficits, behavior disorders, slowed growth, impaired hearing, and possibly high blood pressure and kidney disease later in life. Exposed children who eat a high-fat diet low in calcium, vitamin D, vitamin C, and iron absorb more lead than do those who eat a more healthful diet.

Despite the reduction of lead exposure in children over the last 20 years associated with the decline in lead-based paint, leaded gasoline and lead solder used in homes and in the canning industry, approximately 1.7 million children 1 to 5 years still have elevated blood lead. Medical costs for a child with lead intoxication average $2500 per treatment, and most children require two or more treatments.

Poor African-American children, who reside disproportionately in inner cities, are at increased risk for harmful lead exposure because of the lead-based paint present on the interiors and exteriors of older buildings. As this paint flakes off walls or is abraded from window trim as windows are opened and closed, lead paint chips enter the environment and may be ingested. The American Academy of Pediatrics recommends that physicians screen any child suspected of exposure for lead toxicity. This especially includes areas of the country where much of the housing was built before 1950, as lead-based paint was commonly used before that time.

Other sources of lead include brass fittings on water pumps used in wells, imported wine from areas where leaded gasoline is still used (especially Eastern Europe), and lead caps on wine bottles in general. Wiping the neck of the bottle with a towel limits this type of exposure. An additional risk is posed by acidic products such as fruit juice, sauerkraut, or pickled vegetables stored in galvanized, tin, or other metal containers (except stainless steel). Acid can dissolve the metal, and lead leaches into the food product.

Lead can also leach from solder joints into copper pipes, so it is best to let tap water run a minute or so before drinking it or cooking with it, especially first thing in the morning or when the water has been off for a few hours. In addition, use only cold water for drinking, cooking, and preparing infant formula.

Mercury

FDA first limited mercury in foods in 1969 after 120 people in Japan became ill from eating fish contaminated with high amounts. Birth defects in offspring of some of those people were also blamed on the mercury exposure. The fish most often contaminated was swordfish. Shark may also contain high amounts. Such large predatory fish that live for a long time can accumulate high amounts of mercury. These species are tested more frequently to ensure that the commercial supply is safe. FDA scientists responsible for seafood agree that these fish are safe, provided they are eaten infrequently (no more than once a week). Pregnant women and women of childbearing age who may become pregnant, however, are advised by FDA to limit their consumption of shark and swordfish to no more than once a month. Note that other types of fish and seafood, especially smaller, younger varieties, generally contain little mercury.

Urethane in Alcoholic Beverages

Urethane forms during fermentation of alcoholic beverages. If the fermented product is heated, as in the production of sherry and bourbon, urethane concentration increases. Although urethane causes cancer in laboratory animals, it's unclear whether it causes cancer in humans. A prudent choice is to limit consumption of products such as fruit brandies and sake because these show consistently high amounts of urethane.

Protecting Yourself from Environmental Toxins in Food

Environmental toxins that cause disease can be present in foods. To reduce exposure, find out which foods pose a risk. In addition, emphasize variety and moderation in food selection, and pay attention to any local warnings of risk, especially from local freshwater fish. The presence of mercury may concern you, but it's normally not a health risk unless your diet is dominated by a specific variety of fish. The small amount of mercury in most swordfish or shark isn't harmful if you're exposed to it infrequently. Table 15-5 in the Nutrition Issue offers some other practical tips for limiting pesticide exposure. These apply to reducing exposure to environmental contaminants as well.

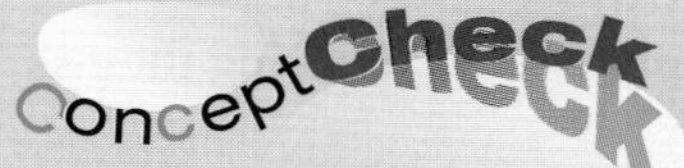

A general program to minimize exposure to environmental contaminants includes knowing which foods pose greater risks and consuming a wide variety of foods in moderation.

Summary

- ➤ Bacteria and other microbes in food pose the greatest risk for foodborne illness. In the past, salt, sugar, smoke, fermentation, and drying were used to protect against foodborne illness. Today careful cooking, pasteurization, and keeping hot foods hot and cold foods cold provide additional insurance.
- ➤ Major causes of foodborne illness today are the bacteria *Salmonella, Staphylococcus aureus, Campylobacter jejuni, and Clostridium perfringens.* In addition, such bacteria as *Clostridium botulinum, Listeria, Yersinia,* and *Escherichia coli* have been found to cause illness.
- ➤ To protect against these bacteria, cover cuts on the hands, do not sneeze or cough on foods, avoid contact between raw meat or poultry products and other food products, and rapidly cool and thoroughly reheat leftovers. Thorough cooking of foods and the use of pasteurized dairy products protect against other bacteria and viruses that scientists are only now beginning to understand.
- ➤ Cross-contamination commonly causes foodborne illness. It occurs particularly when bacteria on raw animal products contact foods that can support bacterial growth. Because of the risk of cross-contamination, no perishable food should be kept at room temperature for more than 1 to 2 hours (depending on the environmental temperature), especially if it may have come in contact with raw animal products.
- ➤ Treatment for foodborne illness usually requires drinking lots of fluids, avoiding touching food while diarrhea is present, thorough handwashing, and bed rest. Antibiotics also may be prescribed. Botulism and hepatitis A infections are types of foodborne illness that require prompt medical attention.
- ➤ Food additives are used primarily to extend shelf life by preventing microbial growth and destruction of food components by oxygen and other processes. Food additives are classified as those intentionally added to foods and those that incidentally end up in foods. An intentional additive is limited to no more than 1/100 of the greatest amount that causes no observed symptoms in animals. The Delaney Clause allows FDA to ban use of any intentional food additive under its jurisdiction that causes cancer.
- ➤ Antioxidants, such as BHA, BHT, vitamins E and C, and sulfites, prevent oxygen and enzyme destruction of food products. Common preservatives include sodium benzoate and sorbic acid, which prevent bacterial growth.
- ➤ Potentially harmful substances occur naturally in a variety of foods, such as green potatoes, raw fish, some types of mushrooms, raw soybeans, and raw egg whites. Cooking foods limits their toxic effects in some cases; other are best to avoid, such as toxic mushroom species and the green parts of potatoes.
- ➤ A variety of environmental contaminants can be found in foods. It's helpful to know which foods pose a special risk and act accordingly to reduce exposure.

Study Questions

1. Identify three major classes of microorganisms that are responsible for foodborne illness.
2. Which kinds of foods are most likely to be involved in foodborne illness? Why are they targets for contamination?
3. What three trends in food purchasing and production have led to a greater number of cases of foodborne illness in recent years?
4. Why is thoroughly cooking food an important practice for reducing the risk of foodborne illness?
5. List four techniques other than thorough cooking that are important in preventing foodborne illness.

6 Define the term *food additive* and give examples of four intentional food additives. What are their specific functions in foods?

7 Describe the federal process that governs the use of food additives, including the Delaney Clause.

8 Put into perspective the benefits and risks of the use of additives in food. Point out any easy way to reduce consumption of food additives. Do you think this is worth the effort in terms of maintaining health? Why or why not?

9 Describe the general recommendations for reducing the risk of toxicity from environmental contaminants.

Read the Nutrition Issue before answering the following question.

10 Outline how various federal agencies work together to monitor the safety of food in the United States.

Further Readings

1 A guide to food additives, *Nutrition Action Health Letter* p. 1, March 1999.
2 American Dietetic Association: Position of the American Dietetic Association: food and water safety, *Journal of the American Dietetic Association* 97:184, 1997.
3 Blaser MJ: How safe is our food? *New England Journal of Medicine* 334:1324, 1996.
4 Buchanan RL, Doyle MP: Foodborne disease significance of *Escherichia coli 0157:H7* and other enterohemorrhagic *E. coli, Food Technology* 51 (10):69, 1997.
5 Centers for Disease Control and Prevention: Multistate outbreak of *Salmonella* serotype agona infections linked to toasted oats cereal—United States, April–May, 1998, *Journal of the American Medical Association* 280:411, 1998.
6 Centers for Disease Control and Prevention: Outbreak of *Campylobacter* enteritis associated with cross-contamination of food—Oklahoma, 1996, *Journal of the American Medical Association* 279:1341, 1998.
7 Clarkson TW: Environmental contaminants in the food chain, *American Journal of Clinical Nutrition* 61:682S, 1995.
8 Eichholzer M, Gutzwiller FG: Dietary nitrates, nitrites, and n-nitroso compounds and cancer risk: a review of the epidemiologic evidence, *Nutrition Reviews* 56:95, 1998.
9 Food Safety: 7 myths, *UC Berkeley Wellness Letter,* p. 3, August 1998.
10 Henneman A: Don't mess with food safety myths, *Nutrition Today* 34(1):23, 1998.
11 Hingley A: Rallying the troops to fight foodborne illness, *FDA Consumer,* p. 7, November–December, 1997.
12 Hutin YJF and others: A multistate foodborne outbreak of hepatitis A, *New England Journal of Medicine* 340:595, 1999.
13 Kurtzweil P: Critical steps toward safer seafood, *FDA Consumer,* p. 10, November–December 1997.
14 Kurtzweil P: Questions keep sprouting about sprouts, *FDA Consumer,* p. 18, January/February 1999.
15 Leonard R: Drugs as feed additives increase risk to health, *CNI Nutrition Week,* p. 4, August 7, 1998.
16 Leonard R: Food safety woes grow as food imports rise, *CNI Nutrition Week,* p. 4, May 15, 1998.
17 Listeria outbreak leads to several deaths and record setting product recalls, *Community Nutrition Institute Nutrition Week,* p. 1, January 29, 1999.
18 Marwick C: New focus on children's environmental health, *Journal of the American Medical Association* 277:871, 1997.
19 McDonough LG: The food safety handbook, *American Health for Women,* p. 56, June 1998.
20 Mushak P, Crocetti AF: Lead and nutrition, *Nutrition Today* 31:12, 1996; II 31:115, 1996.
21 Osterholm MT: Cyclosporiasis and raspberries—lessons for the future, *New England Journal of Medicine* 336:1597, 1997.
22 Raiten DJ and others: Monosodium glutamate, *Food Technology,* p. 8, October 1995.
23 Seafood smart, *Journal of the American Medical Association* 280:760, 1998.
24 Schardt D, Schmidt S: Caffeine: the inside scoop, *Nutrition Action Healthletter* 23(10): 1, 1996.
25 Shewmake RA, Dillon B: Food poisoning, *Postgraduate Medicine* 103(6):125, 1998.

RATE

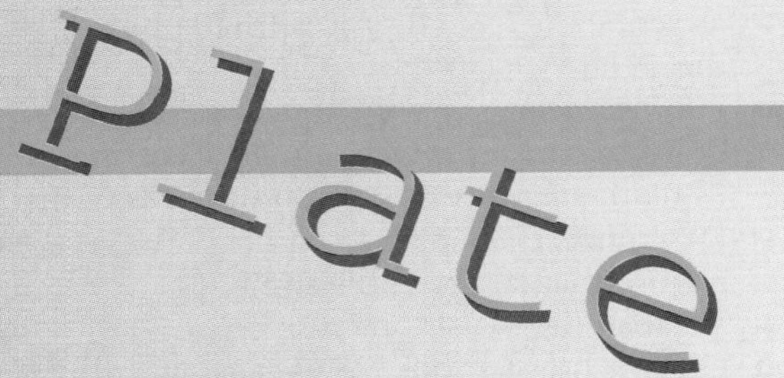

Can you spot the improper food safety practices?

In this chapter you learned the following facts: (1) foodborne illness strikes up to 81 million Americans each year; (2) about 9000 deaths each year in America are caused by foodborne organisms.

Carefully preparing foods to prevent foodborne illness can minimize its occurrence for most of us. Read the excerpt below and find the food safety violations that could contribute to this risk.

I. A Local Health Department Inspector Gives the Following Account of His Visit to a Local Diner

As I walked through the kitchen of the Morningside Diner, I noticed that each food handler washed his or her hands thoroughly with hot, soapy water before handling the food, especially after handling raw meat, fish, poultry, or eggs. Before preparing raw foods they also thoroughly washed the cutting boards, dishes, and other equipment. As they used their cutting boards after cutting foods, they wiped them with a damp rag and used them again to cut more food.

When preparing fresh fruits and vegetables, they washed them but were careful to leave a little dirt on for fear of washing important nutrients from the outside. The cooks generally cooked meats to an internal temperature of 180°F (82°C). However, to preserve the flavor, pork was cooked to an internal temperature of 140°F (60°C). Some cooked foods to be served later were cooled to 40°F (4°C) within 2 hours, and foods like beef stew were cooled in shallow pans.

The diner served canned foods even when the cans were dented. When leftovers were reheated, they were raised to an internal temperature of 150°F (66°C) and served immediately. Food handlers took great care to remove moldy portions of food. The cooks prepared stuffing separately from the poultry. The temperature of refrigerators was approximately 45°F (7°C).

1. Below, list the violations of food safety practices that could contribute to foodborne illness.

____

____

____

____

2. If you were writing a report describing ways to correct these practices, what would you say?

____

____

____

____

II. Food Additives

Evaluate a food label of a convenience food item either in the supermarket or one you may have at home.

1. **Write out the list of ingredients.**

____

____

____

____

2. **Identify the ingredients that you think may be food additives.**

____

____

____

____

3. **Based on the information available in this chapter, what are the functions of these specific food additives?**

____

____

____

____

4. **How might this food product differ without these ingredients?**

____

____

____

____

Share your findings with your classmates.

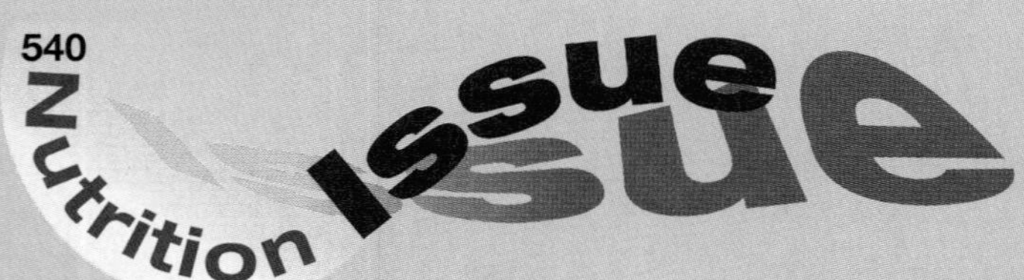

Pesticides in Food

Pesticides used in food production produce both beneficial and unwanted effects. Generally the benefits greatly outweigh the risks for most of us. Pesticides help ensure a safe and adequate food supply and help make foods available at reasonable cost. However, sentiment is growing nationwide that pesticides pose avoidable health risks.

Most concern about pesticide residues in food appropriately focuses on chronic rather than acute toxicity because the amounts of residue present, if any, are extremely small. These low concentrations found in foods are not known to produce adverse effects in the short term, although harm has been caused by the high amounts that occasionally result from accidents or misuse, especially in rural communities. For most of us, pesticides pose a danger mainly in their cumulative effects, so their threats to health are difficult to determine. However, growing evidence, including the problems of contamination of underground water supplies and destruction of wildlife habitats, indicates that we would likely be better off as a nation if we could reduce use of pesticides. Both the federal government and many farmers are working toward that end.

WHAT IS A PESTICIDE?

Federal law defines a *pesticide* as any substance or mixture of substances intended to prevent, destroy, repel, or mitigate any pest. The built-in toxic properties of pesticides lead to the possibility that other, nontarget organisms, including humans, might also be harmed. The term *pesticide* tends to be used as a generic reference to many types of products, including insecticides, herbicides, fungicides, and rodenticides. A pesticide product may be chemical or bacterial, natural or man-made. For agriculture, EPA allows about 10,000 pesticide uses, involving some 300 active ingredients. Pesticide use in general substantially contributes to the chemical load applied intentionally to the earth's surface. About 1.2 billion pounds of pesticides are used each year in the United States, much of which is applied to agricultural crops (Figure 15–4).

Once a pesticide is applied, it can turn up in a number of unintended and unwanted places. It may be carried in the air and dust by wind currents, remain in soil attached to soil particles, be taken up by organisms in the soil, decompose to other compounds, be taken up by plant roots, enter groundwater, or invade aquatic habitats. Each is a route to the food chain; some are more direct than others.

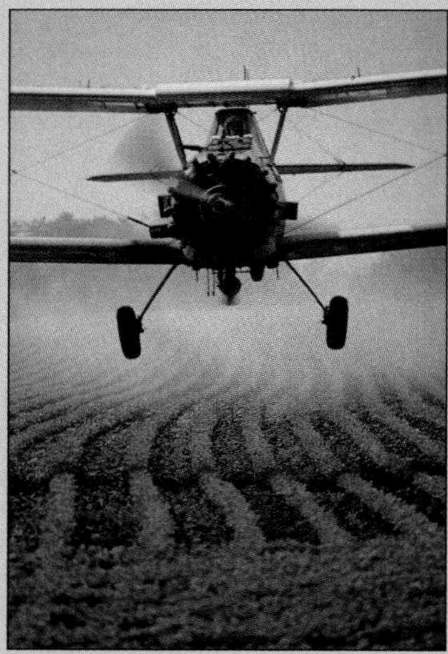

Figure 15–4
Pesticides use poses a risk-versus-benefit question. Each side has points that deserve to be considered. Rural communities, where exposure is more direct, experience the greatest short-term risk.

WHY USE PESTICIDES?

The primary reason for using pesticides is economic—use of agricultural chemicals increases production and lowers the cost of food, at least in the short run. Many farmers believe they would have a tough time staying in business without pesticides. Quick and direct, pesticides help protect farmers from ruinous losses caused by a sudden pest outbreak. Pesticides also can protect against rotting and decay of fresh fruits and vegetables. This is helpful because our food distribution system doesn't usually permit consumer purchase within hours of harvest. In addition, food grown without pesticides can contain naturally occurring organisms that produce carcinogens at concentrations far above current standards for pesticide residues. For example, fungicides help prevent the carcinogen aflatoxin (caused by growth of a fungus) from forming on some crops. Thus the use of pesticides does have important attributes to consider.

Consumer demands also have changed over the years. At one time we wouldn't have thought twice about buying an apple with a worm hole; we simply took it home, cut out the wormy part, and ate the apple. Today consumers find worm holes less acceptable, so farmers rely more and more on pesticides to produce cosmetically attractive fruits and vegetables. Thus, while some pesticide use may improve the appearance of food products, other use helps keep some foods fresher and safer to eat.

TABLE 15-4

U.S. Agencies Responsible for Monitoring the Food Supply

Agency name	Responsibilities	Methods	How to contact
United States Department of Agriculture (USDA)	• Enforces wholesomeness and quality standards for grains and produce (while in the field), meat, poultry, milk, and eggs.	• Inspection • Grading • "Safe Handling Label"	http://www.usda.gov/fsis or http://www.nal.usda.gov/fnic/foodborne/foodborn.htm or call (800) 535-4555
Bureau of Alcohol Tobacco, and Fire Arms (ATF)	• Enforces laws on alcoholic beverages	• Inspection	http://www.atf.trea.gov/
Environmental Protection Agency (EPA)	• Regulates pesticides • Establishes water quality standards	• Approval required for all U.S. pesticides • Sets pesticide residue limits in food	http://www.epa.gov/
Food and Drug Administration (FDA)	• Ensures safety and wholesomeness of all foods in interstate commerce (except meat and poultry) • Regulates seafood • Controls product labels	• Inspection • Food sample studies • Sets standards for specific foods.	http://www.fda.gov/ or http://vm.csfan.fda.gov or call (800) FDA-4010
Centers for Disease Control and Protection (CDC)	• Protects food safety	• Responds to emergencies of foodborne illness • Surveys and studies environmental health problems • Directs/enforces quarantines • National programs for prevention and control of foodborne and other diseases	http://www.cdc.gov/
National Marine Fishery Service	• Overseas fisheries management and harvesting	• Voluntary program for inspecting and grading	http://www.nmfs.gov
State and Local Government	• Milk safety • Monitoring of food industry within their borders	• Inspection of food-related establishments	Government pages of telephone book

REGULATING PESTICIDES

The responsibility for ensuring that residues of pesticides in foods are below amounts that pose a danger to health is shared by FDA, EPA, and the Food Safety and Inspection Service of USDA (see Table 15–4 for the roles of various food protection agencies). FDA is responsible for enforcing pesticide compliance in all foods except meat, poultry, and certain egg products, which are monitored by USDA. A newly proposed pesticide is exhaustively tested, perhaps over 10 years or more, before it is approved for use. In this process, EPA must decide both that the pesticide causes no unreasonable adverse effects on people and the environment and that benefits of use outweigh the risks of using it. However, there is concern about older chemicals registered before 1970, when less stringent testing conditions were permitted. EPA is now asking chemical companies to retest the old compounds using more rigorous tests. Unfortunately, inadequate funding at EPA has hampered the review of older pesticides.

When weighing whether to approve or cancel a pesticide, EPA considers how much more it would cost the farmer to use an alternative pesticide or process and whether cancellation would decrease productivity. After determining the dollar cost to the farmer, EPA then looks at costs to processors and consumers. Once a pesticide is approved for use it must follow the margin of safety provisions required of food additives (see the section on testing food additives in the chapter).

HOW SAFE OR UNSAFE ARE PESTICIDES?

Pesticide use is clearly associated with declining water quality. Accumulating information also links pesticide use to increased cancer rates in farm communities. For rural counties in the United States and Mexico, the incidence of lymph, breast, genital, brain, and digestive tract cancers increases with higher-than-average herbicide use. Developmental problems in children also are noted. Respiratory cancer cases increase with greater insecticide use. In tests using laboratory animals, scientists have found that some pesticide residues cause birth defects, sterility, tumors, organ damage, and injury to the central nervous system. Some pesticides persist in the environment for years.

On the other hand, some researchers argue that the cancer risk from pesticide residues is hundreds of times less than the risk from eating such common foods as peanut butter, brown mustard, and basil. Plants manufacture their own toxic substances to defend themselves against insects, birds, and grazing animals (including humans). When plants are stressed or damaged, they produce even more of these toxins. Because of this, many foods contain naturally occurring chemicals considered toxic, even carcinogenic. Other scientists argue that if natural carcinogens are already in the food supply, then we should reduce the number of added carcinogens whenever possible. In other words, we should do what we can to decrease the problem.

THE RISKS OF PESTICIDES TO CHILDREN

Any discussion of pesticides and associated health risks must focus on children. They are not simply small adults in a biological sense. Children face a higher risk from pesticide exposure than do adults for several reasons.

1. Their exposure is greater; children eat more food in proportion to their body weight than do adults.
2. Children consume more foods that are potential sources of pesticide residues than do adults. For example, they eat more fruit.
3. Exposure at an early age carries a greater risk than does exposure later in life; residues can accumulate to toxic amounts over a longer period. Also, cancer has more time to develop.
4. The effects of carcinogens and neurotoxins in pesticides may be greater; the cells in children are dividing rapidly, and the systems that detoxify chemicals are not fully developed.

EPA now looks at age-related consumption data for approval of new pesticides. Supporting this action is a recent report by the National Academy of Sciences that advocates changes to the current pesticide regulatory system to ensure the safety of foods eaten by children. In addition, its authors stress the value of including fruits and vegetables in children's diets to avoid certain foods. Carefully washing fruits and vegetables and consuming a wide variety are sufficient recommendations. Peeling fruits and vegetables when appropriate is another option (Table 15–5). A final general precaution is to keep children away from lawns, gardens, and flower beds that have recently been treated with pesticides and herbicides.

TABLE 15-5

What You Can Do to Reduce Dietary Exposure to Pesticides

FDA's sampling and testing show that pesticide residues in foods typically do not pose a health hazard. Nevertheless, if you want to reduce dietary exposure to pesticides, follow this advice.

- Thoroughly rinse and scrub (with a brush and dilute dishwashing liquid if possible) fruits and vegetables, especially peaches, potatoes, and carrots if the skin is to be eaten. Other foods to consider are apples and pears. Peel them, if appropriate—though some nutrients will be peeled away.
- Remove outer leaves of leafy vegetables, such as lettuce and cabbage.
  Trim fat from meat and poultry, remove skin (which contains most of the fat) from poultry and fish, and discard fats and oils in broths and pan drippings. Residues of some pesticides in feed concentrate in the animals' fat. Trim skin and fatty deposits from fish.
- Throw back the big fish—the little ones have had less time to take up and concentrate pesticides and other harmful residues. In addition, pay attention to any warnings by local authorities about the high risk for contamination in specific waters or species of fish.
- Eat a variety of foods. The more kinds of food you eat, the less your exposure to any one pesticide.

Adapted from Food and Drug Administration: Safety first: protecting America's food supply, *FDA Consumer,* p. 26, Nov 1988 and other sources.

TESTING AMOUNTS OF PESTICIDES IN FOODS

FDA tests thousands of raw products each year for pesticide residues. (A pesticide is considered illegal in this case if it is not approved for use on the crop in question or if the amount used exceeds the amount allowed.) A 1993 FDA study showed no residues in 64% of domestic samples and 69% of imported samples. Less than 1% of domestic and import samples had residues that were over allowed amounts, and 1% of domestic and 3% of imported samples had residues for which there was no approved use for that specific product. The findings for 1994 continued to demonstrate that pesticide residues in foods are generally well below EPA guidelines, and they confirm the safety of the food supply relative to pesticide residues.

When a problem is identified, FDA takes steps to make sure it's corrected and that the tainted food in question never reaches the consumer. However, of 600 pesticides available on international markets, many are not even detected by any of FDA's current testing procedures. This has raised concern by pesticide critics with regard to imported foods.

PERSONAL ACTION

We often take risks in our own lives, but we prefer to have a choice in the matter after weighing the pros and cons. For instance, we can choose not to immunize a child, but we do so with the understanding that the child might get sick. We can also choose to risk cancer from smoking or to avoid that risk. In regard to pesticides in food, however, someone else is deciding what is acceptable and what is not. Our only choice is whether to buy or avoid pesticide-containing foods. In reality it's almost impossible to avoid pesticides entirely, because even "organic" produce often contains traces of pesticides, probably as the result of cross-contamination from nearby farms.

Short-term studies of the effects of pesticides on laboratory animals cannot pinpoint long-term cancer risks precisely. It should be clearly understood, however, that the presence of minute traces of an environmental chemical in a food doesn't mean that any adverse effect will result from eating that food.

FDA and other scientific organizations believe that the hazards are comparatively low and in the short run are less than the hazards of foodborne illness created in our own kitchens. We can't avoid pesticide risks entirely, but we can limit exposure by following the advice given earlier in this chapter.

We can also encourage farmers to use fewer pesticides to reduce exposure to our foods and water supplies, but we'll have to settle for produce that isn't perfect in appearance. Are you concerned enough about pesticides on food to change your shopping habits or take more political action?

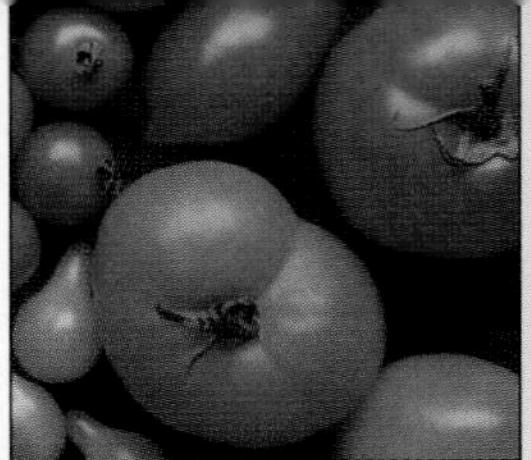

chapter

16 Undernutrition Throughout the World

The images are both vivid and heartrenching. Emaciated children with enormous eyes and stomachs, too weak to cry, stare at us from news photos and television screens. Half of all childhood deaths worldwide are related to undernutrition.

Today, nearly one in five people in the world is chronically undernourished—too hungry to lead a productive, active life. This is twice as many people as a decade ago. Throughout the world the problems of poverty and undernutrition are widespread and growing.

The majority (two-thirds) of undernourished people live in Asia. However the largest increases in numbers of chronically hungry people currently occur in eastern Africa, particularly in Sudan, Ethiopia, Rwanda, Burundi, Kenya, Somalia, and Tanzania. Their eyes haunt us.

This chapter examines the problem of undernutrition and the conditions that create it as well as some possible solutions. If undernutrition is to be eradicated, the world's nations must examine the problem and assume responsibility for supplying some answers. It is important to recognize that many political leaders and citizens worldwide contribute directly and indirectly to the economic and social destruction that spawns world hunger.

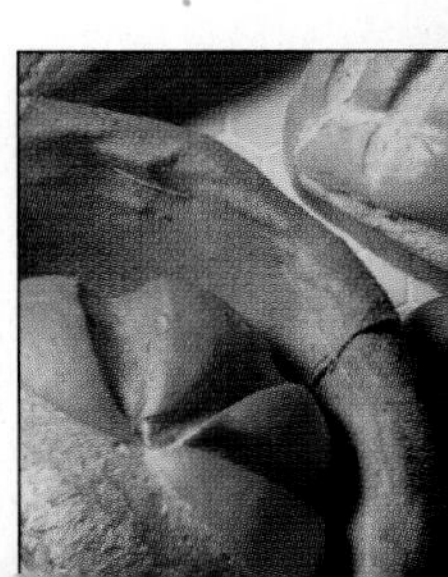

Nutrition Web

Poverty is common wherever people suffer from undernutrition.

The greatest risk of undernutrition occurs during critical periods of growth and development. Low birth weight—often related to undernutrition—is a leading cause of infant deaths worldwide.

Although famine has not existed in the United States since the 1930s, undernutrition is still a problem. In response, soup kitchens, the food stamp program, school lunch and breakfast programs, and the Supplemental Feeding Program for Women, Infants and Children (WIC) have been created to help those in need.

Reducing out-of-wedlock pregnancies and focusing more on the responsibilities of parents are two national priorities for preventing undernutrition, because single parents and their children are likely to live in poverty.

Multiple factors contribute to the problem of undernutrition in the developing world. Food resources may be inadequate. Farming methods often encourage erosion. Naturally occurring devastation from droughts, excessive rainfall, fire, crop infestation, and human causes—such as urbanization, war and civil unrest, debt, and poor sanitation—worsen the problem of undernutrition.

Direct food aid is only a short-term solution to undernutrition in developing countries. A focus on sustainable subsistence-level farming and small-scale industrial development are ways individuals can gain the resources to feed one's family. The world has both the food and the technical expertise to end hunger. What is lacking is the political will and cooperation to do so.

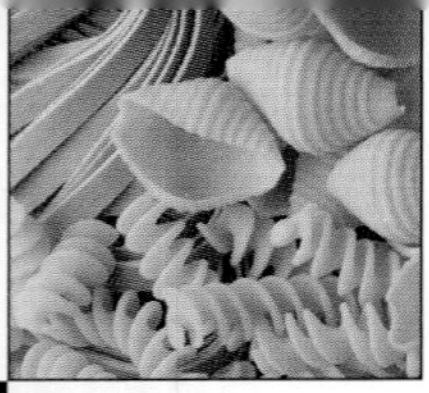

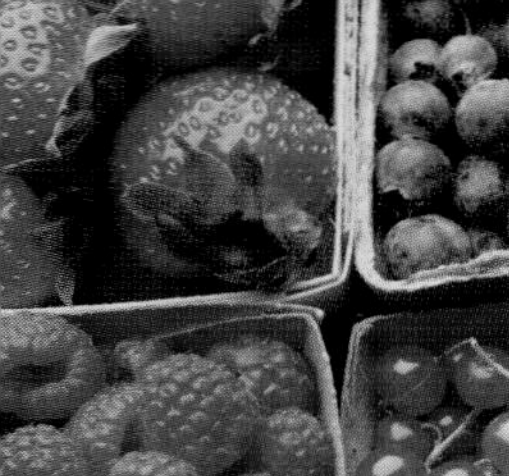

Did You Know?

Consider the following statistics:

- Nearly one in five people in the developing world is chronically undernourished—too hungry to lead a productive, active life. This includes one-third of the world's children.
- About 55,000 people die of hunger each day—two-thirds of them children.
- 3 million newborns in the developing world die in the first week of life.
- Over half of all children who die each year in developing countries do so from causes that could be prevented at low cost.
- Up to 350,000 children are permanently blinded each year simply from lack of sufficient vitamin A intake.
- Poor women in developing countries face a 50- to 200-fold increased risk of death in pregnancy compared with women in the United States.
- In many developing countries, life expectancy of the population is one-half to two-thirds of that in the United States.
- Almost half of the world's people earn less than $200 a year—many use 80% to 90% of that income to obtain food. About $2000 to $3000 each year per person is needed for life expectancy to reach that seen in the United States.
- People in developed countries spent more money on pet food, perfumes, and cosmetics than it would take to provide basic education, water and sanitation, health care, and nutrition for all those now deprived of it.
- Of the nearly 5.8 billion people on earth, more than 1 billion lack access to safe drinking water. In India alone, 300,000 children die each year from drinking contaminated water.
- About 3 billion people in the world are without proper sanitation facilities.
- About 2 billion people have iron deficiency.
- Developing countries have two-thirds of the 30 millions **AIDS** cases worldwide.
- About 28 million people worldwide have developed brain damage from maternal iodide deficiency; currently 1.5 billion people are at risk for iodide deficiency.

Aquired immunodeficiency syndrome (AIDS)
A disorder that takes place when the human immunodeficiency virus (HIV) infects specific immune system cells. This eventually leaves the person quite vulnerable to other infections, typically leading to death. Medical therapy can slow the decline in health in people infected with HIV, but does not cure the disease.

These stark realities should be a call for action. Note that currently 20% of the global population accounts for 86% of worldwide consumption. But to know what to do, it is necessary to understand the roots of the problem. This chapter will help you do so.

World Hunger Is a Continuing Plague

In November 1974 the United Nations World Food conference proclaimed its bold objective "that within a decade no child will go to bed hungry, that no family will fear for its next day's bread, and that no human being's future and capacities will be stunted by malnutrition." Obviously this promise remains unfulfilled: 26 years later hunger looms over many people in the developing world, and even one in nine households in the United States.

Civil wars in Africa and Eastern Europe, coupled with drought in many parts of the world, have brought millions of people to the brink of starvation, about two-thirds of whom live in Africa. Relief aid has been arriving but often with too little, too late, and then often misused by the governments in control. The deadly combination of political corruption/ineptness, war, and poor weather has also recently led to increasing hunger in Bangladesh, Afghanistan, the Philippines, North Korea, and Cambodia.

A recent goal, set at the U.N. Summit at the end of 1996, is to cut the number of hungry people worldwide in half by the year 2015. Some call this goal inadequate, while others call it realistic and attainable. Dr. Norman Meyers, an expert in this field, states that never have we had as rich a resource base to tackle this problem as we have today. Will we take advantage of this opportunity?

Defining World Hunger

Let's begin this look at the problem of world hunger by first defining some key words.

Hunger is the physiological state that results when not enough food is eaten to meet energy needs. It also describes an uneasiness, discomfort, weakness, or pain caused by lack of food. If hunger is not relieved, the resulting medical and social costs from undernutrition are high—preterm births and mental retardation, inadequate growth and development in childhood, poor school performance, decreased work output in adulthood, and chronic disease. Symptoms of chronic hunger are found not only among people in the developing world but also among many people living at or below the poverty level in America. Of any industrialized country, the United States has the largest number of children living in poverty (6.1 million under the age of 6). One out of every four children in this country goes hungry or is at risk for inadequate food intake.

Malnutrition is a condition of impaired development or function caused by either a long-term deficiency or an excess in energy and/or nutrient intake, the latter representing the state of overnutrition described in Chapter 2. When the food supply is ample or overabundant, incorrect food choices coupled with an excessive intake can lead to overnutrition-related chronic diseases, such as Type 2 diabetes.

When food supplies are low and the population is large, undernutrition is common, leading to nutritional deficiency diseases, such as goiter (from an iodide deficiency), xerophthalmia (eye problems caused by poor vitamin A intake), muscle wasting, and a host of other problems (Table 16–1). Undernutrition is the most common form of malnutrition among the poor in both developing and developed countries. Currently half of the 4 million African children under 5 years of age who die annually are undernourished. The most critical micronutrients missing from diets worldwide are iron, vitamin A, and iodide. Zinc intake is also marginal in many areas in the developing world.

Of the 5.8 billion people in the world, up to 2 billion may be affected by some form of micronutrient malnutrition. Death and disease from infections, particularly those causing acute and prolonged diarrhea or acute lower respiratory disease, increase dramatically when the infections are superimposed on a state of chronic undernutrition. Diarrhea alone is the number-one killer of children in developing countries, responsible for over 2 million deaths of children under 5 years of age.

Protein-energy malnutrition (PEM) is a form of undernutrition caused by an extremely deficient intake of energy or protein generally accompanied by an illness. The typically dramatic results of PEM—**kwashiorkor** and **marasmus**—were covered in Chapter 6. This chapter focuses on the more subtle effects of a chronic lack of food.

Famine is not the same thing as chronic hunger. Although both result from poverty and a lack of food, famine is the extreme form of chronic hunger. Periods of famine are characterized by large-scale loss of life, social disruption, and economic chaos that slows food production. As a result of these extreme events, the affected community experiences a downward spiral characterized by human distress; sales of land, livestock, and other important farm assets; migration; division and impoverishment of the poorest families; crime; and the weakening of customary moral codes, as seen recently in Sudan and Rwanda. In the midst of all this, undernutrition rates soar, infectious diseases such as cholera spread, and people die in staggering numbers.

Special efforts are needed to eradicate the fundamental causes of famine. Causes vary by region and decade, but the most common underlying cause is crop failure. The most obvious causes of crop failure are bad weather, war, and civil strife, or all three. War in fact deserves a special focus; this will be specifically addressed in an upcoming section.

Kwashiorkor
A disease occurring primarily in young children who have an existing disease and who consume a marginal amount of energy and considerably insufficient protein in the face of high needs. The child suffers from infections and exhibits edema, poor growth, weakness, and an increased susceptibility to further illness.

Marasmus
A disease that results from consuming a grossly insufficient amount of protein and energy; usually seen in infancy. It is the equivalent of protein-energy malnutrition in adults. The person with marasmus has little or no fat stores and shows muscle wasting. Death from infections is common.

Famine
An extreme shortage of food that leads to massive starvation in a population; often associated with crop failures, war, and political strife.

TABLE 16-1

Effects of Nutrient-Deficiency Diseases That Commonly Accompany Undernutrition

Disease and key nutrient involved	Typical effects	Foods rich in deficient nutrient	Where the problem still exists
XEROPHTHALMIA			
Vitamin A	Blindness from chronic eye infections, poor growth, dryness and eventual blindness	Liver, fortified milk, sweet potatoes, spinach, greens, carrots, cantaloupe, apricots	Asia, Africa
RICKETS			
Vitamin D	Weakened bones, bowed legs, other bone deformities	Fortified milk, fish oils, sun exposure	Asia and Africa where religious practices encourage avoidance of sun exposure for women and children; elderly in developing nations
BERIBERI			
Thiamin	Nerve degeneration, altered muscle coordination heart problems	Sunflower seeds, pork, whole and enriched grains, dried beans	Areas of famine in Africa
ARBOFLAVINOSIS			
Riboflavin	Inflammation of face and oral cavity	Milk, mushrooms, spinach, liver, enriched grains	Areas of famine in Africa
PELLAGRA			
Niacin	Diarrhea, skin inflammation, mental disorders	Mushrooms, bran, tuna, chicken, beef, peanuts, whole and enriched grains	Areas of famine in Africa
SCURVY			
Vitamin C	Delayed wound healing, internal bleeding, abnormal formation of bones and teeth	Citrus fruits, strawberries, broccoli	Areas of famine in Africa
IRON-DEFICIENCY ANEMIA			
Iron	Reduced work output, reduced growth, increased health risk in pregnancy, reduced mental development in early childhood	Meats, spinach, seafood, broccoli, peas, bran, whole-grain and enriched breads	Worldwide
GOITER			
Iodide	Enlarged thyroid gland, poor growth in infancy and childhood, possible mental retardation	Iodized salt, saltwater fish	South America, Eastern Europe, Africa

Often two or more nutrition-deficiency diseases are found in an undernourished person in the developing world. This separate discussion of nutrients just makes it easier to see the important role of each nutrient.

Critical Life Stages When Undernutrition Is Particularly Devastating

Prolonged undernutrition is detrimental to health at all stages of life, but is particularly critical during some periods of growth and old age (Figure 16–1).

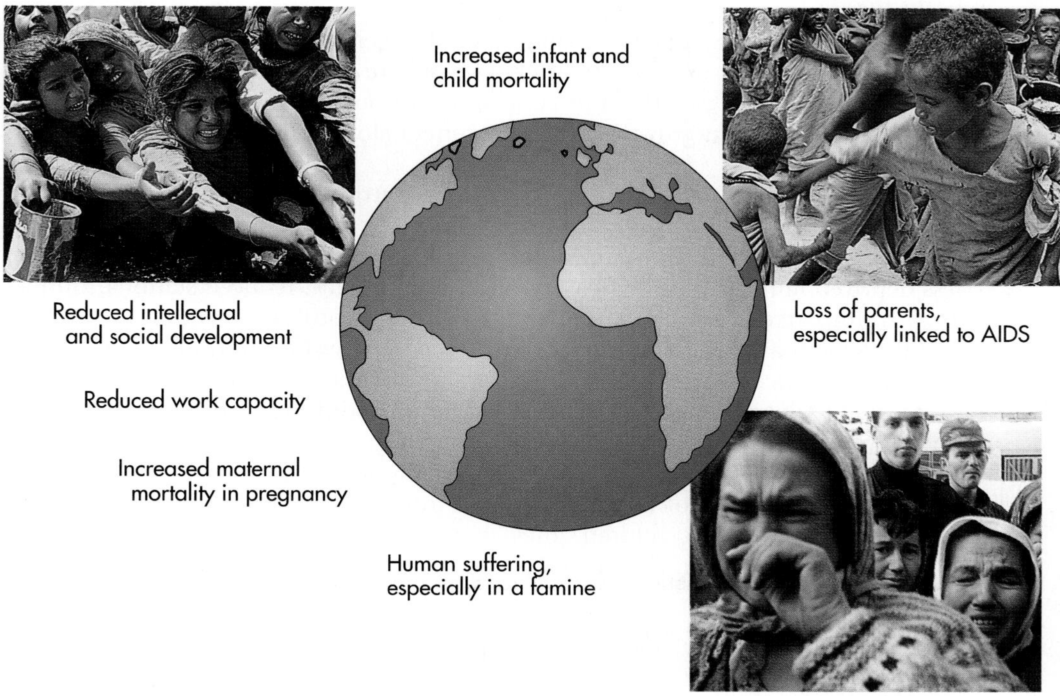

Figure 16–1 *Undernutrition affects many aspects of human health and humanity in general.*

Pregnancy

The period when undernutrition poses the greatest health risk is during pregnancy. A pregnant woman needs extra nutrients to meet both her own needs and those of her developing fetus.

In Africa, women give birth, on average, to more than six live babies. Coupled with chronic undernutrition, these high birth rates create up to a 330 times greater chance that a woman will die from pregnancy-related causes compared to American women. No other social indicator, including literacy, life expectancy, and infant mortality, shows a wider gap between the developing and industrialized world.

More than 3 million people may have perished in the great famine of 1943 in Bengal, India. In 1974, another 1.5 million from that region starved in the new country of Bangladesh. China suffered an almost unbelievable famine from 1959 to 1961—estimates of mortality range from 16 million to 64 million. Most recently up to 2 million people have died from the 3-year famine in North Korea.

Fetal and Infant Stages

The fetus faces major health risks from undernutrition during gestation. To support growth and development of the brain and other body tissues, a growing fetus requires a rich supply of protein, vitamins, and minerals. When these needs are not met, the infant is often born before 37 weeks of gestation, well before the 40 weeks of gestation that is considered ideal. Consequences of preterm birth include reduced lung function and a weakened immune system. These conditions not only compromise health but also increase the likelihood of death. Long-term problems in growth and development can result if the infant survives. In extreme cases, low-birth-weight babies (2500 grams [about 5.5 pounds] or less)—face 5 to 10 times the normal risk of dying before the age of 1 year, primarily because of reduced lung development. Nutritional deprivation, especially in early infancy, also can lead to permanent brain impairment. Chapter 13 pointed out that when low birth weight is accompanied by other physical abnormalities, medical intervention can cost $200,000 or more. Where severe retardation occurs, the lifetime cost of care can exceed $2 million. Currently about 17% of infants show low birth weights, mainly in developing countries.

Childhood

Early childhood, when growth is rapid, is another period when undernutrition is extremely risky. The brain and central nervous system are particularly vulnerable because of their rapid growth from conception through early childhood. After the preschool years, brain growth and development slow dramatically until maturity, when they cease.

About 40% of children in developing countries show evidence of stunting.

In general, poor children experience more nutritional deprivation and overall illness and are more severely affected than other children. For example, iron-deficiency anemia is much more common among poor children than children from less deprived families. This deficiency can lead to fatigue, reduced stamina, stunted growth, impaired motor development and learning problems. Undernutrition in childhood can also weaken resistance to infection, because immune function decreases when such nutrients as protein, vitamin A, and zinc are very low in a diet. Clearly, undernutrition and illness have a cyclical relationship. Not only does undernutrition cause illness, but illness worsens undernutrition, particularly diarrhea and infectious diseases. For this reason, many children in developing countries are dying from the combination of malnutrition and infection. Conversely, when adequate nutrients are restored to children's diets, improvements in health can be obvious.

Later Years

Older people are also at risk for undernutrition. They often require nutrient-dense foods, in amounts depending on their state of health and degree of physical activity. Because many of them have fixed incomes and incur significant medical costs, food often becomes a low-priority item. In addition, older people are often unable to take care of all their own needs, are sometimes isolated, and are more apt to be depressed—all important factors that influence food intake (see chapter 14).

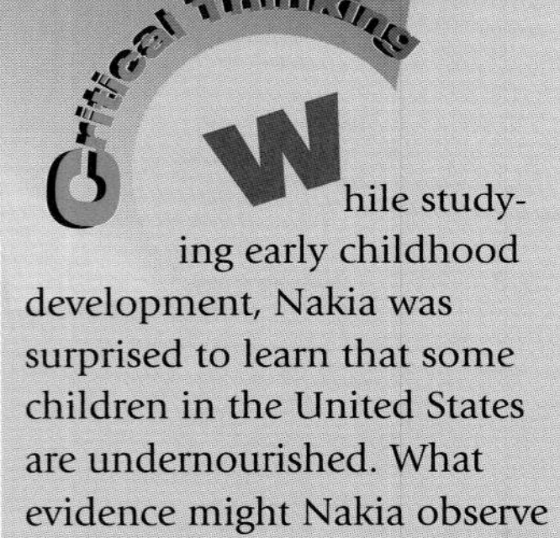

While studying early childhood development, Nakia was surprised to learn that some children in the United States are undernourished. What evidence might Nakia observe in children that would suggest undernourishment?

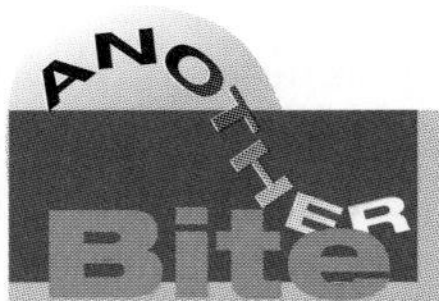

In the 1940s a group of researchers led by Dr. Ansel Keys maintained 32 previously healthy men on a diet averaging about 1600 kcal daily for 6 months. During this time, the men lost an average of 24% of their body weight. After about 3 months the participants complained of fatigue, muscle soreness, irritability, and hunger pains. They exhibited a lack of ambition and self-discipline and poor concentration. They were often moody and depressed. They became less able to laugh heartily, sneeze, and tolerate heat. Heart rate and muscle tone also decreased. When the men were permitted to eat normally again, the desire for more food and a feeling of fatigue continued, even after 12 weeks of rehabilitation. Full recovery required about 33 weeks.

The effects of undernutrition in poor countries are probably even greater than this research indicated because the participants in this study had adequate vitamin and mineral intakes. In addition, the inhabitants of poorer countries must contend with recurrent infections, poor sanitary conditions, extreme weather conditions, and regular exposure to infectious diseases.

General Effects of Semistarvation

In the initial stages the results of undernutrition from semistarvation are often so mild that physical symptoms are absent and blood tests do not usually detect the slight metabolic changes. Even in the absence of clinical symptoms, however, undernourishment may affect reproductive capacity, resistance to and recovery from disease, physical activity and work output, and attitudes and behavior. Recall from Chapter 2 that as tissues continue to be depleted of nutrients, blood tests eventually detect changes, such as a drop in blood hemoglobin concentration. Physical symptoms, such as body weakness, appear with further depletion. Finally, the full-blown symptoms of the predominating deficiency are recognizable, such as when edema accompanies a protein deficiency.

In general, when a few people in a population develop a severe deficiency, this represents only the tip of the iceberg. Typically a much greater number have milder degrees of undernutrition. These deficiencies should not, therefore, be dismissed as trivial, especially in the developing world. It is becoming clear that combined deficiencies of specific vitamins and the minerals iron and zinc can seriously reduce work performance, even when they don't cause obvious physical symptoms. This resulting state of ill health in turn diminishes the ability of individuals, communities, and even whole countries to perform at peak levels of physical and mental capacity, creating a weakening of human resources.

ConceptCheck

Hunger is the uneasiness and pain that result when insufficient food is eaten to meet energy needs. Chronic hunger leads to undernutrition, which can cause growth failure in children and weakness in adults. Risk of infection increases, and nutrient-deficiency diseases result. The primary cause of undernutrition is poverty. The critical periods for undernutrition occur during pregnancy, infancy, childhood, and old age. Chronic undernutrition causes decreased work performance and motivation and compromises immune function. The adverse effects in pregnancy and infancy are quite dramatic, as evidenced by death rates much higher than those of healthy populations.

Undernutrition in the United States

About 50 million Americans live at or near the poverty level for at least part of the year. This is currently estimated at $16,450 annually for a family of four. These poor include about 20% of all Americans; children comprise about half of the poor.

Contrary to popular belief, poor people are not all from minority populations. In fact, 48% of the poor are Caucasian (keep in mind, though, that Caucasians also make up the largest percentage of the total population); 27% of the poor are African-American; and 22% of the poor are Hispanic.

Poor Americans often face difficult choices: whether to buy groceries for the family or pay this month's rent; whether to have dental work done or pay the current utility bill; or whether to replace clothes the children have outgrown or pay for transportation to a job. Food is one of the few flexible items in a poor person's budget. Rents are fixed, utility costs aren't negotiable, the price of medical care and prescription drugs can't be bargained down, and bus drivers won't accept less than the going rate. A person can always eat less, however. The short-term consequences may be less dramatic than having the utilities shut off. The long-term cumulative effects, however, are disturbing.

In sheer numbers, undernutrition in the United States is a troubling problem. Its existence is all the more disturbing because, although the threat of undernutrition for most Americans was virtually eliminated in the 1970s, it reemerged and spread rapidly in the 1980s. The fact that undernutrition and hunger remain in the 1990s indicates that their roots are mainly political and socioeconomic, rather than technical. Clearly, American society is productive enough to generate the resources required to feed all its citizens. In the developing world, far more factors complicate this problem, a subject that will be discussed later in the chapter.

Helping Hungry Americans: A Historical Perspective

Until the twentieth century, individuals and a wide variety of charitable, often church-related organizations provided most of the help to poor, undernourished people in the United States. Very few early efforts distributed direct cash payments to poor people because these were thought to reduce recipients' motivation to improve their circumstances or change behavior, such as excessive drinking, that contributed to their poverty. Beginning in the early 1900s the involvement of local, county, state, and federal governments in providing assistance to the poor has steadily increased.

Depression Era Though the Mid-1970s

The Great Depression of the 1930s marked a decisive change. Studies at the time documented both undernutrition and the existence of widespread pellagra (niacin deficiency) and rickets (vitamin D deficiency). In response, the federal government sponsored soup kitchens and other programs that distributed food commodities throughout the country. During World War II a large percentage of the men rejected for physical reasons by the draft were found to have been undernourished 10 to 12 years earlier, during the Depression era. This practical demonstration of the long-term detrimental effects of childhood undernutrition led Congress to enact legislation setting up the school lunch program in 1946.

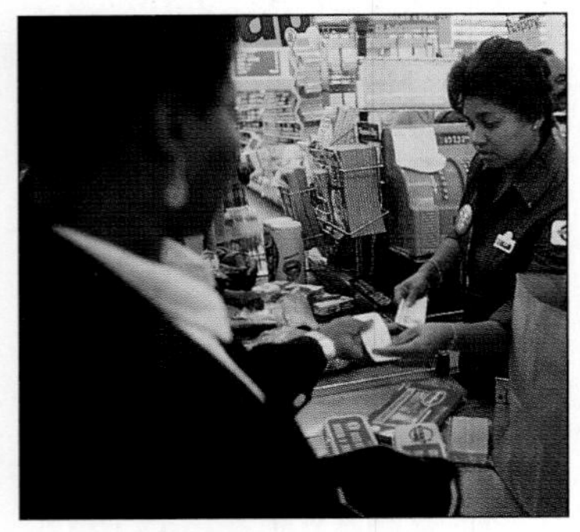

Food stamps are part of the social safety net in the United States.

After observing extensive hunger and poverty during his presidential campaign in the 1960s, John F. Kennedy initiated the Food Stamp program and expanded commodity distribution programs. The Food Stamp program for low-income people allows recipients to use food stamps to purchase food and seeds—but not tobacco, cleaning items, alcoholic beverages, and nonedible products—at stores authorized to accept them. Each household currently receives about \$170 per month, on average. Currently about 1 in 13 Americans participates in this program (Table 16–2). The number of participants has fallen from 1 in 10 just a few years ago due to recent changes in welfare laws that limit eligibility.

Congress established the school breakfast program in 1965 as politicians were made aware of the number of children coming to school hungry. School lunch and breakfast programs still enable low-income students—7 million for breakfast and 25 million for lunch—to receive meals free or at reduced cost if certain income guidelines are met (under \$26,500 annual income for a family of four). In the same year, Congress funded group noontime (called *congregate*) meals and home-delivered meals for all citizens over 60 years of age, regardless of income. Both remain active programs (see Chapter 14). In addition, in 1972 the Special Supplemental Feeding Program for Women, Infants, and Children (WIC) was authorized. This program provides food vouchers and nutrition education to low-income pregnant and lactating women and their young children. Today it serves about 7.4 million people.

A Reevaluation for Our Times

In the 1990s federal funds have fallen short of the amount needed to end hunger in the United States. For instance, the need for WIC services outstrips resources

TABLE 16-2

Some Current Federally Subsidized Programs That Supply Food for Americans

Program	Eligibility	Description
Food Stamps	Low income; employment generally necessary	Coupons are given to purchase food at grocery stores, the amount is based on size of household and income.
Emergency Food System	Low income	Food stamps issued on 24-hour notice for 1 month while eligibility for further use of the program can be investigated.
Commodity Supplemental Food Program	Certain low-income populations, such as pregnant women and young children	USDA surplus foods are distributed by county agencies.
Special Supplemental Feeding Program for Women, Infants and Children (WIC)	Low-income pregnant/lactating women, infants, and children less than 5 years old at nutritional risk	Coupons are given to purchase milk, cheese, fruit juice, cereal, infant formula, and other specific food items at grocery stores.
School Lunch	Low income	Free or reduced-price lunch distributed by the school; meal follows USDA pattern based on the Food Guide Pyramid; cost for the child depends on family income. In schools without a lunch program, special milk programs may be available.
School Breakfast	Low income	Free or reduced-price breakfast distributed by the school; meal follows USDA pattern; cost for the child depends on family income.
Child Care Food Program	Child enrolled in organized child care program; income guidelines are the same as School Lunch Program	Reimbursement given for meals supplied to children at the site; meals must follow USDA guidelines based on the Food Guide Pyramid.
Congregate Meals for for Elderly	Age 60 or over (no income guidelines)	Free noon meal is furnished at a site; meal follows specific pattern based on ⅓ of nutrient needs.
Home-delivered Meals	Age 60 or over, homebound	Noon meal is delivered at no cost or for a fee, depending on income, at least 5 days a week. Sometimes other meals for later consumption are delivered at the same time; private organizations that sponsor these programs often refer to them as "Meals on Wheels."

allocated to the program. This forces children out of the program, because pregnant women and infants are given the highest priority. In addition, the new welfare law that has been hammered out over the past few years generally requires able-bodied recipients to find jobs or risk losing food stamps, and cuts off hundreds of thousands of legal aliens. The government has provided exceptions for some legal aliens—mostly children, the disabled, and older persons—and those who are in training programs or who do volunteer work. Overall, however, it is likely that there are simply not enough jobs in the country to support the current work requirement for the entire population in some areas of the country, especially if the local economy falters.

Privately funded programs augment state and federal efforts to combat hunger in the United States. There are currently more than 180 food banks, 23,000 food pantries, and 3300 soup kitchens helping to cope with this problem. A recent survey found that slightly more than two of every three people requesting such emergency food assistance were members of families—children and their parents. Second Harvest, the largest U.S. food bank, estimates that 26 million people, or more than 1 in 10 of all Americans, rely on food depositories and soup kitchens to feed themselves and their families, and the number is on the rise. Emergency food suppliers do not expect to be able to cover the shortage created by recent welfare law changes.

The presence of undernutrition in the United States raises a broad question for our society at large: Where can people in such situations turn when their own resources fail? The responsibility for helping those in need could lie with the federal, state, and local governments, religious groups, charitable organizations, and in many cases with the individuals themselves. All can be part of the solution.

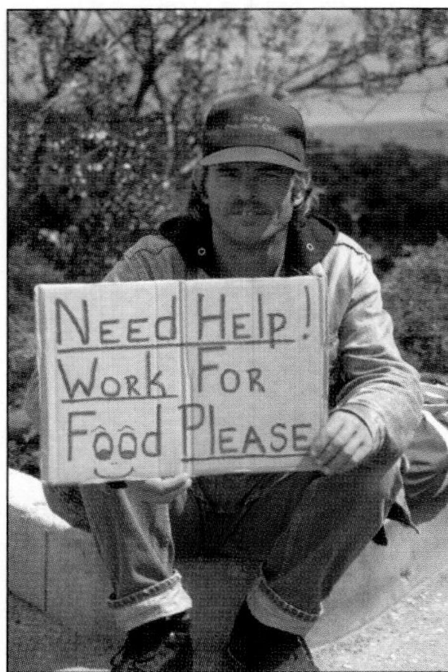

Major job layoffs in blue-collar industries have contributed to the twin problems of hunger and homelessness in the United States.

Socioeconomic Factors Related to Undernutrition

In the United States today, persistent hunger and undernutrition are largely associated with two interrelated conditions: poverty and homelessness. Thus economic, social, and political changes that lead to an increase in the number of poor or homeless people also tend to intensify the problem of undernutrition.

Poverty

Although highly trained people are quite competitive in the increasingly global economy there is a glut of unskilled manual labor available throughout the world. Many families have suffered economic hardship caused by massive layoffs in U.S. manufacturing industries that began in the late 1980s and continue in the 1990s. Furthermore, many jobs created in the 1980s were in the service sector, such as quick-service restaurants. When one or both parents have these low-paying jobs—even full time—their family may still be at or below the poverty level. Note that parents in most poor families do work; nearly two in three contain at least one worker.

A poor family of four in the United States currently has an average income of $10,923. Contrast that with the average earnings of an affluent family:$65,536. Needless to say, the poor family's limited budget must affect food purchases.

Another primary factor contributing to poverty has been the dramatic increase in the number of single-parent families in the United States, the result of high rates of divorce and out-of-wedlock births. Currently, single-parent families constitute about 25% of all families with children. The poverty rate (60%) for the approximately 19 million children in single-parent families is four times higher than the rate for those in two-parent families. Overall, about one in four children lives below the poverty line. They comprise the bulk of the 12% of Americans labeled as "food insecure."

Recent changes in welfare laws have incorporated the assumption that welfare support encourages further reliance on welfare and thus perpetuates poverty. The new law requires able-bodied adults to get jobs, as noted before, limiting future direct support to 3 years in a row and a total of 5 years in a lifetime. It is up to each state to determine how to implement this work requirement.

There has been a dramatic reduction in the number of people on welfare rolls since the implementation of the new laws. There is some evidence, however, that the decline in those receiving welfare has occurred mostly among Caucasians, but not minority populations. Some speculate that the new welfare reform has worked for those most able, but leaves behind peoples with little education and limited support networks. Their state of poverty is likely to worsen. It is also suspected that many families are currently suffering in silence as they try to cope with the cutbacks in welfare.

As with undernutrition in general, there is no one answer to poverty that will serve all people. At minimum more individuals are finding employment and will hopefully achieve better lives, through current welfare reforms. The broader effects will be seen in time.

Many politicians and political writers also point out we need greater wisdom in our approach to illegitimacy and single parenthood when considering poverty. They believe this issue represents a crisis with the potential for disaster and stress the need for solutions we haven't yet found or fully implemented. Some suggestions have been to improve child care, teach parenting skills, and expand job opportunities.

Legislators are taking steps to improve America's hunger problem. Lawmakers from seven states participated in the "Walk-a-Mile" December 1996 in which they were paired with a welfare recipient and were given food stamps to use for a month's worth of food. Most expressed a new appreciation for welfare recipients. In addition, President Clinton recently passed the Good Samaritan Food Donation Act that protects donators from liability (except in cases of deliberate negligence). The law is expected to increase food donations.

Homelessness

The economics of poverty and undernutrition have recently changed in one additional important way. Homelessness is much more evident now than in 1980 and the problem continues to worsen. Families with children currently account for about 43% of the homeless. An estimated 12 million people, or 6.5% of all adults, in the United States have experienced homelessness sometime during their lives. Episodes of homelessness nearly always last for at least 1 week and often for a month or more. The estimated lifetime homelessness rate rises to about 15% of the adult population in the United States when it includes people who have moved into someone else's residence during periods when they had nowhere else to live.

Homelessness exists partly because the cost of housing has substantially increased and partly because federal support for subsidized housing was cut dramatically (by 75%) during the 1980s. The government considers housing costs, which include rent and utilities to be affordable if they consume no more than 30% of a family's income. Today many poor people who rent pay a much larger percentage of their income in rent and utilities. These families, although not homeless, are likely to suffer from undernutrition without direct food assistance. Moreover, even a small change in the economic circumstances of such poor families may force them into actual homelessness, at least temporarily.

Other important causes of homelessness include the widespread release of mentally ill patients from mental institutions in the 1980s, unemployment, substance abuse, and personal crises. The abuse of alcohol and crack cocaine is another notable cause. Nationally, up to 85% of all homeless people in large cities abuse alcohol or drugs or have a mental illness. Most people with such problems are unable to find and hold employment; without support they and their dependents will probably remain homeless. Estimates range from 230,000 to 750,000 people nationwide.

Homeless children suffer higher rates of many medical problems than other children, some of which include:

- **Upper respiratory tract infections**
- **Scabies and lice**
- **Tooth decay**
- **Ear and skin infections**
- **Diaper rash**
- **Conjunctivitis**
- **Developmental delays**
- **Visual problems**
- **Trauma-related injuries**

The availability of cooking facilities affects nutrient intake among the poor. Without cooking facilities, people may buy expensive foods that require no preparation. These are typically processed snack foods, which provide food energy but are often lacking in nutrients.

Possible Solutions to Hunger in the United States

Few would argue the need to support physically and mentally handicapped Americans, as well as the multitude of children in this country. Furthermore, the United States has enough money and food to feed the country. Private emergency-food network systems are also important, as noted earlier, but are not sufficient to meet all food needs in the United States. Progress also requires a cultural shift emphasizing the responsibility of all citizens to provide as best they can for themselves, their families, and the less fortunate around them. Many experts consider an increase in individual responsibility as a critical goal for our society at this time. Government programs can't easily fix poverty and resulting hunger that stem from irresponsible individual behavior. Government programs can, however, help reduce or prevent poverty that results largely from lack of opportunity. We have seen a recent cultural shift against smoking and drunk driving. Could illegitimacy and abandonment of family be similarly discouraged?

Clearly the victims of poverty don't deserve all the blame. Poorer Americans confront substantial difficulties: substandard education and training, poor communication skills, lack of reliable and safe child care, inability to relocate, little employment experience, and no economic reserves to fall back on during crises. Even with a strong desire for a better life, people may get discouraged and apathetic in the face of apparently insurmountable obstacles. Moreover, many poor Americans are unable to meet the demands of a modern, dynamic society—in particular, elderly, sick, and disabled people and young single mothers and their children. Regardless of how repugnant government assistance appears to some people, it will probably always be necessary to some extent.

Because long-term undernutrition and homelessness—especially among children—has both individual and societal consequences, all Americans are affected by this problem, either directly or indirectly. For example, this can contribute to higher health-care premiums for the bulk of Americans, since the poorer among us have higher health-care costs, and use expensive health-care services (e.g., emergency rooms). The next few years are likely to bring further changes in both government

Nutrition Insight

The Human Side of Hunger and Poverty in America

By Susan M. Krueger, M.S., R.D.

As a registered dietitian and college instructor of human nutrition, hunger is a very important issue to me. Good nutrition is vital to the health of our country. Yet, with one in four children living in poverty, estimates of up to 30 million Americans experiencing some degree of hunger on a regular basis, one in 13 Americans using food stamps, and 37 million people still without health insurance, we obviously have problems with the health and well-being of many. All of the nutrition knowledge in the world will not help people if they lack the funds and assistance to purchase healthy foods. This is especially a problem in this country where so many "fun" and "status" foods of low-nutrient density are not only available, but are heavily advertised.

For the past five summers, I, along with my husband and four teenage children, have traveled to the southern Appalachian region of the United States to do volunteer work with the poor. The first time that we left for our destination, I brought with me many ideas, pamphlets, pyramid food guides, coloring books with nutrition themes, and so on, for use in teaching people how to improve their diets and hopefully the quality of their lives. When we got to our destination, I did not use *any* of these things that I had so carefully packed.

Why did I not use any of the teaching tools or share my expertise in nutrition? In the area where we worked, we found people who had greater, or at least more immediate, needs than nutrition education. We found people living in tarpaper shacks. We found people with large holes in their roofs and living in trailers with missing windows and doors. Some of the people had no running water or indoor plumbing facilities. We found children who literally owned no shoes. We found lonely elderly people in nursing homes who rarely had visitors, and others alone in their own homes, which were often in great need of repair.

We also found children craving the attention of adults, many of whom were performing adult responsibilities, especially in regard to child care, as well as household duties. We saw evidence of "silent undernutrition"—adults who looked old beyond their years and children who were very small and thin for their age. We found a food pantry with no food. Food arrived while we were there, but the shelves were soon emptied. When food is available, people are only given food assistance once a month simply because of the lack of donated food available for the great number of people requesting it. In contrast, at the pantry at home where I have been volunteering for the past 7 years in Eau Claire, Wisconsin, recipients can come weekly. The people receive surplus meats and high-protein foods, soups, vegetables, and potatoes from the dietary department of a local hospital. Foods such as canned beans and vegetables, cereal, soup, pasta, fresh produce, and all the bread one can use are also distributed. This pantry receives generous support from individuals, churches, businesses, and grocery stores in the local area.

In our work in Appalachia, we also found people with a strong sense of pride, of wanting to make it on their own without "government handouts." We found others who were in desperate need of assistance but had no idea that they qualified for aid or were unaware of how to obtain it. In many we also found a great love of family. Finally, we found a part of the country that is very beautiful to gaze upon but does not attract industry because of the mountainous terrain, the low attainment of education among many residents, and hazardous two-lane highways that often have no shoulders, just mountains, rivers, or woods on the side.

During our time we performed home repairs of various types, from fixing roofs to painting; visited isolated elderly individuals; and conducted play activities with local children. One of my favorite job sites early on was a very depressed, tiny village where we would play with the local children, three afternoons a week. On some days, 35 or more kids between the ages of 6 months and 15 years would show up! Overall, the children who attended these play groups were eager and trusting.

Over the past 5 years, however, we have also seen smiles change to frowns in too many children. We have seen the toll that poverty and hardship have taken. Some children display despondence, anger, and a sense of hopelessness, especially in situations where their home lives may include abuse, divorce, and parental alcoholism. As they age, their growing awareness of the stark differences between their lives and those of most Americans also plays a role.

What have I learned from my experiences? First, I have confirmed my belief that poor people are not really any different from those who have more. We all have the same basic needs and experience the same basic feelings that are part of being human.

Second, I have learned that people are poor and often hungry for many different reasons. Some of the people I have worked with are poor because they have lost their jobs and have not been able to find new ones. Many of the people who need assistance *work*! Some are working part-time jobs, but many are working full-time jobs that pay minimum wage—which keeps them below poverty level.

Some of the people requiring assistance have problems with alcohol or drug abuse. Others have physical, and many have mental disabilities that greatly diminish their ability to provide for themselves. A great number of people that I have encountered have not had the educational opportunities available to them that can help break the cycle of poverty. Some of the people come from families where there is a lack of academic tradition and knowledge in how to find, finance, and make use of such opportunities.

Many of the people who seek assistance are the heads of single-parent families, who frequently experience difficulty in making ends meet and/or obtaining an education, especially when finding and paying for child care is involved. Finally, many people are poor because of continuing discrimination and economic problems faced by members of our ethnic minority groups.

Finally, I have learned that we all must learn not to judge others in situations that we have not and probably never will encounter. What makes us think that, despite the circumstances, we would have the know-how, confidence, energy, courage, and means (money, skills, and education) to break the cycle of poverty on our own?

Many students have asked how they can get involved in hunger issues. I recommend donating time, money, or food to local food banks and pantries. Even a couple boxes of macaroni and cheese can make a difference and help a family or individual stretch their food supply to the end of the week! Keeping an open mind is also important.

I would recommend becoming aware of poverty and hunger issues in our country, examining the potential solutions that are being offered, exercising your right to vote, and expressing your opinions to your representatives in government.

Susan M. Krueger, M.S., R.D. is a senior lecturer in the Biology Department at the University of Wisconsin-Eau Claire.

and private assistance programs, demanding new initiatives from all Americans. Your contribution to this process as an informed voter and, ideally, an active participant is an important part of the process.

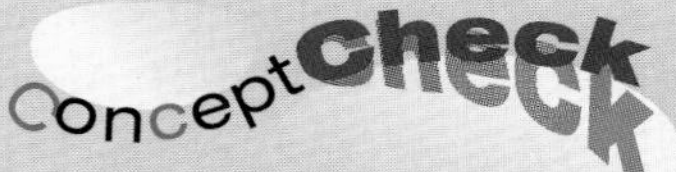

Federal programs designed to reduce hunger and undernutrition began in the 1930s, during the Great Depression. In response to reports of widespread poverty and hunger during the early 1960s, Congress established several new federal food assistance programs and substantially increased funding for already existing programs. Largely as a result of these federal programs, undernutrition decreased substantially. The improvement was short-lived, and the number of Americans experiencing poverty, homelessness, and undernutrition has since grown. The presence of these three interrelated problems is influenced by economic, cultural, and individual factors, as well as government policies. The serious questions about the long-term effectiveness of many government assistance programs are causing major changes in their future administration, funding mechanisms, and program design. All citizens can help to reduce the problem of undernutrition.

Undernutrition in the Developing World: Underlying Causes

Undernutrition in the developing world is also tied to poverty, and any true solution must address this problem. However, these countries have a multitude of problems so complex and interrelated that they cannot be treated separately. Programs that have proved immensely helpful in the United States are only a starting point in this context. The following major obstacles challenge those seeking a solution:

- Extreme imbalances in the food/population ratio in different regions of a country
- War and political/civil unrest
- The rapid depletion of natural resources
- Cultural attitudes toward certain foods
- Poor **infrastructure,** especially poor housing, sanitation and storage facilities, education, communications, and transportation systems
- High external debt

Infrastructure
The basic framework of a system of organization. For a society, this includes roads, bridges, telephones, and other basic technologies.

Each problem deserves individual consideration.

The Food/Population Ratio

Whether the earth can yield enough food for all people has been a long-standing question. As early as 1798, the English clergyman and political economist Thomas Malthus proposed a rather pessimistic view of our prospects. He said that given the passion between the sexes (which he felt should be discouraged), the population would always increase faster than the food supply. Malthus felt that the growing population would therefore be subject to recurring checks imposed by widespread starvation, war, or natural catastrophe brought on by disease.

Malthus's proposals became the object of intense controversy in England and elsewhere, often meeting vigorous opposition. Eminent British scientists pointed out that scientific advances in agriculture would greatly increase food production. In fact, that has proved true. Nevertheless, the aptly named population explosion has undermined this progress. Overall population growth has not slowed significantly through natural checks, disease, or recent human interventions, such as birth control. In the year 1800, 1 billion people inhabited the earth. At the turn of the new century this number will have skyrocketed to more than 7 billion.

Currently, population growth exceeds economic growth in much of the world, and poverty is increasing. Because efforts to speed up economic development have failed, the only remaining way to improve the situation may be slowing down the growth of population, as Malthus recommended. If we want to ensure a decent life for a widening segment of humanity, the growth in the earth's population should slow. According to the World Bank, the world's population increases by 1 billion people every 12 years, mostly in cities and in seacoast and river-basin areas, where the environment is typically under stress. By 2030 the world will have nearly 3 billion more people than today—2 billion of them in countries where the average person earns less than $2 a day. Unless a catastrophe occurs, more than 9 of 10 infants in the next generation will be born in the poorest parts of the world.

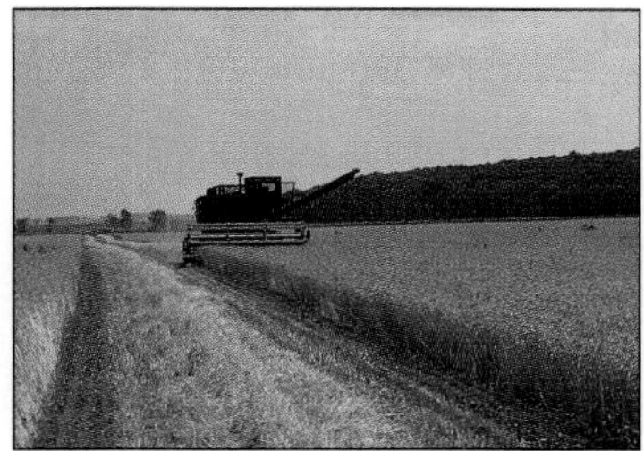

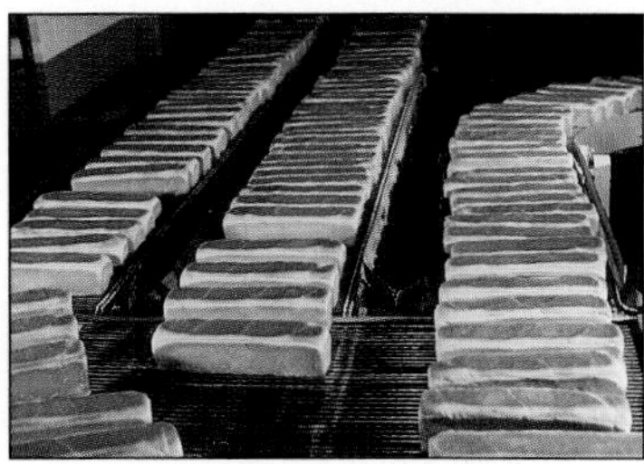

The bounty of food we enjoy in North America relies on its rich agricultural resources. Many underdeveloped countries do not have such resources to employ.

At this time, there are about 5.8 billion people in the world. More than three-quarters live in countries in the developing world, and more than half live in Asia. Many experts believe that the global supply of food would provide adequate nutrition for all 5.8 billion of us, about 2400 kcal each per day. However, food supplies are not distributed equally among consumers. Gross disparities exist between developed and developing countries, among the rich and poor within countries, and even within families.

Food supply and population trends within the developed world also vary greatly. Germany and Japan are facing a large decrease in their populations over the next 50 years unless their birth rates increase. In fact, birth rates have fallen so low that the governments have proposed paying or otherwise providing benefits to couples to have children. Apparently, people there realize the financial strain of increasing numbers of children. On the other hand, the population in Africa will have more than doubled, constituting 19% of the world population.

Economists estimate that world food production will in fact continue to increase more rapidly than the world population in the near future, allowing the food/population ratio to increase through the year 2020. In the short run then, the primary problem appears to be not food production, but distribution and use, especially in poverty-stricken areas of the developing nations.

Eventually, though, food production will probably begin to lag behind population growth, likely by 2025. Most good farmland in the world is already in use, and because of poor farming practices or competing land-use demands, the number of farmable acres worldwide decreases annually. For many reasons, sustainable world food output—an amount that doesn't deplete the earth's resources—is now running well behind food consumption. This discrepancy suggests that food production in less-developed countries will barely keep up with population growth and will soon lag behind.

A Renewed Focus on Population Control

Reproduction is said to be the ultimate driving force behind consumption. Although efforts on the supply side of the food/population ratio are essential, many researchers still emphasize the need to reduce the demand side. They argue that the survival of our civilization depends on limiting reproduction.

For millions of years, maximizing reproduction has been a measure of biological success. Because disease and difficult living conditions often claimed young lives, couples produced many offspring in an attempt to ensure the longevity of the family. These conditions still exist in countries in the developing world, where children also provide the primary means of support to their parents in old age. More children also means more helpers to farm, hunt, and prepare food. In India a rigid class structure that leaves many people destitute encourages large families. Traditionally, poorer people bear more children, contrary to what you might predict.

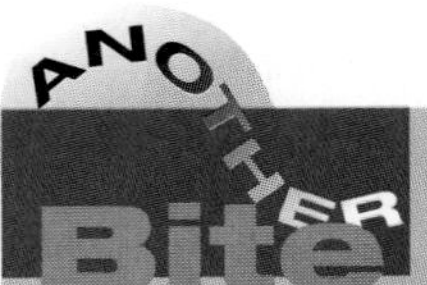

In addition to economics, other obstacles to family-planning programs are ancient cultural, religious, and traditional beliefs. In sub-Saharan Africa, childlessness signifies the end of a line of descent, and women who don't have children are often perceived as evil. The Yoruba believe, for example, that a childless woman made a pact with evil spirits before her own birth to kill her children and, devoid of descendants, will return to join these evil spirits in some otherworldly sphere. These women fear being rendered functionally infertile by the death of all their children almost as much as they fear bearing none. Thus female sterilization and even contraception have not been successful. Even women with four or five children fear, not unreasonably, that all their children may suddenly die. Also, Moslem religious practices typically promote a large, abundant family as a sign of prosperity and health.

In the 1960s, South Korean families averaged six children each. Through economic policies and family-planning programs, this number has been decreased to two. Other countries such as Indonesia and Thailand prove that industrialization is not a prerequisite to population control alone, but rather, family-planning programs can be successful.

Now, in an evolutionary blink of the eye—mere decades—poor people in developing nations are being asked to reverse their attitude toward having children. It is a difficult undertaking.

As one brake on population expansion, birth control programs have been effective in developed countries but relatively ineffective in developing countries that could really benefit from them. Whereas women in the United States average 2.1 live births each, women in some East African countries average 8.5 live births each and women worldwide average 4.0 live births. The poorest countries are increasing the most, further straining their ability to cope. The world's population is likely to exceed 11 billion in 2100. Generally speaking, an ever increasing population stresses existing resources in developing countries; many people's needs are not met, social unrest is intensified, and significant environmental destruction is more likely.

Keys to Successful Family-Planning Programs

Attempts to implement family-planning programs in developing nations have been only partially successful. Some small countries—such as Singapore, Taiwan, Thailand, Bangladesh, Colombia, Costa Rica, and several Caribbean countries—have reduced their birth rates substantially. Larger countries, including India and Mexico, are struggling.

Breastfeeding aids in family planning because it helps space births farther apart. If no supplemental nourishment is given, breastfeeding an infant decreases ovulation—and therefore, the likelihood of fertilization—for an average of about 6 months, although breastfeeding is not a completely reliable form of birth control. When childbirths are more widely spaced, mother and infant are healthier and fewer total births occur. Women who do not breastfeed generally begin to ovulate within a month or so after giving birth.

With its nearly 1.3 billion people, China is seriously overpopulated—22% of the world's population is living on 7% of the world's productive land. Recognizing the gravity of the situation, the Chinese government has imposed the world's most stringent family-planning program, which allows only one child per urban couple—two in rural areas if the first child is a girl. The birth rate now averages 1.8 children in a woman's lifetime. Penalties for having extra children include restricted housing and employment opportunities. Abortion is very common and is sometimes forced on unwilling women, as is sterilization. These policies have lowered China's population growth rate by about one-third. Despite its statistical success, China's program is controversial, and its coercive aspects have been criticized as human rights abuses.

In general, experience with family-planning programs in developing countries and historical changes in birth rates in many industrialized countries suggests an important conclusion: Only when people have enough to eat, basic education, access to health care, and are financially secure do they feel safe having fewer children. Increasing per capita income and improving education, especially for women in developing nations, are currently considered to be the most likely long-term solutions to excessive population growth.

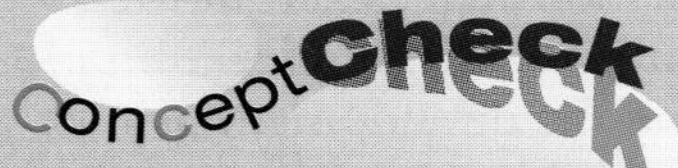

Currently, world food production is sufficient to meet the energy needs of the world's population. Despite adequate food resources, undernutrition exists because of poverty, politics, and unequal distribution. In addition, projected population growth may soon overwhelm food production. Most scientists and world leaders recommend limiting population growth, especially in developing countries where birth rates are high.

War and Political/Civil Unrest

Worldwide military spending has doubled over the past 20 years. In 1994, global military expenditures were estimated at $767 billion—more than the total income of the poorest 45% of the world's population. Although Africa has been ravaged by economic decay and famines for years, military spending in Africa more than doubled in the 1970s and has held firm through the early 1990s. Currently less than one half of 1% of the world's yearly production of goods and services is devoted to economic development assistance, whereas approximately 6% goes to military expenditures.

In the worst cases, civil disruptions and war contribute to massive undernutrition. War-related famine affects millions of people in southern and northeastern Africa. Currently, Sudan, Rwanda, and Somalia are examples of once productive economies now struggling with mass starvation. Most of these people are left without shelter, clothing, food, and any means of obtaining them.

Even when food is available, political divisions may impede distribution to the point that undernutrition will plague many people for years to come. Especially during emergencies, programs designed to help the poor have been undermined by poor administration, corruption, and political influence as noted earlier. In 1996, Sudan's government put a ban on air-drop aid for 10 months because rebels had infiltrated many provinces. The ban caused the near starvation of almost 700,000 innocent people. In 1998, the same conflict put 2.4 million people at risk of starvation.

During such political chaos, relief agencies are often caught between warring factions and those they are trying to help. This was the case recently in Zaire, where Rwandan refugee camps fell under the control of a militant group. The rebels controlled the food coming in and out of the camps and would not allow relief agencies to take census of the inhabitants.

During the 1960s and 1970s the problem of undernutrition in less developed countries was perceived as a technical one: how to produce enough food for the growing world population. The problem is now seen as largely political: how to achieve cooperation among and within nations so that gains in food production and infrastructure are not wiped out by war, and governments seen as fair and representative are the norm. Only a combination of approaches—finding technical solutions that may help with problems of chronic hunger and poverty and solving political crises that push disadvantaged nations into a state of acute hunger and chaos—will help.

The Rapid Depletion of Natural Resources

As we quickly deplete the earth's resources, population control grows increasingly critical. The productive capacity of agriculture is approaching its limits in many areas worldwide. Environmentally unsustainable farming methods undermine food production, especially in parts of the developing world.

Green revolution
This refers to increases in crop yields that accompany the introduction of new agricultural technologies in less developed countries, beginning in the 1960s. The key technologies were high-yielding, disease-resistant strains of rice, wheat, and corn; greater use of fertilizer; and improved cultivation practices.

Ecosystem
A community in nature that includes plants, animals, and their environment.

Cash crop
A crop grown specifically for export so that goods from other countries can be purchased. Cultivation of cash crops diverts agricultural resources necessary to feed a country's own citizens. Examples of cash crops are coffee, tea, cocoa, and bananas.

The term **green revolution** describes a phenomenon that began in the 1960s when crop yields rose dramatically in some countries, such as the Philippines, India, and Mexico. The increased use of fertilizers and the development of superior crops through careful plant breeding made this rise possible. Many of the technologies associated with the green revolution have now achieved most of their potential. For example, rice yield has not increased significantly since the release of superior varieties in 1966, but work on this is ongoing. Future gains in productivity also may be much harder to accomplish because of the need to farm less productive soils. Until the introduction of another superior strain of rice or other grain, developing countries will not benefit greatly from recent, more modest breakthroughs in biotechnology (see the Nutrition Issue at the end of this chapter).

Areas of the world that remain uncultivated or ungrazed are mostly unsuited to farming: rocky, steep, infertile, too dry, too wet, or inaccessible. Much of this land is nonetheless invaluable for the crucial **ecosystem** benefits it provides. This is particularly true for humid tropical areas, such as the Amazon basin rain forests, which significantly influence the earth's climate, most notably through oxygen production. Some nations, such as Brazil, can still expand onto productive land, but such countries are in the minority. Even then, this expansion in Brazil causes further rain forest devastation.

In Africa an area of land twice the size of New Jersey is turned into unproductive desert each year because of soil erosion. The erosion results from over-grazing by livestock, destructive farming techniques, and destruction of mature rain forests. Also, cultivation of many **cash crops** in African countries damages the land, draining the soil of vital nutrients. Then, when the land has been used up, farmers move on to other areas, leaving behind desolate land vulnerable to soil erosion.

Nearly all irrigation water available worldwide is currently being used, and groundwater supplies are becoming depleted at rapid rates in many regions. In developing countries, poultry, swine, and milk production is often overconcentrated around metropolitan areas, in turn polluting and overdrawing groundwater.

The prospects of obtaining substantially more food from the oceans are also poor. In recent years the amount of fish caught worldwide has leveled off. Fish was once considered the poor man's protein. But without actual farming of fish, this is unlikely to be true again.

Clearly, we can exploit the earth's resources only so far—world population probably can't continue to expand as it does today without the potential for serious famine and death. The Food and Agriculture Organization (FAO) of the United Nations works on this principle: "The fight to ensure that all people have enough nutritious food to eat is worthy of our greatest efforts, but it must be fought with the full recognition that it cannot be won unless agricultural, fishery, and forestry production returns to the earth as much as—or more than—it takes." This statement highlights the need for immediate action to protect the earth's already deteriorated environment from further destruction, if food production is to keep up with the expanding population.

Cultural Attitudes Toward Certain Foods

Culture affects food use just as it does family size. In India, for example, the Hindu reverence for cattle has worsened some already significant nutrition problems. These sacred cows consume food rather than provide it; the wandering cows also damage vegetation that could otherwise feed humans. Although the cows provide milk, no attempt is made to improve milk production through selective breeding practices. In certain areas of India a child may not be fed milk curds, because of a superstitious belief that they inhibit growth, or bananas, because they supposedly cause convulsions. These are obstacles, but not barriers, to good nutrition. Given adequate food resources and education, a healthful diet allowing for individual food taboos and prejudices is possible.

Inadequate Shelter and Sanitation

When people die from undernutrition in developing countries, other influences, such as inadequate shelter and sanitation, almost always contribute. Poor sanitation raises the risk of infection, as does undernutrition. Together these represent a lethal combination (Figure 16–2). For example, the 1994 plague that killed almost 5000 people and sparked the panicked exodus of another half a million in Surat, in northwest India, was linked mainly to unsanitary housing conditions.

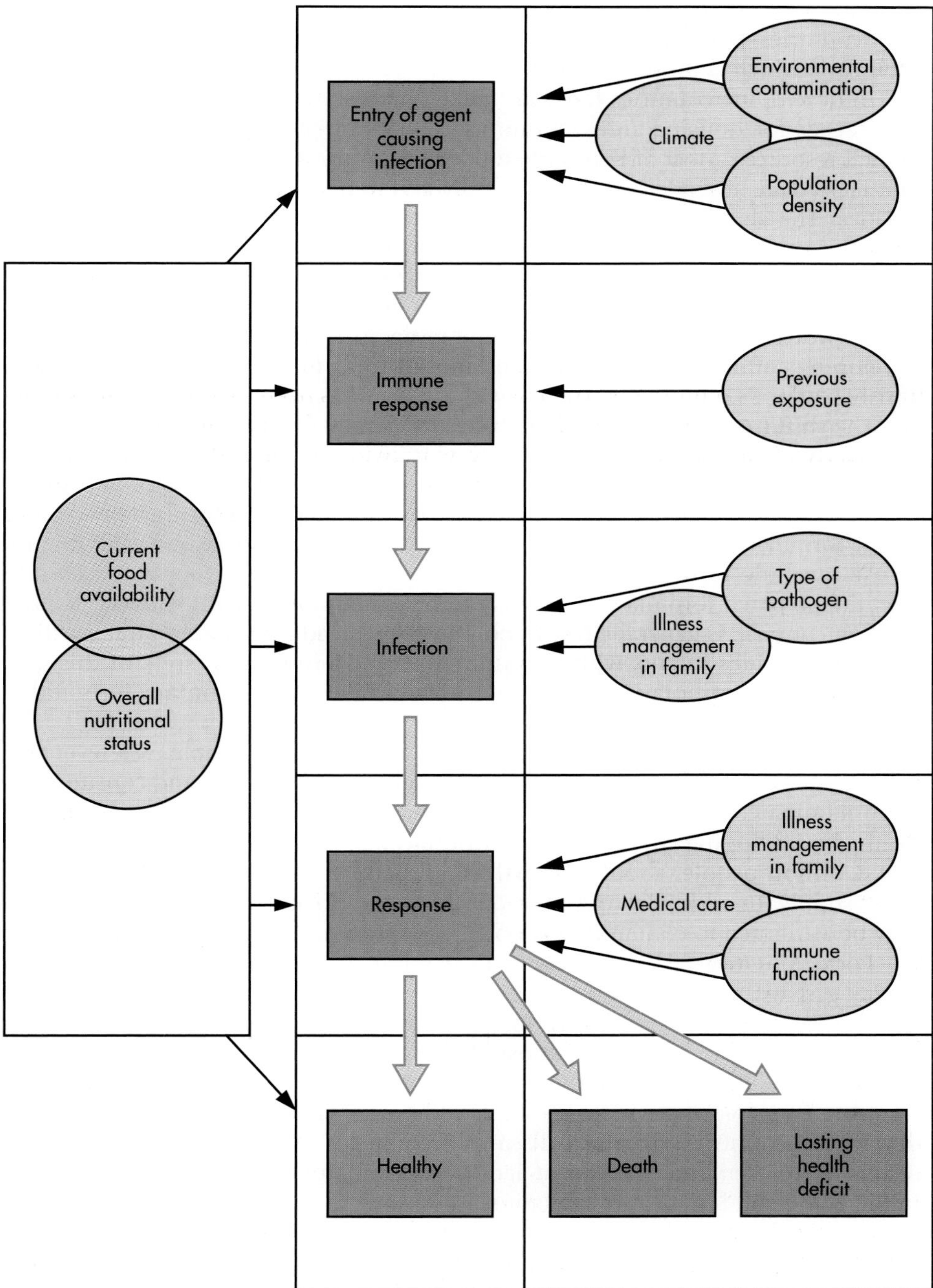

Figure 16–2 *Nutritional status and overall food supply combine with a variety of environmental factors to influence the risk of infection and ultimate outcome.*

In Brazil, migrants displaced by multinational land developers have flooded from the North and Northeast into Rio de Janeiro and São Paulo, attracted by the prospect of jobs. There they have built shantytowns next to apartment towers and affluent suburbs, but the jobs do not materialize, and urban poverty simply replaces rural impoverishment.

Inadequate and deteriorating shelters threaten the lives of more than 500 million people today. Many of the 15 million annual deaths of children—half of them under 5 years old—in developing countries could be prevented by improving standards of environmental hygiene. Urban populations of some developing countries are currently growing at an annual rate of 5% to 7%. Such a skewed population distribution will result in more poverty. The current urban explosion is the result of both high birth rates and continuing migration of people to the cities from the countryside. People come to the cities to find employment and resources the countryside can no longer provide. Worldwide, 38% of people lived in urban areas in 1975. The figure is expected to reach 48% by the turn of the new century and climb to 61% by 2025. Nine of the 10 largest cities 20 years from now will be in poor countries. Los Angeles, which is now the seventh-largest city in the world, and New York, which is third, will drop far down the list.

In developing countries the poor make up most of the urban population, and their needs for housing and community services often outstrip available governmental resources. Most of these urban poor live in overcrowded, self-made shelters that lack a safe and adequate water supply and are only partially served by public utilities. The shantytowns and ghettos of the developing world are often worse than the rural areas the people left behind. Because the urban poor need cash to purchase food, they often subsist on diets that are even more meager than the homegrown rural fare. Making matters worse, haphazard shelters often lack facilities to protect food from spoilage or the ravages of insects and rodents. In some developing countries, food losses can amount to as much as 30% to 40% of the perishable foods.

The shift from rural to urban life takes its greatest toll on infants and children. Infants are often weaned early from the breast, partly because the mother must find employment and partly because she may be influenced by the images of sophisticated, formula-using women promoted in advertisements. Unfortunately, because infant formulas are relatively expensive, poor parents may overdilute the mixture or use too little to meet the baby's needs. Because the water supply may not be safe, the prepared formula is also likely to be contaminated with bacteria. Human milk, in contrast, is generally much more hygienic, readily available, and nutritious and also provides infants with immunity to some ailments. In spite of this grim outlook, major corporations continue to aggressively market infant formulas in these regions.

Overall, the single most effective health advantage for people, wherever they live, is a safe and convenient water supply. Inadequate sanitation and consumption of contaminated water cause 75% of all diseases and more than one-third of all deaths in developing countries. The World Health Organization (WHO) estimates that 1 billion people, about one-sixth of all people, have unsafe and inadequate water supply. In addition, up to 90% of the diseases seen in developing countries may be attributed to contaminated water.

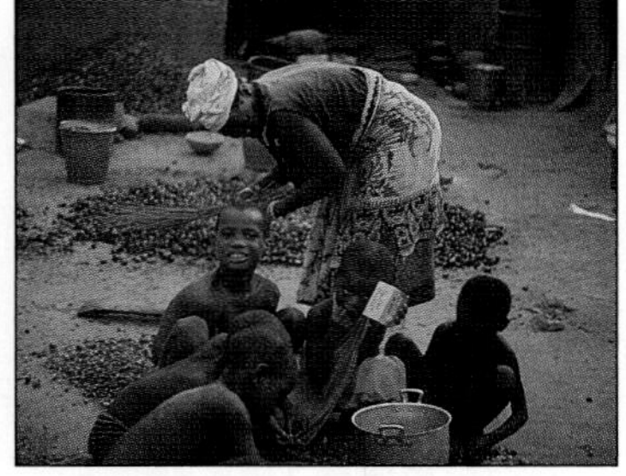

Inadequate sanitation and consumption of contaminated water cause 75% of all diseases, yet more than 1 billion people in developing countries lack access to a safe water supply.

Poor sanitation also creates a critical public health problem. Human feces, rotting garbage, and associated insect and rodent infestations are commonly seen in urban areas of the developing world. Potent sources of disease organisms, human urine and feces are two of the most dangerous substances people encounter in routine daily living. The inability to dispose of the massive numbers of dead people resulting from recent civil wars causes additional sanitation problems. In some developing countries, diarrheal diseases account for as many as one-third of all deaths in children under 5 years of age. WHO estimates that about 3 billion people in the world still lack proper sanitation.

To this already unbalanced equation, add the threat of sickness from acquired immunodeficiency syndrome (AIDS), an essentially incurable disease. Developing countries currently contain the bulk of the world's 30 million cases of human immunodeficiency virus (HIV) infections, and numbers are increasing rapidly. As more people contract AIDS, the economic and social impact will be enormous. In an already undernourished population the long-term effects may rival those of a prolonged war (see the second Nutrition Insight).

High External Debt

During the 1970s and 1980s, many developing countries became trapped in the cycle of borrowing repeatedly from foreign countries. Servicing these external debts, which now total about $2 trillion, has brought several countries to the verge of economic collapse. The external debt of Latin America represents 45% of the region's gross regional output of goods and services. One option is for Latin American nations to form a comprehensive plan aimed at renegotiating the external debt on more realistic terms.

Even the United States is not immune to such national financial problems. Our national debt is now so large that the yearly interest payments account for about 15% of all federal spending. This debt limits our country's ability to help less developed countries.

Many African nations also carry large debt burdens. Recent drops in prices for raw commodities they export, higher prices for imported oil, and embezzlement of funds by high political officials are at the root of this problem. Although the African debts are much smaller in absolute terms than those of Brazil, Argentina, and Mexico, for example, the actual burden is greater when national incomes and export earnings are considered. Nearly half the money African nations earn from exports goes to paying off the continent's multibillion dollar debt. As a result, African nations have had to impose cuts in domestic programs, which can cause widespread undernutrition in many of these poor nations, in part because these countries still need to import—and pay for—machinery, concrete, trucks, and consumer goods. To make up the difference between export income and import expenses, countries have been forced to borrow billions of dollars from international banks.

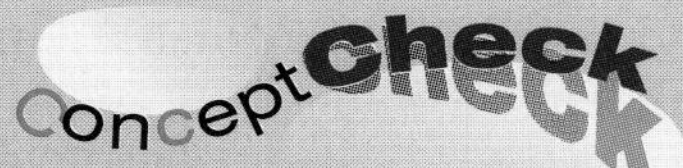

War and civil strife, along with a decline in the world's natural resources, contribute to the difficulty of ending undernutrition in many developing countries. In addition, inadequate housing conditions, impure water, and inadequate sanitation worldwide increase the risk for infection and disease. Infection then combines with undernutrition to further compromise the health of impoverished people. Finally, many developing countries are burdened by extremely high external debts, which severely limit their ability to implement programs to reduce undernutrition.

Reducing Undernutrition in the Developing World

As you have probably guessed, greatly reducing undernutrition in the developing world will be complicated and will take considerable time to accomplish. In the 1980s, it was a common practice for the more affluent nations to supply famished areas with direct food aid. However highly publicized and praised at the time, direct food aid is not a long-term solution. Although it reduces the number of deaths from famine, it can also reduce incentives for local production by driving down local prices. In addition, the affected countries may have little or no means of transporting the food to those who need it most. Furthermore, the donated foods may receive little cultural acceptance.

Nutrition Insight

The Impact of AIDS Worldwide

The Black Plague left its grim mark on civilization by claiming the lives of approximately 25 million people in the fourteenth century. According to the World Health Organization (WHO), 30 million people around the world are currently infected with the human immunodeficiency virus (HIV), and 16,000 new infections take place each day. In the United States alone, it is estimated that up to 1 million people are infected with HIV; this means that as many as 1 out of every 250 Americans may be infected. In more than 60 U.S. cities, acquired immunodeficiency syndrome (AIDS) is the number one killer of men ages 25 to 44.

African-American and Hispanic people account for more cases than whites based on their percentage of the population (101,51, and 17 per 100,000, respectively). Stopping the spread of this disease is imperative for all the nation's citizens, especially in minority communities.

Because no cure essentially exists, the majority of people infected with HIV—the twentieth-century plague—face certain death from it. Current medication regimens can only slow progress of the disease and are expensive. More than 240,000 Americans have already died from AIDS.

The devastating effects of AIDS on our civilization have been very rapid when measured by Earth's scale of time, and the true costs to societies—other than the cost of human lives—have yet to emerge. Though AIDS has not replaced heart disease and stroke as the primary cause of death in America, the very nature of the disease is likely to wreak significant human devastation here and worldwide, partly because its primary route of transmission is a basic human behavior—sexual activity.

The Route of Infection

The vectors, or vehicles of transmission, for HIV are blood and body fluids, including sexual secretions. It is estimated that 75% to 85% of all cases of HIV has been spread through sexual contact, homosexual as well as heterosexual. Intravenous drug use, via shared needles, also accounts for a large number of cases.

Education that ultimately leads to safer sex and use of clean drug needles are known to reduce the spread of the disease and are keys to controlling AIDS. It is unlikely that vaccines will be able to eradicate HIV—at least in the near future—though research with vaccines is under way. A behavioral change currently offers the best hope. After initial contact with HIV, a person may notice no symptoms for as long as 5 to 10 years and may be an unsuspecting carrier. When the immune system can no longer fight off related subsequent infections, such as tuberculosis and pneumonia, the condition of AIDS is well on its way.

Who is Affected?

Though homosexual people currently account for more than half the cases here, the number of AIDS cases in heterosexual people—especially women and the children that HIV-infected women bear—is rapidly increasing.

AIDS needs no passport. Heterosexually transmitted HIV flows freely in Thai sex parlors, along the truck routes of India, around Dominican Republic sugarcane plantations, and in the copper mines of Zambia. It is likely that one-fourth of all adults in Zambia are infected with HIV. Throughout Zambia and the rest of sub-Saharan Africa it is creating numerous orphans as parents die from the disease. Heterosexual contact accounts for the majority of cases of HIV. A recent study warns us that 57 countries risk major HIV outbreaks. Reported HIV cases are increasing rapidly in Africa, Asia, and Russia, with more than 4.5 million men, women, and children becoming infected yearly worldwide. The World Health Organization estimates that 70% of the world's 30 million people infected with the HIV virus are in Africa, with civil war refugees and migration contributing to its spread. The AIDS epicenter, however, is now shifting to Asia, especially India. If the disease continues to progress as it is, the number of cases in Asia will double by the end of the century, bringing the total to 10 million cases in the year 2000. In India alone the number of cases is expected to reach 5 million.

Is There Any Hope?

On a more individual scale, can eating a balanced diet prevent HIV or stave off AIDS? The answer is no. Again, there is no cure for HIV and AIDS. Preventive measures include abstinence or safer sexual practices (especially use of condoms for men) and avoidance of contact with infected blood products and bodily fluids. Breastfeeding poses such a risk for mother-infant transmission, and so its benefits to the infant must be carefully weighed against this risk when counseling HIV positive pregnant women.

Eating a balanced diet helps lessen the impact of infections but does not cure the disease or make it less deadly. A poor nutritional status contributes to quicker onset of such symptoms as body wasting and fever, and ultimately leads to a quicker demise. In addition, many AIDS patients suffer from diarrhea. Eating such foods as applesauce, potatoes without the skin, broth, hot cereal, rice, gelatin, bananas, and crackers may minimize the severity of the diarrhea. Suffers should also stay hydrated with fluids such as fruit juice, sports drinks, water, and ice chips.

Though AIDS patients should consider food an integral part of their treatment regimen, medications are most vital to their survival. A powerful new class of antiviral drugs called protease inhibitors are being combined with previously known drugs (e.g., zidovudine [AZT]) that target genetic material. The HIV infection has been kept to nearly undetectable levels in some patients on this combined therapy. This newer treatment has provided more hope for managing HIV than in the recent past; still the virus can eventually outsmart this protocol. Individuals benefit the most during the first application of this treatment (before the virus has changed in response to therapy); it also must be begun early in the course of the disease if it is to be most effective. This therapy also requires patients to take up to 20 pills a day and costs approximately $14,000 per year, not including any unforeseen hospital stays. (Not many people in the developing world can afford this therapy. People in the United States primarily rely on health insurance to do so.) Note that any less of an effort (or lapse) in therapy allows the virus to readily change, in turn better resisting later attempts at treatment.

Recall from Chapter 12 that AZT treatment reduces mother-infant transmission of HIV at birth. This was recently shown to be true in Africa. Still the same problem just discussed exists—finding the money to pay for such AZT treatment.

What Are the Combined Costs of AIDS?

Though human life can't be tagged with a price, the cost of AIDS research and medical care for AIDS patients, the loss of labor force for industry, and the economic hardship experienced by families of victims can be quantified. By 2000 the AIDS plague could siphon off an estimated $81 to $107 billion from the U.S. economy and may drain $356 to $514 billion from the global economy. This is money that could be spent on goods and services to help maintain stable economies around the world. The impact of AIDS will hit poor countries worst, because their economies are already small and their living standards low.

Hidden Costs

Behind the mind-boggling statistics on AIDS are less obvious costs to businesses, families, and society in general. In India and Thailand, for example, a significant number of the adult male populations will be forfeited to AIDS. Worker productivity will plummet because AIDS victims produce less and demand more, especially as they waste away in the latter stages of the disease. Business productivity drops even further when relatives take time away from work and school to care for family members afflicted with AIDS. Furthermore, AIDS demands a considerable amount of family income. Hard-pressed families that have to devote much of their income to doctors and medicines have little left for living expenses. Other family members must struggle to keep up with daily duties because they must care for orphans left behind in the disease's wake. The number of youngsters orphaned by AIDS could more than double in the next 3 years to reach 3.7 million worldwide.

Individual and Government Response—Has It Been Adequate?

Governments worldwide have come under fire for their slow response in fighting AIDS. At present, neither governments nor the medical profession in developing countries has taken the lead in finding a solution. In India, for example, Bombay's first AIDS clinic, funded by a private interest group, didn't open until January 1993. Governments of developing nations frequently can't afford to supply AIDS counseling or treatment. Even worse, some continue to act as if their countries remain immune to the scourge. The weak response of government leaders and the resignation of citizens will undoubtedly lead to a greater degree of poverty and illness worldwide.

We all must act in concert to stop the spread of HIV. To do any less is to worsen the problem of undernutrition throughout the world. The medical ramifications of caring for those already infected with HIV will be troubling enough, especially in the developing world. If the AIDS epidemic continues to spread at the current rate, the resulting social and economic burdens could very well spark crises that spread beyond national borders. For further information on HIV and AIDS, visit http://www.yahoo.com/Health/Diseases_and_Conditions/AIDS_HIV, or call the CDC National HIV/AIDS hot line at (800) 458-5231. Their web site is http://www.cdcpin.org. Still other useful web sites are http://hivinsite.ucsf.edu, http://www.iapac.org, http://www.niaid.nih.gov/research/daids.htm, http://www.healthcg.com/hiv, and http://www.amfar.org.

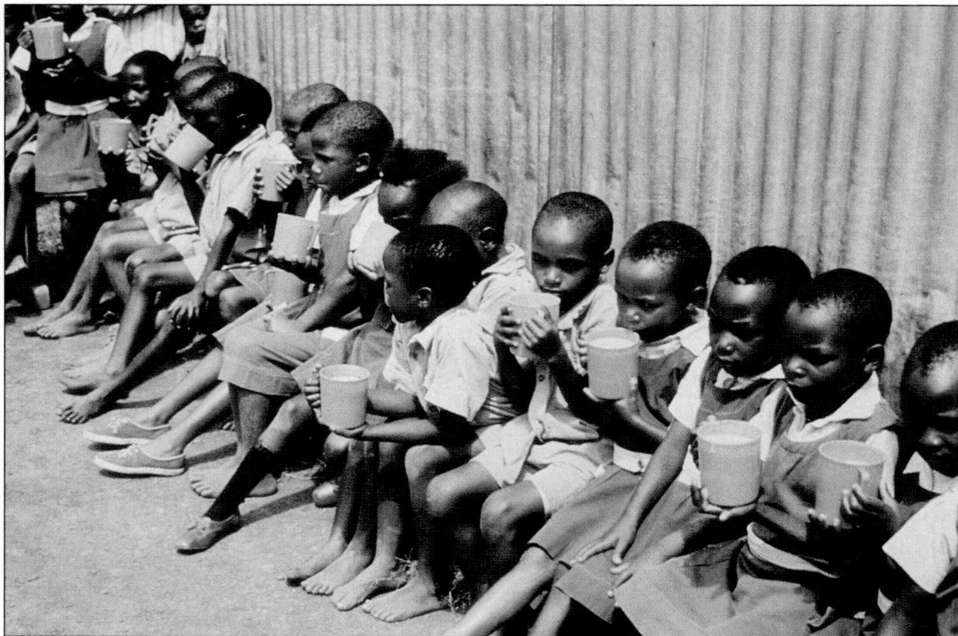

There's no doubt that food aid is important in reducing death from famine, but it isn't a long-term solution.

Since 1950, life expectancy in the developing world has increased 60% and infant mortality has fallen 50%. In the country of Indonesia, xerophthalmia—once a major problem—has been eliminated. This shows that effectively organized health and nutrition programs, such as those directed by the United Nations, can make a difference.

In the short run, there is no choice—aid must be given because people are starving. Still, improving the infrastructure for poor people, especially rural people, needs to be the long-term focus. This long-term approach is necessary because the most significant factor affecting undernutrition of people in impoverished areas of the world is their reliance on outside sources for basic needs. Their dependence makes them constantly vulnerable.

One American program that has helped improve the infrastructure of developing nations is the Peace Corps, which provides education, distributes food and medical supplies, and builds structures for local use. The aim of the Peace Corps is to improve the infrastructure and education of developing countries and thereby help create independent, self-sustaining economies around the world.

Tailoring Development to Local Conditions

There is a growing realization that rural people who own no land will flock to the overcrowded cities unless economic opportunities can be created as part of a plan for sustainable development. In response, careful, small-scale regional development is one option.

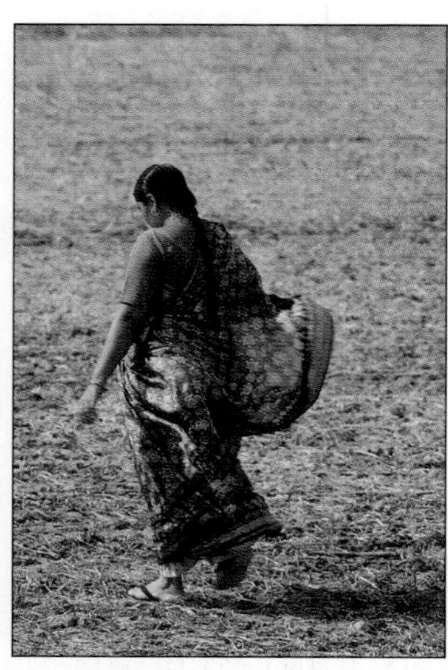

Women are receiving more attention as efforts to improve the health and welfare of the world's people evolve.

Impoverished women are a special concern. In addition to working longer hours than men, they grow most of the food for family consumption and make up three-fourths of the labor force in the informal sector and an increasing proportion in the formal economy. Economic opportunities for women must be augmented. Of the 1.3 billion people living in poverty worldwide, 70% are women. Moreover, among the developing world's 900 million illiterate people, women outnumber men 2 to 1. Thus an important means of propelling nations out of poverty is to end the cycle of female neglect. Providing women with education, entrepreneurship, and political power could pay off in numerous ways, ranging from slower population growth and higher incomes to healthier families.

Suitable technologies for processing, preserving, marketing, and distributing nutritious local staples also need to be encouraged so small farmers can flourish.

Education on how to use these foods to create healthful diets, such as for preparing vitamin A–rich vegetables, adds further benefit. Supplementing indigenous foods with nutrients that are in short supply, such as iron and iodide, also deserves consideration. One current program involves adding iron to sugar in various parts of the world. In addition, advances in water purification using ultraviolet light have the potential to cut energy expenditures by 20,000 times what is used now. This new method would result in a cost of $0.07 for a typical village's annual drinking water bill.

Raising the economic status of impoverished people by employing them is as important as expanding the food supply. If an increase in food supply is achieved without an accompanying rise in employment, there may be no long-term change in the number of undernourished people. Increasing the availability of food is another important part of the solution. If food resources are concentrated among a minority of people, as often happens with unequal land ownership, food won't be equally distributed unless efficient transportation systems are in place. Inequitable distribution then proves a very difficult problem to resolve.

Although food prices may fall with increased mechanization, use of fertilizers and other modern technologies, these same advances can also displace people from jobs. A shipment of high-technology tractors, for example, might put local laborers out of work. From this perspective, it is of little consequence that jobs are technologically primitive by Western standards.

At a recent conference in Rome, the United States touted freer trade policies as the solution to world hunger. At the same time, the United States admitted the need to increase food assistance, grain reserves, and support for agricultural research. Other countries stated that the solution offered by the United States is a simplistic answer to a complicated question. A concerted effort on the part of developed and developing countries' governments, however, to initiate programs such as those discussed above, is a start.

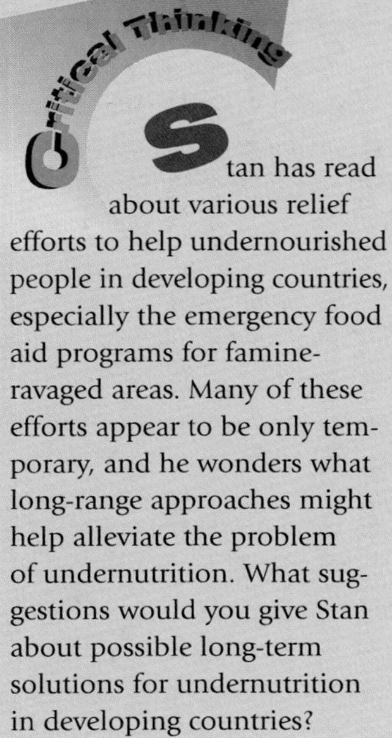

Stan has read about various relief efforts to help undernourished people in developing countries, especially the emergency food aid programs for famine-ravaged areas. Many of these efforts appear to be only temporary, and he wonders what long-range approaches might help alleviate the problem of undernutrition. What suggestions would you give Stan about possible long-term solutions for undernutrition in developing countries?

Some Concluding Thoughts

Clearly the developing world will have to rely largely on its own resources to finance development, especially in light of the current national debt of the United States. For decades, countries in Africa could count on the Cold War as an economic resource. The United States and the former Soviet Union opposed each other through African proxies, pouring in money to prop up pro-Western or pro-Communist governments. Now the big powers' priorities have turned inward. Making full use of the human resources available in the developing world itself is more essential than ever.

Overemphasizing cash crops, such as coffee, tea, rubber, and cocoa—as some developing countries have done, especially in Latin America—is not likely to solve the nutritional problems of poor people. Cash crops are usually grown at the expense of food crops on the assumption that money earned from the cash crops will be used to purchase food for the families of the workers. However, this is not always the case. Food can be bought, but it may not be enough and it is more expensive. In such a situation, poorer families are at greater risk than others, because the money earned from cash crops is often not enough to meet other basic family needs, let alone their food needs. As with poor families in the United States, buying quality foods often takes a secondary position, resulting in nutritional deprivation.

Also detrimental is the economics of drug crops, such as cocaine, marijuana, and opium. Perceiving drugs as valuable cash crops, workers often believe that the large sums of money netted from these crops—which are often more easily grown than food crops—can meet family needs and increase the standard of living. An unfortunate reality is that many workers see little or no cash earnings and become victims of their trade. Cash from drug crops often lines the pockets of criminals and corrupt government officials and results in little incentive to initiate subsistence-level food crops that could provide employment and nourishment for many.

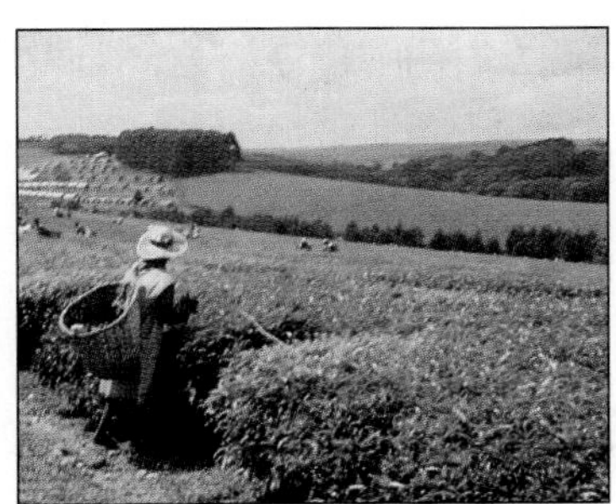

Overreliance on cash crops in developing countries can impede food production for the population as a whole.

ZIGGY®
THE PRESENT IS WHAT SLIPS BY US WHILE WE'RE PONDERING THE PAST AND WORRYING ABOUT THE FUTURE.

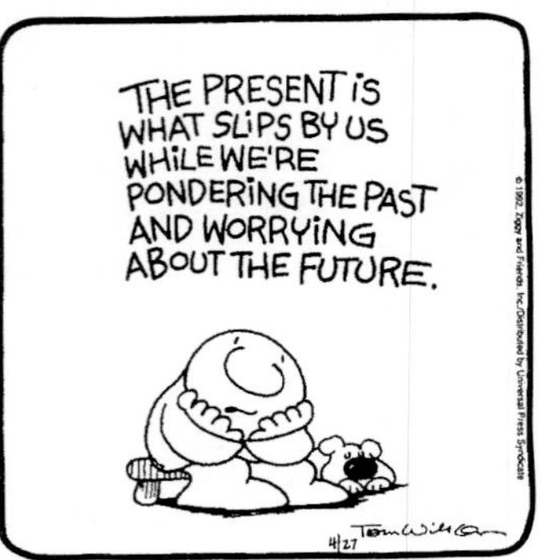

Figure 16–3
Ziggy.
ZIGGY © ZIGGY AND FRIENDS, INC. Reprinted with permission of UNIVERSAL PRESS SYNDICATE. All rights reserved.

With regard to the world food supply, our generation and the next will not likely have to face the absolute limits. Instead, we will have to make difficult choices if the outlook for future generations is to improve. The "live in the now" mentality has the potential to devastate a great part of humanity if it is not corrected.

Today the economic loss from undernutrition is staggering, and the amount of human pain and suffering is incalculable. With all the international relief efforts and assistance from governments and private organizations combined, we are still in the Dark Ages when it comes to our battle against undernutrition (Figure 16–3).

Currently, world leaders are concerned about the "marginalization" of problems in the developing world, fearing rich nations might dismiss war, disease, and famine as a way of life for poorer nations. In a recent survey, Americans identified world famine as less of a concern than violence, drugs, and inflation. Note that U.S. food aid, which averaged $1.9 billion annually in the early 1990s, fell to $1.25 billion in 1995 as the political support for such aid dwindled. Ultimately, however, depletion of world resources, the massive debt incurred by poorer countries, the threat of political unrest, and/or drug resistant diseases (e.g., new forms of tuberculosis) spreading to more prosperous countries nearby, and the toll taken in human lives does affect our world economy and overall well-being.

Leaders of rich and poor nations alike need to come to an agreement on the best possible means to serve all of the world's citizens. Perhaps if we rid ourselves of negative government actions worldwide, the task could become easier. Life is not necessarily fair, but the aim of civilization should be to make it fairer. The world has both the food and the technical expertise to end hunger. What is lacking is the political will and cooperation to do so.

ConceptCheck

Overall, one important solution to reducing undernutrition in the developing world lies in providing sufficient employment so that people can purchase the food their families need or provide access to land and other food production resources. Development programs must be sensitive to regional conditions to ensure that the new technologies introduced don't intensify existing problems for the poorest people.

Summary

- Poverty is a common thread wherever people suffer from undernutrition. Malnutrition can occur when the food supply is either scarce or abundant. The resulting deficiency conditions and degenerative diseases are influenced by genetic makeup.
- Undernutrition is the most common form of malnutrition in developing countries. It results from inadequate intake, absorption, or use of nutrients or food energy by the body. Many deficiency conditions consequently appear, and infectious diseases thrive because the immune system cannot function properly.
- The greatest risk of undernutrition occurs during critical periods of growth and development: gestation, infancy, and childhood. Low birth weight is a leading cause of infant deaths worldwide. Many developmental problems are caused by nutritional deprivation during critical periods of brain growth. Elderly people also experience multiple life changes that can influence intake, putting them at risk.
- In the United States, famine has been nonexistent since the 1930s, but undernutrition remains. Soup kitchens, food stamps, school lunch and breakfast programs, and the Supplemental Feeding Program for Women, Infants, and Children, (WIC) have focused on improving the nutritional health of poor and at-risk people. When adequately funded, these programs have proved effective

in reducing undernutrition. The need to reduce out-of-wedlock pregnancies remains a national priority, because single parents and their children are likely to live in poverty.

- Multiple factors contribute to the problem of undernutrition in the developing world. Food resources, as well as the means for distributing food, may be inadequate. Farming methods often encourage erosion, which deprives the soil of valuable nutrients and thereby hampers future efforts to grow food. Limited water availability limits food production.. Naturally occurring devastation from droughts, excessive rainfall, fire, crop infestation, and human causes—such as urbanization, war and civil unrest, debt, and poor sanitation—all contribute to the major problem of undernutrition.
- Proposed solutions to world undernutrition must include consideration of the interaction of multiple factors, many of which are thoroughly embedded in cultural traditions. Family planning efforts, for example, may not succeed until life expectancy increases. Through education, efforts should be made to upgrade farming methods, encourage breastfeeding, and improve sanitation and hygiene. Direct food aid is only a short-term solution. Many experts recommend sustainable subsistence-level farming, away from the specialization of cash crops, to increase the economic status and education of poor people. Small-scale industrial development is another way to create meaningful employment and purchasing power for vast numbers of the rural poor.

Study Questions

1. Describe the difference between malnutrition and undernutrition.
2. Describe in a short paragraph any evidence of undernutrition that you saw while you were growing up. What are/were the roots of theses problems?
3. What do you believe are the major factors contributing to undernutrition in wealthy nations, such as the United States? What are some solutions to this problem?
4. What three points would you make to a group of seventh-grade girls concerning the economic perils of teenage pregnancy and parenting?
5. Personal responsibility is a common theme in political circles these days. How does this relate to the problem of undernutrition in the United States? Does it apply to all causes of the problem?
6. Outline how war and civil unrest in developing countries have worsened problems of chronic hunger over the last few years.
7. How important is population control in addressing the problem of world hunger? Support your answer with three main points.
8. Why is solving the problem of undernutrition a key factor in development of the full potential of developing countries?
9. Discuss how infrastructure could influence the causes and solutions of chronic hunger in a developing nation.
10. Name three nutrients that are often lacking in the diets of undernourished people. What effects can be expected with each deficiency?

Further Readings

1 American Dietetic Association Reports: Position of the American Dietetic Association: World hunger, *Journal of the American Dietetic Association* 95:1160, 1995.
2 Bassuk EL and others: Single mothers and welfare, *Scientific American*, p. 60, October 1996.
3 Black MM: Zinc deficiency and child development, *American Journal of Clinical Nutrition* 68(suppl):464 S, 1998.
4 Bread for the World Institute: *What governments can do*, Silver Springs, MD, Bread for the World Institute, 1996.
5 Cohen OJ, Fauci AS: HIV/AIDS in 1998—gaining the upper hand? *Journal of the American Medical Association* 280:87, 1998.
6 Cook JT: The Food Stamp Program and low-income legal immigrants, *Nutrition Reviews* 56:218, 1998.
7 Defeating AIDS: What will it take (see entire series of articles), *Scientific American*, p. 81, July 1998.
8 Fawzi WW and others: A prospective study of malnutrition in relation to child mortality in the Sudan, *American Journal of Clinical Nutrition* 65:1062, 1997.
9 Foege WH: Global public health: targeting inequities, *Journal of the American Medical Association* 279:1931, 1998.
10 Katz F: Biotechnology—new tools in food technology's toolbox, *Food Technology*, p. 63, November 1996.
11 Lovgren S: A famine made by man, *U.S. News & World Report*, p. 41, September 14, 1998.
12 Nelson K and others: Hunger in an adult patient population, *Journal of the American Medical Association* 279:1211, 1998.
13 Prasad AS: Zinc deficiency in humans: a neglected problem, *Journal of the American College of Nutrition* 17:542, 1998.
14 Prendergast RM: Hunger and ethics, *Topics in Clinical Nutrition* 13(4):64, 1998.
15 Raloff J: The human numbers crunch, *Science News* 149:396, 1996.
16 Raloff J: Can grain yields keep pace? *Science News* 152:104, 1997.
17 Scheker S.: Genetic engineering poses many questions, *Community Nutrition Institute Nutrition Week*, p. 4, January 15, 1999.
18 Silliman K and others: Evidence of nutritional risk in a population of homeless adults in rural Northern California, *Journal of the American Dietetic Association* 98:908, 1998.
19 Solomons NW, Gross R: Urban nutrition in developing countries, *Nutrition Reviews* 53:90, 1995.
20 Starr P: The homeless and the public household, *New England Journal of Medicine* 338:1761, 1998.
21 State of the world's children 1998: a UNICEF report, *Nutrition Reviews* 56:115, 1998.
22 Underwood BA: Micronutrient malnutrition, *Nutrition Today* 33:121, 1998.

RATE

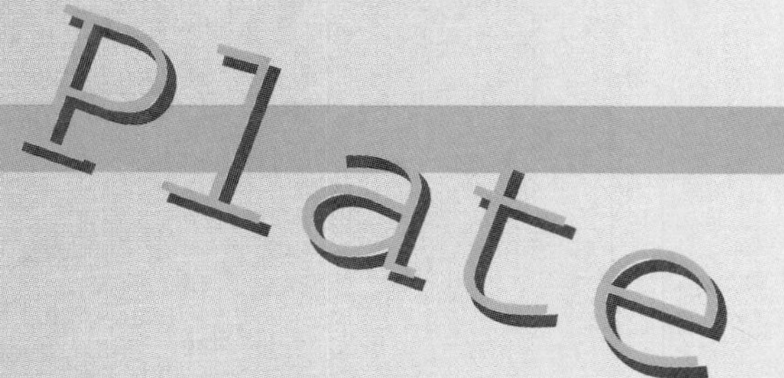

I. Fighting World Undernutrition on a Personal Level

If you want to do something about world and domestic undernutrition, the following activities are suggested. It is a noble act to try to make a difference, even if you make just one small step. As with any change in behavior, don't try to do too many things at once. Try one or two activities that represent your commitment to solving this gigantic problem.

1. Volunteer at a local soup kitchen or homeless shelter for a time-limited period (1 month, for example). What insights did you gain?
2. Donate some money to a voluntary agency that does antihunger work, such as those listed below:

   Bread for the World
   802 Rhode Island Ave., NE
   Washington, DC 20018

   Oxfam America
   115 Broadway
   Boston, MA 02116

   Save the Children Foundation
   P.O. Box 970
   Westport, CT 06881

   Catholic Relief Services
   209 W. Fayette St.
   Baltimore, MD 21201

   CARE
   660 First Ave.
   New York, NY 10016

   Second Harvest
   116 Michigan Ave.
   Suite #4
   Chicago, IL 60603

3. Write a letter to a senator or member of Congress asking what he or she is doing about ending domestic and world undernutrition.
4. Contribute to World Food Day activities each October 16 to stay informed about the issues.
5. Internet users can find information on hunger at several sites, including the following:
   - HungerWeb, at Brown University, which offers information on hunger research, programs, education, and advocacy and an overview of the Alan Shawn Feinstein World Hunger Program at Brown. HungerWeb is a World Wide Web home page that links to Internet sites run by the U.N., U.S. AID, and the World Bank.
     http://www.netspace.org/hungerweb
   - The U.N. Food and Agriculture Organization, which provides an extensive list of publications related to agriculture and global foods security.
     http://www.fao.org
   - Food for the Hungry, which tracks domestic and global hunger issues.
     http://www.fh.org
   - Second Harvest
     http://www.secondharvest.org
   - Bread for the World
     http://www.bread.org
   - CARE
     http://www.care.org
   - World Hunger Year
     http://www.iglou.com/why

II. Joining the Battle Against Undernutrition

Imagine that you recently spent your summer vacation in a developing country and saw evidence of undernutrition and hunger. Then imagine that you are now asking a large corporation to support your efforts to ease hunger and suffering in this area. Develop a two-paragraph statement outlining why addressing hunger issues in this area is important. Address how you think a large corporation could assist you in your efforts.

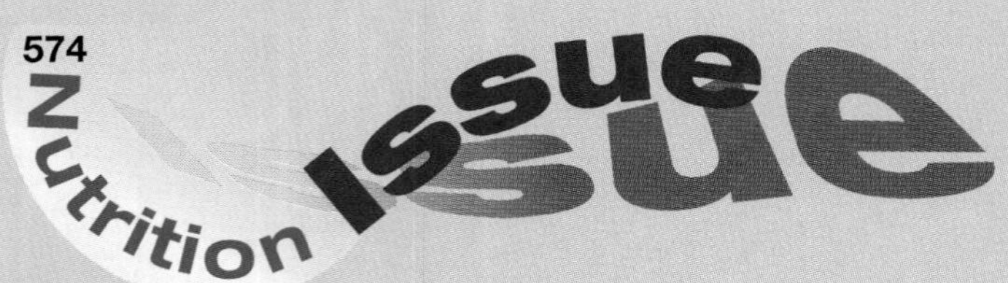

Biotechnology: An Answer to Food Shortages

The ability of humans to manipulate nature has enabled us to improve the production and yield of many important foods. Traditional **biotechnology** is almost as old as agriculture. The first farmer to improve his stock by selectively breeding the best bull with the best cows was implementing biotechnology in a simple sense. The first baker to use yeast to make bread rise took similar advantage of biotechnology.

Biotechnology
A collection of processes that involve the use of biological systems for altering and, ideally, improving the characteristics of plants, animals, and other forms of life.

By the 1930s, biotechnology made possible the selective breeding of better plant hybrids: as a result, corn production in the United Sates quickly doubled. Through similar methods, agricultural wheat was crossed with wild grasses to confer more desirable properties, such as greater yield, increased resistance to mildew and bacterial diseases, and tolerance to salt or adverse climatic conditions.

Another type of biotechnology uses hormones rather than breeding. In the last decade, Canadian salmon have been treated with a hormone that allows them to mature three times faster than normal—without changing the fish in any other way. In general terms, biotechnology can be understood as the use of living things—plants, animals, bacteria—to manufacture products.

THE NEW BIOTECHNOLOGY

The new biotechnology used in agriculture includes several methods that directly modify products. It differs from traditional methods because it directly changes some of the genetic material (DNA) of organisms to improve characteristics. Cross-breeding plants or animals is no longer the only tool. Development of the new process, called **genetic engineering,** began in the 1970s. The field now features a wide range of cell and subcell techniques for the synthesis and placement of genetic material in organisms. This allows access to a wider gene pool, and it permits faster and more accurate production of new and more useful microbial, plant, and animal species. Traditional breeding has had inconsistent results; biotechnology is more precise. Scientists select the traits they want and genetically engineer or introduce the gene that produces the desired trait into animals. It is important to note, however, the genetic engineering doesn't replace conventional breeding practices; both work together.

Genetic engineering
Alteration of genetic material in plants or animals with the intent of improving growth, disease resistance, or other characteristics.

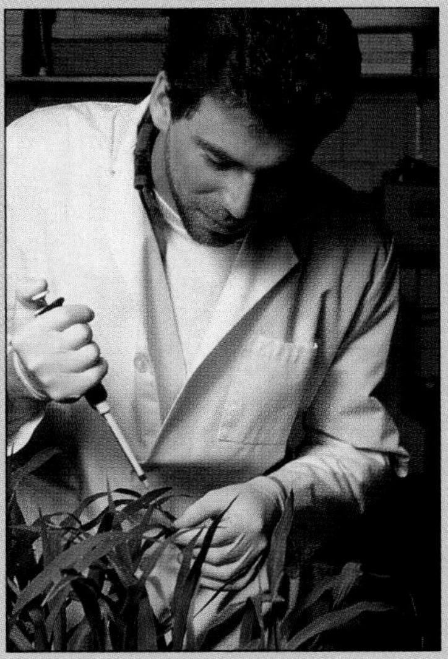
Traditional plant breeding and biotechnology have been combined to produce high-yielding plant varieties.

Already, genetic engineering at the agricultural level has allowed us to make use of new types of seeds, growth hormones, and microbial inoculants to stop pests and frost damage. Biotechnology is also used to develop drought-tolerant crops, as well as to detect *Listeria* and other microbes that cause foodborne illness. Scientists are engineering plants that grow without pesticides and new forms of potatoes that can last without preservatives. In addition, biotechnology can allow scientists to create fruits with more or less sucrose, and greater amounts of vitamin A and C. Researchers are also examining ways to modify the fatty acid makeup of vegetable oils. Because cautious use is the order of the day, these early benefits of the new biotechnology will strike us as only subtly different. The ultimate benefits, however, could be substantial.

Questions surround the use of the new biotechnology. Take, for instance, the Flavr Savr tomato, which was genetically engineered to stay firm longer. Is it still a tomato? It looks the same, feels the same, tastes the same, and even has the same nutritional value. The only change researchers made is to counteract the action of a single gene in the DNA that makes tomatoes rot rapidly. Reversing just one gene out of 10,000 makes the biotech tomato significantly different from the standard garden variety.

Still, the question remains: How many and which properties can be changed in a plant, animal, or bacterium before it becomes something else? A tomato altered in only one specific way still seems to be a tomato, but does it remain one if it is improved in 10 or 20 ways? When traditional methods crossed a tangerine with a grapefruit, the new genetic structure was clearly something else, now commonly known as a *tangelo.*

CONTROVERSY SURROUNDING THE NEW BIOTECHNOLOGY

Public response to use of the new biotechnology has been mixed. Even the scientific community has mixed feelings about this new technology, with supporters as convinced about the benefits as opponents are of the risks. Although the use of genetically modified organisms may reduce the need for environmentally harmful activities, such as spraying crops with insecticides, critics point out that seeds produced with natural insecticides will lead to rapid insect resistance because the insecticides are continuously being emitted. When farmers use insecticides, they use them sparingly and only when needed, in part so the insects do not become resistant.

Although the risks may appear to be momentarily negligible, they may be cumulative and therefore dangerous in the long run. In addition, will allergens, such as those found in peanuts, eggs, milk, wheat, and shellfish, be added to genetically engineered foods that previously did not contain them? Evidence that this can happen has been seen in soybeans. Note, however, that FDA carefully examines all products developed using this technology and will enforce labeling of potential allergens that may be newly present in a biotech food.

The public has long been opposed to processes perceived as harmful to the environment, such as producing unnatural products. Because food reserves are high in the United States, Canada, and Europe, some question the need to increase food production. Skepticism surrounds unnatural products, as exemplified by western Europe's ban of a growth hormone previously used in beef production. Citizens believed the increase in meat supply was not worth the perceived risks associated with the product. In the United States, FDA recently approved the first genetically engineered food product for humans, a substitute for the enzyme renin, called *chymosin.* Renin is traditionally used in making cheese. Both scientists and concerned consumer groups are currently studying other potentially beneficial applications of the new biotechnology. Bovine somatotropin (BST), a hormone produced by cattle, has been known since the 1930s to increase milk production when injected into dairy cattle. Today an identical BST (Posilac) produced through genetic engineering can be used to greatly increase milk yield. Because it is a protein, any BST in the milk produced would be digested and therefore inactivated. People even produce their own form of somatotropin, but its structure differs considerably from that of BST. And because cows produce BST naturally, it has always been present in their milk. Treating the animals with the proposed higher levels of BST doesn't increase the concentration of hormone occurring naturally in the milk, nor will it alter the mik's nutrient composition.

Researchers are interested not only in increasing milk productivity but also in changing its components. Abbot labs and Ciba-Geigy are currently looking at ways to make cow's milk more like human milk. Properties such as substances to increase immune function for disease fighting may improve health in humans.

While FDA is still evaluating the safety of BST with respect to animals and the environment, the agency has determined that milk from treated animals is safe for human consumption. Currently about 1 in 10 dairy farms uses the product. Some critics question whether the increased milk production will stress the health of the cows, leading farmers to use more antibiotics, which can show up in milk. Some of the public already appears to oppose BST, and the European Economic Community has banned its use.

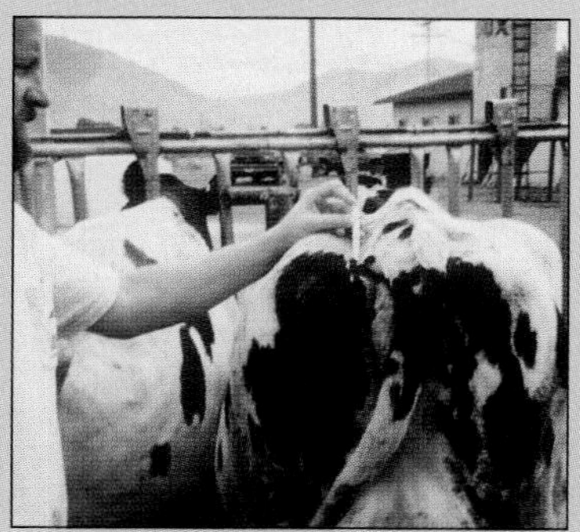

Milk yields can be increased using genetically engineered bovine somatotropin.

Opponents to BST call for labeling of milk from treated cows. The biotech industry opposes labeling as they fear that it may lead to label requirements in all genetically engineered foods, and because studies show no harmful effects from milk of BST-treated cows. FDA has not required such labeling, but the National Organic Standards Board has determined that genetically engineered foods cannot carry an "organic" label.

Again, with a surplus of milk in the United States and Europe, garnering public support will be difficult. Furthermore, dairy farmers in Wisconsin and other dairy-producing regions generally oppose the introduction of the hormone, because they fear negative consumer reaction will lower milk consumption. The industry is also concerned that a sharp increase in milk output will adversely affect prices and thereby harm thousands of small dairy farms facing an already precarious economic situation.

ROLE OF THE NEW BIOTECHNOLOGY IN THE DEVELOPING WORLD

Whether generally engineered applications will help to significantly reduce undernutrition in the developing world remains to be seen. Unless price cuts accompany the increased production, only landowners and suppliers of biotechnology will enjoy the benefits. This point deserves emphasis: The person who couldn't afford a tangelo yesterday probably won't be able to afford one tomorrow. The same can be said for improved tomatoes. As with most innovations, the more successful farmers, often those with larger farms, will adopt the new biotechnology first. Because of this, the present trend of fewer and larger farms will continue in the developing world, a trend that undermines the most pressing undernutrition issues there. Furthermore, biotechnology does not promise dramatic increases in the production of most grains, the primary food resource in the world.

Perhaps the most promising potential of genetically engineered foods is the idea of plant breeding for micronutrients. The dilemma of micronutrient undernutrition may be decreased in developing countries if farmers can afford to use seeds that have these nutrients already added. Still, for the developing world, the focus needs to be on providing people with resources to produce and purchase their own food, not on simply growing more food. Biotechnology is a useful tool against the complex scourge of world undernutrition, but it's no panacea. Improved crops produced by this technology will likely be able to contribute to the battle, together with political and other efforts.

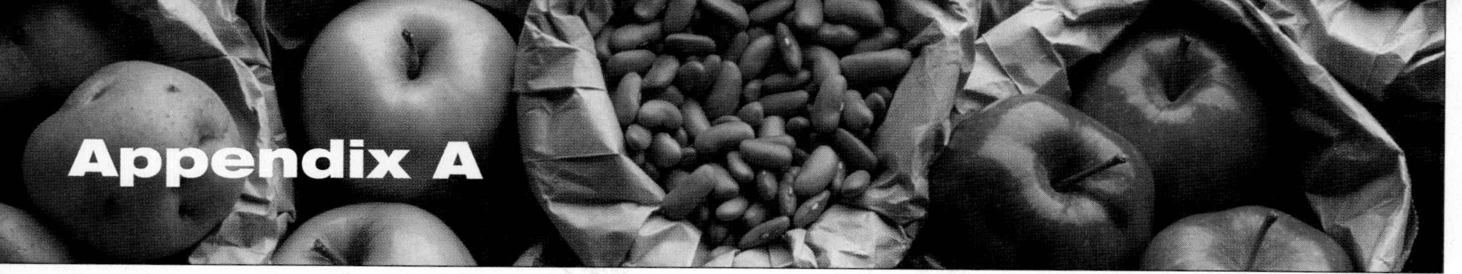

Appendix A

Food Composition Table

The following food composition table includes some of the foods in McGraw-Hill's *NutriQuest*,™ version 2.0—dietary analysis software, which is available as a supplement to this text. (*NutriQuest's* database contains approximately 4,000 foods, so it simply isn't possible to include all of them here.) If you do not find a food in this table, it's likely you will locate it in *NutriQuest*,™ version 2.0.

The following food composition table is handy if you do not have access to a computer or your computer time is limited. The foods in the table are arranged alphabetically. Quick-Service foods ("fast foods," like Wendy's) are listed alphabetically by restaurant name in a separate section toward the end of this appendix (see p. A-62).

The codes in the left-hand column correspond with the numbers in the *NutriQuest*™ database. When working in *NutriQuest*,™ one way to locate a specific food is by entering the appropriate code. More specific instructions for using *NutriQuest*™ are contained in the program's "Help" function and in the User's Guide that accompanies the software.

Code	Name	Amount	Unit	Grams	Energy (kcal)	Carbohydrates (g)	Protein (g)	Fat (g)	Saturated fat (g)	Monounsat... fat (g)
11001	Alfalfa Seeds, Sprouted, Fresh	½	Cup	16.5	5	1	1	0	0	0
19065	Almond Joy Candy Bar	1	Bar	50.0	232	29	2	14	8	3
12067	Almonds, Toasted, Unblanched	½	Cup	71.0	418	16	14	36	3	23
19066	Alpine White Bar w/Almonds	1	Bar	35.0	197	18	4	13	7	5
15002	Anchovy, European, Cnd In Oil	3	Ounce	85.1	179	0	25	8	2	3
55188	Angel Hair Pasta. Lean Cuisine-Stouffer's	1	Each	283.5	240	38	10	5	1	–
18150	Animal Crackers	1	Each	2.5	11	2	0	0	0	0
19294	Apple Butter	1	Tbsp.	18.0	33	9	0	0	–	–
19186	Apple Crisp	1	Cup	282.0	460	91	5	10	2	4
9400	Apple Juice, Unsweetened	¾	Cup	185.8	87	22	0	0	0	0
18302	Apple Pie	1	Slice	155.0	411	58	4	19	5	8
9007	Apples, Cnd, Sweetened	½	Cup	102.0	68	17	0	0	0	0
9009	Apples, Dehydrated, Sulfured	¼	Cup	15.0	52	14	0	0	0	0
9003	Apples, Fresh, w/Skin	1	Medium	138.0	81	21	0	0	0	0
9004	Apples, Fresh, w/o Skin	1	Medium	128.0	73	19	0	0	0	0
9020	Applesauce, Sweetened	½	Cup	127.5	97	1 25	0	0	0	0
9019	Applesauce, Unsweetened	½	Cup	122.0	52	14	0	0	0	0
9403	Apricot Nectar, Cnd, w/Added Vit C	¾	Cup	188.2	105	27	1	0	0	0
9036	Apricot Nectar, Cnd, w/o Added Vit C	¾	Cup	188.2	105	27	1	0	0	0
9028	Apricots, Cnd, Heavy Syrup Pack	½	Cup	129.0	107	28	1	0	0	0
9024	Apricots, Cnd, Juice Pack	½	Cup	124.0	60	15	1	0	0	0
9026	Apricots, Cnd, Light Syrup Pack	½	Cup	126.5	80	21	1	0	0	0
9022	Apricots, Cnd, Water Pack	½	Cup	121.5	33	8	1	0	0	0
9030	Apricots, Dehydrated, Sulfured	¼	Cup	29.8	95	25	1	0	0	0
9032	Apricots, Dried, Sulfured	¼	Cup	32.5	77	20	1	0	0	0
9021	Apricots, Fresh	3	Medium	106.0	51	12	1	0	0	0
9035	Apricots, Frozen, Sweetened	½	Cup	121.0	119	30	1	0	0	0
11705	Asparagus, Ckd	½	Cup	90.0	23	4	2	0	0	0
11015	Asparagus, Cnd	½	Cup	121.0	23	3	3	1	0	0
11011	Asparagus, Fresh	½	Cup	67.0	15	3	2	0	0	0
11019	Asparagus, Frz, Ckd	½	Cup	100.0	28	5	3	0	0	0
9037	Avocados, Fresh	1	Medium	201.0	324	15	4	31	5	19
10124	Bacon	1	Slice	6.0	35	0	2	3	1	1
10131	Bacon, Canadian–style Bacon, Grilled	1	Slice	21.0	39	0	5	2	1	1
62528	Bacon, Turkey	1	Slice	14.0	25	0	3	2	1	–
62631	Bagel Chips	1	Ounce	28.4	150	20	4	6	1	3
18005	Bagels, Cinnamon–raisin	1	3½ In.	71.0	195	39	7	1	0	0
18006	Bagels, Cinnamon–raisin, Toasted	1	3½ In.	66.0	194	39	7	11	0	0
18003	Bagels, Egg	1	3½ In.	71.0	197	38	8	11	0	0
18004	Bagels, Egg, Toasted	1	3½ In.	66.0	197	38	8	1	0	0
18007	Bagels, Oat Bran	1	3½ In.	71.0	181	38	8	1	0	0
18008	Bagels, Oat Bran, Toasted	1	3½ In.	66.0	181	38	8	1	0	0
18001	Bagels, Plain	1	3½ In.	71.0	195	38	7	1	0	0
18409	Bagels, Plain, Toasted	1	3½ In.	66.0	195	38	7	1	0	–
55189	Baked Cheese Ravioli, Lean Cuisine–Stouffer's	1	Each	241.0	240	30	13	8	3	–
41297	Baked Cheese Ravioli–Healthy Choice	1	Each	255.1	250	44	14	12	1	–
55190	Baked Potato w/Sour Cream, Lean Cuisine–Stouffer's	1	Each	294.1	230	38	9	5	2	–
11028	Bamboo Shoots, Cnd	½	Cup	65.5	12	2	1	0	0	0
11026	Bamboo Shoots, Fresh	½	Cup	75.5	20	4	2	0	0	0
19400	Banana Chips	1	Ounce	28.4	147	17	1	10	8	1
18304	Banana Cream Pie	1	Slice	148.0	398	49	7	20	6	8
41240	Banana Nut Muffin–Healthy Choice	1	Each	70.9	180	32	3	6	–	–
19311	Banana Pudding	1	Cup	298.1	379	163	7	11	2	5
9040	Bananas, Fresh	1	Medium	114.0	105	27	1	1	0	0
6150	Barbecue Sauce	½	Cup	125.0	94	16	2	2	0	1
20004	Barley	1	Cup	184.0	651	135	23	14	1	1

Abbreviations: g = grams, mg = milligrams, µg = micrograms.

Polyunsaturated fat (g)	Dietary Fiber (g)	Cholesterol (mg)	Folate (µg)	Vitamin A (RE)	Vitamin B-6 (mg)	Vitamin B-12 (µg)	Vitamin C (mg)	Vitamin E (mg)	Riboflavin (mg)	Thiamin (mg)	Calcium (mg)	Iron (mg)	Magnesium (mg)	Niacin (mg)	Phosphorus (mg)	Potassium (mg)	Sodium (mg)	Zinc (mg)
0	0	0	6	3	0	0	1	0	0	0	5	.2	4	.1	12	13	1	.2
1	–	1	4	2	0	.1	0	–	.1	0	40	.6	33	.2	70	186	67	.4
8	8	0	45	0	.1	0	0	11.4	.4	.1	201	3.5	216	2	390	549	8	3.5
1	2	4	5	9	0	.3	0	–	.1	0	81	.2	13	0	82	146	26	.4
2	0	72	11	18	.2	.7	0	4.3	.3	.1	197	3.9	59	16.9	214	463	3120	2.1
1	–	10	–	250	–	–	6	–	.3	.3	80	1.5	–	2.9	–	500	410	–
0	–	0	0	0	0	0	0	–	0	0	1	.1	0	.1	3	3	10	0
–	0	0	0	0	0	0	0	0	0	0	1	0	1	0	1	16	0	0
3	–	0	14	87	.1	–	6	–	.2	.2	79	2.1	20	2.2	71	274	513	.5
0	–	0	0	0	.1	0	77	0	0	0	13	.7	6	–	13	221	6	.1
5	–	0	6	19	0	0	3	–	.2	.2	11	1.7	11	1.9	43	122	327	.3
0	2	0	0	5	0	0	0	.1	0	0	4	.2	2	.1	5	69	3	0
0	2	0	0	1	0	0	0	.5	0	0	3	.3	3	.1	8	96	19	0
0	4	0	4	7	.1	0	8	.8	0	0	10	.2	7	.1	10	159	0	.1
0	2	0	1	5	.1	0	5	.3	0	0	5	.1	4	.1	9	145	0	.1
0	2	0	1	1	0	0	2	.1	0	0	5	.4	4	.2	9	78	4	.1
0	1	0	1	4	0	0	1	.1	0	0	4	.1	4	.2	9	92	2	0
0	–	0	2	248	0	0	102	–	0	0	13	.7	9	.5	17	215	6	.2
0	1	0	2	248	0	0	1	.2	0	0	13	.7	9	.5	17	215	6	.2
0	–	0	2	160	.1	0	4	–	0	0	12	.6	10	.5	17	173	14	.1
0	2	0	2	210	.1	0	6	1.1	0	0	15	.4	12	.4	25	205	5	.1
0	2	0	2	167	.1	0	3	1.1	0	0	14	.5	10	.4	16	175	5	.1
0	2	0	2	157	.1	0	4	1.1	0	0	10	.4	9	.5	16	233	4	.1
0	–	0	1	377	.2	0	3	–	0	0	18	1.9	19	1.1	47	550	4	.3
0	3	0	3	235	.1	0	1	0	0	0	15	1.5	15	1	38	448	3	.2
0	3	0	9	277	.1	0	11	.9	0	0	15	.6	8	.6	20	314	1	.3
0	2	0	2	203	.1	0	11	1.1	0	0	12	1.1	11	1	23	277	5	.1
0	–	0	88	75	.1	0	24	–	.1	.1	22	.6	17	.9	55	279	216	.4
0	2	0	116	64	.1	0	22	–	.1	.1	19	2.2	12	1.2	52	208	472	.5
0	1	0	86	39	.1	0	9	1.3	.1	.1	14	.6	12	.8	38	183	1	.3
0	–	0	135	82	0	0	24	–	.1	.1	23	.6	13	1	55	218	4	.6
4	12	0	124	123	.6	0	16	2.7	.2	.2	22	2.1	78	3.9	82	1204	20	.8
0	0	5	0	0	0	.1	2	0	0	0	1	.1	1	.4	20	29	96	.2
0	0	12	1	0	.1	.2	5	.1	0	.2	2	.2	4	1.5	62	82	325	.4
–	–	10	–	0	–	–	0	–	–	–	0	0	–	–	–	–	170	–
2	1	0	–	0	–	–	0	–	–	–	0	.4	–	–	–	–	190	–
0	–	0	15	6	0	0	0	–	.2	.3	13	2.7	15	2.2	55	108	229	.5
0	–	0	11	5	0	0	0	–	.2	.2	13	2.7	15	2	55	108	228	.5
0	–	17	16	23	.1	.1	0	–	.2	.4	9	2.8	18	2.4	60	48	359	.5
0	–	17	11	21	.1	.1	0	–	.1	.3	9	2.8	18	2.2	59	48	358	.5
0	–	0	33	0	.1	0	0	–	.2	.2	9	2.2	40	2.1	117	145	360	1.5
0	–	0	23	0	.1	0	0	–	.2	.2	9	2.2	41	1.9	117	145	360	1.5
0	1	0	16	0	0	0	0	–	.2	.4	53	2.5	21	3.2	68	72	379	.6
0	–	0	11	0	0	0	0	–	.2	.3	13	2.5	20	2.9	68	72	379	.6
–	–	55	–	60	–	–	36	–	.3	.1	160	.8	–	1.1	–	380	590	–
–	–	20	–	500	–	–	5	–	.3	.3	200	1.5	–	1.9	240	590	420	–
–	–	15	–	350	–	–	30	–	.3	.2	160	.6	–	1.1	–	900	570	–
0	2	0	2	1	.1	0	1	.2	0	0	5	.2	3	.1	16	52	5	.4
0	2	0	5	2	.2	0	3	.8	.1	.1	10	.4	2	.5	45	402	3	.8
0	2	0	4	2	.1	0	2	1.5	0	0	5	.4	22	.2	16	152	2	.2
5	–	75	16	104	.2	.4	2	–	.3	.2	111	1.5	24	1.6	136	244	355	.7
3	–	0	–	–	–	–	–	–	.1	.2	80	1	–	.8	160	250	80	–
4	–	0	6	89	.1	.5	1	–	.4	.1	253	.4	24	.5	206	328	584	.8
0	3	0	22	9	.7	0	10	.3	.1	.1	7	.4	33	.6	23	451	1	.2
1	1	0	5	109	.1	0	9	1.4	0	0	24	1.1	22	1.1	25	217	1019	.2
2	32	0	35	4	.6	0	0	1	.5	1.2	61	6.6	245	8.5	486	832	22	5.1

Code	Name	Amount	Unit	Grams	Energy (kcal)	Carbohydrates (g)	Protein (g)	Fat (g)	Saturated fat (g)	Monounsaturated fat (g)
15187	Bass, Freshwater, Ckd, Dry Heat	3	Ounce	85.1	124	0	21	14	1	2
15188	Bass, Striped, Ckd, Dry Heat	3	Ounce	85.1	105	0	19	3	1	1
62678	Bean Dip	2	Tbsp.	30.0	20	4	1	0	0	0
11924	Bean Sprouts	½	Cup	66.7	83	6	9	5	–	–
41276	Bean and Ham Soup–Healthy Choice	1	Each	212.6	220	35	12	14	1	–
16006	Beans, Baked, Cnd, Vegetarian	½	Cup	127.0	118	26	6	1	0	0
16007	Beans, Baked, Cnd, w/Beef	½	Cup	133.0	161	22	8	5	2	2
16008	Beans, Baked, Cnd, w/Franks	½	Cup	128.5	182	20	9	8	3	4
16009	Beans, Baked, Cnd, w/Pork	½	Cup	126.5	134	25	7	2	1	1
16005	Beans, Baked, Home Prepared	½	Cup	126.5	191	27	7	7	2	3
16315	Beans, Black, Ckd	½	Cup	86.0	114	20	8	0	0	0
11056	Beans, Green, Cnd	½	Cup	68.0	14	3	1	0	0	0
11052	Beans, Green, Fresh	½	Cup	55.0	17	4	1	0	0	0
11061	Beans, Green, Fzn	½	Cup	67.5	18	4	1	0	0	0
16029	Beans, Kidney, Cnd	½	Cup	128.0	104	19	7	0	0	0
16073	Beans, Lima, Cnd	½	Cup	120.5	95	18	6	0	0	0
11040	Beans, Lima, Fzn	½	Cup	90.0	95	18	6	0	0	0
16039	Beans, Navy, Cnd	½	Cup	131.0	148	27	10	1	0	0
16044	Beans, Pinto, Cnd	½	Cup	120.0	94	17	5	0	0	0
16103	Beans, Refried, Cnd	½	Cup	126.5	135	23	8	1	1	1
11932	Beans, Yellow, Cnd	½	Cup	68.0	14	3	1	0	0	0
11722	Beans, Yellow, Fresh	½	Cup	55.0	17	4	1	0	0	0
14114	Beef Broth and Tomato Juice, Cnd	¾	Cup	183.0	68	16	1	0	0	0
55192	Beef Cannelloni w/Sauce, Lean Cuisine–Stouffer's	1	Each	272.9	200	28	14	3	1	–
62692	Beef Chow Mein	1	Cup	247.0	110	15	10	2	1	–
41249	Beef Enchilada–Healthy Choice	1	Each	379.2	370	66	15	5	2	–
19002	Beef Jerky, Chopped and Formed	3	Ounce	85.1	287	12	34	11	5	5
55149	Beef Pie–Stouffer's	1	Each	283.5	460	37	18	27	–	–
57806	Beef Pot Pie–Swanson	1	Pie	198.5	370	36	12	19	–	–
43405	Beef Ravioli, Micro Cup–Hormel	1	Each	212.6	270	34	9	11	4	5
41251	Beef Sirloin Tips–Healthy Choice	1	Each	318.9	270	29	22	7	3	–
43413	Beef Stew, Micro Cup–Hormel	1	Each	212.6	230	11	13	15	5	4
55158	Beef Stroganoff w/Parsley Noodles–Stouffer's	1	Each	276.4	390	28	24	20	–	–
41335	Beef and Bean Burritos (medium)–Healthy Choice	1	Each	148.8	270	42	12	7	3	0
41334	Beef and Bean Burritos (mild)–Healthy Choice	1	Each	148.8	250	45	11	5	1	–
55191	Beef and Bean Enchiladas, Lean Cuisine–Stouffer's	1	Each	262.2	240	32	15	6	3	–
41270	Beef and Potato Soup–Healthy Choice	1	Each	212.6	110	17	9	1	–	–
13347	Beef, Corned, Brisket, Ckd	3	Ounce	85.1	213	0	15	16	5	8
13353	Beef, Cured, Lunch Meat, Jellied	3	Ounce	85.1	94	0	16	3	1	1
13355	Beef, Cured, Pastrami	3	Ounce	85.1	297	3	15	25	9	12
13357	Beef, Cured, Sausage, Smoked	3	Ounce	85.1	265	2	12	23	10	11
13358	Beef, Cured, Smoked, Chopped Beef	3	Ounce	85.1	105	2	17	4	2	2
13360	Beef, Cured, Thin-sliced Beef	3	Ounce	85.1	151	5	24	3	1	1
13300	Beef, Ground, Extra Lean, Pan-fried	3	Ounce	85.1	217	0	21	14	5	6
13305	Beef, Ground, Lean, Broiled	3	Ounce	85.1	231	0	21	16	6	7
13307	Beef, Ground, Lean, Pan-fried	3	Ounce	85.1	234	0	21	16	6	7
13312	Beef, Ground, Regular, Broiled	3	Ounce	85.1	246	0	20	18	7	8
13314	Beef, Ground, Regular, Pan-fried	3	Ounce	85.1	260	0	20	19	8	8
13326	Beef, Liver, Ckd, Braised	3	Ounce	85.1	137	3	21	4	2	1
13327	Beef, Liver, Ckd, Pan-fried	3	Ounce	85.1	185	7	23	7	2	1
7042	Beef, Loaved, Lunch Meat	1	Slice	28.4	87	1	4	7	3	3
13504	Beef, Steaks and Roasts, Ckd, ½ in. Fat	3	Ounce	85.1	297	0	21	23	9	10
13361	Beef, Steaks and Roasts, Ckd, Fat Trimmed	3	Ounce	85.1	232	0	23	15	6	6
13004	Beef, Steaks and Roasts, Ckd., ¼ in. Fat	3	Ounce	85.1	259	0	22	18	7	8
7043	Beef, Thin Sliced	1	Slice	4.2	7	0	1	0	0	0
14006	Beer, Light	12	Fl Oz	354.0	99	5	1	0	0	0

Polyunsaturated fat (g)	Dietary Fiber (g)	Cholesterol (mg)	Folate (µg)	Vitamin A (RE)	Vitamin B-6 (mg)	Vitamin B-12 (µg)	Vitamin C (mg)	Vitamin E (mg)	Riboflavin (mg)	Thiamin (mg)	Calcium (mg)	Iron (mg)	Magnesium (mg)	Niacin (mg)	Phosphorus (mg)	Potassium (mg)	Sodium (mg)	Zinc (mg)
1	0	74	14	30	.1	2	2	–	.1	.1	88	1.6	32	1.3	218	388	77	.7
1	0	88	9	26	.3	3.8	0	–	0	.1	16	.9	43	2.2	216	279	75	.4
0	1	0	0	0	0	0	0	–	0	0	0	.2	0	0	0	–	150	0
–	–	0	85	1	.1	0	8	–	.1	.3	55	.3	64	.7	144	378	167	1.4
1	–	5	–	60	–	–	2	–	.2	.2	48	1	–	1.1	220	630	480	–
0	6	0	30	22	.2	0	4	–	.1	.2	64	.4	41	.5	132	376	504	1.8
0	–	29	58	28	.1	0	2	–	.1	.1	60	2.1	33	1.3	108	426	632	1.6
1	9	8	39	19	.1	0	3	.6	.1	.1	62	2.2	36	1.2	134	302	553	2.4
0	7	9	46	23	.1	0	3	.7	0	.1	67	2.2	43	.6	137	391	524	1.8
1	7	6	61	0	.1	0	1	.3	.1	.2	77	2.5	54	.5	138	453	534	.9
0	–	0	128	1	.1	0	0	–	.1	.2	23	1.8	60	.4	120	305	204	1
0	1	0	22	24	0	0	3	.1	0	0	18	.6	9	.1	13	74	171	.2
0	2	0	20	37	0	0	9	.2	.1	0	20	.6	14	.4	21	115	3	.1
0	2	0	6	36	0	0	6	.1	0	0	30	.6	14	.3	16	76	9	.4
0	–	0	63	0	.1	0	2	–	.1	.1	35	1.6	40	.6	134	329	444	.7
0	6	0	61	0	.1	0	0	.9	0	.1	25	2.2	47	.3	89	265	405	.8
0	–	0	14	15	.1	0	5	–	0	.1	25	1.8	50	.7	101	370	26	.5
0	7	0	82	0	.1	0	1	.5	.1	.2	62	2.4	62	.6	176	377	587	1
0	4	0	72	0	.1	0	1	–	.1	.1	44	1.9	32	.4	110	361	499	.8
0	7	0	106	0	.1	0	8	0	.1	.1	58	2.2	49	.6	106	497	536	1.7
0	1	0	22	7	0	0	3	.2	0	0	18	.6	9	.1	13	74	171	.2
0	1	0	20	6	0	0	9	0	.1	0	20	.6	14	.4	21	115	3	.1
0	–	0	8	24	0	.1	2	–	.1	0	20	1.1	5	.3	24	176	240	0
–	–	25	–	350	–	–	6	–	.2	.1	120	1.5	–	2.9	–	800	490	–
–	4	10	0	40	0	0	12	–	0	0	24	.4	0	0	0	–	760	0
2	–	30	–	250	–	–	24	–	.3	.3	120	1	–	1.9	260	600	450	–
0	0	96	14	0	.4	3.4	0	.1	.8	.1	9	4.7	43	7.8	323	508	2445	6.9
–	–	–	–	700	–	–	2	–	.4	.3	32	1.5	–	3.8	–	300	1130	–
–	–	–	–	250	–	–	–	–	.2	.2	16	1.5	–	2.9	–	–	730	–
1	–	20	–	100	–	–	11	.5	.3	.2	48	.9	28	2.5	–	359	920	1.1
2	–	65	–	700	–	–	42	–	.2	.2	16	1	–	2.9	190	520	360	–
–	–	45	–	320	–	–	2	.3	.1	0	16	.9	21	2.3	–	487	1140	2.4
–	–	–	–	40	–	–	1	–	.3	.1	48	1.5	–	2.9	–	300	1090	–
3	–	15	–	20	–	–	4	–	.2	.4	48	1.5	–	1.9	180	270	520	–
2	–	10	–	20	–	–	1	–	.2	.4	32	2	–	2.9	130	330	450	–
1	–	45	–	80	–	–	6	–	.3	.2	80	1	–	1.9	–	470	480	–
–	–	20	–	–	–	–	2	–	–	0	–	.2	–	.4	–	100	550	–
1	0	83	5	0	.2	1.4	14	.1	.1	0	7	1.6	10	2.6	106	123	964	3.9
0	0	29	6	0	.2	4.4	15	–	.2	.1	9	2.9	15	4.1	118	342	1124	3
1	0	79	6	0	.2	1.5	3	.2	.1	.1	8	1.6	15	4.3	128	194	1044	3.6
1	0	57	3	0	.1	1.6	10	–	.1	0	6	1.5	11	2.7	89	150	962	2.4
0	0	39	7	0	.3	1.5	18	.1	.1	.1	7	2.4	18	3.9	154	321	1070	3.3
0	0	35	9	0	.3	2.2	12	.1	.2	.1	9	2.3	16	4.5	143	365	1224	3.4
1	0	69	8	0	.2	1.7	0	.2	.2	.1	6	2	18	4	136	265	60	4.6
1	0	74	8	0	.2	2	0	.2	.2	0	9	1.8	18	4.4	134	256	65	4.6
1	0	71	8	0	.2	1.9	0	.2	.2	0	9	1.9	17	4.1	135	254	65	4.4
1	0	77	8	0	.2	2.5	0	.2	.2	0	9	2.1	17	4.9	145	248	71	4.4
1	0	76	8	0	.2	2.3	0	.2	.2	0	9	2.1	17	5	145	255	71	4.3
1	0	331	185	9017	.8	60.4	20	–	3.5	.2	6	5.8	17	9.1	344	200	60	5.2
1	0	410	187	9125	1.2	95.1	20	.5	3.5	.2	9	5.3	20	12.3	392	310	90	4.6
0	0	18	1	0	.1	1.1	4	.1	.1	0	3	.7	4	1	34	59	377	.7
1	0	77	6	0	.3	2	0	–	.2	.1	9	2.2	18	2.9	164	244	50	4.7
1	0	74	6	0	.3	2.1	0	.2	.2	.1	8	2.3	20	3.1	179	275	53	5.2
1	0	75	6	0	.3	2.1	0	.2	.2	.1	9	2.2	19	3.1	173	266	53	5
0	0	2	0	0	0	.1	1	0	0	0	0	.1	1	.2	7	18	60	.2
0	0	0	15	0	.1	0	0	0	.1	0	18	.1	18	1.4	42	64	11	.1

Code	Name	Amount	Unit	Grams	Energy (kcal)	Carbohydrates (g)	Protein (g)	Fat (g)	Saturated fat (g)	Monounsat fat (g)
14003	Beer, Regular	12	Fl Oz	356.4	146	13	1	0	0	0
11081	Beets, Ckd	½	Cup	85.0	37	8	1	0	0	0
18009	Biscuits, Plain or Buttermilk	1	Each	35.0	127	17	2	6	1	2
14008	Bloody Mary	1	Fl Oz	29.7	23	1	0	0	0	0
9052	Blueberries, Cnd, Heavy Syrup	½	Cup	128.0	113	28	1	0	–	–
9050	Blueberries, Fresh	½	Cup	72.5	41	10	0	0	–	–
9055	Blueberries, Frozen, Sweetened	½	Cup	115.0	93	25	0	0	–	–
9054	Blueberries, Frozen, Unsweetened	½	Cup	77.5	40	9	0	0	–	–
41241	Blueberry Muffin–Healthy Choice	1	Each	70.9	190	39	3	4	–	–
18305	Blueberry Pie	1	Slice	125.0	290	44	2	13	2	7
15189	Bluefish, Ckd, Dry Heat	3	Ounce	85.1	135	0	22	5	1	2
10126	Bologna	1	Slice	23.0	57	0	4	5	2	2
7007	Bologna, Beef	1	Slice	28.4	88	0	3	8	3	4
41286	Boneless Beef Ribs w/Barbecue Sauce–Healthy Choice	1	Each	311.8	330	40	28	6	2	–
12078	Brazil Nuts, Dried, Unblanched	½	Cup	70.0	459	9	10	46	11	16
19167	Bread Pudding	1	Cup	252.0	423	62	13	15	6	5
18080	Bread Sticks, Plain	1	Stick	10.0	41	7	1	1	0	0
18083	Bread Stuffing, Plain	1	Cup	232.0	390	52	9	17	3	7
18020	Bread, Banana	1	Slice	60.0	203	33	3	7	2	3
18024	Bread, Cornbread	1	Piece	65.0	173	28	4	5	1	1
18025	Bread, Cracked–wheat	1	Slice	25.0	65	12	2	1	0	0
18344	Bread, Dinner Roll, Egg	1	Each	35.0	107	18	3	2	1	1
18349	Bread, Dinner Roll, French	1	Each	38.0	105	19	3	2	0	1
18345	Bread, Dinner Roll, Oat Bran	1	Each	33.0	78	13	3	2	0	0
18342	Bread, Dinner Roll, Plain	1	Each	35.0	105	18	3	3	1	1
18346	Bread, Dinner Roll, Rye	1	Each	35.0	100	19	4	1	0	0
18347	Bread, Dinner Roll, Wheat	1	Each	33.0	90	15	3	2	1	1
18348	Bread, Dinner Roll, Whole–wheat	1	Each	33.0	88	17	3	2	0	0
18027	Bread, Egg	1	Slice	40.0	115	19	4	2	1	1
18028	Bread, Egg, Toasted	1	Slice	37.0	117	19	4	2	1	1
18029	Bread, French or Vienna	1	Slice	25.0	69	13	2	1	0	0
18033	Bread, Italian	1	Slice	30.0	81	15	3	1	0	0
18049	Bread, Lo Cal, Oat Bran	1	Slice	23.0	46	9	2	1	0	0
18051	Bread, Lo Cal, Oatmeal	1	Slice	23.0	48	10	2	1	0	0
18053	Bread, Lo Cal, Rye	1	Slice	23.0	47	9	2	1	0	0
18055	Bread, Lo Cal, Wheat	1	Slice	23.0	46	10	2	1	0	0
18057	Bread, Lo Cal, White	1	Slice	23.0	48	10	2	1	0	0
18035	Bread, Mixed–grain	1	Slice	26.0	65	12	3	1	0	0
18037	Bread, Oat Bran	1	Slice	30.0	71	12	3	1	0	0
18039	Bread, Oatmeal	1	Slice	27.0	73	13	2	1	0	0
18041	Bread, Pita, White, Enriched	1	Pita	60.0	165	33	5	1	0	0
18042	Bread, Pita, Whole–wheat	1	Pita	64.0	170	35	6	2	0	0
18044	Bread, Pumpernickel	1	Slice	32.0	80	15	3	1	0	0
18046	Bread, Pumpkin	1	Slice	60.0	199	31	2	8	1	2
18047	Bread, Raisin	1	Slice	26.0	71	14	2	1	0	1
18059	Bread, Rice Bran	1	Slice	27.0	66	12	2	1	0	0
18384	Bread, Rice Bran, Toasted	1	Slice	25.0	66	12	2	1	0	0
18353	Bread, Rolls, Hard (includes Kaiser)	1	Each	57.0	167	30	6	2	0	1
18060	Bread, Rye	1	Slice	32.0	83	15	3	1	0	0
18061	Bread, Rye, Toasted	1	Slice	29.0	82	15	3	1	0	0
18064	Bread, Wheat (includes Wheat Berry)	1	Slice	25.0	65	12	2	1	0	0
18066	Bread, Wheat Bran	1	Slice	36.0	89	17	3	1	0	1
18065	Bread, Wheat, Toasted	1	Slice	23.0	65	12	2	1	0	0
18069	Bread, White	1	Slice	25.0	67	12	2	1	0	0
18075	Bread, Whole Wheat	1	Slice	25.0	62	12	2	1	0	0
41348	Breaded Fish–Healthy Choice	1	Stick	9.8	15	2	1	1	–	–

Polyunsaturated fat (g)	Dietary Fiber (g)	Cholesterol (mg)	Folate (µg)	Vitamin A (RE)	Vitamin B-6 (mg)	Vitamin B-12 (µg)	Vitamin C (mg)	Vitamin E (mg)	Riboflavin (mg)	Thiamin (mg)	Calcium (mg)	Iron (mg)	Magnesium (mg)	Niacin (mg)	Phosphorus (mg)	Potassium (mg)	Sodium (mg)	Zinc (mg)
0	1	0	21	0	.2	.1	0	0	.1	0	18	.1	21	1.6	43	89	18	.1
0	1	0	68	3	.1	0	3	.3	0	0	14	.7	20	.3	32	259	65	.3
2	–	0	2	0	0	0	0	–	.1	.1	17	1.2	6	1.2	151	78	368	.2
0	–	0	4	10	0	0	4	–	0	0	2	.1	2	.1	4	43	67	0
–	2	0	2	8	0	0	1	1.3	.1	0	6	.4	5	.1	13	51	4	.1
–	2	0	5	7	0	0	9	.7	0	0	4	.1	4	.3	7	65	4	.1
–	2	0	8	5	.1	0	1	.8	.1	0	7	.4	2	.3	8	69	1	.1
–	2	0	5	6	0	0	2	.8	0	0	6	.1	4	.4	9	42	1	.1
2	–	0	–	–	–	–	4	–	.2	.2	80	.8	–	.8	160	200	110	–
2	–	0	5	43	0	0	3	–	0	0	10	.4	6	.4	26	63	406	.2
1	0	65	2	117	.4	5.3	0	–	.1	.1	8	.5	36	6.2	247	406	65	.9
0	0	14	1	0	.1	.2	8	.1	0	.1	3	.2	3	.9	32	65	272	.5
0	0	16	1	0	0	.4	6	.1	0	0	3	.5	3	.7	25	45	278	.6
2	–	70	–	60	–	–	5	–	.3	.2	48	1	–	2.9	220	670	530	–
17	4	0	3	0	.2	0	0	5.3	.1	.7	123	2.4	158	1.1	420	420	1	3.2
2	–	166	33	164	.2	–	2	–	.6	.2	287	2.8	48	1.6	275	564	582	1.3
0	–	0	3	0	0	0	0	–	.1	.1	2	.4	3	.5	12	12	66	.1
5	–	0	39	160	.1	0	4	–	.3	.4	148	3.8	35	3.7	114	304	1070	.7
2	–	26	7	14	.1	.1	1	–	.1	.1	11	.8	8	.9	34	79	119	.2
2	–	26	12	35	.1	.1	0	–	.2	.2	162	1.6	16	1.5	110	96	428	.4
0	1	0	10	0	.1	0	0	–	.1	.1	11	.7	13	.9	38	44	135	.3
0	1	18	19	8	0	.1	0	–	.2	.2	21	1.2	9	1.2	35	37	191	.3
0	–	0	13	0	0	0	0	–	.1	.2	35	1	8	1.7	32	43	231	.3
1	1	0	10	0	0	0	0	–	.1	.1	28	1.4	10	1.6	34	36	136	.3
0	1	0	11	0	0	0	0	–	.1	.2	42	1.1	8	1.4	41	47	182	.3
0	–	0	8	0	0	0	0	–	.1	.1	11	.9	19	1.4	56	63	312	.4
0	–	0	5	0	0	0	0	–	.1	.1	58	1.2	14	1.3	39	44	112	.3
1	–	0	10	0	.1	0	0	–	.1	.1	35	.8	28	1.2	74	90	158	.7
0	–	20	28	9	0	0	0	–	.2	.2	37	1.2	8	1.9	42	46	197	.3
0	–	21	20	9	0	0	0	–	.2	.1	38	1.2	8	1.8	43	47	200	.3
0	1	0	8	0	0	0	0	–	.1	.1	19	.6	7	1.2	26	28	152	.2
0	1	0	9	0	0	0	0	–	.1	.1	23	.9	8	1.3	31	33	175	.3
0	–	0	8	0	0	0	0	–	0	.1	13	.7	11	.9	28	23	81	.2
0	–	0	8	0	0	–	0	–	.1	.1	26	.5	7	.7	27	35	89	.2
0	–	0	5	0	0	0	0	–	.1	.1	17	.7	4	.6	19	23	93	.2
0	3	0	6	–	0	0	0	–	.1	.1	18	.7	6	.9	–	29	118	.2
0	2	0	8	–	0	.1	0	–	.1	.1	22	.7	6	.8	31	17	104	.3
0	2	0	12	0	.1	0	0	–	.1	.1	24	.9	14	1.1	46	53	127	.3
1	1	0	8	0	0	0	0	–	.1	.2	20	.9	9	1.4	32	34	122	.3
0	1	0	7	1	0	–	0	–	.1	.1	18	.7	10	.8	34	38	162	.3
0	1	0	14	0	0	0	0	–	.2	.4	52	1.6	16	2.8	58	72	322	.5
1	5	0	22	0	.1	0	0	–	.1	.2	10	1.8	44	1.8	115	109	340	1
0	2	0	11	0	0	0	0	–	.1	.1	22	.9	17	1	57	67	215	.5
4	–	26	7	334	0	0	1	–	.1	.1	11	1	8	.8	32	55	188	.2
0	1	0	9	0	0	0	0	–	.1	.1	17	.8	7	.9	28	59	101	.2
0	–	0	8	–	.1	0	0	–	.1	.2	19	1	19	1.8	43	53	119	.3
0	–	0	6	0	.1	0	0	–	.1	.1	19	1	19	1.7	44	53	120	.3
1	–	0	9	0	0	0	0	–	.2	.3	54	1.9	15	2.4	57	62	310	.5
0	2	0	16	0	0	0	–	–	.1	.1	23	.9	13	1.2	40	53	211	.4
0	–	0	11	–	0	0	0	–	.1	.1	23	.9	12	1.1	40	53	210	.4
0	1	0	10	0	0	0	0	–	.1	.1	26	.8	12	1	38	50	133	.3
0	3	0	9	0	.1	0	0	–	.1	.1	27	1.1	29	1.6	67	82	175	.5
0	–	0	7	0	0	0	0	–	.1	.1	26	.8	12	.9	37	50	132	.3
0	1	0	9	0	0	–	0	–	.1	.1	27	.8	6	1	24	30	135	.2
0	2	0	13	0	0	0	0	–	.1	.1	18	.8	22	1	57	63	132	.5
0	–	3	–	–	–	–	–	–	0	0	–	.1	–	.1	–	20	31	–

Code	Name	Amount	Unit	Grams	Energy (kcal)	Carbohydrates (g)	Protein (g)	Fat (g)	Saturated fat (g)	Monounsat… fat (g)
43400	Breast of Chicken w/Spanish Rice, Top Shelf–Hormel	1	Each	283.5	400	38	27	15	7	4
41252	Breast of Turkey–Healthy Choice	1	Each	297.7	290	39	21	5	2	–
62616	Broccoli and Cheese Baked Potato–Weight Watchers	1	Each	283.5	230	34	12	7	2	–
11091	Broccoli, Ckd	½	Cup	78.0	22	4	2	0	0	0
11740	Broccoli, Flower Clusters, Fresh	½	Cup	44.0	12	2	1	0	0	0
11093	Broccoli, Frz, Chopped, Ckd	½	Cup	92.0	26	5	3	0	0	0
18151	Brownies	1	Each	56.0	227	36	3	9	2	5
11099	Brussels Sprouts, Ckd	½	Cup	78.0	30	7	2	0	0	0
62601	Buffalo (Chicken) Wings	4	Each	91.0	190	2	18	12	3	–
18351	Buns, Hamburger or Hot Dog, Mixed–grain	1	Each	43.0	113	19	4	3	1	1
18350	Buns, Hamburger or Hot Dog, Plain	1	Each	43.0	123	22	4	2	1	1
18155	Butter Cookies	1	Each	5.0	23	3	0	1	1	0
1002	Butter, Whipped	1	Tbsp.	11.0	79	0	0	9	6	3
4136	Butter, w/Salt	1	Pat	5.0	36	0	0	4	3	1
1145	Butter, w/o Salt	1	Pat	5.0	36	0	0	4	3	1
19069	Butterfinger Bar	1	Bar	61.0	267	41	5	11	5	4
19070	Butterscotch Candy	1	Piece	6.0	24	6	0	0	0	0
18307	Butterscotch Pudding Pie	1	Slice	127.0	354	42	6	18	5	8
11110	Cabbage, Ckd	½	Cup	75.0	17	3	1	0	0	0
11749	Cabbage, Fresh	1	Cup	70.0	17	4	1	0	0	0
18086	Cake, Angel Food	1	Slice	28.4	73	16	2	0	0	0
18090	Cake, Boston Cream Pie	1	Slice	92.0	232	39	2	8	2	4
18094	Cake, Carrot, w/Cream Cheese Frosting	1	Slice	111.0	484	52	5	29	5	7
18096	Cake, Chocolate w/Chocolate Frosting	1	Slice	64.0	235	35	3	10	3	6
18110	Cake, Fruitcake	1	Piece	43.0	139	26	1	4	0	2
18113	Cake, German Chocolate, w/Frosting	1	Slice	111.0	404	55	4	21	5	9
18115	Cake, Gingerbread	1	Slice	67.0	207	34	3	7	2	4
18119	Cake, Pineapple Upside–down	1	Slice	115.0	367	58	4	14	3	6
18120	Cake, Pound	1	Slice	28.4	110	14	2	6	3	2
18133	Cake, Sponge	1	Slice	38.0	110	23	2	1	0	0
18102	Cake, White, w/Coconut Frosting	1	Slice	112.0	399	71	5	12	4	4
18139	Cake, White, w/o Frosting	1	Slice	74.0	264	42	4	9	2	4
18140	Cake, Yellow, w/Chocolate Frosting	1	Slice	64.0	243	35	2	11	3	6
18141	Cake, Yellow, w/Vanilla Frosting	1	Slice	64.0	239	38	2	9	2	4
55177	Canadian Style Bacon, French Bread Pizzas–Stouffer's	1	Each	163.0	370	40	18	15	–	–
62633	Candy, Candy Corn	26	Each	39.0	140	36	–	–	–	–
19074	Caramels	1	Piece	8.0	31	6	0	1	1	0
11655	Carrot Juice, Cnd	¾	Cup	184.5	74	17	2	0	0	0
11960	Carrots, Baby, Fresh	1	Medium	10.0	4	1	0	0	0	0
11125	Carrots, Ckd	½	Cup	78.0	35	8	1	0	0	0
11128	Carrots, Cnd, Reg Pk	½	Cup	73.0	17	4	0	0	0	0
11124	Carrots, Fresh	1	Medium	60.0	26	6	1	0	0	0
11131	Carrots, Frz, Ckd	½	Cup	73.0	26	6	1	0	0	0
12586	Cashew Oil Roasted	½	Cup	65.0	374	19	10	31	6	18
12585	Cashews, Dry Roasted	½	Cup	68.5	393	22	10	32	6	19
15235	Catfish, Channel, Farmed, Ckd, Dry Heat	3	Ounce	85.1	129	0	16	7	2	4
15233	Catfish, Channel, Wild, Ckd, Dry Heat	3	Ounce	85.1	89	0	16	2	1	1
15011	Catfish, Fried	3	Ounce	85.1	195	7	15	11	3	5
11935	Catsup	1	Tbsp.	15.0	16	4	0	0	0	0
11949	Catsup, Low Sodium	1	Tbsp.	15.0	16	4	0	0	0	0
11136	Cauliflower, Ckd, Boiled	½	Cup	62.0	14	3	1	0	0	0
11135	Cauliflower, Fresh	½	Cup	50.0	13	3	1	0	0	0
11138	Cauliflower, Frz, Ckd	½	Cup	90.0	17	3	1	0	0	0
15012	Caviar, Black and Red, Granular	1	Tbsp.	16.0	40	1	4	3	1	1
11144	Celery, Ckd	½	Cup	75.0	14	3	1	0	0	0
11143	Celery, Fresh	½	Cup	60.0	10	2	0	0	0	0

Polyunsaturated fat (g)	Dietary Fiber (g)	Cholesterol (mg)	Folate (µg)	Vitamin A (RE)	Vitamin B-6 (mg)	Vitamin B-12 (µg)	Vitamin C (mg)	Vitamin E (mg)	Riboflavin (mg)	Thiamin (mg)	Calcium (mg)	Iron (mg)	Magnesium (mg)	Niacin (mg)	Phosphorus (mg)	Potassium (mg)	Sodium (mg)	Zinc (mg)
3	–	75	–	100	–	–	4	.1	.3	.1	80	.4	35	7.6	–	584	810	1.7
–	–	45	–	40	–	–	48	–	.3	.5	32	1	–	5.7	270	540	420	–
–	6	10	–	200	–	–	9	–	–	–	300	.8	–	–	–	830	510	–
0	2	0	39	108	.1	0	58	.4	.1	0	36	.7	19	.4	46	228	20	.3
0	–	0	31	132	.1	0	41	–	.1	0	21	.4	11	.3	29	143	12	.2
0	3	0	52	174	.1	0	37	.4	.1	.1	47	.6	18	.4	51	166	22	.3
1	1	10	7	11	0	.1	0	–	.1	.1	16	1.3	17	1	57	83	175	.4
0	3	0	47	56	.1	0	48	.7	.1	.1	28	.9	16	.5	44	247	16	.3
–	–	100	–	60	–	–	1	–	–	–	24	.4	–	–	–	–	900	–
0	2	0	12	0	0	0	0	–	.1	.2	41	1.7	21	1.9	52	65	197	.5
0	–	0	12	0	0	0	0	–	.1	.2	60	1.4	9	1.7	38	61	241	.3
0	0	4	0	8	0	0	0	–	0	0	1	.1	1	.2	5	6	18	0
0	0	24	0	83	0	0	0	.2	0	0	3	0	0	0	3	3	91	0
0	0	11	0	38	0	0	0	.1	0	0	1	0	0	0	1	1	41	0
0	0	11	0	38	0	0	0	.1	0	0	1	0	0	0	1	1	1	0
2	2	1	19	12	0	.1	2	.8	0	.1	15	.6	27	2	58	129	83	.4
0	0	1	0	2	0	0	0	0	0	0	0	0	0	0	0	0	3	0
4	–	77	14	107	.1	.4	1	–	.3	.2	128	1.6	22	1.3	135	221	335	.7
0	2	0	15	10	.1	0	15	.1	0	0	23	.1	6	.2	11	73	6	.1
0	–	0	40	9	.1	0	36	–	0	0	33	.4	11	.2	16	172	13	.1
0	0	0	1	0	0	–	0	–	.1	0	40	.1	3	.3	66	26	212	0
1	1	34	7	21	0	.1	0	–	.2	.4	21	.3	6	.2	45	36	132	.1
15	–	60	13	426	.1	.1	1	–	.2	.2	28	1.4	20	1.1	79	124	273	.5
1	2	29	5	18	–	.1	0	–	.1	0	28	1.4	22	.4	78	128	214	.4
1	2	2	1	8	0	0	0	–	0	0	14	.9	7	.3	22	66	116	.1
5	–	53	4	23	0	.1	0	–	.1	.1	53	1.2	19	1.1	173	151	369	.5
1	2	23	7	11	0	0	0	–	.1	.1	46	2.2	11	1	113	161	307	.3
4	–	25	8	75	0	.1	1	–	.2	.2	138	1.7	15	1.4	94	129	367	.4
0	–	63	3	44	0	.1	0	–	.1	0	10	.4	3	.4	39	34	113	.1
0	–	39	5	17	0	.1	0	–	.1	.1	27	1	4	.7	52	38	93	.2
2	–	1	6	12	0	.1	0	–	.2	.1	101	1.3	13	1.2	78	111	318	.4
2	–	1	5	12	0	.1	0	–	.2	.1	96	1.1	9	1.1	69	70	242	.2
1	1	35	5	17	0	.1	0	–	.1	.1	24	1.3	19	.8	103	114	216	.4
3	–	36	6	12	0	.1	0	–	0	.1	40	.7	4	.3	92	34	220	.2
–	–	–	–	80	–	–	6	–	.4	.6	160	1	–	3.8	–	300	1070	–
–	–	–	–	0	–	–	0	–	–	–	0	0	–	–	–	–	80	–
0	0	1	0	1	0	0	0	0	0	0	11	0	1	0	9	17	20	0
0	1	0	7	4751	.4	0	16	0	.1	.2	44	.8	26	.7	77	539	54	.3
0	–	0	3	20	0	0	1	–	0	0	2	.1	1	.1	4	28	4	0
0	3	0	11	1915	.2	0	2	.3	0	0	24	.5	10	.4	23	177	51	.2
0	1	0	7	1005	.1	0	2	–	0	0	18	.5	6	.4	18	131	176	.2
0	2	0	8	1688	.1	0	6	.3	0	.1	16	.3	9	.6	26	194	21	.1
0	3	0	8	1292	.1	0	2	.3	0	0	20	.3	7	.3	19	115	43	.2
5	2	0	44	0	.2	0	0	1	.1	.3	27	2.7	166	1.2	277	345	407	3.1
5	2	0	47	0	.2	0	0	.4	.1	.1	31	4.1	178	1	336	387	438	3.8
1	0	54	6	13	.1	2.4	1	–	.1	.4	8	.7	22	2.1	208	273	68	.9
1	0	61	9	13	.1	2.5	1	–	.1	.2	9	.3	24	2	259	356	43	.5
3	–	69	14	7	.2	1.6	0	–	.1	.1	37	1.2	23	1.9	184	289	238	.7
0	0	0	2	15	0	0	2	.2	0	0	3	.1	3	.2	6	72	178	0
0	0	0	2	15	0	0	2	.2	0	0	3	.1	3	.2	6	72	3	0
0	2	0	27	1	.1	0	27	0	0	0	10	.2	6	.3	20	88	9	.1
0	1	0	29	1	.1	0	23	0	0	0	11	.2	8	.3	22	152	15	.1
0	2	0	37	2	.1	0	28	0	0	0	15	.4	8	.3	22	125	16	.1
1	0	94	8	90	.1	3.2	0	1.1	.1	0	44	1.9	48	0	57	29	240	.2
0	1	0	17	10	.1	0	5	.3	0	0	32	.3	9	.2	19	213	68	.1
0	1	0	17	8	.1	0	4	.2	0	0	24	.2	7	.2	15	172	52	.1

Code	Name	Amount	Unit	Grams	Energy (kcal)	Carbohydrates (g)	Protein (g)	Fat (g)	Saturated fat (g)	Monounsaturated fat (g)
8053	Cereals, 100% Bran	1	Cup	66.0	178	48	8	3	1	1
8054	Cereals, 100% Natural Cereal, Plain	1	Cup	104.0	489	65	12	22	15	4
8055	Cereals, 100% Natural Cereal, w/Apple and Cinn.	1	Cup	104.0	477	70	11	20	15	2
8056	Cereals, 100% Natural Cereal, w/Raisins and Dates	1	Cup	110.0	496	72	11	20	14	4
8028	Cereals, 40% Bran Flakes, Kellogg's	1	Cup	39.0	127	31	5	1	–	–
8029	Cereals, 40% Bran Flakes, Post	1	Cup	47.0	152	37	5	1	–	–
8153	Cereals, 40% Bran Flakes, Ralston Purina	1	Cup	49.0	159	39	6	1	–	–
8001	Cereals, All–bran	1	Cup	85.2	212	63	12	2	–	–
8006	Cereals, Bran Chex	1	Cup	49.0	156	39	5	1	–	–
8008	Cereals, C.W. Post, Plain	1	Cup	97.0	432	69	9	15	11	2
8009	Cereals, C.W. Post, w/Raisins	1	Cup	103.0	446	74	9	15	11	2
8010	Cereals, Cap'n Crunch	1	Cup	37.0	156	30	2	3	2	0
8011	Cereals, Cap'n Crunch's Crunchberries	1	Cup	35.0	146	29	2	3	2	0
8012	Cereals, Cap'n Crunch's Peanut Butter	1	Cup	35.0	154	26	3	5	2	1
8013	Cereals, Cheerios	1	Cup	22.7	89	16	3	1	0	1
8014	Cereals, Cocoa Krispies	1	Cup	36.0	139	32	2	1	–	–
8017	Cereals, Cookie–crisp, Choc Chip and Van.	1	Cup	30.0	120	26	2	1	–	–
8018	Cereals, Corn Bran	1	Cup	36.0	125	30	2	1	–	–
8019	Cereals, Corn Chex	1	Cup	28.4	111	25	2	0	–	–
8020	Cereals, Corn Flakes, Kellogg's	1	Cup	22.7	88	20	2	0	–	–
8022	Cereals, Corn Flakes, Low Sodium	1	Cup	25.0	100	22	2	0	–	–
8021	Cereals, Corn Flakes, Ralston Purina	1	Cup	25.0	98	22	2	0	–	–
8023	Cereals, Cracklin' Bran	1	Cup	60.0	229	41	6	9	–	–
8168	Cereals, Cream Of Rice, Ckd	1	Cup	244.0	127	28	2	0	–	–
8171	Cereals, Cream Of Wheat, Instant	1	Cup	241.0	154	32	4	0	–	–
8170	Cereals, Cream Of Wheat, Quick	1	Cup	239.0	129	27	4	0	–	–
8169	Cereals, Cream Of Wheat, Regular	1	Cup	251.0	133	28	4	1	–	–
8024	Cereals, Crisp Rice, Low Sodium	1	Cup	26.0	105	24	1	0	–	–
62634	Cereals, Crispex	1	Cup	30.0	110	26	2	0	0	–
8025	Cereals, Crispy Rice	1	Cup	28.0	111	25	2	0	–	–
8026	Cereals, Crispy Wheats 'n Raisins	1	Cup	43.0	150	35	3	1	–	–
8027	Cereals, Fortified Oat Flakes	1	Cup	48.0	177	35	9	1	–	–
62637	Cereals, Frosted Mini–Wheats	1	Cup	52.0	190	45	–	1	0	–
8030	Cereals, Fruit Loops	1	Cup	28.4	111	25	2	1	–	–
8035	Cereals, Golden Grahams	1	Cup	39.0	150	33	2	1	1	0
8036	Cereals, Graham Crackos	1	Cup	30.0	108	26	2	0	–	–
8037	Cereals, Granola, Homemade	1	Cup	122.0	594	67	15	33	6	9
8038	Cereals, Grape–nuts	1	Cup	113.6	406	93	13	0	–	–
8039	Cereals, Grape–nuts Flakes	1	Cup	32.5	116	27	3	0	–	–
62639	Cereals, Great Grains	1	Cup	79.5	330	57	7	9	1	–
8040	Cereals, Heartland Natural Cereal, Plain	1	Cup	115.0	499	79	12	18	–	–
8041	Cereals, Heartland Natural Cereal, w/Cocnt	1	Cup	105.0	463	71	11	17	–	–
8042	Cereals, Heartland Natural Cereal, w/Raisins	1	Cup	110.0	468	76	11	16	–	–
8045	Cereals, Honey Nut Cheerios	1	Cup	33.0	125	26	4	1	0	0
8043	Cereals, Honey and Nut Corn Flakes	1	Cup	37.9	151	31	2	2	–	–
8044	Cereals, Honeybran	1	Cup	35.0	119	29	3	1	–	–
8046	Cereals, Honeycomb	1	Cup	22.0	86	20	1	0	–	–
62641	Cereals, Just Right	1	Cup	55.0	200	46	4	2	0	–
62642	Cereals, Kellogg's Low–Fat Granola	1	Cup	82.5	315	64	7	4	1	–
8048	Cereals, Kix	1	Cup	18.9	74	16	2	0	0	0
8049	Cereals, Life, Plain and Cinn Products	1	Cup	44.0	162	32	8	1	–	–
8050	Cereals, Lucky Charms	1	Cup	32.0	125	26	3	1	0	0
8178	Cereals, Malt–o–meal, Plain and Choc	1	Cup	240.0	122	26	4	0	–	–
8179	Cereals, Maypo, Ckd w/water, w/Salt	1	Cup	240.0	170	32	6	2	–	–
8119	Cereals, Maypo, Ckd w/water, w/o Salt	1	Cup	240.0	170	32	6	2	–	–
8052	Cereals, Nature Valley Granola	1	Cup	113.0	503	75	12	20	13	3

Polyunsaturated fat (g)	Dietary Fiber (g)	Cholesterol (mg)	Folate (µg)	Vitamin A (RE)	Vitamin B-6 (mg)	Vitamin B-12 (µg)	Vitamin C (mg)	Vitamin E (mg)	Riboflavin (mg)	Thiamin (mg)	Calcium (mg)	Iron (mg)	Magnesium (mg)	Niacin (mg)	Phosphorus (mg)	Potassium (mg)	Sodium (mg)	Zinc (mg)
2	20	0	47	0	2.1	6.3	63	1.5	1.8	1.6	46	8.1	312	20.9	801	824	457	5.7
2	9	1	31	–	.2	.1	0	.7	.6	.3	181	3.1	125	2.4	383	514	45	2.4
1	7	1	17	–	.1	.3	1	.7	.6	.3	157	2.9	72	1.9	350	514	52	2
2	7	1	45	–	.2	.1	0	.8	.6	.3	160	3.1	124	2.1	348	538	47	2.1
–	5	0	138	516	.7	2.1	0	.4	.6	.5	19	24.8	71	6.9	192	248	303	5.1
–	9	0	166	622	.8	2.5	0	.5	.7	.6	21	7.5	102	8.3	296	251	431	2.5
–	7	0	173	649	.9	2.6	26	.6	.7	.6	23	7.8	118	8.6	273	286	456	2
–	30	0	301	1128	1.5	0	45	2	1.3	1.1	69	13.5	318	15	794	1051	961	11.2
–	8	0	173	11	.9	2.6	26	.6	.3	.6	29	7.8	126	8.6	327	394	455	2.1
1	7	0	342	1284	1.7	5.1	0	.7	1.5	1.3	47	15.4	67	17.1	224	198	167	1.6
1	14	0	364	1364	1.9	5.5	0	.7	1.5	1.3	50	16.4	74	18.1	232	261	161	1.6
1	1	0	238	5	1	2.3	0	.1	.7	.7	6	9.8	15	8.6	47	48	278	4
0	1	0	128	5	.9	2.5	0	.1	.7	.6	11	9	14	8.1	47	49	244	3.6
1	0	0	244	6	1	2.3	0	.1	.7	.6	7	9.1	19	9	49	57	268	3.8
1	2	0	5	301	.4	1.2	12	.2	.3	.3	39	3.6	31	4	107	81	246	.6
–	0	0	127	477	.6	0	19	0	.5	.5	6	2.3	12	6.3	47	53	275	1.9
–	0	0	3	397	.5	1.6	16	.1	.4	.4	6	4.8	8	5.3	24	29	207	.3
–	7	0	232	8	.9	1.4	0	.8	.7	.4	41	12.2	18	10.9	52	70	310	4
–	1	0	100	14	.5	1.5	15	.1	.1	.4	3	1.8	4	5	11	23	272	.1
–	1	0	80	301	.4	0	12	.1	.3	.3	1	1.4	3	4	14	21	232	.1
–	0	0	2	10	0	0	0	0	0	0	11	.6	3	.1	12	18	3	.1
–	0	0	2	10	0	0	0	.1	0	.1	2	.6	3	1.1	10	22	239	.1
–	10	0	212	794	1.1	0	32	.7	.9	.8	40	3.8	116	10.6	241	355	487	3.2
–	–	0	7	0	.1	0	0	–	0	0	7	.5	7	1	41	49	422	.4
–	–	0	10	0	0	0	0	–	0	.2	60	12.1	14	1.7	43	48	364	.4
–	–	0	10	0	0	0	0	–	0	.2	50	10.3	12	1.4	100	45	464	.3
–	–	0	10	0	0	0	0	–	0	.3	50	10.3	10	1.5	43	43	336	.3
–	–	0	3	0	0	0	0	–	0	0	17	.8	10	.4	27	20	3	.4
–	1	0	50	150	.5	.5	15	–	.4	.4	0	1	0	4.8	16	–	230	1.5
–	0	0	3	0	0	.1	1	0	0	.1	5	.7	12	2	31	27	206	.5
–	3	0	15	569	.8	2.3	0	11.4	.6	.6	71	6.8	34	7.6	117	174	204	.5
–	1	0	169	636	.9	2.5	0	.3	.7	.6	68	13.7	58	8.4	176	343	429	1.5
–	5	0	50	0	.5	.5	0	–	.4	.4	24	1	35	4.8	120	180	10	1.5
–	1	0	100	376	.5	0	15	.1	.4	.4	3	4.5	7	5	24	26	145	3.7
0	1	0	6	516	.7	2.1	21	.1	.6	.5	24	6.2	16	6.9	56	86	385	.3
–	2	0	106	397	.5	0	16	0	.4	.4	14	1.9	25	5.3	66	108	196	1.6
17	13	0	99	–	.4	0	1	5.7	.3	.7	76	4.8	142	2.1	494	612	12	4.5
–	11	0	401	1504	2	6	0	.3	1.7	1.5	11	4.9	76	20	285	379	790	2.5
–	3	0	115	430	.6	1.7	0	.1	.5	.4	13	9.3	36	5.7	97	113	183	.6
–	6	0	75	375	.7	.7	0	–	.6	.6	36	2.2	52	7.1	180	180	225	1.8
–	7	0	64	–	.2	0	1	.8	.2	.4	75	4.3	147	1.6	416	385	293	3
–	7	0	57	–	.2	0	1	.7	.1	.3	66	5.4	138	1.8	380	384	213	2.7
	6	0	44	–	.2	0	1	.8	.1	.3	66	4	141	1.5	376	415	226	2.8
0	1	0	21	437	.6	1.7	17	.2	.5	.4	23	5.2	39	5.8	122	115	299	.9
–	0	0	134	501	.7	0	20	.1	.6	.5	5	2.4	8	6.7	17	48	301	.1
–	4	0	23	463	.6	1.9	19	.8	.5	.5	16	5.6	46	6.2	132	151	202	.9
–	1	0	78	291	.4	1.2	0	.1	.3	.3	4	2.1	7	3.9	22	70	124	1.2
–	3	0	50	250	.5	.5	0	–	.4	.4	0	9	28	4.8	80	–	250	.6
–	4	0	75	225	.7	.7	0	–	.6	.6	36	1.5	52	7.1	180	255	202	5.6
0	0	0	67	251	.3	1	10	0	.3	.2	24	5.4	8	3.3	26	30	194	.2
–	3	0	37	–	.1	0	–	.3	1	1	154	11.6	14	11.6	238	197	229	1.5
0	1	0	6	424	.6	1.7	17	.2	.5	.4	36	5.1	27	5.6	89	66	227	.6
–	–	0	5	0	0	0	0	–	.2	.5	5	9.6	5	5.8	24	31	324	.2
–	–	0	10	703	1	2.9	29	–	.7	.7	125	8.4	50	9.4	247	211	259	1.5
–	6	0	10	703	1	2.9	29	1.7	.7	.7	125	8.4	50	9.4	247	211	10	1.5
3	6	0	85	–	.1	0	0	3.4	.2	.4	71	3.8	115	.8	354	389	233	2.2

Code	Name	Amount	Unit	Grams	Energy (kcal)	Carbohydrates (g)	Protein (g)	Fat (g)	Saturated fat (g)	Monounsatu... fat (g)
8149	Cereals, Nutri–grain, Barley	1	Cup	41.0	153	34	4	0	–	–
8150	Cereals, Nutri–grain, Corn	1	Cup	42.0	160	35	3	1	–	–
8151	Cereals, Nutri–grain, Rye	1	Cup	40.0	144	34	3	0	–	–
8152	Cereals, Nutri–grain, Wheat	1	Cup	44.0	158	37	4	0	–	–
8123	Cereals, Oats, Instant, Plain	1	Pkt.	177.0	104	18	4	2	–	–
8125	Cereals, Oats, Instant, w/Apples and cinn	1	Pkt.	149.0	136	26	4	2	–	–
8127	Cereals, Oats, Instant, w/bran&rsns	1	Pkt.	195.0	158	30	5	2	–	–
8129	Cereals, Oats, Instant, w/cinn and spice	1	Pkt.	161.0	177	35	5	2	–	–
8131	Cereals, Oats, Instant, w/mapl&brn sug flav	1	Pkt.	155.0	163	32	5	2	–	–
8133	Cereals, Oats, Instant, w/raisins and spice	1	Pkt	158.0	161	32	4	2	–	–
8180	Cereals, Oats, Reg and Quick and Instant	1	Cup	234.0	145	25	6	2	0	1
8058	Cereals, Product 19	1	Cup	33.0	126	27	3	0	–	–
8059	Cereals, Quisp	1	Cup	30.0	124	25	2	2	1	0
8060	Cereals, Raisin Bran, Kellogg's	1	Cup	49.2	154	37	5	1	–	–
8061	Cereals, Raisin Bran, Post	1	Cup	56.8	174	43	5	1	–	–
8062	Cereals, Raisin Bran, Ralston Purina	1	Cup	56.0	178	46	4	0	–	–
8063	Cereals, Raisins, Rice and Rye	1	Cup	46.0	155	39	3	0	–	–
8064	Cereals, Rice Chex	1	Cup	25.2	100	23	1	0	–	–
8065	Cereals, Rice Krispies	1	Cup	28.4	112	25	2	0	–	–
8156	Cereals, Rice, Puffed	1	Cup	14.0	56	13	1	0	–	–
8067	Cereals, Special K	1	Cup	21.3	83	16	4	0	–	–
8068	Cereals, Sugar Corn Pops	1	Cup	28.4	108	26	1	0	–	–
8069	Cereals, Sugar Frosted Flakes	1	Cup	35.0	133	32	2	0	–	–
8074	Cereals, Tasteeos	1	Cup	24.0	94	19	3	1	–	–
8075	Cereals, Team	1	Cup	42.0	164	36	3	1	–	–
8077	Cereals, Total	1	Cup	33.0	116	26	3	1	0	0
8078	Cereals, Trix	1	Cup	28.0	108	25	2	0	–	–
8080	Cereals, Wheat 'n Raisin Chex	1	Cup	54.0	185	43	5	0	–	–
8082	Cereals, Wheat Chex	1	Cup	46.0	169	38	5	1	–	–
8147	Cereals, Wheat, Shredded, Large Biscuit	1	Biscuit	23.6	83	19	3	0	–	–
8148	Cereals, Wheat, Shredded, Small Biscuit	1	Cup	33.1	119	26	4	1	–	–
8143	Cereals, Wheatena, Ckd w/water	1	Cup	243.0	136	29	5	1	–	–
8182	Cereals, Wheatena, Ckd w/water, w/Salt	1	Cup	243.0	136	29	5	1	–	–
8089	Cereals, Wheaties	1	Cup	29.0	101	23	3	0	0	0
8183	Cereals, Whole Wheat Hot Natural Cereal	1	Cup	242.0	150	33	5	1	–	–
55832	Cheddar Cheese Sauce–Stouffer's	1	Cup	283.9	731	22	26	60	–	–
55764	Cheddar Cheese Soup–Stouffer's	1	Cup	283.9	441	18	21	31	–	–
55772	Cheddar Cheese, Heat'n Serve Soup –Stouffer's	1	Cup	307.6	488	22	22	36	–	–
62670	Cheddar Cheese, Non-Fat	1½	Ounce	42.5	68	3	12	0	0	0
62668	Cheerios, Apple Cinnamon	1	Cup	40.0	160	87	3	3	0	0
55196	Cheese Cannelloni, Lean Cuisine–Stouffer's	1	Each	258.7	270	27	23	8	4	–
55108	Cheese Enchiladas–Stouffer's	1	Each	276.4	490	33	23	29	–	–
41331	Cheese French Bread Pizza–Healthy Choice	1	Each	159.5	290	46	19	4	2	–
41300	Cheese Manicotti–Healthy Choice	1	Each	262.2	220	34	15	3	2	–
55796	Cheese Manicotti–Stouffer's	1	Ounce	28.4	29	3	2	1	–	–
55822	Cheese Ravioli–Stouffer's	1	Ounce	28.4	54	6	3	2	–	–
1150	Cheese Spread, Past. Processed, American	2	Ounce	56.7	165	5	9	12	8	4
62671	Cheese Stick, Mozzarella	1	Each	28.0	80	0	8	5	3	0
55808	Cheese Stuffed Shells–Stouffer's	1	Ounce	28.4	28	3	2	1	–	–
55819	Cheese Tortellini w/Egg Pasta–Stouffer's	1	Each	145.3	212	22	11	8	–	–
55821	Cheese Tortellini w/Spinach Pasta–Stouffer's	1	Ounce	28.4	56	6	3	2	–	–
1147	Cheese, American, Pasteurized Processed	2	Ounce	56.7	213	1	13	18	11	5
1004	Cheese, Blue	1½	Ounce	42.5	150	1	9	12	8	3
1005	Cheese, Brick	1½	Ounce	42.5	158	1	10	13	8	4
1006	Cheese, Brie	1½	Ounce	42.5	142	0	9	12	7	3
1008	Cheese, Caraway	1½	Ounce	42.5	160	1	11	12	8	4

Polyunsaturated fat (g)	Dietary Fiber (g)	Cholesterol (mg)	Folate (µg)	Vitamin A (RE)	Vitamin B-6 (mg)	Vitamin B-12 (µg)	Vitamin C (mg)	Vitamin E (mg)	Riboflavin (mg)	Thiamin (mg)	Calcium (mg)	Iron (mg)	Magnesium (mg)	Niacin (mg)	Phosphorus (mg)	Potassium (mg)	Sodium (mg)	Zinc (mg)
–	2	0	145	543	.7	2.2	22	10.8	.6	.5	11	1.4	32	7.2	126	108	277	5.4
–	3	0	148	556	.8	2.2	22	11.1	.6	.5	1	.9	27	7.4	121	98	276	5.5
–	3	0	141	530	.7	2.1	21	10.6	.6	.5	8	1.1	30	7	104	72	272	5.3
–	3	0	155	583	.8	2.3	23	11.6	.7	.6	12	1.2	34	7.7	165	120	299	5.8
–	3	0	150	453	.7	0	0	.2	.3	.5	163	6.3	42	5.5	133	99	285	.9
–	–	0	137	435	.7	0	0	–	.3	.5	158	6.1	34	5.1	118	107	222	.7
–	–	0	156	480	.8	0	0	–	.6	.6	174	7.6	57	8.1	207	236	248	1.3
–	3	0	153	473	.8	0	0	.4	.3	.6	172	6.6	52	5.7	145	105	280	1
–	–	0	146	451	.7	0	0	–	.3	.5	161	6.4	42	5.3	143	102	279	.9
–	2	0	150	441	.7	0	0	.2	.4	.5	166	6.6	36	5.5	133	150	226	.7
1	–	0	9	–	0	0	0	–	0	.3	19	1.6	56	.3	178	131	374	1.1
–	1	0	466	1748	2.3	7	70	34.9	2	1.7	4	21	12	23.3	47	51	378	.5
0	1	0	8	5	.9	2.6	0	.1	.8	.5	9	6.3	12	5.8	25	45	241	.2
–	5	0	133	500	.7	2	0	1.1	.6	.5	17	22.3	63	6.7	183	256	273	5
–	8	0	201	752	1	3	0	1.3	.9	.7	27	9	97	10	238	350	370	3
–	8	0	148	556	.7	2.2	2	1.3	.6	.6	27	27.3	85	7.4	248	287	486	1.7
–	3	0	125	468	.6	1.9	0	.3	.6	.5	10	5.6	20	6.3	50	144	350	4.7
–	0	0	89	2	.5	1.3	13	0	0	.3	4	1.6	6	4.4	25	29	211	.3
–	0	0	100	376	.5	0	15	0	.4	.4	4	1.8	10	5	34	30	341	.5
–	–	0	3	0	0	0	0	–	.3	.4	1	4.4	4	4.9	14	16	0	.1
–	1	0	75	282	.4	0	11	.1	.3	.3	6	3.4	12	3.7	41	37	199	2.8
–	0	0	100	376	.5	0	15	.1	.4	.4	1	1.8	2	5	28	17	104	1.5
–	1	0	124	463	.6	0	19	.1	.5	.5	1	2.2	3	6.2	26	22	284	0
–	3	0	9	318	.4	1.3	13	.2	.4	.3	11	3.8	26	4.2	96	71	183	.7
–	1	0	7	556	.8	2.2	22	.1	.6	.5	6	2.6	18	7.4	65	71	260	.6
0	4	0	466	1748	2.3	7	70	34.9	2	1.7	282	21	37	23.3	137	123	326	.8
–	0	0	3	371	.5	1.5	15	.1	.4	.4	6	4.5	6	4.9	19	26	179	.1
–	4	0	143	0	.7	2.2	2	.3	.6	.5	24	7.7	53	7.1	163	227	306	1.2
–	4	0	162	0	.8	2.4	24	.2	.2	.6	18	7.3	58	8.1	182	173	308	1.2
–	2	0	12	0	.1	0	0	.1	.1	.1	10	.7	40	1.1	86	77	0	.6
–	3	0	17	0	.1	0	0	.2	.1	.1	13	1.4	44	1.7	117	120	3	1.1
–	7	0	17	0	0	0	0	.9	0	0	10	1.4	49	1.3	146	187	5	1.7
–	–	0	17	0	0	0	0	–	0	0	10	1.4	49	1.3	146	187	578	1.7
0	3	0	102	384	.5	1.5	15	.1	.4	.4	44	4.6	32	5.1	100	108	276	.6
–	–	0	27	0	.2	0	0	–	.1	.2	17	1.5	53	2.2	167	172	564	1.2
–	–	130	–	–	–	–	0	–	0	0	6	.1	–	0	–	341	1392	–
–	–	70	–	–	–	–	0	–	0	0	5	0	–	.2	–	511	681	–
–	–	98	–	–	–	–	0	–	0	0	5	.1	–	.2	–	553	770	–
0	0	6	0	91	0	0	0	–	0	0	365	0	0	0	0	–	425	0
0	1	0	67	200	.7	0	20	–	.6	.5	32	3.3	19	6.3	64	87	213	5
–	–	25	–	60	–	–	21	–	.3	.1	240	.4	–	1.5	–	400	590	–
–	–	–	–	150	–	–	6	–	.3	.1	480	.8	–	1.5	–	400	550	–
1	–	15	–	20	–	–	0	–	.3	.5	240	2	–	2.9	240	310	390	–
–	–	30	–	250	–	–	6	–	.3	.3	120	1.5	–	1.9	210	590	310	–
–	–	4	–	–	–	–	2	–	0	0	296	0	–	0	–	45	108	–
–	–	14	–	–	–	–	0	–	0	0	336	0	–	0	–	16	52	–
0	0	31	4	107	.1	.2	0	–	.2	0	319	.2	16	.1	496	137	921	1.5
0	0	15	0	40	0	0	0	–	0	0	240	0	0	0	0	–	170	0
–	–	3	–	–	–	–	1	–	0	0	248	0	–	.1	–	53	59	–
–	–	63	–	–	–	–	0	–	0	0	2	.1	–	.2	–	71	272	–
–	–	19	–	–	–	–	0	–	0	0	0	0	–	.1	–	26	79	–
1	0	54	4	164	0	.4	0	–	.2	0	349	.2	13	0	252	92	369	1.7
0	0	32	15	97	.1	.5	0	.3	.2	0	224	.1	10	.4	165	109	593	1.1
0	0	40	9	128	0	.5	0	.2	.1	0	286	.2	10	.1	192	58	238	1.1
0	0	43	28	77	.1	.7	0	.3	.2	0	78	.2	9	.2	80	65	268	1
0	0	40	8	123	0	.1	0	–	.2	0	286	.3	9	.1	208	40	293	1.3

Code	Name	Amount	Unit	Grams	Energy (kcal)	Carbohydrates (g)	Protein (g)	Fat (g)	Saturated fat (g)	Monounsatu fat (g)
1009	Cheese, Cheddar	1½	Ounce	42.5	171	1	11	14	9	4
62577	Cheese, Cheddar, Reduced Fat	1½	Ounce	42.5	120	2	12	8	5	–
1011	Cheese, Colby	1½	Ounce	42.5	167	1	10	14	9	4
1012	Cheese, Cottage, Creamed	1½	Ounce	42.5	44	1	5	2	1	1
1013	Cheese, Cottage, Creamed, w/Fruit	1½	Ounce	42.5	53	6	4	1	1	0
62690	Cheese, Cottage, Fat Free	½	Cup	113.0	70	0	13	0	0	0
1016	Cheese, Cottage, Lowfat, 1% Fat	1½	Ounce	42.5	31	1	5	0	0	0
1015	Cheese, Cottage, Lowfat, 2% Fat	1½	Ounce	42.5	38	2	6	1	1	0
1014	Cheese, Cottage, Uncreamed, Dry	1½	Ounce	42.5	36	1	7	0	0	0
1017	Cheese, Cream	1½	Ounce	42.5	148	1	3	15	9	4
62554	Cheese, Cream, Fat Free	2	Tbsp.	35.0	35	2	5	0	0	–
62553	Cheese, Cream, Light	2	Tbsp.	32.0	70	2	3	5	4	–
1018	Cheese, Edam	1½	Ounce	42.5	152	1	11	12	7	3
62579	Cheese, Fat Free Slices, White	1	Slice	21.3	30	2	5	0	0	–
62578	Cheese, Fat Free Slices, Yellow	1	Slice	21.3	30	2	5	0	0	–
1019	Cheese, Feta	1½	Ounce	42.5	112	2	6	9	6	2
1156	Cheese, Goat, Hard Type	1½	Ounce	42.5	192	1	13	15	10	3
1157	Cheese, Goat, Semisoft Type	1½	Ounce	42.5	155	1	9	13	9	3
1159	Cheese, Goat, Soft Type	1½	Ounce	42.5	114	0	8	9	6	2
1022	Cheese, Gouda	1½	Ounce	42.5	152	1	11	12	7	3
1023	Cheese, Gruyere	1½	Ounce	42.5	176	0	13	14	8	4
1025	Cheese, Monterey	1½	Ounce	42.5	159	0	10	13	8	4
62576	Cheese, Monterey, Reduced Fat	1½	Ounce	42.5	120	2	12	8	5	–
1028	Cheese, Mozzarella, Part Skim Milk	1½	Ounce	42.5	108	1	10	7	4	2
1161	Cheese, Mozzarella, Substitute	1½	Ounce	42.5	105	10	5	5	2	3
1027	Cheese, Mozzarella, Whole Milk, Low Moisture	1½	Ounce	42.5	135	1	9	10	7	3
1030	Cheese, Muenster	1½	Ounce	42.5	157	0	10	13	8	4
1032	Cheese, Parmesan, Grated	1	Tbsp.	5.0	23	0	2	2	1	0
62608	Cheese, Parmesan, Grated, Fat Free	1	Tbsp.	5.0	5	1	1	0	0	0
1033	Cheese, Parmesan, Piece	1½	Ounce	42.5	167	1	15	11	7	3
1146	Cheese, Parmesan, Shredded	1½	Ounce	42.5	176	1	16	12	7	4
1035	Cheese, Provolone	1½	Ounce	42.5	149	1	11	11	7	3
1037	Cheese, Ricotta, Part Skim Milk	1½	Ounce	42.5	59	2	5	3	2	1
1036	Cheese, Ricotta, Whole Milk	1½	Ounce	42.5	74	1	5	6	4	2
1038	Cheese, Romano	1½	Ounce	42.5	164	2	14	11	7	3
1039	Cheese, Roquefort	1½	Ounce	42.5	157	1	9	13	8	4
1040	Cheese, Swiss, Domestic	1½	Ounce	42.5	160	1	12	12	8	3
1044	Cheese, Swiss, Pasteurized Processed	2	Ounce	56.7	189	1	14	14	9	4
18147	Cheesecake, Commercially Prepared	1	Slice	85.0	273	22	5	19	10	7
18149	Cheesecake, Homemade	1	Slice	85.0	303	21	6	22	12	7
18148	Cheesecake, No–bake Type	1	Slice	80.0	219	28	4	10	6	3
18382	Cheesecake, Plain, w/Cherry Topping	1	Slice	90.0	258	24	5	17	9	5
9066	Cherries, Sour, Red, Cnd, Heavy Syrup Pack	½	Cup	128.0	116	30	1	0	0	0
9065	Cherries, Sour, Red, Cnd, Light Syrup Pack	½	Cup	126.0	95	24	1	0	0	0
9063	Cherries, Sour, Red, Fresh	½	Cup	51.5	26	6	1	0	0	0
9074	Cherries, Sweet, Cnd, Heavy Syrup Pack	½	Cup	128.5	107	27	1	0	0	0
9073	Cherries, Sweet, Cnd, Light Syrup Pack	½	Cup	126.0	84	22	1	0	0	0
9070	Cherries, Sweet, Fresh	½	Cup	72.5	52	12	1	1	0	0
9076	Cherries, Sweet, Frozen, Sweetened	½	Cup	129.5	115	29	1	0	0	0
18308	Cherry Pie	1	Slice	125.0	325	50	3	14	3	7
18444	Cherry Pie, Fried	1	Pie	128.0	404	55	4	21	3	10
19163	Chewing Gum	1	Stick	3.0	10	3	0	0	–	–
62672	Chewing Gum, Sugar–Free	1	Stick	1.7	5	1	–	–	–	–
19033	Chex Mix	1	Cup	42.5	181	28	5	7	–	–
55199	Chicken Cacciatore, Lean Cuisine–Stouffer's	1	Each	308.3	280	31	22	7	2	–
43398	Chicken Cacciatore, Top Shelf–Hormel	1	Each	283.5	210	25	21	3	–	–

Polyunsaturated fat (g)	Dietary Fiber (g)	Cholesterol (mg)	Folate (µg)	Vitamin A (RE)	Vitamin B-6 (mg)	Vitamin B-12 (µg)	Vitamin C (mg)	Vitamin E (mg)	Riboflavin (mg)	Thiamin (mg)	Calcium (mg)	Iron (mg)	Magnesium (mg)	Niacin (mg)	Phosphorus (mg)	Potassium (mg)	Sodium (mg)	Zinc (mg)
0	0	45	8	129	0	.4	0	.2	.2	0	307	.3	12	0	218	42	264	1.3
	0	23	–	90	–	–	0	–	–	–	360	0	–	–	–	35	270	–
0	0	40	8	117	0	.4	0	.1	.2	0	291	.3	11	0	194	54	257	1.3
0	0	6	5	20	0	.3	0	.1	.1	0	26	.1	2	.1	56	36	172	.2
0	0	5	4	15	0	.2	0	0	.1	0	20	0	2	0	44	28	172	.1
0	0	10	0	0	0	0	0	–	0	0	120	0	0	0	0	–	420	0
0	0	2	5	5	0	.3	0	0	.1	0	26	.1	2	.1	57	36	173	.2
0	0	4	6	9	0	.3	0	0	.1	0	29	.1	3	.1	64	41	173	.2
0	0	3	6	3	0	.4	0	0	.1	0	13	.1	2	.1	44	14	5	.2
1	0	47	6	186	0	.2	0	.4	.1	0	34	.5	3	0	44	51	126	.2
–	–	5	–	100	–	–	0	–	–	–	120	0	–	–	–	–	180	–
–	–	15	–	80	–	–	0	–	–	–	48	0	–	–	–	–	150	–
0	0	38	7	108	0	.7	0	.3	.2	0	311	.2	13	0	228	80	410	1.6
–	0	0	–	40	–	–	0	–	–	–	120	0	–	–	–	18	310	–
–	0	0	–	40	–	–	0	–	–	–	120	0	–	–	–	18	310	–
0	0	38	14	54	.2	.7	0	0	.4	.1	209	.3	8	.4	143	26	475	1.2
0	–	45	2	663	0	.1	0	–	.5	.1	381	.8	23	1	310	20	147	.7
0	0	34	1	702	0	.1	0	–	.3	0	127	.7	12	.5	159	67	219	.3
0	0	20	5	578	.1	.1	0	–	.2	0	60	.8	7	.2	109	11	156	.4
0	0	48	9	74	0	.7	0	.1	.1	0	298	.1	12	0	232	51	348	1.7
1	0	47	4	128	0	.7	0	.1	.1	0	430	.1	15	0	257	34	143	1.7
0	0	38	8	108	0	.4	0	.1	.2	0	317	.3	11	0	189	34	228	1.3
–	0	23	–	90	–	–	0	–	–	–	360	0	–	–	–	27	270	–
0	0	25	4	75	0	.3	0	.2	.1	0	275	.1	10	0	197	36	198	1.2
1	0	0	5	186	0	.3	0	–	.2	0	259	.2	17	.1	248	193	291	.8
0	0	38	3	117	0	.3	0	.3	.1	0	244	.1	9	0	175	32	176	1
0	0	41	5	134	0	.6	0	.2	.1	0	305	.2	12	0	199	57	267	1.2
0	0	4	0	9	0	.1	0	0	0	0	69	0	3	0	40	5	93	.2
0	0	2	–	0	–	–	0	–	–	–	16	0	–	–	–	10	15	–
0	0	29	3	63	0	.5	0	.3	.1	0	503	.3	19	.1	295	39	681	1.2
0	0	31	3	74	0	.6	0	–	.1	0	533	.4	22	.1	313	41	721	1.4
0	0	29	4	112	0	.6	0	.1	.1	0	321	.2	12	.1	211	59	372	1.4
0	0	13	6	48	0	.1	0	.1	.1	0	116	.2	6	0	78	53	53	.6
0	0	22	5	57	0	.1	0	.1	.1	0	88	.2	5	0	67	44	36	.5
0	0	44	3	60	0	.5	0	.3	.2	0	452	.3	17	0	323	37	510	1.1
1	0	38	21	127	.1	.3	0	–	.2	0	281	.2	13	.3	167	39	769	.9
0	0	39	3	108	0	.7	0	.2	.2	0	409	.1	15	0	257	47	111	1.7
0	0	48	3	130	0	.7	0	.4	.2	0	438	.3	17	0	432	122	777	2
1	2	47	13	137	0	.1	1	–	.2	0	43	.5	9	.2	79	77	176	.4
2	–	103	10	273	0	.2	0	–	.2	0	49	1.1	7	.3	82	87	241	.5
1	2	34	14	79	0	.2	0	–	.2	.1	138	.4	15	.4	187	169	304	.4
1	–	77	9	217	0	.2	1	–	.1	0	39	1.1	6	.3	64	84	183	.4
0	1	0	10	91	.1	0	3	.2	0	0	13	1.7	8	.2	13	119	9	.1
0	–	0	10	92	.1	0	3	–	0	0	13	1.7	8	.2	13	120	9	.1
0	1	0	4	66	0	0	5	.1	0	0	8	.2	5	.2	8	89	2	.1
0	1	0	5	19	0	0	5	.1	.1	0	12	.4	12	.5	23	186	4	.1
0	1	0	5	20	0	0	5	.2	.1	0	11	.5	11	.5	23	186	4	.1
0	2	0	3	15	0	0	5	.1	0	0	11	.3	8	.3	14	162	0	0
0	1	0	5	25	0	0	1	.2	.1	0	16	.5	13	.2	21	258	1	.1
3	1	0	10	–	.1	0	1	–	0	0	15	.6	10	.3	36	101	308	.2
7	–	–	4	22	0	.1	2	–	.1	.2	28	1.6	13	1.8	55	83	479	.3
–	0	0	0	0	0	0	0	0	0	0	0	0	0	0	0	0	0	0
–	–	–	–	–	–	–	–	–	–	–	–	–	–	–	–	–	–	–
–	–	0	0	6	.7	5.3	20	–	.2	.7	15	10.5	27	7.2	80	114	432	.9
1	–	45	–	100	–	–	9	–	.2	.2	32	.8	–	5.7	–	560	570	–
–	–	50	–	100	–	–	2	.5	.3	.2	80	1	–	6.7	–	–	810	–

Code	Name	Amount	Unit	Grams	Energy (kcal)	Carbohydrates (g)	Protein (g)	Fat (g)	Saturated fat (g)	Monounsatu fat (g)
55200	Chicken Chow Mein w/Rice, Lean Cuisine–Stouffer's	1	Each	255.1	240	34	14	5	1	–
55110	Chicken Chow Mein w/Rice–Stouffer's	1	Each	304.8	250	39	13	5	–	–
41303	Chicken Chow Mein–Healthy Choice	1	Each	241.0	220	31	18	3	1	–
62611	Chicken Chow Mein–Weight Watchers	1	Each	255.2	200	34	12	2	1	–
55807	Chicken Classica –Stouffer's	1	Ounce	28.4	22	2	2	1	–	–
41336	Chicken Con Queso Burritos (mild)–Healthy Choice	1	Each	148.8	280	40	15	8	2	–
41254	Chicken Dijon–Healthy Choice	1	Each	311.8	250	40	21	3	1	–
55111	Chicken Divan–Stouffer's	1	Each	226.8	220	11	24	10	–	–
62618	Chicken Enchiladas Suiza–Weight Watchers	1	Each	255.2	250	28	15	8	3	–
55201	Chicken Enchiladas, Lean Cuisine–Stouffer's	1	Each	280.0	290	34	17	9	3	–
41304	Chicken Enchiladas–Healthy Choice	1	Each	269.3	310	44	14	9	3	–
55112	Chicken Enchiladas–Stouffer's	1	Each	283.5	490	31	21	31	–	–
41305	Chicken Fajitas–Healthy Choice	1	Each	198.5	200	25	17	3	1	–
55203	Chicken Fettucini, Lean Cuisine–Stouffer's	1	Each	255.1	280	33	23	6	3	–
41306	Chicken Fettucini–Healthy Choice	1	Each	241.0	240	29	22	4	2	–
62620	Chicken Fettucini–Weight Watchers	1	Each	233.9	280	25	22	9	3	–
55763	Chicken Gumbo Soup–Stouffer's	1	Cup	283.9	110	9	7	5	–	–
55204	Chicken Italiano, Lean Cuisine–Stouffer's	1	Each	255.1	270	33	22	6	1	–
55789	Chicken Italienne–Stouffer's	1	Ounce	28.4	22	1	2	1	–	–
55755	Chicken Noodle Soup–Stouffer's	1	Cup	283.9	130	10	7	7	–	–
55768	Chicken Noodle, Heat'n Serve Soup–Stouffer's	1	Cup	283.9	320	28	13	17	–	–
55205	Chicken Oriental, Lean Cuisine–Stouffer's	1	Each	255.1	280	31	22	7	2	–
41256	Chicken Oriental–Healthy Choice	1	Each	318.9	200	32	19	1	–	–
41257	Chicken Parmigiana–Healthy Choice	1	Each	326.0	280	45	22	4	2	–
41271	Chicken Pasta Soup–Healthy Choice	1	Each	212.6	100	13	7	2	–	–
55113	Chicken Pie–Stouffer's	1	Each	283.5	440	32	16	27	–	–
57807	Chicken Pot Pie–Swanson	1	Each	198.5	380	35	11	22	–	–
55790	Chicken Primavera–Stouffer's	1	Ounce	28.4	17	1	2	1	–	–
5283	Chicken Salad Sandwich Spread	3	Ounce	85.1	170	6	10	11	3	3
5281	Chicken Spread, Cnd	3	Ounce	85.1	163	5	13	10	3	4
41295	Chicken Stir Fry w/Broccoli–Healthy Choice	1	Each	340.2	280	35	21	6	3	–
55206	Chicken Tenderloins, Lean Cuisine–Stouffer's	1	Each	269.3	240	19	29	5	2	–
55820	Chicken Tortellini w/Egg Pasta–Stouffer's	1	Ounce	28.4	51	6	3	2	–	–
55109	Chicken a la King w/Rice–Stouffer's	1	Each	269.3	270	38	18	5	–	–
43397	Chicken a la King, Top Shelf–Hormel	1	Each	283.5	360	49	18	10	4	4
57799	Chicken a la King–Swanson	1	Each	250.0	319	15	17	20	–	–
55197	Chicken a la Orange, Lean Cuisine–Stouffer's	1	Each	226.8	280	33	27	4	1	–
41301	Chicken a la Orange–Healthy Choice	1	Each	255.1	240	36	20	2	2	–
55792	Chicken and Dumplings–Stouffer's	1	Each	220.0	303	24	15	16	–	–
57801	Chicken and Dumplings–Swanson	1	Each	200.0	207	18	10	10	–	–
41253	Chicken and Pasta Divan–Healthy Choice	1	Each	340.2	300	41	25	4	2	–
55794	Chicken and Veg. Oriental–Stouffer's	1	Each	220.0	186	14	12	9	–	–
55198	Chicken and Veg. w/Vermicelli, Lean Cuisine–Stouffer's	1	Each	333.1	240	30	18	5	1	–
41302	Chicken and Vegetables–Healthy Choice	1	Each	326.0	210	31	20	1	–	–
55202	Chicken in BBQ Sauce, Lean Cuisine–Stouffer's	1	Each	248.1	260	32	20	6	1	–
41248	Chicken w/Barbecue Sauce–Healthy Choice	1	Each	361.5	410	65	24	6	2	–
41277	Chicken w/Rice Soup–Healthy Choice	1	Each	212.6	90	14	5	1	–	–
5063	Chicken, Breast, Meat Only, Ckd, Fried	3	Ounce	85.1	159	0	28	4	1	1
5064	Chicken, Breast, Meat Only, Ckd, Roasted	3	Ounce	85.1	140	0	26	3	1	1
5058	Chicken, Breast, Meat&skin, Ckd, Fried, Batter	3	Ounce	85.1	221	8	21	11	3	5
5060	Chicken, Breast, Meat&skin, Ckd, Roasted	3	Ounce	85.1	168	0	25	7	2	3
5277	Chicken, Cnd.	3	Ounce	85.1	140	0	19	7	2	3
5044	Chicken, Dark Meat, Meat Only, Ckd, Fried	3	Ounce	85.1	203	2	25	10	3	4
5045	Chicken, Dark Meat, Meat Only, Ckd, Roasted	3	Ounce	85.1	174	0	23	8	2	3
5035	Chicken, Dark Meat, Meat&skin, Ckd, Fried, Batter	3	Ounce	85.1	253	8	19	16	4	6
5037	Chicken, Dark Meat, Meat&skin, Ckd, Roasted	3	Ounce	85.1	215	0	22	13	4	5

Polyunsaturated fat (g)	Dietary Fiber (g)	Cholesterol (mg)	Folate (µg)	Vitamin A (RE)	Vitamin B-6 (mg)	Vitamin B-12 (µg)	Vitamin C (mg)	Vitamin E (mg)	Riboflavin (mg)	Thiamin (mg)	Calcium (mg)	Iron (mg)	Magnesium (mg)	Niacin (mg)	Phosphorus (mg)	Potassium (mg)	Sodium (mg)	Zinc (mg)
1	–	30	–	60	–	–	6	–	.2	.2	32	.6	–	4.8	–	350	530	–
–	–	–	–	80	–	–	12	–	.2	0	16	.4	–	1.9	–	340	720	–
1	–	45	–	80	–	–	4	–	.1	.2	16	.8	–	3.8	290	290	440	–
–	3	25	–	300	–	–	36	–	–	–	48	.4	–	–	–	360	430	–
–	–	5	–	–	–	–	1	–	0	0	112	0	–	.1	–	50	83	–
3	–	20	–	20	–	–	6	–	.3	.5	80	1.5	–	2.9	170	260	500	–
–	–	40	–	100	–	–	9	–	.1	.2	16	1	–	9.5	300	350	470	–
–	–	–	–	60	–	–	4	–	.2	.5	200	2	–	3.8	32	490	610	–
–	4	25	–	40	–	–	1	–	–	–	360	.8	–	–	–	470	570	–
2	–	55	–	250	–	–	6	–	.3	.2	120	1.5	–	2.9	–	450	500	–
1	–	35	–	80	–	–	21	–	.2	.2	80	.8	–	4.8	160	380	480	–
–	–	–	–	60	–	–	2	–	.3	.1	240	.6	–	2.9	–	420	860	–
1	–	35	–	150	–	–	9	–	.2	.2	64	1.5	–	3.8	210	360	310	–
–	–	35	–	–	–	–	–	–	.4	.3	120	.8	–	5.7	–	420	500	–
2	–	45	–	–	–	–	–	–	.2	.2	64	1	–	2.9	210	190	370	–
–	2	40	–	40	–	–	0	–	–	–	240	1	–	–	–	730	590	–
–	–	20	–	–	–	–	0	–	0	0	160	.1	–	.2	–	180	1422	–
2	–	40	–	100	–	–	24	–	.3	.3	80	.8	–	5.7	–	600	590	–
–	–	7	–	–	–	–	1	–	0	0	48	0	–	.1	–	57	128	–
–	–	20	–	–	–	–	0	–	0	0	80	.1	–	.2	–	140	1282	–
–	–	60	–	–	–	–	6	–	0	0	240	.2	–	.6	–	310	1793	–
2	–	35	–	40	–	–	6	–	.2	.2	32	1	–	6.7	–	470	480	–
–	–	35	–	250	–	–	36	–	.1	.2	32	.8	–	7.6	200	400	440	–
–	–	45	–	900	–	–	12	–	.2	.2	80	1	–	9.5	260	500	370	–
–	–	15	–	60	–	–	–	–	–	0	–	–	–	.4	–	70	560	–
–	–	–	–	500	–	–	1	–	.4	.3	80	1	–	4.8	–	320	750	–
–	–	–	–	400	–	–	–	–	.2	.2	16	1	–	2.9	–	–	760	–
–	–	5	–	–	–	–	1	–	0	0	48	0	–	.1	–	40	119	–
5	0	26	4	36	.1	.3	1	–	.1	0	9	.5	9	1.4	28	156	321	.9
2	0	44	3	21	.1	.1	0	–	.1	0	106	2	10	2.3	76	90	328	1
–	–	55	–	20	–	–	–	–	.3	.2	48	1.5	–	2.9	260	630	500	–
1	–	60	–	200	–	–	5	–	.3	.2	120	.4	–	7.6	–	750	490	–
–	–	20	–	–	–	–	0	–	0	0	72	0	–	.1	–	31	57	–
–	–	–	–	20	–	–	1	–	.2	.1	160	.8	–	2.9	32	260	800	–
2	–	37	–	250	–	–	1	.2	.2	.1	48	.2	28	8.6	–	476	890	1.2
–	–	–	–	–	–	–	–	–	.2	.1	54	.3	–	3.2	–	–	1159	–
–	–	55	–	80	–	–	12	–	.2	.2	32	.4	–	9.5	–	490	290	–
–	–	45	–	150	–	–	27	–	.1	.2	16	.8	–	5.7	230	430	220	–
–	–	70	–	–	–	–	0	–	0	0	1	.2	–	.4	–	248	660	–
–	–	–	–	75	–	–	–	–	.1	0	15	.4	–	1.8	–	–	922	–
1	–	50	–	800	–	–	72	–	.3	.4	120	1	–	4.8	270	500	520	–
–	–	31	–	–	–	–	5	–	0	0	372	.1	–	.6	–	349	1079	–
1	–	30	–	150	–	–	6	–	.3	.3	64	1	–	5.7	–	500	500	–
–	–	35	–	150	–	–	9	–	.2	.3	32	1.5	–	3.8	190	390	490	–
2	–	50	–	250	–	–	18	–	.2	.2	48	.8	–	5.7	–	650	500	–
2	–	55	–	100	–	–	12	–	.1	.1	48	1.5	–	8.6	250	670	550	–
–	–	10	–	80	–	–	6	–	.1	0	16	.2	–	1.9	70	140	510	–
1	0	77	3	6	.5	.3	0	.4	.1	.1	14	1	26	12.6	209	235	67	.9
1	0	72	3	5	.5	.3	0	.2	.1	.1	13	.9	25	11.7	194	218	63	.9
3	0	72	5	17	.4	.3	0	.9	.1	.1	17	1.1	20	8.9	157	171	234	.8
1	0	71	3	23	.5	.3	0	.2	.1	.1	12	.9	23	10.8	182	208	60	.9
1	0	53	3	29	.3	.2	2	.2	.1	0	12	1.3	10	5.4	94	117	428	1.2
2	0	82	8	20	.3	.3	0	–	.2	.1	15	1.3	21	6	159	215	82	2.5
2	0	79	7	19	.3	.3	0	.2	.2	.1	13	1.1	20	5.6	152	204	79	2.4
4	–	76	8	26	.2	.2	0	–	.2	.1	18	1.2	17	4.8	123	157	251	1.8
3	0	77	6	49	.3	.2	0	–	.2	.1	13	1.2	19	5.4	143	187	74	2.1

Code	Name	Amount	Unit	Grams	Energy (kcal)	Carbohydrates (g)	Protein (g)	Fat (g)	Saturated fat (g)	Monounsaturated fat (g)
5021	Chicken, Giblets, Ckd, Fried	3	Ounce	85.1	236	4	28	11	3	4
5022	Chicken, Giblets, Ckd, Simmered	3	Ounce	85.1	134	1	22	4	1	1
5028	Chicken, Liver, Ckd, Simmered	3	Ounce	85.1	134	1	21	5	2	1
41272	Chili Beef Soup–Healthy Choice	1	Each	212.6	150	22	11	1	–	–
55114	Chili Con Carne w/Beans–Stouffer's	1	Each	248.1	280	28	20	10	–	–
43411	Chili Mac, Micro Cup–Hormel	1	Each	212.6	192	18	10	9	4	4
43408	Chili no Beans, Micro Cup–Hormel	1	Each	209.1	290	15	18	17	8	8
55767	Chili w/Beans Soup–Stouffer's	1	Cup	283.9	240	25	14	9	–	–
16059	Chili w/Beans, Cnd	½	Cup	127.5	143	15	7	7	3	3
43409	Chili w/Beans, Micro Cup–Hormel	1	Each	209.1	250	23	15	11	4	4
43369	Chili w/Beans–Hormel	1	Cup	253.2	357	32	18	18	6	7
43368	Chili w/o Beans–Hormel	1	Cup	253.2	429	17	19	32	13	15
62691	Chili, Fat Free	½	Cup	120.0	80	15	7	0	0	0
18198	Chocolate Chip Cookies, Dietary	1	Each	7.0	32	5	0	1	1	0
18159	Chocolate Chip Cookies, Higher Fat, Enr	1	Each	10.0	48	7	1	2	1	1
18158	Chocolate Chip Cookies, Lower Fat	1	Each	10.0	45	7	1	2	0	1
18160	Chocolate Chip Cookies, Soft-type	1	Each	15.0	69	9	1	4	1	2
18310	Chocolate Creme Pie	1	Slice	113.0	344	38	3	22	6	12
18312	Chocolate Mousse Pie	1	Slice	95.0	247	28	3	15	8	5
19183	Chocolate Pudding	1	Cup	298.1	396	68	8	12	2	5
18157	Chocolate Wafers	1	Each	6.0	26	4	0	1	0	0
19119	Chunky Bar	1	Bar	35.0	173	20	3	10	8	0
43370	Chunky Chili w/Beans–Hormel	1	Cup	253.2	345	30	18	17	–	–
14187	Clam and Tomato Juice, Cnd	¾	Cup	181.1	83	20	1	0	0	0
15158	Clam, Ckd, Breaded and Fried	3	Ounce	85.1	172	9	12	9	2	4
15159	Clam, Ckd, Moist Heat	3	Ounce	85.1	126	4	22	2	0	0
15160	Clam, Cnd, Drained Solids	3	Ounce	85.1	126	4	22	2	0	0
14121	Club Soda	12	Fl Oz	355.2	0	0	0	0	0	0
19219	Coconut Cream Pudding	1	Cup	280.0	291	50	9	7	5	1
18313	Coconut Creme Pie	1	Slice	64.0	191	24	1	11	5	4
18316	Coconut Custard Pie	1	Slice	104.0	270	31	6	14	6	6
15016	Cod, Atlantic, Ckd, Dry Heat	3	Ounce	85.1	89	0	19	1	0	0
15017	Cod, Atlantic, Cnd	3	Ounce	85.1	89	0	19	1	0	0
14209	Coffee, Brewed	6	Fl Oz	177.6	4	1	0	0	0	0
62685	Coffee, Brewed, Decaf.	6	Fl Oz	177.6	4	1	0	0	0	0
14418	Coffee, Instant, Cappuccino Flavor	6	Fl Oz	175.8	56	10	0	2	2	0
14219	Coffee, Instant, Decaffeinated	6	Fl Oz	179.2	4	1	0	0	0	0
14420	Coffee, Instant, Mocha Flavor	6	Fl Oz	175.8	47	8	1	2	2	0
14215	Coffee, Instant, Regular	6	Fl Oz	179.2	4	1	0	0	0	0
18104	Coffeecake	1	Slice	63.0	263	29	4	15	4	8
18106	Coffeecake, Fruit	1	Slice	50.0	156	26	3	5	1	3
14400	Cola	12	Fl Oz	369.6	152	38	0	0	0	–
62530	Cola, Diet	12	Fl Oz	355.2	0	0	0	0	–	–
11159	Coleslaw	½	Cup	64.0	44	8	1	2	0	0
11162	Collards, Ckd	½	Cup	64.0	17	4	1	0	–	–
11161	Collards, Fresh	1	Cup	36.0	11	3	1	0	–	–
11164	Collards, Frz, Chopped, Ckd	½	Cup	85.0	31	6	3	0	–	–
19049	Combos Snacks Cheddar Pretzel	1	Ounce	28.4	136	18	3	6	–	–
55799	Confetti Rice–Stouffer's	1	Ounce	28.4	24	5	1	0	–	–
62656	Corn Chips	13	Chips	29.0	160	15	2	11	2	–
55824	Corn Pudding–Stouffer's	1	Ounce	28.4	38	5	1	2	–	–
55168	Corn Souffle–Stouffer's	1	Each	170.1	240	27	7	11	–	–
20092	Corn, Ckd	½	Cup	70.0	88	20	2	1	0	0
11901	Corn, Sweet, White, Ckd	½	Cup	82.0	89	21	3	1	0	0
11905	Corn, Sweet, White, Cnd	½	Cup	82.0	66	15	2	1	0	0
11906	Corn, Sweet, White, Cnd, Cream Style	½	Cup	128.0	92	23	2	1	0	0

Polyunsaturated fat (g)	Dietary Fiber (g)	Cholesterol (mg)	Folate (µg)	Vitamin A (RE)	Vitamin B-6 (mg)	Vitamin B-12 (µg)	Vitamin C (mg)	Vitamin E (mg)	Riboflavin (mg)	Thiamin (mg)	Calcium (mg)	Iron (mg)	Magnesium (mg)	Niacin (mg)	Phosphorus (mg)	Potassium (mg)	Sodium (mg)	Zinc (mg)
3	0	379	322	3044	.5	11.3	7	–	1.3	.1	15	8.8	21	9.3	243	281	96	5.3
1	0	334	320	1896	.3	8.6	7	1.1	.8	.1	10	5.5	17	3.5	195	134	49	3.9
1	0	537	655	4179	.5	16.5	13	1.2	1.5	.1	12	7.2	18	3.8	265	119	43	3.7
–	–	15	–	20	–	–	6	–	0	.1	16	.6	–	.4	–	290	560	–
–	–	–	–	200	–	–	15	–	.3	.2	64	2	–	2.9	–	700	910	–
–	–	22	–	210	–	–	–	.2	.2	.1	–	1.5	35	2.1	–	443	977	2.1
1	–	60	–	400	–	–	–	0	.2	.1	48	1.6	35	2.5	–	507	830	3.9
–	–	30	–	–	–	–	0	–	0	0	0	.3	–	.6	–	711	991	–
0	6	22	29	43	.2	0	2	.9	.1	.1	60	4.4	57	.5	196	465	666	2.6
–	–	49	–	190	–	–	–	18.9	.2	.1	48	1.9	46	1.7	–	677	977	2.7
1	–	65	–	250	–	–	–	0	.2	.1	57	1.9	58	2	–	913	1226	2.5
1	–	71	–	786	–	–	–	.6	.3	.1	48	1.7	42	2.9	–	592	1024	3.2
0	7	0	0	1000	0	0	12	–	0	0	24	1	0	0	0	–	160	0
0	–	0	0	0	0	0	0	–	0	0	2	.2	2	.2	6	14	1	0
0	0	0	1	0	0	0	0	–	0	0	3	.3	3	.3	11	14	32	.1
0	–	0	1	0	0	0	0	–	0	0	2	.3	3	.3	8	12	38	.1
0	0	0	1	0	0	0	0	–	0	0	2	.4	5	.2	8	14	49	.1
3	2	6	8	–	0	0	0	–	.1	0	41	1.2	24	.8	77	144	154	.3
1	–	21	3	96	0	.2	0	–	.1	0	73	1	30	.6	219	271	437	.6
4	3	9	9	33	.1	0	5	.4	.5	.1	268	1.5	63	1	238	537	385	1.3
0	–	0	1	0	0	0	0	–	0	0	2	.2	3	.2	8	13	35	.1
2	2	4	8	4	0	.1	0	–	.1	0	50	.4	26	.7	73	187	19	.6
–	–	60	–	–	–	–	–	–	–	–	–	–	–	–	–	–	929	–
0	–	0	29	40	.2	55.4	7	–	.1	.1	22	1.1	40	.3	141	163	724	2
2	–	52	15	77	.1	34.2	9	–	.2	.1	54	11.8	12	1.8	160	277	310	1.2
0	0	57	24	145	.1	84.1	19	–	.4	.1	78	23.8	15	2.9	287	534	95	2.3
0	0	57	24	145	.1	84.1	19	.9	.4	.1	78	23.8	15	2.9	287	534	95	2.3
0	0	0	0	0	0	0	0	0	0	0	18	0	4	0	0	7	75	.4
0	–	20	11	140	.4	.7	2	–	.4	.1	316	.6	45	.3	249	445	456	1
1	–	0	3	13	0	–	0	–	.1	0	19	.5	13	.1	54	42	163	.4
1	2	36	4	28	0	.1	0	–	.2	.1	84	.8	19	.4	127	182	348	.7
0	0	47	7	12	.2	.9	1	.3	.1	.1	12	.4	36	2.1	117	208	66	.5
0	0	47	7	12	.2	.9	1	.2	.1	.1	18	.4	35	2.1	221	449	185	.5
0	0	0	0	0	0	0	0	0	0	0	4	.1	9	.4	2	96	4	0
0	0	0	0	0	0	0	0	–	0	0	4	.1	9	.4	2	96	4	0
0	–	0	0	0	0	0	0	–	0	0	7	.1	9	.3	25	109	95	.1
0	–	0	0	0	0	0	0	–	0	0	5	.1	7	.5	5	63	5	.1
0	–	0	0	0	0	0	0	–	0	0	7	.2	9	.2	26	111	33	.1
0	–	0	0	0	0	0	0	–	0	0	5	.1	7	.5	5	64	5	.1
2	2	20	20	18	0	.1	0	–	.1	.1	34	1.2	14	1.1	68	77	221	.5
1	1	11	10	10	0	0	0	–	.1	0	23	1.2	9	1.3	59	45	193	.3
–	0	0	0	0	0	0	0	0	0	0	11	.1	4	0	44	4	15	0
–	0	–	–	–	–	–	–	–	–	–	–	–	–	–	–	–	30	–
1	–	5	17	52	.1	0	21	–	0	0	29	.4	6	.2	20	116	15	.1
–	1	0	4	175	0	0	8	.6	0	0	15	.1	4	.2	5	84	10	.1
–	1	0	4	120	0	0	8	.8	0	0	10	.1	3	.1	4	61	7	0
–	–	0	65	508	.1	0	22	–	.1	0	179	1	26	.5	23	213	43	.2
–	–	3	2	2	0	0	0	–	.2	0	54	.9	6	.9	41	37	317	.2
–	–	1	–	–	–	–	0	–	0	0	24	0	–	0	–	14	136	–
–	1	0	0	0	0	0	0	–	0	0	72	.2	0	0	0	–	200	0
–	–	15	–	–	–	–	1	–	0	0	88	0	–	.1	–	51	125	–
–	–	–	–	60	–	–	–	–	.3	.2	48	.4	–	1.1	–	200	760	–
0	3	0	4	4	0	0	0	.2	0	0	1	.2	25	.4	53	22	0	.4
0	5	0	38	0	0	0	5	.1	.1	.2	2	.5	26	1.3	84	204	14	.4
0	1	0	40	0	0	0	7	.1	.1	0	4	.7	16	1	53	160	265	.3
0	2	0	57	0	.1	0	6	.1	.1	0	4	.5	22	1.2	65	172	365	.7

Code	Name	Amount	Unit	Grams	Energy (kcal)	Carbohydrates (g)	Protein (g)	Fat (g)	Saturated fat (g)	Monounsat… fat (g)
11900	Corn, Sweet, White, Fresh	½	Cup	77.0	66	15	2	1	0	0
11168	Corn, Sweet, Yellow, Ckd	½	Cup	82.0	89	21	3	1	0	0
11172	Corn, Sweet, Yellow, Cnd, Brine Pk	½	Cup	82.0	66	15	2	1	0	0
11174	Corn, Sweet, Yellow, Cnd, Cream Style	½	Cup	128.0	92	23	2	1	0	0
11167	Corn, Sweet, Yellow, Fresh	½	Cup	77.0	66	15	2	1	0	0
43366	Corned Beef Hash–Hormel	1	Cup	253.2	420	18	27	27	9	18
19401	Cornnuts, Barbecue–flavor	1	Ounce	28.4	124	20	3	4	1	2
19402	Cornnuts, Nacho–flavor	1	Ounce	28.4	124	20	3	4	1	2
19009	Cornnuts, Plain	1	Ounce	28.4	124	21	2	4	1	2
41278	Country Vegetable Soup–Healthy Choice	1	Each	212.6	120	23	3	1	–	–
15137	Crab, Alaska King, Ckd, Moist Heat	3	Ounce	85.1	82	0	16	1	0	0
15138	Crab, Alaska King, Imitation	3	Ounce	85.1	87	9	10	1	0	0
15140	Crab, Blue, Ckd, Moist Heat	3	Ounce	85.1	87	0	17	2	0	0
15141	Crab, Blue, Cnd	3	Ounce	85.1	84	0	17	1	0	0
15142	Crab, Blue, Crab Cakes	3	Ounce	85.1	132	0	17	6	1	2
15227	Crab, Queen, Ckd, Moist Heat	3	Ounce	85.1	98	0	20	1	0	0
9077	Crabapples, Fresh	½	Cup	55.0	42	11	0	0	0	0
18214	Crackers, Cheese, Regular	1	Each	1.0	5	1	0	0	0	0
18215	Crackers, Cheese, w/Peanut Butter Filling	1	Each	7.0	34	4	1	2	0	1
18216	Crackers, Crispbread, Rye	1	Each	10.0	37	8	1	0	0	0
18218	Crackers, Matzo, Egg	1	Each	28.4	111	22	3	1	0	0
18217	Crackers, Matzo, Plain	1	Each	28.4	112	24	3	0	0	0
18219	Crackers, Matzo, Whole–wheat	1	Each	28.4	100	22	4	0	0	0
18220	Crackers, Melba Toast, Plain	1	Each	5.0	20	4	1	0	0	0
18424	Crackers, Melba Toast, Plain, w/o Salt	1	Each	5.0	20	4	1	0	0	0
18221	Crackers, Melba Toast, Rye	1	Each	5.0	19	4	1	0	0	0
18222	Crackers, Melba Toast, Wheat	1	Each	5.0	19	4	1	0	0	0
18229	Crackers, Ritz	1	Each	3.0	15	2	0	1	0	0
18427	Crackers, Ritz, Low Sodium	1	Each	3.0	15	2	0	1	0	0
18226	Crackers, Rye, Wafers, Plain	1	Each	25.0	84	20	2	0	0	0
18227	Crackers, Rye, Wafers, Seasoned	1	Each	22.0	84	16	2	2	0	1
18225	Crackers, Rye, w/Cheese Filling	1	Each	7.0	34	4	1	2	0	1
18228	Crackers, Saltines	1	Each	3.0	13	2	0	0	0	0
62688	Crackers, Saltines, Fat Free	1	Each	3.0	12	2	0	0	0	0
18425	Crackers, Saltines, Low Salt	1	Each	3.0	13	2	0	0	0	0
18230	Crackers, Snack–type, w/Cheese Filling	1	Each	7.0	33	4	1	1	0	1
18231	Crackers, Snack–type, w/Peanut Butter Filling	1	Each	7.0	34	4	1	2	0	1
18428	Crackers, Wheat, Low Salt	1	Each	2.0	9	1	0	0	0	0
18232	Crackers, Wheat, Regular	1	Each	2.0	9	1	0	0	0	0
18233	Crackers, Wheat, w/Cheese Filling	1	Each	7.0	35	4	1	2	0	1
18234	Crackers, Wheat, w/Peanut Butter Filling	1	Each	7.0	35	4	1	2	0	1
18235	Crackers, Whole–wheat	1	Each	4.0	18	3	0	1	0	0
18429	Crackers, Whole–wheat, Low Salt	1	Each	4.0	18	3	0	1	0	0
9078	Cranberries, Fresh	½	Cup	47.5	23	6	0	0	–	–
9080	Cranberry Juice Bottled	¾	Cup	189.4	108	27	0	0	–	–
9081	Cranberry Sauce, Cnd, Sweetened	½	Cup	138.5	209	54	0	0	–	–
14238	Cranberry–apple Juice Drink, Bottled	¾	Cup	183.4	123	31	0	0	0	–
14240	Cranberry–apricot Juice Drink, Bottled	¾	Cup	183.4	117	30	0	0	0	–
14241	Cranberry–grape Juice Drink, Bottled	¾	Cup	183.4	103	26	0	0	0	–
9082	Cranberry–orange Relish, Cnd	½	Cup	137.5	245	64	0	0	–	–
15146	Crayfish, Wild, Ckd, Moist Heat	3	Ounce	85.1	75	0	14	1	0	0
18238	Cream Puffs, Shell, w/Custard Filling	1	Each	130.0	335	30	9	20	5	8
14130	Cream Soda	12	Fl Oz	370.8	189	49	0	0	0	0
1067	Cream Substitute, Nondairy, Liquid	1	Tbsp.	15.0	20	2	0	1	0	1
1069	Cream Substitute, Nondairy, Powdered	1	Tsp.	2.0	11	1	0	1	1	0
55762	Cream of Broccoli Soup–Stouffer's	1	Cup	283.9	300	16	12	21	–	–

Polyunsaturated fat (g)	Dietary Fiber (g)	Cholesterol (mg)	Folate (µg)	Vitamin A (RE)	Vitamin B-6 (mg)	Vitamin B-12 (µg)	Vitamin C (mg)	Vitamin E (mg)	Riboflavin (mg)	Thiamin (mg)	Calcium (mg)	Iron (mg)	Magnesium (mg)	Niacin (mg)	Phosphorus (mg)	Potassium (mg)	Sodium (mg)	Zinc (mg)
0	2	0	35	0	0	0	5	.2	0	.2	2	.4	28	1.3	69	208	12	.3
0	2	0	38	18	0	0	5	.1	.1	.2	2	.5	26	1.3	84	204	14	.4
0	2	0	40	13	0	0	7	.1	.1	0	4	.7	16	1	53	160	265	.3
0	2	0	57	13	.1	0	6	.1	.1	0	4	.5	22	1.2	65	172	365	.7
0	2	0	35	22	0	0	5	.1	0	.2	2	.4	28	1.3	69	208	12	.3
–	–	80	–	–	–	–	–	.4	.2	–	71	1.8	31	3.4	–	625	991	4
1	2	0	0	10	.1	0	0	–	0	.1	5	.5	31	.4	80	81	277	.5
1	2	1	4	1	.1	0	4	–	0	.1	10	.5	31	.3	88	88	180	.5
1	2	0	0	0	.1	0	0	.3	0	0	3	.5	32	.5	78	79	156	.5
–	–	0	–	200	–	–	6	–	.1	.1	32	.4	–	1.5	100	380	540	–
0	0	45	43	8	.2	9.8	6	–	0	0	50	.6	54	1.1	238	223	912	6.5
1	0	17	1	17	0	1.4	0	–	0	0	11	.3	37	.2	240	77	715	.3
1	0	85	43	2	.2	6.2	3	.9	0	.1	88	.8	28	2.8	175	276	237	3.6
0	0	76	36	2	.1	.4	2	.9	.1	.1	86	.7	33	1.2	221	318	283	3.4
2	0	128	35	69	.1	5	2	–	.1	.1	89	.9	28	2.5	181	276	281	3.5
0	0	60	36	44	.1	8.8	6	–	.2	.1	28	2.4	54	2.5	109	170	588	3.1
0	–	0	–	2	–	0	4	–	0	0	10	.2	4	.1	8	107	1	–
0	0	0	0	0	0	0	0	–	0	0	2	0	0	0	2	1	10	0
0	0	0	2	–	.1	0	0	–	0	0	6	.2	4	.5	23	17	69	.1
0	2	0	2	0	0	0	0	–	0	0	3	.2	8	.1	27	32	26	.2
0	–	25	8	4	0	.1	0	–	.2	.2	11	.8	7	1.4	45	43	6	.2
0	1	0	4	0	0	0	0	–	.1	.1	4	.9	7	1.1	25	32	1	.2
0	3	0	10	0	0	0	0	–	.1	.1	7	1.3	38	1.5	86	90	1	.7
0	0	0	1	0	0	0	0	–	0	0	5	.2	3	.2	10	10	41	.1
0	–	0	1	0	0	0	0	–	0	0	5	.2	3	.2	10	10	1	.1
0	0	0	1	–	0	0	0	–	0	0	4	.2	2	.2	9	10	45	.1
0	0	0	1	0	0	0	0	–	0	0	2	.2	3	.3	8	7	42	.1
0	0	0	0	0	0	0	0	–	0	0	4	.1	1	.1	7	4	25	0
0	–	0	0	0	0	0	0	–	0	0	4	.1	1	.1	7	11	11	0
0	–	0	11	1	.1	0	0	–	.1	.1	10	1.5	30	.4	84	124	199	.7
0	–	0	11	–	0	0	0	–	0	.1	10	.7	23	.5	68	100	195	.6
0	–	1	1	0	0	0	0	–	0	0	16	.2	3	.2	24	24	73	0
0	0	0	1	0	0	0	0	–	0	0	4	.2	1	.2	3	4	39	0
0	0	0	0	0	0	0	0	–	0	0	0	.1	0	0	0	26	36	0
0	–	0	1	0	0	0	0	–	0	0	4	.2	1	.2	3	22	19	0
0	–	0	1	0	0	0	0	–	0	0	18	.2	3	.3	28	30	98	0
0	–	0	2	0	0	0	0	–	0	0	7	.2	4	.4	17	16	66	.1
0	–	0	0	0	0	0	0	–	0	0	1	.1	1	.1	4	4	6	0
0	0	0	0	0	0	0	0	–	0	0	1	.1	1	.1	4	4	16	0
0	–	0	1	1	0	0	0	–	0	0	14	.2	4	.2	27	21	64	.1
0	–	0	3	0	0	0	0	–	0	0	12	.2	3	.4	24	21	56	.1
0	0	0	1	0	0	0	0	–	0	0	2	.1	4	.2	12	12	26	.1
0	–	0	1	0	0	0	0	–	0	0	2	.1	4	.2	12	12	10	.1
–	2	0	1	2	0	0	6	0	0	0	3	.1	2	0	4	34	0	.1
–	–	0	0	0	0	0	67	–	0	0	6	.3	4	.1	4	34	4	.1
–	1	0	–	3	0	0	3	.1	0	0	6	.3	4	.1	8	36	40	.1
–	0	0	0	0	0	0	59	0	0	0	13	.1	4	.1	6	50	4	.1
–	0	0	1	84	0	0	0	0	0	0	17	.3	6	.2	9	112	4	.1
–	0	0	1	0	.1	0	59	0	0	0	15	0	6	.2	7	44	6	.1
–	–	0	–	10	–	0	25	–	0	0	15	.3	5	.1	11	52	44	–
0	0	113	37	13	.1	1.8	1	1.3	.1	0	51	.7	28	1.9	230	252	80	1.5
5	–	174	20	259	.1	.5	0	–	.4	.2	86	1.5	16	1.1	142	150	443	.8
0	0	0	0	0	0	0	0	0	0	0	19	.2	4	0	0	4	44	.3
0	0	0	0	1	0	0	0	.2	0	0	1	0	0	0	10	29	12	0
0	0	0	0	0	0	0	0	0	0	0	0	0	0	0	8	16	4	0
–	–	60	–	–	–	–	0	–	0	0	2	0	–	0	–	431	791	–

Code	Name	Amount	Unit	Grams	Energy (kcal)	Carbohydrates (g)	Protein (g)	Fat (g)	Saturated fat (g)	Monounsat fat (g)
55765	Cream of Potato Soup–Stouffer's	1	Cup	283.9	300	34	11	13	–	–
1049	Cream, Half and Half, Cream and Milk	1	Tbsp.	15.0	20	1	0	2	1	0
1053	Cream, Heavy Whipping	1	Tbsp.	15.0	52	0	0	6	3	2
1052	Cream, Light Whipping	1	Tbsp.	15.0	44	0	0	5	3	1
1050	Cream, Light, Coffee or Table	1	Tbsp.	15.0	29	1	0	3	2	1
1051	Cream, Medium, 25% Fat	1	Tbsp.	15.0	37	1	0	4	2	1
1054	Cream, Whipped, Pressurized	1	Tbsp.	3.0	8	0	0	1	0	0
55788	Creamed Chicken–Stouffer's	1	Ounce	28.4	48	1	3	4	–	–
55777	Creamed Chipped Beef–Stouffer's	1	Ounce	28.4	45	2	2	3	–	–
55169	Creamed Spinach–Stouffer's	1	Each	127.6	190	8	4	16	–	–
55756	Creamy Chicken Soup–Stouffer's	1	Cup	283.9	240	25	17	8	–	–
14034	Creme De Menthe, 72 Proof	1	Fl Oz	33.6	125	14	0	0	0	0
18240	Croissant, Apple	1	Medium	57.0	145	21	4	5	3	1
18239	Croissant, Butter	1	Medium	57.0	231	26	5	12	7	3
18241	Croissant, Cheese	1	Medium	57.0	236	27	5	12	5	4
18242	Croutons, Plain	½	Cup	15.0	61	11	2	1	0	1
18243	Croutons, Seasoned	½	Cup	20.0	93	13	2	4	1	2
62635	Crystal Lite	8	Fl Oz	236.6	5	–	–	–	–	–
11205	Cucumber, Fresh	½	Cup	52.0	7	1	0	0	0	0
14010	Daiquiri	1	Fl Oz	30.2	56	2	0	0	0	0
14009	Daiquiri, Bottled	1	Fl Oz	30.5	38	5	0	0	0	–
18245	Danish Pastry, Cheese	1	Each	71.0	266	26	6	16	5	8
18244	Danish Pastry, Cinnamon	1	Each	65.0	262	29	5	15	4	8
18246	Danish Pastry, Fruit	1	Each	71.0	263	34	4	13	3	7
18433	Danish Pastry, Lemon	1	Each	71.0	263	34	4	13	3	7
18247	Danish Pastry, Nut	1	Each	65.0	280	30	5	16	4	8
18435	Danish Pastry, Raspberry	1	Each	71.0	263	34	4	13	3	7
9087	Dates, Domestic, Natural and Dry	½	Cup	89.0	245	65	2	0	–	–
1073	Dessert Topping, Nondairy	1	Tbsp.	4.0	13	1	0	1	1	0
43375	Dinty Moore Beef Stew–Hormel	1	Cup	253.2	246	18	12	15	7	6
43376	Dinty Moore Chicken Stew–Hormel	1	Cup	253.2	310	18	13	21	5	7
43377	Dinty Moore Meatball Stew–Hormel	1	Cup	253.2	268	16	12	18	8	8
43378	Dinty Moore Vegetable Stew–Hormel	1	Cup	253.2	173	22	6	7	2	1
19032	Doo Dads Snack Mix, Original Flavor	1	Cup	56.7	259	36	6	10	–	–
62686	Dough Holes	1	Each	15.0	64	8	1	3	1	2
18251	Doughnuts, Chocolate, Sugared or Glazed	1	Each	42.0	175	24	2	8	2	5
18253	Doughnuts, French Crullers, Glazed	1	Each	41.0	169	24	1	8	2	4
18255	Doughnuts, Glazed	1	Each	60.0	242	27	4	14	3	8
18248	Doughnuts, Plain	1	Each	47.0	198	23	2	11	2	5
18249	Doughnuts, Plain, Chocolate–coated or Frosted	1	Each	43.0	204	21	2	13	4	7
18250	Doughnuts, Plain, Sugared or Glazed	1	Each	45.0	192	23	2	10	2	5
18252	Doughnuts, Whole Wheat, Sugared or Glazed	1	Each	45.0	162	19	3	9	1	4
18254	Doughnuts, w/Creme Filling	1	Each	85.0	307	26	5	21	6	11
18256	Doughnuts, w/Jelly Filling	1	Each	85.0	289	33	5	16	4	9
14153	Dr. Pepper	12	Fl Oz	368.4	151	38	0	0	0	–
5142	Duck, Domesticated, Meat Only, Roasted	3	Ounce	85.1	171	0	20	10	4	3
5140	Duck, Domesticated, Meat&skin, Roasted	3	Ounce	85.1	287	0	16	24	8	11
7021	Dutch Brand Loaf, Lunch Meat	1	Slice	28.4	68	2	4	5	2	2
18257	Eclairs, Custard–filled w/Chocolate Glaze	1	Each	62.0	162	15	4	10	3	4
18317	Egg Custard Pie	1	Slice	105.0	221	22	6	12	3	6
19168	Egg Custards	1	Cup	282.0	296	30	14	13	7	4
62636	Egg Roll	1	Each	85.0	160	21	7	5	1	–
1142	Egg Substitute, Frozen	1	Cup	240.0	384	8	27	27	5	6
1143	Egg Substitute, Liquid	1	Cup	251.0	211	2	30	8	2	2
1124	Egg, White Only, w/o Yolk	2	Large	66.8	33	1	7	0	–	–
1057	Eggnog	1	Cup	254.0	342	34	10	19	11	6

Polyunsaturated fat (g)	Dietary Fiber (g)	Cholesterol (mg)	Folate (µg)	Vitamin A (RE)	Vitamin B-6 (mg)	Vitamin B-12 (µg)	Vitamin C (mg)	Vitamin E (mg)	Riboflavin (mg)	Thiamin (mg)	Calcium (mg)	Iron (mg)	Magnesium (mg)	Niacin (mg)	Phosphorus (mg)	Potassium (mg)	Sodium (mg)	Zinc (mg)
–	–	30	–	–	–	–	0	–	0	0	2	.1	–	.2	–	791	1422	–
0	0	6	0	16	0	0	0	0	0	0	16	0	2	0	14	19	6	.1
0	0	21	1	63	0	0	0	.1	0	0	10	0	1	0	9	11	6	0
0	0	17	1	44	0	0	0	.1	0	0	10	0	1	0	9	15	5	0
0	0	10	0	27	0	0	0	0	0	0	14	0	1	0	12	18	6	0
0	0	13	0	35	0	0	0	.1	0	0	14	0	1	0	11	17	6	0
0	0	2	0	6	0	0	0	0	0	0	3	0	0	0	3	4	4	0
–	–	14	–	–	–	–	0	–	0	0	352	0	–	.1	–	37	119	–
–	–	13	–	–	–	–	0	–	0	0	184	0	–	.2	–	57	176	–
–	–	–	–	400	–	–	6	–	.2	0	80	.4	–	–	–	400	400	–
–	–	20	–	–	–	–	0	–	0	0	2	0	–	.2	–	511	1282	–
0	0	0	0	0	0	0	0	0	0	0	0	0	0	0	0	0	2	0
0	1	29	7	42	0	.1	0	–	.1	.1	17	.6	7	.9	33	51	156	.6
1	2	43	16	78	0	.2	0	–	.1	.2	21	1.2	9	1.2	60	67	424	.4
2	2	36	19	89	0	.2	0	–	.2	.3	30	1.2	14	1.2	74	75	316	.5
0	1	0	3	0	0	0	0	–	0	.1	11	.6	5	.8	17	19	105	.1
0	1	1	8	1	0	0	0	–	.1	.1	19	.6	8	.9	28	36	248	.2
–	–	–	0	0	0	0	6	–	0	0	0	0	0	0	0	–	–	0
0	0	0	7	11	0	0	3	0	0	0	7	.1	6	.1	10	75	1	.1
0	0	0	1	0	0	0	0	0	0	0	1	0	1	0	2	6	2	0
–	0	0	0	0	0	0	0	0	0	0	0	0	0	0	1	3	12	0
2	–	32	18	44	0	.2	0	–	.2	.1	25	1.1	11	1.4	77	70	320	.6
2	1	20	21	7	0	.1	0	–	.2	.2	46	1.3	12	1.9	70	81	241	.5
2	1	15	11	11	–	.1	3	–	.2	.2	33	1.3	11	1.4	63	59	251	.4
2	–	–	11	38	–	–	3	–	.1	0	33	.5	11	.5	63	59	251	.4
4	1	30	18	9	.1	.1	1	–	.2	.1	61	1.2	21	1.5	72	62	236	.6
2	–	–	11	43	–	–	3	–	.1	0	33	.5	11	.5	63	59	251	.4
–	7	0	11	4	.2	0	0	.1	.1	.1	28	1	31	2	36	580	3	.3
0	0	0	0	3	0	0	0	0	0	0	0	0	0	0	0	1	1	0
1	–	33	–	815	–	–	3	–	.1	0	27	1	23	2.5	–	588	971	2.8
8	–	95	–	476	–	–	2	–	.3	.1	38	.7	25	3.6	–	610	1012	1.3
1	–	33	–	279	–	–	1	2.6	.2	.1	27	1.2	27	3.2	–	586	1094	2.7
2	–	16	–	714	–	–	2	.6	.1	.1	36	.7	31	1.7	–	509	949	.8
–	4	1	23	24	.1	0	0	–	.1	.2	42	1.4	34	3	168	157	721	1.3
0	–	5	2	0	0	0	0	–	0	0	9	.2	3	.2	18	15	60	.1
1	1	24	7	11	0	.1	0	–	0	0	89	1	14	.2	68	50	143	.2
1	–	5	3	–	0	0	0	–	.1	.1	11	.6	5	.6	50	32	141	.1
2	1	4	13	–	0	.1	0	–	.1	.2	26	1.2	13	1.7	56	65	205	.5
4	1	17	4	8	0	.1	0	–	.1	.1	21	.9	9	.9	126	60	257	.3
2	1	25	7	13	0	.2	0	–	0	.1	15	1.1	17	.6	87	49	184	.3
1	–	14	5	1	0	.1	0	–	.1	.1	27	.5	8	.7	53	46	181	.2
3	–	9	7	9	0	.1	0	–	.1	.1	22	.5	10	.8	47	67	160	.3
3	–	20	12	7	0	.1	0	–	.1	.3	21	1.6	17	1.9	65	68	263	.7
2	–	22	14	7	0	.1	1	–	.1	.3	21	1.5	17	1.8	72	67	249	.6
–	0	0	0	0	0	0	0	0	0	0	11	.1	0	0	41	4	37	.1
1	0	76	9	20	.2	.3	0	.6	.4	.2	10	2.3	17	4.3	173	214	55	2.2
3	0	71	5	54	.2	.3	0	.6	.2	.1	9	2.3	14	4.1	133	174	50	1.6
1	0	13	1	0	.1	.4	5	.1	.1	.1	24	.4	6	.7	46	107	354	.5
2	–	79	9	118	0	.2	0	–	.2	.1	39	.7	9	.5	66	73	209	.4
2	1	35	21	53	.1	.5	0	–	.2	0	84	.6	12	.3	118	111	252	.5
1	–	245	28	169	.1	.9	1	–	.6	.1	316	.8	39	.2	319	431	217	1.5
–	2	10	0	100	0	0	1	–	0	0	24	.2	0	0	0	–	350	0
15	0	5	39	324	.3	.8	1	5.1	.9	.3	175	4.8	36	.3	172	512	479	2.4
4	0	3	37	542	0	.7	0	1.2	.8	.3	133	5.3	22	.3	304	828	444	3.3
–	0	–	2	0	0	.1	0	0	.3	0	4	0	7	.1	9	96	110	0
1	0	149	2	203	.1	1.1	4	.6	.5	.1	330	.5	47	.3	278	420	138	1.2

Code	Name	Amount	Unit	Grams	Energy (kcal)	Carbohydrates (g)	Protein (g)	Fat (g)	Saturated fat (g)	Monounsat fat (g)
62680	Eggnog, Reduced–Fat	1	Cup	246.0	320	48	12	8	5	0
11210	Eggplant, Ckd	½	Cup	48.0	13	3	0	0	0	0
11209	Eggplant, Fresh	½	Cup	41.0	11	2	0	0	0	0
1128	Eggs, Chicken, Whole, Ckd, Fried	1	Large	46.0	92	1	6	7	2	3
1129	Eggs, Chicken, Whole, Ckd, Hard–boiled	1	Large	50.0	78	1	6	5	2	2
1130	Eggs, Chicken, Whole, Ckd, Omelet	1	Large	59.0	90	1	6	7	2	3
1131	Eggs, Chicken, Whole, Ckd, Poached	1	Large	50.0	75	1	6	5	2	2
1132	Eggs, Chicken, Whole, Ckd, Scrambled	½	Cup	110.0	183	2	12	13	4	5
1123	Eggs, Chicken, Whole, Fresh, and Frozen	1	Large	50.0	75	1	6	5	2	2
41242	English Muffin Sandwich–Healthy Choice	1	Each	120.5	200	30	16	3	1	–
18260	English Muffins, Mixed–grain (includes Granola)	1	Each	66.0	155	31	6	1	0	1
18258	English Muffins, Plain	1	Each	57.0	134	26	4	1	0	0
18262	English Muffins, Raisin–cinnamon	1	Each	57.0	139	28	4	2	0	0
18264	English Muffins, Wheat	1	Each	57.0	127	26	5	1	0	0
18266	English Muffins, Whole–wheat	1	Each	66.0	134	27	6	1	0	0
55170	Escalloped Apples–Stouffer's	1	Each	170.1	200	41	0	4	–	–
55117	Escalloped Chicken and Noodles–Stouffer's	1	Each	283.5	420	30	21	24	–	–
62592	Fat Free Cinnamon Graham Snacks–SnackWell	20	Each	13.4	49	12	1	0	0	0
62606	Fat Free Cracked Pepper Crackers–SnackWell	7	Each	15.0	60	13	2	0	0	0
62589	Fat Free Devils Food Cookie Cakes–SnackWell	1	Each	16.0	50	13	1	0	0	0
62591	Fat Free Double Fudge Cookie Cakes–SnackWell	1	Each	16.0	50	12	1	0	0	0
62590	Fat Free Wheat Crackers–SnackWell	5	Each	15.0	60	12	2	0	0	0
62621	Fettucini Alfredo with Broccoli–Weight Watchers	1	Each	241.0	220	24	15	6	3	–
55208	Fettucini Alfredo, Lean Cuisine–Stouffer's	1	Each	255.1	280	41	14	7	3	–
55171	Fettucini Alfredo–Stouffer's	1	Each	141.8	245	22	8	14	–	–
55209	Fettucini Primavera, Lean Cuisine–Stouffer's	1	Each	283.5	260	32	14	8	3	–
55831	Fettucini Sauce (Alfredo Style)–Stouffer's	1	Cup	283.9	701	11	14	67	–	–
41288	Fettucini w/Turkey and Vegetables–Healthy Choice	1	Each	354.4	350	45	29	6	3	–
62612	Fiesta Chicken–Weight Watchers	1	Each	241.0	220	38	12	2	1	–
55773	Fiesta Mexicali Heat'n Serve Soup –Stouffer's	1	Cup	283.9	110	18	3	3	–	–
19098	Fifth Avenue Bar	1	Bar	60.0	280	41	5	13	–	–
18170	Fig Bars	1	Each	16.0	56	11	1	1	0	1
55210	Filet of Fish Divan, Lean Cuisine–Stouffer's	1	Each	294.1	210	13	27	5	2	–
55211	Filet of Fish Florentine, Lean Cuisine–Stouffer's	1	Each	272.9	220	13	26	7	3	–
15027	Fish Fillets and Sticks, Fried	3	Ounce	85.1	231	20	13	10	3	4
15029	Flounder, Ckd, Dry Heat	3	Ounce	85.1	100	0	21	1	0	0
20081	Flour, White	1	Cup	125.0	455	95	13	1	0	0
20080	Flour, Whole Grain	1	Cup	120.0	407	87	16	2	0	0
55178	French Bread Pizza, Cheese–Stouffer's	1	Each	145.3	350	40	16	14	–	–
41332	French Bread Pizza, Deluxe–Healthy Choice	1	Each	180.7	330	41	23	7	3	–
55181	French Bread Pizza, Deluxe–Stouffer's	1	Each	173.6	420	40	21	19	–	–
55180	French Bread Pizza, Double Cheese–Stouffer's	1	Each	166.6	420	43	22	18	–	–
55182	French Bread Pizza, Hamburger–Stouffer's	1	Each	173.6	410	39	23	18	–	–
55183	French Bread Pizza, Pepperoni–Stouffer's	1	Each	159.5	400	39	19	19	–	–
55185	French Bread Pizza, Sausage–Stouffer's	1	Each	170.1	430	40	20	21	–	–
55187	French Bread Pizza, Vegetable Deluxe–Stouffer's	1	Each	180.7	420	41	18	20	–	–
62677	French Onion Dip	2	Tbsp.	30.0	60	2	1	5	3	0
55761	French Onion Soup–Stouffer's	1	Cup	283.9	100	10	4	4	–	–
18268	French Toast, Frozen, Ready–to–heat	1	Slice	59.0	126	19	4	4	1	1
18269	French Toast, Made w/Lowfat (2%) Milk	1	Slice	65.0	149	16	5	7	2	3
18381	French Toast, Made w/Whole Milk	1	Slice	65.0	151	16	5	7	2	3
62638	Frosted Pop Tart, Fruit	1	Each	52.0	200	38	2	5	2	–
19226	Frostings, Chocolate, Creamy	1	Ounce	28.4	113	18	0	5	2	3
19713	Frostings, Cream Cheese–flavor	1	Ounce	28.4	117	19	0	5	1	3
19229	Frostings, Sour Cream–flavor	1	Ounce	28.4	117	19	0	5	1	3
19230	Frostings, Vanilla, Creamy	1	Ounce	28.4	119	20	0	5	1	2

Polyunsaturated fat (g)	Dietary Fiber (g)	Cholesterol (mg)	Folate (µg)	Vitamin A (RE)	Vitamin B-6 (mg)	Vitamin B-12 (µg)	Vitamin C (mg)	Vitamin E (mg)	Riboflavin (mg)	Thiamin (mg)	Calcium (mg)	Iron (mg)	Magnesium (mg)	Niacin (mg)	Phosphorus (mg)	Potassium (mg)	Sodium (mg)	Zinc (mg)
0	0	90	0	160	0	0	2	–	0	0	480	.4	0	0	0	–	280	0
0	1	0	7	3	0	0	1	0	0	0	3	.2	6	.3	11	119	1	.1
0	1	0	8	3	0	0	1	0	0	0	3	.1	6	.2	9	89	1	.1
1	0	211	17	114	.1	.4	0	1.6	.2	0	25	.7	5	0	89	61	162	.5
1	0	212	22	84	.1	.6	0	1	.3	0	25	.6	5	0	86	63	62	.5
1	0	207	17	110	.1	.4	0	1.5	.2	0	25	.7	5	0	87	60	159	.5
1	0	212	18	95	.1	.4	0	.5	.2	0	25	.7	5	0	89	60	140	.6
2	0	387	33	215	.1	.8	0	.9	.5	.1	78	1.3	13	.1	187	152	308	1.1
1	0	213	24	96	.1	.5	0	1	.3	0	25	.7	5	0	89	61	63	.6
1	–	20	–	60	–	–	4	–	.4	.5	120	2	–	2.9	220	200	510	–
0	–	0	23	1	.1	0	0	–	.2	.3	129	2	29	2.4	98	103	275	.6
1	–	0	21	0	0	0	0	–	.2	.3	99	1.4	12	2.2	76	75	264	.4
1	–	0	18	0	0	0	0	–	.2	.2	84	1.4	9	2	44	119	255	.6
0	–	0	22	0	.1	0	0	–	.2	.2	101	1.6	22	1.9	66	106	218	.6
1	4	0	32	0	.1	0	0	–	.1	.2	175	1.6	47	2.3	186	139	420	1.1
–	–	–	–	–	–	–	30	–	–	0	–	–	–	–	–	90	15	–
–	–	–	–	20	–	–	–	–	.3	.2	80	.8	–	3.8	–	300	840	–
0	0	0	–	0	–	–	0	–	–	–	0	.3	–	–	–	–	40	–
0	0	0	–	0	–	–	0	–	–	–	24	.4	–	–	–	–	150	–
0	1	0	–	0	–	–	0	–	–	–	0	0	–	–	–	–	25	–
0	1	0	–	0	–	–	0	–	–	–	0	.2	–	–	–	–	70	–
0	1	0	–	0	–	–	0	–	–	–	24	.4	–	–	–	45	170	–
–	6	15	–	60	–	–	1	–	–	–	300	1.5	–	–	–	510	540	–
–	–	15	–	–	–	–	–	–	.4	.3	200	.8	–	1.5	–	270	570	–
–	–	–	–	–	–	–	–	–	.3	.2	120	.4	–	1	–	100	400	–
–	–	45	–	400	–	–	18	–	.4	.3	240	.8	–	1.5	–	400	510	–
–	–	180	–	–	–	–	0	–	0	0	3	0	–	0	–	341	1813	–
2	–	60	–	150	–	–	–	–	.5	.5	120	1.5	–	3.8	310	450	480	–
–	5	25	–	450	–	–	42	–	–	–	72	1.5	–	–	–	490	480	–
–	–	10	–	–	–	–	6	–	0	0	2	1	–	.2	–	431	711	–
–	–	2	33	5	.1	.1	0	–	.1	0	42	.6	38	2	90	197	112	.6
0	1	0	2	1	0	0	0	–	0	0	10	.5	4	.3	10	33	56	.1
1	–	65	–	20	–	–	27	–	.3	.2	120	.4	–	1.9	–	800	490	–
2	–	65	–	500	–	–	1	–	.3	.2	120	.4	–	1.9	–	780	590	–
3	0	95	15	26	.1	1.5	0	–	.2	.1	17	.6	21	1.8	154	222	495	.6
0	0	58	8	9	.2	2.1	0	–	.1	.1	15	.3	49	1.9	246	293	89	.5
1	4	0	33	0	.1	0	0	.5	.6	1	19	5.8	28	7.4	135	134	3	.9
1	15	0	53	0	.4	0	0	1.5	.3	.5	41	4.7	166	7.6	415	486	6	3.5
–	–	–	–	60	–	–	4	–	.3	.5	200	1.5	–	2.9	–	300	630	–
1	–	35	–	80	–	–	–	–	.3	.5	200	2.5	–	3.8	280	350	500	–
–	–	–	–	100	–	–	6	–	.4	.5	160	1.5	–	3.8	–	350	950	–
–	–	–	–	40	–	–	6	–	.5	.5	360	1.5	–	3.8	–	320	850	–
–	–	–	–	60	–	–	6	–	.3	.4	160	1.5	–	3.8	–	340	650	–
–	–	–	–	100	–	–	6	–	.4	.5	160	1.5	–	3.8	–	300	880	–
–	–	–	–	80	–	–	6	–	.4	.6	160	1.5	–	3.8	–	340	840	–
–	–	–	–	250	–	–	4	–	.4	.5	280	1.5	–	3.8	–	230	830	–
0	0	15	0	40	0	0	1	–	0	0	24	0	0	0	0	–	105	0
–	–	0	–	–	–	–	0	–	0	0	240	0	–	0	–	170	2073	–
1	2	48	14	32	.3	1	0	–	.2	.2	63	1.3	10	1.6	82	79	292	.5
2	–	75	15	86	0	.2	0	–	.2	.1	65	1.1	11	1.1	76	87	311	.4
2	–	76	15	81	0	.2	0	–	.2	.1	64	1.1	11	1.1	76	86	311	.4
–	1	0	20	100	.2	0	0	–	.2	.2	0	1	0	1.9	16	–	170	0
1	–	0	0	56	0	0	0	–	0	0	2	.4	6	0	22	56	52	.1
1	–	0	0	0	0	0	0	–	0	0	1	0	1	0	1	10	11	0
1	–	0	0	35	0	0	0	–	0	0	1	0	1	.2	1	55	58	0
1	–	0	0	64	0	0	0	–	0	0	1	0	0	0	11	10	26	0

Code	Name	Amount	Unit	Grams	Energy (kcal)	Carbohydrates (g)	Protein (g)	Fat (g)	Saturated fat (g)	Monounsaturated fat (g)
41319	Frozen Dessert, Bordeaux Cherry–Healthy Choice	1	Cup	133.0	240	46	6	4	0	–
41320	Frozen Dessert, Butter Pecan Crunch–Healthy Choice	1	Cup	133.0	280	52	6	4	–	–
41321	Frozen Dessert, Chocolate Chip–Healthy Choice	1	Cup	133.0	260	48	6	4	0	–
41322	Frozen Dessert, Coffee Toffee–Healthy Choice	1	Cup	133.0	260	50	6	4	–	–
41323	Frozen Dessert, Cookies 'n Cream–Healthy Choice	1	Cup	133.0	260	48	8	4	0	–
41324	Frozen Dessert, Double Fudge Swirl–Healthy Choice	1	Cup	133.0	260	48	6	4	–	–
41325	Frozen Dessert, Fudge Brownie–Healthy Choice	1	Cup	133.0	280	54	6	4	0	–
41326	Frozen Dessert, Mint Chocolate Chip–Healthy Choice	1	Cup	133.0	280	50	6	4	0	–
41327	Frozen Dessert, Neapolitan–Healthy Choice	1	Cup	133.0	240	44	6	4	0	–
41328	Frozen Dessert, Praline and Caramel–Healthy Choice	1	Cup	133.0	260	52	6	4	0	–
41329	Frozen Dessert, Rocky Road–Healthy Choice	1	Cup	133.0	320	64	6	4	0	–
41330	Frozen Dessert, Vanilla–Healthy Choice	1	Cup	133.0	240	42	8	4	0	–
9100	Fruit cocktail, Hvy Syrup	½	Cup	127.5	93	24	0	0	0	0
9097	Fruit cocktail, Juice Pack	½	Cup	124.0	57	15	1	0	0	0
9099	Fruit cocktail, Lt Syrup	½	Cup	126.0	72	19	1	0	0	0
18319	Fruit Pie, Fried	1	Pie	128.0	404	55	4	21	3	10
14267	Fruit Punch Drink, Cnd	¾	Cup	185.8	87	22	0	0	0	0
9105	Fruit Salad, Hvy Syrup	½	Cup	127.5	93	24	0	0	0	0
9103	Fruit Salad, Juice Pack	½	Cup	124.5	62	16	1	0	0	0
9104	Fruit Salad, Lt Syrup	½	Cup	126.0	73	19	0	0	0	0
9102	Fruit Salad, Water Pack	½	Cup	122.5	37	10	0	0	0	0
9096	Fruit Water Pack	½	Cup	122.5	39	10	1	0	0	0
19263	Fruit and Juice Bars	1	Bar	77.0	63	16	1	0	–	–
9188	Fruit, Mixed, Dried	¼	Cup	37.5	91	24	1	0	0	0
9187	Fruit, Mixed, Hvy Syrup	½	Cup	127.5	92	24	0	0	0	0
19381	Fudge, Brown Sugar w/Nuts	1	Piece	14.0	55	11	0	1	0	0
19100	Fudge, Chocolate	1	Piece	17.0	65	14	0	1	1	0
19101	Fudge, Chocolate w/Nuts	1	Piece	19.0	81	14	1	3	1	1
19102	Fudge, Peanut Butter	1	Piece	16.0	59	13	1	1	0	0
19103	Fudge, Vanilla	1	Piece	16.0	59	13	0	1	1	0
19104	Fudge, Vanilla w/Nuts	1	Piece	15.0	62	11	0	2	1	0
16058	Garbanzo Beans, Cnd	½	Cup	120.0	143	27	6	1	0	0
41337	Garden Potato Casserole–Healthy Choice	1	Each	262.2	180	23	12	4	2	–
55774	Garden Tomato Heat'n Serve Soup–Stouffer's	1	Cup	283.9	110	16	4	3	–	–
41273	Garden Vegetable Soup–Healthy Choice	1	Each	212.6	100	18	3	1	–	–
62687	Gardenburger	1	Each	90.0	140	8	18	4	2	–
19215	Gelatin Pops	1	Each	44.0	31	7	1	0	–	–
14011	Gin and Tonic	1	Fl Oz	30.0	23	2	0	0	0	0
14136	Ginger Ale	12	Fl Oz	366.0	124	32	0	0	0	–
62532	Ginger Ale, Diet	12	Fl Oz	355.2	0	0	0	0	–	–
18172	Gingersnaps	1	Each	7.0	29	5	0	1	0	0
43399	Glazed Breast of Chicken, Top Shelf–Hormel	1	Each	283.5	170	19	19	2	1	1
55212	Glazed Chicken w/Veg. Lean Cuisine–Stouffer's	1	Each	241.0	250	24	21	7	2	–
41307	Glazed Chicken–Healthy Choice	1	Each	241.0	220	27	21	3	1	–
55784	Glazed Chicken–Stouffer's	1	Ounce	28.4	26	1	3	1	–	–
19105	Goobers	1	Piece	1.0	5	0	0	0	0	0
18173	Graham Crackers, Plain or Honey	1	Each	7.0	30	5	0	1	0	0
62684	Granola Bar, Low-Fat	1	Each	28.0	110	21	2	2	0	0
19016	Granola Bars, Hard, Almond	1	Each	28.4	140	18	2	7	4	2
19017	Granola Bars, Hard, Chocolate Chip	1	Each	28.4	124	20	2	5	3	1
19019	Granola Bars, Hard, Peanut	1	Each	28.4	136	18	3	6	1	2
19420	Granola Bars, Hard, Peanut Butter	1	Each	28.4	137	18	3	7	1	2
19015	Granola Bars, Hard, Plain	1	Each	28.4	134	18	3	6	1	1
19404	Granola Bars, Soft, Chocolate Chip	1	Each	28.4	119	20	2	5	3	1
19406	Granola Bars, Soft, Nut and Raisin	1	Each	28.4	129	18	2	6	3	1
19021	Granola Bars, Soft, Peanut Butter	1	Each	28.4	121	18	3	4	1	2

Polyunsaturated fat (g)	Dietary Fiber (g)	Cholesterol (mg)	Folate (µg)	Vitamin A (RE)	Vitamin B-6 (mg)	Vitamin B-12 (µg)	Vitamin C (mg)	Vitamin E (mg)	Riboflavin (mg)	Thiamin (mg)	Calcium (mg)	Iron (mg)	Magnesium (mg)	Niacin (mg)	Phosphorus (mg)	Potassium (mg)	Sodium (mg)	Zinc (mg)
2	–	10	–	–	–	–	–	–	.3	.1	160	–	–	–	200	300	100	–
2	–	10	–	–	–	–	2	–	.3	.1	160	–	–	–	160	300	160	–
2	–	10	–	–	–	–	2	–	.3	.1	160	.4	–	–	160	320	140	–
2	–	10	–	–	–	–	2	–	.3	.1	160	–	–	–	160	320	160	–
2	–	10	–	–	–	–	–	–	.3	.1	240	–	–	–	200	360	160	–
2	–	10	–	–	–	–	–	–	.3	.1	160	.8	–	–	200	420	140	–
2	–	10	–	–	–	–	–	–	.3	.1	160	.4	–	–	160	380	140	–
4	–	10	–	–	–	–	–	–	.3	.1	160	.4	–	–	–	340	160	–
2	–	10	–	–	–	–	–	–	.3	.1	160	–	–	–	200	320	120	–
2	–	10	–	–	–	–	–	–	.3	.1	160	–	–	–	200	320	140	–
2	–	10	–	–	–	–	–	–	.3	.1	160	–	–	–	200	380	140	–
2	–	10	–	–	–	–	–	–	.5	.1	240	–	–	–	200	360	120	–
0	1	0	3	26	.1	0	2	.4	0	0	8	.4	6	.5	14	112	8	.1
0	1	0	3	38	.1	0	3	.2	0	0	10	.3	9	.5	17	118	5	.1
0	1	0	3	26	.1	0	2	.4	0	0	8	.4	6	.5	14	112	8	.1
7	3	0	4	4	0	.1	2	–	.1	.2	28	1.6	13	1.8	55	83	479	.3
0	0	0	2	2	0	0	55	0	0	0	15	.4	4	0	2	46	41	.2
0	1	0	3	64	0	0	3	.6	0	0	8	.4	6	.4	11	102	8	.1
0	–	0	3	75	0	0	4	–	0	0	14	.3	10	.4	17	144	6	.2
0	–	0	3	54	0	0	3	–	0	0	9	.4	6	.5	11	103	8	.1
0	–	0	3	54	0	0	2	–	0	0	9	.4	6	.5	11	96	4	.1
0	1	0	3	31	.1	0	3	.4	0	0	6	.3	9	.4	13	115	5	.1
–	–	0	5	2	0	0	7	–	0	0	4	.1	3	.1	5	41	3	0
0	–	0	1	92	.1	0	1	–	.1	0	14	1	15	.7	29	299	7	.2
0	–	0	4	24	0	0	88	–	.1	0	1	.5	6	.8	13	107	5	.1
1	–	1	2	2	0	0	0	–	0	0	16	.3	7	0	12	52	14	.1
0	0	2	0	8	0	0	0	0	0	0	7	.1	4	0	10	18	11	.1
1	0	3	2	9	0	0	0	.1	0	0	10	.1	9	0	18	30	11	.1
0	–	1	2	2	0	0	0	–	0	0	7	0	4	.2	10	21	12	.1
0	0	3	0	8	0	0	0	0	0	0	6	0	1	0	5	8	11	0
1	0	2	2	7	0	0	0	.1	0	0	7	.1	4	0	11	17	9	.1
1	5	0	80	2	.6	0	5	–	0	0	38	1.6	35	.2	108	206	359	1.3
–	–	20	–	–	–	–	–	–	–	–	–	–	–	–	–	600	360	–
–	–	10	–	–	–	–	0	–	0	0	240	.3	–	.2	–	431	1052	–
–	–	0	–	350	–	–	9	–	.1	.1	16	.4	–	.8	–	230	560	–
1	5	0	–	0	–	–	0	–	–	.3	96	1.5	–	4	–	–	380	7.5
–	0	0	0	0	0	0	0	0	0	0	1	0	0	0	0	1	20	0
0	–	0	0	0	0	0	0	–	0	0	1	0	0	0	0	2	1	0
–	0	0	0	0	0	0	0	0	0	0	11	.7	4	0	0	4	26	.2
–	0	–	–	–	–	–	–	–	–	–	–	–	–	–	–	–	30	–
0	0	0	0	0	0	0	0	–	0	0	5	.4	3	.2	6	24	46	0
1	–	35	–	400	–	–	4	.8	.2	.1	32	.4	35	7.6	–	804	780	1.1
4	–	50	–	20	–	–	4	–	.2	.2	16	.2	–	7.6	–	580	590	–
1	–	45	–	–	–	–	1	–	.1	.2	–	.6	–	6.7	240	370	510	–
–	–	9	–	–	–	–	0	–	0	0	24	0	–	.2	–	45	105	–
0	–	0	0	0	0	0	0	–	0	0	1	0	1	.1	3	5	0	0
0	0	0	1	0	0	0	0	–	0	0	2	.3	2	.3	7	9	42	.1
0	1	0	0	0	0	0	0	–	0	0	0	.2	0	0	0	–	70	0
1	–	0	3	1	0	0	0	–	0	.1	9	.7	23	.2	65	77	73	.4
0	1	0	4	1	0	0	0	–	0	.1	22	.9	20	.2	58	71	98	.5
3	–	0	7	1	0	0	0	–	0	.1	11	.7	31	.4	85	86	79	.6
3	–	0	5	1	0	0	0	–	0	.1	12	.7	16	.6	39	82	80	.4
3	2	0	7	4	0	0	0	–	0	.1	17	.8	27	.4	79	95	83	.6
1	1	0	6	1	0	0	0	–	0	.1	26	.7	22	.3	65	96	77	.4
2	2	0	9	1	0	.1	0	–	.1	.1	24	.6	26	.7	68	111	72	.5
1	1	0	9	1	0	.1	0	–	0	.1	26	.6	24	.9	71	82	116	.5

Code	Name	Amount	Unit	Grams	Energy (kcal)	Carbohydrates (g)	Protein (g)	Fat (g)	Saturated fat (g)	Monounsatu fat (g)
19027	Granola Bars, Soft, Peanut Butter and Choc Chip	1	Each	28.4	122	18	3	6	2	2
19020	Granola Bars, Soft, Plain	1	Each	28.4	126	19	2	5	2	1
19022	Granola Bars, Soft, Raisin	1	Each	28.4	127	19	2	5	3	1
14277	Grape Drink, Cnd	¾	Cup	187.6	84	22	0	0	0	0
14282	Grape Juice Drink, Cnd	¾	Cup	187.6	94	24	0	0	0	0
9135	Grape Juice, Cnd or Bottled, Unsweetened	¾	Cup	189.4	116	28	1	0	0	0
14142	Grape Soda	12	Fl Oz	372.0	160	42	0	0	0	0
9124	Grapefruit Juice, Cnd, Sweetened	¾	Cup	187.0	86	21	1	0	0	0
9123	Grapefruit Juice, Cnd, Unsweetened	¾	Cup	185.2	70	17	1	0	0	0
9404	Grapefruit Juice, Pink, Fresh	¾	Cup	185.3	72	17	1	0	0	0
9128	Grapefruit Juice, White, Fresh	¾	Cup	185.3	72	17	1	0	0	0
9112	Grapefruit, Fresh, Pink&red	1	Medium	146.0	44	11	1	0	0	0
9116	Grapefruit, Fresh, White	1	Medium	136.0	45	11	1	0	0	0
9120	Grapefruit, Sections, Cnd, Juice Pack	¾	Cup	124.5	46	11	1	0	0	0
9121	Grapefruit, Sections, Cnd, Light Syrup Pack	¾	Cup	127.0	76	20	1	0	0	0
9131	Grapes, Fresh	¾	Cup	46.0	29	8	0	0	0	0
6114	Gravy, Au Jus, Cnd	¼	Cup	59.6	10	1	1	0	0	0
6116	Gravy, Beef, Cnd	¼	Cup	58.3	31	3	2	1	1	1
6119	Gravy, Chicken, Cnd	¼	Cup	59.6	47	3	1	3	1	2
6121	Gravy, Mushroom, Cnd	¼	Cup	59.6	30	3	1	2	0	1
6125	Gravy, Turkey, Cnd	¼	Cup	59.6	30	3	2	1	0	1
55172	Green Bean Mushroom Casserole–Stouffer's	1	Each	134.7	160	13	5	10	–	–
55118	Green Pepper Steak w/Rice–Stouffer's	1	Each	297.7	310	35	20	10	–	–
55780	Green Pepper Steak–Stouffer's	1	Ounce	28.4	28	1	3	1	–	–
62617	Grilled Salisbury Steak–Weight Watchers	1	Each	241.0	250	24	19	9	3	–
20030	Grits	½	Cup	80.0	58	11	1	1	0	0
15032	Grouper, Ckd, Dry Heat	3	Ounce	85.1	100	0	21	1	0	0
62534	Guava Juice	¾	Cup	179.9	66	16	–	0	–	–
19106	Gumdrops	1	Each	3.5	14	3	0	0	–	–
15034	Haddock, Ckd, Dry Heat	3	Ounce	85.1	95	0	21	1	0	0
15035	Haddock, Smoked	3	Ounce	85.1	99	0	21	1	0	0
15037	Halibut, Ckd, Dry Heat	3	Ounce	85.1	119	0	23	3	0	1
15196	Halibut, Greenland, Ckd, Dry Heat	3	Ounce	85.1	203	0	16	15	3	9
55159	Ham and Asparagus Bake–Stouffer's	1	Each	269.3	520	32	18	35	–	–
7032	Ham and Cheese Loaf(or Roll), Lunch Meat	1	Slice	28.4	73	0	5	6	2	3
7033	Ham and Cheese Spread, Lunch Meat	1	Tbsp.	15.0	37	0	2	3	1	1
7029	Ham, Approx 11% Fat, Sliced	1	Slice	28.4	52	1	5	3	1	1
7028	Ham, Extra Lean, Appx 5% Fat	1	Slice	28.4	37	0	5	1	0	1
62683	Hamburger Helper, Beef Noodle	1	Cup	220.0	260	23	4	11	4	0
62682	Hamburger Helper, Cheesy Italian	1	Cup	220.0	330	30	5	21	2	0
62681	Hamburger Helper, Chili Mac	1	Cup	220.0	290	30	3	16	4	0
62626	Hamburger Patty, Meatless	1	Each	90.0	140	8	18	4	2	–
55809	Heartland Medley–Stouffer's	1	Ounce	28.4	17	2	1	0	–	–
41279	Hearty Beef Soup–Healthy Choice	1	Each	212.6	120	17	9	1	–	–
41280	Hearty Chicken Soup–Healthy Choice	1	Each	212.6	110	17	7	2	–	–
41258	Herb Roasted Chicken–Healthy Choice	1	Each	347.3	300	50	22	5	2	–
15040	Herring, Ckd, Dry Heat	3	Ounce	85.1	173	0	20	10	2	4
15042	Herring, Kippered	3	Ounce	85.1	185	0	21	11	2	4
15197	Herring, Pacific, Ckd, Dry Heat	3	Ounce	85.1	213	0	18	15	4	7
15041	Herring, Pickled	3	Ounce	85.1	223	8	12	15	2	10
41311	Homestyle Turkey w/Vegetables–Healthy Choice	1	Each	269.3	260	34	26	2	–	–
20330	Hominy, Cnd, Yellow	½	Cup	80.0	58	11	1	1	0	0
19296	Honey	1	Tbsp.	21.0	64	17	0	0	–	–
55214	Honey Mustard Chicken, Lean Cuisine–Stouffer's	1	Each	212.6	230	30	18	4	1	–
41312	Honey Mustard Chicken–Healthy Choice	1	Each	269.3	310	41	26	4	1	–
43371	Hot Chili no Beans–Hormel	1	Each	212.6	360	14	16	27	11	13

Polyunsaturated fat (g)	Dietary Fiber (g)	Cholesterol (mg)	Folate (µg)	Vitamin A (RE)	Vitamin B-6 (mg)	Vitamin B-12 (µg)	Vitamin C (mg)	Vitamin E (mg)	Riboflavin (mg)	Thiamin (mg)	Calcium (mg)	Iron (mg)	Magnesium (mg)	Niacin (mg)	Phosphorus (mg)	Potassium (mg)	Sodium (mg)	Zinc (mg)
1	1	0	9	1	0	.1	0	–	0	0	23	.5	25	.9	74	107	93	.5
2	1	0	7	0	0	.1	0	–	0	.1	30	.7	21	.1	65	92	79	.4
1	1	0	6	0	0	.1	0	–	0	.1	29	.7	20	.3	62	103	80	.4
0	0	0	1	0	0	0	64	0	0	0	6	.3	4	0	2	9	11	.2
0	0	0	2	0	0	0	30	0	0	0	6	.2	8	.2	8	66	2	.1
0	0	0	5	2	.1	0	0	0	.1	0	17	.5	19	.5	21	250	6	.1
0	0	0	0	0	0	0	0	0	0	0	11	.3	4	0	0	4	56	.3
0	0	0	19	0	0	0	50	.1	0	.1	15	.7	19	.6	21	303	4	.1
0	0	0	19	2	0	0	54	.1	0	.1	13	.4	19	.4	20	283	2	.2
0	–	0	19	82	.1	0	70	–	0	.1	17	.4	22	.4	28	300	2	.1
0	0	0	19	2	.1	0	70	.1	0	.1	17	.4	22	.4	28	300	2	.1
0	–	0	18	38	.1	0	56	–	0	0	16	.2	12	.3	13	188	0	.1
0	1	0	14	1	.1	0	45	.3	0	.1	16	.1	12	.4	11	201	0	.1
0	0	0	11	0	0	0	42	.3	0	0	19	.3	14	.3	15	210	9	.1
0	1	0	11	0	0	0	27	.3	0	0	18	.5	13	.3	13	164	3	.1
0	1	0	2	5	.1	0	2	.2	0	0	6	.1	2	.1	5	88	1	0
0	–	0	1	0	0	.1	1	–	0	0	2	.4	1	.5	18	48	30	.6
0	0	2	1	0	0	.1	0	0	0	0	3	.4	1	.4	17	47	326	.6
1	0	1	1	66	0	.1	0	.1	0	0	12	.3	1	.3	17	65	344	.5
1	0	0	7	0	0	0	0	0	0	0	4	.4	1	.4	9	63	340	.4
0	0	1	1	0	0	.1	0	0	0	0	2	.4	1	.8	17	65	344	.5
–	–	–	–	40	–	–	2	–	.2	.1	64	.2	–	.4	–	200	550	–
–	–	–	–	40	–	–	6	–	.2	.2	16	1	–	3.8	–	410	700	–
–	–	7	–	–	–	–	4	–	0	0	48	0	–	.1	–	51	164	–
–	4	30	–	60	–	–	0	–	–	–	120	1.5	–	–	–	450	590	–
0	2	0	1	0	0	0	0	–	0	0	8	.5	13	0	28	7	168	.8
0	0	40	9	43	.3	.6	0	–	0	.1	18	1	31	.3	122	404	45	.4
–	–	0	–	0	–	–	30	–	–	–	0	0	–	–	–	–	18	–
–	0	0	0	0	0	0	0	0	0	0	0	0	0	0	0	0	2	0
0	0	63	11	16	.3	1.2	0	–	0	0	36	1.1	43	3.9	205	339	74	.4
0	0	65	13	19	.3	1.4	0	.3	0	0	42	1.2	46	4.3	213	353	649	.4
1	0	35	12	46	.3	1.2	0	–	.1	.1	51	.9	91	6.1	242	490	59	.5
1	0	50	1	15	.4	.8	0	–	.1	.1	3	.7	28	1.6	179	293	88	.4
–	–	–	–	60	–	–	36	–	.5	.5	160	.8	–	2.9	–	360	1100	–
1	0	16	1	7	.1	.2	7	.1	.1	.2	16	.3	5	1	72	83	381	.6
0	0	9	0	14	0	.1	1	–	0	0	33	.1	3	.3	74	24	180	.3
0	0	16	1	0	.1	.2	8	.1	.1	.2	2	.3	5	1.5	70	94	373	.6
0	0	13	1	0	.1	.2	7	.1	.1	.3	2	.2	5	1.4	62	99	405	.5
0	1	5	0	60	0	0	0	–	.2	.2	24	1	0	3.8	0	240	900	0
0	1	5	0	60	0	0	0	–	.3	.3	120	1.5	0	3.8	0	400	900	0
0	1	4	0	200	0	0	0	–	.3	.3	24	1.5	0	4.8	0	–	900	0
1	5	0	–	0	–	–	0	–	–	.3	96	1.5	–	4	–	–	380	7.5
–	–	3	–	–	–	–	1	–	0	0	40	0	–	.1	–	60	85	–
–	–	20	–	150	–	–	9	–	.1	.1	32	.4	–	1.9	90	280	540	–
–	–	25	–	200	–	–	2	–	.2	.1	32	.4	–	1.9	90	190	520	–
1	–	40	–	250	–	–	24	–	.1	.2	32	.8	–	7.6	280	370	560	–
2	0	65	10	26	.3	11.2	1	1.1	.3	.1	63	1.2	35	3.5	258	356	98	1.1
2	0	70	12	33	.4	15.9	1	.9	.3	.1	71	1.3	39	3.7	276	380	781	1.2
3	0	84	5	30	.4	8.2	0	–	.2	.1	90	1.2	35	2.4	248	461	81	.6
1	0	11	2	219	.1	3.6	0	.9	.1	0	65	1	7	2.8	76	59	740	.5
–	–	30	–	100	–	–	5	–	.1	0	32	–	–	–	–	100	550	–
0	–	0	1	9	0	0	0	–	0	0	8	.5	13	0	28	7	168	.8
–	0	0	0	0	0	0	0	0	0	0	1	.1	0	0	1	11	1	0
1	–	40	–	200	–	–	2	–	.2	.2	16	.4	–	3.8	–	340	540	–
–	–	45	–	100	–	–	4	–	0	.2	16	.8	–	1.5	–	110	520	–
1	–	60	–	330	–	–	–	10.6	.2	0	40	1.4	35	2.5	–	497	860	2.7

Code	Name	Amount	Unit	Grams	Energy (kcal)	Carbohydrates (g)	Protein (g)	Fat (g)	Saturated fat (g)	Monounsat fat (g)
43410	Hot Chili w/Beans, Micro Cup–Hormel	1	Each	209.1	250	24	15	11	4	4
43372	Hot Chili w/Beans–Hormel	1	Each	212.6	300	27	15	15	5	6
7022	Hot Dog, Beef	1	Each	57.0	180	1	7	16	7	8
7024	Hot Dog, Chicken	1	Each	45.0	116	3	6	9	2	4
62605	Hot Dog, Fat Free	1	Each	50.0	40	2	7	0	0	0
7025	Hot Dog, Turkey	1	Each	45.0	102	1	6	8	3	3
16137	Hummus, Fresh	½	Cup	123.0	210	25	6	10	2	4
18270	Hush Puppies	1	Each	22.0	74	10	2	3	0	1
18271	Ice Cream Cones, Cake or Wafer–type	1½	Each	6.0	25	5	0	0	0	0
18272	Ice Cream Cones, Sugar, Rolled–type	1½	Each	15.0	60	13	1	1	0	0
62640	Ice Cream Sandwich	1	Each	63.0	170	27	3	6	3	–
19270	Ice Cream, Chocolate	1½	Cup	198.0	428	56	8	22	13	6
19090	Ice Cream, French Vanilla, Soft–serve	1½	Cup	199.5	429	44	8	26	15	7
19271	Ice Cream, Strawberry	1½	Cup	198.0	380	55	6	17	–	–
19095	Ice Cream, Vanilla	1½	Cup	198.0	398	47	7	22	13	6
19089	Ice Cream, Vanilla, Rich	1½	Cup	199.5	481	45	7	32	20	9
19088	Ice Milk, Vanilla	½	Cup	66.5	92	15	3	3	2	1
19096	Ice Milk, Vanilla, Soft Serve	½	Cup	66.5	84	14	3	2	1	1
19283	Ice Pops	1	Bar	52.0	37	10	0	0	–	–
19717	Ice Pops, w/Added Ascorbic Acid	1	Bar	52.0	37	10	0	0	–	–
62547	Iced Tea, Bottled, All Flavors	1	Cup	236.6	118	29	0	0	0	–
62548	Iced Tea, Bottled, All Flavors, Diet	1	Cup	236.6	0	1	0	0	0	–
62622	Italian Cheese Lasagna–Weight Watchers	1	Each	311.9	300	28	29	8	3	–
43395	Italian Lasagna, Top Shelf–Hormel	1	Each	283.5	350	30	23	16	8	5
55798	Italian Style Vegetables–Stouffer's	1	Ounce	28.4	10	2	0	0	–	–
19297	Jams and Preserves	1	Tbsp.	20.0	48	13	0	0	0	0
19300	Jellies	1	Tbsp.	19.0	51	13	0	0	–	–
19173	Jello	½	Cup	135.0	80	19	2	0	–	–
19108	Jellybeans	1	Each	1.1	4	1	0	0	–	–
19109	Kit Kat Wafer Bar	1	Bar	46.0	235	28	3	13	8	4
9148	Kiwifruit, Fresh	1	Medium	76.0	46	11	1	0	–	–
62643	Kool–Aid	8	Fl Oz	236.6	60	16	–	–	–	–
19110	Krackel Chocolate Bar	1	Bar	47.0	236	29	3	13	6	3
17225	Lamb, Ground, Ckd, Broiled	3	Ounce	85.1	241	0	21	17	7	7
17018	Lamb, Leg, Shank, Meat Only, Ckd, Rstd	3	Ounce	85.1	153	0	24	6	2	2
17016	Lamb, Leg, Shank, Meat and Fat, Ckd, Rstd	3	Ounce	85.1	191	0	22	11	4	4
17022	Lamb, Leg, Sirloin, Meat Only, Ckd, Rstd	3	Ounce	85.1	174	0	24	8	3	3
17020	Lamb, Leg, Sirloin, Meat and Fat, Ckd, Rstd	3	Ounce	85.1	248	0	21	18	7	7
17014	Lamb, Leg, Whole, Meat Only, Ckd, Rstd	3	Ounce	85.1	162	0	24	7	2	3
17012	Lamb, Leg, Whole, Meat and Fat, Ckd, Rstd	3	Ounce	85.1	219	0	22	14	6	6
17027	Lamb, Loin, Meat Only, Ckd, Broiled	3	Ounce	85.1	184	0	26	8	3	4
17028	Lamb, Loin, Meat Only, Ckd, Roasted	3	Ounce	85.1	172	0	23	8	3	3
17024	Lamb, Loin, Meat and Fat, Ckd, Broiled	3	Ounce	85.1	269	0	21	20	8	8
17025	Lamb, Loin, Meat and Fat, Ckd, Roasted	3	Ounce	85.1	263	0	19	20	9	8
17004	Lamb, Meat Only, Ckd	3	Ounce	85.1	175	0	24	8	3	4
17002	Lamb, Meat and Fat, Ckd	3	Ounce	85.1	250	0	21	18	8	8
17033	Lamb, Rib, Meat Only, Ckd, Broiled	3	Ounce	85.1	200	0	24	11	4	4
17034	Lamb, Rib, Meat Only, Ckd, Roasted	3	Ounce	85.1	197	0	22	11	4	5
17030	Lamb, Rib, Meat and Fat, Ckd, Broiled	3	Ounce	85.1	307	0	19	25	11	10
17031	Lamb, Rib, Meat and Fat, Ckd, Roasted	3	Ounce	85.1	305	0	18	25	11	11
4002	Lard	¼	Cup	51.3	462	0	0	51	20	23
62613	Lasagna Florentine–Weight Watchers	1	Each	283.5	210	37	13	2	1	–
55215	Lasagna w/Meat Sauce, Lean Cuisine–Stouffer's	1	Each	290.6	280	36	20	6	3	–
41308	Lasagna w/Meat Sauce–Healthy Choice	1	Each	283.5	260	37	18	5	2	–
62623	Lasagna with Meat Sauce–Weight Watchers	1	Each	290.6	290	34	24	7	3	–
43403	Lasagna, Micro Cup–Hormel	1	Each	212.6	250	25	8	13	6	4

Polyunsaturated fat (g)	Dietary Fiber (g)	Cholesterol (mg)	Folate (µg)	Vitamin A (RE)	Vitamin B-6 (mg)	Vitamin B-12 (µg)	Vitamin C (mg)	Vitamin E (mg)	Riboflavin (mg)	Thiamin (mg)	Calcium (mg)	Iron (mg)	Magnesium (mg)	Niacin (mg)	Phosphorus (mg)	Potassium (mg)	Sodium (mg)	Zinc (mg)
–	–	49	–	190	–	–	–	2	.2	.1	48	1.9	46	1.7	–	677	977	2.7
1	–	55	–	210	–	–	–	0	.2	.1	48	1.8	49	1.7	–	777	1030	2.3
1	0	35	2	0	.1	.9	14	.1	.1	0	11	.8	2	1.4	50	95	585	1.2
2	0	45	2	17	.1	.1	0	.1	.1	0	43	.9	5	1.4	48	38	617	.5
0	0	15	–	0	–	–	0	–	–	–	0	.2	–	–	–	–	460	–
2	0	48	4	0	.1	.1	0	.3	.1	0	48	.8	6	1.9	60	81	642	1.4
4	6	0	73	2	.5	0	10	1.2	.1	.1	61	1.9	36	.5	138	214	300	1.4
2	1	10	4	9	0	0	0	–	.1	.1	61	.7	5	.6	42	32	147	.1
0	0	0	0	0	0	0	0	–	0	0	2	.2	2	.3	6	7	9	0
0	1	0	1	0	0	0	0	–	.1	.1	7	.7	5	.8	15	22	48	.1
–	1	10	0	20	0	0	0	–	0	0	48	.4	0	0	0	–	140	0
1	–	67	32	236	.1	.6	1	–	.4	.1	216	1.8	57	.4	212	493	150	1.1
1	–	182	18	307	.1	1	2	–	.4	.1	261	.4	24	.2	231	353	122	1
–	–	57	24	154	.1	.6	15	–	.5	.1	238	.4	28	.3	198	372	119	.7
1	0	87	10	232	.1	.8	1	0	.5	.1	253	.2	28	.2	208	394	158	1.4
1	0	122	10	367	.1	.7	1	0	.3	.1	233	.1	22	.2	189	317	112	.8
0	0	9	4	31	0	.4	1	0	.2	0	92	.1	10	.1	72	140	57	.3
0	0	8	4	19	0	.3	1	0	.1	0	104	0	9	.1	80	147	47	.4
–	0	0	0	0	0	0	0	0	0	0	0	0	1	0	0	2	6	0
–	–	0	0	0	0	0	6	–	0	0	0	0	1	0	0	2	6	0
–	0	0	–	0	–	–	0	–	–	–	0	0	–	–	–	–	10	–
–	0	0	–	0	–	–	0	–	–	–	0	0	–	–	–	–	0	–
–	7	25	–	350	–	–	15	–	–	–	780	1.5	–	–	–	720	560	–
1	–	60	–	100	–	–	2	.7	.5	.3	240	1.5	49	3.8	–	728	840	3.2
–	–	0	–	–	–	–	2	–	0	0	72	0	–	0	–	62	147	–
0	0	0	7	0	0	0	2	0	0	0	4	.1	1	0	2	15	8	0
–	0	0	0	0	0	0	0	0	0	0	2	0	1	0	1	12	7	0
–	0	0	0	0	0	0	0	0	0	0	3	0	1	0	30	1	57	0
–	0	0	0	0	0	0	0	0	0	0	0	0	0	0	0	0	0	0
0	0	12	0	14	0	.3	1	.4	.1	0	83	.4	20	.2	80	142	46	.5
–	3	0	–	14	–	0	74	.9	0	0	20	.3	23	.4	30	252	4	–
–	–	–	0	0	0	0	6	–	0	0	0	0	0	0	0	–	–	0
3	–	9	4	6	0	.3	0	–	.1	0	84	.4	26	.2	104	161	64	.6
1	0	82	16	0	.1	2.2	–	.2	.2	.1	19	1.5	20	5.7	171	288	69	4
0	0	74	20	0	.1	2.3	0	.2	.2	.1	7	1.8	22	5.4	177	291	56	4.3
1	0	77	19	0	.1	2.3	0	.1	.2	.1	9	1.7	21	5.6	168	277	55	4
1	0	78	18	0	.1	2.2	0	.1	.3	.1	7	1.9	21	5.3	173	283	60	4.1
1	0	82	14	0	.1	2.2	0	.1	.2	.1	9	1.7	19	5.6	156	256	58	3.5
0	0	76	20	0	.1	2.2	0	.2	.2	.1	7	1.8	22	5.4	175	287	58	4.2
1	0	79	17	0	.1	2.2	0	.1	.2	.1	9	1.7	20	5.6	162	266	56	3.7
1	0	81	20	0	.1	2.1	0	.1	.2	.1	16	1.7	24	5.8	192	320	71	3.5
1	0	74	21	0	.1	1.8	0	.1	.2	.1	14	2.1	23	5.8	175	227	56	3.5
1	0	85	15	0	.1	2.1	0	.1	.2	.1	17	1.5	20	6	167	278	65	3
2	0	81	16	0	.1	1.9	0	.1	.2	.1	15	1.8	20	6	153	209	54	2.9
1	0	78	20	0	.1	2.2	0	.2	.2	.1	13	1.7	22	5.4	179	293	65	4.5
1	0	82	15	0	.1	2.2	0	–	.2	.1	14	1.6	20	5.7	160	264	61	3.8
1	0	77	18	0	.1	2.2	0	.2	.2	.1	14	1.9	25	5.6	181	266	72	4.5
1	0	75	19	0	.1	1.8	0	.1	.2	.1	18	1.5	20	5.2	166	268	69	3.8
2	0	84	12	0	.1	2.2	0	.1	.2	.1	16	1.6	20	6	151	230	65	3.4
2	0	82	13	0	.1	1.9	0	.1	.2	.1	19	1.4	17	5.7	141	230	62	3
6	0	49	0	0	0	0	0	.6	0	0	0	0	0	0	0	0	0	.1
–	5	10	–	300	–	–	15	–	–	–	300	1.5	–	–	–	440	420	–
–	–	25	–	100	–	–	6	–	.3	.2	120	1	–	2.9	–	700	560	–
1	–	20	–	150	–	–	2	–	.3	.3	80	1.5	–	1.9	210	500	420	–
–	7	15	–	250	–	–	12	–	–	–	480	1.5	–	–	–	720	580	–
2	–	23	–	100	–	–	2	–	.2	.1	40	.8	25	1.9	–	331	949	1.1

Code	Name	Amount	Unit	Grams	Energy (kcal)	Carbohydrates (g)	Protein (g)	Fat (g)	Saturated fat (g)	Monounsatur- fat (g)
55134	Lasagna–Stouffer's	1	Each	283.5	340	40	18	12	–	–
11247	Leeks, Ckd	½	Cup	52.0	16	4	0	0	0	0
11246	Leeks, Fresh	½	Cup	52.0	32	7	1	0	0	0
18320	Lemon Meringue Pie	1	Slice	113.0	303	53	2	10	2	4
41259	Lemon Pepper Fish–Healthy Choice	1	Each	304.8	300	52	13	5	1	–
18445	Lemon Pie, Fried	1	Pie	128.0	404	55	4	21	3	10
19380	Lemon Pudding	1	Cup	298.1	373	75	0	9	1	4
14145	Lemon–lime Soda	12	Fl Oz	368.4	147	38	0	0	0	0
62529	Lemon–lime Soda, Diet	12	Fl Oz	355.2	0	0	0	0	–	–
14297	Lemonade Flavor Drink	1	Cup	266.0	112	29	0	0	0	0
14543	Lemonade, Pink	1	Cup	247.8	99	26	0	0	0	0
14290	Lemonade, Low Calorie	1	Cup	243.7	5	1	0	0	0	–
14293	Lemonade, White	1	Cup	247.8	99	26	0	0	0	0
9150	Lemons, Fresh, w/o Peel	1	Medium	58.0	17	5	1	0	0	0
41274	Lentil Soup–Healthy Choice	1	Each	212.6	140	23	8	1	–	–
11250	Lettuce, Butterhead, Fresh	1	Cup	56.0	7	1	1	0	0	0
11252	Lettuce, Iceberg, Fresh	1	Cup	56.0	7	1	1	0	0	0
11253	Lettuce, Looseleaf, Fresh	1	Cup	56.0	10	2	1	0	0	0
11251	Lettuce, Romaine, Fresh	1	Cup	56.0	9	1	1	0	0	0
55216	Linguini w/Clam Sauce, Lean Cuisine–Stouffer's	1	Each	272.9	280	36	17	8	2	–
14415	Liqueur, Coffee w/Cream, 34 Proof	1	Fl Oz	31.1	102	6	1	5	3	1
14414	Liqueur, Coffee, 53 Proof	1	Fl Oz	34.8	117	16	0	0	0	0
15148	Lobster, Northern, Ckd, Moist Heat	3	Ounce	85.1	83	1	17	1	0	0
15228	Lobster, Spiny, Ckd, Moist Heat	3	Ounce	85.1	122	3	22	2	0	0
19107	Lollipop	1	Each	6.0	22	6	0	0	–	–
19140	M&M's Peanut	1	Pkg	49.0	243	29	5	13	–	–
19141	M&M's Plain	1	Pkg	48.0	228	33	3	11	–	–
62667	M&M's, Almond	1	Pkg	42.0	230	25	4	13	4	0
12131	Macadamias, Dried	½	Cup	67.0	470	9	6	49	7	39
12633	Macadamias, Oil Roasted	½	Cup	67.0	481	9	5	51	8	40
55217	Macaroni and Beef in Sauce, Lean Cuisine–Stouffer's	1	Each	283.5	250	35	14	6	1	–
55137	Macaroni and Beef w/Tomatoes–Stouffer's	1	Each	326.0	340	38	21	12	–	–
41338	Macaroni and Beef–Healthy Choice	1	Each	241.0	200	32	12	3	1	–
62533	Macaroni and Cheese	1	Cup	111.9	360	44	7	13	8	–
57808	Macaroni and Cheese Pot Pie–Swanson	1	Each	198.5	200	24	7	8	–	–
55218	Macaroni and Cheese, Lean Cuisine–Stouffer's	1	Each	255.1	290	37	15	9	4	–
43406	Macaroni and Cheese, Micro Cup–Hormel	1	Each	212.6	260	28	12	11	6	3
41339	Macaroni and Cheese–Healthy Choice	1	Each	255.1	280	45	12	6	3	–
55155	Macaroni and Cheese–Stouffer's	1	Each	170.1	250	23	11	13	–	–
62624	Macaroni and Cheese–Weight Watchers	1	Each	255.2	260	43	15	6	2	–
20100	Macaroni, Ckd, Enriched	1	Cup	140.0	197	40	7	1	0	0
20400	Macaroni, Ckd, Unenriched	1	Cup	140.0	197	40	7	1	0	0
20106	Macaroni, Vegetable, Ckd, Enriched	1	Cup	134.0	172	36	6	0	0	0
20108	Macaroni, Whole–wheat, Ckd	1	Cup	140.0	174	37	7	1	0	0
41309	Mandarin Chicken–Healthy Choice	1	Each	311.8	260	39	23	2	–	–
62535	Mango Juice	¾	Cup	179.9	66	16	–	0	–	–
9176	Mangos, Fresh	½	Cup	82.5	54	14	0	0	0	0
4128	Margarine, Imitation (appx 40% Fat)	1	Tsp.	4.8	17	0	0	2	0	1
4132	Margarine, Regular, w/Salt Added	1	Tsp.	4.7	34	0	0	4	1	2
4131	Margarine, Regular, w/o Added Salt	1	Tsp.	4.7	34	0	0	4	1	2
4130	Margarine, Soft, w/Salt Added	1	Tsp.	4.7	34	0	0	4	1	1
4129	Margarine, Soft, w/o Added Salt	1	Tsp.	4.7	34	0	0	4	1	2
62645	Margarita Mix, Liquid	1	Fl Oz	29.6	29	5	0	0	–	–
11256	Marinara Sauce	½	Cup	125.0	85	13	2	4	1	2
55830	Marinara Sauce–Stouffer's	1	Cup	283.9	180	18	3	11	–	–
19303	Marmalade, Orange	1	Tbsp.	20.0	49	13	0	0	–	–

Polyunsaturated fat (g)	Dietary Fiber (g)	Cholesterol (mg)	Folate (µg)	Vitamin A (RE)	Vitamin B-6 (mg)	Vitamin B-12 (µg)	Vitamin C (mg)	Vitamin E (mg)	Riboflavin (mg)	Thiamin (mg)	Calcium (mg)	Iron (mg)	Magnesium (mg)	Niacin (mg)	Phosphorus (mg)	Potassium (mg)	Sodium (mg)	Zinc (mg)
–	–	–	–	150	–	–	6	–	.3	.2	200	1	–	6.7	–	570	840	–
0	–	0	13	3	.1	0	2	–	0	0	16	.6	7	.1	9	45	5	0
0	1	0	33	5	.1	0	6	.5	0	0	31	1.1	15	.2	18	94	10	.1
3	1	51	9	59	0	.2	4	–	.2	.1	63	.7	17	.7	119	101	165	.6
2	–	40	–	80	–	–	48	–	.1	.2	32	.6	–	1.1	180	410	370	–
	–	–	4	4	0	.1	0	–	.1	.2	28	1.6	13	1.8	55	83	479	.3
3	–	0	0	0	0	0	0	–	0	0	6	.2	3	0	15	3	417	.1
0	0	0	0	0	0	0	0	0	0	0	7	.3	4	.1	0	4	41	.2
–	0	–	–	–	–	–	–	–	–	–	–	–	–	–	–	–	30	–
0	–	0	0	0	0	0	34	–	0	0	29	.1	3	0	3	3	19	.1
0	–	0	5	0	0	0	10	–	.1	0	7	.4	5	0	5	37	7	.1
–	0	0	0	0	0	0	6	0	0	0	5	.1	2	0	24	0	7	.1
0	–	0	5	5	0	0	10	–	.1	0	7	.4	5	0	5	37	7	.1
0	2	0	6	2	0	0	31	.1	0	0	15	.3	5	.1	9	80	1	0
–	–	0	–	60	–	–	2	–	0	.1	–	.6	–	.4	–	160	480	–
0	1	0	41	54	0	0	4	.2	0	0	18	.2	7	.2	13	144	3	.1
0	1	0	31	18	0	0	2	.1	0	0	11	.3	5	.1	11	88	5	.1
0	1	0	28	106	0	0	10	.2	0	0	38	.8	6	.2	14	148	5	.2
0	1	0	76	146	0	0	13	.2	.1	.1	20	.6	3	.3	25	162	4	.1
2	–	30	–	–	–	–	–	–	.2	.3	32	1.5	–	1.9	–	90	560	–
0	0	5	0	13	0	0	0	0	0	0	5	0	1	0	16	10	29	0
0	0	0	0	0	0	0	0	0	0	0	0	0	1	.1	2	10	3	0
0	0	61	9	22	.1	2.6	0	.9	.1	0	52	.3	30	.9	157	299	323	2.5
1	0	77	1	5	.1	3.4	2	–	0	0	54	1.2	43	4.2	195	177	193	6.2
–	0	0	0	0	0	0	0	0	0	0	0	0	0	0	0	0	2	0
–	2	6	27	4	.1	.2	0	2.7	.1	0	65	.7	40	1.6	134	191	46	.7
–	1	7	4	12	0	.2	0	.6	.1	0	81	.7	32	.3	94	188	49	.6
0	2	5	0	0	0	0	0	–	0	0	72	.4	0	0	0	–	20	0
1	6	0	11	0	.1	0	0	.3	.1	.2	47	1.6	78	1.4	91	247	3	1.1
1	6	0	11	1	.1	0	0	.3	.1	.1	30	1.2	78	1.4	134	220	174	.7
1	–	25	–	100	–	–	4	–	.2	.2	48	1.5	–	2.9	–	450	540	–
–	–	–	–	60	–	–	6	–	.1	.1	32	.8	–	1.9	–	300	1440	–
–	–	15	–	200	–	–	15	–	.3	.3	32	1	–	0	–	530	420	–
–	16	40	–	100	–	–	0	–	–	–	240	1.5	–	–	–	–	1029	–
–	–	–	–	80	–	–	–	–	.2	.1	120	.6	–	.8	–	–	740	–
–	–	30	–	–	–	–	–	–	.4	.3	200	.8	–	1.5	–	160	550	–
1	–	45	–	80	–	–	6	0	.3	.1	80	.6	25	1.1	–	209	650	1.1
1	–	20	–	–	–	–	–	–	.3	.3	120	1	–	1.1	230	220	520	–
–	–	–	–	20	–	–	–	–	.3	.2	160	.4	–	.4	–	140	640	–
–	7	20	–	100	–	–	0	–	–	–	300	1	–	–	–	410	550	–
0	2	0	10	0	0	0	0	0	.1	.3	10	2	25	2.3	76	43	1	.7
0	2	0	10	–	0	0	0	0	0	0	10	.7	25	.6	76	43	1	.7
0	6	0	8	7	0	0	0	.1	.1	.2	15	.7	25	1.4	67	42	8	.6
0	6	0	7	0	.1	0	0	.1	.1	.2	21	1.5	42	1	125	62	4	1.1
–	–	50	–	250	–	–	9	–	.2	.2	16	1	–	4.8	200	400	400	–
–	–	0	–	0	–	–	30	–	–	–	0	0	–	–	–	–	18	–
0	1	0	–	321	.1	0	23	.9	0	0	8	.1	7	.5	9	129	2	0
1	0	0	0	48	0	0	0	.1	0	0	1	0	0	0	1	1	46	0
1	0	0	0	47	0	0	0	.6	0	0	1	0	0	0	1	2	44	0
1	0	0	0	47	0	0	0	.6	0	0	1	0	0	0	1	1	0	0
2	0	0	0	47	0	0	0	.6	0	0	1	0	0	0	1	2	51	0
1	0	0	0	47	0	0	0	.4	0	0	1	0	0	0	1	2	1	0
–	0	–	0	0	0	0	0	–	0	0	0	0	0	0	0	–	12	0
1	–	0	17	120	.3	0	16	–	.1	.1	22	1	30	2	44	530	786	.3
–	–	0	–	–	–	–	66	–	0	0	0	.2	–	.4	–	681	1222	–
–	0	0	7	1	0	0	1	0	0	0	8	0	0	0	1	7	11	0

Code	Name	Amount	Unit	Grams	Energy (kcal)	Carbohydrates (g)	Protein (g)	Fat (g)	Saturated fat (g)	Monounsat... fat (g)
19116	Marshmallows	1	Cup	46.0	146	37	1	0	–	–
14014	Martini	1	Fl Oz	28.2	63	0	0	0	0	0
4018	Mayonnaise	1	Tbsp.	14.7	57	4	0	5	1	1
62610	Mayonnaise, Fat Free	1	Tbsp.	15.0	10	3	0	0	0	–
62609	Mayonnaise, Light	1	Tbsp.	15.0	25	1	0	2	0	–
55219	Meatloaf w/Mac. and Cheese, Lean Cuisine–Stouffer's	1	Each	265.8	280	26	26	8	3	–
41260	Meatloaf–Healthy Choice	1	Each	340.2	340	48	17	8	3	–
55779	Meatloaf–Stouffer's	1	Ounce	28.4	57	2	4	3	–	–
9185	Melon Balls, Frozen, Unthawed	½	Cup	86.5	29	7	1	0	–	–
9181	Melons, Cantaloupe, Fresh	1	Wedge	80.0	28	7	1	0	–	–
9183	Melons, Casaba, Fresh	1	Wedge	164.0	43	10	1	0	–	–
9184	Melons, Honeydew, Fresh	1	Wedge	129.0	45	12	1	0	–	–
55812	Mexicali Chicken–Stouffer's	1	Ounce	28.4	20	2	1	1	–	–
19120	Milk Chocolate	1	Bar	44.0	226	26	3	13	8	4
19126	Milk Chocolate Coated Peanuts	1	Ounce	28.4	147	14	4	9	4	4
19127	Milk Chocolate Coated Raisins	1	Ounce	28.4	111	19	1	4	2	1
19132	Milk Chocolate w/Almonds	1	Bar	41.0	216	22	4	14	7	6
1110	Milk Shakes, Thick Chocolate	1½	Cup	518.2	615	110	16	14	9	4
1111	Milk Shakes, Thick Vanilla	1½	Cup	518.2	579	92	20	16	10	5
1075	Milk Substitutes, Fluid w/hydr Vegetable Oils	1	Cup	244.0	150	15	4	8	2	5
1076	Milk Substitutes, Fluid, w/lauric Acid Oil	1	Cup	244.0	150	15	4	8	7	0
1088	Milk, Buttermilk	1	Cup	245.0	99	12	8	2	1	1
1104	Milk, Chocolate Drink, Lowfat, 1% Fat	1	Cup	250.0	158	26	8	2	2	1
1103	Milk, Chocolate Drink, Lowfat, 2% Fat	1	Cup	250.0	179	26	8	5	3	1
1102	Milk, Chocolate Drink, Whole	1	Cup	250.0	208	26	8	8	5	2
1105	Milk, Chocolate Homemade Hot Cocoa	1	Cup	250.0	218	26	9	9	6	3
1095	Milk, Cnd, Condensed, Sweetened	¼	Cup	76.3	245	42	6	7	4	2
1153	Milk, Cnd, Evaporated	¼	Cup	63.0	85	6	4	5	3	1
1097	Milk, Cnd, Evaporated, Skim	¼	Cup	63.8	50	7	5	0	0	0
1082	Milk, Lowfat, 1% Fat	1	Cup	244.0	102	12	8	3	2	1
1079	Milk, Lowfat, 2% Fat	1	Cup	244.0	121	12	8	5	3	1
1099	Milk, Malted, Beverage	1	Cup	265.0	236	27	10	10	6	3
1085	Milk, Skim	1	Cup	245.0	86	12	8	0	0	0
1077	Milk, Whole, 3.3% Fat	1	Cup	244.0	150	11	8	8	5	2
1078	Milk, Whole, 3.7% Fat	1	Cup	244.0	157	11	8	9	6	3
19135	Milky Way Bar	1	Bar	60.0	251	44	3	9	5	3
18322	Mince Meat Pie	1	Slice	165.0	477	79	4	18	4	8
55770	Minestrone Heat'n Serve Soup–Stouffer's	1	Cup	283.9	130	18	5	4	–	–
41281	Minestrone Soup–Healthy Choice	1	Each	212.6	160	30	6	1	–	–
55760	Minestrone Soup–Stouffer's	1	Cup	283.9	140	20	6	3	–	–
12635	Mixed w/Peanuts, Dry Roasted	½	Cup	68.5	407	17	12	35	5	22
12637	Mixed w/Peanuts, Oil Roasted	½	Cup	71.0	438	15	12	40	6	23
12638	Mixed w/o Peanuts, Oil Roasted	½	Cup	72.0	443	16	11	40	7	24
18177	Molasses Cookies	1	Each	15.0	65	11	1	2	0	1
19142	Mounds Candy Bar	1	Bar	20.0	72	12	1	4	2	1
62659	Mountain Dew	12	Fl Oz	355.2	165	47	–	–	–	–
19143	Mr. Goodbar Chocolate Bar	1	Bar	50.0	257	26	6	16	9	6
18274	Muffins, Blueberry	1	Large	65.0	180	31	4	4	1	2
18279	Muffins, Corn	1	Large	65.0	198	33	4	5	1	2
18283	Muffins, Oat Bran	1	Large	65.0	176	31	5	5	1	1
18273	Muffins, Plain	1	Large	65.0	192	27	4	7	1	2
18287	Muffins, Wheat Bran	1	Large	65.0	184	27	5	8	1	2
15056	Mullet, Striped, Ckd, Dry Heat	3	Ounce	85.1	128	0	21	4	1	1
41313	Mushroom Gravy over Beef Sirloin Tips–Healthy Choice	1	Each	269.3	310	43	22	5	2	–
11261	Mushrooms, Ckd	½	Cup	78.0	21	4	2	0	0	0
11264	Mushrooms, Cnd, Drained Solids	½	Cup	78.0	19	4	1	0	0	0

Polyunsaturated fat (g)	Dietary Fiber (g)	Cholesterol (mg)	Folate (µg)	Vitamin A (RE)	Vitamin B-6 (mg)	Vitamin B-12 (µg)	Vitamin C (mg)	Vitamin E (mg)	Riboflavin (mg)	Thiamin (mg)	Calcium (mg)	Iron (mg)	Magnesium (mg)	Niacin (mg)	Phosphorus (mg)	Potassium (mg)	Sodium (mg)	Zinc (mg)
–	0	0	0	0	0	0	0	0	0	0	1	.1	1	0	4	2	22	0
0	–	0	0	0	0	0	0	–	0	0	1	0	1	0	1	5	1	0
3	0	4	1	12	0	0	0	.6	0	0	2	0	0	0	4	1	104	0
–	0	0	–	0	–	–	0	–	–	–	0	0	–	–	–	10	105	–
–	–	5	–	0	–	–	0	–	–	–	0	0	–	–	–	5	130	–
1	–	55	–	60	–	–	9	–	.4	.2	120	2	–	3.8	–	550	540	–
1	–	40	–	–	–	–	–	–	–	–	–	–	–	–	240	690	560	–
–	–	15	–	–	–	–	0	–	0	0	48	.1	–	.1	–	4	193	–
–	1	0	22	153	.1	0	5	.1	0	.1	9	.3	12	.6	10	242	27	.1
–	1	0	14	258	.1	0	34	.1	0	0	9	.2	9	.5	14	247	7	.1
–	1	0	–	5	–	0	26	.2	0	.1	8	.7	13	.7	11	344	20	–
–	1	0	–	5	.1	0	32	.2	0	.1	8	.1	9	.8	13	350	13	–
–	–	5	–	–	–	–	4	–	0	0	88	0	–	.1	–	68	48	–
0	2	10	3	21	0	.2	0	.5	.1	0	84	.6	26	.1	95	169	36	.6
1	1	3	2	0	.1	.1	0	.7	0	0	29	.4	26	1.2	60	142	12	.5
0	1	1	1	2	0	.1	0	.3	0	0	24	.5	13	.1	41	146	10	.2
1	3	8	5	6	0	.2	0	5.2	.2	0	92	.7	37	.3	108	182	30	.5
1	2	54	25	109	.1	1.6	0	.5	1.2	.2	684	1.6	83	.6	653	1161	575	2.5
1	0	61	34	145	.2	2.7	0	.5	1	.2	757	.5	61	.8	597	947	494	2
1	0	0	0	0	0	0	0	2.6	.2	0	79	1	16	0	181	279	191	2.9
0	0	0	0	0	0	0	0	–	.2	0	79	1	16	0	181	279	191	2.9
0	0	9	12	20	.1	.5	2	.1	.4	.1	285	.1	27	.1	219	371	257	1
0	0	7	12	147	.1	.9	2	–	.4	.1	287	.6	33	.3	256	425	152	1
0	4	17	12	142	.1	.8	2	.1	.4	.1	284	.6	33	.3	254	422	150	1
0	4	30	12	72	.1	.8	2	.2	.4	.1	280	.6	33	.3	251	417	149	1
0	4	33	12	85	.1	.9	2	.3	.4	.1	298	.8	55	.4	270	480	123	1.2
0	0	26	9	62	0	.3	2	.2	.3	.1	216	.1	20	.2	193	284	97	.7
0	0	19	5	34	0	.1	1	–	.2	0	164	.1	15	.1	127	191	67	.5
0	0	2	5	75	0	.2	1	0	.2	0	185	.2	17	.1	124	211	73	.6
0	0	10	12	144	.1	.9	2	.1	.4	.1	300	.1	34	.2	235	381	123	1
0	0	18	12	139	.1	.9	2	.2	.4	.1	297	.1	33	.2	232	377	122	1
1	0	37	22	95	.2	1	3	–	.6	.2	355	.3	53	1.3	302	530	223	1.1
0	0	4	13	149	.1	.9	2	.1	.3	.1	302	.1	28	.2	247	406	126	1
0	0	33	12	76	.1	.9	2	.2	.4	.1	291	.1	33	.2	228	370	120	.9
0	0	35	12	83	.1	.9	4	–	.4	.1	290	.1	33	.2	227	368	119	.9
0	1	12	5	28	0	.3	1	.4	.1	0	78	.5	20	.2	98	145	144	.4
5	–	0	8	3	.1	0	10	–	.2	.2	36	2.5	23	2	69	335	419	.4
–	–	0	–	–	–	–	0	–	0	0	0	.2	–	0	–	310	1192	–
–	–	0	–	60	–	–	15	–	.1	.1	32	.6	–	1.5	130	440	520	–
–	–	10	–	–	–	–	0	–	0	0	0	.2	–	.2	–	371	1282	–
7	6	0	35	1	.2	0	0	4.1	.1	.1	48	2.5	154	3.2	298	409	458	2.6
9	6	0	59	1	.2	0	0	4.3	.2	.4	77	2.3	167	3.6	329	413	463	3.6
8	4	0	41	1	.1	0	0	4.3	.3	.4	76	1.9	181	1.4	323	392	504	3.4
0	–	0	1	0	0	0	0	–	0	.1	11	1	8	.5	14	52	69	.1
0	1	0	1	0	0	0	0	.4	0	0	5	.8	14	0	24	42	25	.2
–	–	–	–	–	–	–	–	–	–	–	–	–	–	–	–	–	75	–
1	2	10	36	5	.1	.2	0	.6	.1	0	56	.6	48	2.4	140	225	17	.9
1	2	20	10	–	0	.4	1	–	.1	.1	37	1	10	.7	128	80	291	.3
2	–	33	22	23	.1	.1	0	–	.2	.2	48	1.8	24	1.3	185	45	339	.5
3	5	0	12	–	.1	0	0	–	.1	.2	41	2.7	102	.3	244	330	255	1.2
4	2	25	8	26	0	.1	0	–	.2	.2	130	1.6	11	1.5	99	79	304	.4
4	–	21	34	163	.2	.1	5	–	.3	.2	122	2.7	51	2.6	185	207	382	1.8
1	0	54	8	36	.4	.2	1	–	.1	.1	26	1.2	28	5.4	208	390	60	.7
–	–	35	–	60	–	–	2	–	0	–	–	.2	–	.4	–	80	500	–
0	2	0	14	0	.1	0	3	.1	.2	.1	5	1.4	9	3.5	68	278	2	.7
0	2	0	10	0	0	0	0	.1	0	.1	9	.6	12	1.2	51	101	332	.6

Code	Name	Amount	Unit	Grams	Energy (kcal)	Carbohydrates (g)	Protein (g)	Fat (g)	Saturated fat (g)	Monounsat fat (g
11950	Mushrooms, Enoki, Fresh	1	Medium	3.0	1	0	0	0	0	0
11260	Mushrooms, Fresh	½	Cup	35.0	9	2	1	0	0	0
11269	Mushrooms, Shiitake, Ckd	½	Cup	72.5	40	10	1	0	0	0
11268	Mushrooms, Shiitake, Dried	1	Medium	3.6	11	3	0	0	0	0
15165	Mussel, Blue, Ckd, Moist Heat	3	Ounce	85.1	146	6	20	4	1	1
62646	Mustard	1	Tbsp.	5.0	0	0	0	0	–	–
62679	Nacho Cheese Dip	2	Tbsp.	33.0	40	4	0	3	1	0
62619	Nacho Grande Chicken Enchiladas–Weight Watchers	1	Each	255.2	290	42	15	8	3	–
41340	Nacho Macaroni and Cheese–Healthy Choice	1	Each	255.1	280	44	13	5	3	–
55754	Navy Bean w/Ham Soup–Stouffer's	1	Cup	283.9	240	31	11	8	–	–
19145	Nestle Crunch	1	Bar	40.0	198	26	2	10	6	4
55757	New England Clam Chowder Soup–Stouffer's	1	Cup	283.9	341	21	14	23	–	–
55829	Newburg Sauce Supreme–Stouffer's	1	Cup	283.9	481	20	7	41	–	–
55804	Noodles Romanoff–Stouffer's	1	Cup	283.9	441	36	17	25	–	–
43407	Noodles and Chicken, Micro Cup–Hormel	1	Each	212.6	174	19	7	7	2	3
20113	Noodles, Chinese, Chow Mein	½	Cup	22.5	119	13	2	7	1	2
20310	Noodles, Egg, Ckd, Enriched	½	Cup	80.0	106	20	4	1	0	0
20510	Noodles, Egg, Ckd, Unenriched	½	Cup	80.0	106	20	4	1	0	0
20112	Noodles, Egg, Spinach, Ckd, Enriched	½	Cup	80.0	106	19	4	1	0	0
20115	Noodles, Japanese, Soba, Ckd	½	Cup	57.0	56	12	3	0	0	0
62647	Noodles, Ramen	1	Each	86.0	380	52	10	16	8	–
18200	Oatmeal Cookies, Dietary	1	Each	7.0	31	5	0	1	1	1
18178	Oatmeal Cookies, Regular	1	Each	18.0	81	12	1	3	1	2
18179	Oatmeal Cookies, Soft–type	1	Each	15.0	61	10	1	2	0	1
3189	Oatmeal, Dry	1	Cup	38.4	153	27	5	3	–	–
3689	Oatmeal, Prepared w/Milk	½	Cup	180.0	209	28	9	7	–	–
15058	Ocean Perch, Atlantic, Ckd, Dry Heat	3	Ounce	85.1	103	0	20	2	0	1
4053	Oil, Olive	1	Tbsp.	13.5	119	0	0	14	2	10
4042	Oil, Peanut	1	Tbsp.	13.5	119	0	0	14	2	6
4058	Oil, Sesame	1	Tbsp.	13.6	121	0	0	14	2	5
4044	Oil, Soybean	1	Tbsp.	13.6	121	0	0	14	2	3
4034	Oil, Soybean, (hydr)	1	Tbsp.	13.6	121	0	0	14	2	6
4543	Oil, Soybean, (hydr)&cttnsd	1	Tbsp.	13.6	121	0	0	14	2	4
4518	Oil, Vegetable, Corn	1	Tbsp.	13.6	121	0	0	14	2	3
4582	Oil, Vegetable, Canola	1	Tbsp.	13.6	121	0	0	14	1	8
4501	Oil, Vegetable, Cocoa Butter	1	Tbsp.	13.6	121	0	0	14	8	4
4502	Oil, Vegetable, Cottonseed	1	Tbsp.	13.6	121	0	0	14	4	2
4055	Oil, Vegetable, Palm	1	Tbsp.	13.6	121	0	0	14	7	5
4513	Oil, Vegetable, Palm Kernel	1	Tbsp.	13.6	118	0	0	14	11	2
4510	Oil, Vegetable, Safflower, Linoleic	1	Tbsp.	13.6	121	0	0	14	1	2
4511	Oil, Vegetable, Safflower, Oleic	1	Tbsp.	13.6	121	0	0	14	1	10
4584	Oil, Vegetable, Sunflower	1	Tbsp.	13.6	121	0	0	14	1	11
11279	Okra, Ckd	½	Cup	80.0	26	6	1	0	0	0
11278	Okra, Fresh	½	Cup	50.0	19	4	1	0	0	0
11281	Okra, Frz, Ckd	½	Cup	92.0	34	8	2	0	0	0
11280	Okra, Frz, Unprepared	½	Cup	71.3	21	5	1	0	0	0
41282	Old Fashioned Chicken Noodle Soup–Healthy Choice	1	Each	212.6	90	11	5	2	–	–
55806	Old–Fashion Stuff'n–Stouffer's	½	Cup	142.0	310	31	6	19	–	–
10161	Olive Loaf, Lunch Meat	1	Slice	28.4	67	3	3	5	2	2
7051	Olive Loaf, Pork, Lunch Meat	1	Slice	28.4	67	3	3	5	2	2
62648	Olives, Green	5	Each	15.0	25	0	0	3	–	–
9194	Olives, Ripe, Canned (jumbo–super colossal)	1	Jumbo	8.3	7	0	0	1	0	0
9193	Olives, Ripe, Canned (small–extra large)	1	Small	3.2	4	0	0	0	0	0
11283	Onions, Ckd	½	Cup	119.9	53	12	2	0	0	0
11285	Onions, Cnd, Sol&liq	½	Cup	112.0	21	4	1	0	0	0
11282	Onions, Fresh	½	Cup	79.9	30	7	1	0	0	0

Polyunsaturated fat (g)	Dietary Fiber (g)	Cholesterol (mg)	Folate (µg)	Vitamin A (RE)	Vitamin B-6 (mg)	Vitamin B-12 (µg)	Vitamin C (mg)	Vitamin E (mg)	Riboflavin (mg)	Thiamin (mg)	Calcium (mg)	Iron (mg)	Magnesium (mg)	Niacin (mg)	Phosphorus (mg)	Potassium (mg)	Sodium (mg)	Zinc (mg)
0	–	0	1	0	0	0	0	–	0	0	0	0	0	.1	3	11	0	0
0	0	0	7	0	0	0	1	0	.2	0	2	.4	4	1.4	36	130	1	.3
0	2	0	15	0	.1	0	0	.1	.1	0	2	.3	10	1.1	21	85	3	1
0	0	0	6	0	0	0	0	0	0	0	0	.1	5	.5	11	55	0	.3
1	0	48	64	77	.1	20.4	12	.7	.4	.3	28	5.7	31	2.6	242	228	314	2.3
–	–	–	0	0	0	0	0	–	0	0	0	0	0	0	0	–	75	0
0	0	0	0	0	0	0	0	–	0	0	24	0	0	0	0	–	200	0
–	4	20	–	300	–	–	12	–	–	–	360	.6	–	–	–	600	560	–
–	–	20	–	0	–	–	0	–	.5	.6	160	.8	–	0	–	420	560	–
–	–	20	–	–	–	–	0	–	0	0	70	3	–	.2	–	571	1252	–
0	1	8	4	6	0	.2	0	–	.1	0	68	.3	18	.2	71	138	59	.4
–	–	40	–	–	–	–	0	–	0	0	2	.1	–	.2	–	571	961	–
–	–	120	–	–	–	–	0	–	0	0	2	0	–	0	–	371	1052	–
–	–	40	–	–	–	–	0	–	0	0	2	.2	–	.2	–	260	1993	–
2	–	29	–	270	–	–	8	–	.1	.1	32	.7	21	1.7	–	254	1009	.8
4	1	0	5	2	0	0	0	0	.1	.1	5	1.1	12	1.3	36	27	99	.3
0	–	26	6	5	0	.1	0	–	.1	.1	10	1.3	15	1.2	55	22	132	.5
0	–	26	6	5	0	.1	0	–	0	0	10	.5	15	.3	55	22	132	.5
0	2	26	17	11	.1	.1	0	0	.1	.2	15	.9	19	1.2	46	30	10	.5
0	–	0	4	0	0	0	0	–	0	.1	2	.3	5	.3	14	20	34	.1
–	2	0	0	0	0	0	0	–	0	0	0	1.6	0	0	0	–	1560	0
0	–	0	1	0	0	0	0	–	0	0	3	.2	2	.1	10	12	1	0
0	1	0	1	0	0	0	0	–	0	0	7	.5	6	.4	25	26	69	.1
0	0	1	1	1	0	0	0	–	0	0	14	.4	5	.3	31	20	52	.1
–	3	–	14	–	.1	0	1	.1	1	1.1	281	28.2	56	13.8	191	180	13	1.4
–	–	–	18	–	.1	.5	–	–	1	.9	396	21.9	63	10.8	288	367	83	1.7
0	0	46	9	12	.2	1	1	–	.1	.1	117	1	33	2.1	236	298	82	.5
1	0	0	0	0	0	0	0	1.6	0	0	0	.1	0	0	0	0	0	0
4	0	0	0	0	0	0	0	1.7	0	0	0	0	0	0	0	0	0	0
6	0	0	0	0	0	0	0	.6	0	0	0	0	0	0	0	0	0	0
8	0	0	0	0	0	0	0	.8	0	0	0	0	0	0	0	0	0	0
5	0	0	0	0	0	0	0	2.2	0	0	0	0	0	0	0	0	0	0
7	0	0	0	0	0	0	0	.6	0	0	0	0	0	0	0	0	0	0
8	0	0	0	0	0	0	0	2.9	0	0	0	0	0	0	0	0	0	0
4	0	–	0	0	0	0	0	–	0	0	0	0	0	0	0	0	0	0
0	0	0	0	0	0	0	0	.2	0	0	0	0	0	0	0	0	0	0
7	0	0	0	0	0	0	0	5.2	–	0	0	0	0	0	0	0	0	0
1	0	0	0	0	0	0	0	3	0	0	0	0	0	0	0	0	0	–
0	0	0	0	0	0	0	0	.5	0	0	0	0	0	0	0	0	0	0
10	0	0	0	0	0	0	0	4.7	0	0	0	0	0	0	0	0	0	0
2	0	0	0	0	0	0	0	4.7	0	0	0	0	0	0	0	0	0	0
1	0	–	0	0	0	0	0	–	0	0	0	0	0	0	0	0	0	0
0	2	0	37	46	.1	0	13	.6	0	.1	50	.4	46	.7	45	258	4	.4
0	1	0	44	33	.1	0	11	.3	0	.1	41	.4	29	.5	32	152	4	.3
0	3	0	134	47	0	0	11	.6	.1	.1	88	.6	47	.7	42	215	3	.6
0	2	0	105	33	0	0	9	.5	.1	.1	58	.4	31	.5	30	150	2	.4
–	–	20	–	80	–	–	12	–	.1	0	16	.2	–	1.9	60	130	540	–
–	–	5	–	–	–	–	0	–	0	0	0	.2	–	.4	–	100	561	–
1	0	11	1	6	.1	.4	2	–	.1	.1	31	.2	5	.5	36	84	421	.4
1	0	11	1	0	.1	.4	3	.1	.1	.1	31	.2	5	.5	36	84	421	.4
–	–	–	0	0	0	0	0	–	0	0	0	0	0	0	0	–	65	0
0	–	0	0	3	0	0	0	–	0	0	8	.3	0	0	0	1	75	0
0	–	–	0	1	0	0	0	–	0	0	3	.1	0	0	0	0	28	0
0	2	0	18	0	.2	0	6	.2	0	.1	26	.3	13	.2	42	199	4	.3
0	1	0	11	0	.2	0	5	.2	0	0	50	.1	7	.1	31	124	416	.3
0	1	0	15	0	.1	0	5	.1	0	0	16	.2	8	.1	26	125	2	.2

Code	Name	Amount	Unit	Grams	Energy (kcal)	Carbohydrates (g)	Protein (g)	Fat (g)	Saturated fat (g)	Monounsat fat (g)
14323	Orange Drink, Cnd	¾	Cup	185.8	95	24	0	0	0	0
9206	Orange Juice, Fresh	¾	Cup	186.0	84	19	1	0	0	0
9215	Orange Juice, From Concentrate	¾	Cup	186.4	84	20	1	0	0	0
62558	Orange Juice, w/Added Calcium	¾	Cup	186.4	84	20	1	0	0	0
14327	Orange and Apricot Juice Drink, Cnd	¾	Cup	187.0	95	24	1	0	0	0
9200	Oranges, Fresh	1	Medium	131.0	62	15	1	0	0	0
18199	Oreos, Dietary	1	Each	10.0	46	7	0	2	1	1
18166	Oreos, Regular	1	Each	10.0	47	7	0	2	0	1
18168	Oreos, w/Extra Creme Filling	1	Each	13.0	65	9	0	3	1	2
55220	Oriental Beef w/Veg., Lean Cuisine–Stouffer's	1	Each	244.5	290	31	20	9	2	–
41314	Oriental Chicken w/Spicy Peanut Sauce–Healthy Choice	1	Each	269.3	340	40	33	5	1	–
19031	Oriental Mix, Rice-based	1	Ounce	28.4	155	9	6	12	5	3
55221	Oven Baked Chicken, Lean Cuisine–Stouffer's	1	Each	226.8	200	21	17	5	2	–
15168	Oyster, Eastern, Breaded and Fried	3	Ounce	85.1	168	10	7	11	3	4
15170	Oyster, Eastern, Cnd	3	Ounce	85.1	59	3	6	2	1	0
15245	Oysters, Raw	3	Ounce	85.1	50	5	4	1	0	0
18288	Pancakes Plain, Frozen	1	4 In.	9.0	21	4	0	0	0	0
18294	Pancakes, Blueberry	1	4 In.	9.5	21	13	1	1	0	0
18390	Pancakes, Buttermilk	1	4 In.	9.5	22	13	1	1	0	0
18298	Pancakes, Dietary	1	3 In.	22.0	44	9	1	0	0	0
18293	Pancakes, Plain	1	4 In.	9.5	22	13	1	1	0	0
18300	Pancakes, Whole-wheat	1	4 In.	44.0	92	13	4	3	1	1
9229	Papaya Nectar, Cnd	¾	Cup	187.0	107	27	0	0	0	0
9226	Papayas, Fresh	1	Medium	304.0	119	30	2	0	0	0
11808	Parsnips, Ckd, w/Salt	½	Cup	78.0	63	15	1	0	0	0
11299	Parsnips, Ckd, w/o Salt	½	Cup	78.0	63	15	1	0	0	0
11298	Parsnips, Fresh	½	Cup	66.5	50	12	1	0	0	0
9232	Passion-fruit Juice, Purple, Fresh	¾	Cup	185.2	94	25	1	0	–	–
9233	Passion-fruit Juice, Yellow, Fresh	¾	Cup	185.2	111	27	1	0	–	–
55800	Pasta Florentine–Stouffer's	½	Cup	142.0	190	16	8	11	–	–
41294	Pasta Italiano–Healthy Choice	1	Each	340.2	350	59	16	5	2	–
55810	Pasta Roma–Stouffer's	½	Cup	142.0	130	16	8	4	–	–
41292	Pasta Shells w/Tomato Sauce–Healthy Choice	1	Each	340.2	330	53	24	3	2	–
55142	Pasta Shells, Cheese w/Sauce–Stouffer's	1	Each	262.2	300	28	17	13	–	–
41287	Pasta w/Cacciatore Chicken–Healthy Choice	1	Each	354.4	310	47	26	3	–	–
41293	Pasta w/Teriyaki Chicken–Healthy Choice	1	Each	357.9	350	58	24	3	1	–
20321	Pasta, Ckd, Enriched, w/Added Salt	½	Cup	70.0	99	20	3	0	0	0
20121	Pasta, Ckd, Enriched, w/o Added Salt	½	Cup	70.0	99	20	3	0	0	0
20094	Pasta, Fresh-refrigerated, Plain, Ckd	½	Cup	73.0	96	18	4	1	0	0
20096	Pasta, Fresh-refrigerated, Spinach, Ckd	½	Cup	73.0	95	18	4	1	0	0
20097	Pasta, Homemade, Made w/Egg, Ckd	½	Cup	73.6	96	17	4	1	0	0
20098	Pasta, Homemade, Made w/o Egg, Ckd	½	Cup	73.6	91	18	3	1	0	0
20127	Pasta, Spinach, Ckd	½	Cup	70.0	91	18	3	0	0	0
20125	Pasta, Whole-wheat, Ckd	½	Cup	70.0	87	19	4	0	0	0
9251	Peach Nectar, Cnd, w/o Added Vit C	¾	Cup	186.4	101	26	1	0	0	0
9241	Peaches, Cnd, Heavy Syrup Pack	½	Cup	128.0	95	26	1	0	0	0
9240	Peaches, Cnd, Light Syrup Pack	½	Cup	125.5	68	18	1	0	0	0
9244	Peaches, Dehydrated, Sulfured	¼	Cup	29.0	94	24	1	0	0	0
9246	Peaches, Dried, Sulfured	¼	Cup	40.0	96	25	1	0	0	0
9236	Peaches, Fresh	1	Medium	87.0	37	10	1	0	0	0
9250	Peaches, Frozen, Sliced, Sweetened	½	Cup	125.0	118	30	1	0	0	0
19147	Peanut Bar	1	Bar	40.0	209	19	6	13	2	7
19148	Peanut Brittle	1	Ounce	28.4	128	20	2	5	1	2
18185	Peanut Butter Cookies, Regular	1	Each	15.0	72	9	1	4	1	1
18186	Peanut Butter Cookies, Soft-type	1	Each	15.0	69	9	1	4	1	2
18201	Peanut Butter Sandwich Cookies, Dietary	1	Each	10.0	54	5	1	3	1	2

Polyunsaturated fat (g)	Dietary Fiber (g)	Cholesterol (mg)	Folate (µg)	Vitamin A (RE)	Vitamin B-6 (mg)	Vitamin B-12 (µg)	Vitamin C (mg)	Vitamin E (mg)	Riboflavin (mg)	Thiamin (mg)	Calcium (mg)	Iron (mg)	Magnesium (mg)	Niacin (mg)	Phosphorus (mg)	Potassium (mg)	Sodium (mg)	Zinc (mg)
0	0	0	4	4	0	0	63	0	0	0	11	.5	4	.1	2	33	30	.2
0	0	0	56	37	.1	0	93	.2	.1	.2	20	.4	20	.7	32	372	2	.1
0	0	0	82	15	.1	0	73	.4	0	.1	17	.2	19	.4	30	354	2	.1
0	0	0	82	15	.1	0	73	–	0	.1	224	.2	19	.4	30	354	2	.1
0	0	0	11	108	.1	0	37	0	0	0	9	.2	7	.4	15	150	4	.1
0	3	0	40	28	.1	0	70	.3	.1	.1	52	.1	13	.4	18	237	0	.1
0	–	0	1	0	0	0	0	–	0	0	6	.5	7	.3	18	30	24	.1
0	0	0	1	0	0	0	0	–	0	0	3	.4	5	.2	10	18	60	.1
0	–	0	1	0	0	0	0	–	0	0	3	.4	4	.2	12	16	64	.1
–	–	40	–	150	–	–	1	–	.2	.1	16	1	–	2.9	–	400	590	–
1	–	45	–	–	–	–	2	–	–	–	–	.2	–	.4	–	50	470	–
3	4	0	25	1	.1	0	0	–	0	.1	22	.8	40	3	112	147	235	1.3
–	–	35	–	350	–	–	6	–	.2	.2	16	.8	–	7.6	–	550	480	–
3	–	69	12	77	.1	13.3	3	–	.2	.1	53	5.9	49	1.4	135	208	355	74.1
1	0	47	8	77	.1	16.3	4	.7	.1	.1	38	5.7	46	1.1	118	195	95	77.4
1	0	21	15	7	.1	13.8	4	–	.1	.1	–	4.9	28	1.1	79	105	151	32.3
0	–	1	1	3	0	0	0	–	0	0	6	.3	1	.4	33	7	46	.1
0	–	5	1	5	0	0	0	–	0	0	20	.2	2	.1	14	13	39	.1
0	–	6	1	3	0	0	0	–	0	0	15	.2	1	.1	13	14	50	.1
0	–	0	1	2	0	0	0	–	0	0	13	.4	6	.4	75	85	58	.2
0	–	6	1	5	0	0	0	–	0	0	21	.2	2	.1	15	13	42	.1
1	–	27	9	28	0	.1	0	–	.2	.1	110	1.4	20	1	164	123	252	.5
0	1	0	4	21	0	0	6	0	0	0	19	.6	6	.3	0	58	9	.3
0	5	0	116	85	.1	0	188	3.4	.1	.1	73	.3	30	1	15	781	9	.2
0	–	0	45	0	.1	0	10	–	0	.1	29	.5	23	.6	54	286	192	.2
0	3	0	45	0	.1	0	10	.8	0	.1	29	.5	23	.6	54	286	8	.2
0	3	0	44	0	.1	0	11	.7	0	.1	24	.4	19	.5	47	249	7	.4
–	0	0	–	133	–	0	55	.1	.2	0	7	.4	31	2.7	24	515	11	–
	0	0	–	446	–	0	34	.1	.2	0	7	.7	31	4.1	46	515	11	–
–	–	25	–	–	–	–	0	–	0	0	2	.1	–	.1	–	200	446	–
3	–	30	–	60	–	–	–	–	.5	.5	48	2	–	2.9	180	540	530	–
–	–	15	–	–	–	–	3	–	0	.1	1	.2	–	.5	–	300	391	–
–	–	35	–	100	–	–	21	–	.4	.5	320	1.5	–	2.9	240	640	470	–
–	–	–	–	150	–	–	9	–	.3	.1	280	1	–	1.9	–	480	820	–
1	–	35	–	100	–	–	6	–	.4	.5	32	1.5	–	6.7	250	660	430	–
2	–	45	–	100	–	–	6	–	.3	.3	48	1.5	–	3.8	200	390	370	–
0	–	0	5	–	0	0	0	–	.1	.1	5	1	13	1.2	38	22	70	.4
0	1	0	5	–	0	0	0	0	.1	.1	5	1	13	1.2	38	22	1	.4
0	–	24	5	4	0	.1	0	–	.1	.2	4	.8	13	.7	46	18	4	.4
0	–	24	13	10	.1	.1	0	–	.1	.1	13	.8	18	.7	42	27	4	.5
0	–	30	14	13	0	.1	0	–	.1	.1	7	.9	10	.9	38	15	61	.3
0	–	0	13	0	0	0	0	–	.1	.1	4	.8	10	1	29	14	54	.3
0	–	0	8	11	.1	0	0	–	.1	.1	21	.7	43	1.1	76	41	10	.8
0	3	0	4	0	.1	0	0	0	0	.1	11	.7	21	.5	62	31	2	.6
0	1	0	3	48	0	0	10	0	0	0	9	.4	7	.5	11	75	13	.1
0	1	0	4	42	0	0	4	1.1	0	0	4	.3	6	.8	14	118	8	.1
0	1	0	4	44	0	0	3	1.1	0	0	4	.5	6	.7	14	122	6	.1
0	–	0	2	41	0	0	3	–	0	0	11	1.6	17	1.4	47	392	3	.2
0	3	0	0	86	0	0	2	0	.1	0	11	1.6	17	1.8	48	398	3	.2
0	2	0	3	47	0	0	6	.6	0	0	4	.1	6	.9	10	171	0	.1
0	2	0	4	35	0	0	118	1.1	0	0	4	.5	6	.8	14	162	7	.1
4	1	3	24	20	0	0	0	.4	.1	0	31	.4	30	3.2	61	163	96	.5
1	1	4	20	13	0	0	0	.5	0	.1	9	.4	14	1	31	59	128	.3
1	–	0	5	1	0	0	0	–	0	0	5	.4	7	.6	13	25	62	.1
1	0	0	1	0	0	0	0	–	0	0	2	.1	5	.3	13	16	50	.1
1	–	0	3	0	0	0	0	–	0	0	5	.2	5	.5	19	29	41	.2

Code	Name	Amount	Unit	Grams	Energy (kcal)	Carbohydrates (g)	Protein (g)	Fat (g)	Saturated fat (g)	Monounsa- fat (g)
18190	Peanut Butter Sandwich Cookies, Regular	1	Each	14.0	67	9	1	3	1	2
16097	Peanut Butter, Chunk Style, w/Salt	2	Tbsp.	32.3	190	7	8	16	3	8
16397	Peanut Butter, Chunk Style, w/o Salt	2	Tbsp.	32.3	190	7	8	16	3	8
62689	Peanut Butter, Reduced Fat	2	Tbsp.	36.0	190	15	8	12	3	–
16098	Peanut Butter, Smooth Style, w/Salt	2	Tbsp.	32.3	190	7	8	16	3	8
16398	Peanut Butter, Smooth Style, w/o Salt	2	Tbsp.	32.3	190	7	8	16	3	8
16088	Peanuts, All Types, Ckd, Boiled, w/Salt	½	Cup	31.5	100	7	4	7	1	3
16090	Peanuts, All Types, Dry–roasted, w/Salt	½	Cup	73.0	427	16	17	36	5	18
16390	Peanuts, All Types, Dry–roasted, w/o Salt	½	Cup	73.0	427	16	17	36	5	18
16087	Peanuts, All Types, Fresh	½	Cup	73.0	414	12	19	36	5	18
16089	Peanuts, All Types, Oil–roasted, w/Salt	½	Cup	72.0	418	14	19	35	5	18
16389	Peanuts, All Types, Oil–roasted, w/o Salt	½	Cup	72.0	418	14	19	35	5	18
16091	Peanuts, Spanish, Fresh	½	Cup	73.0	416	12	19	36	6	16
16092	Peanuts, Spanish, Oil–roasted, w/Salt	½	Cup	73.5	426	13	21	36	6	16
16392	Peanuts, Spanish, Oil–roasted, w/o Salt	½	Cup	73.5	426	13	21	36	6	16
16093	Peanuts, Valencia, Fresh	½	Cup	73.0	416	15	18	35	5	16
16094	Peanuts, Valencia, Oil–roasted, w/Salt	½	Cup	72.0	424	12	19	37	6	17
16394	Peanuts, Valencia, Oil–roasted, w/o Salt	½	Cup	72.0	424	12	19	37	6	17
9340	Pears, Asian, Fresh	1	Medium	122.0	51	13	1	0	0	0
9257	Pears, Cnd, Heavy Syrup Pack	½	Cup	127.5	94	24	0	0	0	0
9254	Pears, Cnd, Juice Pack	½	Cup	124.0	62	16	0	0	0	0
9256	Pears, Cnd, Light Syrup Pack	½	Cup	125.5	72	19	0	0	0	0
9253	Pears, Cnd, Water Pack	½	Cup	122.0	35	10	0	0	0	0
9252	Pears, Fresh	1	Medium	166.0	98	25	1	1	0	0
11318	Peas and Carrots, Cnd	½	Cup	76.0	29	6	2	0	0	0
11323	Peas and Carrots, Frz, Ckd	½	Cup	80.0	38	8	2	0	0	0
11324	Peas and Onions, Cnd	½	Cup	60.0	31	5	2	0	0	0
11327	Peas and Onions, Frz, Ckd	½	Cup	90.0	41	8	2	0	0	0
11305	Peas, Green, Ckd	½	Cup	80.0	67	13	4	0	0	0
11308	Peas, Green, Cnd	½	Cup	85.0	59	11	4	0	0	0
11310	Peas, Green, Cnd, Seasoned	½	Cup	85.0	43	8	3	0	0	0
11304	Peas, Green, Fresh	½	Cup	72.5	59	10	4	0	0	0
11313	Peas, Green, Frz, Ckd	½	Cup	80.0	62	11	4	0	0	0
18324	Pecan Pie	1	Slice	113.0	452	65	5	21	4	12
12142	Pecans, Dried	½	Cup	54.0	360	10	4	37	3	23
41333	Pepperoni French Bread Pizza–Healthy Choice	1	Each	170.1	310	38	20	7	3	–
62625	Pepperoni Pizza–Weight Watchers	1	Each	157.6	390	46	23	12	4	–
11329	Peppers, Hot Chili, Green, Cnd	1	Each	73.0	18	4	1	0	0	0
11670	Peppers, Hot Chili, Green, Fresh	1	Each	45.0	18	4	1	0	0	0
11820	Peppers, Hot Chili, Red, Cnd	1	Each	73.0	18	4	1	0	0	0
11819	Peppers, Hot Chili, Red, Fresh	1	Each	45.0	18	4	1	0	0	0
11632	Peppers, Jalapeno, Cnd	¼	Cup	34.0	8	2	0	0	0	0
11333	Peppers, Sweet, Green, Fresh	1	Medium	74.0	20	5	1	0	0	0
11821	Peppers, Sweet, Red, Fresh	1	Medium	74.0	20	5	1	0	0	0
11951	Peppers, Sweet, Yellow, Fresh	1	Medium	74.0	20	5	1	0	–	–
15061	Perch, Ckd, Dry Heat	3	Ounce	85.1	100	0	21	1	0	0
55827	Pesto Sauce–Stouffer's	¼	Cup	71.0	193	5	9	15	–	–
11958	Pickle Relish, Hamburger	1	Tbsp.	15.0	19	5	0	0	0	0
11944	Pickle Relish, Hot Dog	1	Tbsp.	15.0	14	4	0	0	0	0
11945	Pickle Relish, Sweet	1	Tbsp.	15.0	19	5	0	0	0	0
10162	Pickle and Pimento Loaf, Lunch Meat	1	Slice	28.4	74	2	3	6	2	3
7058	Pickle and Pimiento Loaf, Pork, Lunch Meat	1	Slice	28.4	74	2	3	6	2	3
11941	Pickle, Cucumber ,Sour	1	Slice	7.0	1	0	0	0	0	0
11937	Pickle, Cucumber, Dill	1	Slice	6.0	1	0	0	0	0	0
11947	Pickle, Cucumber, Dill, Low Sodium	1	Slice	6.0	1	0	0	0	0	0
11946	Pickle, Cucumber, Sour, Low Sodium	1	Slice	7.0	1	0	0	0	0	0

Polyunsaturated fat (g)	Dietary Fiber (g)	Cholesterol (mg)	Folate (µg)	Vitamin A (RE)	Vitamin B-6 (mg)	Vitamin B-12 (µg)	Vitamin C (mg)	Vitamin E (mg)	Riboflavin (mg)	Thiamin (mg)	Calcium (mg)	Iron (mg)	Magnesium (mg)	Niacin (mg)	Phosphorus (mg)	Potassium (mg)	Sodium (mg)	Zinc (mg)
1	–	0	2	0	0	0	0	–	0	0	7	.4	7	.5	26	27	52	.1
5	2	0	30	0	.1	0	0	3.2	0	0	13	.6	51	4.4	102	241	157	.9
5	2	0	30	0	.1	0	0	3.2	0	0	13	.6	51	4.4	102	241	5	.9
–	2	–	12	0	.1	0	0	–	0	0	0	.4	53	4.8	0	721	250	.9
5	2	0	25	0	.1	0	0	3.2	0	0	11	.5	51	4.2	104	233	154	.8
5	–	0	25	0	.1	0	0	–	0	0	11	.5	51	4.2	104	233	5	.8
11	6	0	91	0	.2	0	0	5.3	.1	.2	63	1.3	133	10.3	372	491	312	4.8
2	3	0	23	0	0	0	0	1	0	.1	17	.3	32	1.7	62	57	237	.6
11	6	0	106	0	.2	0	0	5.4	.1	.3	39	1.6	128	9.9	261	480	593	2.4
11	6	0	106	0	.2	0	0	5.7	.1	.3	39	1.6	128	9.9	261	480	4	2.4
11	6	0	175	0	.3	0	0	6.7	.1	.5	67	3.3	123	8.8	274	515	13	2.4
11	7	0	91	0	.2	0	0	5.3	.1	.2	63	1.3	133	10.3	372	491	4	4.8
13	7	0	175	0	.3	0	0	–	.1	.5	77	2.9	137	11.6	283	543	16	1.5
13	–	0	93	0	.2	0	0	–	.1	.2	74	1.7	123	11	284	570	318	1.5
13	–	0	93	0	.2	0	0	–	.1	.2	74	1.7	123	11	284	570	4	1.5
12	–	0	179	0	.2	0	0	–	.2	.5	45	1.5	134	9.4	245	242	1	2.4
13	–	0	90	0	.2	0	0	–	.1	.1	39	1.2	115	10.3	230	441	556	2.2
13	–	0	90	0	.2	0	0	–	.1	.1	39	1.2	115	10.3	230	441	4	2.2
0	4	0	10	0	0	0	5	.6	0	0	5	0	10	.3	13	148	0	0
0	3	0	2	0	0	0	1	.6	0	0	6	.3	5	.3	9	83	6	.1
0	2	0	1	1	0	0	2	.6	0	0	11	.4	9	.2	15	119	5	.1
0	3	0	2	0	0	0	1	.6	0	0	6	.4	5	.2	9	83	6	.1
0	2	0	1	0	0	0	1	.6	0	0	5	.3	5	.1	9	65	2	.1
0	4	0	12	3	0	0	7	.8	.1	0	18	.4	10	.2	18	208	0	.2
0	3	0	14	438	.1	0	5	.3	0	.1	17	.6	11	.4	35	76	197	.4
0	3	0	21	621	.1	0	6	.3	.1	.2	18	.8	13	.9	39	126	54	.4
0	–	0	16	10	.1	0	2	–	0	.1	10	.5	10	.8	31	58	265	.3
0	3	0	18	32	.1	0	6	.1	.1	.1	13	.8	12	.9	31	105	33	.3
0	4	0	51	48	.2	0	11	.3	.1	.2	22	1.2	31	1.6	94	217	2	1
0	3	0	38	65	.1	0	8	.3	.1	.1	17	.8	14	.6	57	147	186	.6
0	–	0	24	37	.1	0	10	–	.1	.1	13	1	13	.6	46	104	216	.6
0	4	0	47	46	.1	0	29	.3	.1	.2	18	1.1	24	1.5	78	177	4	.9
0	4	0	47	54	.1	0	8	.1	.1	.2	19	1.3	23	1.2	72	134	70	.8
3	4	36	7	53	0	.1	1	–	.1	.1	19	1.2	20	.3	87	84	479	.6
9	4	0	21	7	.1	0	1	1.7	.1	.5	19	1.2	69	.5	157	212	1	3
1	–	30	–	150	–	–	–	–	.3	.5	160	2.5	–	3.8	240	350	470	–
–	4	45	–	80	–	–	5	–	–	–	540	1	–	–	–	320	650	–
0	1	0	7	45	.1	0	50	.5	0	0	5	.4	10	.6	12	137	856	.1
0	1	0	11	35	.1	0	109	.3	0	0	8	.5	11	.4	21	153	3	.1
0	1	0	7	868	.1	0	50	.3	0	0	5	.4	10	.6	12	137	856	.1
0	1	0	11	484	.1	0	109	.3	0	0	8	.5	11	.4	21	153	3	.1
0	–	0	5	58	.1	0	4	–	0	0	9	1	4	.2	6	46	497	.1
0	1	0	16	47	.2	0	66	.5	0	0	7	.3	7	.4	14	131	1	.1
0	2	0	16	422	.2	0	141	.5	0	0	7	.3	7	.4	14	131	1	.1
–	–	0	19	18	.1	0	136	–	0	0	8	.3	9	.7	18	157	1	.1
0	0	98	5	9	.1	1.9	1	–	.1	.1	87	1	32	1.6	219	293	67	1.2
–	–	18	–	–	–	–	3	–	0	0	1	.1	–	.1	–	155	341	–
0	0	0	0	4	0	0	0	–	0	0	1	.2	1	.1	3	11	164	0
0	–	0	0	3	0	0	0	–	0	0	1	.2	3	.1	6	12	164	0
0	–	0	0	2	0	0	0	–	0	0	0	.1	1	0	2	4	122	0
1	0	10	1	2	.1	.3	4	–	.1	.1	27	.3	5	.6	40	96	394	.4
1	0	10	1	8505	.1	.3	4	.1	.1	.1	27	.3	5	.6	40	96	394	.4
0	0	0	0	1	0	0	0	0	0	0	0	0	0	0	1	2	85	0
0	0	0	0	2	0	0	0	0	0	0	1	0	1	0	1	7	77	0
0	–	0	0	2	0	0	0	–	0	0	1	0	1	0	1	7	1	0
0	0	0	–	1	–	0	0	0	0	0	0	0	0	0	1	2	1	0

Code	Name	Amount	Unit	Grams	Energy (kcal)	Carbohydrates (g)	Protein (g)	Fat (g)	Saturated fat (g)	Monounsatu fat (g)
11940	Pickle, Cucumber, Sweet	1	Slice	6.0	7	2	0	0	0	0
11948	Pickle, Cucumber, Sweet, Low Sodium	1	Slice	6.0	7	2	0	0	0	0
15063	Pike, Northern, Ckd, Dry Heat	3	Ounce	85.1	96	0	21	1	0	0
15204	Pike, Walleye, Ckd, Dry Heat	3	Ounce	85.1	101	0	21	1	0	0
14017	Pina Colada	1	Fl Oz	31.4	58	9	0	1	0	0
12147	Pine Nuts	1	Tbsp.	10.0	52	1	2	5	1	2
9273	Pineapple Juice, Cnd	¾	Cup	187.6	105	26	1	0	0	0
14334	Pineapple and Grapefruit Juice Drink, Cnd	¾	Cup	187.6	88	22	0	0	0	0
14341	Pineapple and Orange Juice Drink, Cnd	¾	Cup	187.6	94	22	2	0	0	0
9270	Pineapple, Cnd, Heavy Syrup Pack	½	Cup	127.5	99	26	0	0	0	0
9269	Pineapple, Cnd, Light Syrup Pack	½	Cup	126.0	66	17	0	0	0	0
9266	Pineapple, Fresh	1	Slice	84.0	41	10	0	0	0	0
12151	Pistachios, Dried	½	Cup	64.0	369	16	13	31	4	21
12652	Pistachios, Dry Roasted	½	Cup	64.0	388	18	10	34	4	23
9284	Plums, Cnd, Purple, Heavy Syrup Pack	½	Cup	129.0	115	30	0	0	0	0
9283	Plums, Cnd, Purple, Light Syrup Pack	½	Cup	126.0	79	21	0	0	0	0
9279	Plums, Fresh	1	Medium	66.0	36	9	1	0	0	0
15205	Pollock, Atlantic, Ckd, Dry Heat	3	Ounce	85.1	100	0	21	1	0	0
19034	Popcorn, Air–popped	1	Cup	8.0	31	6	1	0	0	0
19036	Popcorn, Cakes	1	Cake	10.0	38	8	1	0	0	0
19038	Popcorn, Caramel–coated, w/Peanuts	1	Cup	35.2	141	28	2	3	0	1
19039	Popcorn, Caramel–coated, w/o Peanuts	1	Cup	35.2	152	28	1	5	1	1
19040	Popcorn, Cheese–flavor	1	Cup	11.0	58	6	1	4	1	1
62649	Popcorn, Microwave	4	Cup	56.0	170	17	3	12	3	–
62650	Popcorn, Microwave, Low–Fat	4	Cup	56.0	93	15	3	4	1	–
19035	Popcorn, Oil–popped	1	Cup	11.0	55	6	1	3	1	1
62602	Popsicles	1	Each	56.0	40	11	0	0	0	0
19408	Pork Skins, Barbecue–flavor	1	Ounce	28.4	153	0	16	9	3	4
9041	Pork Skins, Plain	1	Ounce	28.4	155	0	17	9	3	4
10193	Pork, Backribs	3	Ounce	85.1	315	0	21	25	9	11
10127	Pork, Braunschweiger	3	Ounce	85.1	305	3	11	27	9	13
7045	Pork, Cnd, Lunch Meat	1	Slice	21.0	70	0	3	6	2	3
10220	Pork, Ground, Ckd	3	Ounce	85.1	253	0	22	18	7	8
10154	Pork, Ham and Cheese Loaf or Roll	3	Ounce	85.1	220	1	14	17	6	8
10143	Pork, Ham, Chopped, Cnd	3	Ounce	85.1	203	0	14	16	5	8
10138	Pork, Ham, Cnd, Extra Lean (appx 4% Fat), Roasted	3	Ounce	85.1	116	0	18	4	1	2
10140	Pork, Ham, Cnd, Regular (approx 13% Fat), Roasted	3	Ounce	85.1	192	0	17	13	4	6
10134	Pork, Ham, Extra Lean (5% Fat), Roasted	3	Ounce	85.1	123	1	18	5	2	2
10153	Pork, Ham, Meat Only, Roasted	3	Ounce	85.1	134	0	21	5	2	2
10151	Pork, Ham, Meat and Fat, Roasted	3	Ounce	85.1	207	0	18	14	5	7
10136	Pork, Ham, Regular (11% Fat), Roasted	3	Ounce	85.1	151	0	19	8	3	4
10135	Pork, Ham, Regular (11% Fat), Unheated	3	Ounce	85.1	155	3	15	9	3	4
10172	Pork, Smoked Link Sausage, Grilled	3	Ounce	85.1	331	2	19	27	10	12
10089	Pork, Spareribs, Meat and Fat, Ckd, Braised	3	Ounce	85.1	338	0	25	26	9	11
10223	Pork, Tenderloin, Meat Only, Ckd, Broiled	3	Ounce	85.1	159	0	26	5	2	2
10221	Pork, Tenderloin, Meat and Fat, Ckd, Broiled	3	Ounce	85.1	171	0	25	7	2	3
19042	Potato Chips, Barbecue–flavor	1	Ounce	28.4	139	15	2	9	2	2
19421	Potato Chips, Cheese–flavor	1	Ounce	28.4	141	16	2	8	2	2
19422	Potato Chips, Light	1	Ounce	28.4	134	19	2	6	1	1
19411	Potato Chips, Plain, Salted	1	Ounce	28.4	152	15	2	10	3	3
19811	Potato Chips, Plain, Unsalted	1	Ounce	28.4	152	15	2	10	3	3
19045	Potato Chips, Pringles, Light	1	Ounce	28.4	142	18	2	7	1	2
19410	Potato Chips, Pringles, Plain	1	Ounce	28.4	158	14	2	11	3	2
19043	Potato Chips, Sour–cream–and–onion–flavor	1	Ounce	28.4	151	15	2	10	3	2
11920	Potato Chips, w/o Salt Added	1	Ounce	28.4	148	15	2	10	3	2
11672	Potato Pancakes, Home–prepared	1	Ounce	28.4	77	8	2	4	1	1

Polyunsaturated fat (g)	Dietary Fiber (g)	Cholesterol (mg)	Folate (µg)	Vitamin A (RE)	Vitamin B-6 (mg)	Vitamin B-12 (µg)	Vitamin C (mg)	Vitamin E (mg)	Riboflavin (mg)	Thiamin (mg)	Calcium (mg)	Iron (mg)	Magnesium (mg)	Niacin (mg)	Phosphorus (mg)	Potassium (mg)	Sodium (mg)	Zinc (mg)
0	0	0	0	1	0	0	0	0	0	0	0	0	0	0	1	2	56	0
0	0	0	0	1	0	0	0	0	0	0	0	0	0	0	1	2	1	0
0	0	43	15	20	.1	2	3	–	.1	.1	62	.6	34	2.4	240	282	42	.7
0	0	94	14	20	.1	2	0	–	.2	.3	120	1.4	32	2.4	229	424	55	.7
0	–	0	3	0	0	0	1	–	0	0	3	.1	3	0	2	22	2	0
2	0	0	6	0	0	0	0	.4	0	.1	3	.9	23	.4	51	60	0	.4
0	0	0	43	0	.2	0	20	0	0	.1	32	.5	24	.5	15	251	2	.2
0	0	0	20	8	.1	0	86	0	0	.1	13	.6	11	.5	11	114	26	.1
0	0	0	20	99	.1	0	42	0	0	.1	9	.5	11	.4	8	86	6	.1
0	1	0	6	1	.1	0	9	.1	0	.1	18	.5	20	.4	9	133	1	.2
0	1	0	6	1	.1	0	9	.1	0	.1	18	.5	20	.4	9	132	1	.2
0	1	0	9	2	.1	0	13	.1	0	.1	6	.3	12	.4	6	95	1	.1
5	7	0	37	15	.2	0	5	3.3	.1	.5	86	4.3	101	.7	322	700	4	.9
5	7	0	38	15	.2	0	5	4.1	.2	.3	45	2	83	.9	305	621	499	.9
0	1	0	3	34	0	0	1	.9	0	0	12	1.1	6	.4	17	117	25	.1
0	1	0	3	33	0	0	1	.9	0	0	11	1.1	6	.4	16	117	25	.1
0	1	0	1	21	.1	0	6	.4	.1	0	3	.1	5	.3	7	114	0	.1
1	0	77	3	10	.3	3.1	0	–	.2	0	65	.5	73	3.4	241	388	94	.5
0	1	0	2	2	0	0	0	0	0	0	1	.2	10	.2	24	24	0	.3
0	0	0	2	1	0	0	0	0	0	0	1	.2	16	.6	28	33	29	.4
1	1	0	6	2	.1	0	0	.5	0	0	23	1.4	28	.7	45	125	104	.4
2	2	2	1	4	0	0	0	.4	0	0	15	.6	12	.8	29	38	73	.2
2	1	1	1	5	0	.1	0	0	0	0	12	.2	10	.2	40	29	98	.2
–	3	0	0	0	0	0	0	–	0	0	0	.2	0	0	0	–	290	0
–	2	0	0	0	0	0	0	–	0	0	0	.3	0	0	0	–	220	0
1	1	0	2	2	0	0	0	0	0	0	1	.3	12	.2	27	25	97	.3
0	0	0	–	0	–	–	1	–	–	–	0	0	–	–	–	–	10	–
1	–	33	9	52	0	0	0	–	.1	0	12	.3	0	1	62	51	756	.2
1	–	27	0	11	0	.2	0	–	.1	0	9	.2	3	.4	24	36	521	.2
2	–	100	3	3	.3	.5	0	–	.2	.4	38	1.2	18	3	166	268	86	2.9
3	0	133	37	3589	.3	17.1	8	–	1.3	.2	8	8	9	7.1	143	169	972	2.4
1	0	13	1	0	0	.2	0	–	0	.1	1	.2	2	.7	17	45	271	.3
2	0	80	5	2	.3	.5	1	–	.2	.6	19	1.1	20	3.6	192	308	62	2.7
2	0	48	3	20	.2	.7	21	–	.2	.5	49	.8	14	2.9	215	250	1142	1.7
2	0	42	1	0	.3	.6	2	–	.1	.5	6	.8	11	2.7	118	242	1161	1.6
0	0	26	4	0	.4	.6	23	.2	.2	.9	5	.8	18	4.2	178	296	965	1.9
2	0	53	4	0	.3	.9	12	–	.2	.7	7	1.2	14	4.5	207	304	800	2.1
0	0	45	3	0	.3	.6	18	.2	.2	.6	7	1.3	12	3.4	167	244	1023	2.4
1	0	47	3	0	.4	.6	–	.2	.2	.6	6	.8	19	4.3	193	269	1129	2.2
2	0	53	3	0	.3	.5	–	.2	.2	.5	6	.7	16	3.8	182	243	1010	2
1	0	50	3	0	.3	.6	19	.2	.3	.6	7	1.1	19	5.2	239	348	1276	2.1
1	0	48	3	0	.3	.7	24	.2	.2	.7	6	.8	16	4.5	210	282	1120	1.8
3	0	58	4	0	.3	1.4	2	.3	.2	.6	26	1	16	3.9	138	286	1276	2.4
2	0	103	3	3	.3	.9	–	.2	.3	.3	40	1.6	20	4.7	222	272	79	3.9
0	–	80	5	2	.4	.9	1	–	.3	.8	4	1.2	31	4.4	251	384	55	2.5
1	–	80	5	2	.4	.8	1	–	.3	.8	4	1.2	30	4.3	247	378	54	2.5
5	1	0	24	6	.2	0	10	1.4	.1	.1	14	.5	21	1.3	53	357	213	.3
3	–	1	0	2	.1	0	15	–	0	0	20	.5	21	1.4	85	433	225	.3
3	–	0	8	0	.2	0	7	–	.1	.1	6	.4	25	2	55	494	139	0
3	1	0	13	0	.2	0	9	1.4	.1	0	7	.5	19	1.1	47	361	168	.3
3	–	0	13	0	.2	0	9	–	.1	0	7	.5	19	1.1	47	361	2	.3
4	1	0	7	0	.2	0	3	1.4	0	.1	10	.4	18	1.2	44	285	121	.2
6	1	0	2	0	0	0	2	1.4	0	.1	7	.4	16	.9	45	286	186	.2
5	1	2	18	6	.2	.3	11	–	.1	.1	20	.5	21	1.1	50	377	177	.3
5	1	0	13	0	.1	0	12	2.2	0	0	7	.3	17	1.2	43	368	2	.3
2	1	27	7	4	.1	.1	6	0	0	0	7	.4	9	.6	31	223	144	.2

Code	Name	Amount	Unit	Grams	Energy (kcal)	Carbohydrates (g)	Protein (g)	Fat (g)	Saturated fat (g)	Monounsaturated fat (g)
11414	Potato Salad	½	Cup	125.0	179	14	3	10	2	3
19415	Potato Sticks	1	Ounce	28.4	148	15	2	10	3	2
55174	Potatoes Au Gratin–Stouffer's	1	Each	163.0	170	17	5	9	–	–
11843	Potatoes, Au Gratin, Home–prepared	½	Cup	122.5	162	14	6	9	4	3
11363	Potatoes, Baked w/o Skin	1	Medium	202.0	188	44	4	0	0	0
11364	Potatoes, Baked, Skin only	1	Each	58.0	115	27	2	0	0	0
11674	Potatoes, Baked, w/Skin	1	Medium	202.0	220	51	5	0	0	0
11365	Potatoes, Boiled, Ckd In Skin w/o Skin	1	Medium	202.0	176	41	4	0	0	0
11367	Potatoes, Boiled, Ckd w/o Skin	1	Medium	202.0	174	40	3	0	0	0
11366	Potatoes, Boiled, Skin only	1	Each	34.0	27	6	1	0	0	0
11376	Potatoes, Cnd, Drained Solids	½	Cup	90.0	54	12	1	0	0	0
11374	Potatoes, Cnd, Solids and Liquids	½	Cup	150.0	60	13	2	0	0	0
11370	Potatoes, Hashed Brown	½	Cup	78.0	119	6	2	11	4	5
11657	Potatoes, Mashed, Home–prepared	½	Cup	105.0	81	18	2	1	0	0
11930	Potatoes, Mashed, Prepared From Flakes	½	Cup	105.0	119	16	2	6	2	2
11368	Potatoes, Microwaved w/o Skin	½	Cup	78.0	78	18	2	0	0	0
11369	Potatoes, Microwaved, Skin only	1	Each	58.0	77	17	3	0	0	0
11675	Potatoes, Microwaved, w/Skin	1	Medium	202.0	212	49	5	0	0	0
11671	Potatoes, O'brien, Home–prepared	½	Cup	97.0	79	15	2	1	1	0
11844	Potatoes, Scalloped	½	Cup	122.5	105	13	4	5	2	2
62693	Power Bar	1	Each	65.0	230	45	10	3	1	2
19047	Pretzels, Hard, Plain, Salted	1	Ounce	28.4	108	22	3	1	0	0
19814	Pretzels, Hard, Plain, Unsalted	1	Ounce	28.4	108	22	3	1	0	0
19050	Pretzels, Hard, Whole–wheat	1	Ounce	28.4	103	23	3	1	0	0
9294	Prune Juice, Cnd	¾	Cup	191.8	136	33	1	0	0	0
9289	Prunes, Dehydrated	¼	Cup	33.0	112	29	1	0	0	0
9291	Prunes, Dried, Uncooked	¼	Cup	40.3	96	25	1	0	0	0
19072	Pudding Pops, Chocolate	1	Each	47.0	72	12	2	2	–	–
19073	Pudding Pops, Vanilla	1	Each	47.0	75	13	2	2	–	–
18326	Pumpkin Pie	1	Slice	109.0	229	30	4	10	2	5
11423	Pumpkin, Ckd	½	Cup	122.5	24	6	1	0	0	0
11424	Pumpkin, Cnd, w/o Salt	½	Cup	122.5	42	10	1	0	0	0
11429	Radishes, Fresh	½	Cup	58.0	10	2	0	0	0	0
11431	Radishes, Oriental, Ckd	½	Cup	73.5	12	3	0	0	0	0
11432	Radishes, Oriental, Dried	½	Cup	58.0	157	37	5	0	0	0
11430	Radishes, Oriental, Fresh	½	Cup	44.0	8	2	0	0	0	0
19149	Raisinets	10	Piece	10.0	41	7	0	2	1	1
9297	Raisins, Golden Seedless	½	Cup	72.5	219	58	2	0	0	0
9299	Raisins, Seeded	½	Cup	72.5	215	57	2	0	0	0
9298	Raisins, Seedless	½	Cup	72.5	218	57	2	0	0	0
9304	Raspberries, Cnd, Red, Heavy Syrup Pack	½	Cup	128.0	116	30	1	0	0	0
9302	Raspberries, Fresh	½	Cup	61.5	30	7	1	0	0	0
9306	Raspberries, Frozen, Red, Sweetened	½	Cup	125.0	129	33	1	0	0	0
62536	Ravioli, Beef	1	Cup	243.9	230	36	9	5	2	–
62537	Ravioli, Cheese	1	Cup	243.9	220	38	9	3	1	–
62557	Red Beans and Rice	2	Ounce	56.7	189	40	8	1	0	–
62607	Reduced Fat Chocolate Chip Cookies	13	Each	5.8	26	4	0	1	0	0
62595	Reduced Fat Chocolate Sandwich Cookies–SnackWell	2	Each	25.0	100	–	1	3	1	1
62593	Reduced Fat Classic Golden Crackers–SnackWell	6	Each	14.0	60	11	1	1	0	0
62594	Reduced Fat Creme Sandwich Cookies–SnackWell	2	Each	26.0	110	21	1	3	1	1
62597	Reduced Fat French Onion Snack Crackers–SnackWell	32	Each	30.0	120	23	2	2	0	1
62598	Reduced Fat Oatmeal Raisin Cookies–SnackWell	2	Each	27.0	110	20	2	3	0	1
62525	Reduced Fat Zesty Cheese Snack Crackers–SnackWell	32	Each	30.0	120	23	3	2	1	1
19150	Reese's Peanut Butter Cups	1	Each	7.0	34	3	1	2	2	0
19151	Reese's Pieces Candy	1	Pkg	55.0	258	34	7	11	–	–
62632	Refried Beans, Fat Free	½	Cup	134.0	120	21	8	0	0	–

Polyunsaturated fat (g)	Dietary Fiber (g)	Cholesterol (mg)	Folate (µg)	Vitamin A (RE)	Vitamin B-6 (mg)	Vitamin B-12 (µg)	Vitamin C (mg)	Vitamin E (mg)	Riboflavin (mg)	Thiamin (mg)	Calcium (mg)	Iron (mg)	Magnesium (mg)	Niacin (mg)	Phosphorus (mg)	Potassium (mg)	Sodium (mg)	Zinc (mg)
5	–	85	8	41	.2	0	12	–	.1	.1	24	.8	19	1.1	65	317	661	.4
5	1	0	11	0	.1	0	13	1.4	0	0	5	.6	18	1.4	49	351	71	.3
–	–	–	–	20	–	–	4	–	.1	–	48	.8	–	.8	–	260	670	–
1	–	18	10	47	.2	0	12	–	.1	.1	146	.8	24	1.2	138	485	530	.8
0	3	0	18	0	.6	0	26	.1	0	.2	10	.7	51	2.8	101	790	10	.6
0	2	0	13	0	.4	0	8	0	.1	.1	20	4.1	25	1.8	59	332	12	.3
0	5	0	22	0	.7	0	26	.1	.1	.2	20	2.7	55	3.3	115	844	16	.6
0	4	0	20	0	.6	0	26	.1	0	.2	10	.6	44	2.9	89	766	8	.6
0	4	0	18	0	.5	0	15	.1	0	.2	16	.6	40	2.7	81	663	10	.5
0	–	0	3	0	.1	0	2	–	0	0	15	2.1	10	.4	18	138	5	.1
0	–	0	6	0	.2	0	5	–	0	.1	4	1.1	13	.8	25	206	234	.3
0	2	0	7	0	.2	0	19	.1	0	.1	45	1.5	21	1.3	33	364	451	.6
1	2	–	6	0	.2	0	4	.1	0	.1	6	.6	16	1.6	33	250	19	.2
0	2	2	9	20	.2	0	7	.1	0	.1	27	.3	19	1.2	50	314	318	.3
2	–	4	8	22	0	0	10	–	.1	.1	51	.2	19	.7	59	245	349	.2
0	–	0	10	0	.2	0	12	–	0	.1	4	.3	20	1.3	85	321	5	.3
0	–	0	10	0	.3	0	9	–	0	0	27	3.4	21	1.3	48	377	9	.3
0	–	0	24	0	.7	0	31	–	.1	.2	22	2.5	55	3.5	212	903	16	.7
0	–	4	8	55	.2	0	16	–	.1	.1	35	.5	17	1	49	258	210	.3
1	–	7	11	23	.2	0	13	–	.1	.1	70	.7	23	1.3	77	463	410	.5
1	3	0	200	0	2	2	0	–	1.7	1.5	360	3.5	123	19	280	–	90	5.3
0	1	0	24	0	0	0	0	.1	.2	.1	10	1.2	10	1.5	32	41	486	.2
0	1	0	24	0	0	0	0	.1	.2	.1	10	1.2	10	1.5	32	41	82	.2
0	–	0	15	0	.1	0	0	–	.1	.1	8	.8	9	1.9	35	122	58	.2
0	2	0	1	0	.4	0	8	0	.1	0	23	2.3	27	1.5	48	529	8	.4
0	–	0	1	58	.2	0	0	–	.1	0	24	1.2	21	1	37	349	2	.2
0	3	0	1	80	.1	0	1	.6	.1	0	21	1	18	.8	32	300	2	.2
–	0	1	1	16	0	.3	0	0	.1	0	66	.2	10	.1	53	105	78	.2
–	0	1	2	24	0	.2	0	0	.1	0	61	0	5	0	47	65	50	.2
2	3	22	16	523	.1	.4	2	–	.2	.1	65	.9	16	.2	77	168	307	.5
0	–	0	10	132	.1	0	6	–	.1	0	18	.7	11	.5	37	282	1	.3
0	3	0	15	2702	.1	0	5	1.3	.1	0	32	1.7	28	.4	43	252	6	.2
0	1	0	16	1	0	0	13	0	0	0	12	.2	5	.2	10	135	14	.2
0	1	0	13	0	0	0	11	0	0	0	12	.1	7	.1	18	209	10	.1
0	–	0	171	0	.4	0	0	–	.4	.2	365	3.9	99	2	118	2027	161	1.2
0	1	0	12	0	0	0	10	0	0	0	12	.2	7	.1	10	100	9	.1
0	–	0	1	1	0	0	0	–	0	0	11	.1	5	0	14	51	4	.1
0	3	0	2	3	.2	0	2	.5	.1	0	38	1.3	25	.8	83	541	9	.2
0	5	0	2	0	.1	0	4	.5	.1	.1	20	1.9	22	.8	54	598	20	.1
0	3	0	2	1	.2	0	2	.5	.1	.1	36	1.5	24	.6	70	544	9	.2
0	4	0	13	4	.1	0	11	.6	0	0	14	.5	15	.6	12	120	4	.2
0	4	0	16	8	0	0	15	.3	.1	0	14	.4	11	.6	7	93	0	.3
0	5	0	32	7	0	0	21	.6	.1	0	19	.8	16	.3	21	142	1	.2
–	4	20	–	150	–	–	2	–	–	–	0	1.5	–	–	–	–	1150	–
–	4	15	–	60	–	–	1	–	–	–	24	1.5	–	–	–	–	1280	–
–	7	0	–	99	–	–	6	–	–	.2	48	1.5	–	2.8	–	–	786	–
0	0	0	–	0	–	–	0	–	–	–	0	.1	–	–	–	–	34	–
0	1	0	–	0	–	–	0	–	–	–	0	.4	–	–	–	–	190	–
0	0	0	–	0	–	–	0	–	–	–	24	.4	–	–	–	–	140	–
0	1	0	–	0	–	–	0	–	–	–	24	.2	–	–	–	–	95	–
–	1	23	–	0	–	–	0	–	–	–	48	.6	–	–	–	–	290	–
1	1	0	–	0	–	–	0	–	–	–	24	.4	–	–	–	–	135	–
0	1	5	0	0	0	0	0	0	0	0	48	.6	0	0	0	0	350	0
0	0	1	2	1	0	0	0	.1	0	0	5	.1	6	.3	17	28	20	.1
–	2	2	31	2	.1	.2	0	.7	.1	0	73	.8	45	3.1	127	242	83	.6
–	7	0	–	0	–	–	0	–	–	–	0	1	–	–	–	–	480	–

Code	Name	Amount	Unit	Grams	Energy (kcal)	Carbohydrates (g)	Protein (g)	Fat (g)	Saturated fat (g)	Monounsat fat (g)
19052	Rice Cakes, Brown Rice, Buckwheat	1	Cake	9.0	34	7	1	0	0	0
19817	Rice Cakes, Brown Rice, Buckwheat, Unsalted	1	Cake	9.0	34	7	1	0	0	0
19413	Rice Cakes, Brown Rice, Corn	1	Cake	9.0	35	7	1	0	0	0
19414	Rice Cakes, Brown Rice, Multigrain	1	Cake	9.0	35	7	1	0	0	0
19818	Rice Cakes, Brown Rice, Multigrain, Unsalted	1	Cake	9.0	35	7	1	0	0	0
19051	Rice Cakes, Brown Rice, Plain	1	Cake	9.0	35	7	1	0	0	0
19816	Rice Cakes, Brown Rice, Plain, Unsalted	1	Cake	9.0	35	7	1	0	0	0
19416	Rice Cakes, Brown Rice, Rye	1	Cake	9.0	35	7	1	0	0	0
62669	Rice Krispie Treats	1	Cup	40.0	160	33	1	2	0	1
19193	Rice Pudding	1	Cup	298.1	486	66	6	22	3	10
20037	Rice, Brown, Long–grain, Ckd	½	Cup	97.5	108	22	3	1	0	0
20041	Rice, Brown, Medium–grain, Ckd	½	Cup	97.5	109	23	2	1	0	0
20045	Rice, White, Long–grain, Ckd	½	Cup	79.0	103	22	2	0	0	0
20049	Rice, White, Long–grain, Instant, Enriched	½	Cup	82.5	81	18	2	0	0	0
20051	Rice, White, Medium–grain, Ckd	½	Cup	93.0	121	27	2	0	0	0
20053	Rice, White, Short–grain, Ckd	½	Cup	93.0	121	27	2	0	0	0
20057	Rice, White, w/Pasta, Ckd	½	Cup	101.0	123	22	3	3	1	1
62662	Rice–a–Roni Wild Rice	1	Cup	56.0	240	43	5	1	0	0
55222	Rigatoni Bake, Lean Cuisine–Stouffer's	1	Each	276.4	250	27	18	8	3	–
41341	Rigatoni in Meat Sauce–Healthy Choice	1	Each	269.3	260	34	16	6	2	–
55782	Rigatoni w/Meat Sauce–Stouffer's	½	Cup	142.0	145	16	8	6	–	–
62614	Roast Turkey Medallions–Weight Watchers	1	Each	241.0	190	34	10	2	1	–
41310	Roasted Turkey & Mushrooms in Gravy–Healthy Choice	1	Each	241.0	200	26	18	3	1	–
15071	Rockfish, Pacific, Ckd, Dry Heat	3	Ounce	85.1	103	0	20	2	0	0
14157	Root Beer	12	Fl Oz	369.6	152	39	0	0	0	0
62531	Root Beer, Diet	12	Fl Oz	355.2	0	0	0	0	–	–
15232	Roughy, Orange, Ckd, Dry Heat	3	Ounce	85.1	76	0	16	1	0	1
62541	Salad Dressing, Blue Cheese	2	Tbsp.	32.0	90	5	1	7	4	–
62542	Salad Dressing, Blue Cheese, Fat Free	2	Tbsp.	35.0	50	12	1	0	0	–
4120	Salad Dressing, French	2	Tbsp.	31.3	134	5	0	13	3	3
62545	Salad Dressing, French, Fat Free	2	Tbsp.	35.0	50	12	0	0	0	–
4020	Salad Dressing, French, Lo Fat	2	Tbsp.	32.5	44	7	0	2	0	0
4114	Salad Dressing, Italian	2	Tbsp.	29.4	137	3	0	14	2	3
62543	Salad Dressing, Italian, Fat Free	2	Tbsp.	31.0	10	2	0	0	0	–
4021	Salad Dressing, Italian, Lo Cal	2	Tbsp.	30.0	32	1	0	3	0	1
62539	Salad Dressing, Ranch	2	Tbsp.	29.0	170	2	0	18	3	–
62540	Salad Dressing, Ranch, Fat Free	2	Tbsp.	35.0	50	11	0	0	0	–
4015	Salad Dressing, Russian	2	Tbsp.	30.7	151	3	0	16	2	4
4022	Salad Dressing, Russian, Low Cal	2	Tbsp.	32.5	46	9	0	1	0	0
4016	Salad Dressing, Sesame Seed	2	Tbsp.	30.7	136	3	1	14	2	4
4017	Salad Dressing, Thousand Island	2	Tbsp.	31.3	118	5	0	11	2	3
62544	Salad Dressing, Thousand Island, Fat Free	2	Tbsp.	35.0	45	11	0	0	0	–
4023	Salad Dressing, Thousand Island, Lo Cal	2	Tbsp.	30.7	49	5	0	3	0	1
4135	Salad Dressing, Vinegar and Oil	2	Tbsp.	31.3	140	1	0	16	3	5
41290	Salisbury Steak w/Mushroom Gravy–Healthy Choice	1	Each	311.8	280	35	21	6	3	–
43402	Salisbury Steak, Top Shelf–Hormel	1	Each	283.5	320	22	25	15	7	8
15209	Salmon, Atlantic, Wild, Ckd, Dry Heat	3	Ounce	85.1	155	0	22	7	1	2
15210	Salmon, Chinook, Ckd, Dry Heat	3	Ounce	85.1	196	0	22	11	3	5
15211	Salmon, Chum, Ckd, Dry Heat	3	Ounce	85.1	131	0	22	4	1	2
15087	Salmon, Cnd	3	Ounce	85.1	130	0	17	6	1	2
15239	Salmon, Coho, Farmed, Ckd, Dry Heat	3	Ounce	85.1	151	0	21	7	2	3
15247	Salmon, Coho, Wild, Ckd, Dry Heat	3	Ounce	85.1	118	0	20	4	1	1
15082	Salmon, Coho, Wild, Ckd, Moist Heat	3	Ounce	85.1	156	0	23	6	1	2
15212	Salmon, Pink, Ckd, Dry Heat	3	Ounce	85.1	127	0	22	4	1	1
62546	Salsa	2	Tbsp.	33.0	20	5	0	0	0	–
41262	Salsa Chicken–Healthy Choice	1	Each	318.9	240	36	20	2	1	–

Polyunsaturated fat (g)	Dietary Fiber (g)	Cholesterol (mg)	Folate (µg)	Vitamin A (RE)	Vitamin B-6 (mg)	Vitamin B-12 (µg)	Vitamin C (mg)	Vitamin E (mg)	Riboflavin (mg)	Thiamin (mg)	Calcium (mg)	Iron (mg)	Magnesium (mg)	Niacin (mg)	Phosphorus (mg)	Potassium (mg)	Sodium (mg)	Zinc (mg)
0	0	0	2	0	0	0	0	–	0	0	1	.1	14	.7	34	27	10	.2
0	–	0	2	0	0	0	0	–	0	0	1	.1	14	.7	34	27	0	.2
0	0	0	2	0	0	0	0	–	0	0	1	.1	10	.6	29	25	26	.2
0	0	0	2	0	0	0	0	–	0	0	2	.2	12	.6	33	26	23	.2
0	–	0	2	0	0	0	0	–	0	0	2	.2	12	.6	33	26	0	.2
0	0	0	2	0	0	0	0	.1	0	0	1	.1	12	.7	32	26	29	.3
0	0	0	2	0	0	0	0	0	0	0	1	.1	12	.7	32	26	2	.3
0	0	0	0	0	0	0	0	–	0	0	2	.2	13	.6	34	28	10	.3
0	0	0	0	200	.7	.7	20	–	.6	.5	0	1.3	0	6.3	21	27	227	0
8	–	3	9	104	.1	.6	1	–	.2	.1	155	.9	24	.5	203	179	253	1.5
0	2	0	4	0	.1	0	0	.7	0	.1	10	.4	42	1.5	81	42	5	.6
0	–	0	4	0	.1	0	0	–	0	.1	10	.5	43	1.3	75	77	1	.6
0	0	0	2	0	.1	0	0	0	0	.1	8	.9	9	1.2	34	28	1	.4
0	0	0	3	0	0	0	0	0	0	.1	7	.5	4	.7	12	3	2	.2
0	0	0	2	0	0	0	0	–	0	.2	3	1.4	12	1.7	34	27	0	.4
0	–	0	2	0	.1	0	0	–	0	.2	1	1.4	7	1.4	31	24	0	.4
1	4	1	7	0	.1	.1	0	–	.1	.1	8	.9	12	1.8	37	42	574	.3
0	1	0	0	80	0	0	6	–	.1	.2	48	.8	0	1.5	0	–	1110	0
1	–	25	–	200	–	–	6	–	.3	.2	160	1.5	–	3.8	–	620	430	–
–	–	30	–	200	–	–	2	–	.3	.3	120	1.5	–	2.9	200	700	540	–
–	–	15	–	–	–	–	24	–	0	0	1	.2	–	.4	–	310	426	–
–	4	20	–	100	–	–	5	–	–	–	24	1	–	–	–	220	530	–
1	–	40	–	200	–	–	–	–	.1	.1	16	.8	–	2.9	150	260	380	–
1	0	37	9	56	.2	1	0	–	.1	0	10	.5	29	3.3	194	442	65	.5
0	0	0	0	0	0	0	0	0	0	0	18	.2	4	0	0	4	48	.3
–	0	–	–	–	–	–	–	–	–	–	–	–	–	–	–	–	30	–
0	0	22	7	20	.3	2	0	–	.2	.1	32	.2	32	3.1	218	327	69	.8
–	0	10	–	0	–	–	0	–	–	–	24	0	–	–	–	–	470	–
–	0	0	–	0	–	–	0	.4	–	–	0	0	–	–	–	–	340	–
7	0	18	1	6	0	0	0	2.6	0	0	3	.1	0	0	4	25	428	0
–	0	0	–	100	–	–	0	–	–	–	0	0	–	–	–	–	300	–
1	0	2	0	0	0	0	0	.5	0	0	4	.1	0	0	5	26	256	.1
8	0	0	1	7	0	0	0	3	0	0	3	.1	0	0	1	4	231	0
–	0	0	–	0	–	–	0	–	–	–	0	0	–	–	–	–	290	–
2	0	2	0	0	0	0	0	.5	0	0	1	.1	0	0	2	5	236	0
–	0	5	–	0	–	–	0	–	–	–	0	0	–	–	–	–	270	–
–	0	0	–	0	–	–	0	.6	–	–	0	0	–	–	–	–	310	–
9	0	6	3	63	0	.1	2	3.1	0	0	6	.2	0	.2	11	48	266	.1
1	0	2	1	5	0	0	2	.2	0	0	6	.2	0	0	12	51	282	0
8	–	0	0	63	0	0	0	1.5	0	0	6	.2	0	0	11	48	307	0
6	1	8	2	30	0	.1	0	.4	0	0	3	.2	1	0	5	35	219	0
–	0	0	–	0	–	–	0	–	–	–	0	0	–	–	–	–	300	–
2	0	5	2	29	0	.1	0	2.3	0	0	3	.2	0	0	5	35	307	0
8	0	0	0	0	0	0	0	2.8	0	0	0	0	0	0	0	2	0	0
–	–	55	–	–	–	–	–	–	–	–	–	–	–	–	260	630	500	–
1	–	70	–	0	–	–	4	0	.3	0	16	1.5	35	4.8	–	801	910	5.7
3	0	60	25	11	.8	2.6	0	–	.4	.2	13	.9	31	8.6	218	534	48	.7
2	0	72	30	127	.4	2.4	3	–	.1	0	24	.8	104	8.5	316	430	51	.5
1	0	81	4	29	.4	2.9	0	–	.2	.1	12	.6	24	7.3	309	468	54	.5
2	0	37	8	45	.3	.3	0	1.4	.2	0	203	.9	25	4.7	277	321	458	.9
2	0	54	12	50	.5	2.7	1	–	.1	.1	10	.3	29	6.3	282	391	44	.4
1	0	47	11	33	.5	4.3	1	–	.1	.1	–	.5	28	6.8	274	369	49	.5
2	0	48	8	27	.5	3.8	1	–	.1	.1	39	.6	30	6.6	253	387	45	.4
1	0	57	4	35	.2	2.9	0	–	.1	.2	14	.8	28	7.3	251	352	73	.6
–	0	0	–	80	–	–	4	–	–	–	0	0	–	–	–	–	240	–
–	–	50	–	200	–	–	66	–	.2	.2	64	.6	–	3.8	200	540	450	–

Code	Name	Amount	Unit	Grams	Energy (kcal)	Carbohydrates (g)	Protein (g)	Fat (g)	Saturated fat (g)	Monounsatur fat (g)
62651	Salt Substitute	¼	Tsp.	1.2	0	–	–	0	–	–
2047	Salt, Table	1	Tsp.	6.0	0	0	0	0	0	0
15088	Sardine, Atlantic, Cnd In Oil	3	Ounce	85.1	177	0	21	10	1	3
6313	Sauce, White	½	Cup	131.9	120	11	5	7	3	2
11439	Sauerkraut, Cnd, Sol&liq	½	Cup	118.0	22	5	1	0	0	0
7003	Sausage, Beerwurst, Pork	1	Slice	23.0	55	0	3	4	1	2
7006	Sausage, Bockwurst	1	Link	65.0	200	0	9	18	7	8
7013	Sausage, Bratwurst	1	Link	85.0	256	2	12	22	8	10
7089	Sausage, Italian, Ckd	1	Link	83.0	268	1	17	21	8	10
7037	Sausage, Kielbasa, Kolbassy	1	Link	85.0	264	2	11	23	8	11
7038	Sausage, Knockwurst	1	Link	68.0	209	1	8	19	7	9
7075	Sausage, Link, Pork and Beef	1	Link	68.0	228	1	9	21	7	10
16107	Sausage, Meatless	1	Link	25.0	64	2	5	5	1	1
7057	Sausage, Pepperoni	1	Slice	5.5	27	0	1	2	1	1
7059	Sausage, Polish–style	1	Each	227.0	740	4	32	65	23	31
7064	Sausage, Pork, Links or Bulk, Ckd	1	Link	13.0	48	0	3	4	1	2
7072	Sausage, Salami, Beef and Pork, Dry	1	Slice	10.0	42	0	2	3	1	2
7068	Sausage, Salami, Beef, Ckd	1	Slice	23.0	60	1	3	5	2	2
7074	Sausage, Smoked Link, Pork	1	Link	68.0	265	1	15	22	8	10
62661	Sausage, Turkey	3	Ounce	85.1	135	5	12	8	4	0
15173	Scallop, Breaded and Fried	3	Ounce	85.1	183	9	15	9	2	4
15174	Scallop, Imitation	3	Ounce	85.1	84	9	11	0	0	0
43412	Scalloped Potatoes and Ham, Micro Cup–Hormel	1	Each	212.6	260	21	8	16	6	8
55175	Scalloped Potatoes–Stouffer's	1	Each	163.0	130	16	4	6	–	–
62652	Scallops, Sauteed	3	Ounce	85.1	150	2	29	1	0	–
14018	Screwdriver	1	Fl Oz	30.4	25	3	0	0	0	0
15092	Sea Bass, Ckd, Dry Heat	3	Ounce	85.1	105	0	20	2	1	0
12036	Seeds, Sunflower, Dried	½	Cup	72.0	410	14	16	36	4	7
12537	Seeds, Sunflower, Dry Roasted, w/Salt added	½	Cup	64.0	372	15	12	32	3	6
12037	Seeds, Sunflower, Dry Roasted, w/o Salt	½	Cup	64.0	372	15	12	32	3	6
12538	Seeds, Sunflower, Oil Roasted, w/Salt added	½	Cup	67.5	415	10	14	39	4	7
12038	Seeds, Sunflower, Oil Roasted, w/o Salt	½	Cup	67.5	415	10	14	39	4	7
12539	Seeds, Sunflower, Toasted, w/Salt added	½	Cup	67.0	415	14	12	38	4	7
12039	Seeds, Sunflower, Toasted, w/o Salt	½	Cup	67.0	415	14	12	38	4	7
19418	Sesame Sticks, Wheat–based, Salted	1	Ounce	28.4	153	13	3	10	2	3
19820	Sesame Sticks, Wheat–based, Unsalted	1	Ounce	28.4	153	13	3	10	2	3
14346	Shake, Chocolate	1½	Cup	339.6	431	70	12	13	8	4
14428	Shake, Strawberry	1½	Cup	339.6	384	64	12	10	6	–
14347	Shake, Vanilla	1½	Cup	339.6	377	61	12	10	6	3
11640	Shallots, Freeze–dried	½	Cup	7.2	25	6	1	0	0	0
11677	Shallots, Fresh	½	Cup	79.9	58	13	2	0	0	0
15096	Shark, Ckd, Batter–dipped and Fried	3	Ounce	85.1	194	5	16	12	3	5
19097	Sherbet, All Flavors	1	Cup	192.0	265	58	2	4	2	1
18193	Shortbread Cookies, Pecan	1	Each	14.0	76	8	1	5	1	3
18192	Shortbread Cookies, Plain	1	Each	8.0	40	5	0	2	0	1
41263	Shrimp Marinara–Healthy Choice	1	Each	297.7	260	51	10	1	–	–
62615	Shrimp Marinara–Weight Watchers	1	Each	255.2	190	35	9	2	1	–
15150	Shrimp, Ckd, Breaded and Fried	3	Ounce	85.1	206	10	18	10	2	3
15151	Shrimp, Ckd, Moist Heat	3	Ounce	85.1	84	0	18	1	0	0
15152	Shrimp, Cnd	3	Ounce	85.1	102	1	20	2	0	0
15149	Shrimp, Fresh	3	Ounce	85.1	90	1	17	1	0	0
15153	Shrimp, Imitation	3	Ounce	85.1	86	8	11	1	0	0
55143	Single Serving Stuffed Pepper–Stouffer's	1	Each	283.5	220	28	10	8	–	–
41264	Sirloin Beef w/Barbecue Sauce–Healthy Choice	1	Each	311.8	280	44	17	4	2	–
19370	Skittles Bite Size Candies	1	Pkg	65.0	255	62	0	2	–	–
41291	Sliced Turkey Breast w/Gravy and Dressing–Healthy Choice	1	Each	283.5	270	30	27	4	2	–

Polyunsaturated fat (g)	Dietary Fiber (g)	Cholesterol (mg)	Folate (µg)	Vitamin A (RE)	Vitamin B-6 (mg)	Vitamin B-12 (µg)	Vitamin C (mg)	Vitamin E (mg)	Riboflavin (mg)	Thiamin (mg)	Calcium (mg)	Iron (mg)	Magnesium (mg)	Niacin (mg)	Phosphorus (mg)	Potassium (mg)	Sodium (mg)	Zinc (mg)
–	–	–	0	0	0	0	0	–	0	0	0	0	0	0	0	610	0	0
0	0	0	0	0	0	0	0	–	0	0	3	0	0	0	0	0	2325	0
4	0	121	10	57	.1	7.6	0	.3	.2	.1	325	2.5	33	4.5	417	338	430	1.1
1	–	17	8	46	0	.5	1	–	.2	0	212	.1	132	.3	128	222	398	.3
0	3	0	28	2	.2	0	17	.1	0	0	35	1.7	15	.2	24	201	780	.2
1	0	14	1	0	.1	.2	7	.1	0	.1	2	.2	3	.7	24	58	285	.4
2	0	38	4	4	.1	.5	0	.1	.1	.3	10	.4	12	2.7	95	176	718	1
2	0	51	2	0	.2	.8	1	.2	.2	.4	37	1.1	13	2.7	127	180	473	2
3	0	65	4	0	.3	1.1	2	.2	.2	.5	20	1.2	15	3.5	141	252	765	2
3	0	57	4	0	.2	1.4	18	.2	.2	.2	37	1.2	14	2.4	126	230	915	1.7
2	0	39	1	0	.1	.8	18	.4	.1	.2	7	.6	7	1.9	67	135	687	1.1
2	0	48	1	0	.1	1	13	.1	.1	.2	7	1	8	2.2	73	129	643	1.4
2	1	0	7	16	.2	0	0	.5	.1	.6	16	.9	9	2.8	56	58	222	.4
0	0	4	0	0	0	.1	0	0	0	0	1	.1	1	.3	7	19	112	.1
7	0	159	5	0	.4	2.2	2	–	.3	1.1	27	3.3	32	7.8	309	538	1989	4.4
0	0	11	0	0	0	.2	0	0	0	.1	4	.2	2	.6	24	47	168	.3
0	0	8	0	0	.1	.2	3	0	0	.1	1	.2	2	.5	14	38	186	.3
0	0	15	0	0	0	.7	4	0	0	0	2	.5	3	.7	26	52	270	.5
3	0	46	3	0	.2	1.1	1	.2	.2	.5	20	.8	13	3.1	110	228	1020	1.9
0	0	45	0	30	0	0	18	–	0	0	36	5.3	0	0	0	–	900	0
2	–	52	15	19	.1	1.1	2	–	.1	0	36	.7	50	1.3	201	283	395	.9
0	0	19	1	17	0	1.4	0	–	0	0	7	.3	37	.3	240	88	676	.3
2	–	33	–	–	–	–	11	.4	.1	.1	32	.4	21	2.1	–	425	768	.9
–	–	–	–	–	–	–	2	–	.1	0	80	.2	–	.8	–	375	610	–
–	–	60	0	0	0	0	2	–	0	0	24	0	0	0	0	–	275	0
0	–	0	11	2	0	0	9	–	0	0	2	0	2	0	4	47	0	0
1	0	45	5	54	.4	.3	0	–	.1	.1	11	.3	45	1.6	211	279	74	.4
24	8	0	164	4	.6	0	1	36.2	.2	1.6	84	4.9	255	3.2	508	496	2	3.6
21	4	0	152	0	.5	0	1	32.2	.2	.1	45	2.4	83	4.5	739	544	499	3.4
21	6	0	152	0	.5	0	1	32.2	.2	.1	45	2.4	83	4.5	739	544	2	3.4
26	5	0	158	3	.5	0	1	27	.2	.2	38	4.5	86	2.8	769	326	407	3.5
26	5	0	158	3	.5	0	1	33.9	.2	.2	38	4.5	86	2.8	769	326	2	3.5
25	–	0	159	0	.5	0	1	–	.2	.2	38	4.6	86	2.8	776	329	411	3.6
25	–	0	159	0	.5	0	1	–	.2	.2	38	4.6	86	2.8	776	329	2	3.6
5	1	0	6	3	0	0	0	1.1	0	0	48	.2	13	.4	39	50	422	.3
5	–	0	6	3	0	0	0	–	0	0	48	.2	13	.4	39	50	8	.3
0	–	44	12	78	.2	1.2	1	–	.8	.2	384	1.1	58	.5	346	679	329	1.4
–	–	37	10	98	.1	1.1	3	–	.7	.2	384	.4	44	.6	340	618	282	1.2
0	–	37	11	109	.2	1.2	3	–	.6	.2	414	.3	41	.6	346	591	278	1.2
0	–	0	8	404	.1	0	3	–	0	0	13	.4	7	.1	21	119	4	.1
0	–	0	27	998	.3	0	6	–	0	0	30	1	17	.2	48	267	10	.3
3	0	50	4	46	.3	1	0	–	.1	.1	43	.9	37	2.4	165	132	104	.4
0	–	10	8	27	.1	.2	8	–	.1	0	104	.3	15	.2	77	184	88	.9
1	0	5	1	0	0	0	0	–	0	0	4	.3	3	.3	12	10	39	.1
0	–	2	1	1	0	0	0	–	0	0	3	.2	1	.3	9	8	36	0
–	–	60	–	100	–	–	114	–	.1	.2	48	1.5	–	1.1	130	390	320	–
–	4	40	–	150	–	–	6	–	–	–	120	1	–	–	–	440	400	–
4	–	151	7	48	.1	1.6	1	–	.1	.1	57	1.1	34	2.6	185	191	293	1.2
0	0	166	3	56	.1	1.3	2	3.1	0	0	33	2.6	29	2.2	117	155	191	1.3
1	0	147	2	15	.1	1	2	2.1	0	0	50	2.3	35	2.3	198	179	144	1.1
1	0	129	3	46	.1	1	2	2.4	0	0	44	2	31	2.2	174	157	126	.9
1	0	31	1	17	0	1.4	0	–	0	0	16	.5	37	.1	240	76	600	.3
–	–	–	–	20	–	–	6	–	.2	.2	32	1	–	2.9	–	400	1010	–
1	–	25	–	–	–	–	–	–	–	–	–	–	–	–	190	630	240	–
–	0	0	0	0	0	0	0	0	0	0	2	.1	1	0	2	15	30	0
1	–	50	–	150	–	–	–	–	.3	.3	48	1	–	7.6	310	590	530	–

Code	Name	Amount	Unit	Grams	Energy (kcal)	Carbohydrates (g)	Protein (g)	Fat (g)	Saturated fat (g)	Monounsat fat (g
41296	Sliced Turkey Breast w/Gravy–Healthy Choice	1	Each	340.2	290	46	19	3	1	–
55225	Sliced Turkey w/Dressing, Lean Cuisine–Stouffer's	1	Each	223.3	200	23	16	5	1	–
19407	Slim Jims, Smoked	1	Ounce	28.4	156	2	6	14	6	6
15100	Smelt, Rainbow, Ckd, Dry Heat	3	Ounce	85.1	105	0	19	3	0	1
15102	Snapper, Ckd, Dry Heat	3	Ounce	85.1	109	0	22	1	0	0
19155	Snickers Bar	1	Bar	61.0	278	37	6	14	7	4
62599	Sorbet, All Flavors	½	Cup	90.0	100	25	0	0	0	–
6474	Soup, Bean w/Bacon	1	Cup	264.9	106	16	5	2	1	1
6007	Soup, Bean w/Ham	1	Cup	243.0	231	27	13	9	3	4
6406	Soup, Bean w/Hot Dogs	1	Cup	250.0	187	22	10	7	2	3
6404	Soup, Bean w/Pork	1	Cup	253.0	172	23	8	6	2	2
6008	Soup, Beef Broth or Bouillon	1	Cup	240.0	17	0	3	1	0	0
6547	Soup, Beef Mushroom	1	Cup	244.0	73	6	6	3	1	1
6409	Soup, Beef Noodle	1	Cup	244.0	83	9	5	3	1	1
6070	Soup, Beef, Chunky	1	Cup	240.0	170	20	12	5	3	2
6402	Soup, Black Bean	1	Cup	247.0	116	20	6	2	0	1
6478	Soup, Cauliflower	1	Cup	256.1	69	11	3	2	0	1
6411	Soup, Cheese	1	Cup	247.0	156	11	5	10	7	3
6480	Soup, Chicken Broth or Bouillon	1	Cup	244.0	22	1	1	1	0	0
6417	Soup, Chicken Gumbo	1	Cup	244.0	56	8	3	1	0	1
6549	Soup, Chicken Mushroom	1	Cup	244.0	132	9	4	9	2	4
6419	Soup, Chicken Noodle	1	Cup	241.0	75	9	4	2	1	1
6018	Soup, Chicken Noodle, Chunky	1	Cup	240.0	175	17	13	6	1	3
6485	Soup, Chicken Rice	1	Cup	252.8	61	9	2	1	0	1
6022	Soup, Chicken Rice, Chunky	1	Cup	240.0	127	13	12	3	1	1
6425	Soup, Chicken Vegetable	1	Cup	241.0	75	9	4	3	1	1
6024	Soup, Chicken Vegetable, Chunky	1	Cup	240.0	166	19	12	5	1	2
6412	Soup, Chicken w/Dumplings	1	Cup	241.0	96	6	6	6	1	3
6423	Soup, Chicken w/Rice	1	Cup	241.0	60	7	4	2	0	1
6015	Soup, Chicken, Chunky	1	Cup	251.0	178	17	13	7	2	3
6426	Soup, Chili Beef	1	Cup	250.0	170	21	7	7	3	3
6027	Soup, Clam Chowder, Manhattan Style	1	Cup	240.0	134	19	7	3	2	1
6230	Soup, Clam Chowder, New England	1	Cup	248.0	164	17	9	7	3	2
6034	Soup, Crab	1	Cup	244.0	76	10	5	2	0	1
6201	Soup, Cream Of Asparagus	1	Cup	248.0	161	16	6	8	3	2
6210	Soup, Cream Of Celery	1	Cup	248.0	164	15	6	10	4	2
6216	Soup, Cream Of Chicken	1	Cup	248.0	191	15	7	11	5	4
6243	Soup, Cream Of Mushroom	1	Cup	248.0	203	15	6	14	5	3
6246	Soup, Cream Of Onion	1	Cup	248.0	186	18	7	9	4	3
6253	Soup, Cream Of Potato	1	Cup	248.0	149	17	6	6	4	2
6256	Soup, Cream Of Shrimp	1	Cup	248.0	164	14	7	9	6	3
6501	Soup, Cream Of Vegetable	1	Cup	260.1	107	12	2	6	1	3
6036	Soup, Gazpacho	1	Cup	244.0	56	1	9	2	0	1
6037	Soup, Lentil w/ham	1	Cup	248.0	139	20	9	3	1	1
6440	Soup, Minestrone	1	Cup	241.0	82	11	4	3	1	1
6039	Soup, Minestrone, Chunky	1	Cup	240.0	127	21	5	3	1	1
6493	Soup, Mushroom	1	Cup	253.0	96	11	2	5	1	2
6445	Soup, Onion	1	Cup	241.0	58	8	4	2	0	1
6249	Soup, Pea, Green	1	Cup	254.0	239	32	13	7	4	2
6451	Soup, Pea, Split w/Ham	1	Cup	253.0	190	28	10	4	2	2
6050	Soup, Pea, Split w/Ham, Chunky	1	Cup	240.0	185	27	11	4	2	2
6359	Soup, Tomato	1	Cup	248.0	161	22	6	6	3	2
6461	Soup, Tomato Beef w/noodle	1	Cup	244.0	139	21	4	4	2	2
6463	Soup, Tomato Rice	1	Cup	247.0	119	22	2	3	1	1
6499	Soup, Tomato Vegetable	1	Cup	253.0	56	10	2	1	0	0
6465	Soup, Turkey Noodle	1	Cup	244.0	68	9	4	2	1	1

Polyunsaturated fat (g)	Dietary Fiber (g)	Cholesterol (mg)	Folate (µg)	Vitamin A (RE)	Vitamin B-6 (mg)	Vitamin B-12 (µg)	Vitamin C (mg)	Vitamin E (mg)	Riboflavin (mg)	Thiamin (mg)	Calcium (mg)	Iron (mg)	Magnesium (mg)	Niacin (mg)	Phosphorus (mg)	Potassium (mg)	Sodium (mg)	Zinc (mg)
1	–	20	–	150	–	–	27	–	.1	.2	16	.6	–	1.5	–	360	520	–
2	–	25	–	500	–	–	6	–	.3	.2	32	.8	–	4.8	–	400	590	–
1	–	38	0	48	.1	.3	2	–	.1	0	19	1	6	1.3	51	73	420	.7
1	0	77	4	14	.1	3.4	0	–	.1	0	65	1	32	1.5	251	316	65	1.8
1	0	40	5	30	.4	3	1	–	0	0	34	.2	31	.3	171	444	48	.4
1	2	7	24	19	.1	.3	0	3.4	.1	0	70	.5	37	1.8	129	199	163	.7
–	1	0	–	0	–	–	12	–	–	–	0	0	–	–	–	–	10	–
0	9	3	8	5	0	0	1	.3	.3	.1	56	1.3	29	.4	90	326	927	.7
1	11	22	29	396	.1	.1	4	.1	.1	.1	78	3.2	46	1.7	143	425	972	1.1
2	–	12	30	87	.1	.1	1	–	.1	.1	87	2.3	47	1	165	477	1092	1.2
2	9	3	32	89	0	.1	2	.1	0	.1	81	2	46	.6	132	402	951	1
0	0	0	5	0	0	.2	0	0	.1	0	14	.4	5	1.9	31	130	782	0
0	–	7	10	0	0	.2	5	–	.1	0	5	.9	10	1	34	154	942	1.5
0	1	5	4	63	0	.2	0	0	.1	.1	15	1.1	5	1.1	46	100	952	1.5
0	1	14	13	262	.1	.6	7	.2	.2	.1	31	2.3	5	2.7	120	336	866	2.6
0	4	0	25	49	.1	0	1	.1	.1	.1	44	2.1	42	.5	106	274	1198	1.4
1	–	0	3	0	0	.2	3	–	.1	.1	10	.5	3	.5	51	105	843	.3
0	–	30	5	109	0	0	0	–	.1	0	141	.7	5	.4	136	153	958	.6
0	0	0	2	12	0	0	0	0	0	0	15	.1	5	.2	12	24	1484	0
0	2	5	5	15	.1	0	5	0	0	0	24	.9	5	.7	24	76	954	.4
2	–	10	0	112	0	0	0	–	.1	0	29	.9	10	1.6	27	154	942	1
1	1	7	2	72	0	.1	0	.1	.1	.1	17	.8	5	1.4	36	55	1106	.4
2	4	19	5	122	0	.3	0	.8	.2	.1	24	1.4	10	4.3	72	108	850	1
0	1	3	1	0	0	.1	0	0	0	0	8	0	0	.4	10	10	981	.1
1	1	12	4	586	0	.3	4	.1	.1	0	34	1.9	10	4.1	72	108	888	1
1	1	10	5	265	0	.1	1	.1	.1	0	17	.9	7	1.2	41	154	945	.4
1	–	17	12	600	.1	.2	6	–	.2	0	26	1.5	10	3.3	106	367	1068	2.2
1	1	34	2	53	0	.2	0	.1	.1	0	14	.6	5	1.8	60	116	860	.4
0	1	7	1	65	0	.1	0	.1	0	0	17	.7	0	1.1	22	101	815	.3
1	2	30	5	131	.1	.3	1	.2	.2	.1	25	1.7	8	4.4	113	176	889	1
0	9	12	17	150	.2	.3	4	.2	.1	.1	42	2.1	30	1.1	147	525	1035	1.4
0	3	14	9	329	.3	7.9	12	.1	.1	.1	67	2.6	19	1.8	84	384	1001	1.7
1	1	22	10	40	.1	10.2	3	.1	.2	.1	186	1.5	22	1	156	300	992	.8
0	1	10	15	51	.1	.2	0	.1	.1	.2	66	1.2	15	1.3	88	327	1235	1.5
2	1	22	30	84	.1	.5	4	.8	.3	.1	174	.9	20	.9	154	360	1042	.9
3	1	32	8	67	.1	.5	1	1	.2	.1	186	.7	22	.4	151	310	1009	.2
2	0	27	8	94	.1	.5	1	.2	.3	.1	181	.7	17	.9	151	273	1047	.7
5	0	20	10	37	.1	.5	2	1.3	.3	.1	179	.6	20	.9	156	270	1076	.6
2	1	32	12	67	.1	.5	2	.1	.3	.1	179	.7	22	.6	154	310	1004	.6
1	0	22	9	67	.1	.5	1	.1	.2	.1	166	.5	17	.6	161	322	1061	.7
0	0	35	10	55	.4	1	1	.9	.2	.1	164	.6	22	.5	146	248	1037	.8
1	1	0	8	3	0	.1	4	1.2	.1	1.2	31	.5	10	.5	55	96	1170	.3
1	4	0	10	20	.1	0	3	.5	0	0	24	1	7	.9	37	224	1183	.2
0	–	7	50	35	.2	.3	4	–	.1	.2	42	2.7	22	1.4	184	357	1319	.7
1	1	2	16	234	.1	0	1	.1	0	.1	34	.9	7	.9	55	313	911	.7
0	2	5	31	434	.2	0	5	.7	.1	.1	60	1.8	14	1.2	110	612	864	1.4
2	1	0	5	0	0	.3	1	.6	.1	.3	66	.5	5	.5	76	200	1020	.1
1	1	0	15	0	0	0	1	.3	0	0	27	.7	2	.6	12	67	1053	.6
1	3	18	8	58	.1	.4	3	.2	.3	.2	173	2	56	1.3	239	376	1046	1.8
1	–	8	3	46	.1	.3	2	–	.1	.1	23	2.3	48	1.5	213	400	1007	1.3
1	4	7	5	487	.2	.2	7	.1	.1	.1	34	2.1	38	2.5	178	305	965	3.1
1	0	17	21	109	.2	.4	68	2.6	.2	.1	159	1.8	22	1.5	149	449	932	.3
1	1	5	7	54	.1	.2	0	.8	.1	.1	17	1.1	7	1.9	56	220	917	.8
1	1	2	14	77	.1	0	15	.8	0	.1	22	.8	5	1.1	35	331	815	.5
0	1	0	10	20	.1	0	6	.8	0	.1	8	.6	20	.8	30	104	1146	.2
0	1	5	2	29	0	.1	0	.1	.1	.1	12	1	5	1.4	49	76	815	.6

Code	Name	Amount	Unit	Grams	Energy (kcal)	Carbohydrates (g)	Protein (g)	Fat (g)	Saturated fat (g)	Monounsa fat (g)
6466	Soup, Turkey Vegetable	1	Cup	241.0	72	9	3	3	1	1
6064	Soup, Turkey, Chunky	1	Cup	236.0	135	14	10	4	1	2
6500	Soup, Vegetable Beef	1	Cup	253.1	53	8	3	1	1	0
6067	Soup, Vegetable, Chunky	1	Cup	240.0	122	19	4	4	1	2
6468	Soup, Vegetarian Vegetable	1	Cup	241.0	72	12	2	2	0	1
1056	Sour Cream	1	Tbsp.	12.0	26	1	0	3	2	1
62556	Sour Cream, Fat Free	1	Tbsp.	16.0	13	3	1	0	0	–
1074	Sour Cream, Imitation, Nondairy, Cultured	1	Tbsp.	14.4	30	1	0	3	3	0
62555	Sour Cream, Light	1	Tbsp.	16.0	16	1	1	1	1	–
62660	Sour Cream, Non–Fat	2	Tbsp.	32.0	25	5	1	0	0	0
41265	Southwestern Style Chicken–Healthy Choice	1	Each	354.4	340	51	25	5	2	–
6134	Soy Sauce	1	Tbsp.	18.0	10	2	1	0	0	0
16109	Soybeans, Boiled	½	Cup	86.0	149	9	14	8	1	2
16111	Soybeans, Dry Roasted	½	Cup	86.0	387	28	34	19	3	4
11455	Spaghetti Sauce	½	Cup	124.5	136	20	2	6	1	3
62666	Spaghetti Sauce, Healthy Choice	1	Cup	146.0	59	13	2	1	0	0
62665	Spaghetti Sauce, Prego	1	Cup	146.0	154	26	4	4	1	0
62664	Spaghetti Sauce, Ragu	1	Cup	146.0	131	20	4	5	2	0
43404	Spaghetti and Meatballs, Micro Cup–Hormel	1	Each	212.6	210	27	10	7	3	3
55226	Spaghetti w/Meat Sauce, Lean Cuisine–Stouffer's	1	Each	326.0	290	45	15	6	2	–
43396	Spaghetti w/Meat Sauce, Top Shelf–Hormel	1	Each	283.5	260	37	14	6	2	2
41342	Spaghetti w/Meat Sauce–Healthy Choice	1	Each	283.5	280	42	14	6	2	–
55247	Spaghetti w/Meat Sauce–Stouffer's	1	Each	365.0	320	38	16	12	–	–
55150	Spaghetti w/Meatballs–Stouffer's	1	Each	276.4	290	37	14	9	–	–
19164	Special Dark Sweet Chocolate Bar	1	Bar	79.0	376	49	4	24	–	–
55176	Spinach Souffle–Stouffer's	1	Each	170.1	220	11	9	15	–	–
11458	Spinach, Ckd	½	Cup	90.0	21	3	3	0	0	0
11461	Spinach, Cnd, Drained Solids	½	Cup	107.0	25	4	3	1	0	0
11459	Spinach, Cnd, Reg Pk, Sol&liq	½	Cup	117.0	22	3	2	0	0	0
11457	Spinach, Fresh	1	Cup	56.0	12	2	2	0	0	0
11464	Spinach, Frz, Ckd	½	Cup	95.0	27	5	3	0	0	0
11463	Spinach, Frz, Unprepared	½	Cup	78.0	19	3	2	0	0	0
55766	Split Pea Soup w/Ham–Stouffer's	1	Cup	283.9	220	35	15	3	–	–
41283	Split Pea and Ham Soup–Healthy Choice	1	Each	212.6	170	25	10	3	1	–
11483	Squash, Acorn, Ckd. w/o Salt	½	Cup	102.5	57	15	1	0	0	0
11486	Squash, Butternut, Ckd. w/o Salt	½	Cup	102.5	41	11	1	0	0	0
11493	Squash, Spaghetti, Ckd. w/o Salt	½	Cup	77.5	22	5	1	0	0	0
11642	Squash, Summer, Ckd	½	Cup	90.0	18	4	1	0	0	0
11641	Squash, Summer, Fresh	½	Cup	65.0	13	3	1	0	0	0
11644	Squash, Winter, Baked	½	Cup	102.5	40	9	1	1	0	0
11643	Squash, Winter, Fresh	½	Cup	58.0	21	5	1	0	0	0
11953	Squash, Zucchini, Baby, Fresh	1	Medium	11.0	2	0	0	0	0	0
15176	Squid, Fried	3	Ounce	85.1	149	7	15	6	2	2
9316	Strawberries, Fresh	½	Cup	74.5	22	5	0	0	0	0
9320	Strawberries, Frozen, Sweetened	½	Cup	127.5	122	33	1	0	0	0
9318	Strawberries, Frozen, Unsweetened	½	Cup	74.5	26	7	0	0	0	0
14351	Strawberry Flavor Beverage	1	Cup	266.0	234	33	8	8	5	2
18354	Strudel, Apple	1	Each	71.0	195	29	2	8	2	4
55781	Stuffed Cabbage no Sauce–Stouffer's	1	Ounce	28.4	39	3	2	2	–	–
55228	Stuffed Cabbage w/Meat, Lean Cuisine–Stouffer's	1	Each	269.3	210	26	13	6	2	–
55778	Stuffed Cabbage–Stouffer's	1	Ounce	28.4	29	3	1	1	–	–
55157	Stuffed Green Peppers–Stouffer's	1	Each	219.7	200	22	9	8	–	–
18203	Sugar Cookies, Dietary	1	Each	7.0	30	5	1	1	0	1
18204	Sugar Cookies, Regular (includes Vanilla)	1	Each	15.0	72	10	1	3	1	2
19334	Sugar, Brown	1	Tsp.	5.0	19	5	0	0	–	–
19335	Sugar, Granulated	1	Tsp.	4.0	15	4	0	0	–	–

Polyunsaturated fat (g)	Dietary Fiber (g)	Cholesterol (mg)	Folate (µg)	Vitamin A (RE)	Vitamin B-6 (mg)	Vitamin B-12 (µg)	Vitamin C (mg)	Vitamin E (mg)	Riboflavin (mg)	Thiamin (mg)	Calcium (mg)	Iron (mg)	Magnesium (mg)	Niacin (mg)	Phosphorus (mg)	Potassium (mg)	Sodium (mg)	Zinc (mg)
1	0	2	5	243	0	.2	0	.1	0	0	17	.8	5	1	41	176	906	.6
1	–	9	11	715	.3	2.1	6	–	.1	0	50	1.9	24	3.6	104	361	923	2.1
0	1	0	8	23	.1	.3	1	0	0	0	13	.9	23	.5	35	76	1002	.3
1	1	0	17	588	.2	0	6	.6	.1	.1	55	1.6	7	1.2	72	396	1010	3.1
1	0	0	11	301	.1	0	1	.8	0	.1	22	1.1	7	.9	34	210	822	.5
0	0	5	1	23	0	0	0	.1	0	0	14	0	1	0	10	17	6	0
–	–	3	–	30	–	–	0	–	–	–	36	0	–	–	–	–	18	–
0	0	0	0	0	0	0	0	0	0	0	0	.1	1	0	6	23	15	.2
–	–	5	–	18	–	–	0	–	–	–	22	0	–	–	–	27	9	–
0	0	5	0	60	0	0	0	–	0	0	72	0	0	0	0	–	35	0
2	–	60	–	–	–	–	–	–	–	–	–	–	–	–	260	560	550	–
0	0	0	3	0	0	0	0	0	0	0	3	.4	6	.6	20	32	1029	.1
4	5	0	46	1	.2	0	1	1.7	.2	.1	88	4.4	74	.3	211	443	1	1
10	7	0	176	2	.2	0	4	1.7	.6	.4	232	3.4	196	.9	558	1173	2	4.1
2	4	0	27	153	.4	0	14	3.1	.1	.1	35	.8	30	1.9	45	478	618	.3
0	2	0	0	119	0	0	6	–	0	0	57	.7	0	0	0	–	463	0
0	4	0	0	356	0	0	21	–	0	0	85	.7	0	0	0	–	724	0
0	4	0	0	178	0	0	1	–	0	0	57	.7	0	0	0	–	653	0
1	–	20	–	140	–	–	4	0	.3	.1	32	1.1	25	2.3	–	341	930	1.1
2	–	20	–	100	–	–	6	–	.3	.3	48	2	–	3.8	–	500	500	–
1	–	20	–	100	–	–	2	.1	.3	.2	48	1.5	46	3.8	–	879	980	2.4
2	–	20	–	250	–	–	5	–	.3	.4	48	2	–	1.9	160	540	480	–
12	–	–	–	150	–	–	6	–	.2	.2	80	1.5	–	3.8	–	800	560	–
–	–	–	–	100	–	–	6	–	.3	.3	64	1.5	–	3.8	–	550	790	–
–	4	0	3	2	0	0	0	.8	.2	0	15	1.7	91	.5	126	269	8	1.2
–	–	–	–	200	–	–	6	–	.3	.1	120	.4	–	.4	–	345	820	–
0	2	0	131	737	.2	0	9	.9	.2	.1	122	3.2	78	.4	50	419	63	.7
0	–	0	105	939	.1	0	15	–	.1	0	136	2.5	81	.4	47	370	29	.5
0	3	0	68	752	.1	0	16	1.1	.1	0	97	1.8	66	.3	37	269	373	.5
0	2	0	109	376	.1	0	16	1.1	.1	0	55	1.5	44	.4	27	312	44	.3
0	3	0	102	739	.1	0	12	.9	.2	.1	139	1.4	66	.4	46	283	82	.7
0	2	0	93	605	.1	0	19	.7	.1	.1	87	1.6	45	.3	32	252	58	.3
–	–	10	–	–	–	–	0	–	0	0	240	.2	–	.4	–	571	1192	–
–	–	10	–	100	–	–	6	–	.1	.2	16	.6	–	1.9	190	450	460	–
0	–	0	19	44	.2	0	11	–	0	.2	45	1	44	.9	46	448	4	.2
0	–	0	20	718	.1	0	15	–	0	.1	42	.6	30	1	28	291	4	.1
0	1	0	6	9	.1	0	3	.1	0	0	16	.3	9	.6	11	91	14	.2
0	1	0	18	26	.1	0	5	.1	0	0	24	.3	22	.5	35	173	1	.4
0	1	0	17	13	.1	0	10	.1	0	0	13	.3	15	.4	23	127	1	.2
0	3	0	29	365	.1	0	10	.1	0	.1	14	.3	8	.7	21	448	1	.3
0	1	0	13	235	0	0	7	.1	0	.1	18	.3	12	.5	19	203	2	.1
0	–	0	2	5	0	0	4	–	0	0	2	.1	4	.1	10	50	0	.1
2	0	221	5	9	0	1	4	–	.4	0	33	.9	32	2.2	213	237	260	1.5
0	2	0	13	2	0	0	42	.1	0	0	10	.3	7	.2	14	124	1	.1
0	2	0	19	3	0	0	53	.2	.1	0	14	.8	9	.5	17	125	4	.1
0	2	0	13	3	0	0	31	.2	0	0	12	.6	8	.3	10	110	1	.1
0	–	32	12	74	.1	.9	2	–	.4	.1	293	.2	32	.2	229	370	128	.9
1	2	20	4	6	0	.1	1	–	0	0	11	.3	6	.2	23	69	191	.1
–	–	5	–	–	–	–	1	–	0	0	72	0	–	.1	–	48	150	–
1	–	30	–	80	–	–	6	–	.2	.1	64	1.5	–	3.8	–	600	560	–
–	–	4	–	–	–	–	3	–	0	0	48	0	–	.1	–	51	145	–
–	–	–	–	60	–	–	6	–	.1	.1	32	.8	–	2.9	–	380	650	–
0	–	0	0	0	0	0	0	–	0	0	2	.3	1	.2	6	7	0	0
0	–	8	2	4	0	0	0	–	0	0	3	.3	2	.4	12	9	54	.1
–	0	0	0	0	0	0	0	0	0	0	4	.1	1	0	1	17	2	0
–	0	0	0	0	0	0	0	0	0	0	0	0	0	0	0	0	0	0

Code	Name	Amount	Unit	Grams	Energy (kcal)	Carbohydrates (g)	Protein (g)	Fat (g)	Saturated fat (g)	Monounsatur fat (g)
19336	Sugar, Powdered	1	Tbsp.	8.0	31	8	0	0	–	–
15218	Sunfish, Ckd, Dry Heat	3	Ounce	85.1	97	0	21	1	0	0
55229	Swedish Meatballs w/Pasta, Lean Cuisine–Stouffer's	1	Each	258.7	290	31	23	8	3	–
55148	Swedish Meatballs w/Pasta–Stouffer's	1	Each	262.2	420	32	24	21	–	–
18359	Sweet Rolls w/Raisins and Nuts	1	Each	57.0	196	30	4	7	1	3
18355	Sweet Rolls, Cheese	1	Each	66.0	238	29	5	12	4	6
18356	Sweet Rolls, Cinnamon w/Raisins	1	Each	60.0	223	31	4	10	3	5
41266	Sweet and Sour Chicken–Healthy Choice	1	Each	326.0	280	52	20	2	–	–
11508	Sweet Potatoes, Baked In Skin	½	Cup	100.0	103	24	2	0	0	0
11510	Sweet Potatoes, Boiled, w/o Skin	½	Cup	164.0	172	40	3	0	0	0
11659	Sweet Potatoes, Candied	½	Cup	113.4	155	32	1	4	2	1
11514	Sweet Potatoes, Mashed	½	Cup	127.5	129	30	3	0	0	0
11647	Sweet Potatoes, Syrup Pack, Drained Solids	½	Cup	98.0	106	25	1	0	0	0
15111	Swordfish, Ckd, Dry Heat	3	Ounce	85.1	132	0	22	4	1	2
19093	Symphony Milk Chocolate Bar	1	Bar	68.0	355	39	5	22	–	–
19348	Syrup, Chocolate, Fudge–type	1	Tbsp.	21.0	73	12	1	3	1	1
19349	Syrup, Corn, Dark	1	Tbsp.	20.0	56	15	0	0	–	–
19351	Syrup, Corn, High–fructose	1	Tbsp.	19.0	53	14	0	0	–	–
19350	Syrup, Corn, Light	1	Tbsp.	20.0	56	15	0	0	–	–
19352	Syrup, Malt	1	Tbsp.	24.0	76	17	1	0	–	–
19353	Syrup, Maple	1	Tbsp.	20.0	52	13	0	0	–	–
19128	Syrup, Pancake, Lo Cal	1	Tbsp.	20.0	33	9	0	0	–	–
19360	Syrup, Pancake, w/2% Maple	1	Tbsp.	20.0	53	14	0	0	–	–
19113	Syrup, Pancake, w/Butter	1	Tbsp.	20.0	59	15	0	0	0	0
62653	Tabouli	1	Ounce	28.4	30	2	1	2	0	–
18360	Taco Shells, Baked	1	Medium	13.0	61	8	1	3	0	1
18448	Taco Shells, Baked, w/o Added Salt	1	Medium	13.0	61	8	1	3	0	1
43438	Taco Shells, Chi–Chi's–Hormel	1	Each	20.0	99	12	1	5	–	–
19382	Taffy	1	Piece	15.0	56	14	0	0	0	0
9223	Tangerine Juice, Cnd, Sweetened	¾	Cup	186.4	93	22	1	0	0	0
9221	Tangerine Juice, Fresh	¾	Cup	185.2	80	19	1	0	0	0
9219	Tangerines, Cnd, Juice Pack	½	Cup	124.5	46	12	1	0	0	0
9220	Tangerines, Cnd, Light Syrup Pack	½	Cup	126.0	77	20	1	0	0	0
9218	Tangerines, Fresh	1	Medium	84.0	37	9	1	0	0	0
19218	Tapioca Pudding	1	Cup	298.1	355	58	6	11	2	5
19524	Taro Chips	1	Ounce	28.4	141	19	1	7	2	1
62654	Tator Tots	10	Each	28.4	140	20	3	5	1	–
14355	Tea, Brewed	8	Fl Oz	236.8	2	1	0	0	0	0
14381	Tea, Herb, Brewed	8	Fl Oz	236.8	2	0	0	0	0	0
14371	Tea, Instant, Sweetened	8	Fl Oz	259.0	88	22	0	0	0	0
14367	Tea, Instant, Unsweetened	8	Fl Oz	236.8	2	0	0	0	0	0
43401	Tender Beef Roast, Top Shelf–Hormel	1	Each	283.5	240	19	28	6	2	2
14020	Tequila Sunrise	1	Fl Oz	31.2	34	3	0	0	0	0
41267	Teriyaki Chicken–Healthy Choice	1	Each	347.3	290	39	24	4	1	–
6112	Teriyaki Sauce	1	Tbsp.	18.0	15	3	1	0	0	0
55811	Three Bean Chili–Stouffer's	1	Cup	283.9	210	32	10	5	–	–
19159	Three Musketeers Bar	1	Bar	60.0	250	46	2	8	4	3
18361	Toaster Pastries, Brown–sugar–cinn.	1	Each	52.0	214	35	3	7	2	4
18362	Toaster Pastries, Fruit	1	Each	52.0	204	37	2	5	1	2
19383	Toffee	1	Piece	12.0	65	8	0	4	2	1
16126	Tofu, Fresh, Firm	1	Ounce	28.4	41	1	4	2	0	1
16127	Tofu, Fresh, Regular	1	Ounce	28.4	22	1	2	1	0	0
16129	Tofu, Fried	1	Ounce	28.4	77	3	5	6	1	1
16429	Tofu, Fried, Prepared w/Calcium Sulfate	1	Ounce	28.4	77	3	5	6	1	1
16130	Tofu, Okara	1	Ounce	28.4	22	4	1	0	0	0
16132	Tofu, Salted and Fermented (fuyu)	1	Ounce	28.4	33	1	2	2	0	1

Polyunsaturated fat (g)	Dietary Fiber (g)	Cholesterol (mg)	Folate (μg)	Vitamin A (RE)	Vitamin B-6 (mg)	Vitamin B-12 (μg)	Vitamin C (mg)	Vitamin E (mg)	Riboflavin (mg)	Thiamin (mg)	Calcium (mg)	Iron (mg)	Magnesium (mg)	Niacin (mg)	Phosphorus (mg)	Potassium (mg)	Sodium (mg)	Zinc (mg)
–	0	0	0	0	0	0	0	0	0	0	0	0	0	0	0	0	0	0
0	0	73	14	14	.1	2	1	–	.1	.1	88	1.3	32	1.2	196	382	88	1.7
1	–	55	–	20	–	–	–	–	.3	.2	48	1.5	–	3.8	–	450	550	–
–	–	–	–	20	–	–	1	–	.3	.2	48	1.5	–	2.9	–	350	740	–
3	–	13	18	60	.1	.1	0	–	.2	.2	36	1.5	16	1.3	63	123	185	.4
1	–	37	20	41	0	.1	0	–	.1	.1	78	.5	13	.5	65	87	236	.4
1	1	40	14	38	.1	.1	1	–	.2	.2	43	1	10	1.4	46	67	230	.4
–	–	35	–	250	–	–	30	–	.2	.2	32	1	–	8.6	220	480	320	–
0	3	0	23	2182	.2	0	25	4.6	.1	.1	28	.4	20	.6	55	348	10	.3
0	4	0	18	2796	.4	0	28	7.5	.2	.1	34	.9	16	1	44	302	21	.4
0	–	9	13	475	0	0	8	–	0	0	29	1.3	12	.4	29	214	79	.2
0	–	0	14	1929	.3	0	7	–	.1	0	38	1.7	31	1.2	66	268	96	.3
0	–	0	8	702	.1	0	11	–	0	0	17	.9	12	.3	25	189	38	.2
1	0	43	2	35	.3	1.7	1	–	.1	0	5	.9	29	10	287	314	98	1.3
–	–	19	5	9	0	.3	0	–	.3	.1	160	.7	37	.2	170	262	58	.8
1	0	3	1	5	0	.1	0	0	0	0	21	.3	10	0	36	45	27	.2
–	0	0	0	0	0	0	0	0	0	0	4	.1	2	0	2	9	31	0
–	0	0	0	0	0	0	0	0	0	0	0	0	0	0	0	0	0	0
–	–	0	0	0	0	0	0	–	0	0	1	0	0	0	0	1	24	0
–	–	0	3	0	.1	0	0	–	.1	0	15	.2	17	1.9	57	77	8	0
–	0	0	0	0	0	0	0	0	0	0	13	.2	3	0	0	41	2	.8
–	0	0	0	0	0	0	0	0	0	0	0	0	0	0	9	1	40	0
–	0	0	0	0	0	0	0	0	0	0	1	0	0	0	2	1	12	0
0	–	1	0	3	0	0	0	–	0	0	0	0	0	0	2	1	20	0
–	1	0	0	100	0	0	12	–	0	0	0	.4	0	0	0	–	75	0
1	1	0	1	5	0	0	0	–	0	0	21	.3	14	.2	32	23	48	.2
1	–	0	1	–	–	0	0	–	0	0	21	.3	14	.2	32	23	2	.2
–	–	0	–	–	–	–	–	.1	.1	.1	–	.1	–	.5	–	–	4	–
0	–	1	0	5	0	0	0	–	0	0	0	0	0	0	0	1	13	0
0	0	0	9	78	.1	0	41	.2	0	.1	34	.4	15	.2	26	332	2	.1
0	0	0	9	78	.1	0	57	.2	0	.1	33	.4	15	.2	26	330	2	.1
0	1	0	6	106	.1	0	43	.6	0	.1	14	.3	14	.6	12	166	6	.6
0	1	0	6	106	.1	0	25	.4	.1	.1	9	.5	10	.6	13	98	8	.3
0	2	0	17	77	.1	0	26	.2	0	.1	12	.1	10	.1	8	132	1	.2
4	0	3	12	0	.3	.3	2	.3	.3	.1	250	.7	24	.9	236	310	352	.8
4	2	0	6	0	.1	0	1	1.4	0	0	17	.3	24	.1	37	214	97	.1
–	3	0	0	0	0	0	0	–	0	0	0	0	0	0	0	240	240	0
0	0	0	12	0	0	0	0	0	0	0	0	0	7	0	2	88	7	0
0	0	0	1	0	0	0	0	0	0	0	5	.2	2	0	0	21	2	.1
0	–	0	10	0	0	0	0	–	0	0	5	.1	5	.1	3	49	8	.1
0	0	0	1	0	0	0	0	0	0	0	5	0	5	.1	2	47	7	.1
1	–	60	–	400	–	–	2	0	.4	.8	16	1.5	42	5.7	–	933	880	4.5
0	–	0	3	3	0	0	6	–	0	0	2	.1	2	.1	3	32	1	0
2	–	55	–	20	–	–	6	–	.1	.1	32	.8	–	7.6	250	520	560	–
0	0	0	4	0	0	0	0	0	0	0	5	.3	11	.2	28	41	690	0
–	–	20	–	–	–	–	6	–	0	0	1	.4	–	.6	–	891	861	–
0	1	7	0	16	0	.1	0	.3	.1	0	50	.4	17	.1	55	80	116	.3
1	–	0	42	116	.2	.1	0	–	.3	.2	18	2.1	12	2.4	69	59	220	.3
2	–	0	42	55	.2	0	0	–	.2	.2	14	1.8	9	2	58	58	218	.3
0	–	13	0	38	0	0	0	–	0	0	4	0	0	0	4	6	22	0
1	1	0	8	5	0	0	0	–	0	0	58	3	27	.1	54	67	4	.4
1	0	0	4	3	0	0	0	0	0	0	30	1.5	29	.1	27	34	2	.2
3	1	0	8	0	0	0	0	0	0	0	105	1.4	17	0	81	41	5	.6
3	–	0	8	0	0	0	0	–	0	0	272	1.4	27	0	81	41	5	.6
0	–	0	7	0	0	0	0	–	0	0	23	.4	7	0	17	60	3	.2
1	–	0	8	5	0	0	0	–	0	0	13	.6	15	.1	21	21	814	.4

Code	Name	Amount	Unit	Grams	Energy (kcal)	Carbohydrates (g)	Protein (g)	Fat (g)	Saturated fat (g)	Monounsaturated fat (g)
14023	Tom Collins	1	Fl Oz	29.6	16	0	0	0	0	0
11954	Tomatillos, Fresh	1	Medium	34.0	11	2	0	0	–	–
41284	Tomato Garden Soup–Healthy Choice	1	Each	212.6	130	22	4	3	1	–
11540	Tomato Juice, Cnd, w/Salt	¾	Cup	183.0	31	8	1	0	0	0
11886	Tomato Juice, Cnd, w/o Salt	¾	Cup	183.0	31	8	1	0	0	0
11883	Tomatoes, Cherry	1	Each	10.0	2	0	0	0	0	0
11530	Tomatoes, Ckd, Boiled	½	Cup	120.0	32	7	1	0	0	0
11660	Tomatoes, Ckd, Stewed	½	Cup	50.5	40	7	1	1	0	1
11533	Tomatoes, Cnd, Stewed	½	Cup	127.5	33	8	1	0	0	0
11535	Tomatoes, Cnd, Wedges In Tomato Juice	½	Cup	130.5	34	8	1	0	0	0
11531	Tomatoes, Cnd, Whole, Reg Pk	½	Cup	120.0	24	5	1	0	0	0
11537	Tomatoes, Cnd, w/Green Chilies	½	Cup	120.5	18	4	1	0	0	0
11529	Tomatoes, Fresh	1	Medium	123.0	26	6	1	0	0	0
11527	Tomatoes, Green, Fresh	1	Medium	123.0	30	6	1	0	0	0
11955	Tomatoes, Sun–dried	¼	Cup	13.5	35	8	2	0	0	0
11956	Tomatoes, Sun–dried, Packed In Oil	¼	Cup	27.5	59	6	1	4	1	2
14155	Tonic Water	12	Fl Oz	366.0	124	32	0	0	0	0
19364	Toppings, Butterscotch or Caramel	1	Tbsp.	20.5	52	14	0	0	0	0
62550	Toppings, Caramel	1	Tbsp.	16.7	52	13	0	–	–	–
62549	Toppings, Hot Fudge	1	Tbsp.	19.0	70	11	1	2	1	–
19365	Toppings, Marshmallow Cream	1	Tbsp.	20.5	64	16	0	0	–	–
19367	Toppings, Nuts in Syrup	1	Tbsp.	20.5	84	11	1	5	0	1
19366	Toppings, Pineapple	1	Tbsp.	21.3	54	14	0	0	–	–
19137	Toppings, Strawberry	1	Tbsp.	21.3	54	14	0	0	–	–
62538	Tortellini, Beef	1	Cup	257.9	230	46	5	1	0	–
55160	Tortellini–Cheese in Alfredo Sauce–Stouffer's	1	Each	251.6	580	35	26	37	–	–
55161	Tortellini–Cheese w/Tomato Sauce–Stouffer's	1	Each	262.2	360	39	18	15	–	–
62655	Tortilla Chips, Low–Fat, Baked	13	Chips	28.4	110	24	3	1	–	–
19057	Tortilla Chips, Nacho–flavor	1	Ounce	28.4	141	18	2	7	1	4
19424	Tortilla Chips, Nacho–flavor, Light	1	Ounce	28.4	126	20	2	4	1	3
19056	Tortilla Chips, Plain	1	Ounce	28.4	142	18	2	7	1	4
19058	Tortilla Chips, Ranch–flavor	1	Ounce	28.4	139	18	2	7	1	4
19063	Tortilla Chips, Taco–flavor	1	Ounce	28.4	136	18	2	7	1	4
18363	Tortillas, Corn	1	Medium	25.0	56	12	1	1	0	0
18449	Tortillas, Corn, w/o Added Salt	1	Medium	25.0	56	12	1	1	0	0
18364	Tortillas, Flour	1	Medium	35.0	114	19	3	2	0	1
18450	Tortillas, Flour, w/o Added Salt	1	Medium	35.0	114	19	3	2	0	1
19059	Trail Mix, Regular	1	Cup	150.0	693	67	21	44	8	19
19821	Trail Mix, Regular, Unsalted	1	Cup	150.0	693	67	21	44	8	19
19062	Trail Mix, Regular, w/Chocolate Chips	1	Cup	146.0	707	66	21	47	9	20
19061	Trail Mix, Tropical	1	Cup	140.0	570	92	9	24	12	3
62673	Triscuits	7	Each	31.0	140	21	3	5	1	1
62674	Triscuits, Low–Fat	8	Each	32.0	130	24	3	3	1	0
14269	Tropical Fruit Juice, Blend	¾	Cup	185.2	85	22	0	0	0	0
15219	Trout, Ckd, Dry Heat	3	Ounce	85.1	162	0	23	7	1	4
15241	Trout, Rainbow, Farmed, Ckd, Dry Heat	3	Ounce	85.1	144	0	21	6	2	2
15116	Trout, Rainbow, Wild, Ckd, Dry Heat	3	Ounce	85.1	128	0	19	5	1	1
19138	Truffles	1	Piece	12.0	59	5	1	4	3	1
55162	Tuna Noodle Casserole–Stouffer's	1	Each	283.5	280	33	17	15	–	–
15128	Tuna Salad	3	Ounce	85.1	159	8	14	8	1	2
15183	Tuna, Light Meat, Cnd In Oil	3	Ounce	85.1	168	0	25	7	1	3
15184	Tuna, Light Meat, Cnd In Water	3	Ounce	85.1	111	0	25	0	0	0
15121	Tuna, Light, Cnd In Water	3	Ounce	85.1	99	0	22	1	0	0
15185	Tuna, White Meat, Cnd In Oil	3	Ounce	85.1	158	0	23	7	1	2
15186	Tuna, White Meat, Cnd In Water	3	Ounce	85.1	116	0	23	2	1	1
15221	Tuna, Yellowfin, Ckd, Dry Heat	3	Ounce	85.1	118	0	25	1	0	0

Polyunsaturated fat (g)	Dietary Fiber (g)	Cholesterol (mg)	Folate (µg)	Vitamin A (RE)	Vitamin B-6 (mg)	Vitamin B-12 (µg)	Vitamin C (mg)	Vitamin E (mg)	Riboflavin (mg)	Thiamin (mg)	Calcium (mg)	Iron (mg)	Magnesium (mg)	Niacin (mg)	Phosphorus (mg)	Potassium (mg)	Sodium (mg)	Zinc (mg)
0	–	0	0	0	0	0	1	–	0	0	1	0	0	0	0	2	5	0
–	1	0	2	4	0	0	4	.1	0	0	2	.2	7	.6	13	91	0	.1
–	–	5	–	100	–	–	6	–	.1	.1	32	.4	–	1.1	70	440	510	–
0	1	0	36	102	.2	0	33	1.7	.1	.1	16	1.1	20	1.2	35	403	661	.3
0	1	0	36	102	.2	0	33	1.7	.1	.1	16	1.1	20	1.2	35	403	18	.3
0	–	0	2	6	0	0	3	0	0	0	1	0	1	.1	2	22	1	0
0	1	0	16	89	.1	0	27	.5	.1	.1	7	.7	17	.9	37	335	13	.1
	1	0	6	34	0	0	9	.6	0	.1	13	.5	8	.6	19	125	230	.1
0	–	0	7	70	0	0	17	–	0	.1	42	.9	15	.9	26	305	324	.2
0	–	0	13	76	.2	0	19	–	0	.1	34	.6	14	.9	30	328	283	.2
0	1	0	9	72	.1	0	18	.4	0	.1	31	.7	14	.9	23	265	196	.2
0	–	0	11	47	.1	0	7	–	0	0	24	.3	13	.8	17	129	483	.2
0	1	0	18	76	.1	0	23	.5	.1	.1	6	.6	14	.8	30	273	11	.1
0	2	0	11	79	.1	0	29	.5	0	.1	16	.6	12	.6	34	251	16	.1
0	2	0	9	12	0	0	5	0	.1	.1	15	1.2	26	1.2	48	463	283	.3
1	–	0	6	35	.1	0	28	–	.1	.1	13	.7	22	1	38	430	73	.2
0	0	0	0	0	0	0	0	0	0	0	4	0	0	0	0	0	15	.4
0	–	0	0	6	0	0	0	–	0	0	11	0	1	0	10	17	72	0
–	–	–	–	–	–	–	0	–	0	0	2	–	–	–	5	6	11	0
–	–	0	–	0	–	–	0	–	–	–	36	.2	–	–	–	–	35	–
–	–	0	0	0	0	0	0	–	0	0	1	0	0	0	2	1	9	0
3	0	0	4	1	0	0	0	.2	0	0	8	.2	13	.1	23	43	9	.2
–	0	0	1	0	0	0	12	0	0	0	5	.1	0	0	2	67	13	.1
–	0	0	0	0	0	0	5	0	0	0	5	.2	1	.1	3	16	4	.1
–	9	15	–	150	–	–	4	–	–	–	96	1.5	–	–	–	–	770	–
–	–	–	–	40	–	–	4	–	.5	.3	320	.8	–	1.9	–	270	830	–
–	–	–	–	150	–	–	6	–	.3	.2	240	1	–	1.9	–	420	720	–
–	2	0	0	0	0	0	0	–	0	0	48	0	0	0	0	–	140	0
1	2	1	4	12	.1	0	1	–	.1	0	42	.4	23	.4	69	61	201	.3
1	–	1	7	12	.1	0	0	–	.1	.1	45	.5	27	.1	90	77	284	–
1	2	0	3	6	.1	0	0	.4	.1	0	44	.4	25	.4	58	56	150	.4
1	–	0	5	8	.1	0	0	–	.1	0	40	.4	25	.4	68	69	174	.4
1	–	1	6	26	.1	0	0	–	.1	.1	44	.6	25	.6	68	62	223	.4
0	1	0	4	6	.1	0	0	–	0	0	44	.4	16	.4	79	39	40	.2
0	–	0	4	–	.1	0	0	–	0	0	44	.4	16	.4	79	39	3	.2
1	1	0	4	0	0	0	0	–	.1	.2	44	1.2	9	1.3	43	46	167	.2
1	–	0	4	0	0	0	0	–	.1	.2	14	1.2	9	1.3	43	46	167	.2
14	–	0	107	3	.4	0	2	–	.3	.7	117	4.6	237	7.1	518	1028	344	4.8
14	–	0	107	3	.4	0	2	–	.3	.7	117	4.6	237	7.1	518	1028	15	4.8
16	–	6	95	7	.4	0	2	–	.3	.6	159	4.9	235	6.4	565	946	177	4.6
7	–	0	59	7	.5	0	11	–	.2	.6	80	3.7	134	2.1	260	993	14	1.6
2	4	0	0	0	0	0	0	–	0	0	0	.8	0	0	80	–	170	0
1	4	0	0	0	0	0	0	–	0	0	0	1	0	0	120	–	180	0
0	–	0	2	2	0	0	81	–	0	0	7	.2	4	0	2	24	7	.1
2	0	63	13	16	.2	6.4	0	–	.4	.4	47	1.6	24	4.9	267	394	57	.7
2	0	58	20	73	.3	4.2	3	–	.1	.2	–	.3	27	7.5	226	375	36	.4
2	0	59	16	13	.3	5.4	2	–	.1	.1	–	.3	26	4.9	229	381	48	.4
0	–	6	0	17	0	0	0	–	0	0	19	.1	6	0	21	37	9	.1
–	–	–	–	20	–	–	–	–	.3	.2	120	.6	–	3.8	–	380	1090	–
4	0	11	6	23	.1	1	2	–	.1	0	14	.9	16	5.7	151	151	342	.5
2	0	15	5	20	.1	1.9	0	1	.1	0	11	1.2	26	10.5	265	176	43	.8
0	0	15	4	20	.3	1.9	0	.5	.1	0	10	2.7	25	10.5	158	267	43	.4
0	0	26	3	14	.3	2.5	0	.5	.1	0	9	1.3	23	11.3	139	202	287	.7
3	0	26	4	20	.4	1.9	0	–	.1	0	3	.6	29	9.9	227	283	43	.4
1	0	36	3	20	.4	1.9	0	–	0	0	3	.5	29	4.9	227	241	43	.4
0	0	49	2	17	.9	.5	1	–	0	.4	18	.8	54	10.2	208	484	40	.6

Code	Name	Amount	Unit	Grams	Energy (kcal)	Carbohydrates (g)	Protein (g)	Fat (g)	Saturated fat (g)	Monounsaturated fat (g)
5297	Turkey Bologna	1	Slice	21.0	42	0	3	3	1	1
7079	Turkey Breast Meat	1	Slice	21.0	23	0	5	0	0	0
55232	Turkey Dijon, Lean Cuisine–Stouffer's	1	Each	269.3	210	20	20	6	2	–
55791	Turkey Dijonnaise–Stouffer's	1	Each	260.0	113	7	8	5	–	–
5287	Turkey Lunch Meat	1	Slice	28.4	36	0	5	1	0	0
5289	Turkey Pastrami	1	Slice	28.4	40	0	5	2	1	1
5292	Turkey Patties, Breaded, Battered, Fried	3	Ounce	85.1	241	13	12	15	4	6
55163	Turkey Pie–Stouffer's	1	Each	283.5	410	33	16	24	–	–
57809	Turkey Pot Pie–Swanson	1	Each	198.0	191	18	6	11	–	–
5296	Turkey Roast, Roasted	3	Ounce	85.1	132	3	18	5	2	1
5290	Turkey Roll, Light Meat	3	Ounce	85.1	125	0	16	6	2	2
5291	Turkey Roll, Light and Dark Meat	3	Ounce	85.1	127	2	15	6	2	2
5299	Turkey Salami	1	Slice	28.4	56	0	5	4	1	1
41243	Turkey Sausage Omelet on English Muffin–Healthy Choice	1	Each	134.7	210	30	16	4	2	–
5300	Turkey Sticks, Breaded, Battered, Fried	3	Ounce	85.1	237	14	12	14	4	6
41268	Turkey Tetrazzini–Healthy Choice	1	Each	357.9	340	49	23	6	3	–
55164	Turkey Tetrazzini–Stouffer's	1	Each	283.5	400	26	22	23	–	–
5294	Turkey Thigh, Prebasted, Meat&skin, Ckd, Roasted	3	Ounce	85.1	134	0	16	7	2	2
41275	Turkey Vegetable Soup–Healthy Choice	1	Each	212.6	110	17	4	3	1	–
55814	Turkey and Gravy–Stouffer's	1	Each	255.0	78	2	12	2	–	–
5190	Turkey, Back, Meat&skin, Ckd, Roasted	3	Ounce	85.1	207	0	23	12	4	4
5192	Turkey, Breast, Meat&skin, Ckd, Roasted	3	Ounce	85.1	161	0	24	6	2	2
5164	Turkey, Ckd, Roasted, Meat&skin&giblets&neck	3	Ounce	85.1	174	0	24	8	2	3
5188	Turkey, Dark Meat, Ckd, Roasted	3	Ounce	85.1	159	0	24	6	2	1
5184	Turkey, Dark Meat, Meat&skin, Ckd, Roasted	3	Ounce	85.1	188	0	23	10	3	3
5172	Turkey, Giblets, Ckd, Simmered, Some Giblet Fat	3	Ounce	85.1	142	2	23	4	1	1
5306	Turkey, Ground, Ckd	3	Ounce	85.1	200	0	23	11	3	4
5194	Turkey, Leg, Meat&skin, Ckd, Roasted	3	Ounce	85.1	177	0	24	8	3	2
5186	Turkey, Light Meat, Ckd, Roasted	3	Ounce	85.1	134	0	25	3	1	0
5182	Turkey, Light Meat, Meat&skin, Ckd, Roasted	3	Ounce	85.1	168	0	24	7	2	2
5168	Turkey, Meat Only, Ckd, Roasted	3	Ounce	85.1	145	0	25	4	1	1
5166	Turkey, Meat&skin, Ckd, Roasted	3	Ounce	85.1	177	0	24	8	2	3
5288	Turkey, Thin Sliced	3	Ounce	85.1	94	0	19	1	0	0
5196	Turkey, Wing, Meat&skin, Ckd, Roasted	3	Ounce	85.1	195	0	23	11	3	4
11565	Turnips, Ckd	½	Cup	78.0	14	4	1	0	0	0
11564	Turnips, Fresh	½	Cup	65.0	18	4	1	0	0	0
19160	Twix	1	Each	57.0	272	37	3	13	–	–
19112	Twizzlers Strawberry Candy	1	Pkg	71.0	263	66	2	1	–	–
62663	Uncle Ben's Wild Rice	1	Cup	56.0	190	41	6	1	0	0
62644	V8, Low Salt	8	Fl Oz	240.0	60	11	2	0	0	–
18328	Vanilla Cream Pie	1	Slice	126.0	350	41	6	18	5	8
19201	Vanilla Pudding	1	Cup	298.1	388	65	7	11	2	5
18210	Vanilla Sandwich Cookies w/Creme Filling	1	Each	10.0	48	7	0	2	0	1
18213	Vanilla Wafers, Higher Fat	1	Each	6.0	28	4	0	1	0	1
18212	Vanilla Wafers, Lower Fat	1	Each	4.0	18	3	0	1	0	0
17091	Veal, Meat Only, Ckd	3	Ounce	85.1	167	0	27	6	2	2
17089	Veal, Meat and Fat, Ckd	3	Ounce	85.1	196	0	26	10	4	4
41285	Vegetable Beef Soup–Healthy Choice	1	Each	212.6	130	21	8	1	–	–
55759	Vegetable Beef w/Barley Soup–Stouffer's	1	Cup	283.9	190	15	4	13	–	–
55797	Vegetable Chow Mein–Stouffer's	1	Ounce	28.4	14	2	0	1	–	–
11578	Vegetable Juice Cnd	¾	Cup	181.5	34	8	1	0	0	0
55166	Vegetable Lasagna–Stouffer's	1	Each	274.0	400	33	23	20	–	–
41343	Vegetable Pasta Italiano–Healthy Choice	1	Each	283.5	220	46	7	1	–	–
11581	Vegetables, Mixed, Cnd	½	Cup	81.5	38	8	2	0	0	0
11584	Vegetables, Mixed, Frz	½	Cup	91.0	54	12	3	0	0	0
55758	Vegetarian Vegetable Soup–Stouffer's	1	Cup	283.9	120	20	6	2	–	–

Polyunsaturated fat (g)	Dietary Fiber (g)	Cholesterol (mg)	Folate (μg)	Vitamin A (RE)	Vitamin B-6 (mg)	Vitamin B-12 (μg)	Vitamin C (mg)	Vitamin E (mg)	Riboflavin (mg)	Thiamin (mg)	Calcium (mg)	Iron (mg)	Magnesium (mg)	Niacin (mg)	Phosphorus (mg)	Potassium (mg)	Sodium (mg)	Zinc (mg)
1	0	21	1	0	0	.1	0	–	0	0	18	.3	3	.7	28	42	184	.4
0	0	9	1	0	.1	.4	0	–	0	0	1	.1	4	1.7	48	58	301	.2
–	–	45	–	400	–	–	2	–	.3	.2	120	.4	–	4.8	–	640	590	–
–	–	28	–	–	–	–	1	–	0	0	0	.1	–	.3	–	176	356	–
0	0	16	2	0	.1	.1	0	.2	.1	0	3	.8	5	1	54	92	282	.8
0	0	15	1	0	.1	.1	0	.1	.1	0	3	.5	4	1	57	74	296	.6
4	0	53	7	9	.2	.2	0	2	.2	.1	12	1.9	13	2	230	234	680	1.2
–	–	–	–	250	–	–	–	–	.4	.3	80	1	–	3.8	–	290	750	–
–	–	–	–	176	–	–	–	–	.1	.1	8	.5	–	1.4	–	–	363	–
1	0	45	4	0	.2	1.3	–	.3	.1	0	4	1.4	19	5.3	208	253	578	2.2
1	0	37	3	0	.3	.2	0	–	.2	.1	34	1.1	14	6	156	213	416	1.3
2	0	47	4	0	.2	.2	0	.3	.2	.1	27	1.1	15	4.1	143	230	498	1.7
1	0	23	1	0	.1	.1	0	–	0	0	6	.5	4	1	30	69	285	.5
1	–	20	–	60	–	–	–	–	.5	.4	160	2	–	2.9	250	590	470	–
4	–	54	8	10	.2	.2	0	–	.2	.1	12	1.9	13	1.8	199	221	713	1.2
2	–	40	–	–	–	–	72	–	.3	.2	80	1	–	3.8	250	510	490	–
–	–	–	–	20	–	–	–	–	.4	.2	80	.8	–	2.9	–	300	960	–
2	0	53	5	0	.2	.2	0	–	.2	.1	7	1.3	14	2	145	205	372	3.5
1	–	15	–	150	–	–	5	–	0	0	16	.2	–	.4	–	140	540	–
–	–	23	–	–	–	–	0	–	0	0	85	0	–	.9	–	406	296	–
3	0	77	7	0	.3	.3	0	.5	.2	0	28	1.9	19	2.9	161	221	62	3.3
2	0	63	5	0	.4	.3	0	–	.1	0	18	1.2	23	5.4	179	245	54	1.7
2	0	81	17	58	.3	1.1	0	–	.2	0	22	1.7	20	4.2	170	231	57	2.7
2	0	72	8	0	.3	.3	0	.5	.2	.1	27	2	20	3.1	174	247	67	3.8
3	0	76	8	0	.3	.3	0	.5	.2	0	28	1.9	20	3	167	233	65	3.5
1	0	356	293	1527	.3	20.4	1	1.2	.8	0	11	5.7	14	3.8	174	170	50	3.1
3	0	87	6	0	.3	.3	0	.3	.1	0	21	1.6	20	4.1	167	230	91	2.4
2	0	72	8	0	.3	.3	0	.5	.2	.1	27	2	20	3	169	238	65	3.6
1	0	59	5	0	.5	.3	0	.1	.1	.1	16	1.1	24	5.8	186	259	54	1.7
2	0	65	5	0	.4	.3	0	.1	.1	0	18	1.2	22	5.3	177	242	54	1.7
1	0	65	6	0	.4	.3	0	.3	.2	.1	21	1.5	22	4.6	181	253	60	2.6
2	0	70	6	0	.3	.3	0	.3	.2	0	22	1.5	21	4.3	173	238	58	2.5
0	0	35	3	0	.3	1.7	0	.1	.1	0	6	.3	17	7.1	195	236	1217	1
3	0	69	5	0	.4	.3	0	.1	.1	0	20	1.2	21	4.9	168	226	52	1.8
0	2	0	7	0	.1	0	9	0	0	0	17	.2	6	.2	15	105	39	.2
0	1	0	9	0	.1	0	14	0	0	0	20	.2	7	.3	18	124	44	.2
–	1	5	4	18	0	.2	0	.4	.1	0	67	.4	17	.2	76	117	115	.4
–	–	0	0	0	0	0	0	–	0	0	25	.4	4	.1	220	45	197	.1
0	1	0	0	0	0	0	2	–	0	0	24	1	0	0	0	–	620	0
–	2	0	0	500	0	0	60	–	0	0	48	.6	0	0	0	740	140	0
4	–	78	14	107	.1	.4	1	–	.3	.2	113	1.3	16	1.2	131	159	328	.7
4	0	21	0	18	0	.3	0	.4	.4	.1	262	.4	24	.8	203	337	402	.7
0	0	0	0	0	–	0	0	–	0	0	3	.2	1	.3	8	9	35	0
0	–	0	0	–	0	0	0	–	0	0	2	.1	1	.2	4	6	18	0
0	–	2	0	1	0	0	0	–	0	0	2	.1	1	.1	4	4	12	0
1	0	100	14	0	.3	1.4	0	.4	.3	.1	20	1	24	7.2	213	287	76	4.3
1	0	97	13	0	.3	1.3	0	.3	.3	.1	19	1	22	6.8	203	276	74	4
–	–	15	–	150	–	–	15	–	.1	.1	32	.4	–	1.9	120	360	530	–
–	–	10	–	–	–	–	0	–	0	0	240	.1	–	.2	–	341	1252	–
–	–	0	–	–	–	–	1	–	0	0	24	0	–	0	–	26	156	–
0	1	0	38	212	.3	0	50	.6	.1	.1	20	.8	20	1.3	31	350	662	.4
–	–	–	–	250	–	–	–	–	.4	.1	160	.6	–	.8	–	350	760	–
–	–	0	–	250	–	–	0	–	.3	.5	32	2.5	–	1.5	–	380	330	–
0	–	0	19	949	.1	0	4	–	0	0	22	.9	13	.5	34	237	121	.3
0	5	0	17	389	.1	0	3	.3	.1	.1	23	.7	20	.8	46	154	32	.4
–	–	0	–	–	–	–	0	–	0	0	0	.1	–	.2	–	401	911	–

Code	Name	Amount	Unit	Grams	Energy (kcal)	Carbohydrates (g)	Protein (g)	Fat (g)	Saturated fat (g)	Monounsat fat (g)
55828	Veloute Sauce Supreme–Stouffer's	1	Cup	307.6	564	21	9	50	–	–
17165	Venison, Ckd, Roasted	3	Ounce	85.1	134	0	26	3	1	1
62629	Vitamin Supplement, Centrum	1	Each	1.0	–	–	–	–	–	–
62628	Vitamin Supplement, One-A-Day	1	Each	1.0	–	–	–	–	–	–
62630	Vitamin Supplement, StressTab	1	Each	1.0	–	–	–	–	–	–
18392	Waffles, Buttermilk	1	Each	75.0	217	25	6	10	2	3
18367	Waffles, Plain	1	Each	75.0	218	25	6	11	2	3
18403	Waffles, Plain, Frozen, Toasted	1	Each	33.0	87	13	2	3	0	1
12154	Walnuts, Black, Dried	½	Cup	62.5	379	8	15	35	2	8
12155	Walnuts, English, Dried	½	Cup	60.0	385	11	9	37	3	9
9326	Watermelon	½	Cup	80.0	26	6	0	0	–	–
55167	Welsh Rarebit–Stouffer's	1	Each	141.8	270	9	13	20	–	–
41244	Western Style Omelet on English Muffin–Healthy Choice	1	Each	134.7	200	29	16	3	2	–
62675	Wheat Thins	16	Each	29.0	140	19	2	6	1	1
62676	Wheat Thins, Low-Fat	18	Each	29.0	120	21	2	4	0	0
55826	Whipped Sweet Potatoes–Stouffer's	½	Cup	142.0	205	30	2	9	–	–
14032	Whiskey Sour	1	Fl Oz	29.9	41	2	0	0	0	0
15223	Whitefish, Ckd, Dry Heat	3	Ounce	85.1	146	0	21	6	1	2
15131	Whitefish, Smoked	3	Ounce	85.1	92	0	20	1	0	0
20089	Wild Rice, Ckd	½	Cup	82.0	83	17	3	0	0	0
14536	Wine, Dessert, Dry	3	Fl Oz	90.0	113	4	0	0	0	0
14057	Wine, Dessert, Sweet	3	Fl Oz	90.0	138	11	0	0	0	0
14084	Wine, Table, All	3	Fl Oz	88.5	62	1	0	0	0	0
14096	Wine, Table, Red	3	Fl Oz	88.5	64	2	0	0	0	0
14104	Wine, Table, Rose	3	Fl Oz	88.5	63	1	0	0	0	0
14106	Wine, Table, White	3	Fl Oz	88.5	60	1	0	0	0	0
11602	Yam, Baked	½	Cup	68.0	79	19	1	0	0	0
41269	Yankee Pot Roast–Healthy Choice	1	Each	311.8	260	36	19	4	2	–
15225	Yellowtail, Ckd, Dry Heat	3	Ounce	85.1	159	0	25	6	–	–
15135	Yellowtail, Fresh	3	Ounce	85.1	124	0	20	4	1	2
62657	Yogurt, Frozen	½	Cup	74.0	160	24	3	6	2	–
62552	Yogurt, Frozen, Fat Free	½	Cup	67.0	100	22	4	0	0	–
62658	Yogurt, Frozen, Low-Fat	½	Cup	74.0	140	24	3	3	2	–
62604	Yogurt, Fruit, Fat Free	1	Cup	248.0	233	48	10	0	0	0
62627	Yogurt, Fruit, Fat Free, Light	1	Cup	248.0	110	19	10	0	0	0
1121	Yogurt, Fruit, Lowfat, 10 Gm Protein Per 8 Oz	1	Cup	227.0	231	43	10	2	2	1
1122	Yogurt, Fruit, Lowfat, 11 Gm Protein Per 8 Oz	1	Cup	227.0	239	42	11	3	2	1
1120	Yogurt, Fruit, Lowfat, 9 Gm Protein Per 8 Oz	1	Cup	227.0	225	42	9	3	2	1
62603	Yogurt, Plain, Fat Free	1	Cup	248.0	120	17	13	0	0	0
1117	Yogurt, Plain, Lowfat, 12 Gm Protein Per 8 Oz	1	Cup	227.0	144	16	12	4	2	1
1118	Yogurt, Plain, Skim Milk, 13 Gm Protein Per 8 Oz	1	Cup	227.0	127	17	13	0	0	0
1116	Yogurt, Plain, Whole Milk, 8 Gm Protein Per 8 Oz	1	Cup	227.0	139	11	8	7	5	2
19393	Yogurt, Soft-serve, Chocolate	1	Cup	144.1	231	36	6	9	5	3
19293	Yogurt, Soft-serve, Vanilla	1	Cup	144.1	229	35	6	8	5	2
1119	Yogurt, Vanilla, Lowfat, 11 Gm Protein Per 8 Oz	1	Cup	227.0	194	31	11	3	2	1
19091	York Peppermint Pattie	1	Sm Patty	11.0	38	9	0	1	–	–
55233	Zucchini Lasagna, Lean Cuisine–Stouffer's	1	Each	311.8	260	34	17	6	2	–
41344	Zucchini Lasagna–Healthy Choice	1	Each	326.0	250	41	14	3	2	–

Polyunsaturated fat (g)	Dietary Fiber (g)	Cholesterol (mg)	Folate (µg)	Vitamin A (RE)	Vitamin B-6 (mg)	Vitamin B-12 (µg)	Vitamin C (mg)	Vitamin E (mg)	Riboflavin (mg)	Thiamin (mg)	Calcium (mg)	Iron (mg)	Magnesium (mg)	Niacin (mg)	Phosphorus (mg)	Potassium (mg)	Sodium (mg)	Zinc (mg)
–	–	98	–	–	–	–	0	–	0	0	2	0	–	0	–	369	1410	–
1	0	95	–	0	–	–	0	–	.5	.2	6	3.8	20	5.7	192	285	46	2.3
–	–	–	400	1000	2	6	60	10	1.7	1.5	162	18	100	20	109	40	–	15
–	–	–	400	1000	2	6	60	10	1.7	1.5	–	–	–	20	–	–	–	–
–	–	–	400	–	5	12	500	10	–	10	–	18	–	100	–	–	–	–
5	–	50	11	26	0	.2	0	–	.3	.2	137	1.6	14	1.5	124	128	451	.6
5	–	52	11	49	0	.2	0	–	.3	.2	191	1.7	14	1.6	143	119	383	.5
1	–	8	12	120	.3	.8	0	–	.2	.1	77	1.5	7	1.5	139	42	260	.2
23	3	0	41	19	.3	0	2	1.6	.1	.1	36	1.9	126	.4	290	328	1	2.1
23	3	0	40	7	.3	0	2	1.6	.1	.2	56	1.5	101	.6	190	301	6	1.6
–	0	0	2	30	.1	0	8	.1	0	.1	6	.1	9	.2	7	93	2	.1
–	–	–	–	40	–	–	–	–	.3	0	280	.2	–	–	–	140	460	–
–	–	15	–	100	–	–	4	–	.5	.5	160	2	–	1.9	240	220	480	–
3	2	0	0	0	0	0	0	–	0	0	24	.4	0	0	0	–	170	0
2	2	0	0	0	0	0	0	–	0	0	24	.4	0	0	80	–	220	0
–	–	30	–	–	–	–	0	–	0	0	0	.1	–	.1	–	200	556	–
0	–	0	2	0	0	0	4	–	0	.1	2	0	1	0	2	16	3	0
2	0	65	14	33	.3	.8	0	–	.1	.1	28	.4	36	3.3	294	345	55	1.1
0	0	28	6	48	.3	2.8	0	.2	.1	0	15	.4	20	2	112	360	867	.4
0	1	0	21	0	.1	0	0	–	.1	0	2	.5	26	1.1	67	83	2	1.1
0	0	0	0	0	0	0	0	0	0	0	7	.2	8	.2	8	83	8	.1
0	0	0	0	0	0	0	0	0	0	0	7	.2	8	.2	8	83	8	.1
0	0	0	1	0	0	0	0	0	0	0	7	.4	9	.1	12	79	7	.1
0	–	0	2	0	0	0	0	–	0	0	7	.4	12	.1	12	99	4	.1
0	–	0	1	0	0	0	0	–	0	0	7	.3	9	.1	13	88	4	.1
0	–	0	0	0	0	0	0	–	0	0	8	.3	9	.1	12	71	4	.1
0	3	0	11	0	.2	0	8	3.1	0	.1	10	.4	12	.4	33	456	5	.1
–	–	55	–	100	–	–	9	–	.2	.2	32	1	–	1.5	150	350	400	–
–	0	60	3	26	.2	1.1	2	–	0	.1	25	.5	32	7.4	171	458	43	.6
1	0	47	3	25	.1	1.1	2	–	0	.1	20	.4	26	5.8	134	357	33	.4
–	–	10	0	20	0	0	0	–	0	0	96	0	0	0	0	–	50	0
–	–	0	–	20	–	–	0	–	–	–	96	0	–	–	–	–	70	–
–	–	10	0	20	0	0	0	–	0	0	96	0	0	0	0	–	50	0
0	0	7	–	0	–	–	0	–	–	–	438	0	–	–	–	423	153	–
0	0	5	–	0	–	–	15	–	–	–	420	.2	–	–	–	510	160	–
0	0	10	21	25	.1	1.1	1	.1	.4	.1	345	.2	33	.2	271	442	133	1.7
0	0	12	24	34	.1	1.2	2	–	.4	.1	383	.2	37	.2	301	491	147	1.9
0	0	10	19	27	.1	1	1	.1	.4	.1	314	.1	30	.2	247	402	121	1.5
0	0	5	–	0	–	–	4	–	.2	–	480	0	–	–	0	600	170	–
0	0	14	25	36	.1	1.3	2	.1	.5	.1	415	.2	40	.3	326	531	159	2
0	0	4	28	5	.1	1.4	2	0	.5	.1	452	.2	43	.3	355	579	174	2.2
0	0	29	17	68	.1	.8	1	.2	.3	.1	274	.1	26	.2	215	351	105	1.3
0	–	7	16	62	.1	.4	0	–	.3	.1	212	1.8	39	.4	200	376	141	.7
0	0	3	9	82	.1	.4	1	.1	.3	.1	206	.4	20	.4	186	304	125	.6
0	0	11	24	30	.1	1.2	2	.1	.5	.1	389	.2	37	.2	306	498	149	1.9
–	–	0	0	0	0	0	0	–	0	0	2	.2	7	.1	10	13	4	.1
–	–	20	–	150	–	–	6	–	.3	.2	200	.8	–	1.9	–	650	520	–
–	–	15	–	350	–	–	6	–	.3	.4	200	1.5	–	1.9	250	830	400	–

Code	Name	Amount	Unit	Grams	Energy (kcal)	Carbohydrates (g)	Protein (g)	Fat (g)	Saturated fat (g)	Monounsatu fat (g)
	Arby's Roast Chicken Delux	1	Each	195	276	33	20	6	2	2
32391	Arby's–Beef'N Cheddar Sandwich	1	Each	194	443.1	29.7	35.2	19.8	9.9	4
32433	Arby's–Boston Clam Chowder	1	Each	226.7	207	18	10	11	4	5
32400	Arby's–Chicken Breast Fillet Sandwich	1	Each	204	546.5	53.2	25.5	27.7	5.6	10.6
	Arby's–Chicken Cordon Bleu	1	Each	240	623	46	38	33	5.6	10.6
	Arby's–Chicken Fingers	1	Each	102	290	20	16	16	2	4
32434	Arby's–Cream of Broccoli Soup	1	Each	226.7	180	19	9	8	5	2
32413	Arby's–Curly Fries	1	Each	99.2	337	43.2	4.2	17.7	7.4	7.6
32405	Arby's–Fish Fillet Sandwich	1	Each	221	526	50	23	27	7	9.2
32411	Arby's–French Fries	1	Each	70.8	246	29.8	2.1	13.2	3	5.5
	Arby's–Grilled Chicken BBQ	1	Each	201	388	47	23	13	3	2
	Arby's–Grilled Chicken Delux	1	Each	230	430	47	23	20	4	2
32406	Arby's–Ham'N Cheese Sandwich	1	Each	170	411.2	38.4	24.4	18.6	7.4	7.8
32390	Arby's–Regular Roast Beef	1	Each	155.9	388.1	38.1	24.6	15.7	4	7.6
32393	Arby's–Super Roast Beef	1	Each	240.9	515.9	51.4	25.7	22.6	8.7	8.4
32410	Arby's–Turkey Sub	1	Each	277	598.6	53.9	32.8	28.1	6.2	7
32438	Arby's–Wisconsin Cheese Soup	1	Each	226.7	287	19	9	19	8	8
	Burger King Barbecue Dipping Sauce	1	Each	28	35	9	0	0	0	0
	Burger King Biscuit With Bacon, Egg and Cheese	1	Each	171	280	39	19	31	10	0
	Burger King Biscuit with Sausage	1	Each	151	360	41	16	40	13	0
	Burger King BK Big Fish sandwich	1	Each	255	700	56	26	41	6	0
	Burger King BK Broiler– chicken sandwich	1	Each	248	550	41	30	29	6	0
	Burger King Broiled Chicken Salad	1	Each	302	90	7	21	10	4	0
	Burger King Chicken Sandwich	1	Each	229	710	54	26	43	9	0
	Burger King Chicken Tenders – 8 piece	1	Piece	117	310	19	21	17	4	0
	Burger King Chicken Tenders – 8 piece	1	Each	117	310	19	21	17	4	0
	Burger King Chocolate Shake – Medium	1	Each	397	440	75	12	10	6	0
	Burger King Coated French Fries, medium, salted	1	Each	102	340	43	3	17	5	0
	Burger King Coca Cola Classic – medium	1	Each	360	280	70	0	0	0	0
	Burger King Croissan'Wich, w/sausage, egg and cheese	1	Each	176	600	25	22	46	16	0
	Burger King Diet Coke – medium	1	Each	360	1	0	0	0	0	0
	Burger King Double Whopper	1	Each	351	730	46	33	46	16	0
	Burger King Double Whopper w/cheese	1	Each	375	960	46	52	63	24	0
	Burger King Dutch Apple Pie	1	Each	113	300	39	3	15	3	0
	Burger King French Dressing	1	Each	30	140	11	0	10	2	0
	Burger King French Fries, medium, salted	1	Each	116	180	43	5	20	5	0
	Burger King French Toast Sticks	1	Each	141	500	60	4	27	27	0
	Burger King Garden Salad	1	Each	255	100	8	6	5	3	0
	Burger King Grape Jam	1	Each	12	30	8	0	0	0	0
	Burger King Hash Browns	1	Each	71	110	25	2	12	3	0
	Burger King Honey Dipping Sauce	1	Each	28	80	21	0	0	0	0
	Burger King Ketchup	1	Each	14	15	4	0	0	0	0
	Burger King Onion Rings	1	Each	124	310	41	4	14	2	0
	Burger King Ranch Dressing	1	Each	30	180	2	0	19	4	0
	Burger King Reduced Calorie light Italian Dressing	1	Each	30	15	3	0	0.5	0	0
	Burger King Side Salad	1	Each	133	60	4	3	3	2	0
	Burger King Strawberry Jam	1	Each	12	30	8	0	0	0	0
	Burger King Sweet & Sour Dipping Sauce	1	Each	28	45	11	0	0	0	0
	Burger King Thousand Island Dressing	1	Each	30	140	7	0	12	3	0
	Burger King Vanilla Shake – medium	1	Each	397	430	73	13	9	5	0
	Burger King Whopper Jr.	1	Each	164	420	29	21	24	8	0
	Burger King Whopper Jr. with cheese	1	Each	177	460	29	23	28	10	0
34858	Burger King–Bacon Double Cheeseburger	1	Each	218	640	28	44	39	18	14.5
34856	Burger King–Cheeseburger	1	Each	138	380	28	23	16	9	0
34857	Burger King–Double Cheeseburger	1	Each	210	600	28	41	36	17	12.2
34855	Burger King–Hamburger	1	Each	126	330	28	20	15	6	0

Polyunsaturated fat (g)	Dietary Fiber (g)	Cholesterol (mg)	Folate (µg)	Vitamin A (RE)	Vitamin B-6 (mg)	Vitamin B-12 (µg)	Vitamin C (mg)	Vitamin E (mg)	Riboflavin (mg)	Thiamin (mg)	Calcium (mg)	Iron (mg)	Magnesium (mg)	Niacin (mg)	Phosphorus (mg)	Potassium (mg)	Sodium (mg)	Zinc (mg)
1	4	33	35.4	16.6	0.7	0.3	0	0	0.4	0.5	123	3.8	51	16.4	321.5	365.8	777	1.8
3.8	1.2	84.8	45.1	63.9	0.3	2.2	1.3	0.4	0.5	0.4	201.7	5.6	44	6.5	442	380.2	1801.1	5.9
2	1.4	28	9	100	0.1	9.3	4	0.1	0.2	0	170	1.4	20	0.9	143	319	1157	0.7
11.4	1.7	100.8	35.4	16.6	0.7	0.3	0	2.8	0.4	0.5	123	3.8	51	16.4	321.5	365.8	1129.7	1.8
11.4	5	77	35.4	16.6	0.7	0.3	0	2.8	0.4	0.5	123	3.8	51	16.4	321.5	365.8	1594	1.8
4.1	0.5	32	17	2.6	0	0.1	0	1.4	0	0	92	1.9	22	0	140	190	677	0.3
1	1.8	3	46	50	0.1	0.5	9	1.4	0.4	0.1	237	0.8	55	0.8	193	455	1113	0.7
1.5	0	0	0	0	0	0	0	0	0	0	16	0.8	0	1.9	0	724	167	0
10.6	0	43.8	0	0	0	0	1.2	0	0.3	0.3	72	2.1	0	5.3	0	450	872	0
4.7	0	0	0	0	0	0	3.6	0	0	0	0	0.6	0	1.9	0	240	114	0
1	2	43	35.4	16.6	0.7	0.3	0	0	0.4	0.5	123	3.8	51	16.4	321.5	365.8	1002	1.8
1	3	61	35.4	16.6	0.7	0.3	0	0	0.4	0.5	123	3.8	51	16.4	321.5	365.8	848	1.8
1.6	1.1	67.5	82.7	111.8	0.2	0.6	3.5	1.2	0.5	0.3	151.4	3.8	18.6	3.1	177	337.8	899.4	1.6
1.9	1.1	58.3	44.8	70.6	0.3	1.3	2.2	0.2	0.3	0.4	60.5	4.7	34.7	6.6	268	354.4	888.4	3.8
5.5	1.6	41.1	42.2	0	0.4	4.4	0	0.4	0.6	0.6	118.4	6.5	59.7	9.6	413.9	517.9	821.7	11
8.2	0	82.1	0	0	0	0	0	0	0.4	0.5	93.9	3.1	0	9.3	0	0	1431.9	0
3	1.8	31	7	90	0	0	2	0.4	0.2	0	252	1.3	7	0.7	241	441	1129	1.1
0	0	0	0	0	0	0	0	0	0	0	0	0	0	0	0	0	400	0
0	1	225	0	0	0	0	0	0	0	0	0	0	0	0	0	0	1530	0
0	1	45	0	0	0	0	0	0	0	0	0	0	0	0	0	0	1390	0
0	3	90	0	0	0	0	0	0	0	0	0	0	0	0	0	0	980	0
0	2	80	0	0	0	0	0	0	0	0	0	0	0	0	0	0	4803	0
0	3	60	0	0	0	0	0	0	0	0	0	0	0	0	0	0	110	0
0	2	60	0	0	0	0	0	0	0	0	0	0	0	0	0	0	1400	0
0	3	50	0	0	0	0	0	0	0	0	0	0	0	0	0	0	710	0
0	3	50	0	0	0	0	0	0	0	0	0	0	0	0	0	0	710	0
0	4	30	0	0	0	0	0	0	0	0	0	0	0	0	0	0	330	0
0	3	0	0	0	0	0	0	0	0	0	0	0	0	0	0	0	680	0
0	0	0	0	0	0	0	0	0	0	0	0	0	0	0	0	0	0	0
0	1	260	0	0	0	0	0	0	0	0	0	0	0	0	0	0	1140	0
0	0	0	0	0	0	0	0	0	0	0	0	0	0	0	0	0	0	0
0	3	115	0	0	0	0	0	0	0	0	0	0	0	0	0	0	1350	0
0	3	195	0	0	0	0	0	0	0	0	0	0	0	0	0	0	1420	0
0	2	0	0	0	0	0	0	0	0	0	0	0	0	0	0	0	230	0
0	0	0	0	0	0	0	0	0	0	0	0	0	0	0	0	0	190	0
0	3	0	0	0	0	0	0	0	0	0	0	0	0	0	0	0	240	0
0	1	0	0	0	0	0	0	0	0	0	0	0	0	0	0	0	490	0
0	4	15	0	0	0	0	0	0	0	0	0	0	0	0	0	0	115	0
0	0	0	0	0	0	0	0	0	0	0	0	0	0	0	0	0	0	0
0	2	0	0	0	0	0	0	0	0	0	0	0	0	0	0	0	320	0
0	0	0	0	0	0	0	0	0	0	0	0	0	0	0	0	0	20	0
0	0	0	0	0	0	0	0	0	0	0	0	0	0	0	0	0	180	0
0	6	0	0	0	0	0	0	0	0	0	0	0	0	0	0	0	810	0
0	0	10	0	0	0	0	0	0	0	0	0	0	0	0	0	0	170	0
0	0	0	0	0	0	0	0	0	0	0	0	0	0	0	0	0	50	0
0	2	5	0	0	0	0	0	0	0	0	0	0	0	0	0	0	55	0
0	0	0	0	0	0	0	0	0	0	0	0	0	0	0	0	0	5	0
0	0	0	0	0	0	0	0	0	0	0	0	0	0	0	0	0	50	0
0	0	15	0	0	0	0	0	0	0	0	0	0	0	0	0	0	190	0
0	2	30	0	0	0	0	0	0	0	0	0	0	0	0	0	0	330	0
0	2	60	0	0	0	0	0	0	0	0	0	0	0	0	0	0	530	0
0	2	75	0	0	0	0	0	0	0	0	0	0	0	0	0	0	770	0
6.2	1	145	32.1	73.5	0.3	3.3	8.2	1.5	0.4	0.3	161.5	4.1	39.3	8.3	386.3	479.5	1240	6.6
0	1	65	0	0	0	0	0	0	0	0	0	0	0	0	0	0	770	0
2.2	1	135	34.4	111.2	0.2	2	6.6	2	0.3	0.2	210.2	3.3	34.4	5.4	339.3	382.7	1060	4.4
0	1	55	0	0	0	0	0	0	0	0	0	0	0	0	0	0	530	0

Code	Name	Amount	Unit	Grams	Energy (kcal)	Carbohydrates (g)	Protein (g)	Fat (g)	Saturated fat (g)	Monounsaturated fat (g)
34843	Burger King–Salad w/1000 Island	1	Each	176	145	9	2	12	0	0
34842	Burger King–Salad w/Bleu Cheese	1	Each	176	184	7	3	16	0	0
34844	Burger King–Salad w/French	1	Each	176	152	13	2	11	0	0
34845	Burger King–Salad w/Golden Italian	1	Each	176	162	7	2	14	0	0
34841	Burger King–Salad w/House Dressing	1	Each	176	159	8	3	13	0	0
34846	Burger King–Salad w/Reduced–Calorie Italian	1	Each	176	42	7	2	1	0	0
34859	Burger King–Whopper	1	Each	270	640	45	27	39	11	14.9
37167	Dunkin' Donuts–Almond Croissant	1	Each	105	420	38	8	27	0	0
37146	Dunkin' Donuts–Apple Filled w/Cinnamon Sugar	1	Each	79	250	33	5	11	0	0
37160	Dunkin' Donuts–Apple 'n Spice Muffin	1	Each	100	300	52	6	8	0	0
37159	Dunkin' Donuts–Banana Nut Muffin	1	Each	103	310	49	7	10	0	0
37147	Dunkin' Donuts–Bavarian Filled /w Chocolate	1	Each	79	240	32	5	11	0	0
37149	Dunkin' Donuts–Blueberry Filled	1	Each	67	210	29	4	8	0	0
37156	Dunkin' Donuts–Blueberry Muffin	1	Each	101	280	46	6	8	0	0
37157	Dunkin' Donuts–Bran Muffin w/Raisins	1	Each	104	310	51	6	9	0	0
37151	Dunkin' Donuts–Cake Ring, Plain	1	Each	62	270	25	4	17	0	0
37163	Dunkin' Donuts–Chocolate Chunk Cookie	1	Each	43	200	25	3	10	0	0
37164	Dunkin' Donuts–Chocolate Chunk Cookie w/Nuts	1	Each	43	210	23	3	11	0	0
37168	Dunkin' Donuts–Chocolate Croissant	1	Each	94	440	38	7	29	0	0
37145	Dunkin' Donuts–Chocolate Frosted Yeast Ring	1	Each	55	200	25	4	10	0	0
37158	Dunkin' Donuts–Corn Muffin	1	Each	96	340	51	7	12	0	0
37161	Dunkin' Donuts–Cranberry Nut Muffin	1	Each	98	290	44	6	9	0	0
37166	Dunkin' Donuts–Croissant, Plain	1	Each	72	310	27	7	19	0	0
37153	Dunkin' Donuts–Glazed Buttermilk Ring	1	Each	74	290	37	4	14	0	0
37152	Dunkin' Donuts–Glazed Chocolate Rings	1	Each	71	324	34	3.5	21	0	0
37144	Dunkin' Donuts–Glazed Coffee Roll	1	Each	81	280	37	5	12	0	0
37155	Dunkin' Donuts–Glazed French Cruller	1	Each	38	140	16	2	8	0	0
37143	Dunkin' Donuts–Glazed Yeast Ring	1	Each	55	200	26	4	9	0	0
37150	Dunkin' Donuts–Jelly Filled	1	Each	67	220	31	4	9	0	0
37148	Dunkin' Donuts–Lemon Filled	1	Each	79	260	33	4	12	0	0
37162	Dunkin' Donuts–Oat Bran Muffin	1	Each	100	330	50	7	11	0	0
37165	Dunkin' Donuts–Oatmeal Pecan Raisin Cookie	1	Each	46	200	28	3	9	0	0
21002	Fast Food–Biscuit w/Egg	1	Each	136	315.5	24.1	11.1	20.2	6.1	8.1
21003	Fast Food–Biscuit w/Egg and Bacon	1	Each	150	457.5	28.5	17	31.1	9.9	13.2
21004	Fast Food–Biscuit w/Egg and Ham	1	Each	192	441.6	30.3	20.4	27	8.3	11.3
21005	Fast Food–Biscuit w/Egg and Sausage	1	Each	180	581.4	41.1	19.1	38.7	14.9	16.4
21007	Fast Food–Biscuit w/Egg, Cheese, and Bacon	1	Each	144	476.6	33.4	16.2	31.3	11.4	14.2
21008	Fast Food–Biscuit w/Ham	1	Each	113	386.4	43.7	13.3	18.4	11.4	4.8
21009	Fast Food–Biscuit w/Sausage	1	Each	124	484.8	40	12.1	31.7	14.2	12.8
21010	Fast Food–Biscuit w/Steak	1	Each	141	455.4	44.3	13.1	25.9	6.9	11
21001	Fast Food–Biscuit, Plain	1	Each	74	276	34.4	4.3	13.3	8.7	3.4
21027	Fast Food–Brownie	1	Each	60	243	38.9	2.7	10.1	3.1	3.8
21060	Fast Food–Burrito w/Beans	1	Each	108.5	223.5	35.7	7	6.7	3.4	2.3
21061	Fast Food–Burrito w/Beans and Cheese	1	Each	93	188.7	27.4	7.5	5.8	3.4	1.2
21062	Fast Food–Burrito w/Beans and Chili Peppers	1	Each	102	206	29	8.1	7.3	3.8	2.6
21063	Fast Food–Burrito w/Beans and Meat	1	Each	115.5	254.1	33	11.2	8.9	4.1	3.5
21064	Fast Food–Burrito w/Beans, Cheese, and Beef	1	Each	101.5	165.4	19.8	7.2	6.6	3.5	2.2
21065	Fast Food–Burrito w/Beans, Cheese, and Chili Peppers	1	Each	167	328.9	42.3	16.5	11.4	5.5	4.2
21066	Fast Food–Burrito w/Beef	1	Each	110	261.8	29.2	13.3	10.4	5.2	3.7
21067	Fast Food–Burrito w/Beef and Chili Peppers	1	Each	100.5	213	24.7	10.7	8.2	4	3
21068	Fast Food–Burrito w/Beef, Cheese, and Chili Peppers	1	Each	152	316.1	31.8	20.4	12.3	5.2	4.9
21069	Fast Food–Burrito w/Fruit (Apple or Cherry)	1	Each	74	230.8	34.9	2.5	9.5	4.5	3.4
21100	Fast Food–Cheeseburger, Large, Double Patty	1	Each	258	704.3	39.6	37.9	43.6	17.6	17.3
21098	Fast Food–Cheeseburger, Large, Single Patty	1	Each	219	562.8	38.3	28.1	32.9	15	12.6
21097	Fast Food–Cheeseburger, Large, Single Patty w/Bcn&cond	1	Each	195	608.4	37.1	32	36.7	16.2	14.4
21096	Fast Food–Cheeseburger, Large, Single Patty, Plain	1	Each	185	608.6	47.4	30.1	32.9	14.8	12.7

Polyunsaturated fat (g)	Dietary Fiber (g)	Cholesterol (mg)	Folate (µg)	Vitamin A (RE)	Vitamin B-6 (mg)	Vitamin B-12 (µg)	Vitamin C (mg)	Vitamin E (mg)	Riboflavin (mg)	Thiamin (mg)	Calcium (mg)	Iron (mg)	Magnesium (mg)	Niacin (mg)	Phosphorus (mg)	Potassium (mg)	Sodium (mg)	Zinc (mg)
0	0	17	0	0	0	0	25.8	0	0	0	336	0.1	98	0.1	528	405	251	0
0	0	22	0	0	0	0	25.2	0	0	0	528	0.1	101.5	0.1	664	382	333	0
0	0	0	0	0	0	0	25.8	0	0	0	320	0.1	98	0.1	480	410	330	0
0	0	0	0	0	0	0	25.2	0	0	0	320	0.1	98	0.1	480	389	292	0
0	0	11	0	0	0	0	25.2	0	0	0	352	0.1	94.5	0.1	592	402	293	0
0	0	0	0	0	0	0	25.2	0	0	0	320	0.1	105	0.1	472	390	430	0
2.3	3	90	33.6	208.5	0.3	3	14.1	4.2	0	0	112.9	6.5	54.3	5.6	338.8	564.8	870	5.7
0	3	0	0	0	0	0	0	0	0	0	0	0	0	0	0	0	280	0
0	1	0	0	0	0	0	0	0	0	0	0	0	0	0	0	0	280	0
0	2	25	0	0	0	0	0	0	0	0	0	0	0	0	0	0	360	0
0	3	30	0	0	0	0	0	0	0	0	0	0	0	0	0	0	410	0
0	2	0	0	0	0	0	0	0	0	0	0	0	0	0	0	0	260	0
0	2	0	0	0	0	0	0	0	0	0	0	0	0	0	0	0	240	0
0	2	30	0	0	0	0	0	0	0	0	0	0	0	0	0	0	340	0
0	4	15	0	0	0	0	0	0	0	0	0	0	0	0	0	0	560	0
0	1	0	0	0	0	0	0	0	0	0	0	0	0	0	0	0	330	0
0	1	30	0	0	0	0	0	0	0	0	0	0	0	0	0	0	110	0
0	2	30	0	0	0	0	0	0	0	0	0	0	0	0	0	0	100	0
0	3	0	0	0	0	0	0	0	0	0	0	0	0	0	0	0	220	0
0	1	0	0	0	0	0	0	0	0	0	0	0	0	0	0	0	190	0
0	1	40	0	0	0	0	0	0	0	0	0	0	0	0	0	0	560	0
0	2	25	0	0	0	0	0	0	0	0	0	0	0	0	0	0	360	0
0	2	0	0	0	0	0	0	0	0	0	0	0	0	0	0	0	240	0
0	1	10	0	0	0	0	0	0	0	0	0	0	0	0	0	0	370	0
0	1.9	0	0	0	0	0	0	0	0	0	0	0	0	0	0	0	383	0
0	2	0	0	0	0	0	0	0	0	0	0	0	0	0	0	0	310	0
0	0	30	0	0	0	0	0	0	0	0	0	0	0	0	0	0	130	0
0	1	0	0	0	0	0	0	0	0	0	0	0	0	0	0	0	230	0
0	1	0	0	0	0	0	0	0	0	0	0	0	0	0	0	0	230	0
0	1	0	0	0	0	0	0	0	0	0	0	0	0	0	0	0	280	0
0	3	0	0	0	0	0	0	0	0	0	0	0	0	0	0	0	450	0
0	1	25	0	0	0	0	0	0	0	0	0	0	0	0	0	0	100	0
4.2	0	232.5	29.9	178.1	0	0.7	0	0	0.3	0.3	153.6	3.1	20.4	0.7	184.9	160.4	654.1	1.1
5.7	0	352.5	30	52.5	0.1	1	2.7	0	0.2	0.1	189	3.7	24	2.4	238.5	250.5	999	1.6
5.1	0	299.5	32.6	240	0.2	1.1	0	0	0.6	0.6	220.8	4.5	30.7	2	316.8	318.7	1382.4	2.2
4.4	0	302.4	39.6	163.8	0.2	1.3	0	0	0.4	0.5	154.8	3.9	25.2	3.6	489.6	320.4	1141.2	2.1
3.4	0	260.6	37.4	165.6	0.1	1	1.5	0	0.4	0.3	164.1	2.5	20.1	2.3	459.3	230.4	1260	1.5
1	0	24.8	7.9	33.9	0.1	0	0.1	0	0.3	0.5	160.4	2.7	22.6	3.4	553.7	196.6	1432.8	1.6
3	1.3	34.7	8.6	13.6	0.1	0.5	0.1	3	0.2	0.4	127.7	2.5	19.8	3.2	446.4	198.4	1071.3	1.5
6.4	0	25.3	11.2	15.5	0.1	0.9	0.1	0	0.3	0.3	115.6	4.3	26.7	4.1	204.4	234	795.2	2.6
0.5	0	5.1	5.9	24.4	0	0.1	0	0	0.1	0.2	89.5	1.6	8.8	1.6	260.4	86.5	583.8	0.2
2.6	0	9.6	4.2	2.4	0	0.1	3.1	0	0.1	0	25.2	1.2	16.2	0.5	87.6	83.4	153	0.5
0.6	0	2.1	58.5	16.2	0.1	0.5	0.9	0	0.3	0.3	56.4	2.2	43.4	2	48.8	326.5	492.5	0.7
0.8	0	13.9	40.9	119	0.1	0.4	0.8	0	0.3	0.1	106.9	1.1	39.9	1.7	90.2	248.3	583.1	0.8
0.4	0	16.3	59.1	10.2	0.1	0.5	0.6	0	0.3	0.2	49.9	2.2	35.7	2.1	57.1	289.6	522.2	1.7
0.6	0	24.2	36.9	32.3	0.1	0.8	0.9	0	0.4	0.2	53.1	2.4	41.5	2.7	70.4	328	667.5	1.9
0.5	0	61.9	30.4	75.1	0.1	0.5	2.5	0	0.3	0.1	64.9	1.8	25.3	1.9	70	205	495.3	1.1
0.6	0	78.4	71.8	190.3	0.2	0.9	3.3	0	0.6	0.2	143.6	3.8	48.4	3.8	141.9	402.4	1023.7	3
0.4	0	31.9	19.8	14.3	0.1	0.9	0.5	0	0.4	0.1	41.8	3	40.7	3.2	86.9	369.6	745.8	2.3
0.4	0	27.1	18	23.1	0.1	0.6	0.8	0	0.4	0.2	43.2	2.2	30.1	2.5	70.3	249.2	557.7	2.1
1.1	0	85.1	28.8	56.2	0.1	1	1.8	0	0.6	0.3	110.9	3.9	34.9	4.1	158	332.8	1045.7	3.9
1	0	3.7	3.7	37	0	0.5	0.7	0	0.1	0.1	15.5	1	7.4	1.8	14.8	104.3	211.6	0.4
4.7	0	141.9	49	54.1	0.4	3.4	1	0	0.4	0.3	239.9	5.9	51.6	7.2	394.7	595.9	1148.1	6.6
2	0	87.6	28.4	129.2	0.2	2.5	7.8	1.1	0.4	0.3	205.8	4.6	43.8	7.3	310.9	444.5	1108.1	4.6
2.7	0	111.1	33.1	79.9	0.3	2.3	2.1	0	0.4	0.3	161.8	4.7	44.8	6.6	399.7	331.5	1043.2	6.8
2.4	0	96.2	38.8	148	0.2	2.5	0	0	0.5	0.4	90.6	5.4	38.8	11.1	421.8	643.8	1589.1	5.5

Code	Name	Amount	Unit	Grams	Energy (kcal)	Carbohydrates (g)	Protein (g)	Fat (g)	Saturated fat (g)	Monounsaturated fat (g)
21095	Fast Food–Cheeseburger, Regular, Double Patty	1	Each	228	649.8	53.1	29.7	35.2	12.7	12.6
21091	Fast Food–Cheeseburger, Regular, Single Patty	1	Each	154	358.8	28.1	17.8	19.7	9.1	7.1
21089	Fast Food–Cheeseburger, Regular, Single Patty, Plain	1	Each	102	319.2	31.7	14.7	15.1	6.4	5.7
21101	Fast Food–Cheeseburger, Triple Patty, Plain	1	Each	304	796.4	26.6	56	50.9	21.7	21.5
21103	Fast Food–Chicken Fillet Sandwich w/Cheese	1	Each	228	631.5	41.5	29.4	38.7	12.4	13.6
21102	Fast Food–Chicken Fillet Sandwich, Plain	1	Each	182	515	38.6	24.1	29.4	8.5	10.4
21037	Fast Food–Chicken Nuggets, Plain	1	Each	17	48.2	2.5	2.8	2.9	0.9	1.4
21038	Fast Food–Chicken Nuggets, w/Barb. Sauce	1	Each	17	43.1	3.2	2.2	2.3	0.7	1.1
21039	Fast Food–Chicken Nuggets, w/Honey	1	Each	17	48.6	3.9	2.4	2.5	0.8	1.2
21040	Fast Food–Chicken Nuggets, w/Must. Sauce	1	Each	17	42.1	2.7	2.2	2.4	0.7	1.1
21041	Fast Food–Chicken Nuggets, w/Sweet and Sour	1	Each	17	45.2	3.7	2.2	2.3	0.7	1.1
21042	Fast Food–Chili Con Carne	1	Cup	252.9	255.5	21.9	24.6	8.2	3.4	3.4
21070	Fast Food–Chimichanga, w/Beef	1	Each	174	424.5	42.8	19.6	19.6	8.5	8
21071	Fast Food–Chimichanga, w/Beef and Cheese	1	Each	183	442.8	39.3	20	23.4	11.1	9.4
21030	Fast Food–Chocolate Chip Cookies	1	Box	55	232.6	36.2	2.8	12.1	5.3	5
21043	Fast Food–Clams, Breaded and Fried	1	Ounce	28.3	111.1	9.5	3.1	6.5	1.6	2.8
21128	Fast Food–Corn On The Cob w/Butter	1	Each	146	154.7	31.9	4.4	3.4	1.6	1
21045	Fast Food–Crab, Soft-shell, Fried	1	Each	125	333.7	31.2	10.9	17.8	4.4	7.6
21011	Fast Food–Croissant w/Egg and Cheese	1	Each	127	368.3	24.3	12.7	24.7	14	7.5
21012	Fast Food–Croissant w/Egg, Cheese, and Bacon	1	Each	129	412.8	23.6	16.2	28.3	15.4	9.1
21013	Fast Food–Croissant w/Egg, Cheese, and Ham	1	Each	152	474.2	24.2	18.9	33.5	17.4	11.3
21014	Fast Food–Croissant w/Egg, Cheese, and Sausage	1	Each	160	523.2	24.7	20.3	38.1	18.2	14.2
21015	Fast Food–Danish Pastry, Cheese	1	Each	91	353	28.6	5.8	24.6	5.1	15.6
21016	Fast Food–Danish Pastry, Cinnamon	1	Each	88	349.3	46.8	4.8	16.7	3.4	10.5
21017	Fast Food–Danish Pastry, Fruit	1	Each	94	334.6	45	4.7	15.9	3.3	10.1
21104	Fast Food–Egg and Cheese Sandwich	1	Each	146	340.1	25.9	15.6	19.4	6.6	8.2
21018	Fast Food–Egg, Scrambled	1	Eggs	47	175	2.5	13.2	14.7	2.8	2.7
21074	Fast Food–Enchilada w/Cheese	1	Each	163	319.4	28.5	9.6	18.8	10.5	6.3
21075	Fast Food–Enchilada w/Cheese and Beef	1	Each	192	322.5	30.4	11.9	17.6	9	6.1
21076	Fast Food–Enchirito w/Cheese, Beef, and Beans	1	Each	193	343.5	33.7	17.8	16	7.9	6.5
21019	Fast Food–Eng. Muffin w/Butter	1	Each	63	189	30.3	4.8	5.7	2.4	1.5
21020	Fast Food–Eng. Muffin w/Cheese and Sausage	1	Each	115	393.3	29.1	15.3	24.2	9.8	10
21021	Fast Food–Eng. Muffin w/Egg, Cheese, and Can. Bacon	1	Each	146	382.5	31.4	19.8	19.7	9	6.7
21022	Fast Food–Eng. Muffin w/Egg, Cheese, and Sausage	1	Each	165	486.7	30.9	21.6	30.8	12.4	12.7
21047	Fast Food–Fish Fillet, Battered and Fried	1	Each	91	211.1	15.4	13.3	11.1	2.5	2.3
21105	Fast Food–Fish Sandwich w/Tartar Sauce	1	Each	158	431.3	41	16.9	22.7	5.2	7.6
21106	Fast Food–Fish Sandwich w/Tartar Sauce and Cheese	1	Each	183	523.3	47.6	20.6	28.6	8.1	8.9
21023	Fast Food–French Toast w/Butter	1	Slice	67.5	178.2	18	5.1	9.3	0	0
21031	Fast Food–Fried Pie, Fruit (Apple, Cherry, or Lemon)	1	Each	85	266	33	2.4	14.3	6.5	5.8
21077	Fast Food–Frijoles w/Cheese	1	Ounce	28.3	38.2	4.8	1.9	1.3	0.6	0.4
21116	Fast Food–Ham and Cheese Sandwich	1	Each	146	351.8	33.3	20.6	15.4	6.4	6.7
21117	Fast Food–Ham, Egg, and Cheese Sandwich	1	Each	143	347.4	30.9	19.2	16.3	7.4	5.7
21114	Fast Food–Hamburger, Double Patty w/Cond and Veg	1	Each	226	540.1	40.2	34.2	26.5	10.5	10.3
21111	Fast Food–Hamburger, Double Patty w/Condiments	1	Each	215	576.2	38.7	31.8	32.4	12	14.1
21110	Fast Food–Hamburger, Double Patty, Plain	1	Each	176	543.8	42.9	29.9	27.9	10.3	12.1
21113	Fast Food–Hamburger, Large, Single Patty w/Cond&veg	1	Each	218	512.3	40	25.8	27.3	10.4	11.4
21112	Fast Food–Hamburger, Large, Single Patty, Plain	1	Each	137	426	31.7	22.6	22.9	8.3	9.8
21108	Fast Food–Hamburger, Single Patty w/Condiments	1	Each	107	274.9	32.6	13.6	10.2	3.5	3.7
21107	Fast Food–Hamburger, Single Patty, Plain	1	Each	90	274.5	30.5	12.3	11.8	4.1	5.4
21115	Fast Food–Hamburger, Triple Patty w/Condiments	1	Each	259	691.5	28.5	49.9	41.4	15.9	18.2
21119	Fast Food–Hot Dog w/Chili	1	Each	114	296.4	31.2	13.5	13.4	4.8	6.5
21120	Fast Food–Hot Dog w/Corn Flour Coating (corndog)	1	Each	175	460.2	55.7	16.8	18.9	5.1	9.1
21118	Fast Food–Hot Dog, Plain	1	Each	98	242	18	10.3	14.5	5.1	6.8
21028	Fast Food–Ice Milk, Vanilla, Soft-serve w/Cone	1	Each	103	163.7	24.1	3.8	6.1	3.5	1.8
21078	Fast Food–Nachos w/Cheese	1	Ounce	28.3	86.7	9.1	2.2	4.7	1.9	2
21079	Fast Food–Nachos w/Cheese and Jalapeno Peppers	1	Ounce	28.3	84.4	8.3	2.3	4.7	1.9	2

Polyunsaturated fat (g)	Dietary Fiber (g)	Cholesterol (mg)	Folate (µg)	Vitamin A (RE)	Vitamin B-6 (mg)	Vitamin B-12 (µg)	Vitamin C (mg)	Vitamin E (mg)	Riboflavin (mg)	Thiamin (mg)	Calcium (mg)	Iron (mg)	Magnesium (mg)	Niacin (mg)	Phosphorus (mg)	Potassium (mg)	Sodium (mg)	Zinc (mg)
6.3	0	93.4	34.2	84.3	0.2	2	2.7	1.9	0.4	0.5	168.7	4.7	36.4	8.3	348.8	389.8	921.1	4.1
1.4	0	52.3	21.5	70.8	0.1	1.2	2.3	0	0.2	0.3	181.7	2.6	26.1	6.3	215.6	229.4	976.3	2.6
1.5	0	49.9	26.5	36.7	0	0.9	0	0	0.4	0.4	140.7	2.4	21.4	3.7	195.8	164.2	499.8	2.3
3.1	0	161.1	51.6	85.1	0.6	5.9	2.7	0	0.6	0.6	282.7	8.3	60.8	11.4	541.1	820.8	1212.9	10.8
9.9	0	77.5	45.6	127.6	0.4	0.4	2.9	0	0.4	0.4	257.6	3.6	43.3	9	405.8	332.8	1238	2.9
8.3	0	60	29.1	30.9	0.2	0.3	8.9	0	0.2	0.3	60	4.6	34.5	6.8	232.9	353	957.3	1.8
0.3	0	10.2	1.8	5.1	0	0	0	0.3	0	0	2.7	0.2	3.4	1.1	34	41.8	90.4	0.1
0.3	0	7.9	3.5	6.1	0	0	0.1	0	0	0	2.7	0.1	3.2	0.9	28	41.6	108.4	0.1
0.3	0	9	1.7	4.4	0	0	0	0	0	0	2.5	0.2	2.8	1	29.9	37.7	79.3	0.1
0.3	0	7.9	1.5	4.2	0	0	0	0	0	0	3.2	0.1	3.4	0.9	28.5	36.5	103.3	0.1
0.2	0	7.9	1.5	9.5	0	0	0.1	0	0	0	2.7	0.1	3	0.9	27.5	36.2	88.5	0.1
0.5	0	134	30.3	166.9	0.3	1.1	1.5	0	1.1	0.1	68.3	5.1	45.5	2.4	197.3	690.6	1006.9	3.5
1.1	0	8.7	31.3	15.6	0.2	1.5	4.7	0	0.6	0.4	62.6	4.5	62.6	5.7	123.5	586.3	910	4.9
0.7	0	51.2	32.9	126.2	0.2	1.3	2.7	0	0.8	0.3	237.9	3.8	60.3	4.6	186.6	203.1	957	3.3
1	0	11.5	15.9	14.8	0	0.1	0.5	0.3	0.1	0	19.8	1.4	16.5	1.3	52.2	81.9	188.1	0.3
1.6	0	21.5	2.2	9	0	0.2	0	0	0	0	5.1	0.7	7.6	0.7	58.6	65.4	205.5	0.4
0.6	0	5.8	43.8	96.3	0.3	0	6.8	0	0.1	0.2	4.3	0.8	40.8	2.1	108	359.1	29.2	0.9
4.8	0	45	20	3.7	0.1	4.4	0.7	0	0	0.1	55	1.8	25	1.7	131.2	162.5	1117.5	1
1.3	0	215.9	36.8	255.2	0.1	0.7	0.1	0	0.3	0.1	243.8	2.2	21.5	1.5	347.9	173.9	551.1	1.7
1.7	0	215.4	34.8	119.9	0.1	0.8	2.1	0	0.3	0.3	150.9	2.1	23.2	2.1	276	201.2	888.8	1.9
2.3	0	212.8	36.4	117	0.2	1	11.4	0	0.3	0.5	144.4	2.1	25.8	3.1	335.9	272	1080.7	2.1
3	0	216	38.4	108.8	0.1	0.9	0.1	0	0.3	0.9	144	3	24	4	289.6	283.2	1115.2	2.1
2.4	0	20	14.5	42.7	0	0.2	2.6	0	0.2	0.2	70	1.8	15.4	2.5	80	116.4	319.4	0.6
1.6	0	27.2	14	5.2	0	0.2	2.5	0	0.1	0.2	36.9	1.8	14	2.2	73.9	95.9	326.4	0.4
1.5	0	18.8	15	24.4	0	0.2	1.6	0	0.2	0.2	21.6	1.4	14.1	1.8	68.6	109.9	332.7	0.4
2.5	0	290.5	36.5	181	0.1	1.1	1.4	0	0.5	0.2	224.8	2.9	21.9	2	302.2	188.3	804.4	1.6
0.9	0	346	63	125.9	0.1	0.9	1	0.4	0.6	0	60	2.5	13	0.3	230	154	226	1.6
0.8	0	44	34.2	185.8	0.3	0.7	0.9	0	0.4	0	324.7	1.3	50.5	1.9	133.6	239.6	784	2.5
1.3	0	40.3	192	142	0.2	1	1.3	0	0.4	0.1	228.4	3	82.5	2.5	167	574	1319	2.6
0.3	0	50.1	252.8	133.1	0.2	1.6	4.6	0	0.6	0.1	218	2.3	71.4	2.9	223.8	559.7	1250.6	2.7
1.3	0	12.6	17	33.3	0	0	0.7	0.1	0.3	0.2	102.6	1.5	13.2	2.6	85	69.3	386.1	0.4
2.6	0	58.6	18.4	86.2	0.1	0.6	1.2	0	0.2	0.7	167.9	2.2	24.1	4.1	186.3	215	1036.1	1.6
2	0	233.6	43.8	157.6	0.1	0.8	1.3	0.6	0.5	0.4	207.3	3.2	33.5	3.9	319.7	213.1	784	1.8
3.3	0	273.9	54.4	171.6	0.2	1.3	1.4	0	0.5	0.8	196.3	3.4	29.7	4.4	287.1	293.7	1135.2	2.3
5.7	0	30.9	50.9	10.9	0	1	0	0	0.1	0.1	16.3	1.9	21.8	1.9	155.6	291.2	484.1	0.4
8.2	0	55.3	44.2	30	0.1	1	2.8	0.8	0.2	0.3	83.7	2.6	33.1	3.4	211.7	339.7	614.6	1
9.4	0	67.7	31.1	96.9	0.1	1	2.7	1.8	0.4	0.4	184.8	3.5	36.6	4.2	311.1	353.1	938.7	1.1
0	0	58	14.8	72.9	0	0.1	0	0	0.2	0.2	36.4	0.9	8.1	1.9	72.9	88.4	256.5	0.3
1.1	0	12.7	4.2	33.1	0	0	1.1	0.3	0	0.1	12.7	0.8	7.6	0.9	37.4	51	324.7	0.1
0.1	0	6.2	18.9	11.9	0	0.1	0.2	0	0	0	32	0.3	14.4	0.2	29.7	102.6	149.6	0.2
1.3	0	58.4	71.5	75.9	0.2	0.5	2.7	0.2	0.4	0.3	129.9	3.2	16	2.6	151.8	290.5	770.8	1.3
1.6	0	245.9	42.9	148.7	0.1	1.2	2.7	0	0.5	0.4	211.6	3.1	25.7	4.2	346	210.2	1005.2	1.9
2.8	0	122	27.1	11.3	0.5	4	1.1	0	0.3	0.3	101.7	5.8	49.7	7.5	314.1	569.5	791	5.6
2.7	0	103.2	45.1	4.3	0.3	3.3	1	0	0.4	0.3	92.4	5.5	45.1	6.7	283.8	526.7	741.7	5.8
2.3	0	98.5	36.9	0	0.3	2.9	0	1.3	0.3	0.3	86.2	4.5	36.9	8.2	234	362.5	554.4	5.7
2.2	0	87.2	37	32.7	0.3	2.3	2.6	0	0.3	0.4	95.9	4.9	43.6	7.2	233.2	479.6	824	4.8
2.1	0	71.2	31.5	0	0.2	2	0	0	0.2	0.2	73.9	3.5	27.4	6.2	175.3	267.1	474	4.1
1.7	0	42.8	17.1	12.8	0.1	0.8	2.5	0.4	0.3	0.2	51.3	2.4	22.4	4.7	110.2	215	563.8	2
0.9	0	35.1	25.2	0	0	0.8	0	0.5	0.2	0.3	63	2.4	18.9	3.7	102.6	144.9	387	2
2.7	0	142.4	31.0	15.5	0.6	4.9	1.3	0	0.5	0.3	64.7	8.3	54.3	10.9	393.6	784.7	712.2	10.7
1.1	0	51.3	50.1	5.7	0	0.3	2.7	0	0.4	0.2	19.3	3.2	10.2	3.7	191.5	166.4	479.9	0.7
3.5	0	78.7	59.5	36.7	0	0.4	0	0	0.7	0.2	101.5	6.1	17.5	4.1	166.2	262.5	973	1.3
1.7	0	44.1	29.4	0	0	0.5	0.1	0	0.2	0.2	23.5	2.3	12.7	3.6	97	143	670.3	1.9
0.3	0	27.8	5.1	51.5	0	0.2	1.1	0.3	0.2	0	153.4	0.1	15.4	0.3	139	168.9	91.6	0.5
0.5	0	4.5	2.5	22.9	0	0.2	0.3	0	0	0	68.3	0.3	13.8	0.3	69.1	43	204.6	0.4
0.5	0	11.6	2.5	65.4	0	0.1	0.1	0	0	0	86.1	0.3	15	0.3	54.7	40.8	241.2	0.4

Code	Name	Amount	Unit	Grams	Energy (kcal)	Carbohydrates (g)	Protein (g)	Fat (g)	Saturated fat (g)	Monounsat fat (g)
21080	Fast Food–Nachos w/Cheese, Beans, Ground Beef	1	Ounce	28.3	63.2	6.2	2.2	3.4	1.3	1.2
21081	Fast Food–Nachos w/Cinnamon and Sugar	1	Ounce	28.3	153.9	16.4	1.8	9.3	4.7	3
21130	Fast Food–Onion Rings, Breaded and Fried	1	Each	10	33.2	3.7	0.4	1.8	0.8	0.8
21048	Fast Food–Oysters, Battered or Breaded, and Fried	1	Ounce	28.3	75.1	8.1	2.5	3.6	0.9	1.4
21025	Fast Food–Pancakes w/Butter and Syrup	1	Each	74	165.7	28.9	2.6	4.4	1.8	1.6
21049	Fast Food–Pizza w/Cheese	1	Slice	63	140.4	20.5	7.6	3.2	1.5	0.9
21050	Fast Food–Pizza w/Cheese, Sausage, and Vegetables	1	Slice	79	184	21.2	13	5.3	1.5	2.5
21051	Fast Food–Pizza w/Pepperoni	1	Slice	71	181	19.8	10.1	6.9	2.2	3.1
21131	Fast Food–Potato, Baked w/Cheese Sauce	1	Each	296	473.6	46.5	14.6	28.7	10.5	10.7
21132	Fast Food–Potato, Baked w/Cheese Sauce and Bacon	1	Each	299	451.4	44.4	18.4	25.8	10.1	9.7
21133	Fast Food–Potato, Baked w/Cheese Sauce and Broccoli	1	Each	339	403.4	46.5	13.6	21.4	8.5	7.6
21134	Fast Food–Potato, Baked w/Cheese Sauce and Chili	1	Each	395	481.9	55.8	23.2	21.8	13	6.8
21135	Fast Food–Potato, Baked w/Sour Cream and Chives	1	Each	302	392.6	50	6.6	22.3	10	7.8
21136	Fast Food–Potato, French Fried In Beef Tallow	1	Large	115	358.8	44.3	4.5	18.5	8.5	8
21137	Fast Food–Potato, French Fried In Beef Tallow and Veg Oil	1	Large	115	357.6	44.3	4.5	18.5	7.6	8.2
21138	Fast Food–Potato, French Fried In Vegetable Oil	1	Large	115	355.3	44.3	4.5	18.5	5.7	9.1
21139	Fast Food–Potato, Mashed	1	Cup	240	199.2	38.6	5.5	2.9	1.1	0.8
21026	Fast Food–Potatoes, Hashed Brown	1	Cup	144	302.4	32.3	3.8	18.4	8.6	7.7
21122	Fast Food–Roast Beef Sandwich w/Cheese	1	Each	176	473.4	45.3	32.2	18	9	3.6
21121	Fast Food–Roast Beef Sandwich, Plain	1	Each	139	346.1	33.4	21.5	13.7	3.6	6.8
21052	Fast Food–Salad, w/o Dressing	1	Cup	138.6	22.1	4.4	1.7	0.1	0	0
21053	Fast Food–Salad, w/o Dressing, w/Cheese and Egg	1	Cup	144.6	67.9	3.1	5.8	3.8	1.9	1.1
21054	Fast Food–Salad, w/o Dressing, w/Chicken	1	Cup	145.3	69.7	2.4	11.6	1.4	0.3	0.4
21055	Fast Food–Salad, w/o Dressing, w/Pasta and Seafood	1	Cup	277.9	252.9	21.3	10.9	13.9	1.7	3.2
21056	Fast Food–Salad, w/o Dressing, w/Shrimp	1	Cup	157.3	70.8	4.4	9.6	1.6	0.4	0.5
21058	Fast Food–Scallops, Breaded and Fried	1	Each	24	64.3	6.4	2.6	3.2	0.8	2
21059	Fast Food–Shrimp, Breaded and Fried	1	Ounce	28.3	78.5	6.9	3.2	4.3	0.9	3
21123	Fast Food–Steak Sandwich	1	Each	140	315	35.6	20.8	9.6	2.6	3.6
21124	Fast Food–Submarine Sandwich w/Coldcuts	1	Each	228	456	51	21.8	18.6	6.8	8.2
21125	Fast Food–Submarine Sandwich w/Roast Beef	1	Each	216	410.4	44.3	28.6	12.9	7	1.8
21126	Fast Food–Submarine Sandwich w/Tuna Salad	1	Each	256	583.6	55.3	29.7	27.9	5.3	13.4
21032	Fast Food–Sundae, Caramel	1	Each	155	303.8	49.3	7.3	9.2	4.5	3
21033	Fast Food–Sundae, Hot Fudge	1	Each	158	284.4	47.6	5.6	8.6	5	2.3
21034	Fast Food–Sundae, Strawberry	1	Each	153	267.7	44.6	6.2	7.8	3.7	2.6
21082	Fast Food–Taco	1	Large	263	568	41.1	31.7	31.6	17.4	10.1
21083	Fast Food–Taco Salad	1	Cup	132	186.1	15.7	8.8	9.8	4.5	3.4
21084	Fast Food–Taco Salad w/Chili Con Carne	1	Cup	174	193.1	17.7	11.6	8.7	4	3
21088	Fast Food–Tostada w/Guacamole	1	Ounce	28.3	39.1	3.4	1.3	2.5	1	0.9
21085	Fast Food–Tostada, w/Beans and Cheese	1	Each	144	223.2	26.5	9.6	9.8	5.3	3
21086	Fast Food–Tostada, w/Beans, Beef, and Cheese	1	Each	225	333	29.6	16	16.9	11.4	3.5
21087	Fast Food–Tostada, w/Beef and Cheese	1	Each	163	314.5	22.7	18.9	16.3	10.3	3.3
40349	Hardee's–Big Cheese	1	Each	141.7	495	28	30	30	0	0
40350	Hardee's–Big Deluxe	1	Each	248.1	675	46	31	41	0	0
40356	Hardee's–Big Fish Sandwich	1	Each	191.3	514	49	20	26	0	0
40353	Hardee's–Big Roast Beef	1	Each	163	364.9	38.9	21.9	13.3	6	6
40351	Hardee's–Big Twin	1	Each	141.7	368.7	27.8	18.8	20.4	9	7.3
40358	Hardee's–Biscuit	1	Each	77.9	275	35	5	13	0	0
40348	Hardee's–Cheeseburger	1	Each	100.6	335	29	17	17	0	0
40357	Hardee's–Chicken Fillet	1	Each	191.3	510	42	27	26	0	0
40347	Hardee's–Hamburger	1	Each	100	305	29	17	13	0	0
40354	Hardee's–Hot Dog	1	Each	50	346	26	11	22	0	0
40355	Hardee's–Hot Ham & Cheese	1	Each	141.7	376	37	23	15	0	0
40352	Hardee's–Roast Beef Sandwich	1	Each	141.7	323.2	38.5	18.6	11.1	4.9	4.9
44118	Jack In The Box–Bacon Cheeseburger	1	Each	242	705	41	35	45	14.9	15.7
44101	Jack In The Box–Breakfast Jack	1	Each	126	313.4	29.1	18.7	13.5	5.3	5.2
44141	Jack In The Box–Cheesecake	1	Each	99	309	29	8	18	9.4	7.4

Polyunsaturated fat (g)	Dietary Fiber (g)	Cholesterol (mg)	Folate (µg)	Vitamin A (RE)	Vitamin B-6 (mg)	Vitamin B-12 (µg)	Vitamin C (mg)	Vitamin E (mg)	Riboflavin (mg)	Thiamin (mg)	Calcium (mg)	Iron (mg)	Magnesium (mg)	Niacin (mg)	Phosphorus (mg)	Potassium (mg)	Sodium (mg)	Zinc (mg)
0.6	0	2.2	4.2	52.1	0	0.1	0.5	0	0	0	42.8	0.3	10.7	0.3	43	50.1	200.1	0.4
1	0	10.2	1.9	2.8	0	0.4	2	0	0.1	0	22.1	0.7	5.1	1	8.5	20.4	114.2	0.1
0	0	1.7	1.4	0.1	0	0	0	0	0	0	8.8	0.1	1.9	0.1	10.4	15.6	51.8	0
0.9	0	22.1	2.5	22.1	0	0.2	0.8	0	0	0	5.6	0.9	4.8	0.9	39.9	37.1	138	3.1
0.6	0	18.5	11.1	22.2	0	0	1.1	0.4	0.1	0.1	40.7	0.8	15.5	1	151.7	79.9	352.2	0.3
0.4	0	9.4	58.5	73.7	0	0.3	1.2	0	0.1	0.1	116.5	0.5	15.7	2.4	112.7	109.6	335.7	0.8
0.9	0	20.5	26.8	101.1	0.	0.3	1.5	0	0.1	0.2	101.1	1.5	18.1	1.9	131.1	178.5	382.3	1.1
1.1	0	14.2	52.5	54.6	0	0.1	1.6	0	0.2	0.1	64.6	0.9	8.5	3	75.2	152.6	266.9	0.5
6	0	17.7	26.6	227.9	0.7	0.1	26	0	0.2	0.2	310.8	3	65.1	3.3	319.6	1166.2	381.8	1.8
4.7	0	29.9	29.9	173.4	0.7	0.3	28.7	0	0.2	0.2	307.9	3.1	68.7	3.9	346.8	1178	971.7	2.1
4.1	0	20.3	61	277.9	0.7	0.3	48.4	0	0.2	0.2	335.6	3.3	77.9	3.5	345.7	1440.7	484.7	2
0.9	0	31.6	51.3	173.8	0.9	0.2	31.6	0	0.3	0.2	410.8	6.1	110.6	4.1	497.7	1572.1	699.1	3.7
3.3	0	24.1	33.2	277.8	0.7	0.2	33.8	0	0.1	0.2	105.7	3.1	69.4	3.7	184.2	1383.1	181.2	0.9
0.9	0	20.7	37.9	3.4	0.3	0.1	6.1	0	0	0.1	18.4	1.5	37.9	2.6	152.9	818.8	187.4	0.6
1.9	0	16.1	37.9	3.4	0.3	0.1	6.1	0	0	0.1	18.4	1.5	37.9	2.6	152.9	818.8	187.4	0.6
2.8	0	0	37.9	3.4	0.3	0.1	6.1	0.2	0	0.1	18.4	1.5	37.9	2.6	152.9	818.8	187.4	0.6
0.7	0	4.8	19.2	24	0.5	0.1	0.9	0	0.1	0.2	50.4	1.1	43.2	2.8	132	705.6	544.8	0.7
0.9	0	18.7	15.8	5.7	0.3	0	10.9	0.2	0	0.1	14.4	0.9	31.6	2.1	138.2	534.2	580.3	0.4
3.5	0	77.4	40.4	45.7	0.3	2	0	0	0.4	0.3	183	5	40.4	5.9	401.2	344.9	1633.2	5.3
1.7	0	51.4	40.3	20.8	0.2	1.2	2	0	0.3	0.3	54.2	4.2	30.5	5.8	239	315.5	792.3	3.3
0	0	0	51.3	158	0.1	0	32.1	0	0	0	18	0.8	15.2	0.7	54	238.5	36	0.2
0.3	0	65.1	56.4	76.6	0	0.2	6.5	0	0.1	0	66.5	0.4	15.9	0.6	88.2	247.3	79.5	0.6
0.3	0	47.9	45	63.9	0.2	0.1	11.6	0	0	0	24.7	0.7	21.8	3.9	113.3	297.9	139.5	0.6
6	0	33.3	66.7	425.3	0.2	1.1	25.5	0	0.1	0.1	47.2	2.1	33.3	2.3	136.2	400.3	1048	1.1
0.3	0	119.5	58.2	51.9	0	2.5	6.1	0	0.1	0	39.3	0.6	25.1	0.7	106.9	269	325.6	0.8
0.1	0	18	6.7	6.9	0	0	0	0	0.1	0	3.1	0.3	5.2	0	48.7	48.9	153.1	0.1
0.1	0	34.5	8.2	6.2	0	0	0	0	0.1	0	14.4	0.5	6.8	0	59.5	31.7	250	0.2
2.3	0	50.4	61.6	30.8	0.2	1	3.7	0	0.2	0.2	63	3.5	33.6	5	204.4	359.8	547.4	3.1
2.2	0	36.4	54.7	79.8	0.1	1	12.3	0	0.8	1	189.2	2.5	68.4	5.4	287.2	394.4	1650.7	2.5
2.6	0	73.4	45.3	49.6	0.3	1.8	5.6	0	0.4	0.4	41	2.8	66.9	5.9	192.2	330.4	844.5	4.3
7.3	0	48.6	56.3	40.9	0.2	1.6	3.5	0	0.3	0.4	74.2	2.6	79.3	11.3	220.1	335.3	1292.8	1.8
1	0	24.8	12.4	68.2	0	0.6	3.4	0.9	0.2	0	189.1	0.2	27.9	0.9	217	317.7	195.3	0.8
0.8	0	20.5	9.4	56.8	0.1	0.6	2.3	0.6	0.3	0	206.9	0.5	33.1	1	227.5	395	181.7	0.9
1	0	21.4	18.3	58.1	0	0.6	1.9	0.7	0.2	0	160.6	0.3	24.4	0.9	154.5	270.8	91.8	0.6
1.4	0	86.7	36.8	226.1	0.3	1.6	3.4	0	0.6	0.2	339.2	3.7	107.8	4.9	312.9	728.5	1233.4	6.0
1.1	0	29	26.4	51.4	0.1	0.4	2.3	0	0.2	0	128	1.5	34.3	1.6	95	277.2	508.2	1.8
1	0	3.4	41.7	142.6	0.3	0.4	2.2	0	0.3	0.1	163.5	1.7	34.8	1.6	102.6	261	589.8	2.1
0.3	0	4.2	11.9	23.5	0	0.1	0.4	0	0	0	45.9	0.1	7.9	0.2	25.2	70.5	86.7	0.4
0.7	0	30.2	74.8	84.9	0.1	0.6	1.3	0	0.3	0.1	210.2	1.8	59	1.3	116.6	403.2	542.8	1.9
0.6	0	74.2	96.7	173.2	0.2	1.1	4	0	0.5	0	189	2.4	67.5	2.8	173.2	490.5	870.7	3.1
0.97	0	40.7	14.6	96.1	0.2	1.1	2.6	0	0.55	0.1	216.7	2.8	63.5	3.1	179.3	572.1	896.5	3.6
0	0	0	0	0	0	0	0	0	0	0	0	0	0	0	0	0	1251	0
0	0	0	0	0	0	0	0	0	0	0	0	0	0	0	0	0	1063	0
0	0	0	0	0	0	0	0	0	0	0	0	0	0	0	0	0	314	0
2.4	1	54.7	29.2	0	0.3	2.9	0	0.2	0.4	0.3	80.2	4.5	40.1	6.5	279.7	389.2	1070.5	7.4
4.1	1.3	45	27.8	13.9	0.2	1.8	2.4	0.7	0.2	0.2	65.5	3.2	28.6	5.4	161.4	229.4	475.2	3.7
0	0	0	0	0	0	0	0	0	0	0	0	0	0	0	0	0	650	0
0	0	0	0	0	0	0	2	0	0.3	0.5	0	0	0	5.5	0	0	789	0
0	0	0	0	0	0	0	0	0	0	0	0	0	0	0	0	0	360	0
0	0	0	0	0	0	0	2	0	0.5	0.5	0	0	0	6.4	0	0	682	0
0	0	0	0	0	0	0	0	0	0	0	0	0	0	0	0	0	744	0
0	0	0	0	0	0	0	0	0	0	0	0	0	0	0	0	0	1067	0
2.4	0.9	43.5	24.8	0	0.3	2.6	0	0.2	0.3	0.3	69.6	3.8	34.8	5.7	243.7	323.2	907.6	6.4
8.7	0	113	0	70	0	0	7.8	0.6	0.4	0.2	200	2.8	0	8.3	0	0	1240	0
2.6	0	189.5	0	138.5	0.5	1.1	3.1	0.1	0.4	0.4	184.3	2.6	24.9	5.3	322.8	197.8	1079.8	1.8
1.6	0	63	0	0	0	0	0	0.3	0.2	0	88	0.3	0	1.9	0	0	208	0

Code	Name	Amount	Unit	Grams	Energy (kcal)	Carbohydrates (g)	Protein (g)	Fat (g)	Saturated fat (g)	Monounsat fat (g)
44115	Jack In The Box–Jumbo Jack	1	Each	222	497.2	40.6	25.2	26.1	10.2	11.3
44116	Jack In The Box–Jumbo Jack w/Cheese	1	Each	242	558.7	40	28.4	31.1	13.3	11.2
44136	Jack In The Box–Regular French Fries	1	Each	109	351	45	4	17	4	7
44135	Jack In The Box–Small French Fries	1	Each	68	219	28	3	11	2.5	7
47265	K.F.C.–Colonel's Chicken Sandwich	1	Each	166	482	39	20.8	27	6	3.9
47261	K.F.C.–French Fries	1	Each	77	244	31	3.2	12	3	7
47260	K.F.C.–Mashed Potatoes and Gravy	1	Each	98	71	12	2.4	2	1	0
47239	K.F.C.–Original Recipe Center Breast	1	Each	103	260.9	9.1	25.1	15.2	3.8	3.5
47240	K.F.C.–Original Recipe Drumstick	1	Each	57	168.5	4.9	11.5	11.5	2.4	3
47241	K.F.C.–Original Recipe Thigh	1	Each	95	324.1	11.1	15.9	23.9	6.3	5.5
47237	K.F.C.–Original Recipe Wing	1	Each	53	172	5	11.8	11	3	6
	Kraft Macaroni & Cheese	1	Serving	70	420	50	12	18.5	5	0
	Kraft Macaroni & Cheese Deluxe – Light	1	Serving	90	290	48	14	4.5	2.5	0
48215	McDonald's–Apple Danish	1	Each	105	360	51	5	16	4	11
	McDonald's–Arch Deluxe	1	Each	239	550	39	28	31	11	0
	McDonald's–Arch Deluxe w/Bacon	1	Each	247	590	39	32	34	12	0
48204	McDonald's–Bacon, Egg and Cheese Biscuit	1	Each	153	470	36	18	28	8	15.7
48174	McDonald's–Big Mac	1	Each	215	560	43	25	32	10.1	20.1
48205	McDonald's–Biscuit w/Spread	1	Each	75	260	32	5	13	3	9
	McDonald's–Breakfast Burrito	1	Each	117	320	23	13	19	7	0
48170	McDonald's–Cheeseburger	1	Each	116	320	35	15	13	5	7.7
48181	McDonald's–Chicken McNuggets	1	Each	18.5	45	2.8	3.3	2.5	0.5	1.6
48226	McDonald's–Chocolate Lowfat Milk Shake	1	Each	294.1	321.2	66.2	11	1.7	0.7	0.9
	McDonald's–Cinnamon Roll	1	Each	95	400	47	7	20	5	0
	McDonald's–Crispy Chicken Deluxe	1	Each	223	0	43	26	25	4	0
48198	McDonald's–Egg McMuffin	1	Each	135	283.7	27.3	17.6	10.7	3.7	5.9
48201	McDonald's–English Muffin w/Spread	1	Each	58	170	26	5	4	2.4	2
48175	McDonald's–Fish Filet Deluxe	1	Each	141	560	54	27	28	5.1	10.1
48188	McDonald's–Garden Salad	1	Each	189	50	6	4	2	0.6	1
	McDonald's–Grilled Chicken Deluxe	1	Each	223	300	38	27	20	1	0
	McDonald's–Grilled Chicken Sld Deluxe	1	Each	257	120	7	21	1.5	0	0
48169	McDonald's–Hamburger	1	Each	102	260	34	13	9	3.5	5
48209	McDonald's–Hash Brown Potatoes	1	Each	53	130	15	1	7	1	4
48210	McDonald's–Hotcakes w/Margarine and Syrup	1	Each	174	570	100	13	19	3	5
48216	McDonald's–Iced Cheese Danish	1	Each	110	410	47	7	22	6	13
48180	McDonald's–Large French Fries	1	Each	122	450	57	6	22	5	15
	McDonald's–Lowfat Apple Bran Muffin	1	Each	114	300	61	6	3	0.5	0
48223	McDonald's–McDonaldland Cookies	1	Each	56.6	180	32	3	5	1	7
48171	McDonald's–Quarter Pounder	1	Each	166	420	37	23	21	8	11
	McDonald's–Quarter Pounderw/Chse	1	Each	200	530	38	28	30	13	0
48207	McDonald's–Sausage Biscuit	1	Each	118	470	35	11	31	8	17
48203	McDonald's–Sausage Biscuit w/Egg	1	Each	175	440	27	19	28	10	20
48199	McDonald's–Sausage McMuffin	1	Each	135	345	27	15	20	7	11
48200	McDonald's–Sausage McMuffin w/Egg	1	Each	159	430	27	21	25	8	14
48208	McDonald's–Scrambled Eggs	1	Each	100	140	1	12	10	3	5
48178	McDonald's–Small French Fries	1	Each	68	220	26	3	12	2.5	8
48227	McDonald's–Strawberry Lowfat Milk Shake	1	Each	294.1	360	60	11	9	0.6	0.6
	McDonald's–Super Size Fries	1	Each	176	540	68	8	26	4.5	0
48225	McDonald's–Vanilla Lowfat Milk Shake	1	Each	294.1	360	60	11	9	0.6	0.6
	McDonald's–Vanilla RF Ice Crm Cone	1	Each	90	150	23	4	4.5	3	0
52366	Pizza Hut–Cheese Pizza, Hand Tossed	1	Slice	70	259	27.5	17	10	6.8	3.2
52359	Pizza Hut–Cheese Pizza, Pan	1	Slice	70	246	28.5	15	9	4.5	4.5
53322	Pizza Hut–Cheese Pizza, Thin'n Crispy	1	Slice	70	199	18.5	14	8.5	5.2	3.3
52370	Pizza Hut–Pepperoni Personal Pan Pizza	1	Each	250	675	76	37	29	12.5	16.5
52367	Pizza Hut–Pepperoni Pizza, Hand Tossed	1	Slice	70	250	25	14	11.5	6.4	5
52360	Pizza Hut–Pepperoni Pizza, Pan	1	Slice	70	270	31	14.5	11	4.5	6.5

Polyunsaturated fat (g)	Dietary Fiber (g)	Cholesterol (mg)	Folate (µg)	Vitamin A (RE)	Vitamin B-6 (mg)	Vitamin B-12 (µg)	Vitamin C (mg)	Vitamin E (mg)	Riboflavin (mg)	Thiamin (mg)	Calcium (mg)	Iron (mg)	Magnesium (mg)	Niacin (mg)	Phosphorus (mg)	Potassium (mg)	Sodium (mg)	Zinc (mg)
2.1	0	72.2	0	66.7	0.2	2.4	3.6	0.1	0.3	0.4	120.9	4	39.7	10.4	235.5	444	1023.3	3.7
1.7	0	97.8	0	195.7	0.2	2.7	4.4	0.2	0.3	0.4	242.8	4	43.6	10	365.6	443.9	1482.2	4.2
0	0	0	0	0	0	0	25.8	5.3	0	0.1	0	0.7	0	3.6	0	0	194	0
0	0	0	0	0	0	0	16.2	10.3	0	0.1	0	0.4	0	2.2	0	0	121	0
9	1.4	47	29	14	0.5	0.3	0	2.3	0.2	0.3	100	3.1	41	10.6	261	297	1060	1.5
1	0	2	0	0	0	0	15.6	0	0	0.1	0	0.3	0	1.9	0	0	139	0
0	0	0	0	0	0	0	0	0	0	0	16	0.2	0	1.1	0	0	339	0
1.5	0	86.9	3.8	15.2	0.5	0.3	0	0.4	0.1	0	16	1.2	30.5	14	238	264.7	602.7	1.1
1.6	0	58.6	4.9	14	0.2	0.1	0	0.4	0.1	0	6.6	0.7	13.2	3.3	99.1	129.7	267.6	1.6
3.1	0	102.9	7.9	27.9	0.3	0.2	0	0.4	0.2	0	12.7	1.4	23.1	6.5	176.4	223.5	549.2	2.3
2	0	59	0	0	0	0	0	0	0	0	24	0.3	0	2.8	0	0	383	0
0	0	15	0	0	0	0	0	0	0	0	120	1.5	0	0	0	0	760	0
0	0	15	0	0	0	0	0	0	0	0	160	1.5	0	0	0	0	810	0
2	1.6	25	3	35	0	0	15	3.8	0.1	0.3	14	1.4	8	2.2	31	69	290	0.2
0	4	90	0	10	0	0	0	0	0	0	6	25	0	0	0	0	1010	0
0	4	100	0	10	0	0	0	0	0	0	6	6	0	0	0	0	1150	0
1.9	1	235	17.6	156.9	0.1	0.5	0	1.4	0.3	0.3	181.4	2.5	30.4	2.4	442.3	232.4	1250	1.6
1.5	0	103	21	106	0.2	1.8	2	0	0.4	0.4	256	4	38	6.8	314	237	950	4.7
1	1	1	6	0	0	0.1	0	1.8	0.1	0.2	75	1.3	14	1.5	168	100	730	0.7
0	1	195	0	10	0	0	15	0	0	0	8	10	0	0	0	0	600	0
1	0	50	18	118	0.1	0.9	2	0.5	0.2	0.2	199	2.3	21	3.9	177	223	750	2.1
0.2	0	9.1	0	0	0	0	0	0	0	0	0	0.1	0	1.2	0	0	96.6	0
0.1	0	10	0	92.3	0	0	0	0	0.5	0.1	333.2	0.8	0	0.4	0	0	240.9	0
0	2	75	0	10	0	0	0	0	0	0	8	8	0	0	0	0	340	0
0	3	55	0	6	0	0	8	0	0	0	6	15	0	0	0	0	1060	0
1.2	1.3	221	43	146.7	0.1	0.7	0.9	1.7	0.3	0.4	250.4	2.7	32.2	3.6	312	208.3	723.9	1.7
1	1.6	9	51	37	0.1	0	0	0.1	0.1	0.3	151	1.6	12	2.5	60	74	285	0.4
10.7	1	49.6	19.8	43.6	0.1	0.8	0	0	0.1	0.3	163.8	1.7	26.8	2.6	227.3	148.9	1060	0.8
0.4	0	65	0	900	0	0	21	0	0.1	0	32	0.8	0	0.3	0	0	70	0
0	3	50	0	6	0	0	8	0	0	0	6	15	0	0	0	0	930	0
0	0	45	0	120	0	0	40	0	0	0	4	8	0	0	0	0	240	0
1	0	30	0	40	0	0	4	0	0.1	0.3	15	1.5	0	3.8	0	0	580	0
2	0	0	0	0	0	0	1.2	0	0	0	0	0	0	0.7	0	0	330	0
5	0	15	0	40	0	0	0	0	0.3	0.3	80	1	0	2.8	0	0	750	0
2	0	47	0	40	0	0	0	0	0.2	0.3	32	0.8	0	1.9	0	0	420	0
2	0	0	0	0	0	0	15	0	0	0.2	0	0.6	0	2.8	0	0	290	0
0	3	0	0	0	0	0	0	0	0	0	10	8	0	0	0	0	380	0
1	0	0	0	0	0	0	0	0	0.1	0.2	0	1	0	1.9	0	0	190	0
1	0	85	0	40	0	0	3.6	0	0.2	0.3	120	2	0	6.6	0	0	645	0
0	2	95	0	10	0	0	4	0	0	0	15	25	0	0	0	0	1290	0
3	0	44	0	0	0	0	0	0	0.1	0.4	64	1	0	3.8	0	0	1080	0
3	0	260	0	60	0	0	0	0	0.3	0.4	80	2	0	3.8	0	0	1210	0
2	0	57	0	40	0	0	0	0	0.2	0.5	160	1.5	0	4.7	0	0	770	0
3	0	270	0	100	0	0	0	0	0.4	0.5	200	2	0	4.7	0	0	920	0
2	0	425	0	100	0	0	0	0	0.2	0	48	1	0	0	0	0	290	0
1	0	0	0	0	0	0	9	0	0	0.1	0	0.2	0	1.9	0	0	110	0
0.1	0	10	0	60	0	0	0	0	0.5	0.1	280	0	0	0.3	0	0	170	0
0	6	0	0	0	0	0	0	0	0	0	35	8	0	0	0	0	350	0
0.1	0	10	0	60	0	0	0	0	0.5	0.1	280	0	0	0	0	0	170	0
0	0	20	0	6	0	0	2	0	0	0	10	2	0	0	0	0	75	0
0	0	27.5	0	50	0	0.3	4.8	0	0.2	0.2	300	1.5	31.5	2.5	220	198	638	2.3
0	0	17	0	45	0	0.3	3.6	0	0.3	0.2	252	1.5	26.2	2.4	188	160	470	2
0	0	16.5	0	35	0	0.2	2.4	0	0.2	0.2	264	0.9	21	2.2	188	130.5	433.5	1.8
0	0	53	0	120	0	0.4	10.2	0	0.6	0.5	584	3.2	52.5	7.7	360	408	1335	3.7
0	0	25	0	50	0	0.3	3.6	0	0.2	0.2	176	1.4	26.2	2.6	156	207.5	633.5	1.8
0	0	21	0	50	0	0.3	4.2	0	0.2	0.3	208	1.7	24.5	2.5	176	202.5	563.5	2.1

Code	Name	Amount	Unit	Grams	Energy (kcal)	Carbohydrates (g)	Protein (g)	Fat (g)	Saturated fat (g)	Monounsatu- fat (g)
52363	Pizza Hut–Pepperoni Pizza, Thin'n Crispy	1	Slice	70	206.5	18	13	10	5.3	4.7
52365	Pizza Hut–Super Sprm Pizza, Thin'n Crispy	1	Slice	70	231.5	22	14.5	10.5	5.1	5.3
52362	Pizza Hut–Super Supreme Pizza, Pan	1	Slice	70	281.5	26.5	16.5	13	6	7
52369	Pizza Hut–Super Supreme, Hand Tossed	1	Slice	70	278	27	16.5	12.5	6.5	6
52371	Pizza Hut–Supreme Personal Pan Pizza	1	Each	250	647	76	33	28	11.2	16.8
52368	Pizza Hut–Supreme Pizza, Hand Tossed	1	Slice	70	270	25	16	13	6.1	6.9
52361	Pizza Hut–Supreme Pizza, Pan	1	Slice	70	294.5	26.5	16	15	7	8
52364	Pizza Hut–Supreme Pizza, Thin'n Crispy	1	Slice	70	229.5	20.5	14	11	5.5	5.5
54494	Red Lobster–Atlantic Ocean Perch, Lunch	1	Each	141.7	130	1	24	4	1.1	0
54506	Red Lobster–Calamari, Brded and Fried, Lunch	1	Each	141.7	360	30	13	21	5.6	0
54486	Red Lobster–Catfish, Lunch Portion	1	Each	141.7	170	0	20	10	2.5	0
54514	Red Lobster–Chicken Breast, Skinless, Lunch	1	Each	113.3	140	0	26	3	1	0
54487	Red Lobster–Cod, Atlantic, Lunch Portion	1	Each	141.7	100	0	23	1	0.3	0
54510	Red Lobster–Deep Sea Scallops, Lunch Portion	1	Each	141.7	130	2	26	2	0.4	0
54488	Red Lobster–Flounder, Lunch Portion	1	Each	141.7	100	1	21	1	0.3	0
54489	Red Lobster–Grouper, Lunch Portion	1	Each	141.7	110	0	26	1	0.3	0
54490	Red Lobster–Haddock, Lunch Portion	1	Each	141.7	110	2	24	1	0.3	0
54491	Red Lobster–Halibut, Lunch Portion	1	Each	141.7	110	1	25	1	0.3	0
54513	Red Lobster–Hamburger, Lunch Portion	1	Each	151.1	410	0	37	28	11	0
54504	Red Lobster–King Crab Legs, Lunch Portion	1	Each	453.5	170	6	32	2	0.5	0
54507	Red Lobster–Langostino, Lunch Portion	1	Each	141.7	120	2	26	1	0.2	0
54500	Red Lobster–Lemon Sole, Lunch Portion	1	Each	141.7	120	1	27	1	0.3	0
54524	Red Lobster–Live Maine Lobster	1	Each	510.2	240	5	36	8	1.9	0
54492	Red Lobster–Mackerel, Lunch Portion	1	Each	141.7	190	1	20	12	3.6	0
54493	Red Lobster–Monkfish, Lunch Portion	1	Each	141.7	110	0	24	1	0.2	0
54498	Red Lobster–Norwegian Salmon, Lunch	1	Each	141.7	230	3	27	12	2.7	0
54495	Red Lobster–Pollock, Lunch Portion	1	Each	141.7	120	1	28	1	0.3	0
54502	Red Lobster–Rainbow Trout, Lunch Portion	1	Each	141.7	170	0	23	9	2.5	0
54496	Red Lobster–Red Rockfish, Lunch Portion	1	Each	141.7	90	0	21	1	0.3	0
54497	Red Lobster–Red Snapper, Lunch Portion	1	Each	141.7	110	0	25	1	0.4	0
54509	Red Lobster–Rock Lobster, Lunch Portion	1	Each	368.5	230	2	49	3	0.7	0
54511	Red Lobster–Shrimp, Lunch Portion	1	Each	198.4	120	0	25	2	0.5	0
54505	Red Lobster–Snow Crab Legs, Lunch Portion	1	Each	453.5	150	1	33	2	0.6	0
54499	Red Lobster–Sockeye Salmon, Lunch Portion	1	Each	141.7	160	3	28	4	1.1	0
54512	Red Lobster–Strip Steak, Lunch Portion	1	Each	255.1	560	0	47	40	17	0
54501	Red Lobster–Swordfish, Lunch Portion	1	Each	141.7	100	0	17	4	1.2	0
54503	Red Lobster–Yellow Fin Tuna, Lunch Portion	1	Each	141.7	180	6	32	2	0.5	0
	Subway B.L.T. – 6″ white	1	Each	191	311	38	14	10	3	0
	Subway Bologna – Deli Sandwich	1	Each	171	292	38	10	12	4	0
	Subway Chicken Taco Sub – 6″ white	1	Each	286	421	43	24	16	5	0
	Subway Classic Italian B.M.T. – 6″ white	1	Each	246	445	39	21	21	8	0
	Subway Club – 6″ white	1	Each	246	297	40	21	5	1	0
	Subway Club Salad	1	Each	331	126	12	14	3	1	0
	Subway Cold Cut Trio – 6″ white	1	Each	246	362	39	19	13	4	0
	Subway Cold Cut Trio Salad	1	Each	330	191	11	13	11	3	0
	Subway Ham – 6″ white	1	Each	232	287	39	18	5	1	0
	Subway Ham – Deli Sandwich	1	Each	171	234	37	11	4	1	0
	Subway Meatballs – 6″ white	1	Each	260	404	44	18	16	6	0
	Subway Melt – 6″ white	1	Each	251	366	40	22	12	5	0
	Subway Pizza Sub – 6″ white	1	Each	250	448	41	19	22	9	0
	Subway Roast Beef – 6″ white	1	Each	232	288	39	19	5	1	0
	Subway Roast Beef – Deli Sandwich	1	Each	180	245	38	13	4	1	0
	Subway Roast Beef Salad	1	Each	316	117	11	12	3	1	0
	Subway Roasted Chicken Breast – 6″ hot	1	Each	246	332	41	26	6	1	0
	Subway Seafood & Crab – 6″ white	1	Each	246	415	38	19	19	3	0
	Subway Seafood & Crab Salad	1	Each	331	244	10	13	17	3	0

Polyunsaturated fat (g)	Dietary Fiber (g)	Cholesterol (mg)	Folate (µg)	Vitamin A (RE)	Vitamin B-6 (mg)	Vitamin B-12 (µg)	Vitamin C (mg)	Vitamin E (mg)	Riboflavin (mg)	Thiamin (mg)	Calcium (mg)	Iron (mg)	Magnesium (mg)	Niacin (mg)	Phosphorus (mg)	Potassium (mg)	Sodium (mg)	Zinc (mg)
0	0	23	0	35	0	0.2	3	0	0.2	0.2	180	0.9	19.2	2.4	148	143.5	493	1.7
0	0	28	0	50	0	0.3	4.2	0	0.2	0.2	184	1.3	26.2	2.5	168	231.5	668	2.2
0	0	27.5	0	60	0	0.4	5.4	0	0.3	0.3	216	1.8	31.5	3	188	266	723.5	2.7
0	0	27	0	55	0	0.4	6	0	0.2	0.3	176	1.9	33.2	3.5	168	258	824	2.4
0	0	49	0	120	0	0.4	10.8	0	0.6	0.5	416	3.7	52.5	7.6	320	487	1313	3.7
0	0	27.5	0	55	0	0.4	6	0	0.2	0.3	192	2.2	35	3.4	184	289	735	2.8
0	0	24	0	60	0	0.3	4.8	0	0.4	0.4	200	1.4	33.2	2.8	184	290	831.5	2.7
0	0	21	0	50	0	0.3	4.8	0	0.2	0.3	172	1.6	29.7	2.5	160	272	664	2.3
1.2	0	75	0	0	0	0.3	0	0	0.1	0	0	0	21	1.5	160	0	190	0.3
1.5	0	140	0	0	0	2	0	0	0.1	0.2	0	0.6	21	1.5	360	0	1150	0.9
1.9	0	85	0	0	0	0	0	0	0.1	0.3	0	0	21	1.9	160	0	50	0.3
1	0	70	0	0	0	0	0	0	0.1	0	0	0.4	21	11.4	160	0	60	0.9
0.6	0	70	0	0	0	0.6	0	0	0	0	0	0	28	0.7	200	0	200	0.3
1.5	0	50	0	0	0	0.4	0	0	0.1	0	0	0	52.5	1.9	240	0	260	1.5
0.7	0	70	0	0	0	0.3	0	0	0	0	16	0	21	1.5	48	0	95	0.3
0.5	0	65	0	0	0	0	0	0	0	0	32	0	28	1.5	200	0	70	0.3
1.1	0	85	0	0	0	0.2	0	0	0	0	0	0	21	2.8	160	0	180	0.3
0.7	0	60	0	0	0	0.3	0	0	0	0.1	0	0	28	2.8	240	0	105	0
1	0	130	0	0	0	1.2	0	0	0.3	0	0	1.5	28	7.6	200	0	115	7.5
1.6	0	100	0	0	0	1.6	0	0	0.1	0	48	0	70	1.9	320	0	900	6
0.6	0	210	0	0	0	2	0	0	0	0.1	16	0.8	35	1.1	160	0	410	1.5
0.4	0	65	0	0	0	0.4	0	0	0.1	0	0	0	21	0.3	64	0	90	0.3
4.1	0	310	0	0	0	2	0	0	0.1	0.1	320	0.8	52.5	2.8	320	0	550	6.7
5.4	0	100	0	0	0	0.8	0	0	0.4	0.1	16	0.8	21	5.7	200	0	250	1.2
0.7	0	80	0	40	0	0.2	0	0	0.1	0	0	1	14	0.7	64	0	95	0.3
4.6	0	80	0	0	0	0.2	0	0	0	0.2	16	0	35	6.6	240	0	60	0.3
1	0	90	0	0	0	1	0	0	0.1	0	0	0	28	0.3	160	0	90	0.3
4	0	90	0	0	0	1	0	0	0.1	0.1	80	0	21	2.8	200	0	90	0.9
0.5	0	85	0	0	0	0.6	0	0	0.1	0	0	0	21	0.7	120	0	95	0.3
0.6	0	70	0	0	0	0.3	0	0	0	0	0	0	21	4.7	120	0	140	0.3
1.4	0	200	0	0	0	0.5	0	0	0	0	48	0	87.5	3.8	400	0	1090	6
1.1	0	230	0	0	0	0.5	0	0	0	0	32	0	35	1.9	120	0	110	1.5
1.8	0	130	0	0	0	1.6	0	0	0.1	0	80	0.2	70	1.9	200	0	1630	6
1.8	0	50	0	0	0	2	0	0	0.1	0.3	0	0	35	7.6	280	0	60	0.3
2	0	150	0	0	0	1.2	0	0	0.3	0.1	0	2	35	7.6	280	0	115	9
1	0	100	0	20	0	0.3	0	0	0	0	0	0	28	3.8	80	0	140	0.6
1.6	0	70	0	0	0	1.6	0	0	0	0	0	0.6	35	13.3	240	0	70	0.3
0	3	16	0	601	0	0	15	0	0	0	27	3	0	0	0	0	945	0
0	2	20	0	565	0	0	14	0	0	0	39	3	0	0	0	0	744	0
0	3	52	0	1044	0	0	18	0	0	0	118	4	0	0	0	0	1264	0
0	3	56	0	753	0	0	15	0	0	0	44	4	0	0	0	0	1652	0
0	3	26	0	601	0	0	15	0	0	0	29	4	0	0	0	0	1341	0
0	1	26	0	1363	0	0	32	0	0	0	26	2	0	0	0	0	1067	0
0	3	64	0	649	0	0	16	0	0	0	49	4	0	0	0	0	1401	0
0	1	64	0	1412	0	0	33	0	0	0	46	2	0	0	0	0	1127	0
0	3	28	0	601	0	0	15	0	0	0	28	3	0	0	0	0	1308	0
0	2	14	0	565	0	0	14	0	0	0	24	3	0	0	0	0	773	0
0	3	33	0	712	0	0	16	0	0	0	32	4	0	0	0	0	1035	0
0	3	42	0	777	0	0	15	0	0	0	93	4	0	0	0	0	1735	0
0	3	50	0	1190	0	0	16	0	0	0	103	4	0	0	0	0	1609	0
0	3	20	0	601	0	0	15	0	0	0	25	4	0	0	0	0	928	0
0	2	13	0	565	0	0	14	0	0	0	23	3	0	0	0	0	638	0
0	1	20	0	1363	0	0	32	0	0	0	23	2	0	0	0	0	654	0
0	3	48	0	617	0	0	15	0	0	0	35	3	0	0	0	0	967	0
0	3	34	0	604	0	0	15	0	0	0	28	3	0	0	0	0	849	0
0	2	34	0	1366	0	0	32	0	0	0	25	2	0	0	0	0	575	0

Code	Name	Amount	Unit	Grams	Energy (kcal)	Carbohydrates (g)	Protein (g)	Fat (g)	Saturated fat (g)	Monounsat fat (g)
	Subway Spicy Italian – 6″ white	1	Each	232	467	38	20	24	9	0
	Subway Steak & Cheese – 6″ white	1	Each	257	383	41	29	10	6	0
	Subway Tuna – 6″ white	1	Each	246	527	38	18	32	5	0
	Subway Tuna – Deli Sandwich, lite mayo	1	Each	178	279	38	11	9	2	0
	Subway Turkey Breast – 6″ white	1	Each	232	273	40	17	4	1	0
	Subway Turkey Breast – Deli sandwich	1	Each	180	235	38	12	4	1	0
	Subway Turkey Breast & Ham – 6″ white	1	Each	232	280	39	18	5	1	0
	Subway Turkey Breast Salad	1	Each	316	316	12	11	2	1	0
	Subway Veggie Delight – 6″ white	1	Each	175	222	38	9	3	0	0
	Subway Veggie Delite – 6″ wheat	1	Each	182	237	44	9	3	0	0
	Subway Veggie Delite Salad	1	Each	260	51	10	2	1	0	0
	Subway–BMT – 6″ Italian	1	Each	213	982	83	44	55	20	24
	Subway–BMT – 6″ Wheat	1	Each	253	460	45	21	22	7	25
	Subway–Club Sandwich – 12″ Italian	1	Each	213	693	83	46	22	7	8
	Subway–Club Sandwich – 12″ Wheat	1	Each	220	722	89	47	23	7	9
	Subway–Cold Cut Combo – 12″ Italian	1	Each	184	853	83	46	40	12	15
	Subway–Cold Cut Combo – 12″ Wheat	1	Each	184	853	88	48	41	12	15
	Subway–Ham and Cheese – 12″ Italian	1	Each	184	643	81	38	18	7	8
	Subway–Ham and Cheese – 12″ Italian	1	Each	239	302	45	19	5	1	8
	Subway–Meat Ball Sandwich – 12″ Italian	1	Each	215	918	96	42	44	17	17
	Subway–Meat Ball Sandwich – 12″ Wheat	1	Each	224	947	101	44	45	17	18
	Subway–Roast Beef – 12″ Italian	1	Each	184	689	84	42	23	8	9
	Subway–Roast Beef – 12″ Wheat	1	Each	189	717	89	41	24	8	9
	Subway–Seafood – 12″ Italian	1	Each	210	986	94	29	57	11	15
	Subway–Seafood – 12″ Wheat	1	Each	219	1015	100	31	58	11	16
	Subway–Spicy Italian – 12″ Italian	1	Each	213	1043	83	42	63	23	28
	Subway–Steak and Cheese – 12″ Italian	1	Each	213	765	83	43	32	12	12
	Subway–Turkey Breast – 12″ Wheat	1	Each	192	674	88	42	20	6	7
58318	Taco Bell–Bean Burrito	1	Each	206	387	63	15	14	4	0
58319	Taco Bell–Beef Burrito	1	Each	206	431	48	25	21	8	0
58321	Taco Bell–Burrito Supreme	1	Each	198	440	55	20	22	8	0
62585	Taco Bell–Light 7–Layer Burrito	1	Each	276	440	67	19	9	0	0
62583	Taco Bell–Light Bean Burrito	1	Each	198	330	55	14	6	0	0
62586	Taco Bell–Light Burrito Supreme	1	Each	248	350	50	20	8	0	0
62584	Taco Bell–Light Chicken Burrito	1	Each	170	290	45	12	6	0	0
62587	Taco Bell–Light Chicken Burrito Supreme	1	Each	248	410	62	18	10	0	0
62582	Taco Bell–Light Chicken Soft Taco	1	Each	120	180	26	9	5	0	0
62575	Taco Bell–Light Soft Taco	1	Each	99	180	19	13	5	4	0
62581	Taco Bell–Light Soft Taco Supreme	1	Each	128	200	23	14	5	0	0
62574	Taco Bell–Light Taco	1	Each	78	140	11	11	5	4	0
62588	Taco Bell–Light Taco Salad	1	Each	464	330	35	30	9	0	0
62580	Taco Bell–Light Taco Supreme	1	Each	106	160	23	14	5	0	0
58328	Taco Bell–Mexican Pizza	1	Each	223	575	40	21	37	11	0
58325	Taco Bell–Nachos	1	Each	106	346	37	7	18	6	0
58323	Taco Bell–Nachos Bell Grande	1	Each	287	649	61	22	35	12	0
58329	Taco Bell–Pintos 'N Cheese	1	Each	128	190	19	9	9	4	0
58337	Taco Bell–Salsa	1	Each	10	18	4	1	0	0	0
58314	Taco Bell–Soft Taco	1	Each	92	225	18	12	12	5	0
58313	Taco Bell–Taco	1	Each	78	183	11	10	11	5	0
58332	Taco Bell–Taco Salad	1	Each	575	905	55	34	61	19	0
58333	Taco Bell–Taco Salad w/o Shell	1	Each	520	484	22	28	31	14	0
58316	Taco Bell–Tostada	1	Each	156	243	27	9	11	4	0
	Wendy's Big Bacon Classic	1	Each	285	580	46	34	30	12	0
	Wendy's Breaded Chicken Sandwich	1	Each	208	440	44	28	18	3.5	0
	Wendy's Cheesburger, Kids' Meal	1	Each	123	320	33	17	13	6	0
	Wendy's Grilled Chicken Sandwich	1	Each	189	310	35	27	8	1.5	0

Polyunsaturated fat (g)	Dietary Fiber (g)	Cholesterol (mg)	Folate (µg)	Vitamin A (RE)	Vitamin B-6 (mg)	Vitamin B-12 (µg)	Vitamin C (mg)	Vitamin E (mg)	Riboflavin (mg)	Thiamin (mg)	Calcium (mg)	Iron (mg)	Magnesium (mg)	Niacin (mg)	Phosphorus (mg)	Potassium (mg)	Sodium (mg)	Zinc (mg)
0	3	57	0	845	0	0	15	0	0	0	40	4	0	0	0	0	1592	0
0	3	70	0	877	0	0	18	0	0	0	88	5	0	0	0	0	1106	0
0	3	36	0	627	0	0	15	0	0	0	32	3	0	0	0	0	875	0
0	2	16	0	628	0	0	14	0	0	0	26	3	0	0	0	0	583	0
0	3	19	0	601	0	0	15	0	0	0	30	4	0	0	0	0	1391	0
0	2	12	0	565	0	0	14	0	0	0	26	3	0	0	0	0	944	0
0	3	24	0	601	0	0	15	0	0	0	29	3	0	0	0	0	1350	0
0	1	19	0	1363	0	0	32	0	0	0	28	2	0	0	0	0	1117	0
0	3	0	0	601	0	0	15	0	0	0	25	0	0	0	0	0	3	0
0	3	0	0	601	0	0	15	0	0	0	32	3	0	0	0	0	593	0
0	1	0	0	1363	0	0	32	0	0	0	23	1	0	0	0	0	308	0
7	5	133	63	67	0.4	2.3	5	5.1	0.3	0.2	64	4.3	66	5.1	308	917	3139	6.1
7	3	56	0	753	0	0	15	0	0	0	44	4	0	0	0	1002	3199	0
4	5	84	47	74	0.5	0.9	20	1.3	0.3	0.4	58	3.1	66	12.5	384	971	2717	2.5
4	6	84	43	83	0.4	0.4	15	4.2	0.3	0.4	96	3.2	40	9.3	247	1055	2777	1.4
10	5	166	39	87	0.2	1.2	17	0.9	0.3	0.3	227	2.9	28	3.8	315	876	2218	2.7
10	6	166	41	90	0.2	1.2	18	0.9	0.3	0.3	235	3	29	3.9	327	1010	2278	2.8
4	5	73	45	174	0.3	0.7	17	3.8	0.3	0.5	304	2.2	50	3.6	527	834	1710	2.8
4	3	28	0	0	0	0	0	0	0	0	35	3	0	0	0	918	1319	0
4	3	88	35	72	0.4	3.21	19	1	0.3	0.3	78	5	47	9.4	263	1210	2022	6.2
4	0	88	0	0	0	0	0	0	0	0	0	0	0	0	0	1498	2082	0
4	5	83	54	58	0.4	2	5	4.4	0.2	0.2	55	3.7	57	4.4	266	910	2288	5.3
4	6	75	56	59	0.4	2	5	4.5	0.3	0.2	56	3.8	59	4.5	273	994	2348	5.4
28	0	56	91	107	0.2	6.5	5	2.5	0.3	0.5	230	4.4	32	7	336	641	2027	5.3
28	2.5	56	0	0	0	0	0	0	0	0	0	0	0	0	0	557	1967	0
7	5	137	0	0	0	0	0	0	0	0	0	0	0	0	0	880	2282	0
4	6	82	36	119	0.3	2.5	6	0.8	0.4	0.3	231	4.2	43	5.1	456	909	1556	6.8
7	7	67	0	0	0	0	0	0	0	0	0	0	0	0	0	605	2520	0
2	3	9	0	0	0	0	53	0	2	0.4	190	4	0	2.8	0	495	1148	0
2	2	57	0	0	0	0	2	0	0.3	0.4	150	3	0	3.2	0	380	1311	0
2	3	33	0	0	0	0	26	0	2.1	0.4	190	4	0	3.6	0	501	1181	0
0	0	5	0	350	0	0	4.8	0	0	0	300	2.5	0	0	0	0	1130	0
0	0	5	0	300	0	0	2.4	0	0	0	120	2	0	0	0	0	1340	0
0	0	25	0	600	0	0	9	0	0	0	96	1.5	0	0	0	0	1160	0
0	0	30	0	200	0	0	3.6	0	0	0	72	1.5	0	0	0	0	900	0
0	0	65	0	250	0	0	4.8	0	0	0	72	1.5	0	0	0	0	1190	0
0	0	30	0	150	0	0	4.8	0	0	0	48	0.8	0	0	0	0	570	0
1	2	25	0	40	0	0	0	0	0.2	0.4	48	0.6	0	2.8	0	196	554	0
0	0	25	0	100	0	0	2.4	0	0	0	48	0.6	0	0	0	0	610	0
1	1	20	0	40	0	0	0	0	0.1	0.1	0	0	0	1.2	0	159	276	0
0	0	50	0	1200	0	0	27	0	0	0	120	1.5	0	0	0	0	1610	0
0	0	20	0	100	0	0	2.4	0	0	0	0	0	0	0	0	0	340	0
10	3	52	0	0	0	0	31	0	0.3	0.3	257	4	0	3	0	408	1031	0
2	1	9	0	0	0	0	2	0	0.2	0	191	1	0	0.6	0	159	399	0
3	4	36	0	0	0	0	58	0	0.3	0.1	297	3	0	2.2	0	674	997	0
1	2	16	0	0	0	0	52	0	0.2	0.1	156	1	0	0.4	0	384	642	0
0	0.4	0	0	0	0	0	0	0	0.1	0	36	1	0	0	0	376	376	0
1	2	32	0	0	0	0	1	0	0.2	0.4	116	2	0	2.8	0	196	554	0
1	1	32	0	0	0	0	1	0	0.1	0.1	84	1	0	1.2	0	159	276	0
12	4	80	0	0	0	0	75	0	0.6	0.5	320	6	0	4.8	0	673	910	0
2	3	80	0	0	0	0	74	0	0.4	0.2	290	4	0	3.2	0	612	680	0
1	2	16	0	0	0	0	45	0	0.2	0.1	180	2	0	0.6	0	401	596	0
0	3	100	0	15	0	0	25	0	0	0	25	30	0	0	0	0	1460	0
0	2	60	0	4	0	0	10	0	0	0	10	16	0	0	0	0	840	0
0	2	45	0	6	0	0	0	0	0	0	17	18	0	0	0	0	830	0
0	2	65	0	4	0	0	10	0	0	0	10	15	0	0	0	0	790	0

Code	Name	Amount	Unit	Grams	Energy (kcal)	Carbohydrates (g)	Protein (g)	Fat (g)	Saturated fat (g)	Monounsaturated fat (g)
	Wendy's Hamburger, Kids' Meal	1	Each	111	270	33	15	10	3.5	0
	Wendy's Jr. Bacon Cheesburger	1	Each	166	380	34	20	19	7	0
	Wendy's Jr. Cheesburger	1	Each	130	320	34	17	13	6	0
	Wendy's Jr. Cheesburger Deluxe	1	Each	180	360	36	18	17	6	0
	Wendy's Jr. Hamburger	1	Each	118	270	34	15	10	3.5	0
	Wendy's Spicy Chicken Sandwich	1	Each	213	410	43	28	15	2.5	0
61273	Wendy's–Big Classic	1	Each	251	480	44	27	23	7	8
62322	Wendy's–Bkd Potato w/Bacon and Cheese	1	Each	380	510	75	17	17	4	3
61287	Wendy's–Bkd Potato w/Broccoli and Cheese	1	Each	411	450	77	9	14	2	3
62524	Wendy's–Bkd Potato w/Cheese	1	Each	383	550	74	14	24	8	6
61281	Wendy's–Chicken Club Sandwich	1	Each	216	470	44	31	20	4	7
61292	Wendy's–Chili, Large	1	Each	340	290	31	28	9	4	2
61291	Wendy's–Chili, Small	1	Each	227	190	21	19	6	2	1
61285	Wendy's–French Fries, Biggie	1	Each	170	450	61	7	23	5	15
61284	Wendy's–French Fries, Medium	1	Each	136	360	50	5	17	4	12
61283	Wendy's–French Fries, Small	1	Each	91	240	33	3	12	2	8
61302	Wendy's–Frosty Dairy Dessert, Large	1	Each	402.2	570	91	15	17	9	4
61301	Wendy's–Frosty Dairy Dessert, Medium	1	Each	321.7	460	76	12	13	7	3
61300	Wendy's–Frosty Dairy Dessert, Small	1	Each	241.3	340	57	9	10	5	3
61271	Wendy's–Plain Single	1	Each	133	360	31	24	16	6	7
61272	Wendy's–Single w/everything	1	Each	219	420	37	25	20	6	7
62477	White Castle–Cheeseburger Sandwich	1	Each	64.8	199.5	15.5	7.8	11.2	0	0
62481	White Castle–Chicken Sandwich	1	Each	63.7	185.7	20.4	7.9	7.4	0	0
62478	White Castle–Fish Sandwich, w/o Tartar	1	Each	59.3	155.4	20.8	5.7	4.9	0	0
62483	White Castle–French Fries	1	Each	96.8	301.1	37.7	2.4	14.7	0	0
62476	White Castle–Hamburger Sandwich	1	Each	58.5	161.2	15.3	5.8	7.9	0	0
62484	White Castle–Onion Rings	1	Each	60.1	245.4	26.6	2.9	13.3	0	0
62479	White Castle–Sausage and Egg Sandwich	1	Each	96.2	322.3	16	12.5	22	0	0
62480	White Castle–Sausage Sandwich	1	Each	48.6	196.1	13.3	6.6	12.2	0	0

Polyunsaturated fat (g)	Dietary Fiber (g)	Cholesterol (mg)	Folate (µg)	Vitamin A (RE)	Vitamin B-6 (mg)	Vitamin B-12 (µg)	Vitamin C (mg)	Vitamin E (mg)	Riboflavin (mg)	Thiamin (mg)	Calcium (mg)	Iron (mg)	Magnesium (mg)	Niacin (mg)	Phosphorus (mg)	Potassium (mg)	Sodium (mg)	Zinc (mg)
0	2	30	0	2	0	0	0	0	0	0	11	17	0	0	0	0	610	0
0	2	60	0	8	0	0	10	0	0	0	17	19	0	0	0	0	850	0
0	2	45	0	6	0	0	2	0	0	0	17	18	0	0	0	0	830	0
0	3	50	0	10	0	0	10	0	0	0	18	19	0	0	0	0	890	0
0	2	30	0	2	0	0	2	0	0	0	11	17	0	0	0	0	610	0
0	2	65	0	4	0	0	10	0	0	0	11	15	0	0	0	0	1280	0
7	0	75	0	60	0	0	12	0	0.2	0.4	120	3.5	0	6.6	0	500	850	0
8	0	15	0	100	0	0	36	0	0.1	0.4	80	2.5	0	6.6	0	1370	1170	0
7	0	0	0	200	0	0	60	0	0.1	0.3	80	2.5	0	4.7	0	1310	450	0
7	0	30	0	150	0	0	36	0	0.1	0.3	240	2	0	3.8	0	1210	640	0
9	2	70	0	20	0	0	9	0	0.4	0.6	80	8	0	15.2	0	470	970	0
1	0	60	0	150	0	0	12	0	0.1	0.1	80	4.5	0	2.8	0	660	1000	0
1	0	40	0	100	0	0	6	0	0.1	0	64	3	0	1.9	0	440	670	0
1	0	0	0	0	0	0	12	0	0	0.3	16	0.8	0	3.8	0	950	280	0
1	0	0	0	0	0	0	9	0	0	0.2	16	0.6	0	2.8	0	760	220	0
1	0	0	0	0	0	0	6	0	0	0.1	0	0.4	0	1.9	0	510	150	0
1	0	70	0	100	0	0	0	0	1.3	0.2	400	1	0	0.7	0	1040	330	0
1	0	55	0	100	0	0	0	0	1	0.1	320	0.8	0	0.7	0	830	260	0
0	0	40	0	80	0	0	0	0	0.7	0.1	240	0.6	0	0.3	0	630	200	0
2	2	65	0	0	0	0	0	0	0.1	0.3	80	3	0	5.7	0	280	580	0
7	3	70	0	60	0	0	9	0	0.1	0.3	80	3	0	6.6	0	430	920	0
0	2.7	0	0	0	0	0	0	0	0	0	0	0	0	0	0	0	361	0
0	1.7	0	0	0	0	0	0	0	0	0	0	0	0	0	0	0	497	0
0	1.4	0	0	0	0	0	0	0	0	0	0	0	0	0	0	0	201	0
0	4.6	0	0	0	0	0	0	0	0	0	0	0	0	0	0	0	193	0
0	2.1	0	0	0	0	0	0	0	0	0	0	0	0	0	0	0	266	0
0	2.6	0	0	0	0	0	0	0	0	0	0	0	0	0	0	0	566	0
0	3	0	0	0	0	0	0	0	0	0	0	0	0	0	0	0	698	0
0	1.9	0	0	0	0	0	0	0	0	0	0	0	0	0	0	0	488	0

Appendix B

Nutrition Advice for Canadians

Canada has its own version of the RDAs, called Recommended Nutrient Intakes (RNIs), published by the Minister of National Health and Welfare. Note that the current DRI revisions of the 1989 RDA revisions will apply to both Americans and Canadians, as this is a joint scientific venture.

Summary of Examples of Recommended Nutrients Based on Energy Expressed as Daily Rates

Age	Gender	Energy (kcal)	Thiamin (mg)	Riboflavin (mg)	Niacin (Ne)†	ω-3 PUFA* (g)	ω-6 PUFA (g)
MONTHS							
0–4	Both	600	0.3	0.3	4	0.5	3
5–12	Both	900	0.4	0.5	7	0.5	3
YEARS							
1	Both	1100	0.5	0.6	8	0.6	4
2–3	Both	1300	0.6	0.7	9	0.7	4
4–6	Both	1800	0.7	0.9	13	1.0	6
7–9	M	2200	0.9	1.1	16	1.2	7
	F	1900	0.8	1.0	14	1.0	6
10–12	M	2500	1.0	1.3	18	1.4	8
	F	2200	0.9	1.1	16	1.2	7
13–15	M	2800	1.1	1.4	20	1.5	9
	F	2200	0.9	1.1	16	1.2	7
16–18	M	3200	1.3	1.6	23	1.8	11
	F	2100	0.8	1.1	15	1.2	7
19–24	M	3000	1.2	1.5	22	1.6	10
	F	2100	0.8	1.1	15	1.2	7
25–49	M	2700	1.1	1.4	19	1.5	9
	F	1900	0.8	1.0	14	1.1	7
50–74	M	2300	0.9	1.2	16	1.3	8
	F	1800	0.8‡	1.0‡	14‡	1.1‡	7‡
75+	M	2000	0.8	1.0	14	1.1	7
	F§	1700	0.8‡	1.0‡	14	1.1‡	7‡
PREGNANCY (ADDITIONAL)							
1st trimester		100	0.1	0.1	1	0.05	0.3
2nd trimester		300	0.1	0.3	2	0.16	0.9
3rd trimester		300	0.1	0.3	2	0.16	0.9
Lactation		450	0.2	0.4	3	0.25	1.5

Abbreviations: g = grams, mg = milligrams
*Niacin equivalents.
†PUFA, polyunsaturated fatty acids.
‡Level below which intake should not fall.
§Assumes moderate physica1 activity.

From Scientific Review Committee: *Nutrition recommendations.* Ottawa, Canada, 1990. Health and Welfare.

Summary of Examples of Recommended Nutrient Intake Based on Age and Body Weight Expressed as Daily Rates

Age	Gender	Weight (kg)	Protein (g)	Vit. A (RE)*	Vit. D (μg)	Vit. E (mg)	Vit. C (mg)	Folate (μg)	Vit. B-12 (μg)	Calcium (mg)	Phosphorus (mg)	Magnesium (mg)	Iron (mg)	Iodine (μg)	Zinc (mg)
MONTHS															
0–4	Both	6	12†	400	10	3	20	25	0.3	250‡	150	20	0.3§	30	2
5–12	Both	9	12	400	10	3	20	40	0.4	400	200	32	7	40	3
YEARS															
1	Both	11	13	400	10	3	20	40	0.5	500	300	40	6	55	4
2–3	Both	14	16	400	5	4	20	50	0.6	550	350	50	6	65	4
4–6	Both	18	19	500	5	5	25	70	0.8	600	400	65	8	85	5
7–9	M	25	26	700	2.5	7	25	90	1.0	700	500	100	8	110	7
	F	25	26	700	2.5	6	25	90	1.0	700	500	100	8	95	7
10–12	M	34	34	800	2.5	8	25	120	1.0	900	700	130	8	125	9
	F	36	36	800	2.5	7	25	130	1.0	1100	800	135	8	110	9
13–15	M	50	49	900	2.5	9	30	175	1.0	1100	900	185	10	160	12
	F	48	46	800	2.5	7	30	170	1.0	1000	850	180	13	160	9
16–18	M	62	58	1000	2.5	10	40‖	220	1.0	900	1000	230	10	160	12
	F	53	47	800	2.5	7	30‖	190	1.0	700	850	200	12	160	9
19–24	M	71	61	1000	2.5	10	40‖	220	1.0	800	1000	240	9	160	12
	F	58	50	800	2.5	7	30‖	180	1.0	700	850	200	13	160	9
25–49	M	74	64	1000	2.5	9	40‖	230	1.0	800	1000	250	9	160	12
	F	59	51	800	2.5	6	30‖	185	1.0	700	850	200	13	160	9
50–74	M	73	63	1000	5	7	40‖	230	1.0	800	1000	250	9	160	12
	F	63	54	800	5	6	30‖	195	1.0	800	850	210	8	160	9
75+	M	69	59	1000	5	6	40‖	215	1.0	800	1000	230	9	160	12
	F	64	55	800	5	5	30‖	200	1.0	800	850	210	8	160	9
PREGNANCY (ADDITIONAL)															
1st trimester			5	0	2.5	2	0	200	1.2	500	200	15	0	25	6
2nd trimester			20	0	2.5	2	10	200	1.2	500	200	45	5	25	6
3rd trimester			24	0	2.5	2	10	200	1.2	500	200	45	10	25	6
Lactation			20	400	2.5	3	25	100	0.2	500	200	65	0	50	6

Abbreviations: μg = micrograms, kg = kilograms, g = grams, mg = milligrams
*Retinol equivalents.
†Protein is assumed to be from breast milk and must be adjusted for infant formula.
‡Infant formula with high phosphorus should contain 375 mg calcium.
§Breast milk is assumed to be the source of the mineral.
‖Smokers should increase vitamin C values by 50%.

From Scientific Review Committee: *Nutrition recommendations.* Ottawa, Canada, 1990. Health and Welfare.

Summary of the Desired Characteristics of the Canadian Diet

Excellent world wide web resources for Canadians are: Health Canada (http:\\www.hwc.ca), Dietitians of Canada (http:\\www.dietitians.ca), and the National Institute of Nutrition (http:\\www.nin.ca).

1. **The Canadian diet should provide energy consistent with the maintenance of body weight within the recommended range.** Physical activity should be appropriate to circumstances and capabilities. Although the importance of maintaining some activity throughout life can be stressed, it is not possible to specify a level of physical activity for the whole population. As a general guideline it is desirable that adults, for as long as possible, maintain an activity level that permits an energy intake of at least 1800 kcal while keeping weight within the recommended range.
2. **The Canadian diet should include essential nutrients in amounts recommended in this report.** Although it is important that the diet provide the recommended amounts of nutrients, it should be understood that no evidence was found that intakes in excess of the RNI confer any health benefit. There is no general need for supplements except for vitamin D for infants and folate during pregnancy. Vitamin D supplementation might be required for elderly persons not exposed to the sun, and iron for pregnant women with low iron stores.
3. **The Canadian diet should include no more than 30% of energy as fat (33 grams per 1000 kcal) and no more than 10% as saturated fat (11 grams per 1000 kcal).** Dietary cholesterol, though not as influential in affecting blood cholesterol, is not without importance. A reduction in cholesterol intake normally will accompany a reduction in total fat and saturated fat. The recommendation to reduce total fat intake does not apply to children under the age of 2 years.
4. **The Canadian diet should provide 55% of energy as carbohydrate (138 grams per 1000 kcal) from a variety of sources.** Sources should be selected that provide complex carbohydrates, a variety of dietary fiber, and beta-carotene.
5. **The sodium content of the Canadian diet should be reduced.** The present food supply provides sodium in an amount greatly exceeding requirements. Although insufficient evidence exists to support a precise recommendation, potential benefit would be expected from a reduction in current sodium intake.
6. **The Canadian diet should include no more than 5% of total energy as alcohol, or two drinks daily, whichever is less.** The harmful influence of alcohol on blood pressure provides a more urgent reason for moderation. During pregnancy it is prudent to abstain from alcoholic beverages because a safe intake is not known with certainty.

7. **The Canadian diet should contain no more caffeine than the equivalent of four regular cups of coffee per day.** This is a prudent measure in view of the increased risk for cardiovascular disease associated with high intakes of caffeine.
8. **Community water supplies containing less fluoride than 1 milligram per liter should be fluoridated to that level.** Fluoridation of community water supplies has proven to be a safe, effective, and economical method of improving dental health.

In essence, suggested actions toward healthful eating as listed in Canada's *Guidelines for Healthy Eating* include the following:

- Enjoy a variety of foods.
- Emphasize cereals, breads, other grain products, vegetables, and fruits.
- Choose low-fat dairy products, lean meats, and foods prepared with little or no fat.
- Achieve and maintain a healthful body weight by enjoying regular physical activity and healthful eating.
- Limit salt, alcohol, and caffeine.

More details are available on RNI and diet recommendations in the 1990 publication *Nutrition Recommendations: The Report of the Scientific Review Committee.*

A separate Canadian food guide, illustrated on the following pages, provides a plan to meet these nutrient needs.

Canada's Basic Labeling Requirements: Under the Food and Drugs Act and the Consumer Packaging and Labeling Act

In general, prepackaged products must show the following basic label information:

1. THE COMMON NAME. This is either the name by which the food is generally known (e.g., orange drink, vanilla cookies, chocolate candies) or the name prescribed by a regulation (e.g., orange juice from concentrate, 60% whole wheat bread, milk chocolate, mayonnaise).
   When a prescribed common name is used, the product must conform to the compositional standard set forth in the regulations.
   The common name is to be shown on the principal display panel (i.e., main panel) in English and French in a minimum type height of 1.6 mm, based on the lower case letter "o."

The Canadian Food Inspection Agency is responsible for the safety and quality of all foods sold in Canada (http:\\www.cfia-acia.agr.ca).

2. A Metric Net Quality declaration by volume (e.g., milliliters, liters), weight (e.g., grams, kilograms) or by count, as applicable. The net quantity declaration is to be shown on the principal display panel in English and French. The following symbols are considered to be bilingual:
   grams - g
   kilograms - k
   milliliters - ml or mL
   liters - l or L

   A minimum type height of 1.6 mm, based on the lower case letter "o," is required for all information in the net declaration except for the numbers which are to be shown in bold face type of not less than the following height:
   a) 1/16 inch (1.6 millimeters), where the principal display surface of the container is not more than 5 square inches (32 square centimeters);
   b) 1.8 inch (3.2 millimeters), where the principal display surface of the container is more than 5 square inches (32 centimeters) but not more than 40 square inches (258 square centimeters);
   c) 1/4 inch (6.4 millimeters), where the principal display surface of the container is more than 40 square inches (258 square centimeters) but not more than 100 square inches (645 square centimeters);
   d) 3/8 inch (9.5 milliliters), where the principal display surface of the container is more than 100 square inches (645 square centimeters) but not more than 400 square inches (25.8 square decimeters); and
   e) 1/2 inch (12.7 milliliters), where the principal display surface of the container is more than 400 square inches (25.8 square decimeters).

   Additional non-metric declarations (e.g., fluid ounces, pounds) are not required but may be shown grouped with the metric statement provided they are not false or misleading.
3. A LIST OF INGREDIENTS and their components (i.e., ingredients of ingredients) in descending order of proportion by weight. Spices, seasonings and herbs except salt, natural and artificial flavors, flavor enhancers, food additives, vitamin and mineral nutrients, may be shown at the end of the list in any order. Some components are completely exempt from a component declaration, while others are exempt depending on the amount used.

   Components of natural or artificial flavoring preparations, seasonings and spice or herb mixtures that are:
   a) flavor enhancers
   b) salt

c) food additives which affect the finished product, and
d) food additives listed in Table X of Division 16 of the Food and Drug Regulations must be shown in the ingredient list as if they were an ingredient of the finished food.

An ingredient or component must be shown in the list of ingredients by its common name.

The list of ingredients is to be shown in English and French on any label panel except the bottom. It is required to be displayed clearly and prominently and be readily discernible. A minimum type height of 1.6 mm based on the lower case letter "o" will usually satisfy this requirement.

4. THE NAME AND ADDRESS declaration of the responsible company. The company name must be the legal registered company name. The address should be complete enough for postal purposes and include the name of the country, if other than Canada or USA.

   This information is to be shown in either English or French on any label panel except the bottom, in a minimum type height of 1.6 mm based on the lower case letter "o."

   If only a Canadian company name and address is shown on an imported product that has been wholly manufactured outside of Canada, the Canadian declaration must be preceded by the appropriate terms "imported by/importé par" or "imported from/importé pour." Alternatively, the country of origin may be declared adjacent to the Canadian company name and address.
5. When a food has a DURABLE LIFE of 90 days or less, a "best before" date and storage instructions if they differ from normal room storage conditions must be declared. Additional information is available upon request.
6. When artificial flavors are used whether alone or with natural flavoring agents and a vignette on the label indicates a natural flavor source (e.g., picture of an apple) information that the added flavoring ingredient is imitation, artificial, or simulated must appear on or adjacent to the vignette in French and English in at least the same type height as required for the numbers in the net quantity.
7. Standard container sizes are specified for wine, glucose and refined sugar syrups, peanut butter, cookies, and biscuits. Specific information is available upon request.

Healthy Canada

Health and Welfare Canada   Santé et Bien-être social Canada

CANADA'S

Food Guide

TO HEALTHY EATING

Enjoy a variety of foods from each group every day.

Choose lower-fat foods more often.

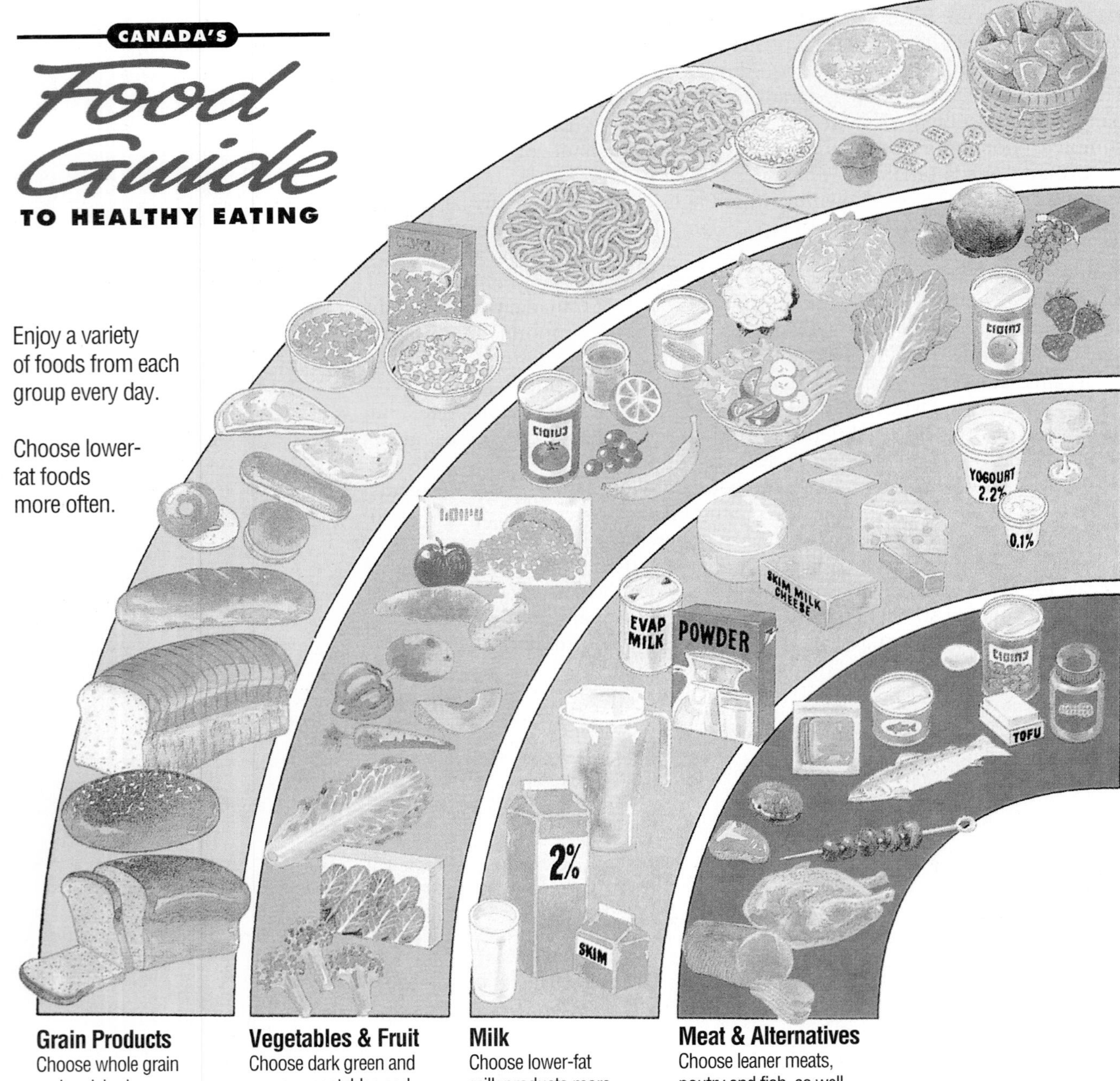

Grain Products
Choose whole grain and enriched products more often.

Vegetables & Fruit
Choose dark green and orange vegetables and orange fruit more often.

Milk
Choose lower-fat milk products more often.

Meat & Alternatives
Choose leaner meats, poutry and fish, as well as dried peas, beans and lentils more often.

Canada

CANADA'S
Food Guide
TO HEALTHY EATING
FOR PEOPLE FOUR YEARS AND OVER

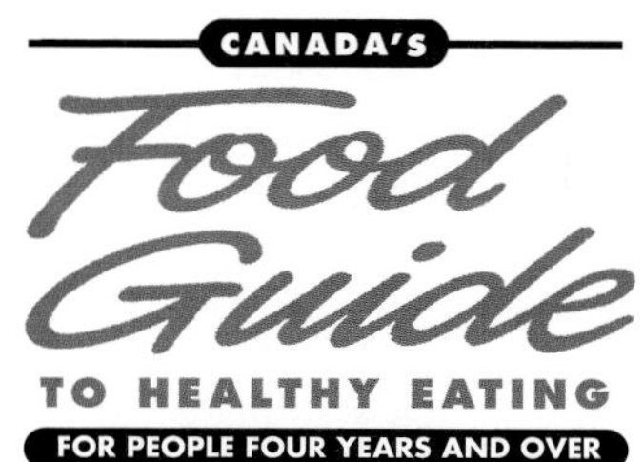

Different People Need Different Amounts of Food

The amount of food you need every day from the four food groups and other foods depends on your age, body size, activity level, whether you are male or female and if you are pregnant or breastfeeding. That's why the Food Guide gives a lower and higher number of servings for each food group. For example, young children can choose the lower number of servings, while male teenagers can go to the higher number. Most other people can choose servings somewhere in between.

Grain Products

5–12 SERVINGS PER DAY

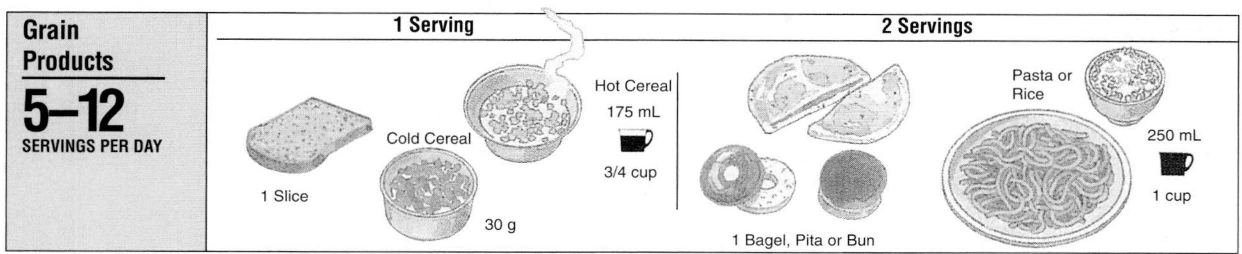

Vegetables & Fruit

5–10 SERVINGS PER DAY

1 Serving
1 Medium Size Vegetable or Fruit
Fresh, Frozen or Canned Vegetables or Fruit
125 mL
1/2 cup
Salad
250 mL
1 cup
Juice
125 mL
1/2 cup

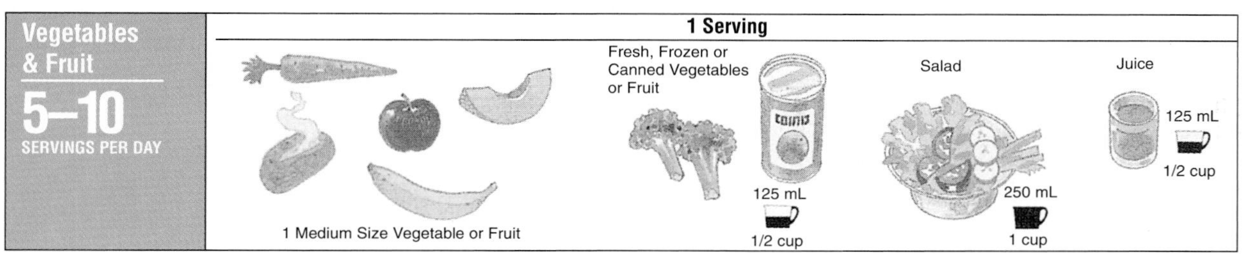

Milk Products

SERVINGS PER DAY
Children 4–9 years: 2-3
Youth 10–16 years: 3–4
Adults: 2-4
Pregnant & Breast-feeding Women: 3-4

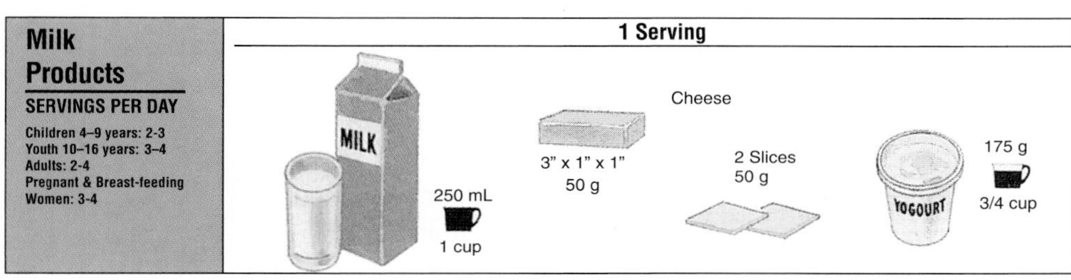

Meat & Alternatives

2–3 SERVINGS PER DAY

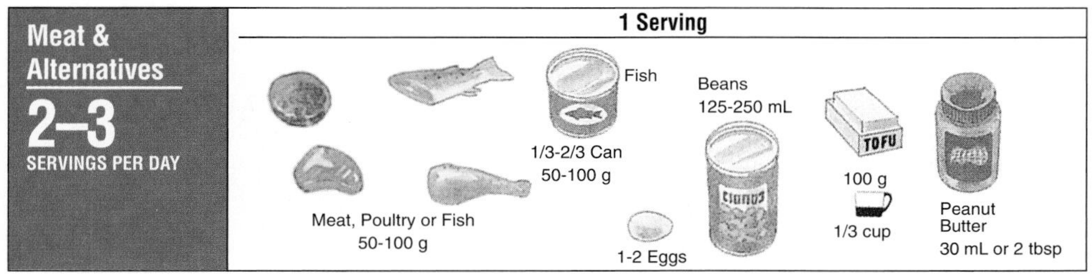

Other Foods

Taste and enjoyment can also come from other foods and beverages that are not part of the 4 food groups. Some of these foods are higher in fat or Calories, so use these foods in moderation.

Enjoy eating well, being active, and feeling good about yourself. That's VITALIT®

ISBN 0-662-19648-1

HOW TO READ A CANADIAN NUTRITION INFORMATION LABEL

Nutrition information is expressed per **suggested serving.** The serving size will vary according to food type and brand. Consider this fact when comparing foods.

Gives the calorie content (Cal).

Indicates the quantity of naturally occurring and added sugars as well as dietary fibre.

Indicates the level of sodium from salt and all other sources.

Vitamins and minerals are expressed as a percentage of the highest recommended amount.

millilitres:
5 mL = 1 teaspoon

kilojoules:
metric unit of energy
1 Cal = 4.18kJ

grams: 28 g = 1 ounce

LASAGNA
Nutrition Information
per 275 g serving
(1 cup/250 mL)

Energy	275	Cal
	1140	kJ
Protein	19	g
Fat	7	g
Polyunsaturates	0.8	g
Monounsaturates	1.9	g
Saturates	2.5	g
Cholesterol	46	mg
Carbohydrate	34	g
Starch	29	g
Sugars	5	g
Dietary Fibre	0.2	g
Sodium	850	mg
Potassium	675	mg

Percentage of Recommended Daily Intake

Thiamine	20%
Riboflavin	19%
Niacin	18%
Calcium	12%
Iron	28%

Appendix C

The Exchange System: A Helpful Menu-Planning Tool

The Exchange System is a tool for quickly estimating the energy, protein, carbohydrate, and fat content of a food or meal. Although learning to use the Exchange System is a bit tedious, much like learning a foreign language, it greately simplifies menu planning. The Exchange System organizes many details of the nutrient compositon of foods into a manageable framework. By using the Exchange System, you can plan daily menus without having to look up or memorize the nutrient values of numerous foods. So the time you spend now becoming familiar with the Exchange System will pay dividends in the future.

In the Exchange System, individual foods are placed into three broad groups: carbohydrate, meat and meat substitutes, and fat. Within these groups are lists that contain foods of similar macronutrient composition: various types of milk; fruit; vegetables; starch; other carbohydrates; various types of meat and meat substitutes; and fat. These lists are designed so that when the proper serving size is observed, each food on a list provides about the same amount of carbohydrate, protein, fat, and energy. This equality allows the exchange of foods on each list. Hence the term *Exchange System*.

The Exchange System was originally developed for planning diabetic diets. Diabetes is easier to control if the person's diet has about the same composition day after day. If a certain number of "exchanges" from each of the various lists is eaten each day, that regularity is easier to achieve. However, because the Exchange System provides a quick way to estimate the energy, carbohydrate, protein, and fat content in any food or meal, it is a valuable menu-planning tool.

Becoming Familiar with the Exchange System

To use the Exchange System, you must know which foods are on each list and the serving sizes for each food.

Table C–1 gives the serving sizes for foods on each exchange list, as well as the carbohydrate, protein, fat, and energy content per exchange. Note that the meat and milk lists are divided into subclasses that vary in fat content and hence in the number of calories they provide. Foods on the meat and fat lists contain essentially no carbohydrate; those on the fruit and fat lists lack appreciable amounts of protein; and those on the vegetable, fruit, and other carbohydrates lists contain no fat. You need to study Table C–1 and Figure C–1 to become familiar with the sizes of the exchanges (i.e., serving sizes) on each list and the amounts of carbohydrate, protein, fat, and energy per exchange.

Before you can turn a group of exchanges into a daily meal plan, you must be aware of which foods are on each exchange list. The entire U.S. Exchange System is presented in Appendix D, which you should consult frequently while exploring the system to discover its various peculiarities. For example, the starch list includes not only bread, dry cereal, cooked cereal, rice, and pasta, but also baked beans, corn on the cob, and potatoes. The Exchange System, unlike the Food Guide Pyramid, is not concerned with the origin, whether animal or vegetable. Instead, it is primarily

TABLE C-1

Nutrient Composition of Exchange System Lists (1995 Edition)

Groups/lists	Household measures*	Carbohydrate (grams)	Protein (grams)	Fat (grams)	Energy (kcal)
CARBOHYDRATE GROUP					
Starch	1 slice, ¾ cup raw, or ½ cup cooked	15	3	1 or less†	80
Fruit	1 small/medium piece	15	—	—	60
Milk	1 cup				
Skim/very low-fat		12	8	0–3†	90
Low-fat		12	8	5	120
Whole		12	8	8	150
Other carbohydrates	Varies	15	Varies	Varies	Varies
Vegetables	1 cup raw or ½ cup cooked	5	1	—	25
MEAT AND MEAT SUBSTITUTES GROUP	1 oz				
Very lean		—	7	0–1	35
Lean		—	7	3	55
Medium-fat		—	7	5	75
High-fat		—	7	8	100
FAT GROUP					
	1 tsp	—	—	5	45

The American Diabetes Association and American Dietetic Association: *Exchange lists for meal planning,* 1995.
*Just an estimate. See exchange lists for actual amounts.
†Calculated as 1 gram for purposes of energy contribution.

concerned with the macronutrients carbohydrate, protein, and fat in each food on a specific list. For example, the carbohydrate composition of potatoes resembles that of bread more than that of broccoli, although potatoes are vegetables.

The very lean–meat list contains the white meat of chicken and turkey (without skin), water-packed tuna, shrimp, nonfat cottage cheese, and fat-free cheese. The lean-meat list contains round steak, lean ham, veal, the dark meat of chicken and turkey (without skin), fish, cottage cheese, and low-fat luncheon meat. The medium-fat meat list contains T-bone steak, pork loin roast, lamb rib roast, any fried fish, mozzarella cheese, and eggs. The high-fat meat list contains ribs, sausage, most luncheon meats (full fat), cheddar cheese, and peanut butter. Note that several foods on the meat and meat substitutes list are not meats, again demonstrating that origin is not important in clasifying foods in the Exchange System.

The vegetable list contains most vegetables, but some starchy vegetables are on the starch list. Most vegetables, such as cabbage, celery, mushrooms, lettuce, and zucchini, can be considred "free foods"; their minimal energy contribution need not count in the calculations when they are eaten in moderation (1 to 2 servings per meal or snack). The fruit list contains fruits and fruit juices. The list of other carbohydrates includes jam, angel food cake, fat-free frozen yogurt, and foods such as frosted cake that count as both other carbohydrate exchanges and fat exchanges.

The milk exchange list contains milk, plain yogurt, and buttermilk. The amount of fat in a product determines whether the serving is skim/very low fat, low fat, or whole.

Starch exchange choices

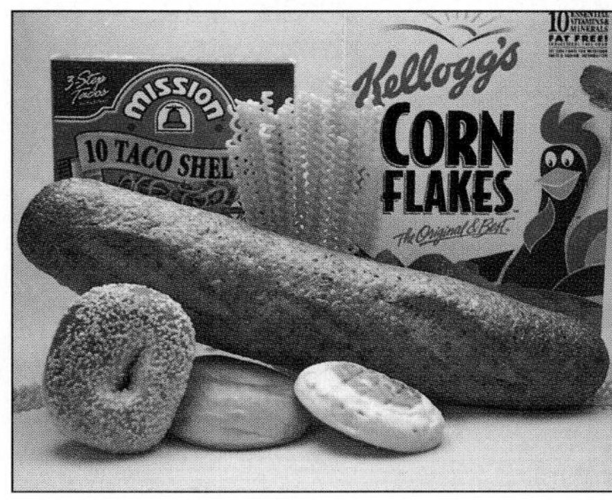

Meat and meat substitutes exchange choices

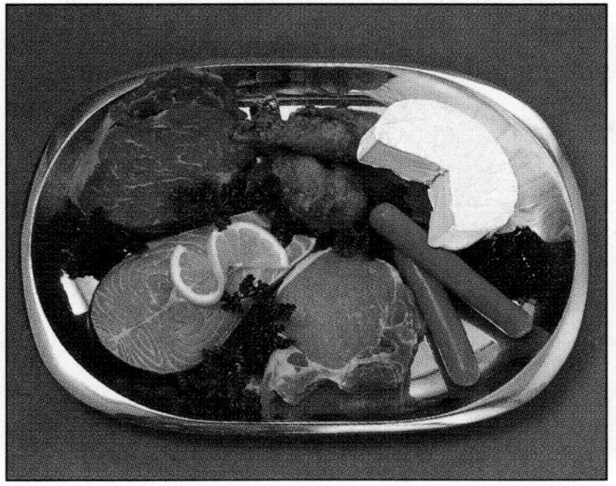

Vegetable exchange choices

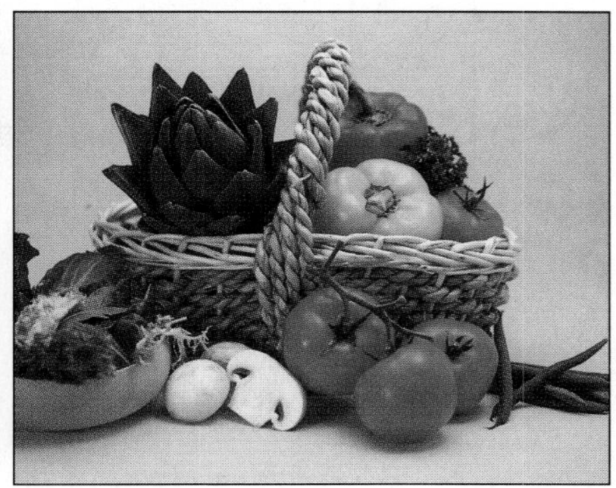

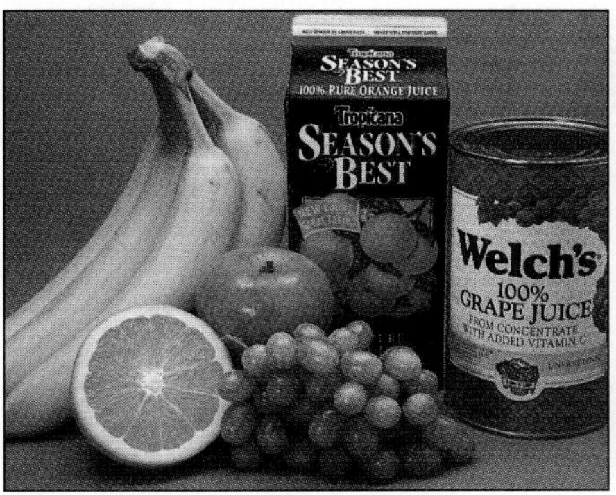

Fruit exchange choices

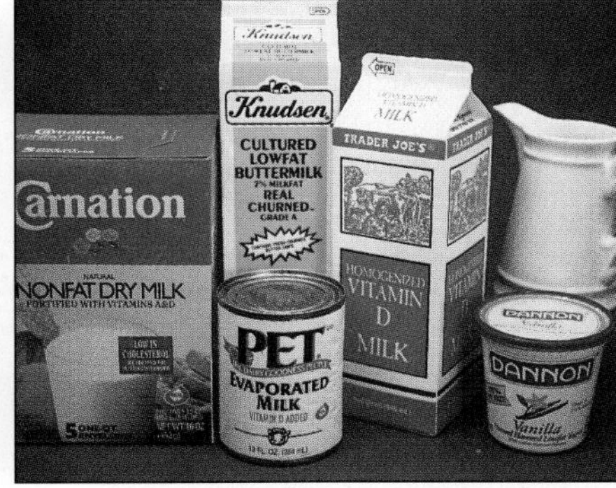

Milk exchange choices

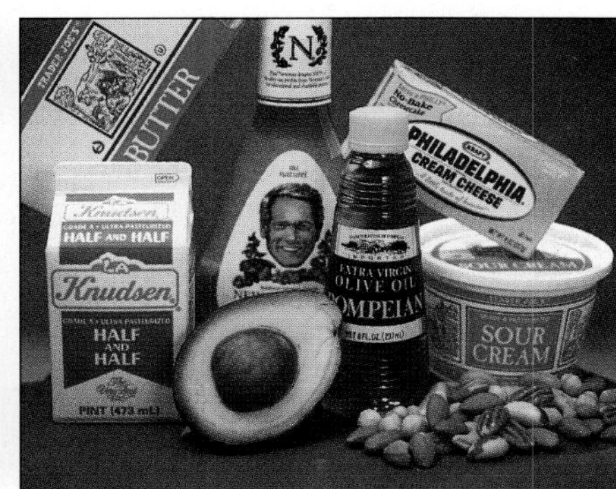

Fat exchange choices

Figure C–1 *Foods arranged according to the exchange lists.*

The fat list contains margarine, mayonnaise, nuts and seeds, salad oils, olives, and full-fat sour cream and cream cheese. Bacon is listed as a fat, rather than as a high-fat meat.

Free foods, other than a moderate intake of most vegetables, include bouillon, diet soda, coffee, tea, dill pickles, and vinegar, as well as herbs and spices.

Using the Exchange System to Develop Daily Menus

Now let's use the Exchange System to plan a 1-day menu. We will target an energy content of 2000 kcal, with 55% coming from carbohydrates (1100 kcal), 15% from protein (300 kcal), and 30% from fat (600 kcal). This can be translated into 2 low-fat milk exchanges, 3 vegetable exchanges, 5 fruit exchanges, 11 starch exchanges, 4 lean meat exchanges, and 6 fat exchanges (Table C–2). Note that this is only one of many possible combinations; the Exchange System offers great flexibility.

Table C–3 arbitrarily separates these exchanges into breakfast, lunch, dinner, and a snack. Breakfast includes 1 low-fat milk exchange, 2 fruit exchanges, 2 starch exchanges, and 1 fat exchange. This total corresponds to ¾ cup of cold cereal, 1 cup of 2% milk, 1 slice of bread with 1 teaspoon margarine, and 1 cup of orange juice.

Lunch consists of 2 fat exchanges, 5 starch exchanges, 1 vegetable exchange, 1 low-fat milk exchange, and 2 fruit exchanges. This translates into 1 slice of bacon with 1 teaspoon mayonnaise on two slices of bread, with tomato. In other words, a bacon and tomato sandwich. You can also add lettuce to the sandwich. This can be considered a "free vegetable" choice. Add to this meal a 9-inch banana (1 exchange = 1 small banana), 1 cup of 2% milk, and 24 animal cookies.

TABLE C-2

Possible Exchange Patterns That Yield 55% of Energy as Carbohydrate; 30% as Fat; and 15% as Protein for Energy Intakes ≥ 2000 Kcal

Kcal/day	1200*	1600*	2000	2400	2800	3200	3600
EXCHANGE LIST							
Milk (low fat)	2	2	2	2	2	2	2
Vegetable	3	3	3	4	4	4	4
Fruit	3	4	5	6	8	9	9
Starch	5	8	11	13	15	18	21
Meat (lean)	4	4	4	5	6	7	8
Fat	2	4	6	8	10	11	13

This is just one set of options. More meat could be included if less milk is used, for example.
*Energy intakes of 1200 and 1600 kcal contain 19% of energy as protein and less carbohydrate to allow for greater flexibility in diet planning.

TABLE C-3

Sample 1-Day Menu Based on the Exchange System Plan*

BREAKFAST	
1 low-fat milk exchange	1 cup 2% milk (put some on cereal)
2 fruit exchanges	1 cup orange juice
2 starch exchanges	¾ cup cold cereal, 1 piece whole-wheat toast
1 fat exchange	1 tsp margarine on toast
LUNCH	
5 starch exchanges	2 slices whole-wheat bread, 24 animal cookies
2 fat exchanges	1 slice bacon, 1 tsp mayonnaise
1 vegetable exchange	1 sliced tomato
2 fruit exchanges	1 banana (9 inches)
1 low-fat milk exchange	1 cup 2% milk
DINNER	
4 lean meat exchanges	4 oz lean ham
2 starch exchanges	1 medium baked potato
1 fat exchange	1 tsp margarine
2 vegetable exchanges	1 cup cooked broccoli
1 fruit exchange	1 kiwi fruit
	Coffee (if desired)
SNACK	
2 starch exchanges	1 bagel
2 fat exchanges	2 tbsp regular cream cheese

*The target plan was a 2000 kcal energy intake, with 55% from carbohydrate, 15% from protein, and 30% from fat. Computer analysis indicated that this menu yielded 2050 kcal, with 55% from carbohydrate, 16% from protein, and 29% from fat—in close agreement with the targeted goals.

Dinner consists of 4 lean meat exchanges, 1 fruit exchange, 2 vegetable exchanges, 1 fat exchange, and 2 starch exchanges. This total corresponds to 4 ounces of lean ham, 1 medium baked potato (1 exchange = 1 small baked potato) with 1 teaspoon of margarine, 1 cup of cooked broccoli, and 1 kiwi fruit. Coffee (if desired) is not counted because it contains no appreciable energy.

Finally, there is a snack containing 2 starch exchanges and 2 fat exchanges. This translates into 1 bagel and 2 tablespoons of regular cream cheese.

This 1-day menu is only one of many that are possible with the exchange lists we selected as an example. Apple juice could replace the orange juice; two apples could be exchanged for the banana. The lean ham could be 4 ounces of flank steal. The choices are endless. Notice that an exchange diet is much easier to plan if you use individual foods; however, the Exchange Sytem tables list some combination foods to help you (see Appendix D). Using combination foods, such as pizza or lasagna, however, makes it more difficult to calculate the number of exchanges in a serving. For instance, lasagna typically has meat exchanges, vegetables exchanges, and starch exchanges. With experience, you will be able to tackle this system (Figure C–2). For now, start by using individual foods as this makes learning the Exchange System much easier. Finally, you might want to prove to yourself that our food choices really meet the exchange plan. This demonstration will give you practice turning exchanges into actual food servings.

Exchange List	Total Exchanges to be Consumed Daily	Exchanges Consumed at Each Meal		
		Breakfast	Lunch	Dinner
MILK				
VEGETABLE				
FRUIT				
STARCH				
MEAT AND SUBSTITUTES				
FAT				

Figure C–2 *Record the Exchange System pattern you have chosen in the left-hand column. Then distribute the exchanges throughout the day, noting the food to be used and the serving size.*

Appendix D

Exchange System Lists

Milk Exchange List

Skim and Very-Low-Fat Milk (12 grams carbohydrate, 8 grams protein, 0–3 grams fat, 90 kcal)

1 cup	skim or nonfat milk (½% and 1%)
⅓ cup	powdered (nonfat dry, before adding liquid)
½ cup	canned, evaporated skim milk
1 cup	buttermilk made from nonfat or low-fat milk
¾ cup	yogurt made from nonfat milk (plain, unflavored)
1 cup	nonfat or low-fat fruit-flavored yogurt sweetened with aspartame or nonnutritive sweeener

Low-Fat Milk (12 grams carbohydrate, 8 grams protein, 5 grams fat, 120 kcal)

1 cup	2% milk
¾ cup	plain low-fat yogurt (added milk solids)
1 cup	sweet acidophilus milk

Whole Milk (12 grams carbohydrate, 8 grams protein, 8 grams fat, 150 kcal)

1 cup	whole milk
½ cup	evaporated whole milk
1 cup	goat's milk
1 cup	kefir

Vegetable Exchange List

(5 grams carbohydrate, 2 grams protein, 0 grams fat, 25 kcal)
1 vegetable exchange equals:

½ cup cooked vegetables or vegetable juice
1 cup raw vegetables

artichoke
artichoke hearts
asparagus
beans (green, wax, Italian)
bean sprouts
beets
broccoli
brussels sprouts
cabbage
carrots
cauliflower
celery
cucumber
eggplant
green onions or scallions
green pepper
greens (e.g., collard)
kohlrabi
leeks
mixed vegetables (without corn, peas, or pasta)
mushrooms
okra
onions
pea pods
peppers
radishes
salad greens
sauerkraut
spinach
squash (summer)
tomato (fresh, canned, sauce)
tomato/vegetable juice
turnips
water chestnuts
watercress
zucchini

The Exchange Lists are the basis of a meal planning system designed by a committee of the American Diabetes Association and The American Dietetic Association. While designed primarily for people with diabetes and others who must follow special diets, the Exchange Lists are based on principles of good nutrition that apply to everyone.

Fruit Exchange List

Fruit (15 grams carbohydrate, 0 grams protein, 0 grams fat, 60 kcal)

1 fruit exchange equals:

1	apple (small)
4 rings	apple, dried
½ cup	applesauce (unsweetened)
4	apricots, fresh
8 halves	apricots, dried
1	banana (small)
¾ cup	blackberries
¾ cup	blueberries
⅓ melon	cantaloupe (small)
1 cup cubes	cantaloupe
12	cherries (3 oz)
½ cup	cherries, canned
3	dates
2	figs, fresh (3½ oz)
1½	figs, dried
½ cup	fruit cocktail
½	grapefruit
¾ cup	grapefruit sections
17	grapes (small)
1 slice	honeydew melon (or 1 cup cubes)
1	kiwi
¾ cup	mandarin orange sections
½	mango (or ½ cup cubes)
1	nectarine (small)
1	orange (small)
½	papaya (or 1 cup cubes)
1	peach, fresh (medium)
½ cup	peaches, canned
½	pear, fresh
½ cup	pear, canned
¾ cup	pineapple, fresh
½ cup	pineapple, canned
2	plums (small)
½ cup	plums, canned
3	prunes, dried
2 tbsp	raisins
1 cup	raspberries
1¼ cup	strawberries (raw, whole)
2	tangerines
1 slice	watermelon (or 1¼ cups cubes)

Fruit Juice

½ cup	apple juice/cider
⅓ cup	cranberry juice cocktail
1 cup	cranberry juice cocktail, reduced-calorie
⅓ cup	fruit juice blends, 100% juice
⅓ cup	grape juice
½ cup	grapefruit juice
½ cup	orange juice
½ cup	pineapple juice
⅓ cup	prune juice

Starch Exchange List

(15 grams carbohydrate, 3 grams protein, 0–1 grams fat, 80 kcal)
1 starch exchange equals:

Bread

½ (1 oz)	bagel
2 slices (1½ oz)	bread, reduced-calorie
1 slice (1 oz)	bread, white, whole-wheat, pumpernickel, or rye
2 (⅔ oz)	bread sticks, crisp, 4 in. long × 3½ in.
½	English muffin
½ (1 oz)	hot dog or hamburger bun
½	pita, 6 in. across
1 slice (1 oz)	raisin bread, unfrosted
1 (1 oz)	roll, plain (small)
1	tortilla, corn, 6 in. across
1	tortilla, flour, 7–8 in. across
1	waffle, 4½ in. square, reduced-fat

Cereals and Grains

½ cup	bran cereal
½ cup	bulgur
½ cup	cereal
¾ cup	cereal, unsweetened, ready-to-eat
3 tbsp	cornmeal (dry)
⅓ cup	couscous
3 tbsp	flour (dry)
¼ cup	granola, low-fat
¼ cup	Grape-Nuts
½ cup	grits
½ cup	kasha
¼ cup	millet
¼ cup	muesli
½ cup	oats
½ cup	pasta
1½ cup	puffed cereal
½ cup	rice milk
⅓ cup	rice, white or brown
½ cup	Shredded Wheat
½ cup	sugar-frosted cereal
3 tbsp	wheat germ

Starchy Vegetables

⅓ cup	baked beans
½ cup	corn
1 (5 oz)	corn on the cob (medium)
1 cup	mixed vegetables with corn, peas, or pasta
½ cup	peas, green
½ cup	plantain
1 (3 oz)	potato, baked or boiled (small)
½ cup	potato, mashed
1 cup	squash, winter (acorn, butternut)
½ cup	yam, sweet potato, plain

Crackers and Snacks

8	animal crackers
3	graham crackers, 2½ in. square
¾ oz	matzoh
4 slices	melba toast
24	oyster crackers
3 cups	popcorn (popped, no fat added or low-fat microwave)
¾ oz	pretzels
2	rice cakes, 4 in. across
6	saltine-type crackers
15–20 (¾ oz)	snack chips, fat-free (tortilla, potato)
2–5 (¾ oz)	whole-wheat crackers, no fat added

Dried Beans, Peas, and Lentils

(counts as 1 starch exchange plus 1 very-lean-meat exchange)

½ cup	beans and peas (garbanzo, pinto, kidney, white, split, black-eyed).
⅔ cup	lima beans
½ cup	lentils
3 tbsp	miso

Starchy Foods Prepared with Fat

(counts as 1 starch exchange plus 1 fat exchange)

1	biscuit, 2½ in. across
½ cup	chow mein noodles
1 (2 oz)	corn bread, 2 in. cube
6	crackers, round butter type
1 cup	croutons
16–25 (3 oz)	french-fried potatoes
¼ cup	granola
1 (1½ oz)	muffin (small)
2	pancakes, 4 in. across
3 cups	popcorn, microwave
3	sandwich crackers, cheese or peanut butter filling
⅓ cup	stuffing, bread (prepared)
2	taco shells, 6 in. across
1	waffle, 4½ in. square
4–6 (1 oz)	whole-wheat crackers, fat added

Other Carbohydrates Exchange List

One exchange equals 15 g carbohydrate, or 1 starch, or 1 fruit, or 1 milk

Exchanges per serving

1/12th cake	angel food cake, unfrosted	2 carbohydrates
2 in. square	brownie, unfrosted (small)	1 carbohydrate, 1 fat
2 in. square	cake, unfrosted	1 carbohydrate, 1 fat
2 in. square	cake, frosted	2 carbohydrates, 1 fat
2	cookies, fat-free (small)	1 carbohydrate
2	cookies or sandwich cookies with creme filling (small)	1 carbohydrate, 1 fat
¼ cup	cranberry sauce, jellied	1½ carbohydrates
1	cupcake, frosted (small)	2 carbohydrates, 1 fat
1 (1½ oz)	doughnut, plain cake (medium)	1½ carbohydrates, 2 fats
3¾ in. across (2 oz)	doughnuts, glazed	2 carbohydrates, 2 fats
1 bar (3 oz)	fruit juice bars, frozen, 100% juice	1 carbohydrate
1 roll (¾ oz)	fruit snacks, chewy (puréed fruit concentrate)	1 carbohydrate

Other Carbohydrates Exchange List—cont'd

Exchanges per serving

1 tbsp	honey	1 carbohydrate
1 tbsp	sugar	1 carbohydrate
1 tbsp	fruit spread, 100% fruit	1 carbohydrate
½ cup	gelatin, regular	1 carbohydrate
3	gingersnaps	1 carbohydrate
1 bar	granola bar	1 carbohydrate, 1 fat
1 bar	granola bar, fat-free	2 carbohydrates
⅓ cup	hummus	1 carbohydrate, 1 fat
½ cup	ice cream	1 carbohydrate, 2 fats
½ cup	ice cream, light	1 carbohydrate, 1 fat
½ cup	ice cream, fat-free, no sugar added	1 carbohydrate
1 tbsp	jam or jelly, regular	1 carbohydrate
1 cup	milk, chocolate, whole	2 carbohydrates, 1 fat
⅙ pie	pie, fruit, 2 crusts	3 carbohydrates, 2 fats
⅛ pie	pie, pumpkin or custard	1 carbohydrate, 2 fats
12–18 (1 oz)	potato chips	1 carbohydrate, 2 fats
½ cup	pudding, regular (made with low-fat milk)	2 carbohydrates
½ cup	pudding, sugar-free (made with low-fat milk)	1 carbohydrate
¼ cup	salad dressing, fat-free	1 carbohydrate
½ cup	sherbet, sorbet	2 carbohydrates
½ cup	spaghetti or pasta sauce, canned	1 carbohydrate, 1 fat
1 (2½ oz)	sweet roll or Danish	2½ carbohydrates, 2 fats
2 tbsp	syrup, light	1 carbohydrate
1 tbsp	syrup, regular	1 carbohydrate
6–12 (1 oz)	tortilla chips	1 carbohydrate, 2 fats
5	vanilla wafers	1 carbohydrate, 1 fat
⅓ cup	yogurt, frozen, low-fat or fat-free	1 carbohydrate, 0–1 fat
½ cup	yogurt, frozen, fat-free, no sugar added	1 carbohydrate
1 cup	yogurt, low-fat, with fruit	3 carbohydrates, 0–1 fat

Meat and Meat Substitutes Exchange List

Very Lean Meat and Substitutes List (0 grams carbohydrate, 7 grams protein, 0–1 grams fat, and 35 kcal)

One very lean meat exchange equals:

Poultry

1 oz	chicken or turkey (white meat, no skin), Cornish hen (no skin)

Fish

1 oz	fresh or frozen cod, flounder, haddock, halibut, trout; tuna, fresh or canned in water

Shellfish

1 oz	clams, crab, lobster, scallops, shrimp, imitation shellfish

Game

1 oz	duck or pheasant (no skin), venison, buffalo, ostrich

Cheese with 1 gram or less fat per ounce

¼ cup	nonfat or low-fat cottage cheese
1 oz	fat-free cheese

Other

1 oz	processed sandwich meats with 1 gram or less fat per ounce, such as deli thin, shaved meats, chipped beef, turkey ham
2	egg whites
¼ cup	egg substitute, plain
1 oz	hot dogs with 1 gram or less fat per ounce
1 oz	kidney (high in cholesterol)
1 oz	sausage with 1 gram or less fat per ounce

Counts as one very lean meat and one starch exchange:

½ cup	dried beans, peas, lentils (cooked)

Lean Meat and Substitutes List (0 grams carbohydrate, 7 grams protein, 3 grams fat, and 55 kcal)

One lean meat exchange equals:

Beef

1 oz	USDA Select or Choice grades of lean beef trimmed of fat, such as round, sirloin, and flank steak; tenderloin; roast (rib, chuck, rump); steak (T-bone, porterhouse, cubed), ground round

Pork

1 oz	lean pork, such as fresh ham; canned, cured, or boiled ham; Canadian bacon; tenderloin, center loin chop

Lamb

1 oz	roast, chop, leg

Veal

1 oz	lean chop, roast

Poultry

1 oz	chicken, turkey (dark meat, no skin), chicken white meat (with skin), domestic duck or goose (well drained of fat, no skin)

Fish

1 oz	herring (uncreamed or smoked)
6	oysters (medium)
1 oz	salmon (fresh or canned), catfish
2	sardines (canned, medium)
1 oz	tuna (canned in oil, drained)

Game

1 oz	goose (no skin), rabbit

Cheese

¼ cup	4.5%-fat cottage cheese
2 tbsp	grated Parmesan
1 oz	cheeses with 3 grams or less fat per ounce

Other

1½ oz	hot dogs with 3 grams or less fat per ounce
1 oz	processed sandwich meat with 3 grams or less fat per ounce, such as turkey pastrami or kielbasa
1 oz	liver, heart (high in cholesterol)

Medium-Fat Meat and Substitutes List (0 grams carbohydrate, 7 grams protein, 5 grams fat, and 75 kcal)

One medium-fat meat exchange equals:

	Beef
1 oz	Most beef products fall into this category (ground beef, meatloaf, corned beef, short ribs, prime grades of meat trimmed of fat, such as prime rib)
	Pork
1 oz	top loin, chop, Boston butt, cutlet
	Lamb
1 oz	rib roast, ground
	Veal
1 oz	cutlet (ground or cubed, unbreaded)
	Poultry
1 oz	chicken dark meat (with skin), ground turkey or ground chicken, fried chicken (with skin)
	Fish
1 oz	any fried fish product
	Cheese (with 5 grams or less fat per ounce)
1 oz	feta
1 oz	mozzarella
¼ cup (2 oz)	ricotta
	Other
1	egg (high in cholesterol, limit to 3 per week)
1 oz	sausage with 5 g or less fat per ounce
1 cup	soy milk
¼ cup	tempeh
4 oz or ½ cup	tofu

High-Fat Meat and Substitutes List (0 grams carbohydrate, 7 grams protein, 8 grams fat, and 100 kcal)

One high-fat meat exchange equals:

	Pork
1 oz	spareribs, ground pork, pork sausage
	Cheese
1 oz	all regular cheeses, such as American, cheddar, Monterey Jack, Swiss
	Other
1 oz	processed sandwich meats with 8 grams or less fat per ounce, such as bologna, pimento loaf, salami
1 oz	sausage, such as bratwurst, Italian, knockwurst, Polish, smoked
1 (10/lb)	hot dog (turkey or chicken)
3 slices (20 slices/lb)	bacon

Counts as one high-fat meat plus one fat exchange:

1 (10/lb)	hot dog (beef, pork, or combination)
2 tbsp	peanut butter (contains unsaturated fat)

Fat Exchange List

Monosaturated Fats List (5 grams fat and 45 kcal)

One exchange equals:

⅛ (1 oz)	avocado (medium)
1 tsp	oil (canola, olive, peanut)
	olives:
8	ripe, black (large)
10	green, stuffed (large)
6 nuts	almonds, cashews
6 nuts	mixed (50% peanuts)
10 nuts	peanuts
4 halves	pecans
2 tsp	peanut butter, smooth or crunchy
1 tbsp	sesame seeds
2 tsp	tahini paste

Polyunsaturated Fats List (5 grams fat and 45 kcal)

One exchange equals:

	margarine:
1 tsp	stick, tub, or squeeze
1 tbsp	lower-fat (30% to 50% vegetable oil)
	mayonnaise:
1 tsp	regular
1 tbsp	reduced-fat
4 halves	nuts, walnuts, English
1 tsp	oil (corn, safflower, soybean)
	salad dressing:
1 tbsp	regular
2 tbsp	reduced-fat
	Miracle Whip Salad Dressing®:
2 tsp	regular
1 tbsp	reduced-fat
1 tbsp	seeds: pumpkin, sunflower

Saturated Fats List (5 grams fat and 45 kcal)

One exchange equals:

1 slice (20 slices/lb)	bacon, cooked
1 tsp	bacon, grease
	butter:
1 tsp	stick
2 tsp	whipped
1 tbsp	reduced-fat
2 tbsp (½ oz)	chitterlings, boiled
2 tbsp	coconut, sweetened, shredded
2 tbsp	cream, half and half
	cream cheese:
1 tbsp (½ oz)	regular
2 tbsp (1 oz)	reduced-fat
	fatback or salt pork, see below*
1 tsp	shortening or lard
	sour cream:
2 tbsp	regular
3 tbsp	reduced-fat

*Use a piece 1 in. × 1in. × ¼ in. if you plan to eat the fatback cooked with vegetables. Use a piece 2 in. × 1 in. × ½ in. when eating only the vegetables with the fatback removed.

Free Foods List

A *free food* is any food or drink that contains less than 20 kcal or less than 5 grams of carbohydrate per serving. Foods with a serving size listed should be limited to 3 servings per day. Foods listed without a serving size can be eaten as often as you like.

Fat-Free or Reduced-Fat Foods

1 tbsp	cream cheese, fat-free
1 tbsp	creamers, nondairy, liquid
2 tsp	creamers, nondairy, powdered
1 tbsp	mayonnaise, fat-free
1 tsp	mayonnaise, reduced-fat
4 tbsp	margarine, fat-free
1 tsp	margarine, reduced-fat
1 tbsp	Miracle Whip®, nonfat
1 tsp	Miracle Whip®, reduced-fat
	nonstick cooking spray
1 tbsp	salad dressing, fat-free
2 tbsp	salad dressing, fat-free, Italian
¼ cup	salsa
1 tbsp	sour cream, fat-free, reduced-fat
2 tbsp	whipped topping, regular or light

Sugar-Free or Low-Sugar Foods

1 candy	candy, hard, sugar-free
	gelatin dessert, sugar-free
	gelatin, unflavored
	gum, sugar-free
2 tsp	jam or jelly, low-sugar, or light
	sugar substitutes†
2 tbsp	syrup, sugar-free

†Sugar substitutes, alternatives, or replacements that are approved by the Food and Drug Administration (FDA) are safe to use. Common brand names include:
Equal® (aspartame)
Sprinkle Sweet® (saccharin)
Sweet One® (acesulfame-K)
Sweet-10® (saccharin)
Sugar Twin® (saccharin)
Sweet `n Low® (saccharin)

Drinks

	bouillon, broth, consommé
	bouillon or broth, low-sodium
	carbonated or mineral water
	club soda
1 tbsp	cocoa powder, unsweetened
	coffee
	diet soft drinks, sugar-free
	drink mixes, sugar-free
	tea
	tonic water, sugar-free

Condiments

1 tbsp	catsup
	horseradish
	lemon juice
	lime juice
	mustard
1½	pickles, dill (large)
	soy sauce, regular or light
1 tbsp	taco sauce
	vinegar

Seasonings

flavoring extracts
garlic
herbs, fresh or dried
pimento
spices
Tabasco® or hot pepper sauce
wine, used in cooking
worcestershire sauce

Combination Foods List

	Entrées	**Exchanges per serving**
1 cup (8 oz)	tuna noodle casserole, lasagna, spaghetti with meatballs, chili with beans, macaroni and cheese	2 carbohydrates, 2 medium-fat meats
2 cups (16 oz)	chow mein (without noodles or rice)	1 carbohydrate, 2 lean meats
¼ of 10 in. (5 oz)	pizza, cheese, thin crust	2 carbohydrates, 2 medium-fat meats, 1 fat
¼ of 10 in. (5 oz)	pizza, meat topping, thin crust	2 carbohydrates, 2 medium-fat meats, 2 fats
1 (7 oz)	pot pie	2 carbohydrates, 1 medium-fat meat, 4 fats
	Frozen entrées	
1 (11 oz)	salisbury steak with gravy, mashed potato	2 carbohydrates, 3 medium-fat meats, 3–4 fats
1 (11 oz)	turkey with gravy, mashed potato, dressing	2 carbohydrates, 2 medium-fat meats, 2 fats
1 (8 oz)	entrée with less than 300 kcal	2 carbohydrates, 3 lean meats
	Soups	
1 cup	bean	1 carbohydrate, 1 very lean meat
1 cup (8 oz)	cream (made with water)	1 carbohydrate, 1 fat
½ cup (4 oz)	split pea (made with water)	1 carbohydrate
1 cup (8 oz)	tomato (made with water)	1 carbohydrate
1 cup (8 oz)	vegetable beef, chicken noodle, or other broth-type	1 carbohydrate

Fast (Quick-Service) Foods

		Exchanges per serving
2	burritos with beef	4 carbohydrates, 2 medium-fat meats, 2 fats
6	chicken nuggets	1 carbohydrate, 2 medium-fat meats, 1 fat
1 each	chicken breast and wing, breaded and fried	1 carbohydrate, 4 medium-fat meats, 2 fats
1	fish sandwich/tartar sauce	3 carbohydrates, 1 medium-fat meat, 3 fats
20–25	french fries, thin	2 carbohydrates, 2 fats
1	hamburger (regular)	2 carbohydrates, 2 medium-fat meats
1	hamburger (large)	2 carbohydrates, 3 medium-fat meats, 1 fat
1	hot dog with bun	1 carbohydrate, 1 high-fat meat, 1 fat
1	individual pan pizza	5 carbohydrates, 3 medium-fat meats, 3 fats
1	soft-serve cone (medium)	2 carbohydrates, 1 fat
1 sub (6 in.)	submarine sandwich	3 carbohydrates, 1 vegetable, 2 medium-fat meats, 1 fat
1 (6 oz)	taco, hard shell	2 carbohydrates, 2 medium-fat meats, 2 fats
1 (3 oz)	taco, soft shell	1 carbohydrate, 1 medium-fat meat, 1 fat

Appendix E

Dietary Intake and Energy Expenditure Assessment

Although it may seem overwhelming at first, it is actually very easy to track the foods you eat. One tip is to record foods and beverages consumed as soon as possible after the actual time of consumption.

I. Fill in the food record form that follows. This appendix contains a blank copy (see the completed example in Table E-1). Then, to estimate the nutrient values of the foods you are eating, consult food labels and the food composition table in Appendix A or use the nutrition software package available with this book. If these resources do not have the serving size you need, adjust the value. If you drink ½ cup of orange juice, for example, but a table has values only for 1 cup, halve all values before you record them. Then, consider pooling all the same food to save time; if you drink a cup of 1% milk three times throughout the day, enter your milk consumption only once as 3 cups. As you record your intake for use on the nutrient analysis form that follows, consider the following tips:

- Measure and record the amounts of foods eaten in portion sizes of cups, teaspoons, tablespoons, ounces, slices, or inches (or convert metric units to these units).
- Record brand names of all food products, such as "Quick Quaker Oats."
- Measure and record all those little extras, such as gravies, salad dressings, taco sauces, pickles, jelly, sugar, ketchup, and margarine.
- For beverages
  - —List the type of milk, such as whole, skim, 2%, evaporated, chocolate, or reconstituted dry.
  - —Indicate whether fruit juice is fresh, frozen, or canned.
  - —Indicate type for other beverages, such as fruit drink, fruit-flavored drink, Kool-Aid, and hot chocolate made with water or milk.
- For fruits
  - —Indicate whether fresh, frozen, dried, or canned.
  - —If whole, record number eaten and size with approximate measurements (such as 1 apple—3 in. in diameter).
  - —Indicate whether processed in water, light syrup, or heavy syrup.
- For vegetables
  - —Indicate whether fresh, frozen, dried, or canned.
  - —Record as portion of cup, teaspoon, or tablespoon, or as pieces (such as carrot sticks—4 in. long, ½ in. thick).
  - —Record preparation method.
- For cereals
  - —Record cooked cereals in portions of tablespoon or cup (a level measurement after cooking).
  - —Record dry cereal in level portions of tablespoon or cup.
  - —If margarine, milk, sugar, fruit, or something else is added, measure and record amount and type.
- For breads
  - —Indicate whether whole wheat, rye, white, and so on.
  - —Measure and record number and size of portion (biscuit—2 in. across, 1 in. thick; slice of homemade rye bread—3 in. by 4 in., ¼ in. thick).
  - —Sandwiches: list *all* ingredients (lettuce, mayonnaise, tomato, and so on).

- For meat, fish, poultry, and cheese
  - —Give size (length, width, thickness) in inches or weight in ounces after cooking for meat, fish, and poultry (such as cooked hamburger patty—3 in. across, ½ in. thick).
  - —Give size (length, width, thickness) in inches or weight in ounces for cheese.
  - —Record measurements only for the cooked edible part—without bone or fat that is left on the plate.
  - —Describe how meat, poultry, or fish was prepared.
- For eggs
  - —Record as soft or hard cooked, fried, scrambled, poached, or omelet.
  - —If milk, butter, or drippings are used, specify kinds and amount.
- For desserts
  - —List commercial brand or "homemade" or "bakery" under brand.
  - —Purchased candies, cookies, and cakes: specify kind and size.
  - —Measure and record portion size of cakes, pies, and cookies by specifying thickness, diameter, and width or length, depending on the item.

Time	Minutes spent eating	M or S*	H† (0–3)	Activity while eating	Place of eating	Food and quantity	Others present	Reason for choice

*M or S: Meal or snack
†H: Degree of hunger (0 = none; 3 = maximum).

TABLE E-1

One Day's Food Record—this Activity Can Help You Understand More About Your Food Habits

Time	Minutes spent eating	M or S*	H†	Activity while eating	Place of eating	Food and quantity	Others present	Reason for choice
7:10 AM	15	M	2	Standing, fixing lunch	Kitchen	Orange juice, 1 cup Crispix, 1 cup 2% milk, ½ cup Sugar, 2 tsp Black coffee	–	Health Habit Health Taste Habit
10:00 AM	4	S	1	Sitting, taking notes	Classroom	Diet cola, 12 oz	Class	Weight control
12:15 PM	40	M	2	Sitting, talking	Student union	Chicken sandwich with lettuce and mayonnaise Pear, 1 2% milk, 1 cup	Friends	Taste Health Health
2:30 PM	10	S	1	Sitting, studying	Library	Regular cola, 12 oz	Friend	Hunger
6:30 PM	35	M	3	Sitting, talking	Kitchen	Pork chop, 1 Baked potato, 1 Margarine, 2 tbsp Lettuce and tomato salad Ranch dressing, 2 tbsp Peas, ½ cup Whole milk, 1 cup Cherry pie, 1 piece	Boyfriend	Convenience Health Taste Health Taste Health Habit Taste
9:10 PM	10	S	2	Sitting, studying	Living room	Apple, 1 Glass mineral water, 1	–	Weight control Weight control

*M or S: Meal or snack
†H: Degree of hunger (0 = none; 3 = maximum).

II. Now complete the nutrient analysis form as shown, using your food record. A blank copy of this form is printed 3 pages ahead for your use. Note that the NutriQuest software available with this book will create such a table for you if you simply enter all food eaten.

Nutrient Analysis Form (Sample)

Name	Quantity	Kcal	Carbohydrates (g)	Protein (g)	Total fat (g)	Saturated fat (g)	Monounsaturated fat (g)	Polyunsaturated fat (g)	Dietary fiber (g)	Cholesterol (mg)	Folate (µg)	Vitamin A (RE)
Egg bagel, 3.5 inch diameter	1 ea.	180	34.7	7.45	1.00	0.171	0.286	0.400	0.748	44.0	16.3	7.00
Jelly	1 tbsp	49.0	12.7	0.018	0.018	0.005	0.005	0.005	–	–	2.00	0.200
Orange juice, prepared fresh or frozen	1½ cup	165	40.2	2.52	0.210	0.025	0.037	0.045	1.49	–	163	28.5
Cheeseburger, McDonald's	2 ea.	636	57.0	30.2	32.0	13.3	12.2	2.18	0.460	80.0	42.0	134
French fries, McDonald's	1 order	220	26.1	3.00	11.5	4.61	4.37	0.570	4.19	8.57	19.0	5.00
Cola beverage, regular	1½ cup	151	38.5	–	–	–	–	–	–	–	–	–
Pork loin chop, broiled, lean	4 oz	261	–	36.2	11.9	4.09	5.35	1.43	–	112	6.77	3.15
Baked potato with skin	1 ea.	220	51.0	4.65	0.200	0.052	0.004	0.087	3.90	–	22.2	
Peas, frozen, cooked	½ cup	63.0	11.4	4.12	0.220	0.039	0.019	0.103	3.61	–	46.9	53.4
Margarine, regular or soft, 80% fat	20 g	143	0.100	0.160	16.1	2.76	5.70	6.92	–	–	0.211	199
Iceberg lettuce, chopped	2 cup	14.6	2.34	1.13	0.212	0.028	0.008	0.112	1.68	–	62.8	37.0
French dressing	2 oz	300	3.63	0.318	32.0	4.94	14.2	12.4	0.431	–	–	0.023
2% low-fat milk	1 cup	121	11.7	8.12	4.78	2.92	1.35	0.170	–	22.0	12.0	140
Graham crackers	2 ea.	60.0	10.8	1.04	1.46	0.400	0.600	0.400	1.40	–	1.80	
Totals		2584	300	99.0	112	33.4	44.1	24.8	17.9	266	395	607
RDA or related nutrient standard		2900		58					–		400	1000
% of nutrient needs		89		170					–		99	61

Abbreviations: g = grams, mg = milligrams, µg = micrograms.

*Values from inside cover. The values listed are for a male age 19 years. Note that number of kcal is just a rough estimate. It is better to base energy needs on actual energy output.

Nutrient Analysis Form (Sample)—cont'd

Vitamin B-6 (mg)	Vitamin B-12 (µg)	Vitamin C (mg)	Vitamin E (mg)	Riboflavin (mg)	Thiamin (mg)	Calcium (mg)	Iron (mg)	Magnesium (mg)	Niacin (mg)	Phosphorus (mg)	Potassium (mg)	Sodium (mg)	Zinc (mg)
0.030	0.065	–	1.80	0.197	2.58	20.0	2.10	18.0	2.40	61.0	65.0	300	0.612
0.005	–	0.710	0.016	0.005	0.002	2.00	0.120	0.720	0.036	1.00	16.0	4.00	–
0.165	–	145	0.714	0.060	0.300	33.0	0.411	36.0	0.750	60.0	711	3.00	0.192
0.230	1.82	4.10	0.560	0.480	0.600	338	5.68	45.8	8.66	410	314	1460	5.20
0.218	0.027	12.5	0.203	0.020	0.122	9.10	0.605	26.7	2.26	101	564	109	0.320
–	–	–	–	–	–	9.00	0.120	3.00	–	46.0	4.00	15.0	0.049
0.535	0.839	0.454	0.405	0.350	1.30	5.67	1.04	34.0	6.28	277	476	88.2	2.54
0.701	–	26.1	0.100	0.067	0.216	20.0	2.75	55.0	3.32	115	844	16.0	0.650
0.090	–	7.90	0.400	0.140	0.226	19.0	1.25	23.0	1.18	72.0	134	70.0	0.750
0.002	0.017	0.028	2.19	0.006	0.002	5.29	–	0.467	0.004	4.06	7.54	216	0.041
0.044	–	4.36	0.120	0.034	0.052	21.2	0.560	10.1	0.210	22.4	177	10.1	0.246
0.006	–		15.9	–	–	7.10	0.227	5.81	–	3.63	7.03	666	0.045
0.105	0.888	2.32	0.080	0.403	0.095	297	0.120	33.0	0.210	232	377	122	0.963
0.011	–			0.030	0.020	6.00	0.367	6.00	0.600	20.0	36.0	86.0	0.113
2.14	3.65	204	22.5	1.79	5.52	792	15.4	298	25.9	1425	3732	3165	11.7
1.3	2.4	60	10	1.3	1.2	1000	10	400	16	700	2000	500	15
160	152	340	225	138	450	79	154	75	162	204	187	633	78

Nutrient Analysis Form (Sample)

Name	Quantity	Kcal	Carbohydrates (g)	Protein (g)	Total fat (g)	Saturated fat (g)	Monounsaturated fat (g)	Polyunsaturated fat (g)	Dietary fiber (g)	Cholesterol (mg)	Folate (µg)	Vitamin A (RE)
Totals												
RDA or related nutrient standard*												
% of nutrient needs												

*Values from inside cover. Note that number of kcals is just a rough estimate. It is better to base energy needs on actual energy output.

Nutrient Analysis Form (Sample)—cont'd

Vitamin B-6 (mg)	Vitamin B-12 (µg)	Vitamin C (mg)	Vitamin E (mg)	Riboflavin (mg)	Thiamin (mg)	Calcium (mg)	Iron (mg)	Magnesium (mg)	Niacin (mg)	Phosphorus (mg)	Potassium (mg)	Sodium (mg)	Zinc (mg)

III. Complete the following table as you summarize your dietary intake.

Percentage of kcal from Protein, Fat, Carbohydrate, and Alcohol

Intake				
Protein (P):	____ g/day × 4 kcal/g	=	(P)________	kcal/day
Fat (F):	____ g/day × 9 kcal/g	=	(F)________	kcal/day
Carbohydrate (C):	____ g/day × 4 kcal/g	=	(C)________	kcal/day
Alcohol (A):			(A)________	kcal/day*
	Total kcal (T)/day	=	(T)________	kcal/day

Percentage of kcal from protein:

$\frac{(P)}{(T)}$ × 100 = ____ % of total kcal

Percentage of kcal from fat:

$\frac{(F)}{(T)}$ × 100 = ____ % of total kcal

Percentage of kcal from carbohydrate:

$\frac{(C)}{(T)}$ × 100 = ____ % of total kcal

Percentage of kcal from alcohol:

$\frac{(A)}{(T)}$ × 100 = ____ % of total kcal

NOTE: The four percentages can total 99, 100, or 101, depending on the way in which figures were rounded off earlier.

*To calculate how many kcal in a beverage are from alcohol, look up the beverage in Appendix A. Determine how many kcal are from carbohydrate (multiply carbohydrate grams times 4), fat (fat grams times 9), and protein (protein grams times 4). The remaining kcal are from alcohol.

IV. Use the following table to again record your food intake for one day, placing each food item in the correct category of the Food Guide Pyramid, with the correct number of servings (see Table 2–5). Note that a food such as toast with margarine would contribute to two categories—namely, to the bread, cereal, rice, and pasta group and to the fats, oils, and sweets group. You can expect that many food choices will contribute to more than one group. Indicate the number of servings from the Food Guide Pyramid that each food yields.

Indicate the Number of Servings from the Food Guide Pyramid That Each Food Yields

Food or beverage	Amount eaten	Milk, yogurt, and cheese	Meat, poultry, fish, dry beans, eggs, and nuts	Fruits	Vegetables	Bread, cereal, rice, and pasta	Fats, oils, and sweets
bagel	one					2	
milk	8 oz	1					
turkey " "							
cheese slice	1 oz	1					
apple w/skin	1 piece						
peas	cup						
salad							
1 banana							
roll							
Water	8 oz						
Group totals							
Recommended servings		2-4	2-3	2-4	3-5	8-11	In moderation
Shortages in numbers of servings							

V. Evaluation. Are there weaknesses suggested in your nutrient intake that correspond to missing servings in the Food Guide Pyramid? Consider replacing the missing servings to improve your nutrient intake.

VI. For the same day you keep your food record, also keep a 24-hour record of your activities. Include sleeping, sitting, and walking, as well as the obvious forms of exercise. Calculate your energy expenditure for these activities using Table 9–6 in Chapter 9 or the software available with this book. Try to substitute a similar activity if your particular activity is not listed. Calculate the total kcal you used for the day (total for column 3). Below is an example of an activity record. A blank form follows for your use. Ask your professor whether you are to turn in the form or the activity printout from the software.

Weight (kg)*: 70 kg

		Energy cost		
Activity	Time (minutes); Convert to hours	Column I kcal/kg/hr (from Table 9-6)	Column 2 (Column 1 × Time)	Column 3 (Column 2 × Weight in kg)
Brisk walking	(60 min.) 1 hr	4.4	(× 1) = 4.4	(× 70) = 308

*lbs/2.2

Weight (kg)*:

		Energy cost		
Activity	Time (minutes); Convert to hours	Column I kcal/kg/hr (from Table 9-6)	Column 2 (Column 1 × Time)	Column 3 (Column 2 × Weight in kg)

Total kcal used (from adding all of column 3)

*lbs/2.2

Appendix F

The Human Cell—Primary Site for Metabolism

The cell is the basic unit of body structure, and it is where most metabolic reactions occur (Figure F–1). The cell is surrounded by a semipermeable membrane that controls the passage of nutrients and other substances in and out of it. Within the cell is fluid called the cytosol. Within the cytosol are small bodies called organelles that perform specific metabolic functions. The name and activities of the various cell parts are given below:

Nucleus: This spherical structure is bound by its own double membrane. Within the nucleus are chromosomes, which are long threads of DNA (also called chromatin) that contain hereditary information for directing cell protein synthesis and cell division. Although most cell types have only one nucleus, muscle cells contain many nuclei.

Mitochondria: These have their own outer membrane, as well as an inner membrane that is highly folded. The mitochondria are the major sites of energy production in the cell. Muscle cells contain many mitochondria.

Endoplasmic reticulum: This network of internal membranes serves as a communication network within the cell. Small granules called ribosomes are attached to parts of the outside of the endoplasmic reticulum, which is known as the rough endoplasmic reticulum. Ribosomes are the site for protein synthesis. Fat is synthesized in other areas of the endoplasmic reticulum where there are no ribosomes—namely, the smooth endoplasmic reticulum. In muscles, this organelle (called sarcoplasmic reticulum) plays a key role in muscle contraction.

Golgi complex: This consists of stacks of flattened structures that both package proteins for export from the cell and help form other cell organelles (Figure F–2).

Lysosomes: These small bodies contain digestive enzymes that break down worn-out cell parts and other cell debris. When a lysosome fuses with a particle that is to be digested, the digestive activity begins.

Storage forms of energy: These occur in the cell as glycogen granules and lipid droplets.

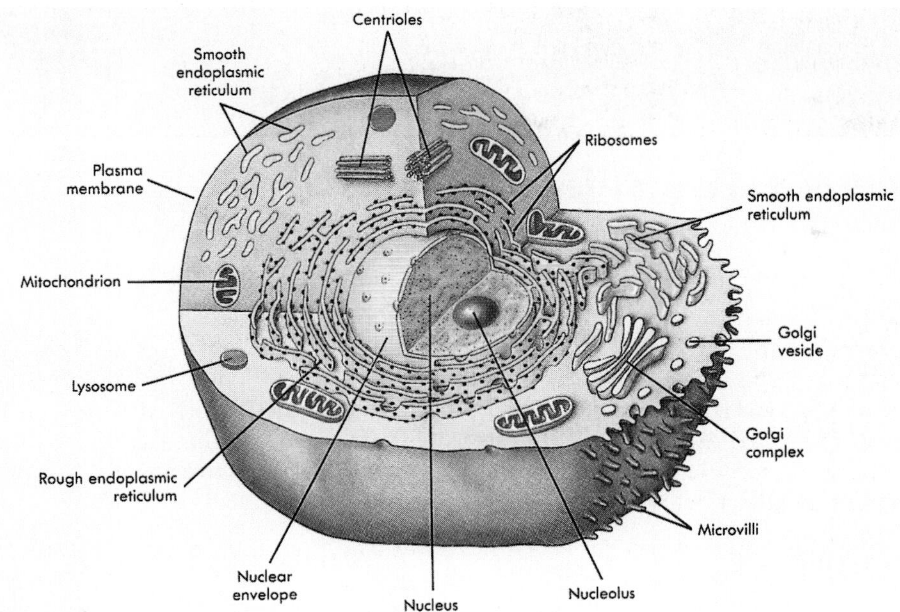

Figure F–1 *An animal cell. Almost all human cells contain these various organelles.*

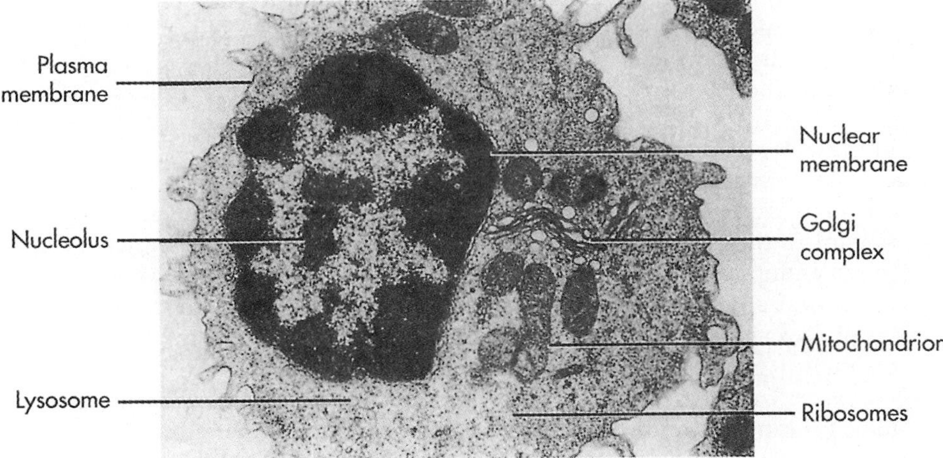

Figure F–2 *Electron micrograph of a cell, magnified 40,500 times. Our understanding of the structures in cells is based mainly on such pictures as this. (From Raven PH, Johnson GB:* Biology, *St. Louis, 1992, Mosby–Year Book.)*

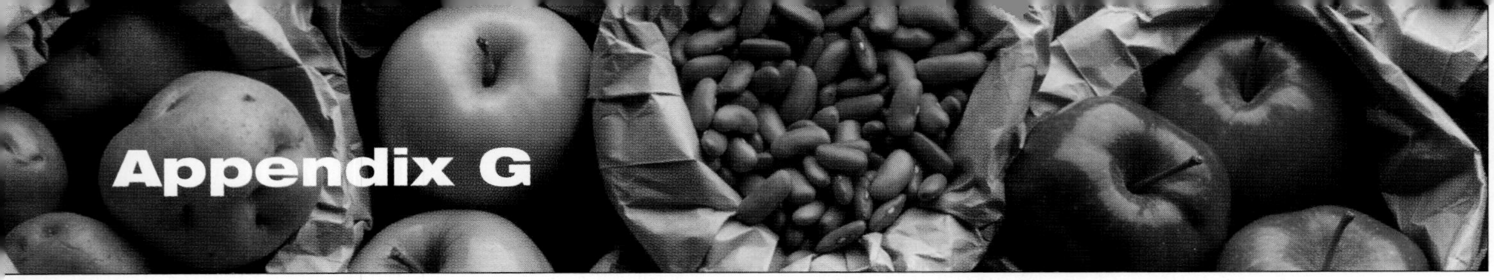

Appendix G

Important Chemical Structures in Nutrition

Amino Acids

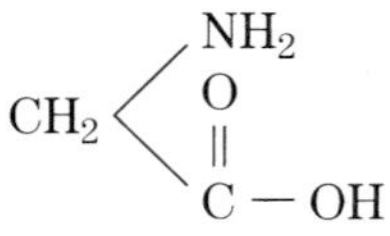

NH_2
CH_2 ⟨ O ‖ C — OH

Glycine

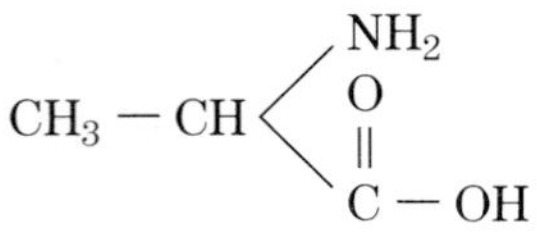

NH_2
$CH_3 - CH$ ⟨ O ‖ C — OH

Alanine

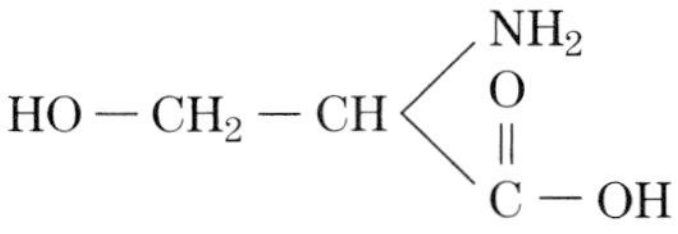

NH_2
$HO - CH_2 - CH$ ⟨ O ‖ C — OH

Serine

CH_3 ⟩ $CH - CH_2 - CH$ ⟨ NH_2 / O ‖ C — OH
CH_3

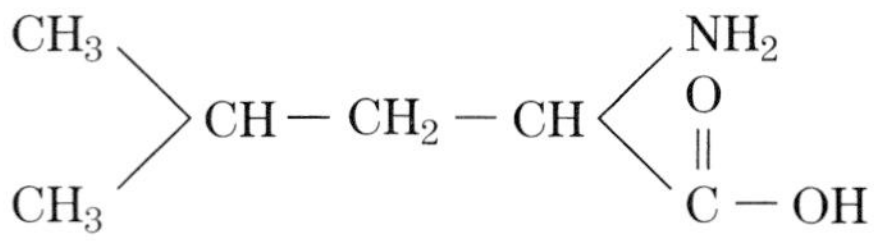

Leucine
(essential)

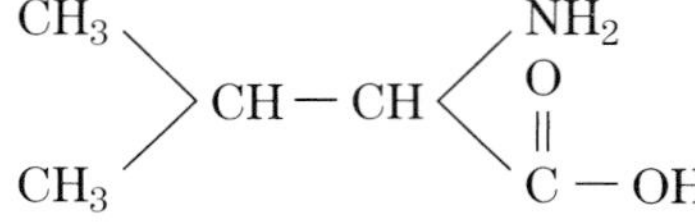

Valine
(essential)

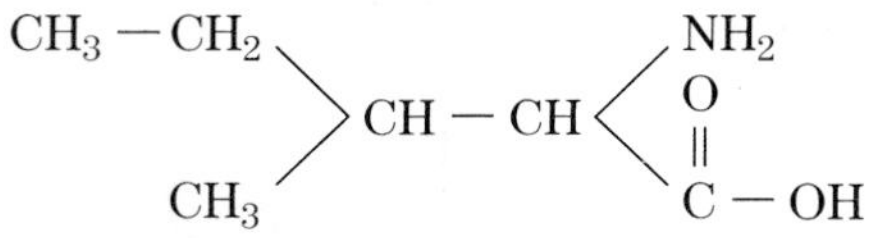

$CH_3 - CH_2$ ⟩ $CH - CH$ ⟨ NH_2 / O ‖ C — OH
CH_3

Isoleucine
(essential)

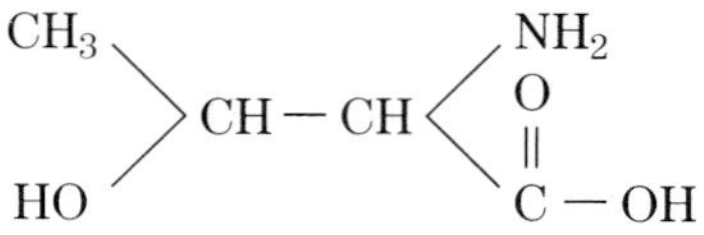

CH_3 ⟩ $CH - CH$ ⟨ NH_2 / O ‖ C — OH
HO

Threonine
(essential)

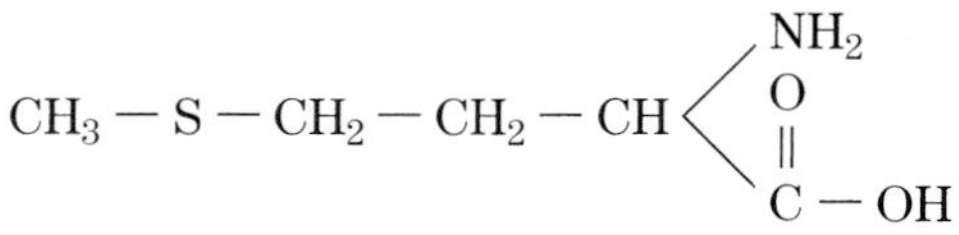

NH_2
$CH_3 - S - CH_2 - CH_2 - CH$ ⟨ O ‖ C — OH

Methionine
(essential)

NH_2
$HS - CH_2 - CH$ ⟨ O ‖ C — OH

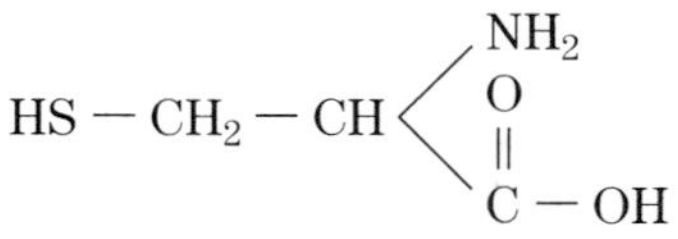

Cysteine

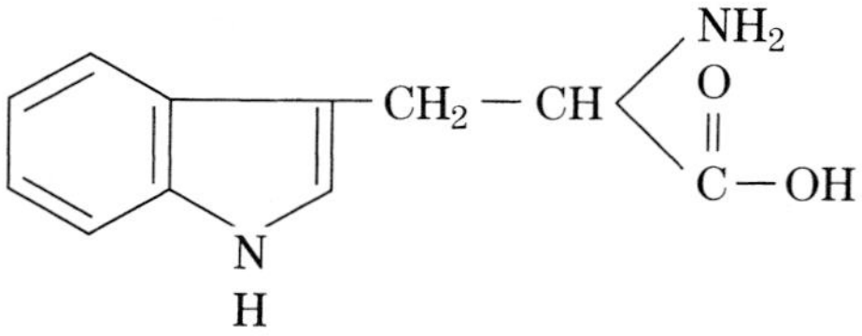

Tryptophan
(essential)

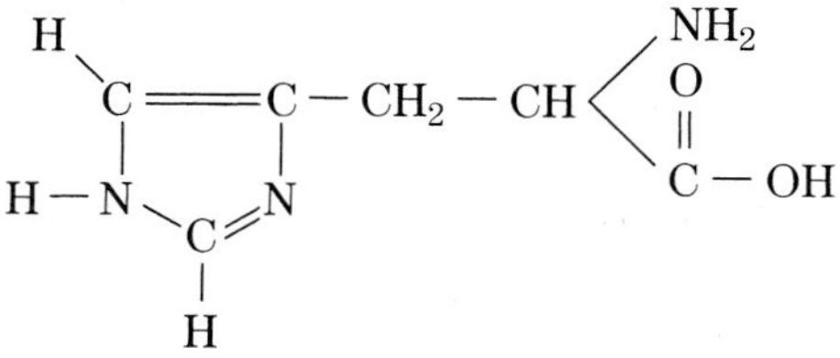

Histidine
(essential)

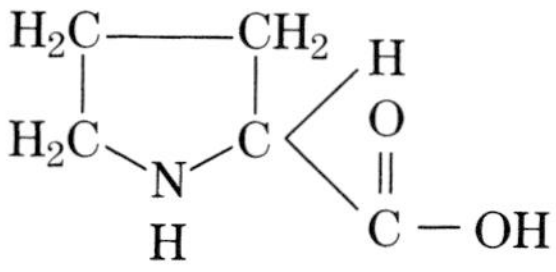

Proline

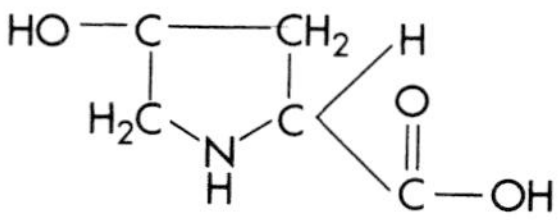

Hydroxyproline

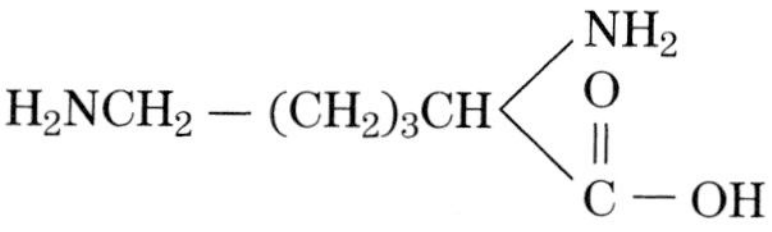

Lysine
(essential)

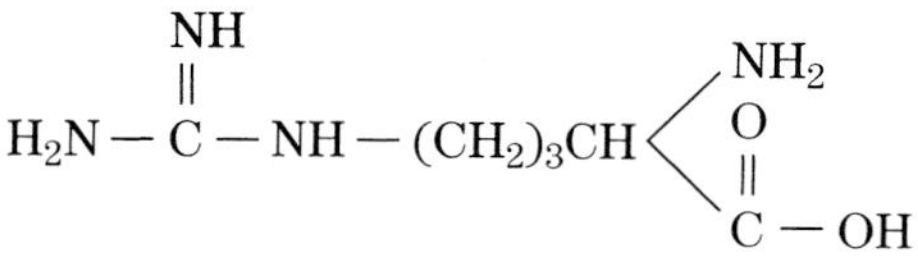

Arginine
(essential)

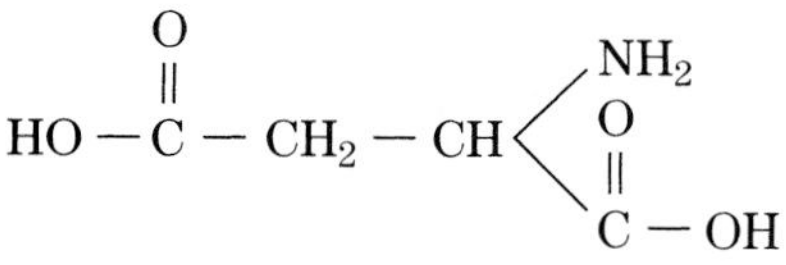

Aspartic Acid

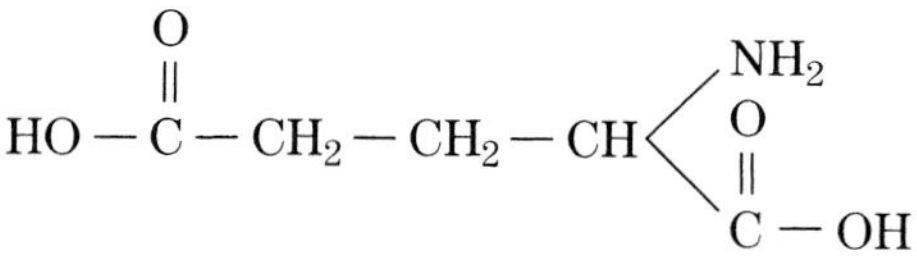

Glutamic acid

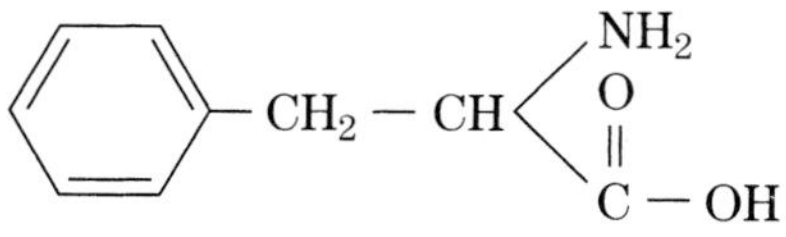

Phenylalanine
(essential)

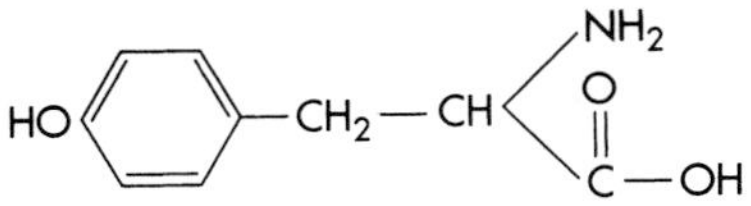

Tyrosine

Vitamins

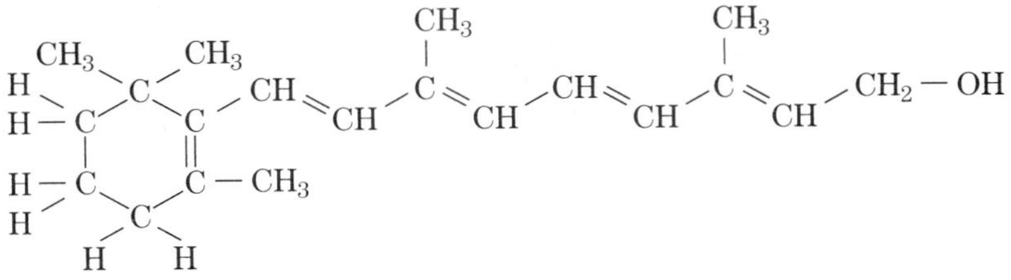

Vitamin A: retinol

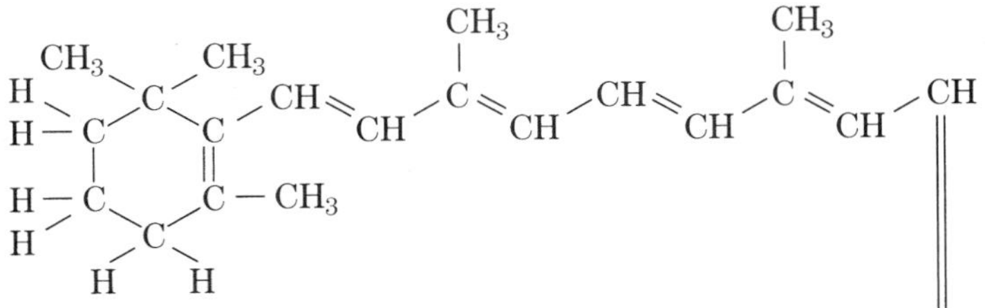

Beta-carotene

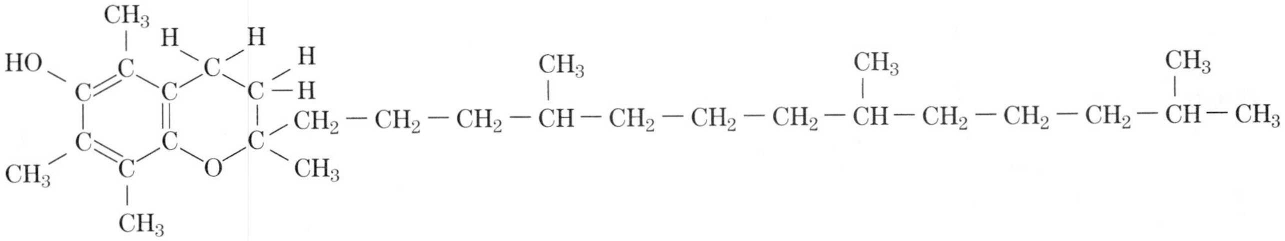

Vitamin E

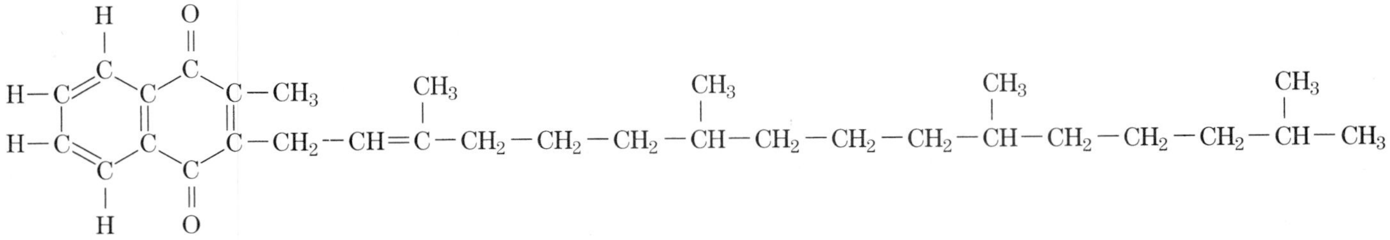

Vitamin K

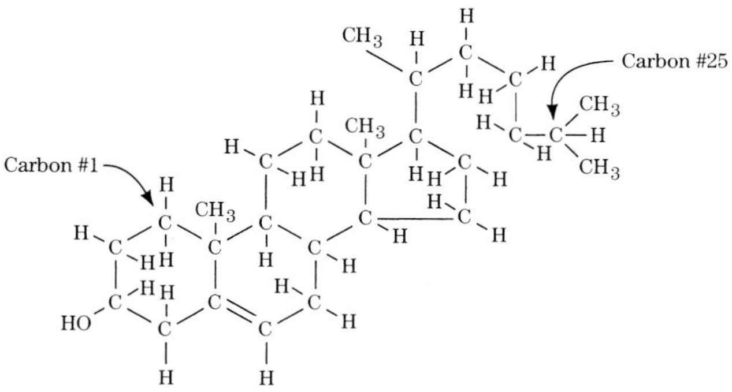

Carbon #1

Carbon #25

7-dehydrocholesterol

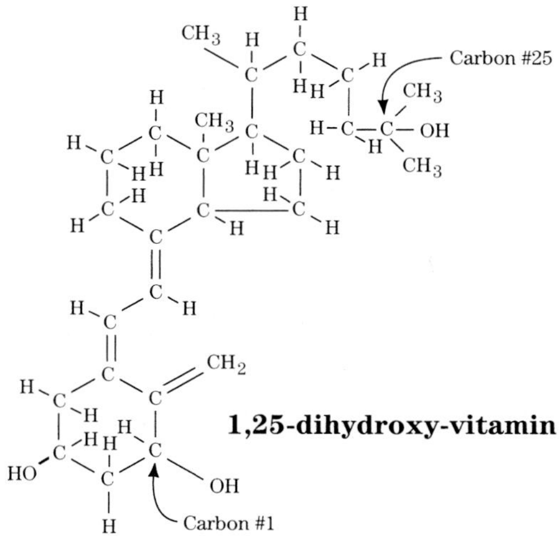

Carbon #25

Carbon #1

1,25-dihydroxy-vitamin D_3 (calcitriol)

Active vitamin D (calcitriol) and its precursor 7-dehydrocholesterol

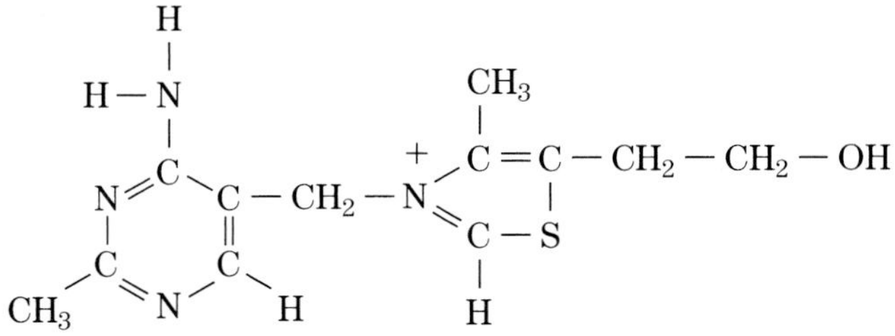

Thiamin

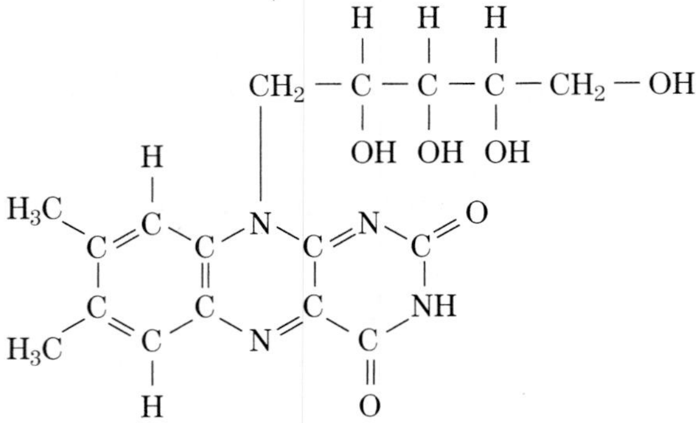

Riboflavin

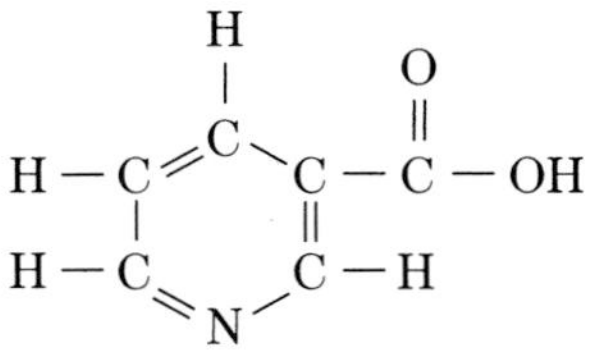

Nicotinic acid

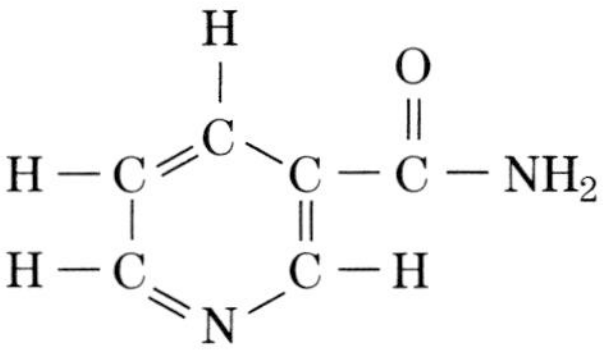

Nicotinamide

Niacin (nicotinic acid and nicotinamide)

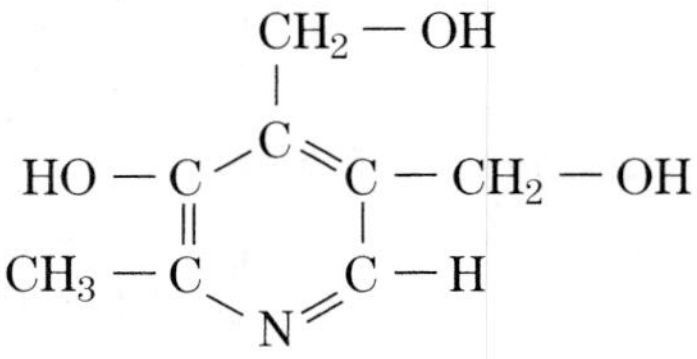

Pyridoxine

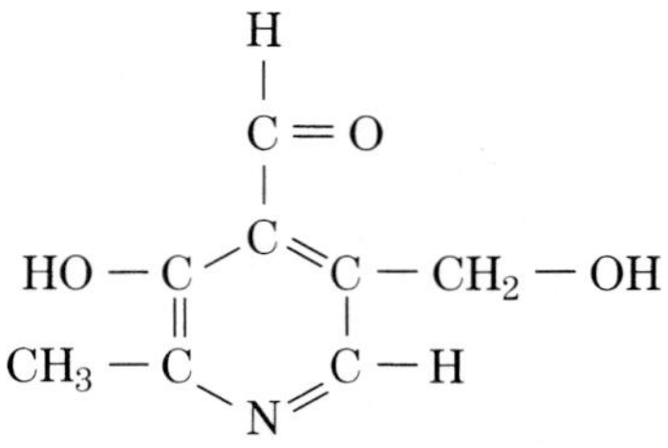

Pyridoxal

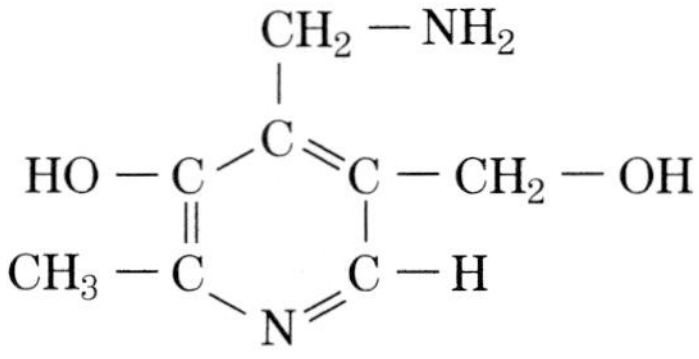

Pyridoxamine

Vitamin B-6 (a general name for three compounds—pyridoxine, pyridoxal, and pyridoxamine).

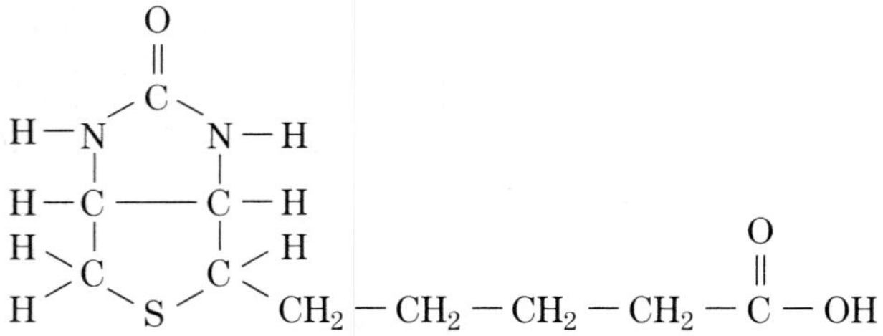

Biotin

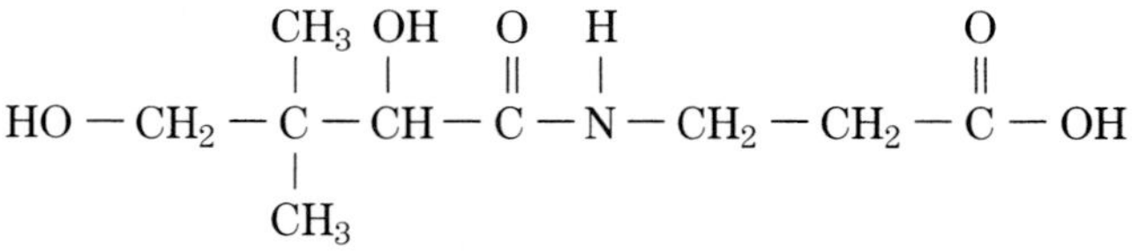

Pantothenic acid

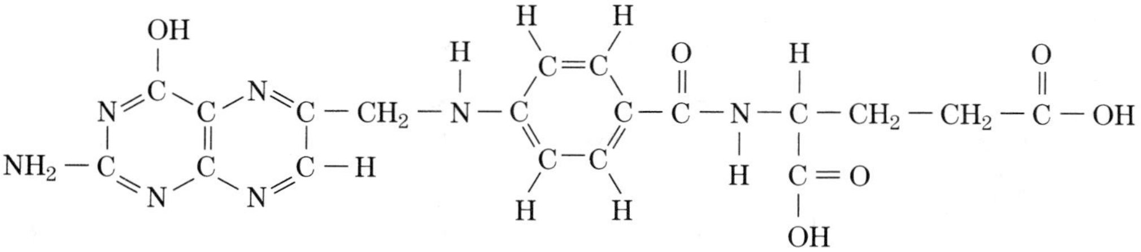

Folate (folacin or folic acid)

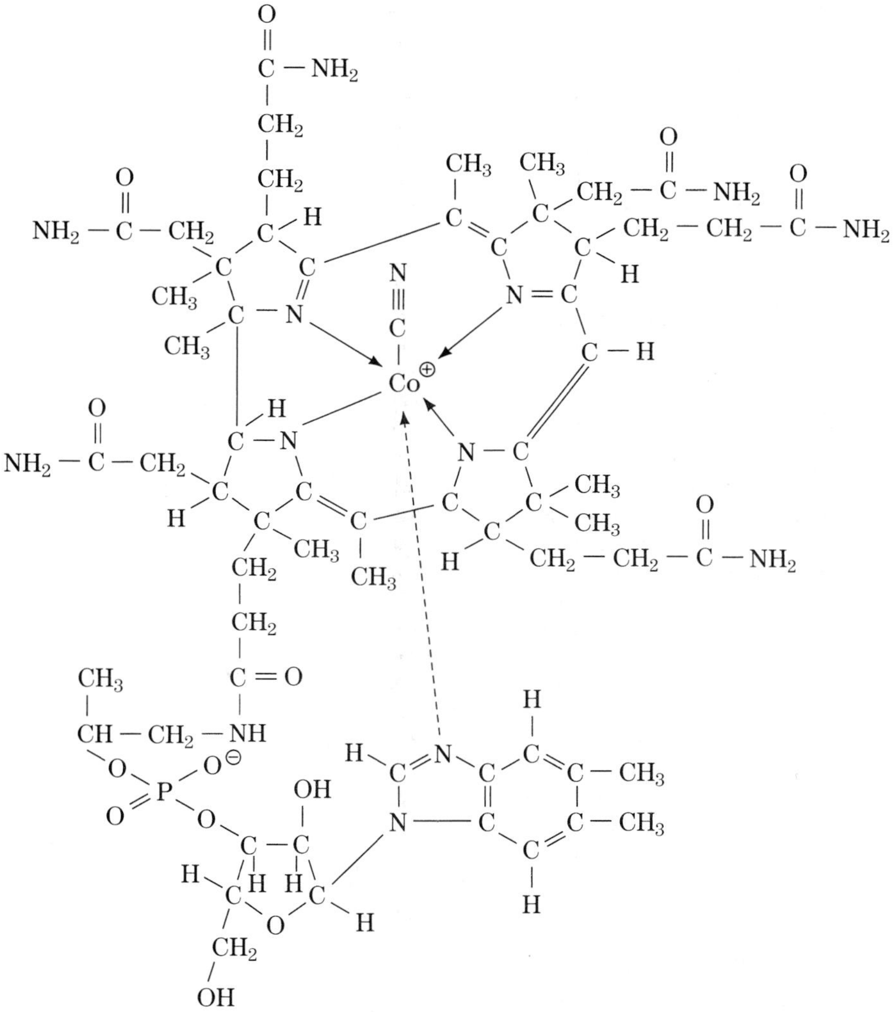

Vitamin B-12 (cyanocobalamin). The arrows in this diagram indicate that the spare electrons on the nitrogens attract them to the cobalt atom.

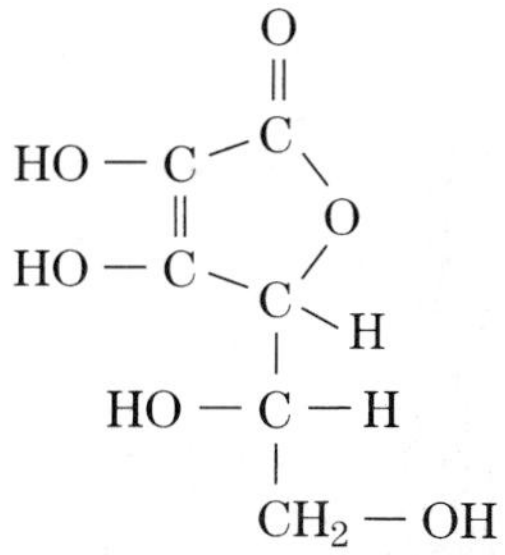

Vitamin C

Vitamin C (ascorbic acid)

Ketone Bodies

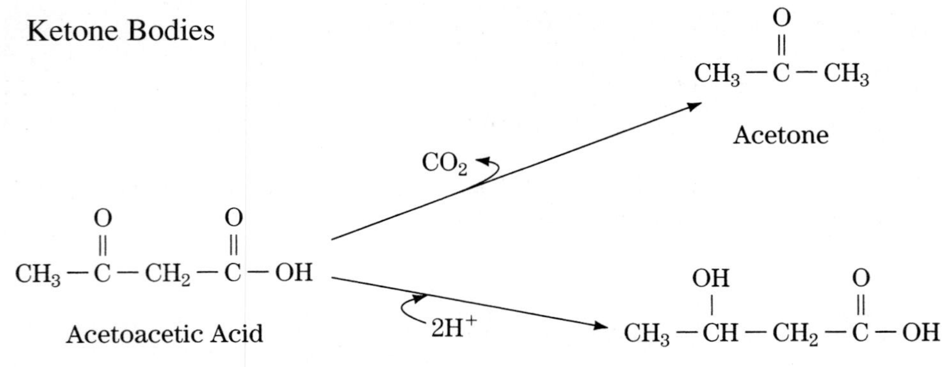

Adenosine Triphosphate (ATP)

Point of cleavage to yield ADP and energy release

Triphosphate

Adenine

Ribose (a sugar)

Appendix H

The 1983 Metropolitan Life Insurance Company Height-Weight Tables and Determination of Frame Size

1983 Metropolitan Life Insurance Company Height-Weight Table*†

Height		WOMEN Frame*			Height		MEN Frame*		
Ft	In.	Small	Medium	Large	Ft	In.	Small	Medium	Large
4	10	102–111	109–121	118–131	5	2	128–134	131–141	138–150
4	11	103–113	111–123	120–134	5	3	130–136	133–143	140–153
5	0	104–115	113–126	122–137	5	4	132–138	135–145	142–156
5	1	106–118	115–129	125–140	5	5	134–140	137–148	144–160
5	2	108–121	118–132	128–143	5	6	136–142	139–151	146–164
5	3	111–124	121–135	131–147	5	7	138–145	142–154	149–168
5	4	114–127	124–138	134–151	5	8	140–148	145–157	152–172
5	5	117–130	127–141	137–155	5	9	142–151	148–160	155–176
5	6	120–133	130–144	140–159	5	10	144–154	151–163	158–180
5	7	123–136	133–147	143–163	5	11	146–157	154–166	161–184
5	8	126–139	136–150	146–167	6	0	149–160	157–170	164–188
5	9	129–142	139–153	149–170	6	1	152–164	160–174	168–192
5	10	132–145	142–156	152–173	6	2	155–168	164–178	172–197
5	11	135–148	145–159	155–176	6	3	158–172	167–182	176–202
6	0	138–151	148–162	158–179	6	4	162–176	171–187	181–207

*Based on a weight-height mortality study conducted by the Society of Actuaries and the Association of Life Insurance Medical Directors of America, Metropolitan Life Insurance Medical Directors of America, Metropolitan Life Insurance Company, revised 1983.
†Weights at ages 25 to 59 based on lowest mortality. Height includes 1-in. heel. Weight for women includes 3 lb for indoor clothing. Weight for men includes 5 lb for indoor clothing.
Reprinted courtesy of Metropolitan Life Insurance Company, *Statistical Bulletin.*
Permission granted courtesy of Metropolitan Life Insurance Company, *Statistical Bulletin.*

Using the Metropolitan Life Insurance Table to Estimate Healthy Weight

The Metropolitan Life Insurance Table is a common method for estimating healthy weight. The table lists for any height the weight that is associated with a maximum life span. The table does not tell the healthiest weight for a living person; it simply lists the weight associated with longevity.

There are many criticisms of this table. These stem from the inclusion of some people and the exclusion of others. For example, only policyholders of life insurance are included. In addition, smokers are included, but anyone over the age of 60 is excluded. Weight is only measured at the time of purchase, and there is no follow-up. All of these factors contribute to the fact that this table is to be used only as a rough screening tool; not meeting the exact recommendations should not be cause for alarm.

To diagnose overweight or obesity using the table, calculate the percentage of the Metropolitan Life Insurance Table weight. Use the midpoint of a weight range for a specific height.

$$\frac{\text{(Current wt. − wt. from table)}}{\text{Weight from table}} \times 100$$

Example:

$$\frac{140 - 120}{120} \times 100 = \text{17\% over standard}$$

Overweight can be defined as weighing at least 10% more than the weight listed on the table. Obesity weighs in at 20% more than that listed on the table. Moreover, this measure of obesity comes in degrees. Whereas mild obesity carries little risk, severe obesity raises overall risk twelvefold.

Degrees of obesity

% Over healthy body weight	Form of obesity
20%–40%	MILD
41%–99%	MODERATE
100%+	SEVERE

Determination of Frame Size

Method 1

Height is recorded without shoes.

Wrist circumference is measured just beyond the bony (styloid) process at the wrist joint on the right arm, using a tape measure.

The following formula is used:

$$r = \frac{\text{height (cm)}}{\text{wrist circumference (cm)}}$$

Frame size can be determined as follows:

Males	Females
$r > 10.4$ small	$r > 11$ small
$r = 9.6–10.4$ medium	$r = 10.1–11$ medium
$r < 9.6$ large	$r < 10.1$ large

*From Grant JP: *Handbook of total parenteral nutrition.* Philadelphia: WB Saunders, 1980.

Method 2

The patient's right arm is extended forward perpendicular to the body, with the arm bent so the angle at the elbow forms 90 degrees, with the fingers pointing up and the palm turned away from the body. The greatest breadth across the elbow joint is measured with a sliding caliper along the axis of the upper arm, on the two prominent bones on either side of the elbow. This is recorded as the elbow breadth. The following tables give elbow breadth measurements for medium-framed men and women of various heights. Measurements lower than those listed indicate a small frame size; higher measurements indicate a large frame size.

Men

Height in 1″ heels	Elbow breadth
5′2″–5′3″	2½–2⅞″
5′4″–5′7″	2⅝–2⅞″
5′8″–5′11″	2¾–3″
6′0″–6′3″	2¾–3¼″
6′4″ and over	2⅞–3¼″

Women

Height in 1″ heels	Elbow breadth
4′10″–4′11″	2¼–2½″
5′0″–5′3″	2¼–2½″
5′4″–5′7″	2⅜–2⅝″
5′8″–5′11″	2⅜–2⅝″
6′0″ and over	2½–2¾″

*From Metropolitan Life Insurance Co., 1983.

Appendix I

Caffeine Content of Foods

BEVERAGES	mg
Carbonated beverages*	
Cherry Coke, Coca-Cola—12 fl oz (370 g)	46
cherry cola, Slice—12 fl oz (360 g)	48
Cherry RC—12 fl oz (360 g)	12
Coca-Cola—12 fl oz (370 g)	46
Coca-Cola Classic—12 fl oz (369 g)	46
Cola, RC—12 fl oz (360 g)	18
Mello Yello—12 fl oz (372 g)	52
Mr. Pibb—12 fl oz (369 g)	40
Mountain Dew—12 fl oz (360 g)	54
Dr. Pepper-type soda—12 fl oz (368 g)	41
Pepsi Cola—12 fl oz (360 g)	38
Carbonated beverages, low calorie*	
Diet Cherry Coke, Coca-Cola—12 fl oz (354 g)	46
Diet cherry cola, Slice—12 fl oz (360 g)	41
Diet Coke, Coca-Cola—12 fl oz (354 g)	46
Diet cola, aspartame-sweetened—12 fl oz (355 g)	50
Diet Pepsi—12 fl oz (360 g)	36
Diet RC—12 fl oz (360 g)	48
Coffee	
Brewed—6 fl oz (177 g)	103
Instant powder—1 tsp (1.8 g)	57
Decaffeinated—1 rounded tsp (1.8 g)	2
With chicory—1 tsp (1.8 g)	37
Prepared from instant powder—6 fl oz & 1 tsp powder (179 g)	57
Amaretto, General Foods—6 fl oz & 11.5 g powder (189 g)	60
Amaretto, sugar-free, General Foods—6 fl oz water & 7.7 g powder (185 g)	60

Abbreviations: g = grams, mg = milligrams.
*Caffeine-free carbonated beverages and most noncarbonated beverages contain no caffeine.

Data from Pennington JAT, *Bowes and Church's Food Values of Portions Commonly Consumed,* ed. 17, 1998, JB Lippincott. Reprinted with permission.

Continued

Coffee cont'd	
Decaffeinated—6 fl oz water & 1 tsp powder (179 g)	2
Francais, General Foods—6 fl oz water & 11.5 g powder (189 g)	53
Francais, sugar-free, General Foods—6 fl oz water & 7.7 g powder (185 g)	59
Irish creme, General Foods—6 fl oz water & 12.8 g powder (190 g)	53
Irish creme, sugar free, General Foods—6 fl oz water & 7.1 g powder (185 g)	48
Irish mocha mint, General Foods—6 fl oz water & 11.5 g powder (189 g)	27
Irish mocha mint, sugar-free, General Foods—6 fl oz water & 6.4 g powder (189 g)	25
Orange cappuccino, General Foods—6 fl oz water & 14 g powder (191 g)	73
Orange cappuccino, sugar-free, General Foods—6 fl oz water & 6.7 g powder (184 g)	71
Suisse mocha, General Foods—6 fl oz water & 11.5 g powder (189 g)	41
Suisse mocha, sugar-free, General Foods—6 fl oz water & 6.4 g powder (184 g)	40
Vienna, General Foods—6 fl oz water & 14 g powder (191 g)	56
Vienna, sugar-free, General Foods—6 fl oz water & 6.7 g powder (184 g)	55
with chicory—6 fl oz water & 1 tsp powder (179 g)	38
Tea, hot/iced	
Brewed 3 min—6 fl oz water (178 g)	36
Instant powder—1 tsp (0.7 g)	31
With lemon flavor—1 rounded tsp (1.4 g)	25
With sugar & lemon flavor—3 tsp (23 g)	29
With sodium saccharin & lemon flavor—2 tsp (1.6 g)	36
Prepared from instant powder	
1 tsp powder in 8 fl oz water (237 g)	31
Crystal Light—8 fl oz (238 g)	11
With lemon flavor—1 tsp powder in 8 fl oz water (238 g)	26
With sugar & lemon flavor—3 tsp powder in 8 fl oz water (259 g)	29
With sodium, saccharin & lemon flavor—2 tsp powder in 8 fl oz water (238 g)	36
CANDY	
Chocolate	
German sweet, Bakers—1 oz square (28 g)	8
Semi-sweet, Bakers—1 oz square (28 g)	13
Chocolate chips	
Bakers—1⁄4 cup (43 g)	12
German sweet, Bakers—¼ cup (43 g)	15
Semi-sweet, Bakers—¼ cup (43 g)	14
DESSERTS	
Frozen desserts	
Pudding pops, Jell-O	
Chocolate—1 pop (47 g)	2
Chocolate caramel swirl—1 pop (47 g)	1
Chocolate fudge—1 pop (47 g)	3
Chocolate vanilla swirl—1 pop (47 g)	2
Chocolate with chocolate coating—1 pop (49 g)	3
Double chocolate swir1 pop (47 g)	2
Milk chocolate—1 pop (47 g)	2

Pies	
Chocolate mousse, from mix, Jell-O—⅛ pie (95 g)	6
Puddings, from instant mix	
Chocolate	
Jell-O—½ cup (150 g)	5
sugar-free, D-Zerta—½ cup (130 g)	4
sugar-free, Jell-O—½ cup (133 g)	4
Chocolate fudge	
Jell-O—½ cup (150 g)	8
Chocolate fudge mousse, Jell-O—½ cup (86 g)	12
Chocolate mousse, Jell-O—½ cup (86 g)	9
Chocolate tapioca, Jell-O—½ cup (147 g)	8
Milk chocolate, Jell-O—½ cup (150 g)	5
MILK BEVERAGES	
Chocolate flavor mix in whole milk—2–3 tsp powder in 8 fl oz milk (266 g)	8
Chocolate malted milk flavor powder	
In whole milk—3 tsp powder in 8 fl oz milk (265 g)	8
With added nutrients in whole milk—4–5 tsp powder in 8 fl oz milk (265 g)	5
Chocolate syrup in whole milk—2 tbsp syrup in 8 fl oz milk (282 g)	6
Cocoa/hot chocolate, prepared with water from mix—3–4 tsp powder in 6 fl oz water (206 g)	4
Milk beverage mixes	
Chocolate flavor mix, powder—2–3 tsp (22 g)	8
Chocolate malted milk flavor mix, powder—¾ oz (3 tsp) (21 g)	8
Chocolate malted milk flavor mix with added nutrients, powder—¾ oz (4–5 tsp) (21 g)	6
Chocolate syrup—2 tbsp (1 fl oz) (38 g)	5
Cocoa mix powder—1 oz pkt (3–4 tsp) (28 g)	5
MISCELLANEOUS	
Baking chocolate, unsweetened, Bakers—1 oz (28 g)	25

Appendix J

Sources of Nutrition Information

Consider the following reliable sources of food and nutrition information:

Journals that regularly cover nutrition topics

American Family Physician*
American Journal of Clinical Nutrition http://www.faseb.org/ajcn
American Journal of Epidemiology
American Journal of Medicine
American Journal of Nursing
American Journal of Obstetrics and Gynecology
American Journal of Physiology
American Journal of Public Health
American Scientist
Annals of Internal Medicine
Annual Reviews of Medicine
Annual Reviews of Nutrition
Archives of Disease in Childhood
Archives of Internal Medicine
British Journal of Nutrition
BMJ (British Medical Journal)
Cancer
Cancer Research
Circulation
Diabetes
Diabetes Care
Disease-a-Month
FASEB Journal
FDA Consumer* http://www.fda.gov
Food Chemical Toxicology
Food Engineering
Gastroenterology
Geriatrics
Gut
Human Nutrition: Applied Nutrition
Human Nutrition: Clinical Nutrition
Journal of the American College of Nutrition*
Journal of The American Dietetic Association* http://www.eatright.org
Journal of The American Geriatric Society
JAMA (Journal of the American Medical Association) http://www.ama-assn.org
Journal of Applied Physiology
Journal of Canadian Dietetic Association*
Journal of Clinical Investigation
Journal of Food Service
Journal of Food Technology
JNCI (Journal of the National Cancer Institute)
Journal of Nutrition
Journal of Nutritional Education*
Journal of Nutrition for the Elderly
Journal of Nutrition Research
Journal of Pediatrics
Lancet
Mayo Clinic Proceedings http://www.mayohealth.org
Medicine and Science in Sports and Exercise
Nature
New England Journal of Medicine http://www.nejm.org
Nutrition
Nutrition Reviews
Nutrition Today*
Pediatrics
The Physician and Sports Medicine http://www.physsportsmed.com/
Postgraduate Medicine*
Proceedings of the Nutrition Society
Science
Science News*
Scientific American*

The majority of these journals are available in college or university libraries or in a specialty library on campus, such as one designated for health services or home economics. As indicated, a few journals will be filed under their abbreviations, rather than the first word in their full name. A reference librarian can help you locate any of these sources. The asterisked (*) journals are ones you may find especially interesting and useful because of the number of nutrition articles presented each month or the less technical nature of the presentation.

Magazines for the consumer that cover nutrition topics

American Health for Women
Better Homes and Gardens
Good Housekeeping
Health
Parents
Self

Textbooks and other sources for advanced study of nutrition topics

Brody T: *Nutritional biochemistry,* San Diego, 1994, Academic Press.
Food and Nutrition Board: *Recommended dietary allowances.,* 10th ed., Washington, D.C., 1989, National Academy of Sciences.
Groff JL, Gropper SS, Hunt SM: *Advanced human nutrition and metabolism,* St. Paul, MN, 1995, West.
International Life Sciences Institute: *Present knowledge in nutrition,* 7th ed., 1996, The Nutrition Foundation.
Mahan LK, Escott-Stump: *Krause's food, nutrition, and diet therapy,* Philadelphia, 1996, WB Saunders.
Murray RK and others: *Harper's biochemistry,* 24th ed., Norwalk, CT, 1996, Appleton & Lange.
Schils ME, Olson JA, Shike M, Ross AC: *Modern nutrition in health and disease,* 9th ed., Philadelphia, 1999, Lea & Febiger.

Newsletters that cover nutrition issues on a regular basis

American Institute for Cancer Research
(AICR) Washington, DC 20069
http://www.icr.ac.uk/

CNI Nutrition Week
Community Nutrition Institute
910 17th St. N.W., Suite 413
Washington, DC 20006

Dairy Council Digest
National Dairy Council
10255 West Higgins Road, Suite 900
Rosemont, IL 60018
(inexpensive)
http://www.national/dairycouncil.com/

Dietetic Currents
Ross Laboratories
Director of Professional Services
625 Cleveland Ave.
Columbus, OH 43216
(free)

Egg Nutrition Center
1819 H St. N.W., No. 510
Washington, DC 20009
(free)
http://www.enc-online.org/

Environmental Nutrition
52 Riverside Dr.
New York, NY 10024

Food and Nutrition News
National Cattlemen's Beef Association
444 Michigan Ave.
Chicago, IL 60611
(free)

Harvard Medical School Health Letter
Department of Continuing Education
25 Shattuck St.
Boston, MA 02115
http://www.hms.harvard.edu/news/index.html

Mayo Clinic Health Letter
P.O. Box 53889
Boulder, CO 80322-3889
http://mayohealth.org

National Council Against Health Fraud Newsletter (NCAHF)
P.O. Box 1276
Loma Linda, CA 92354
http://www.ncahf.org/

Nutrition Action Healthletter
1875 Connecticut Ave.
Washington, DC 20009-5728
http://www.cspinet.org

Nutrition Forum
George Stickley Co.
210 Washington Square
Philadelphia, PA 19106
http://www.quackwatch.com

Nutrition & the M.D.
Raven Press
1185 Avenue of the Americas
New York, NY 10036

Nutrition Research Newsletter
P.O. Box 700
Pallisades, NY 10964

Tufts University Diet & Nutrition Letter
P.O. Box 10948
Des Moines, IA 50940
http://www.healthletter.tufts.edu/

University of California at Berkeley
Wellness Letter
P.O. Box 420148
Palm Coast, FL 32142
http://magazines.enews.com/magazines/vcbw

Soy Connection
United Soybean Board
16305 Swingley Ridge Drive
Suite 110
Chesterfield, MO 63017
(free)
http://smartsoy.ag.uiuc.edu/~usb/speced.html/

Professional organizations with a commitment to nutrition issues

American Academy of Pediatrics
P.O. Box 1034
Evanston, IL 60204
http://www.aap.org

American Cancer Society
90 Park Ave.
New York, NY 10016
http://www.cancer.org

American College of Sports Medicine
P.O. Box 1440
Indianapolis, IN 46204
http://www.acsm.org/

American Dental Association
211 E. Chicago Ave.
Chicago, IL 60611
http://www.ada.org

American Diabetes Association
2 Park Ave.
New York, NY 10016
http://www.diabetes.org

American Dietetic Association
216 W. Jackson Blvd.
Suite 800
Chicago, IL 60606
http://www.eatright.org

American Geriatrics Society
770 Lexington Ave.
Suite 400
New York, NY 10021
http://www.americangeriatrics.org

American Heart Association
7272 Greenville Ave.
Dallas, TX 75231
http://www.amhrt.org

American Home Economics Association
2010 Massachusetts Ave. N.W.
Washington, DC 20036

American Society for Nutritional Sciences
9650 Rockville Pike
Bethesda, MD 20014
http://www.faseb.org/asns

American Medical Association
Nutrition Information Section
535 N. Dearborn St.
Chicago, IL 60610
http://www.ama-assn org/

American Public Health Association
1015 Fifteenth St. N.W.
Washington, DC 20005
http://www.apha.org

American Society for Clinical Nutrition
9650 Rockville Pike
Bethesda, MD 20014
http://www.faseb.org/ajcn

The Canadian Diabetes Association
15 Toronto St.
Suite 1001
Toronto, Ontario M5C 2E3 Canada
http://www.diabetes.ca

The Canadian Dietetic Association
480 University Ave.
Suite 601
Toronto, Ontario M5G 1V2 Canada

The Canadian Society for Nutritional Sciences
Department of Foods and Nutrition
University of Manitoba
Winnipeg, Manitoba, R3T 2N2 Canada

Food and Nutrition Board
National Research Council
National Academy of Sciences
2101 Constitution Ave. N.W.
Washington, DC 20418
http://www.nas.edu/fnb/

Institute of Food Technologies
221 N. LaSalle St.
Chicago, IL 60601
http://www.ift.org

National Council on the Aging
1828 L St. N.W.
Washington, DC 20036

National Institute of Nutrition
1335 Carling Ave.
Suite 210
Ottawa, Ontario K1Z OL2 Canada
http://www.nines.com

National Osteoporosis Foundation
1150 Seventeenth St. N.W., Suite 500
Washington, DC 20036
http://www.nof.org

Nutrition Foundation, Inc.
1126 Sixteenth St. N.W.
Suite 111
Washington, DC 20036

Nutrition Today Society
428 E. Preston St.
Baltimore, MD 21202

Society for Nutrition Education
2001 Killebrew Dr., Suite 340
Minneapolis, MN 55425

Professional or lay organizations concerned with nutrition issues

Bread for the World Institute
1100 Wayne Ave.
Silver Springs, MD 20910
http://www.bread.org

California Council Against Health Fraude, Inc.
P.O. Box 1276
Loma Linda, CA 92354
http://www.ncahf.org

Children's Foundation
1420 New York Ave. N.W.
Suite 800
Washington, DC 20005
http://www.chiildrenfoundation.com

Food Research and Action Center (FRAC)
1875 Connecticut Ave. N.W. #540
Washington, DC 20009
http://www.iglou.com/why/resource/1100.htm

Institute for Food and Development Policy
1885 Mission St.
San Francisco, CA 94103

La Leche League International, Inc.
9616 Minneapolis Ave.
Franklin Park, IL 60131
http://www.lalecheleague.org

March of Dimes Birth Defects Foundation
(National Headquarters)
1275 Mamaroneck Ave.
White Plains, NY 10605
http://www.modimes.org

Overeaters Anonymous (OA)
2190 190th St.
Torrance, CA 90504
http://www.overeatersanonymous.org

Oxfam America
115 Broadway
Boston, MA 02116
http://www.oxfamamerica.org

Local resources for advice on nutrition issues

Cooperative extension agents in county extension offices
Dietitians (Contact the state or local Dietetics Association.)
Nutrition faculty affiliated with departments of food and nutrition, home economics, and dietetics
Registered Dietitians (RDs) in city, county, or state agencies

Government agencies that are concerned with nutrition issues or that distribute nutrition information

United States
The Consumer Information Center
Department 609K
Pueblo, CO 81009

Food and Drug Administration (FDA)
5600 Fishers Lane
Rockville, MD 20852
http://www.fda.gov

Food and Nutrition Information and Education Resources Center
National Library of Congress
Beltsville, MD 20705

Human Nutrition Research Division
Agricultural Research Center
Beltsville, MD 20705
http://www.usda.gov

National Center for Health Statistics
3700 East-West
Hyattsville, MD 20782
http://www.cdc.gov/nchswww

National Heart, Lung, and Blood Institute
9000 Rockville Pike, Building 31, Room 4A21
Bethesda, MD 20892
http://www.nhlbi.gov

National Institute on Aging
Information Office
Building 31, Room 5C35
Bethesda, MD 20205
http://www.nih.gov/nia/

Office of Cancer Communications
National Cancer Institute
Building 31, Room 10A18
90 Rockville Pike
Bethesda, MD 20205
http://www.nci.nih.gov

USDA, Agricultural Research Service
6505 Belcrest Rd., Room 344
Hyattsville, MD 20782
http://www.usda.gov

USDA, Food Safety & Inspection Service
Room 1180 South, 14th and Independence Ave. S.W.
Washington, DC 20250
http://www.usda.gov

U.S. Government Printing Office
The Superintendent of Documents
Washington, DC 20402
http://www.printgovt.org

Canada
Department of Community Health
1075 Ste-Foy Rd.
Quebec, Quebec G1S 2M1

Health and Welfare Canada
Canadian Government Publishing Center
Minister of Supply and Services
Ottawa, Ontario K1A 0S9

Home Economics Directorate
880 Portage Ave.
Second Floor
Winnepeg, Manitoba R3G 0P1

Nutrition Programs
446 Jeanne Mance Building
Tunney's Pasture
Ottawa, Ontario K1A 1B4

Nutrition Services
P.O. Box 488
Halifax, Nova Scotia B3J 3R8

Nutrition Services
P.O. Box 6000
Fredericton, New Brunswick E3B 5H1

Public Health Resource Service
15 Overlea Blvd.
Fifth Floor
Toronto, Ontario M4H 1A9

United Nations
Food and Agriculture Organization (FAO)
North American Regional Office
1001 22nd St. N.W.
Washington, DC 20437
or
Via della Terma di Caracella
0100 Rome, Italy
http://.www.fao.org

World Health Organization (WHO)
1211 Geneva 27
Switzerland
http://www.who.org

Trade organizations and companies that distribute nutrition information

American Institute of Baking
P.O. Box 1148
Manhattan, KS 66502
http://www.aibonline.org

American Meat Institute
P.O. Box 3556
Washington, DC 20007
http://www.meatami.org

Beech-Nut Nutrition Corporation
Booth 1414
Checkerboard Square
St. Louis, MO 63164
http://www.beech-nut.com/index.htm

Best Foods
Consumer Service Department
Division of CPC International
International Plaza
Englewood Cliffs, NJ 07632
http://www.bestfoods.com

Campbell Soup Co.
Food Service Products Division
Campbell Plaza
Camden, NJ 08103
http://www.campbellsoups.com

Continental Baking Company
Checkerboard Square
St. Louis, MO 63164

The Dannon Company, Inc.
120 White Plains Rd.
Tarrytown, NY 10591-5536
http://www.dannon.com

Del Monte Foods
One Market Plaza
San Francisco, CA 94105
http://www.delmonte-international.com

Fleischman's Margarines
Standard Brands, Inc.
625 Madison Ave.
New York, NY 10022

General Foods Consumer Center
250 North St.
White Plains, NY 10625

General Mills
P.O. Box 1113
Minneapolis, MN 55440
http://www.generalmills.com

Gerber Products Co.
445 State St.
Fremont, MI 49413
http://www.gerber.com/home1.html

H.J. Heinz
Consumer Relations
P.O. Box 57
Pittsburgh, PA 15230
http://www.heinzbaby.com

Idaho Potato Commission
P.O. Box 1968
Boise, ID 83701

Kellogg Co.
Department of Home Economics Services
Battle Creek, MI 49016
http://www.kellog.com

Kraft General Foods
Three Lakes Dr.
Northfield, IL 60093
http://www.kraftfoods.com

Mead Johnson Nutritionals
2404 Pennsylvania Ave.
Evansville, IN 47721
http://www.meadjohnson.com

National Dairy Council
10255 W. Higgins Rd.
Rosemont, IL 60018-4233
http://wwwnatdairycoun.org

The NutraSweet Kelco Company
1751 Lake Cook Rd.
Deerfield, IL 60015
http://www.nutrasweetkelco.com/default.htm

Pillsbury Co.
1177 Pillsbury Building
608 Second Ave. S.
Minneapolis, MN 55402
www.pillsbury.com

Rice Council
P.O. Box 740123
Houston, TX 77274

Ross Laboratories
Director of Professional Services
625 Cleveland Ave.
Columbus, OH 43216

Sunkist Growers, Inc.
14130 Riverside Dr.
Sherman Oaks, CA 91423
http://www.sunkist.com/index.html

United Fresh Fruit and Vegetables
Association
727 N. Washington St.
Alexandria, VA 22314

Vitamin Nutrition Information Service
(VNIS)
Hoffmann-LaRoche
340 Kingsland Ave.
Nutley, NJ 07110

Appendix K

English-Metric Conversions and Metric Units

Metric-English Conversions

LENGTH **English (USA)**	**= Metric**
inch (in.)	= 2.54 cm, 25.4 mm
foot (ft)	= 0.30 m, 30.48 cm
yard (yd)	= 0.91 m, 91.4 cm
mile (statute) (5280 ft)	= 1.61 km, 1609 m
mile (nautical) (6077 ft, 1.15 statute mi)	= 1.85 km, 1850 m

Metric	**= English (USA)**
millimeter (mm)	= 0.039 in. (thickness of a dime)
centimeter (cm)	= 0.39 in.
meter (m)	= 3.28 ft, 39.37 in.
kilometer (km)	= 0.62 mi, 1091 yd, 3273 ft

WEIGHT **English (USA)**	**= Metric**
grain	= 64.80 mg
ounce (oz)	= 28.35 g
pound (lb)	= 453.60 g, 0.45 kg
ton (short—2000 lb)	= 0.91 metric ton (907 kg)

Metric	**= English (USA)**
milligram (mg)	= 0.002 grain (0.000035 oz)
gram (g)	= 0.04 oz (1/28 of an oz)
kilogram (kg)	= 35.27 oz, 2.20 lb
metric ton (1000 kg)	= 1.10 tons

VOLUME **English (USA)**	**= Metric**
cubic inch	= 16.39 cc
cubic foot	= 0.03 m^3
cubic yard	= 0.765 m^3
ounce	= 0.03 liter (30 ml)*
pint (pt)	= 0.47 liter
quart (qt)	= 0.95 liter
gallon (gal)	= 3.79 liters

Metric	**= English (USA)**
milliliter (ml)	= 0.03 oz
liter (L)	= 2.12 pt
liter	= 1.06 qt
liter	= 0.27 gal

1 liter ÷ 1000 = 1 milliliter or 1 cubic centimeter (10^{-3} liter)
1 liter ÷ 1,000,000 = 1 microliter (10^{-6} liter)
*Note: 1 ml = 1 cc.

Fahrenheit-Celsius Temperature Conversion Scale

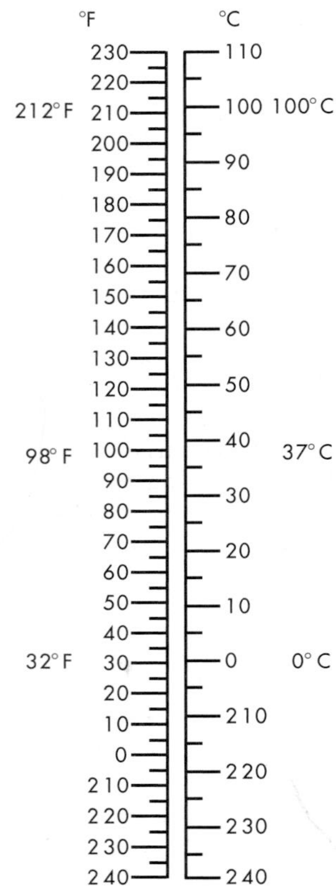

To convert temperature scales:
Fahrenheit to Celsius °C = (°F − 32) × 5/9
Celsius to Fahrenheit °F = 9/5 (°C) + 32

Additional Metric and Other Units Commonly Used in Nutrition

Unit/Abbreviation	Other Equivalent Measure
milligram (mg)	1/1000 of a gram
microgram (μg)	1/1,000,000 of a gram
deciliter (dl)	1/10 of a liter (about ½ cup)
milliliter (ml)	1/1000 of a liter (5 ml is about 1 tsp)
International Unit (IU)	Crude measure of vitamin activity generally based on growth rate seen in animals

Overall, it is important to know what meter, gram, and liter represent, as well as the prefixes micro (1/1,000,000), milli (1/1000), centi (1/100), and kilo (1000).

Answers to Critical Thinking Questions

Chapter 1

1 Flavor and texture are the primary influences on one's diet. Keeping this in mind, it takes deliberate effort to moderate one's intake of sweet, fatty foods. As a college student, Sarah is also influenced by social factors, as well as convenience, economics, and habits. To overcome all of these factors, Sarah will have to set aside time to deliberately plan ways of incorporating more fruit, vegetable, and grain sources.
2 Early man lived only 30 years or so. Today our life expectancy is more than double that. History can give us clues to improve our diets, but only actual studies—such as double-blind research—can establish the actual advantages of any diet.

Chapter 2

1 A diet consisting primarily of foods derived from animal sources contains mostly proteins and fats, with a high percentage of fats as saturated fats. Saturated fats reduce cholesterol clearance by the liver. High blood cholesterol increases the risk for heart disease. A diet high in fat is also related to increased risk of colon, breast, and prostate cancer. Fruits and vegetables are rich in dietary fiber, which helps decrease blood cholesterol and increase the passage of wastes in the gastrointestinal tract. Fruits and vegetables, for the most part, contain low amounts of fats, if any, and are also low in energy, thus helping to maintain healthy body weight.
2 Because the typical American diet consists of many foods high in fat and low in dietary fiber, Devan should assess his diet with respect to these components. He should list all of the foods he eats, preferably for a whole week, and estimate how much fat and dietary fiber he consumes. He then should change his eating habits to obtain recommended amounts of fat and dietary fiber. Most likely, Devan will need to decrease fat intake as well as increase fiber in his diet.

Chapter 3

1 Although taste sensors for sweet, salty, sour, and bitter flavors are located on the tongue, there are sensors associated with the nose that help us taste various flavors. These cells in the nose detect combinations of chemical molecules that, along with the taste sensors on the tongue, allow us to perceive the flavors in our foods. When you have a cold, your nose secretes excess mucus, which prevents the molecules from exciting the sensors. Hence, your sense of taste is inhibited.
2 The small intestine is the most important absorption site in the digestive system because of its large surface area. Because much of the young girl's small intestine was removed, many of the nutrients she consumes are escaping absorption. Only a highly refined (liquid) diet or intravenous therapy is likely to succeed in keeping her adequately nourished.

Chapter 4

1 Diverticulosis is a condition in which tiny pouches form in the wall of the large intestine (colon). When foods are eaten that are not easily digestible, like large pieces of nuts, these may become trapped in the pouches. Bacteria then metabolize these foodstuffs into acids and gases that irritate the diverticula, causing them to swell; this condition is called *diverticulitis.* The acids and gases in the swollen pouches cause cramping and abdominal pain.
2 Foods that remain in the mouth, usually caught between the teeth, are a source of food that bacteria can metabolize. As a by-product of this metabolism, bacteria produce acids that can decay tooth enamel, causing dental caries. Chewing sugarless gum after meals decreases the risk of caries because chewing stimulates the secretion of saliva, which helps to dislodge foods that remain in the mouth. In addition, saliva helps to neutralize the acids produced by the bacteria. Sugar-free gums also contain sugar substitutes which bacteria can't metabolize.

Chapter 5

1 The general term *fats* refers to lipids in foods without reference to their structure. Only dietary fats with a high proportion of saturated fatty acids have been associated with heart disease. In the body, fat (primarily in the form of triglycerides) has many beneficial functions. Triglycerides form the main energy stores in the body and can release fatty acids, which serve as fuel for many cells, such as those in muscles. Stored fat insulates the body and protects vital organs. Absorption of fat-soluble vitamins from the small intestine is aided by dietary fats. In addition, the two essential fatty acids, linoleic acid and alpha-linolenic acid, are not synthesized by the body and must be in the diet to maintain health. Thus some fat is needed in the diet; moderation, not elimination, of intake is the goal.
2 The amount of cholesterol carried in HDL (high-density lipoprotein) also indicates the risk of heart disease. If HDL is greater than 60 milligrams per deciliter, the risk of heart disease is low. If it's less than 35 milligrams per deciliter, the risk is high. The ratio of total serum cholesterol to HDL cholesterol is also a good indicator of one's risk. If the ratio exceeds 4 to 1, the risk is high. Since his total

cholesterol was only slightly elevated and HDL cholesterol was high, the ratio is not elevated. Thus his overall heart disease risk is not increased with regard to these factors.

Chapter 6

1 PKU is the abbreviation for the disease phenylketonuria. The liver of a person with phenylketonuria cannot readily convert phenylalanine, an essential amino acid, to tyrosine. This defect is caused by insufficient enzyme action. Because phenylalanine cannot be sufficiently degraded, tyrosine must be considered an essential amino acid for people with PKU.

The inability to metabolize excess phenylalanine to tyrosine leads to the formation of abnormal products that arise from alternative metabolism; these products can cause mental retardation. Thus determining which infants have PKU is vital, because the phenylalanine content in their diets must be monitored. However, because phenylalanine is an essential amino acid, some must be consumed.

2 Protein synthesis is a complex process by which a specific sequence and number of amino acids determine the structure of a protein. If enough of a given amino acid is not present during protein synthesis, production will stop. In other words, protein is an all-or-none process: all of the amino acids necessary to make the protein must be available, or the protein will not be made at all. A mixed diet of plant products will contain enough of all 9 essential amino acids, so the all-or-none principle won't typically be an issue in diet planning, even in vegetarianism.

Chapter 7

1 People with alcoholism usually have unbalanced diets, which can impair absorption of vitamins and minerals from the GI tract. An associated problem is poor metabolism. The B vitamins are essential for energy metabolism.

Alcohol consumption decreases the absorption of many B vitamins, such as thiamin and folate. These vitamins are important in maintaining proper metabolic and nervous system function.

2 Humans must obtain vitamin C from foods because the body cannot synthesize it. An important function of this vitamin is to promote the formation of connective tissue, bone, skin, and blood vessels. Thus a low intake of vitamin C will impair wound healing. Deficiency can also lead to scurvy, the symptoms of which include bleeding gums and pinpoint hemorrhages on the skin.

Vitamin C is an antioxidant. It works with vitamin E against free radicals and helps "reactivate" vitamin E so that it can continue to function. Vitamin C also deters certain forms of cancer and enhances iron absorption.

In addition, vitamin C is essential for immune system activity. However, vitamin C does not cure the common cold.

Chapter 8

1 Calcium is needed for normal bone growth and development. Bones serve as stores of calcium for the bloodstream. Regulation of blood calcium may necessitate the breakup of bone mineral deposits for the release of calcium from bone. Bone mineralization is maximal before and during adolescence. Manuela is already an adult, but she should still consume calcium in amounts sufficient to decrease bone demineralization.

The best sources of calcium are milk and fish, which Manuela, a vegan, will not eat. She should therefore acquaint herself with alternative sources—vegetables and nuts that contain calcium, such as spinach and almonds, respectively. She should also choose calcium-fortified foods, such as some brands of orange juice. However, if she cannot meet her calcium needs by modifying her diet, based on a nutrient analysis of her current intake, calcium supplements are advised.

2 The mineral selenium aids in the activity of the enzyme that participates in a system that metabolizes peroxides into less toxic alcohol derivatives and water. Peroxides tend to become free radicals, which in turn can attack and break down cell membranes, causing cell damage.

Selenium is important in protecting heart cells and other cells against oxidative damage. In addition, because this enzyme reduces the amount of free-radical damage to cells, selenium helps protect against certain forms of cancer.

Chapter 9

1 Although Hal has seen a steady decrease in his weight for the duration of his diet thus far, his body has built-in mechanisms that tend to fight weight loss. One of those factors is basal metabolism. This tends to decrease to conserve energy as the number of calories in the diet decreases. Also fat uptake by adipose (fat) cells increases. The increase allows the body to take up fats more efficiently from the blood after the dieting has stopped.

Thus, the body resists weight loss by physiological means; however, it may finally "surrender" to persistent dieting, and Hal will continue to lose weight as long as he continues to diet. He may consider increasing physical activity to aid in success.

2 The young woman would be advised to focus first on weight maintenance as she tries to organize the other aspects of her life. Then, possibly in 6 months or so, when she has time to focus on dieting, she can provide enough attention to this goal to make success more likely.

Chapter 10

1 Marty has enhanced his cardiovascular fitness, a laudable goal. In addition, after a period of training, muscle cells worked on a regular basis will make more mitochondria. Because mitochondria are the sites of aerobic metabolism, more ATP can be generated. ATP is a necessary component for muscle contraction, so a greater amount of ATP production allows a greater amount of muscle contraction.

2 Many wrestlers and other athletes lose weight quickly by losing large amounts of body fluid, usually by sweating. By doing so, an athlete can compete in a lower weight class and thus theoretically gain an advantage over an opponent. However, losing weight this way can significantly impede performance. Over time, repeated dehydration episodes can lead to serious complications, such as kidney failure and even death.

Chapter 11

1 Signs that could indicate an eating disorder include the following:

(1) Compulsive behavior patterns

(2) Obsession with being and looking thin
(3) Obsession with counting calories
(4) Anxiety about eating with others (for example, refusing to go to a restaurant)
(5) Continual self-criticism and frequent comparisons of self with others, especially slender people.
(6) Belief that one is fat.

2 One of the most important topics Tom should discuss is proper nutrition. Using the concepts of variety, balance, and moderation, he can teach students about their diets. He should also present case studies of real people who have anorexia nervosa and bulimia nervosa so that his students can better understand the outcome of these diseases. Tom should also focus on increasing the self-esteem of young adults. The prepuberty and teenage years are a time of self-evaluation and criticism. It is important for Tom to help his students feel good about themselves by emphasizing the importance of self-worth—regardless of physical appearance. Finally, Tom can teach his students how to cope with difficult situations by showing them how to alleviate stress in positive and constructive ways.

Chapter 12

1 It is important to assess a woman's nutritional and health status before she begins trying to become pregnant. The dietary habits of the mother-to-be can affect the health of the newborn. Good nutrition is critical during a woman's childbearing years. Nutritional deficiencies have been shown to result in improper fetal development. An adequate vitamin and mineral intake in the months before conception and during the pregnancy, such as with the vitamin folate, can prevent certain fetal defects.

2 As the pregnancy advances, the uterus will continue to grow to accommodate the growing fetus. As the uterus enlarges, it presses against the stomach and intestines. Also, hormones produced in increased amounts during pregnancy relax muscles. This explains why heartburn may occur; the lower esophageal sphincter relaxes allowing some foods and acid to regurgitate back into the esophagus causing heartburn. Ingesting smaller quantities of foods and not reclining after eating are recommended. High amounts of fats also decrease the rate of stomach emptying; therefore decreasing fat in the diet should also help. Because hormones relax muscles, the rate of peristalsis may also decrease and constipation may develop. Gradually increasing the amounts of dietary fiber and fluid in Sandy's diet to improve her digestive system's activity would be wise

Chapter 13

1 Human milk is low in iron. Although it provides the baby with many essential nutrients, it doesn't meet all of a baby's needs after about 6 months, because iron stores are depleted by this time. This iron deficiency can lead to anemia. Tatiana should have started feeding her infant iron-fortified cereal between 4 and 6 months of age to prevent iron-deficiency anemia. In addition, some pediatricians recommend giving iron supplements to breastfed infants, beginning shortly after birth.

2 Typical breakfast foods include cereal, eggs, toast, and pancakes, but any food can be a breakfast, lunch, or dinner food as long as it is nutrient dense. If Tim doesn't like the traditional breakfast foods but enjoys a sandwich, macaroni and cheese, or yogurt, his parents can offer these instead. These foods are no more beneficial at lunch time than they are at 7 AM. The depletion of carbohydrate stores that occurs during the night can cause children to be lethargic and inattentive in the morning. Eating early in the morning replenishes carbohydrate stores. Many experts believe that the nutrients consumed stimulate attention in children, allowing them to perform better in school.

Chapter 14

1 Science has established a considerable link between nutrition (diet) and health. For example, low-fat vegan diets have been shown to reverse atherosclerosis and weight-loss diets improve Type 2 diabetes control in some people by reducing body fat. Although body cells will age no matter what health practices are followed, much of the risk for disease can be decreased through diet and lifestyle. A consistently healthful diet and a regimen of regular physical activity have proved effective in maintaining a healthy body: muscles are firmer, bone fractures are less likely, and the person looks and feels better. Overall, the secret to enjoying "youth" throughout life is to establish a healthy physical, mental, and social framework.

2 Many older people have experienced the death of a lifelong companion. Men and women who have lived with another person for 20, 30, and sometimes over 50 years find the loss of their loved one traumatic. If they have no means to cope with this overwhelming loss, they may become depressed. Depressed people often eat decreased amounts of food, show little interest in meals, and stop eating altogether. In addition, many older people depended on their loved ones for planing, buying, and preparing meals. The surviving partner may feel indifferent or overwhelmed by these tasks.

As the body ages, the senses lose their acuity. People lose some sensors on the tongue and some in the nose. This loss of taste and smell contributes to apathy about eating (consider your appetite when you have a cold and can't smell or taste as well).

Chapter 15

1 John's boss should have emphasized that animal products are a likely source of bacterial contamination in the kitchen. These products should be cut on boards reserved for that task. If that is not possible, any non-animal products should be cut first; the animal products should be cut next. Careful sanitizing of the cutting board is also important after any contact with animal products. Raw fruits and vegetables also should be washed as they can contain bacterial contamination on the outer covering. A final point to make is that any food can support bacterial contamination; thus all foods pose a risk and need to be handled carefully, and not remain at room temperature for more than 1 to 2 hours if perishable.

2 Bacteria thrive at room temperature, especially between 60° and 110°F. Some bacteria causes foodborne illness. Cooling by refrigeration slows down bacterial growth, but it does not stop it or destroy toxins already produced by the bacteria. Foods left at room temperature for 2 hours, or even 1 hour in hot weather, give bacteria the opportunity to grow. Refrigeration after that time is too late. Diana is correct in wanting to discard the food.

Chapter 16

1 Undernourished children (and adults) often show short stature, apathy, muscular weakness, and decreased physical activity and work capability. Because undernutrition decreases resistance to disease, undernourished children are likely to have more frequent infections and recover more slowly from illness than well-fed children.

2 Where extreme food shortages exist, there is no choice but to supply hungry people with food—they are starving and dying. However, reliance on outside help is not a long-range solution. Rather, developing countries need to improve their economies and infrastructures so that people are able to produce or buy sufficient amounts of nutritious food to meet their needs. Appropriate development includes many aspects: education, availability of machinery and other agricultural tools, and alternative employment opportunities. Small farms and businesses should be encouraged. As the economy expands, more people will be able to afford nutritious food. Agricultural production should focus on basic food crops to be consumed by a country's own citizens, rather than primarily on cash crops for export.

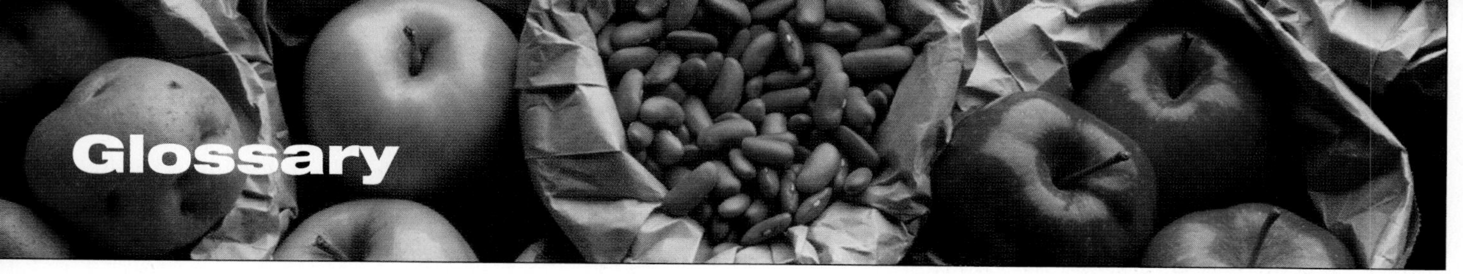

Glossary

Medical Terminology to Aid in the Study of Nutrition

Term Meaning

a- Without, from
acyl A carbon chain
aden-, adeno- Gland
-algia Pain
aliment Food
-amine Containing nitrogen
andr-, andro- Man or male
apo-, ap- Detached
arteri-, arterio- Artery
arthr-, arthro- Joint
-ase Enzyme
-blast Immature form, embryonic
brady- Slow
buli- Ox
canc-, carcino- Malignancy
cardi-, cardio- Heart
centi- Divided into 100 parts
chol-, chole-, cholo- Bile, gall
cholecyst- Gallbladder
chondr-, chondri-, chondro- Cartilage
chrom-, chromo- Color, colored
-clast Something that breaks
col-, coli-, colo- Colon
cyano-, cyan- Blue
cyt-, cyto- Cell
derm-, dermato- Skin
dextr-, dextro- Right, on or toward the right
duoden-, duodeno- Duodenum
dys- Difficult, painful
ect-, ecto- Without, outside, external
-ectomy Excision of
-ein A protein
em- Blood
-emia In blood
encephal-, encephalo- Brain
endo-, ento-, end-, ent- Within
enter-, entero- Intestine
erythr-, erythro- Red
esophag-, esophago- Esophagus
eu- Well, easy, good
gastr-, gastro-, gastri- Stomach
gen- To become or produce
gloss-, glosso- Tongue
glyco-, glyc- Sugar
gynec-, gyn-, gyne- Women or female (especially female reproductive organs)
hem-, hemat- Blood
hepat-, hepato- Liver
hexa-, hex- Six
histo-, hist- Tissue
homeo-, homoeo-, homoio- Sameness, similarity
hydr-, hydro- Water
hyper- Excessive, above, beyond
hypo-, hyp- Under, beneath, deficient
hyster-, hystero- Uterus
idio- One's own, peculiar to, separate, distinct
ile-, ileo- Ileum
inter- Between, among
intra- Within, during, between layers of
-itis Inflammation of
jenun-, jejuno- Jejunum
kilo- One thousand
lact-, lacti-, lacto- Milk
leuc-, leuk- White, colorless
lev-, levo- Left, toward the left
lip-, lipo- Fat, lipid
litho-, lith- Stone
lymph-, lympho- Waterlike
lysis Destruction
mal- Bad, badly
malac-, malaco- Soft, a condition of abnormal softness
mega-, meg- Large, great
meta- After, later; change, exchange
metallo- Containing metal
micro- Divided into 1 million parts
milli- Divided into 1,000 parts
mono- One
morph-, morpho- Form, shape
my-, myo- Muscle
myel-, myelo- Marrow, spinal cord
nas-, naso- Nose, nasal
necr-, necro- Dead
nephr-, nephro- Kidney
neur-, neuro- Nerve
-oid Formed like, resembling
-ol Alcohol
olig-, oligo- Few, scant
-oma Tumor
ophthalmo-, ophthalm- Eye, eyeball
-orex Mouth
-orexis Desire, appetite
-ose Sugar, carbohydrate
-osis Action, process, result, usually abnormal or diseased
ost-, osteo-, oste- Bone
ot- Ear
ovari-, ovario- Ovary
ovo-, ovi- Eggs
pan- All
pancreat-, pancreato- Pancreas
para- Beside
parieto- Wall of a cavity, parietal bone
patho-, path- Disease
ped- Child, foot
-penia Without, lack of
-phobia Fear of
-plasm, -plasma Formative, formed, cell or tissue substance
pneum-, pneumo-, pneumono- Lung
-poiesis Production, format
poly- Many, much
post- After
pre- Before
prot-, proto- First
pseud-, pseudo- False
pulmo-, pulmon-, pulmono- Lung
pyel-, pyelo- Pelvis
pyr- Fever, fire
rect-, recto- Rectum
reni-, reno- Kidney
rhin-, rhino- Nose
-rrhagia Rupture, excessive fluid discharge
-rrhea Flow, discharge
sate To fill
scler-, sclero- Hard, hardness
-scopy Viewing
seb-, sebi-, sebo- Hard fat sebum, sebaceous glands
semi- Half

-soma, somat-, somato- Body
-stasia, -stasis Slowing or stopping of
stenosis Narrowing of
stomat-, stomato- Mouth, stoma
-stomy Surgical opening
sub- Under, below
super- Over, above
tachy- Swift, fast
thi-, thio- Containing sulfur
thromb-, thrombo- Blood clot
tox-, toxi-, toxo- Poison
trache-, tracheo- Trachea
-trophy Growth or mutation
ure-, urea-, ureo- Urine
uter-, utero- Uterus
vas-, vaso- Blood vessel
ven-, veni-, veno- Vein
vita- Life
xer-, xero- Dry

Glossary Terms

absorption The process by which substances are taken up by the GI tract and enter the bloodstream.

absorptive cells A class of cells, also called *enterocytes,* that line the villi; fingerlike projections in the small intestine that participate in nutrient absorption.

acesulfame-K (ay-SUL-fame) An alternate sweetener that yields no energy to the body; it is about 200 times sweeter than sucrose.

acetic acid A two-compound fatty acid that is used in the synthesis of lipids.

acquired immunodeficiency syndrome (AIDS) A disorder in which a virus (human immunodeficiency virus [HIV]) infects one type of immune system cell. This leaves the person with reduced immune function and in turn defenseless against numerous infectious agents; typically contributes to the person's death.

active absorption Absorption using a carrier protein and expending energy. In this way the absorptive cell absorbs nutrients, such as glucose, when a high concentration of the nutrient is already present in the absorptive cells.

adaptive thermogenesis Adaptive energy expended in heat production, such as when subjected to cold environmental conditions or overfeeding

adenosine diphosphate (ADP) A breakdown product of ATP. ADP is synthesized into ATP using energy from foodstuffs and a phosphate group (abbreviated Pi).

adenosine triphosphate (ATP) (ah-DEN-o-sin try-FOS-fate) The main energy currency for cells. ATP energy is used to promote ion pumping, enzyme activity, and muscular contraction.

adequate intake (AI) Recommendations for nutrient intake when not enough information is available to establish an RDA. AIs are based on observed or experimentally determined estimates of the average nutrient intake that appears to maintain a defined nutritional state (e.g., bone health) in a specific population.

adipose tissue (ADD-ih-pos) A group of fat-storing cells.

aerobic (air-ROW-bic) Requiring oxygen.

alcohol Refers to ethyl alcohol or ethanol, CH_3CH_2OH; yields 7 kcal per gram.

aldosterone (al-DOS-ter-own) A powerful hormone produced by the adrenal glands that acts on the kidneys to cause sodium reabsorption and, in turn, water conservation.

allergen A foreign protein, or antigen, that induces excess production of certain immune system antibodies; subsequent exposure to the same protein leads to allergic symptoms. While all allergens are antigens, not all antigens are allergens.

allergy A hypersensitive immune response that occurs when antibodies produced by the body react with a protein foreign to the body (antigen).

alpha-linolenic acid (AL-fah-lin-oh-LE-nik) An essential acid with 18 carbon atoms and 3 double bonds (omega-3).

amenorrhea (A-men-or-ee-a) The absence of three or more consecutive menstrual cycles; the absence of menses in a female.

amino acid (ah-MEE-noh) The building block for proteins containing a central carbon atom with a nitrogen atom and other chemical elements attached.

amniotic fluid (am-nee-OTT-ik) Fluid contained in a sac within the uterus. This fluid surrounds and protects the fetus during development.

amylopectin A branched-chain type of starch composed of glucose units.

amylose (AM-uh-los) A digestible straight-chain polysaccharide made of glucose units; primary component of starch in foods.

anabolic/anabolism (an-AH-bol-iz-um) Building compounds.

anabolic steroids A general term for hormones that stimulate development in male sex organs and such male characteristics as facial hair (for example, testosterone).

anaerobic (AN-ah-ROW-bic) Not requiring oxygen.

analog A chemical compound that differs slightly from another, usually natural, compound. Analogs generally contain extra or altered chemical groups and may have similar or opposite metabolic effects compared with the native compound.

anaphylactic shock (an-ah-fih-LAK-tic) A severe allergic response that results in lowered blood pressure and respiratory and gastrointestinal distress. This can be fatal.

anemia Generally refers to a decreased oxygen-carrying capacity of the blood. This can be caused by many factors.

angiotensin I (an-jee-oh-TEN-sin) An intermediary compound produced during the body's attempt to conserve water and sodium; it is converted in the lungs to angiotensin II.

angiotensin II A compound produced from angiotensin I, which increases blood vessel constriction and triggers production of the hormone aldosterone.

animal model Study of disease in animals that duplicates human disease. This can be used to understand more about human disease.

anorexia nervosa (an-oh-REX-ee-uh ner-VOH-sah) An eating disorder involving a psychological loss of appetite and self-starvation, related in part from a distorted body image and to various social pressures; commonly associated with puberty.

anthropometrry (an-throw-PO-meh-tree) The measurement of weight, lengths, circumferences, and thicknesses of parts of or the whole body.

antibody (AN-tih-bod-ee) Blood proteins that inactivate foreign proteins found in the body. This helps prevent and control infections.

antidiuretic hormone (ADH) (an-tie-dye-u-RET-ik) A hormone secreted by the pituitary gland that acts on the kidney to cause a decrease in water excretion.

antigen (AN-ti-jen) Any substance that induces a state of sensitivity and/or resistance to microbes or toxic substances after a lag period; substance that stimulates a specific aspect of the immune system.

antioxidant Generally a compound that prevents the oxidation of substances in food or the body, particularly lipids. Antioxidants are especially important in preventing the oxidation of polyunsaturated lipids in the membranes of cells. An antioxidant is able to donate electrons to electron-seeking compounds. This in turn reduces electron loss and thus breakdown of unsaturated fatty acids and other cell components by oxidizing agents. Vitamin E is one antioxidant cells use for protection. Some compounds have antioxidant capabilities (i.e., stop oxidation) but are not electron donors per se.

appetite The external (psychological) influences that encourage us to find and eat food, often in the absence of obvious hunger.

arachidonic acid (ar-a-kih-DON-ik) A fatty acid with 20 carbon atoms and four double bonds (omega-6).

aseptic processing (ah-SEP-tik) A method by which food and container are simultaneously sterilized; it allows manufacturers to produce boxes of milk that can be stored at room temperature. Variations of this process are also known as *ultrahigh temperature* (UHT) packaging.

aspartame (AH-spar-tame) An alternate sweetener made of two amino acids and methanol; it is about 200 times sweeter than sucrose.

atherosclerosis (ath-e-roh-scle-ROH-sis) A buildup of fatty material (plaque) in the arteries, including those surrounding the heart.

autoimmune Immune reactions against normal body cells; self against self.

avidin (AV-ih-din) A protein found in raw egg whites that can bind biotin and inhibit its absorption. Avidin is destroyed by cooking.

bacteria A group of single-cell microorganisms, some of which produce poisonous substances called toxins that lead to ill health in humans. They contain only one chromosome and lack many organelles found in human cells. Bacteria produce enzymes that can digest substances around them. Some can live without oxygen and survive harsh conditions by means of spore formation.

baryophobia (bear-ee-oh-FO-bee-ah) A disorder of young children and young adults characterized by stunted growth resulting from underfeeding by caregivers in an attempt to prevent development of obesity and heart disease.

basal metabolism The minimal energy the body requires to support itself when resting and awake. It amounts to roughly 1 kcal/minute, or about 1400 kcal per day.

benign Noncancerous; tumors that do not spread.

beriberi (BEAR-ee-BEAR-ee) Thiamin deficiency disorder characterized by muscle weakness, loss of appetite, nerve degeneration, and sometimes edema.

BHA Butylated hydroxyanisol, a synthetic antioxidant added to food.

BHT Butylated hydroxytoluene, a synthetic antioxidant added to food.

bile A substance made in the liver and stored in the gallbladder; it is released into the small intestine to aid fat absorption by suspending fat into tiny droplets within a watery fluid.

binge-eating disorder An eating disorder characterized by recurrent binge eating and feelings of loss of control over eating that has lasted at least 6 months. Binge episodes can be triggered by frustration, anger, depression, anxiety, permission to eat forbidden foods, and excessive hunger.

bioavailability The degree to which the amount of an ingested nutrient is absorbed and is available to the body.

bioelectrical impedance A method to estimate total body fat that uses a low-energy electrical current. The more fat storage a person has, the more impedance (resistance) to electrical flow will be exhibited.

biotechnology A collection of processes that involve use of advanced scientific techniques to alter and, ideally, improve characteristics of animals, plants, and other forms of life.

bisphosphonates Compounds primarily composed of carbon and phosphorus that bind to bone mineral and in turn reduce bone breakdown.

blood doping A technique by which an athlete's red blood cell count is increased. Blood is taken from the athlete, and the red blood cells are concentrated and then later reinjected into the athlete. An alternate method uses a medication to increase red blood cell production.

body mass index (BMI) Weight (in kilograms) divided by height squared (in meters). A value of 25 or greater indicates a higher risk for obesity-related health disorders.

bomb calorimeter (kal-oh-RIM-eh-ter) An instrument used to determine the energy content of a food.

bond A sharing of electrons, charges, or attractions linking two atoms.

bone mass Total mineral substance (such as calcium or phosphorus) in a cross section of bone, generally expressed as grams per centimeter of length.

bone mineral density Total mineral content of bone at a specific bone site divided by the width of the bone at that site, generally expressed as grams per cubic centimeter.

brown adipose tissue (ADD-ih-pose) A specialized form of adipose tissue that produces large amounts of heat by metabolizing energy-yielding nutrients inefficiently. The energy released mostly just forms heat.

buffer A compound that helps a solution resist changes in acid-base balance. This is generally done by either having the compound take up or release hydrogens.

bulimia nervosa (boo-LEEM-ee-uh) An eating disorder in which large quantities of food are eaten at one time (binge eating) and then purged from the body by vomiting, use of laxatives, or other means.

calcitriol (kal-sih-TRIH-ol) The active hormone form of vitamin D

(1,25-dihydroxy-vitamin D). It contains a derivative of cholesterol as part of its structure.

cancer A condition characterized by uncontrolled growth of abnormal body cells.

cancer initiation The step in the process of cancer development that begins with alterations in DNA, the genetic material in a cell. This may cause the cell to no longer respond to normal physiological controls.

cancer progression The final stage in the cancer process in which the cancer cell grows to a sufficient mass so it will significantly affect body metabolism.

cancer promotion The step in the cancer process when cell division increases, in turn decreasing the time available for repair enzymes to act on altered DNA, and encouraging cells with altered DNA to develop and grow. Anything that increases the rate of cell division decreases the chance that the repair enzymes will find the altered part of the DNA in time to do their work.

carbohydrate (kar-bow-HIGH-drate) A compound containing carbon, hydrogen, and oxygen; most are known as *sugars, starches,* and *dietary fibers.* They yield on average 4 kcal per gram.

carbohydrate loading A process in which a very high carbohydrate intake is consumed for 6 days before an athletic event while tapering exercise duration in an attempt to increase muscle glycogen stores.

carcinogens Compounds that have potential to cause cancer.

cardiac output (CARD-ee-ack) The amount of blood pumped by the heart.

cardiovascular disease Disease of the heart and blood vessels.

carnitine (CAR-nih-teen) A compound used to shuffle fatty acids from the interior fluid of the cell into mitochondria.

carotenoids (kah-ROT-en-oyds) Plant pigments, some of which can yield vitamin A. Of the 600 or so carotenoids found in nature, about 50 yield vitamin A activity and thus are called provitamin A. Many have antioxidant properties as well. One example is beta-carotene.

carpal tunnel syndrome (CAR-pull) (SIN-drom) A disease in which nerves that travel to the wrist are pinched as they pass through a narrow opening in a bone in the wrist.

casein (KAY-seen) Protein found in milk that forms curds when exposed to acid and is difficult for infants to digest.

cash crop A crop grown by a country specifically for export, to gain the ability to purchase goods from other countries. Cultivation of cash crops diverts needed agricultural resources from production of crops needed to feed a country's own citizens. Examples are coffee, tea, cocoa, and bananas.

catabolic/catabolism (cat-ah-BOL-ik) Breaking down compounds.

catalyst (CAT-ul-ist) A compound that speeds reaction rates but is not altered by the reaction.

cell A minute structure; the living basis of plant and animal organization. In animals it is bounded by a cell membrane. Cells contain both genetic material and systems for synthesizing energy-yielding compounds. Cells have the ability to take up compounds from and excrete compounds into their surroundings.

Celsius A centigrade measure of temperature. For conversion: (degrees in Fahrenheit $-$ 32) $\times$ 5/9 = C°; (degrees in Celsius $\times$ 9/5) + 32 = F°.

chain-breaking Breaking the link between two or more actions that encourage problem behavior, such as snacking while watching television.

chemical bond An attachment or strong attraction between two atoms based on the sharing of electrons (attachment) or interaction of positive and negative charges (attraction).

cholecystokinin (CCK) (ko-la-sis-toe-KY-nin) A hormone that stimulates enzyme release from the pancreas, bile release from the gallbladder, and helps regulate hunger.

cholesterol (ko-LES-te-rol) A waxy lipid found in all body cells; it has a structure containing multiple chemical rings (steroid structure). Cholesterol is found only in foods that contain animal products.

chronic (KRON-ik) Long-standing, developing over time; slow to develop or resolve. When referring to disease, this indicates that the disease progress, once developed, is slow and tends to remain; a good example is heart disease.

chylomicrons (kye-lo-MY-krons) Lipoprotein made of dietary fat surrounded by a shell of cholesterol, phospholipids, and protein. These are made in the intestine after fat absorption and travel through the lymphatic system to the bloodstream.

chyme (KIME) A mixture of stomach secretions and partially digested food.

cirrhosis (see-ROH-sis) A loss of functioning liver cells, which are replaced by nonfunctioning connective tissue. Any substance that poisons liver cells can lead to cirrhosis. The most common cause is a chronic, excessive alcohol intake.

cis isomer (sis EYE-so-mer) An isomer form seen in compounds with double bonds, such as fatty acids, in which the hydrogens on both ends of the double bond lie on the same side of the plane of that bond.

clinical symptoms Generally, a change in health status noted by the individual (such as stomach pain) or noticed by a clinician during physical examination (the latter is technically called a clinical sign).

***Clostridium botulinum* (klo-STRID-ee-um BOT-you-LY-num)** A bacterium that can cause a fatal type of foodborne illness.

coenzyme The active form of many vitamins; the coenzyme aids enzyme function.

cognitive behavior therapy Psychological therapy in which the person's assumptions about dieting, body weight, and related issues are challenged. New ways of thinking are explored and then practiced by the person. In this way the person can learn new ways to control eating disorders behaviors and related life stress.

cognitive restructuring Changing negative, self-defeating, or pessimistic thoughts that undermine weight control efforts to those that are positive, optimistic, and supportive of weight control. For one example, instead of using a difficult day as an excuse to overeat, substituting other pleasures for rewards, such as a relaxing walk with a friend could be done.

colic (KOL-ik) Periodic, inconsolable crying in a healthy young infant associated with sharp abdominal pain.

colostrum (ko-LAHS-trum) The first fluid secreted by the breast during late pregnancy and the first few days after birth. This thick fluid is rich in immune factors and protein.

complementarity of proteins Two food protein sources that make up for each other's insufficient contribution of specific essential amino acids, so that together they yield a high-quality (complete) protein diet.

complete proteins Proteins that contain ample amounts of all nine essential amino acids.

compound A group of different types of atoms bonded together in definite proportion (see **molecule**). Not all chemical compounds exist as molecules. Some compounds are made up of ions attracted to each other, such as Na^+Cl^- (table salt).

connective tissue Protein tissue that holds different structures in the body together. Some structures are made up of connective tissue, notably tendons and cartilages. Connective tissue also forms part of bone and the nonmuscular structures of arteries and veins.

constipation A condition in which bowel movements are infrequent.

contingency management Forming a plan of action for responding to an environment in which overeating is likely, such as when snacks are within easy reach at a party.

control group Participants in an experiment who are not given the treatment being tested.

cortical bone (KORT-ih-kal) Dense, compact bone that comprises the outer surface and shafts of bone.

cortisol (KORT-ih-sol) A hormone made by the adrenal gland that, among other functions, stimulates the production of glucose from amino acids and increases the desire to eat.

cretinism (KREET-in-ism) Stunting of body growth and poor mental development in the offspring that results from inadequate maternal intake of iodide during pregnancy.

cystic fibrosis (SIS-tik figh-BRO-sis) A disease that often leads to overproduction of mucus. Mucus can invade the pancreas, decreasing enzyme output. The lack of lipase enzyme output then contributes to severe fat malabsorption.

Daily Reference Values (DRV) Standards of intake for certain components of a diet (such as carbohydrate, fat, protein, saturated fat, cholesterol, sodium, potassium, and dietary fiber) set by FDA for which no RDAs exist. These values are intended to be used for comparing intakes of these factors to desirable (or maximum) intakes. DRVs help consumers evaluate individual food choices and determine how they fit into a total diet as they form part of the Daily Values. The DRVs for cholesterol, sodium, and potassium are constant; those for other nutrients increase as energy intake increases. The DRVs constitute part of the Daily Values used in food labeling.

Daily Values A set of standard nutrient-intake values developed by the FDA and used as a reference for expressing nutrient content on nutrition labels. The Daily Values include two types of standards—RDIs and DRVs.

Delaney Clause A clause to the 1958 Food Additives Amendment of the Pure Food and Drug Act in the United States that prevents the intentional (direct) addition to foods of a compound that has been shown to cause cancer in laboratory animals or man.

dementia (de-MEN-sha) General persistent loss or decrease in mental function.

denature (dee-NAY-ture) Alteration of the three dimensional structure of a protein, usually as a result of treatment by heat, acid, base, or agitation.

dental caries (KARE-ees) Erosions in the surface of a tooth caused by acids made by bacteria as they metabolize sugars.

deoxyribonucleic acid (DNA) The site of hereditary information in cells; DNA directs the synthesis of cell proteins.

dermatitis Inflammation of the skin.

DEXA bone scan Method to measure bone density that uses small amounts of x-ray radiation. The ability of a bone to block the path of the radiation is used as a measure of bone density at that bone site. DEXA stands for dual energy x-ray absorptiometry.

diabetes (DYE-uh-BEET-eez) A disease characterized by high blood glucose (hyperglycemia), resulting from insufficient insulin action in the body (see **Type I diabetes** and **Type 2 diabetes**). Although this disease is commonly refereed to as "diabetes," its technical name is *diabetes mellitus.*

diastolic blood pressure (dye-ah-STOL-ik) The pressure in the arterial blood vessels when the heart is between beats.

dietary fiber Substances in food (essentially from plants) that are not digested by the processes that take place in the stomach or small intestine. These add bulk to feces.

Dietary Guidelines General goals for nutrient intake and diet composition set by government agencies—USDA and DHHS.

Dietary Reference Intakes (DRIs) The overarching framework for nutrient recommendations being made as part of revision of the 1989 RDA.

dietitian See **Registered Dietitian.**

digestibility (dye-JES-tih-bil-it-ee) The proportion of food substances eaten that can be broken down in the intestinal tract for absorption into the bloodstream.

digestion The process by which food is mechanically and chemically broken down to produce smaller forms that can be absorbed by the GI tract.

direct calorimetry (kal-oh-RIM-eh-tree) A method to determine energy use by the body by measuring heat that emanates from the body, usually using an insulated chamber.

disaccharides (dye-SACK-uh-rides) Class of sugars formed by chemically linking two monosaccharides.

diuretic (dye-u-RET-ik) A substance that, when ingested, increases the flow of urine.

diverticula (DYE-ver-TIK-you-luh) Pouches that protrude through the wall of the large intestine to the outside of the intestine.

diverticulitis (DYE-ver-tik-you-LITE-us) An inflammation of the diverticula caused by acids produced by bacterial metabolism inside the diverticula.

diverticulosis (DYE-ver-tik-you-LOW-sus) The condition of having many diverticula in the large intestine.

docosahexaenoic acid (DHA) (DOE-co-sa-hex-ee-no-ik) An omega-3 fatty acid with 22 carbons and six carbon-carbon double bonds. DHA is present in fish oils and is also synthesized from alpha-linolenic acid.

double-blind study An experiment in which the participants and researchers are unaware of the participant's assignment (test or placebo) or the outcome of the study until it is completed. An independent third party holds the code and the data until the study is completed.

ecosystem A "community" in nature that includes plants and animals and the environment associated with them.

ectomorph (EK-tuh-morf) A body type associated with very long, thin bones and very long, thin fingers.

edema (uh-DEE-muh) The buildup of excess fluid outside body cells (technically called extracellular spaces).

eicosanoids (eye-KOH-san-oyds) Hormonlike compounds synthesized from polyunsaturated fatty acids. Within this class of compounds are prostaglandins, thromboxanes, and leukotrienes.

eicosapentaenoic acid (EPA) (eye-KOH-sah-pen-tah-ee-NO-ik) An omega-3 fatty acid with 20 carbon atoms and five double bonds; present in fish oils and is made from alpha-linolenic acid as well.

electrolytes (ih-LEK-tro-lites) Substances that break down into ions in water and, in turn, are able to conduct an electrical current. These include sodium, chloride, and potassium.

elements Substances that cannot be broken down further by using ordinary chemical procedures.

elimination diet A restrictive diet that systematically tests foods that may cause an allergic response by first eliminating them for 1 to 2 weeks and then adding them back, one at a time.

embryo (EM-bree-oh) In humans, the developing human life form from about the third to eighth week after conception.

emulsifier (ee-MULL-sih-fire) A compound that can suspend fat in water by isolating individual fat drops using a shell of water molecules or other substances to prevent the fat from coalescing.

endometrium (en-doh-ME-tree-um) The membrane that lines the inside of the uterus. It increases in thickness during the menstrual cycle until ovulation occurs. The surface layers are shed during menstruation if conception does not take place.

endomorph (EN-doh-morf) A body type characterized by short, stubby bones, a short trunk, and short fingers.

endorphins (en-DOR-fins) Natural body tranquilizers that may be involved in the feeding response and function in pain reduction.

energy balance A state in which the energy intake, in the form of food or alcohol, matches the energy expended, primarily through basal metabolism and physical activity.

enriched A term generally meaning that the vitamins thiamin, niacin, riboflavin, and folate, and the mineral iron have been added to a grain product to improve nutritional quality.

enzyme (EN-zime) A compound that speeds the rate of a chemical process but is not altered by the process. Almost all enzymes are proteins.

epidemiology (ep-uh-dee-me-OLL-uh-gee) The study of how disease patterns vary between different population groups, such as the cases of stomach cancer in Japan compared with that in Germany.

epinephrine (ep-ih-NEF-rin) Also known as *adrenaline.* This hormone is released by the adrenal gland. A related form, norepinephrine, is released from various nerve endings in the body. Both hormones act to increase glycogen breakdown in the liver, among other functions.

epithelial cells (ep-ih-THEE-lee-ul) The surface cells that line the outside of the body and all external passages within it.

ergogenic (ur-go-JEN-ic) Work producing. An ergogenic acid is a physical, mechanical, nutritional, psychological, or pharmacological substance or treatment that is intended to directly improve exercise performance.

erythrocyte Mature red blood cell. This has no nucleus, and a lifespan of about 120 days; contains hemoglobin, which transports oxygen and carbon dioxide.

essential (indispensable) amino acids Amino acids not synthesized efficiently by humans. They therefore must be included in the diet. There are nine essential amino acids.

essential fatty acids Fatty acids that must be present in the diet to maintain health. These are linoleic acid and alpha-linolenic acid.

essential nutrient In nutritional terms, this represents a substance that, when left out of a diet, leads to signs of poor health. The body either can't produce these nutrients or can't produce them fast enough to meet its needs. Then, if added back to a diet before permanent damage occurs, the affected aspects of health are restored.

estimated average requirements (EARs) An amount of nutrient intake that is estimated to meet the needs of 50% of the individuals in a specific age and gender group.

estimated safe and adequate daily dietary intake (ESADDI) Nutrient intake recommendations made by the Food and Nutrition Board where a range for intake for some nutrients is given, because not enough information is available to set a more specific RDA.

Exchange System A system for classifying foods into numerous lists based on their macronutrient composition and establishing serving sizes so that one serving of each food on a list contains the same amount of carbohydrate, protein, fat, and energy content.

experiment A test made to examine the validity of a hypothesis.

failure to thrive Inadequate gains in height and weight in infancy, often due to an inadequate food intake.

famine An extreme shortage of food that leads to massive starvation; often associated with crop failures, war, and political strife.

fasting hypoglycemia (HIGH-po-gligh-SEE-me-ah) Low blood glucose that follows about a day or so of fasting; generally caused by pancreatic cancer.

fat-soluble vitamins Vitamins that dissolve in such substances as ether and benzene, but not readily in water. These vitamins are A, D, E, and K.

fatty acids Major part of most lipids, composed of carbon flanked by hydrogen with an acid group

$$\overset{\text{O}}{\underset{\|}{}}$$

(–C–OH) at one end and a methyl group (–CH_3) at the other.

feces (FEE-seas) Substances discharged from the bowel during defecation, consisting of the undigested residue of food, dead GI tract cells, mucus, bacteria, and other waste material. Another term for feces is *stool.*

feeding center A group of cells in the hypothalamus that, when stimulated, causes hunger.

female athlete triad A condition characterized by disordered eating, lack of menstrual periods, and low age-adjusted bone density.

fermentation The conversion, without use of oxygen, of carbohydrates to alcohols, acids, and carbon dioxide.

fetal alcohol syndrome (FAS) (FEET-al) A group of physical and mental abnormalities in the infant that result from the mother consuming alcohol during pregnancy.

fetus (FEET-us) The developing life form from about the beginning of the ninth week after conception until birth.

fluorosis A condition caused by excessive fluoride intake, characterized by poor tooth structure and discoloration.

foodborne illness Sickness caused by ingestion of foods containing toxic substances produced by microorganisms.

food diary A written record of sequential food intake for a period of time. Details associated with the food intake are often recorded as well.

food intolerance An adverse reaction to food that does not involve an allergic reaction.

food sensitivity A mild reaction to a substance in a food that might be expressed as slight itching or redness of the skin.

fortified A term generally meaning that vitamins, minerals, or both have been added to a food product in excess of what was originally found in the product.

fraternal twins Offspring that develop from two separate ova and sperm and therefore have separate genetic identities, although they develop simultaneously in the mother.

free radical Short-lived form of compounds that exist with an unpaired electron in the outer electron shell. This causes an electron-seeking nature, which can be very destructive to electron-dense areas of a cell, such as DNA and cell membranes.

fructose (FROOK-tose) A monosaccharide with six carbons that form a five-membered or six-membered ring with oxygen in the ring; found in fruits and honey.

fruitarian (froot-AIR-een-un) A person who eats primarily fruits, nuts, honey, and vegetable oils.

functional food A food that contains substances that provide health benefits beyond those supplied by traditional nutrients. An example is a tomato: this contains the phytochemical lycopene.

fungi Simple parasitic life forms including molds, mildews, yeasts, and mushrooms. They live on dead or decaying organic matter. Fungi can grow as single cells, like yeast, or as multicellular colonies, as seen with molds.

galactose A six-carbon monosaccharide; an isomer of glucose.

galactosemia (gah-LAK-toh-SEE-mee-ah) A rare, genetic disease characterized by the buildup of the single sugar galactose in the bloodstream resulting from the inability of the liver to metabolize it. If present at birth and left untreated, this disease causes severe mental and growth retardation in the infant.

gastroesophageal reflux disease (GERD) Disease that results from stomach acid backing up into the esophagus. The acid irritates the lining of the esophagus, causing pain.

gastrointestinal (GI) tract The main sites in the body used for digestion and absorption of nutrients. It consists of the mouth, esophagus, stomach, small intestine, large intestine, rectum, and anus.

gastroplasty (GAS-troh-plas-tee) Surgery performed on the stomach to limit its volume to approximately 50 milliliters, the size of a shot glass.

gene (JEAN) The genetic material on chromosomes that makes up DNA. Genes provide the blueprint for the production of cell proteins.

generally recognized as safe (GRAS) A list of food additives that in 1958 were considered safe for consumption. Manufacturers were allowed to continue to use those additives, without special clearance, when needed for food products. FDA bears responsibility for proving they are not safe, but can remove unsafe products from the list.

genetic engineering Alteration of genetic material in plants or animals with the intent of improving growth, disease resistance, or other characteristics.

gestation (jes-TAY-shun) The period of the development of the offspring from conception to birth; this lasts about 40 weeks after the woman's last menstrual period.

gestational diabetes (jes-TAY-shun-al) Elevated blood glucose that develops during pregnancy but returns to normal after birth; one cause is placental production of hormones that antagonize blood glucose regulation.

glucagon (GLOO-kuh-gon) A hormone made by the pancreas that stimulates the breakdown of glycogen in the liver into glucose; this raises blood glucose. Glucagon also performs other functions.

gluconeogenesis (gloo-ko-nee-oh-JEN-uh-sis) The production of new glucose molecules by metabolic pathways in the cell. The source of the carbon for these new glucose molecules is usually amino acids.

glucose (GLOO-kos) A six-carbon atom carbohydrate found in blood and in table sugar bound to fructose; also known as *dextrose,* it is one of the simple sugars.

glucose polymer A carbohydrate source used in some sports drinks that consists of a few glucose molecules bonded together.

glycerol A three-carbon alcohol used to form triglycerides.

glycogen A carbohydrate made of multiple units of glucose with a highly branched structure; sometimes known as animal starch. It is the storage form of glucose in humans and is synthesized (and stored) in the liver and muscles.

glycosylation The process by which glucose attaches to other compounds, such as proteins.

goiter An enlargement of the thyroid gland, which can be caused by a lack of iodide in the diet.

green revolution Increases in crop yields accompanying the introduction of new agricultural technologies in less developed countries, beginning in the 1960s. The key technologies were high-yielding, disease-resistant strains of rice, wheat, and corn; greater use of fertilizer; and improved cultivation practices.

growth hormone A pituitary hormone that stimulates body growth and release of fat from storage, and has other effects.

gum A dietary fiber containing chains of galactose, glucuronic acid, and other monosaccharides; characteristically found between plant cell walls.

heart attack Rapid fall in heart function caused by reduced blood flow through the heart's blood vessels. Often part of the heart dies in the process. Technically called a myocardial infarction.

heartburn A pain arising from the esophagus, caused by stomach acid backing up into the esophagus and irritating its tissue.

heart disease A disease usually caused by the deposition of fatty material in the blood vessels in the heart. This in turn reduces blood flow to the heart, thereby reducing heart function, which in turn can lead to death.

heat cramps Heat cramps are a frequent complication of heat exhaustion. They usually occur in individuals exercising for several hours in a hot climate who have experienced large sweat losses and have consumed a large volume of unsalted water. The cramps occur in skeletal muscles and consist of contractions for one to three minutes at a time.

heat exhaustion Heat illness that occurs when heat stress causes depletion of blood volume from fluid loss by the body. This increases body temperature and can lead to headache, dizziness, muscle weakness, and visual disturbances, among other effects.

heatstroke Heatstroke can occur when internal body temperature reaches 105° F. Sweating generally ceases if left untreated, and blood circulation is greatly reduced. Nervous system damage may ensue and death is likely. Oftentimes in individuals who suffer heatstroke the skin is hot and dry.

hematocrit (hee-MAT-oh-krit) The percentage of total blood volume made up of red blood cells.

heme iron (HEEM) Iron provided from animal tissues as hemoglobin and myoglobin. Approximately 40% of the iron in meat is heme iron; it is readily absorbed.

hemicellulose (hem-ih-SELL-you-los) A dietary fiber containing xylose, galactose, glucose, and other monosaccharides bonded together.

hemochromatosis (heem-oh-krom-ah-TOE-sis) A disorder of iron metabolism characterized by increased iron absorption and deposition in the liver and heart tissue. This eventually poisons the cells in those organs.

hemoglobin (HEEM-oh-glow-bin) The iron-containing part of the red blood cell that carries oxygen to the cells and some carbon dioxide away from the cells. It is also responsible for the red color of blood.

hemolysis (hee-MOL-ih-sis) Destruction of red blood cells caused by the breakdown of the red blood cell membranes. This allows the cell contents to leak into the fluid portion of the blood.

hemorrhoid (HEM-or-oyd) A pronounced swelling in a large vein, particularly veins found in the anal region.

herbicide (ERB-ih-side) A compound that reduces the growth and reproduction of plants.

high blood pressure A condition in which blood pressure remains persistently elevated, especially when the heart is between beats; also called hypertension.

high-density lipoprotein (HDL) The lipoprotein synthesized primarily by the liver and intestine that picks up cholesterol from dying cells and other sources and transfers it to the other lipoproteins in the bloodstream, as well as directly to the liver. A low blood HDL value increases the risk for heart disease.

high-fructose corn syrup A corn syrup that has been manufactured to contain between 40% and 90% fructose.

high-quality (complete) proteins Dietary proteins that contain ample amounts of all nine essential amino acids.

hormone A compound secreted into the bloodstream that acts to control the function of distant target organ cells. Hormones can be either amino acidlike (epinephrine), proteinlike (insulin), or fatlike (estrogen).

hunger The primary physiological (internal) drive to find and eat food, mostly regulated by internal cues to eating.

hydrogenation (high-dro-jen-AY-shun) The addition of hydrogen atoms to the double bonds of polyunsaturated and monounsaturated fatty acids to reduce the extent of unsaturation. This process turns liquid vegetable oils into solid fats and is used to make margarine and shortening. Trans fatty acids are a by-product of this process.

hydroxyapatite (high-drox-ee-APP-uh-tite) A compound, composed primarily of calcium and phosphate, that is deposited into the bone protein matrix to give bone strength and rigidity ($Ca_{10}[PO_4]_6OH_2$).

hyperglycemia (HIGH-per-gligh-SEE-me-uh) High blood glucose, above 125 milligrams per 100 milliliters (dl) of blood.

hypergymnasia Exercising beyond the amount required for good physical fitness or maximum performance in a sport; excessive exercise.

hypoglycemia (HIGH-po-gligh-SEE-me-uh) Low blood glucose, below 40 to 50 milligrams per 100 milliliters (dl) of blood.

hypothalamus (high-po-THALL-uh-mus) A region at the base of the brain that contains cells that play a role in the regulation of hunger, respiration, body temperature, and other body functions.

hypothesis (high-POTH-eh-sis) An "educated guess" by a scientist to explain a phenomenon.

hysterectomy Surgical removal of the uterus.

identical twins Two offspring that develop from a single ovum and sperm and, consequently, have the same genetic makeup.

ileum (ILL-ee-um) Essentially, the area consisting of the last half of the small intestine.

incidental food additives Additives that appear in food products indirectly, from environmental contamination of food ingredients or during the manufacturing process.

incomplete (lower-quality) protein Food protein that lacks ample amount of one or more of the essential amino acids needed to support human protein needs.

indirect calorimetry (kal-oh-RIM-eh-tree) A method to measure the energy use by the body by measuring oxygen uptake. Formulas are then used to convert this gas exchange value into energy use.

infectious disease (in-FEK-shus) Any disease caused by an invasion of the body by microorganisms, such as bacteria, fungi, or viruses.

infrastructure The basic framework of a system or organization. For society, this includes roads, bridges, telephones, and other basic technologies.

inorganic Anything that is free of carbon atoms bonded to hydrogen atoms in the chemical structure.

insoluble fiber Fiber that mostly does not dissolve in water and is not metabolized by bacteria in the large intestine. Such fiber includes cellulose, some hemicelluloses, and lignins.

insulin A hormone produced by the beta cells of the pancreas. Insulin increases the synthesis of glycogen in the liver and the movement of glucose from the bloodstream into muscle and adipose cells, among other processes.

intentional food additive Additives manufacturers knowingly (directly) incorporate into food products.

international unit (IU) A crude measure of vitamin activity, often based on the growth rate of animals. Today these units have generally been replaced by precise measurement of actual quantities in milligrams or micrograms.

intravenous nutrition Nutrition that is supplied directly into the veins, rather than via the GI tract. This is generally called total parenteral nutrition in health-care settings.

intrinsic factor A substance present in gastric juice that enhances vitamin B-12 absorption.

in utero (in YOU-ter-oh) "In the uterus" or, during pregnancy.

ion An atom with an unequal number of electrons and protons. Negative ions have more electrons than protons; positive ions have more protons than electrons.

irradiation (ir-RAY-dee-AY-shun) A process whereby radiation energy is applied to foods, creating compounds (free radicals) within the food that destroy cell membranes, break down genetic material, link proteins together, limit enzyme activity, and alter a variety of other proteins and cell functions that would otherwise lead to food spoilage. This process does not make the food radioactive.

isomers (EYE-so-mers) Different chemical structures for compounds that share the same chemical formula.

ketone (KEE-tone) Incomplete breakdown product of fat containing three or four carbons. An example is acetoacetic acid.

ketosis (kee-TOE-sis) The condition of having a high concentration of ketones in the bloodstream.

kidney nephrons (NEF-rons) Units of kidney cells that filter wastes from the bloodstream and deposit them in the urine.

kilocalorie (kill-oh-KAL-oh-ree) (kcal) The heat needed to raise the temperature of 1000 grams (1 liter) of water 1 degree Celsius.

kilojoule (KIL-oh-jool) (kj) A measure of work in which kilojoule equals the work needed to move 1 kilogram a distance of 1 meter with the force of 1 newton. One kcal equals 4.18 kilojoules.

kwashiorkor (kwash-ee-OR-core) A disease occurring primarily in young children who have an existing disease and who consume a marginal amount of energy and considerably insufficient protein in the face of high needs. The child suffers from infections and exhibits edema, poor growth, weakness, and an increased susceptibility to further illness.

lactase An enzyme made by cells of the intestinal wall; this enzyme digests lactose into glucose and galactose.

lactic acid (LAK-tik) A three-carbon acid; also called lactate, formed during anaerobic cell metabolism; a partial breakdown product of glucose.

***Lactobacillus bifidus* factor (lak-toe-bah-SIL-us BIFF-id-us)** A protective factor secreted in the colostrum that encourages growth of beneficial bacteria in the newborn's intestines.

lacto-ovo-pesco vegetarian A person who consumes only plant products, dairy products, eggs, and fish.

lacto-ovo vegetarian A person who consumes only plant products, dairy products, and eggs.

lactose (LAK-tose) A sugar made up of glucose linked to galactose.

lactose intolerance (primary and secondary) Primary lactose intolerance occurs when lactase production declines for no apparent reason. Secondary lactose intolerance occurs when a specific cause, like long-standing diarrhea, results in a decline in lactase production.

lactovegetarian (lak-toe-vej-eh-TEAR-ree-an) A person who consumes only plant products and dairy products.

lanugo (lah-NEW-go) Downlike hair that appears on a person who has lost much body fat during semistarvation. The hair stands erect and traps air, which acts as insulation to the body, replacing the insulation properties usually supplied by body fat. Fetuses also have lanugo.

larvae (LAR-va) An early developmental stage in the life history of some microorganisms, such as parasites. Larvae is the plural form of Larva.

laxative A medication or other substance that stimulates evacuation of the intestinal tract.

lean body mass The part of the human body that is free of all but essential body fat. About 2% of body weight as fat is essential. The rest of the fat in the body represents storage and so is not part of lean body mass. Lean body mass includes brain, muscle, bone, organs, connective tissue, skin, and other body parts, including body fluids such as blood.

lecithin (LESS-uh-thin) Any of several phospholipids containing two fatty acids, a phosphate group, and a choline-molecule.

leptin A hormone made by adipose cells that in turn influences food intake by communicating the degree of fat stores in the person (or laboratory animal).

let-down reflex A reflex stimulated by infant suckling that causes the release (ejection) of milk from milk ducts in the mother's breast.

life expectancy The average length of life for a given group of people born in a certain year, such as this year.

life span The potential oldest age to which a person can reach.

lignins (LIG-nins) Insoluble fiber made up of a multiringed alcohol (non-carbohydrate) structure.

limiting amino acid The essential amino acid in the lowest concentration in a food in proportion to body needs.

linoleic acid (lin-oh-LEE-ik) An essential fatty acid with 18 carbon atoms and two carbon-carbon double bonds; omega-6.

lipid (LIP-id) A compound containing much carbon and hydrogen, little oxygen, and sometimes other chemical elements. Lipids dissolve in ether or benzene and include fats, oils, and cholesterol. Yields on average 9 kcals per gram.

lipoprotein (ly-poh-PRO-teen) A compound found in the bloodstream containing a core of lipids with a shell of protein, phospholipid, and cholesterol.

liter (LEE-ter) (L) A measure of volume in the metric system. One liter equals 0.96 quarts.

long-chain fatty acids Fatty acids that contain 12 or more carbon atoms.

low birth weight (LBW) Infant weight at birth of less than 2.5 kilograms (5.5 pounds); usually caused by preterm birth; these infants are at higher risk for health problems.

low-density lipoprotein (LDL) The product of the VLDL containing primarily cholesterol; elevated LDL is strongly linked to heart disease risk.

lower-body obesity The type of obesity, also called gynoid, in which fat storage is primarily located in the buttocks and thigh area.

lower-quality (incomplete) proteins Dietary proteins that are low in or lack an ample amount of one or more of the amino acids essential for human protein needs.

lumen (LOO-men) The inside cavity of a tube, such as the GI tract.

lymphatic system (lim-FAT-ick) System of vessels that can accept fluid surrounding cells and large particles, such as products of fat absorption. This lymph fluid eventually passes into the bloodstream via the lymphatic system.

lysosome (LYE-so-som) A cellular organelle that contains digestive enzymes for use inside the cell for turnover of cell parts.

lysozyme (LYE-so-zime) A set of enzyme substances produced by a variety of cells; it can destroy bacteria by rupturing cell membranes.

macrocytic anemia Anemia characterized by the presence of abnormally large red blood cells. A typical cause is folate or vitamin B-12 deficiency.

major mineral A mineral vital to health that is required in the diet in amounts greater than 100 mg/day.

malignant Essentially to do anything malicious. In reference to a tumor, the property of spreading locally and to distant sites.

malnutrition Failing health that results from long-standing dietary practices that do not coincide with nutritional needs.

maltose Glucose bonded to glucose.

mannitol An alcohol derivative of fructose.

marasmus A disease that results from consuming grossly insufficient amounts of energy and protein: one of the diseases classed as protein-energy malnutrition. Victims will have little or no fat stores, little muscle mass, and poor strength. Death from infection is common.

meconium The first thick, mucuslike stool passed by the infant after birth.

medium-chain fatty acid A fatty acid that contains 6 to 10 carbons.

megadose Intake of a nutrient in excess of 10 times that of human need.

megaloblast (MEG-ah-low-blast) A large, nucleated, immature red blood cell that results from an inability for cell division during red blood cell development.

menarche (men-AR-kee) The onset of menstruation. Menarche usually occurs around age 13, 2 or 3 years after the first signs of puberty start to appear.

menopause (MEN-oh-paws) The cessation of menses in women, usually beginning at about 50 years of age.

mesomorph (MEZ-oh-morf) A body type associated with average bone size, trunk size, and finger length.

metabolism (meh-TAB-oh-lizm) Chemical processes that occur in the body, enabling cells to release energy from foods, convert one substance into another, and prepare end products for excretion. In sum the processes allow for life.

metastasis Spread of cancerous cells from their site of origin to other areas of the body.

meter A measure of length in the metric system. One meter equals 39.4 in.

minerals The basic chemical elements used in the body to help form body structures and promote chemical reactions. Examples are calcium and iron.

miscarriage Termination of pregnancy that occurs before the fetus can survive; also called *spontaneous abortion.*

mitochondria The main sites of energy production in a cell. Mitochondria also contain the pathway for burning fat for fuel, among other metabolic pathways.

molecule A group of atoms chemically linked together; that is, tightly connected by attractive forces (see **compound**).

monoglyceride (mon-oh-GLIS-er-ide) A breakdown product of a triglyceride consisting of one fatty acid bonded to a glycerol backbone.

monosaccharide (mon-oh-SACK-uh-ride) A class of simple sugars, such as glucose, that is not broken down further during digestion.

monounsaturated fatty acid A fatty acid containing one carbon-carbon double bond.

mortality This represents a population's death rate. The term *morbidity* refers to the amount of sickness present.

mottling (MOT-ling) Discoloration or marking of the surface of teeth from fluorosis.

mucilage (MYOU-sih-laj) A dietary fiber consisting of chains of galactose, mannose, and other monosaccharides; characteristically found in seaweed.

mucus (MYOO-cuss) A thick fluid secreted by glands throughout the body. It contains a compound that has both carbohydrate and protein parts. It acts as a lubricant and means of protection for cells.

mutation A permanent change in a cell's DNA; includes changes in sequence, alteration of gene position, gene loss or duplication, and insertion of foreign gene sequences.

mycotoxin (MY-ko-tok-sin) A group of toxic compounds produced by molds, such as aflatoxin B-1 found on moldy grains.

myocardial infarction (MY-oh-CARD-ee-ahl in-FARK-shun) Death of part of the heart muscle.

myoglobin (my-oh-GLOW-bin) Iron-containing compound that binds oxygen (O_2) in muscle.

negative energy balance The state in which the energy intake is less than the energy expended. The result of this is a decrease in body weight.

neural tube defect A defect in the formation of the neural tube occurring during early fetal development. These are seen in about 2500 infants per year in the United States. The defect results in various nervous system disorders, such as spina bifida.

Folate deficiency in the pregnant woman increases the risk of the fetus developing this disorder.

neurotransmitter A compound made by a nerve cell that allows for communication between it and other cells.

night blindness A vitamin A deficiency condition in which the retina in the eye cannot adjust to low amounts of light.

nitrate A nitrogen-containing compound used to cure meats. Its use contributes a pink color to meats and confers some resistance to bacterial growth.

nitrosamines A carcinogen formed from nitrates and breakdown products of amino acids; can lead to stomach cancer.

nonessential (dispensable) amino acids Amino acids the body readily make in sufficient amounts. There are 11 nonessential amino acids.

nonheme iron Iron provided from plant sources and animal tissues other than hemoglobin and myoglobin. Nonheme iron is less efficiently absorbed than heme iron, as absorption is also more closely dependent on body needs.

nutrient density The ratio formed by dividing a food's contribution to the needs for a nutrient by its contribution to energy needs. When the contribution to nutrient needs exceeds that to energy needs, the food is considered to have a favorable nutrient density for that nutrient.

nutrients Chemical substances in food that nourish the body by providing energy, building materials, and factors to regulate needed chemical reactions in the body.

nutrition The Council on Food and Nutrition of the American Medical Association defines nutrition as "the science of food; the nutrients and the substances therein; their action, interaction, and balance in relation to health and disease; and the process by which the organism (i.e., body) ingests, digests, absorbs, transports, utilizes, and excretes food substances."

nutrition label A label containing "Nutrition Facts" that must be included on most foods. It depicts nutrient content in comparison to the Daily Values set by FDA.

nutrition state The nutritional health of a person as determined by anthropometric measures (height, weight, circumferences, and so on), biochemical measures of nutrients or their by—products in blood and urine, a clinical (physical) examination, and a dietary analysis (ABCD).

obesity (oh-BEES-ih-tee) A condition characterized by excess body fat, often defined as a body mass index of 30 or above, or being 20% or more over healthy weight.

omega-3 (ω-3) fatty acid An unsaturated fatty acid with its first double bond starting just after the third carbon from the methyl end ($—CH_3$).

omega-6 (ω-6) fatty acid An unsaturated fatty acid with its first double bond just after the sixth carbon atom from the methyl end ($—CH_3$).

omnivor (AHM-nih-voor) A person who consumes foods from both plant and animal sources.

opportunistic infection An infection that arises primarily in people who are already ill because of another disease.

organ A group of tissues designed to perform a specific function; for example, the heart. It contains muscle tissue, nerve tissue, and so on.

organic Anything that contains carbon atoms bonded to hydrogen atoms in the chemical structure.

organism A living thing. The human body is an organism consisting of many organs that act in a coordinated manner to support life.

osteoblasts Cells in bone that secrete mineral and bone matrix (e.g., collagen).

osteoclasts Bone cells that arise originally from a type of white blood cell. Osteoclasts secrete substances that lead to bone erosion. This erosion can set the stage for subsequent bone mineralization.

osteomalacia (OS-tee-oh-mal-AY-shuh) Adult form of rickets. This results from a vitamin D deficiency disease, leading to weak bones and increased fracture risk.

osteoporosis (os-tee-oh-po-ROH-sis) Decreased bone density where no outward causes can be found. Related to effects of aging, poor diet, and hormonal effects of menopause in women.

overnutrition A state in which nutritional intake exceeds the body's needs.

ovum An egg; female germ cell released from the ovary at ovulation.

oxalic acid (or oxalate) An organic acid found in spinach, rhubarb, and other leafy green vegetables that can depress the absorption of certain minerals, such as calcium.

oxidation Loss of an electron by an atom or molecule. In metabolism, often associated with a gain of oxygen or loss of hydrogen. Oxidation (loss of an electron) and reduction (gain of an electron) take place simultaneously in metabolism, because an electron that is lost by one atom is accepted by another.

oxidize (ox-ih-dize) In the most basic sense, this means a chemical substance has either lost an electron or gained an oxygen. This then typically alters the substance. An oxidizing agent is a substance capable of capturing an electron from a source that is rich in them.

oxytocin A hormone secreted by the posterior part of the pituitary gland. It causes contraction of the musclelike cells surrounding the ducts of the breasts, and muscles of the uterus.

parathyroid hormone (PTH) A hormone made by the parathyroid glands that increases synthesis of the vitamin D hormone and aids calcium release from bone and calcium uptake by the kidneys, among other functions.

passive absorption Absorption that uses no energy. It requires permeability for the substance through the wall of the small intestine and a concentration gradient higher in the lumen of the intestine than in the absorptive cell. The higher concentration of the substance in the lumen of the intestine in comparison with that in the absorptive cells promotes the absorption of the nutrient.

pasteurizing (PAS-tur-i-zing) The process of rapidly heating food products to kill disease-causing microorganisms. One method heats milk at 161°F for at least 20 seconds.

peer-reviewed journal A journal that publishes research only after two or three scientists who were not part of the study agree it was well conducted and the results are fairly represented. Thus the research has been approved by peers of the research team.

pellagra (peh-LAHG-rah) A disease characterized by inflammation of the skin, diarrhea, and eventual mental incapacity; results from an insufficient amount of the vitamin niacin in the diet.

peptide bond A chemical bond formed to link amino acids in a protein.

percentile Classification of a measurement of a unit into divisions of 100 units.

peristalsis (per-ih-STALL-sis) A coordinated muscular contraction that is used to propel food down the gastrointestinal tract.

pernicious anemia (per-NISH-us ah-NEE-mee-ah) The anemia that results from a lack of vitamin B-12 absorption. It is pernicious (deadly) because of the associated nerve degeneration that can result in eventual paralysis and death.

pesticide A general term for an agent that can destroy bacteria, fungi, insects, rodents, or other pests.

pH A measure of the hydrogen ion concentration in a solution.

phenylketonuria (PKU) (fen-ihl-kee-toh-NEW-ree-ah) A disease caused by a defect in the ability of the liver to metabolize the animo acid phenylalanine into the amino acid tyrosine. Toxic by-products of phenylalanine can then build up in the body and lead to mental retardation.

phenylpropanolamine (fen-ihl-pro-pan-OL-ah-meen) An over-the-counter decongestant that has a mild appetite-reducing effect.

phosphocreatine (PCr) (fos-fo-CREE-a-tin) A high-energy compound that can be used to re-form adenosine triphosphate (ATP) from adenosine diphosphate (ADP). It is used primarily during short bursts of energy, such as lifting and jumping.

phospholipid Any of a class of fat-related substances that contain phosphorus, fatty acids, and a nitrogen-containing base. The phospholipids are an essential part of every cell.

photosynthesis (foto-SIN-tha-sis) The process by which plants use solar energy from the sun to produce energy-yielding compounds, such as glucose.

phylloquinone (fil-oh-KWIN-own) A form of vitamin K that comes from plants.

phytic acid (phytate) (FY-tick, FY-tate) A constituent of plant fibers that binds positive ions to its multiple phosphate groups.

phytochemical A chemical found in plants. Some phytochemicals may contribute to a reduced risk of cancer or heart disease in people who consume them regularly.

pica (PIE-kah) The practice of eating nonfood items such as dirt, laundry starch, or clay.

placebo (plah-SEE-bo) A fake medicine used to disguise the roles of participants in an experiment.

placenta (plah-SEN-tah) An organ formed in a woman only during pregnancy that secretes hormones to maintain the pregnant state and makes possible the transfer of oxygen and nutrients from the mother's blood to the fetus, as well as removal of fetal wastes.

plaque (PLACK) In terms of heart disease, a cholesterol-rich substance deposited in the blood vessels. It also contains various white blood cells and smooth muscle cells, cholesterol and other lipids, and eventually calcium. Sometimes called *atherosclerotic plaque* to distinguish it from bacterial plaque, which forms on teeth.

polysaccharide (POL-ee-SACK-uh-ride) Carbohydrate containing many glucose units, up to 3000 or more; also known as complex carbohydrates.

polyunsaturated fatty acid A fatty acid containing two or more carbon-carbon double bonds.

portal vein A large vein that distributes blood from the intestine to the liver through capillaries.

positive balance A state in which nutrient intake exceeds losses. This causes a net gain of the nutrient in the body, such as when tissue protein is gained during growth.

positive energy balance State in which energy intake is greater than energy expended, generally resulting in weight gain.

precursor A compound that comes before; to precede.

pregnancy-induced hypertension A serious disorder that can include high blood pressure, kidney failure, convulsion, and even death of the mother and the fetus. Mild cases are known as *preeclampsia;* more severe cases are call *eclampsia* (formally called *toxemia*).

premenstrual syndrome A disorder (also referred to as *PMS*) found in some women a few days before the onset of menses and characterized by depression, headache, bloating, and mood swings. Severe cases are currently termed premenstrual dysphoric disorder (PDD).

preservatives Compounds that extend the shelf life of foods by inhibiting microbial growth or minimizing the destructive effect of oxygen and metals.

preterm An infant born before 37 weeks of gestation; also known as premature.

prevalence The number of people at any one time who have a specific disease, such as obesity or cancer.

primary disease A disease process that is not simply caused by another disease process.

prognosis (prog-NO-sis) A forecast of the course and end of a disease.

prolactin (pro-LACK-tin) A hormone secreted by the mother that stimulates the synthesis of milk.

prostate gland A solid, chestnut-shaped organ surrounding the first part of the urethra in the male. The prostate gland is situated immediately under the bladder and in front of the rectum. The prostate gland secretes substances into the semen as the fluid passes through ducts leading from the seminal vesicles into the urethra.

protein Food components made of amino acids; contain carbon, hydrogen, oxygen, nitrogen, and sometimes other chemical elements, in a specific configuration. Proteins contain the form of nitrogen most easily used by the human body. Yields on average 4 kcals per gram.

protein-energy malnutrition (PEM) A condition resulting from regularly consuming insufficient amounts of energy and protein. The deficiency eventually results in body wasting and an increased susceptibility to infection.

psyllium (SIL-ee-um) A mostly soluble type of dietary fiber found in the seeds of the plantain plant.

radiation Literally; energy that is emitted from a center in all directions. Various forms of radiation energy include X-rays and ultraviolet rays from the sun.

rancid (RAN-sid) Containing products of decomposed fatty acids; these yield off-flavors and odors.

reactive hypoglycemia (HIGH-po-gligh-SEE-mee-uh) Low blood glucose that may follow a meal high in simple sugars, with corresponding symptoms of irritability, headache, nervousness, and sweating. The actual number of cases of this disease in the population is low.

receptor A site in a cell at which compounds (such as hormones) bind. Cells that contain receptors for a specific compound are partially controlled by that compound.

Recommended Dietary Allowances (RDAs) Recommended intakes of nutrients that meet the needs of almost all healthy people of similar age and gender. These are established by the Food and Nutrition Board of the National Academy of Sciences.

Recommended Nutrient Intake (RNI) The Canadian version of RDA.

reduction In chemical terms the gain of an electron by an atom; takes place simultaneously with oxidation (loss of an electron by an atom) in metabolism because an electron that is lost by one atom is accepted by another. In metabolism reduction is often associated with the gain of hydrogen.

Reference Daily Intake (RDI) Standards established by FDA for expressing nutrient content on nutrient labels. RDIs are generally based on the maximum 1968 RDA values set for a nutrient that span a particular age range, such as children over 4 years through adults. *RDI* replaced the term *U.S. RDA*. The RDIs constitute part of the Daily Values used in food labeling.

Registered Dietitian (RD) (dye-eh-TISH-shun) A person who has completed a baccalaureate degree program approved by The American Dietetic Association, performed at least 900 hours of supervised professional practice, and passed a registration examination.

requirement The amount of a nutrient required by one person to maintain health. This varies between individuals. We do not know our individual requirements for each nutrient.

reserve capacity The extent to which an organ can preserve essentially normal function despite decreasing cell number or cell activity.

respiration The utilization of oxygen; in the human organism, the inhalation of oxygen and the exhalation of carbon dioxide; in cells, the oxidation (electron removal) of food molecules, particularly in the mitochondria, to obtain energy.

resting metabolic rate The amount of energy used during rest, without stringently controlling recent physical activity. Essentially the same as the basal metabolic rate, but the subject does not need to meet the strict conditions used for a basal metabolic rate determination. Today, both terms are often used interchangeably.

retinoids (RET-ih-noyds) Chemical forms of preformed vitamin A; one source is animal foods, like liver. Forms include retinol, retinal, and retinoic acid.

ribose (RIGH-bos) A five-carbon sugar found in genetic material, specifically RNA.

rickets A disease characterized by softening of the bones because of poor calcium content. This deficiency disease arises in infancy and childhood from insufficient vitamin D activity in the body.

risk factor A characteristic or a behavior that contributes to the chances of developing an illness, such as smoking as a risk factor for developing lung cancer.

runner's anemia (ah-NEE-me-ah) A decrease in the blood's ability to carry oxygen, found in athletes, which may be caused by iron loss through perspiration and feces, red blood cell destruction due to the impact of exercise as the foot strikes the ground, or increased blood volume.

saccharin (SACK-ah-rin) An alternate sweetener that yields no energy to the body; it is 300 times sweeter than sucrose.

saliva (sah-LIGH-vah) A water fluid produced by the salivary glands in the mouth that contains lubricants, enzymes, and other substances.

salt Generally refers to a compound of sodium and chloride in a 40:60 ratio.

satiety (suh-TIE-uh-tee) State in which there is no longer a desire to eat; a feeling of satisfaction.

saturated fatty acid A fatty acid containing no carbon-carbon double bonds.

scurvy (SKER-vee) The deficiency disease that results after a few weeks to months of consuming a diet that lacks vitamin C; pinpoint hemorrhages on the skin are an early sign.

secondary disease A disease process that develops as a result of another disease.

secrete To produce a useful substance by a cell and then deliver that substance to the bloodstream or body cavity.

secretin (SEE-kreh-tin) A hormone that causes bicarbonate ion release from the pancreas.

self-monitoring A process of tracking foods eaten and conditions affecting eating; actions are usually recorded in a diary, along with location, time, and state of mind. This is a tool to help a person understand more about his or her eating habits.

self-talk The internal dialogue that each one of us carries on in our heads as we sort out beliefs, feelings, attitudes, and events happening in our lives.

sequesterants (see-KWES-ter-ants) Compound that binds free metal ions. By so doing, they reduce the ability of ions to cause rancidity in foods containing fat.

serotonin (ser-oh-TONE-in) A neurotransmitter synthesized from the amino acid tryptophan that appears to both decrease the desire to eat carbohydrates and induce sleep.

serum The portion of the blood fluid remaining after (1) the blood is allowed to clot and (2) the red and white blood cells are removed by centrifugation.

set point Often refers to the close regulation of body weight. It is not known what cells control this set point nor how it actually functions in weight regulation. There is evidence, however, that mechanisms exist that help regulate weight.

short-chain fatty acids Fatty acids that contain fewer than eight carbon atoms.

sickle cell disease (sickle cell anemia) An anemia that results from a malformation of the red blood cell because of an incorrect primary structure in part of its hemoglobin protein chains. The disease can lead to episodes of severe bone and joint pain, abdominal pain, headache, convulsions, paralysis, and even death.

sign A change in health status that is apparent on physical examination.

slough To shed or cast off.

small for gestational age (SGA) (jes-TAY-shun-al) Referring to infants who weight less than the expected weight for their length of gestation. This corresponds to less than 2.5 kilograms (5.5 pounds) in a full-term newborn. A preterm infant who is also SGA will most likely develop some medical complications.

sodium bicarbonate An alkaline substance made basically of sodium and carbon dioxide ($NaHCO_3$).

soluble fibers (SOL-you-bull) Fibers that either dissolve or swell when put into water and are metabolized (fermented) by bacteria in the large intestine. These include pectins, gums, mucilages, and some hemicelluloses.

solvent A substance that other substances dissolve in.

sorbitol (SOR-bih-tol) An alcohol derivative of glucose that yields about 3 kcal per gram but is slowly absorbed from the small intestine. It is used in some sugarless gums and dietetic foods.

sphincter (SFINK-ter) A muscular valve that controls flow of foodstuff in the GI tract.

spontaneous abortion Any cessation of pregnancy and expulsion of the embryo or nonviable fetus as the result of natural causes, such as a genetic defect or developmental problem; also called *miscarriage.*

spore A dormant reproductive cell capable of forming into an adult organism without the help of another cell. Various fungi and bacteria form spores.

starch A carbohydrate made of multiple units of glucose attached together in a form the body can digest; also known as *complex carbohydrate.*

sterol A compound containing a multiring (steroid) structure and a hydroxyl group (–OH).

stimulus control Altering the environment to minimize the stimuli for eating; for example, removing foods from sight and storing them in kitchen cabinets.

stomach distention Expansion of the walls of the stomach (intestines as well) from the pressure caused by the presence of gases, food, drink, or other factors.

stress fracture A fracture that occurs from repeated jarring of a bone. Common sites include bones of the foot.

stroke Damage to part of the brain caused by interruption if its blood supply or leakage of blood outside vessel walls. Sensation, movement, or function controlled by the damaged area is then impaired.

subclinical Not seen on a clinical (physical) examination.

sucralose A sweetener made by substituting 3 chlorines for 3 hydroxyl (–OH) groups on sucrose; 600 times sweeter than sucrose.

sucrose (SOO-kros) Fructose bonded to glucose; table sugar.

sugar Simple carbohydrate form with a chemical composition ratio of CH_2O. Most sugars form ringed structures when in solution.

superoxide dismutase (soo-per-OX-ide DISS-myoo-tase) An enzyme that can quench (deactivate) a superoxide negative free radical ($^{\cdot}O_2^{-}$). This can contain the minerals manganese, copper or zinc.

sympathetic nervous system Part of the nervous system that regulates involuntary vital functions, including the activity of the heart, smooth muscles, and adrenal glands. The sympathetic nervous system specifically accelerates heart rate, constricts blood vessels, and raises blood pressure. The parasympathetic nervous system slows heart rate, increases intestinal peristalsis and gland activity, and relaxes sphincters.

symptom A change in health status noted by the person with the problem, such as a stomach pain.

systolic blood pressure (sis-TOL-lik) The pressure in the arterial blood vessels associated with the pumping of blood from the heart.

tetany (TET-ah-nee) A state marked by sharp contraction of muscles with failure to relax afterward; usually caused by abnormal calcium metabolism.

theory An explanation for a phenomenon that has numerous lines of evidence to support it.

thermic effect of food The increase in metabolism that occurs during the digestion, absorption, and metabolism of energy-yielding nutrients; also called diet-induced thermogenes. This represents about 5% to 10% of energy consumed.

thrifty metabolism A metabolism that characteristically uses less energy than normal, such that the risk of weight gain and obesity is enhanced.

tissue A group of cells designed to perform a specific function; muscle tissue is an example.

tocopherol (tuh-KOFF-er-all) The chemical name for some forms of vitamin E. The alpha form is most potent.

tocotrienol (toe-co-TRY-en-ol) Compound related to tocopherol, but differs in the fatty acid side chain on the molecules, in that they contain more carbon-carbon double bonds.

tolerable upper intake level (UL) Maximum chronic daily intake of a nutrient that is unlikely to cause adverse health effects in almost all people in a population. This number applies to a chronic daily use.

toxic Poisonous; caused by a poison.

toxicity The capacity of a substance to produce injury or illness at some dosage.

toxin A poisonous compound that can cause disease. Some toxins are produced by organisms.

trabecular bone (trah-BEK-you-lar) The spongy, inner matrix of bone, found primarily in the spine, pelvis, and ends of bones.

trace mineral A mineral vital to health that is required in the diet in amounts less than 100 mg per day.

***trans* fatty acids** A form of unsaturated fatty acids that, when found in food, is usually a monounsaturated fatty acid. In a *trans* fatty acid, the hydrogens of both carbons that form the double bond lie on opposite sides of that bond. A *cis* fatty acid has the hydrogens lying on the same side of the carbon-carbon double bond. *Trans* fatty acids are by-products of hydrogenation of vegetable oils.

triglyceride (try-GLISS-uh-ride) The major form of lipid in the body and in food. It is composed of three fatty acids linked to glycerol, an alcohol.

trimester The normal pregnancy of 38 to 42 weeks is divided into three 13- to 14-week periods called *trimesters.* Development of the embryo and fetus, however, is continuous throughout pregnancy with no specific physiological markers demarcating the transition from one trimester to the next.

tumor Mass of cells; may be cancerous (malignant) or noncancerous (benign).

Type 1 diabetes A form of diabetes in which the person with the disease is prone to ketosis and requires insulin therapy.

Type 2 diabetes A form of diabetes in which ketosis is not commonly seen. Insulin therapy can be used, but often is not required; often associated with obesity.

ulcer (UL-sir) Erosion of the tissue lining usually in the stomach (gastric ulcer) or the upper small intestine (duodenal ulcer). These are generally referred to as peptic ulcers.

umani A brothy, meaty, savory flavor in some foods. Monosodium glutamate enhances this flavor when added to foods.

undernutrition Failing health that results from a longstanding dietary intake that does not meet nutritional needs.

underwater weighing A method to estimate total body fat by weighing the individual first normally and then when submerged in water. The loss of weight when submerged in water is used to estimate total body fat.

underweight Body weight for height about 15% to 20% below healthy weight, or a body mass index below about 19. These cutoffs are less precise than for obesity because less study of this condition has been undertaken.

upper-body obesity The type of obesity, also called android, in which fat is stored primarily in the abdominal area; defined as a waist-to-hip circumference ratio of greater than 1.0 in men and 0.8 in women; closely associated with a high risk of heart disease, high blood pressure, and diabetes.

urea Nitrogen-containing waste product found in urine. Most nitrogen excreted from the body leaves in this form.

vegan (VEE-gun) A person who eats only plant foods.

vegetarian A person who avoids eating animal products to a varying degree, ranging from consuming no animal products to simply not consuming four-footed animal products.

very low-calorie diet (VLCD) Known also as *protein-sparing modified fast* (PSMF), this diet allows a person 400 to 800 kcal per day, often in liquid form. Of this, 120 to 480 kcal is carbohydrate, while the rest is mostly high–biological value protein.

very-low-density lipoprotein (VLDL) The lipoprotein that initially leaves the liver. It carries both the cholesterol and lipid newly synthesized by the liver.

villi (VIL-eye) Fingerlike protrusions into the small intestine that participate in digestion and absorption of foodstuff.

virus The smallest known type of infectious agent, many of which cause disease in humans. They do not metabolize, grow, or move by themselves. They reproduce by the aid of a living cellular host. Viruses are essentially a piece of genetic material surrounded by a coat of protein.

vitamins Carbon-containing compounds needed in very small amounts in the diet to help regulate and support chemical reactions in the body. Absence from the diet must result in a disease that timely replacement of the vitamin will cure.

water The solvent of life; chemically H_2O. The body is composed of about 60% water. Water (fluid) needs are about 6 to 8 cups per day.

water-soluble vitamins Vitamins that dissolve in water. These vitamins are the B vitamins and vitamin C.

whey (WAY) Proteins, such as lactalbumin, that are found in great amounts in human milk and are easy to digest.

whole grains Grains containing the entire seed of the plant, including the bran, germ, and endosperm (starchy interior). Examples are whole wheat and brown rice.

xerophthalmia (zer-op-THAL-mee-uh) Literally "dry eye." This is a cause of blindness that results from infection of the eye coupled with a vitamin A deficiency. The specific cause is linked to a lack of mucus production by the eye, which then leaves it more vulnerable to damage from surface dirt and bacteria.

yo-yo dieting The practice of losing weight and then regaining it, only to lose it and regain it again. This practice has been shown to lead to an increased risk for heart disease in some studies.

zygote The fertilized ovum; the cell resulting from union of an egg cell (ovum) and sperm until it divides.

Credits

Table of Contents.

p. vi. Ohio State University Extension/Jodi Miller.
p. vii. USA Rice Federation.
p. viii. Ohio State University Extension/Jodi Miller.
p. ix. Ohio State University Extension/Jodi Miller.

Chapter 1

p. 2 & 4. (all) PhotoDisc.
p. 5. James Mulligan.
p. 8, Fig. 1-1. (top) Wheat Foods Council/(middle) Photo from National Sunflower Association/(bottom) Photo courtesy of the National Fisheries Institute.
p. 11, Fig. 1-2. (left) PhotoDisc/(right) David Frasier Photo Library.
p. 11. Ken Halfmann/Photographix.
p. 13. Greg Kidd & Joanne Scott.
p. 14. Cherry Marketing Institute.
p. 19. Ohio State University Extension.
p. 21. Gordon Wardlaw.
p. 22. Gordon Wardlaw.
p. 22. Ohio State University Extension.
p. 30. USDA.
p. 31. Ohio State University Extension.

Chapter 2

p. 36. (both) PhotoDisc.
p. 38. USA Rice Federation.
p. 45. Quaker® Oats.
p. 46. Ohio State University/Malcolm W. Emmons.
p. 48. Ohio State University Extension/Jodi Miller.
p. 53. William Wardlaw.
p. 56. Gordon Wardlaw.
p. 54. Mark Kempf.
p. 55. William Wardlaw.
p. 57. Greg Kidd & Joanne Scott.
p. 65. Joanne Scott.
p. 68. Photo courtesy of National Cattlemen's Beef Association.
p. 70. William Wardlaw.

Chapter 3

p. 74. PhotoDisc.
p. 75, Fig. 3-1. (top left) H. Armstrong Roberts/(middle right) Ed Reschke.
p. 76. PhotoDisc.
p. 78. PhotoDisc.
p. 83. William Wardlaw.
p. 84. Ohio State University Extension.
p. 86. Photo courtesy of National Cattlemen's Beef Association.
p. 90. Science Photo Library/Photo Researchers.
p. 91. PhotoDisc.
p. 99. Gordon Wardlaw.
p. 100. California Prune Board.

Chapter 4

p. 104. PhotoDisc.
p. 105. Washington State Fruit Commission.
p. 106. Greg Kidd & Joanne Scott.
p. 109. Photo courtesy of The Sugar Association, Inc., Washington, D.C.
p. 112. Wheat Foods Council.
p. 114. Ohio State University Extension/Jodi Miller.
p. 120. Ohio State University Extension.
p. 117, Fig. 4-8. Gregg Kidd/Joanne Scott.
p. 121. Gordon Wardlaw.
p. 123. USA Rice Federation.

Chapter 5

p. 136. (both) PhotoDisc.
p. 138. Gregg Kidd & Joanne Scott.
p. 139. American Egg Board.
p. 140. William Wardlaw.
p. 143. William Wardlaw.
p. 150. Photo courtesy of the National Fisheries Institute.
p. 141. Mark Kempf.
p. 147, Fig. 5-7. Gregg Kidd & Joanne Scott.
p. 155. Ventura Foods.
p. 157. National Cancer Institute.
p. 169. Gordon Wardlaw.
p. 171. California Avocado Commission.

Chapter 6

p. 176. (top two) PhotoDisc.
p. 176. Ohio State University Extension.
p. 178. Gregg Kidd & Joanne Scott.
p. 182. National Cancer Institute.
p. 183. Walnut Marketing Board.
p. 183. Beano® is a registered trademark of AkPharma Inc.
p. 184, Fig. 6-5. Joanne Scott/Gregg Kidd.
p. 188. Peanut Advisory Board.
p. 190. Florida Tomato Committee.
p. 192. Gordon Wardlaw.
p. 204. Gordon Wardlaw.

Chapter 7

p. 208. (both) PhotoDisc.
p. 212. William Wardlaw.
p. 220. William Wardlaw.
p. 214. Gordon Wardlaw.
p. 216. Courtesy of NATIONAL DAIRY COUNCIL®.
p. 221. William Wardlaw.
p. 228. (top) Reproduced with permission. ©Culinary Hearts Kitchen, 1982. Copyright American Heart Association.
p. 228. (bottom) Courtesy of National Pork Producers Council.

p. 231. Mark Kempf.
p. 232. American Egg Board.
p. 233. Photo courtesy of National Cattlemen's Beef Association.
p. 239. Gordon Wardlaw.
p. 241, (top). Ohio State University Extension/(bottom) California Strawberry Commission.
p. 252. Gregg Kidd/Joanne Scott.

Chapter 8

p. 258. (both) PhotoDisc.
p. 263. Gordon Wardlaw.
p. 265. Ohio State University Extension/Malcolm W. Emmons.
p. 268. Ohio State University Extension.
p. 270. PhotoDisc.
p. 272. Mark Kempf.
p. 275. USDA.
p. 278. William Wardlaw.
p. 279. Courtesy of NATIONAL DAIRY COUNCIL®.
p. 281. Florida Tomato Committee.
p. 284. Photo courtesy of National Cattlemen's Beef Association.
p. 288. PhotoDisc.
p. 292. Raw Peeled & Deveined Tail/On Shrimp. Fishery Products International, Danvers, MA.
p. 293. Gordon Wardlaw.
p. 295. Photo courtesy of Almond Board of California.
p. 305. James Mulligan.

Chapter 9

p. 310. (top two) PhotoDisc.
p. 313. USA Rice Federation.
p. 315. Gordon Wardlaw.
p. 316, Fig. 9-3. Medical Graphics, Inc.
p. 321, Fig. 9-6. (A) Diana Linsley/Linsley Photographics.
p. 323, Fig. 9-8. Robert Jones, Jr.
p. 325, Fig. 9-9. Ohio State University Extension/Jodi Miller.
p. 329. PhotoDisc.
p. 333. The Ohio State University Communications Photo Service.
p. 333. Ohio State University Extension.
p. 334. Gordon Wardlaw.
p. 339. Gordon Wardlaw.

Chapter 10

p. 358. (both) PhotoDisc.
p. 359. OSU Photo Archives.
p. 361. The Ohio State University Communications Photo Service.
p. 362. David R. Frasier, PhotoLibrary Inc.
p. 363. PhotoDisc.
p. 364. David R. Frasier, PhotoLibrary Inc.
p. 367. James Mulligan.
p. 370. Shore Grilled® Shrimp. Fishery Products International, Danvers, MA.
p. 372. James Mulligan.
p. 375. Gordon Wardlaw.
p. 381. Ohio State University Extension.

Chapter 11

p. 386. PhotoDisc.
p. 386, Fig. 11-1. Bill Hall.
p. 387. David Frasier PhotoLibrary, Inc.
p. 388, Fig. 11-3. Gordon Wardlaw.
p. 389. David Frasier PhotoLibrary, Inc.
p. 391. PhotoDisc.
p. 393. Barros/Barros/The Image Bank, Chicago.
p. 394. Gordon Wardlaw.
p. 395, Fig. 11-5. James Mulligan.
p. 398, Fig. 11-7. Paul Casamassimo, DDS, MS.
p. 398. Gordon Wardlaw.
p. 400. (top) Ohio State University Extension/(bottom) Ohio State University Extension.
p. 402. PhotoDisc.
p. 410, Fig. 11-9. (A) Culver Pictures/(B) Kobal Collection/Superstock/(C) Gilles Caron/Gamma Liaison/(D) ©Daniel Simon/GAMMA.

Chapter 12

p. 414. (top two) PhotoDisc.
p. 414. Joanne Scott.
p. 416. Gordon Wardlaw.
p. 417, Fig. 12-3. Gregg Wolff.
p. 419. Gordon Wardlaw.
p. 420. Gordon Wardlaw.
p. 421. Sunkist Growers.
p. 435. PhotoDisc.
p. 442. George Steinmetz.

Chapter 13

p. 446. (top two) PhotoDisc.
p. 446. Joanne Scott.
p. 447. PhotoDisc.
p. 449. PhotoDisc.
p. 454. Gordon Wardlaw.
p. 456. ©1993 Gerber Products Company. Reprinted with permission of Gerber Products Company. All rights reserved.
p. 457. Gordon Wardlaw.
p. 458, Fig. 13-3. Paul Casamassimo, DDS, MS.
p. 461. Joanne Scott.
p. 462. Washington Apple Commission.
p. 466. Digital Stock.
p. 467. PhotoDisc.
p. 467. Ohio State University Extension/Jodi Miller.
p. 470. Gordon Wardlaw.
p. 477. Gregg Kidd/Joanne Scott.

Chapter 14

p, 482. (top two) PhotoDisc.
p. 482. David Craddock.
p. 487. PhotoDisc.
p. 489. Gordon Wardlaw.
p. 492. PhotoDisc.
p. 494. PhotoDisc.
p. 498. Courtesy of St. Louis District Dairy Council.
p. 499. Ohio State University Extension.
p. 506. Gregg Kidd/Joanne Scott.
p. 507. James Mulligan.

Chapter 15

p. 516. (both) PhotoDisc.
p. 519. Ohio State University Extension.
p. 523. Northwest Cherry Growers.
p. 523. Greg Wolff.
p. 525. Gregg Kidd/Joanne Scott.
p. 526. National Fisheries Institute.
p. 531. Gregg Kidd/Joanne Scott.
p. 532. Gordon Wardlaw.
p. 533, Fig. 15-3. (a) Gordon Wardlaw/(b) Gordon Wardlaw.

p. 534. Ohio State University Extension.
p. 540, Fig. 15-4. Ohio State University Extension/ Lloyd Lemmermann.

Chapter 16

p. 546. (both) PhotoDisc.
p. 549, Fig. 16-1. AP/Wide World Photos.
p. 552. USDA.
p. 554. David R. Frasier, PhotoLibrary, Inc.
p. 559. (top) Ohio State University Extension/(bottom) Ohio State University Extension.
p. 564. Ohio State University Extension.
p. 568. Ohio State University Extension.
p. 569. Ohio State University Extension.
p. 574. Ohio State University Extension/Jodi Miller.
p. 575. Provita/Monsanto.

Appendices

p. A-89, C-1. (all photos) Gregg Kidd/ Joanne Scott.
p. A-113, Fig. F-2.

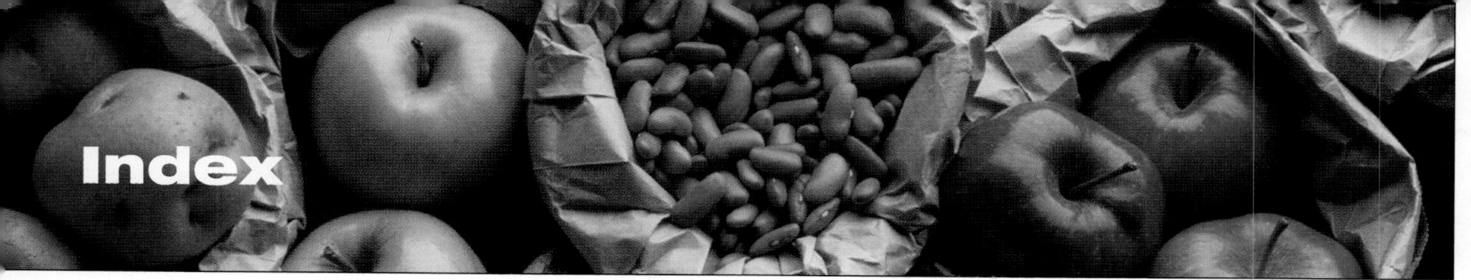

Index

Page numbers followed by a "t" indicate tables; numbers followed by an "f" indicate figures.

Estimated minimum sodium, chloride, and potassium requirements for healthy persons

Age	Weight (kg)	Sodium (mg)*†	Chloride (mg)*†	Potassium (mg)‡
Months				
0–5	4.5	120	180	500
6–11	8.9	200	300	700
Years				
1	11	225	350	1000
2–5	16	300	500	1400
6–9	25	400	600	1600
10–18	50	500	750	2000
>18§	70	500	750	2000

mg = milligram; kg = kilogram (2.2 pounds)
*No allowance has been included for large, prolonged losses from the skin through sweat.
†There is no evidence that higher intakes confer any additional health benefit.
‡Desirable intakes of potassium may considerably exceed these values (~3500 mg for adults).
§No allowance has been included for growth. Values given for people under 18 years of age assume a growth rate corresponding to the 50th percentile reported by the National Center for Health Statistics and averaged for males and females

Estimated safe and adequate daily dietary intakes (ESADDIs) of selected minerals*

Category	Age (years)	Trace Elements† Copper (mg)	Manganese (mg)	Chromium (μg)	Molybdenum (μg)
Infants	0–0.5	0.4–0.6	0.3–0.6	10–40	15–30
	0.5–1	0.6–0.7	0.6–1	20–60	20–40
Children and adolescents	1–3	0.7–1	1–1.5	20–80	25–50
	4–6	1–1.5	1.5–2	30–120	30–75
	7–10	1–2	2–3	50–200	50–150
	11+	1.5–2.5	2–5	50–200	75–250
Adults		1.5–3	2–5	50–200	75–250

μg = microgram; mg = milligram
*Because there is less information on which to base recommendations for allowances of minerals, these figures are not given in the main table of RDAs and are provided here in the form of ranges of recommended intakes.
†Since toxic levels for many trace elements may be reached with only several times usual intakes, the upper levels for the trace elements given in this table should not be habitually exceeded.